MW01101804

ATLAS OF CLINICAL OPHTHALMOLOGY

ATLAS OF CLINICAL OPHTHALMOLOGY

DANIEL M. ALBERT, M.D.
Frederick A. Davis Professor and Chair,
Department of Ophthalmology,
University of Wisconsin Medical School,
Madison, Wisconsin

FREDERICK A. JAKOBIEC, M.D., D.Sc. (Med.)
Henry Willard Williams Professor of Ophthalmology,
Professor of Pathology, and Chairman,
Department of Ophthalmology,
Harvard Medical School;
Chief, Department of Ophthalmology, and
Surgeon in Ophthalmology,
Massachusetts Eye and Ear Infirmary,
Boston, Massachusetts

Managing Editors:
NANCY L. ROBINSON, A.B.
University of Wisconsin Medical School
RICHARD A. BAINS, M.D.
Massachusetts Eye and Ear Infirmary

W.B. SAUNDERS COMPANY
A Division of Harcourt Brace & Company
Philadelphia London Toronto Montreal Sydney Tokyo

W.B. SAUNDERS COMPANY

A Division of Harcourt Brace & Company

The Curtis Center
Independence Square West
Philadelphia, Pennsylvania 19106

Library of Congress Cataloging-in-Publication Data

Albert, Daniel M.
Atlas of clinical ophthalmology/Daniel M. Albert, Frederick A. Jakobiec.—1st ed.

p. cm.

ISBN 0-7216-3417-6

1. Ophthalmology—Atlases. I. Jakobiec, Frederick A. II. Title.
[DNLM: 1. Eye Diseases—atlases. 2. Eye—atlases. WW 17 A333a 1996]

RE71.A43 1996
617.7′1—dc20

DNLM/DLC 95-1015

Atlas of Clinical Ophthalmology ISBN 0-7216-3417-6

Copyright © 1996 by W.B. Saunders Company

All rights reserved. No part of this publication may be reproduced or transmitted in any form or by any means, electronic or mechanical, including photocopy, recording, or any information storage and retrieval system, without permission in writing from the publisher.

Printed in the United States of America

Last digit is the print number: 9 8 7 6 5 4 3 2 1

This book is dedicated to the memory of David Glendenning Cogan, consummate teacher and friend to my generation of ophthalmologists.

D.M.A.

To the past and present faculty and trainees of the Departments of Ophthalmology of the Harvard Medical School and the Massachusetts Eye and Ear Infirmary, and to our distinguished colleagues from other institutions, whose coruscating contributions made the **Principles and Practice of Ophthalmology** *a success and this* **Atlas of Clinical Ophthalmology** *possible.*

F.A.J.

Contributors

SECTION 1

Cornea, Conjunctiva, and Sclera

Mark B. Abelson, MD, CM, FRCS(C)
Anthony P. Adamis, MD
Daniel M. Albert, MD
Eduardo C. Alfonso, MD
Mathea R. Allansmith, MD
Ann M. Bajart, MD, FACS
S. Arthur Boruchoff, MD
M. Ronan Conlon, MB, BCh
Claes H. Dohlman, MD, PhD
C. Stephen Foster, MD, FACS
Gary N. Foulks, MD
Jeffrey P. Gilbard, MD
Jack V. Greiner, DO, PhD
Peter S. Hersh, MD
Kenneth R. Kenyon, MD
David Miller, MD
Deborah Pavan-Langston, MD, FACS
Mark A. Pavilack, MD
Michael B. Raizman, MD
Oliver D. Schein, MD, MPH
Tomy Starck, MD
Roger F. Steinert, MD
Jonathan H. Talamo, MD
Richard A. Thoft, MD
Ira J. Udell, MD
Michael D. Wagoner, MD

SECTION 2

Uvea and Lens

Thomas M. Aaberg, MD
Usha Andley, PhD
Charles J. Bock, BS
Robert J. Brockhurst, MD
Henry G. Brown, MD, PhD
Antonio Capone, Jr., MD
Leo T. Chylack, Jr., MD
Thomas A. Deutsch, MD, FACS
Ralph C. Eagle, Jr., MD
C. Stephen Foster, MD, FACS
Alan H. Friedman, MD
George E. Garcia, MD
Ahmed A. Hidayat, MD
David G. Hunter, MD, PhD
Frederick A. Jakobiec, MD, DSc(Med)
Lee M. Jampol, MD
Patricia M. Khu, MD
David L. Knox, MD
J.R. Kuszak, PhD
J. Wallace McMeel, MD
E. Mitchel Opremcak, MD
Susanna S. Park, MD, PhD
Henry Perry, MD
Michael B. Raizman, MD
Gary A. Rankin, MD
Shiyoung Roh
Allan R. Rutzen, BS, MD
Roger F. Steinert, MD
Paul P. Svitra, MD
King W. To, MD
John J. Weiter, MD, PhD
Lorenz E. Zimmerman, MD, DSc

SECTION 3

Retina and Vitreous

Lloyd M. Aiello, MD
George K. Asdourian, MD
Mark W. Balles, MD
Eliot L. Berson, MD
Norman P. Blair, MD
Mark S. Blumenkranz, MD
Neil M. Bressler, MD
Susan B. Bressler, MD
Alfred Brini, MD
Norman E. Byer, MD

Nabil G. Chedid, MD
Donald J. D'Amico, MD
Monica A. De La Paz, MD
Maryanna Destro, MD
Jay S. Duker, MD
Bishara M. Fairs, MD
C. Stephen Foster, MD, FACS
Thomas R. Friberg, MS, MD
Alexander R. Gaudio, MD
Stephen C. Gieser, MD
Evangelos S. Gragoudas, MD
David R. Guyer, MD
Robert Haimovici, MD
Lawrence S. Halperin, MD
Gary D. Haynie, MD
Thomas R. Hedges, III, MD
Tatsuo Hirose, MD
David G. Hunter, MD, PhD
Henry J. Kaplan, MD
Shalom J. Kieval, MD
Sang H. Kim, MD
Arnold J. Kroll, MD
John S. Lean, MD, FRCS
Carol M. Lee, MD
Marc R. Levin, MD
John I. Loewenstein, MD
Peter L. Lou, MD
John C. Madigan, Jr., MD
Raymond R. Margherio, MD
W. Wynn McMullen, MD
Joan W. Miller, MD
Eric Mukai, BS
Shizuo Mukai, MD
Robert P. Murphy, MD
Don H. Nicholson, MD
Stuart W. Noorily, MD
R. Joseph Olk, MD
E. Mitchel Opremcak, MD
Andrew J. Packer, MD
Samir C. Patel, MD
Michael K. Pinnolis, MD
Ronald C. Pruett, MD
Carmen A. Puliafito, MD
Charles D.J. Regan, MD
Elias Reichel, MD
Steven J. Rose, MD
Michael A. Sandberg, PhD
Johanna M. Seddon, MD, MS
John A. Sorenson, MD
Richard R. Tamesis, MD
David V. Weinberg, MD
Lawrence A. Yannuzzi, MD
Lucy H.Y. Young, MD, PhD

SECTION 4
Glaucoma

R. Rand Allingham, MD
C. Davis Belcher, III, MD
A. Robert Bellows, MD
David G. Campbell, MD
David M. Chacko, MD, PhD
Jean-Bernard Charles, MD
Marshall N. Cyrlin, MD
Michael V. Drake, MD
David A. Echelman, MD
Philip M. Fiore, MD
Linda J. Greff, MD
Eve Juliet Higginbotham, MD, SM
Douglas H. Johnson, MD
Murray A. Johnstone, MD
Kathleen A. Lamping, MD
Mark A. Latina, MD
Paul P. Lee, MD, JD
Robert A. Lytle, MD
Peter J. McDonnell, MD
Randall Ozment, MD
Thomas M. Richardson, MD
Claudia U. Richter, MD
Robert C. Rosenquist, MD
Joel S. Schuman, MD, FACS
M. Bruce Shields, MD
Bradford J. Shingleton, MD
Omah S. Singh, MD
Sandra J. Sofinski, MD
David P. Tingey, MD
Martin Wand, MD
David P. Wellington, MD
A. Sydney Williams, MD

SECTION 5
Eyelids

Charles K. Beyer-Machule, MD
M. Ronan Conlon, MB, BCh
Richard K. Dortzbach, MD, FACS
Craig E. Geist, MD
A. Tyrone Glover, MD
Ahmed A. Hidayat, MD
Frederick A. Jakobiec, MD, DSc(Med)
Jemshed A. Khan, MD
Jan W. Kronish, MD
David B. Lyon, MD
Curtis E. Margo, MD
Marlon Maus, MD
Klaus G. Riedel, MD

I. Rand Rodgers, MD
Peter A.D. Rubin, MD
Joseph W. Sassani, MD
Kevin R. Scott, MD
Francis C. Sutula, MD
William L. White, MD
Janey L. Wiggs, MD, PhD
John J. Woog, MD

SECTION 6

Orbit

Daniel M. Albert, MD
Ann Sullivan Baker, MD
Gary E. Borodic, MD
Richard L. Dallow, MD
Ramon L. Font, MD
Arthur S. Grove, Jr., MD
Frederick A. Jakobiec, MD, DSc(Med)
Leonard A. Levin, MD, PhD
Marlon Maus, MD
Peter A. Netland, MD, PhD
Steven G. Pratt, MD
I. Rand Rodgers, MD
Peter A.D. Rubin, MD
John W. Shore, MD, FACS
Neal G. Snebold, MD
Francis C. Sutula, MD
Daniel J. Townsend, MD
Nicholas J. Volpe, MD
Christopher T. Westfall, MD, FACS

SECTION 7

Neuroophthalmology

Don C. Bienfang, MD
James J. Corbett, MD
Steven E. Feldon, MD
Joel S. Glaser, MD
G. Michael Halmagyi, MD
Thomas R. Hedges, III, MD
Robert S. Hepler, MD
Barrett Katz, MD
Nancy J. Newman, MD
Joseph F. Rizzo, III, MD
Alfredo A. Sadun, MD, PhD
Shirley H. Wray, MD, PhD, FRCP

SECTION 8

Pediatric Ophthalmology

William P. Boger, III, MD
Anthony J. Fraioli, MD
Stephen J. Fricker, ScD, MD
Anne B. Fulton, MD
David G. Hunter, MD, PhD
Carl Cordes Johnson, MD, FACS
Shizuo Mukai, MD
Robert A. Peterson, MD, DrMedSci
Richard M. Robb, MD
Lois Hodgson Smith, MD, PhD
David S. Walton, MD

SECTION 9

The Eye and Systemic Disease

Robin K. Avery, MD
Ann Sullivan Baker, MD
Irmgard Behlau, MD
H. Richard Christlieb, MD
Richard L. Dallow, MD
Donald J. D'Amico, MD
Mary De Groot, EdM
Donald S. Fong, MD
C. Stephen Foster, MD
Richard D. Granstein, MD
David G. Hunter, MD, PhD
Deborah S. Jacobs, MD
Frederick A. Jakobiec, MD, DSc(Med)
R. Paul Johnson, MD
Jeffrey C. Lamkin, MD
Dennis M. Marcus, MD
W. Wynn McMullen, MD
Peter A. Netland, MD, PhD
Annabelle A. Okada, MD
Ronald C. Pruett, MD
Michael B. Raizman, MD
Chittaranjan V. Reddy, MD
Anil K. Rustgi, MD
Edward T. Ryan, AB, MD
Michele Trucksis, MD, PhD
Scott M. Whitcup, MD

SECTION 10

Ocular Oncology

Daniel M. Albert, MD
William P. Boger, III, MD
James R. Cassady, MD
Devron H. Char, MD
Victor T. Curtin, MD
Thaddeus P. Dryja, MD
Eleanore Ebert, MD, MPH
Evangelos S. Gragoudas, MD
Frederick A. Jakobiec, MD, DSc(Med)
Dennis M. Marcus, MD
Shizuo Mukai, MD
Karl R. Olsen, MD

Robert A. Petersen, MD, DrMedSci
José Alain Sahel, MD
Charles S. Specht, MD
Nicholas J. Volpe, MD
Janey L. Wiggs, MD, PhD
Lucy H.Y. Young, MD

SECTION 11

Trauma

J. Paul Dieckert, MD
Peter S. Hersh, MD
Darren L. Hoover, MD
Kenneth R. Kenyon, MD
Mariana D. Mead, MD
Peter A.D. Rubin, MD
Oliver D. Schein, MD, MPH
Bradford J. Shingleton, MD
John W. Shore, MD, FACS
Lois Hodgson Smith, MD, PhD
Neal G. Snebold, MD
Paul F. Vinger, MD
Michael J. Yaremchuk, MD, FACS

Preface

The purpose of this **Atlas** is to provide ophthalmologists and other physicians concerned with eye disease with a comprehensive and carefully selected collection of quality color illustrations that review the spectrum of eye diseases seen in general ophthalmologic practice. It is our primary goal in this work to instruct and inform the reader with regard to the diagnosis and treatment of these disorders. These illustrations are drawn from the **Principles and Practice of Ophthalmology** and were contributed by the authors and editors. At the time that book was conceived, the intent was to select and structure the illustrations used in it so that they could stand alone as an atlas. This is consistent with the long-standing realization in medicine that an atlas is a highly effective teaching tool, which in ophthalmology has a particular relevance and adaptability to cases encountered in the clinic.

The desire to go beyond words in the teaching of medicine goes far back in history. In the 11th and 12th centuries at Salerno, medical practice was systematized in the form of verses to make it more easily committed to memory than prose. Around 1500, Leonardo da Vinci, then actively studying and recording human anatomy, observed in his notebook: "I counsel you not to cumber yourself with words unless you are speaking to the blind." In fact, ancient pictures and sculptures of men and women with ocular and other diseases may still be seen both at their sites of origin and in museums and libraries. It has been suggested that some of the medical and anatomic illustrations made during the Middle Ages arc derived from figures prepared in the Alexandrian school from as early as 300 BC. If indeed there were Alexandrian illustrations, these were drawn on papyrus sheets that were rolled into scrolls. Papyrus proved a poor format, however, for the long-term preservation of illustrations. The codex, or book with leaves bound together, appeared in the first century AD. The pages were made of vellum or other animal-derived materials and lent themselves well to illustration. Paper made of vegetable fiber was introduced into Europe around the 11th century. Descriptions of wonderful collections of medical illustrations from manuscripts preceding the printed page are given by Herrlinger[1] and by Roberts and Tomlinson.[2]

With the introduction of printing in 1466, medical illustrations, particularly anatomic and surgical ones, became widely disseminated. These early works are well described by Choulant.[3] The first drawing of an eye was published in the *Margarita Philosophica*—the earliest "modern" encyclopedia to appear in print—written by Gregor Reisch and published in Freiburg by Johann Schott in 1503. This illustration is reproduced in Figure 1. Georg Bartisch's *Ophthalmodouleia,* published in 1583, is not only the first systematic work on eye disease and ophthalmic surgery but also the first ophthalmic atlas to be published. Herrlinger notes that the 91 woodcuts for this work were produced after watercolors painted by Bartisch himself. The woodcuts were executed by Hans Hewamaul and illustrate pathologic conditions, operations, and surgical instruments. The figures of the eye and brain contain superimposed flaps to show the anatomy at various levels. Many additional useful atlases of the anatomy, of clinical pathology, and of surgery of the eye appeared during the 17th and 18th centuries. Notable among these were the *Opticorum* of François Aguilon (1613), a landmark of baroque book illustration with drawings contributed by Peter Paul Rubens, and Johann Zinn's great *Atlas of the Human Eye*, published in 1755.

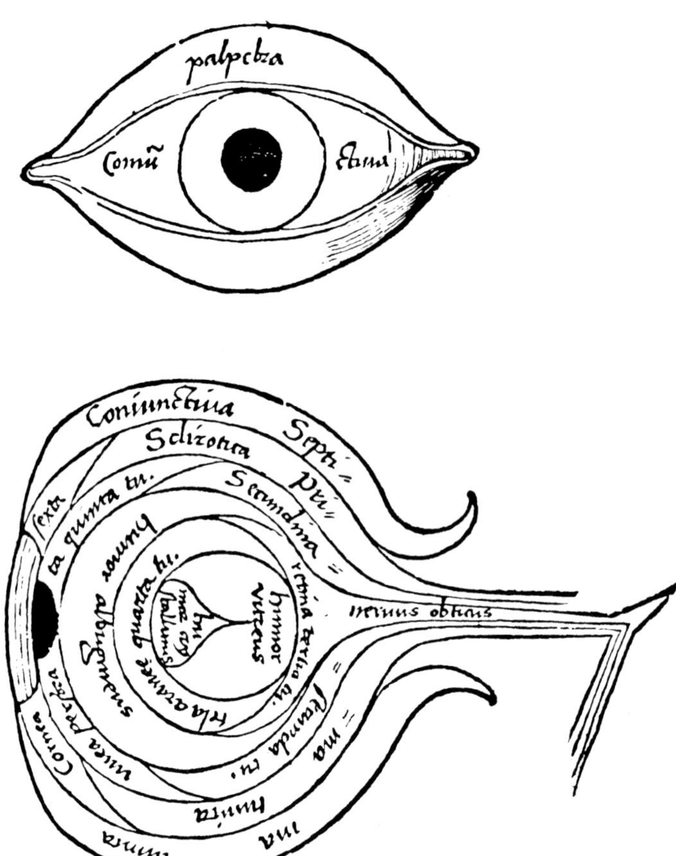

FIGURE 1 First drawing of the eye ever published. From Gregor Reisch: *Margarita Philosophica,* published in Freiburg by Johann Schott in 1503.

The full potential of the atlas in ophthalmic instruction was realized following Helmholtz's invention of the ophthalmoscope in 1850. The importance of this instrument and its usefulness in interpreting diseases of the fundus oculi were appreciated to only a very limited degree for the first 10 years after its invention. It was the appearance of various atlases illustrating the instrument's use and interpreting the observed fundus changes that led to the widespread use of the ophthalmoscope and to the development of ophthalmology as a specialty in the United States. Key among these atlases were those by Adrian van Trigt, Richard Liebreich, and Eduard von Jaeger. A fine history of the atlases of ophthalmology in the first hundred years following the invention of the ophthalmoscope has been written by C. Wilber Rucker and Thomas E. Keys.[4] The most influential of these atlases was Eduard Jaeger's *Ophthalmoskopischer Hand-atlas,* published in 1869 and republished in revised editions in 1870, 1890, and 1894.

It was my good fortune to locate in 1963, after nearly a century, the 184 paintings executed by Eduard Jaeger on which his atlas was based, together with his case books. In 1972 I published a new English edition of Jaeger's *Atlas of Diseases of the Ocular Fundus with New Descriptions, Revisions, and Additions* under W.B. Saunders' imprint. This whet my appetite to participate in the production of a major modern atlas. Simultaneously with this effort, Harold G. Scheie and I undertook the eighth edition of *Adler's Textbook of Ophthalmology,* the predecessor of **Principles and Practice of Ophthalmology**. In the course of totally rewriting this work, we added 565 new illustrations, 275 of which were in color. This work, also published by W.B. Saunders Company in 1969, perhaps had the seeds of an atlas in it. These proved a useful preparatory exercise for the present work.

Many fine atlases have appeared in recent years. I hope that the **Atlas of Clinical Ophthalmology** will be distinguished by the scope of pathology it presents and the quality of the illustrations.

We owe warm thanks to the many contributors of **Principles and Practice of Ophthalmology** who provided this striking material. In addition, we extend our particular appreciation to Nancy Robinson, the Managing Editor at the University of Wisconsin-Madison, and Dr. Rick Bains at the Massachusetts Eye and Ear Infirmary; also to Hazel Hacker, Developmental Editor, and Linda R. Garber, Production Manager, both at W.B. Saunders.

Although the purpose of this book is to present outstanding diagnostic points regarding the practice of ophthalmology, the **Atlas of Clinical Ophthalmology** demonstrates to this author and it is hoped to the reader what a "fearfully and wonderfully made" structure the eye is.

DANIEL M. ALBERT, M.D.
Madison, Wisconsin

---

1. Herrlinger, R: *History of Medical Illustration from Antiquity to 1600.* New York, Editions Medicina Rara Ltd, 1970.
2. Roberts KB, Tomlinson JDW: *The Fabric of the Body: European Traditions of Anatomical Illustration.* Oxford, Clarendon Press, 1992.
3. Choulant L: *A History and Bibliography of Anatomic Illustration,* edited by M. Frank. New York, Schuman, 1945.
4. Rucker CW, Keys TE: *The Atlases of Ophthalmology: 1850–1950.* no publisher, 1950.

Preface

Atlas was first employed as a book title for a collection of maps by Gerhardus Mercator (Gerhard Kremer), a Flemish cartographer who died in 1594 and whose mapbook appeared posthumously in 1595. Atlas was a titan of Greek mythology depicted as carrying the heavens on his shoulders, and his likeness was contained on the title page of early cartographic collections. Over the ensuing centuries, ''atlas'' has become associated with all kinds of richly illustrated treatises on virtually every subject with a relative sparsity of discursive text; it is a seductive format for portraying medical information. With respect to ophthalmology, a review of atlases in the Library of Congress either previously published or in preparation reveals that there are 172 in the English language covering myriad topics (from surgery to feline ophthalmology) and another 65 in other languages.

In my own career two textbooks had a seminal and portentous influence in shaping my professional interests and development. When I was an intern in internal medicine at the Stanford University Medical Center during 1968–1969, on those evenings when I was still able to stay awake I would repair to an alcove in the medical library that had several shelves of ophthalmology textbooks. Two caught my fancy. The first was David Barsky's *Color Atlas of Pathology of the Eye* (McGraw-Hill, 1966). This compact but extraordinarily attractive and valuable treatise consisted of 135 pages of color plates (totaling 393 individual color illustrations) and 95 pages of dense text devoted to various topics in ophthalmic pathology. This may well have been the first color atlas of ophthalmic pathology. I was transfixed not only by the ineffable beauty of the eye but also by the distinctive features of its diseases. This monograph confirmed my early interest in studying ophthalmic pathology, which led eventually to a fellowship at the Armed Forces Institute of Pathology and my obtaining board qualification in general anatomic pathology as well as ophthalmology. The second ensorcelling textbook that I found in the Stanford medical library was the late Algernon Reese's capaciously illustrated *Tumors of the Eye* (2nd ed, Hoeber, 1963; 593 pages, 367 figures), which further focused my interests on ophthalmic oncology. At the end of my internship I went to the Harkness Eye Institute of the Columbia–Presbyterian Medical Center in New York to do my residency training. There I was privileged to meet Dr. Reese, and after going on staff at the Institute, to share a suite of offices with him. Much of the content of my waking hours over the past 25 years has been determined by my early encounters with these two books. Such is the potential and actual power of books to transform our lives.

The illustrations in this **Atlas of Clinical Ophthalmology** have been culled from the best of those that appeared in the 5-volume **Principles and Practice of Ophthalmology**. There are 1,603 figures, many of which have several parts. The figure legends were rewritten to enhance their didactic value when they were initially sparse, substitutions were made when better illustrations could be found, and supplemental blocks of illustrations were added where lacunae existed in the initial textbook. For the breadth of coverage of clinical entities and findings, including juxtaposed pathologic and radiographic findings and those of other ancillary diagnostic tests (ultrasonography, angiography, etc.), this **Atlas** probably has no peer. Although it is not exhaustive, there is more than enough fodder to kindle the novice's wonderment or to resupply the intellectual entrepôt of the expert. One can conveniently peruse a broad spectrum of material in any of the clinical subspecialties of ophthalmology in about an hour to an hour and a half, thereby gaining a matchless conspectus of the area. Special interests and cravings that might be stirred by this kind of lambent review can be satiated by returning to the **Principles and Practice** textbook in order to deepen one's knowledge.

We have been gratified that the **Principles and Practice of Ophthalmology** has enjoyed an extremely favorable academic reception and a widespread dissemination among our colleagues; it has recently been selected by the Association of American Publishers as the outstanding textbook in the medical sciences for 1994. This **Atlas** is yet another systematic and somewhat museologic approach to studying ophthalmology, and we hope it will enjoy a wide readership with many repeat visits to the morbid but heuristically invaluable treasures of our field.

From an ethical fascination with disease there must come an expansion of humankind's health. This will occur to the extent that all scholarly efforts, including this **Atlas of Clinical Ophthalmology** and the **Principles and Practice of Ophthalmology**, stimulate critical reflection, teaching, and research. It is our fondest hope that our academic labors will advance in some measurable way the causes of medical idealism, probity, and efficacy.

FREDERICK A. JAKOBIEC, M.D., D. SC. (MED.)
Boston, Massachusetts

Acknowledgment

The editors and publishers wish to credit the contributors to **Principles and Practice of Ophthalmology** as the original source for many of the illustrations to be found in this **Atlas of Clinical Ophthalmology.** Those illustrations borrowed from other sources have been individually credited. The list of contributors has been arranged by sections so that the contributing authors to each section can be identified.

Contents

SECTION 1

Cornea, Conjunctiva, and Sclera

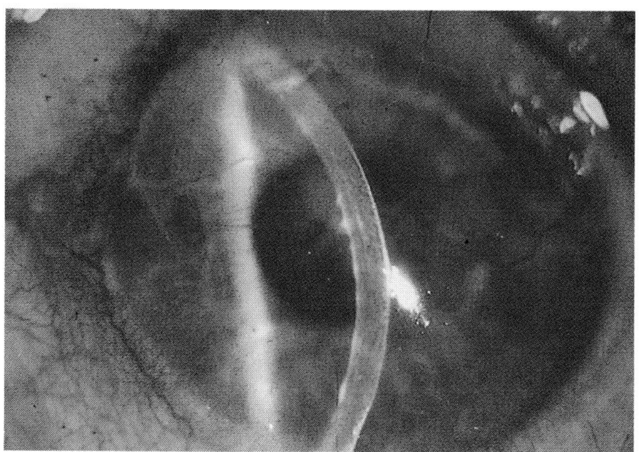

FIGURE 1–1 **Slit-lamp examination.** The slit-lamp beam strikes the cornea in an oblique fashion. The scattering properties of the cornea give the viewer an optical cross section. In this case, folds in Descemet's membrane can be seen. Using the fine slit beam, one can get an appreciation of the level of corneal lesions as well as the thickness of the cornea.

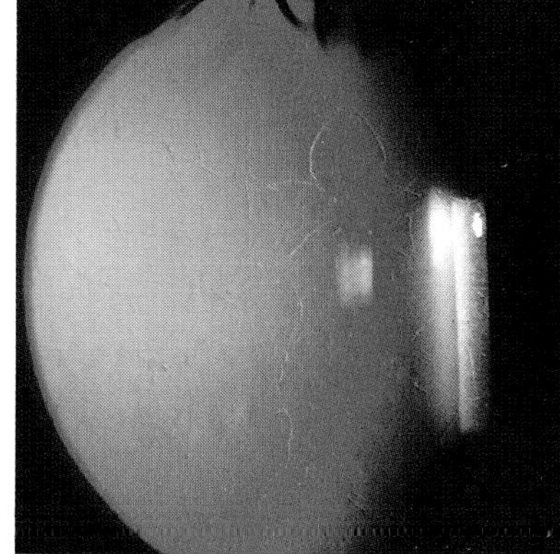

FIGURE 1–2 **Slit-lamp examination.** Retroillumination from the fundus provides an orange background, which allows subtle corneal lesions to become silhouetted and much easier to see. In this case, early signs of lattice dystrophy of the cornea can be seen.

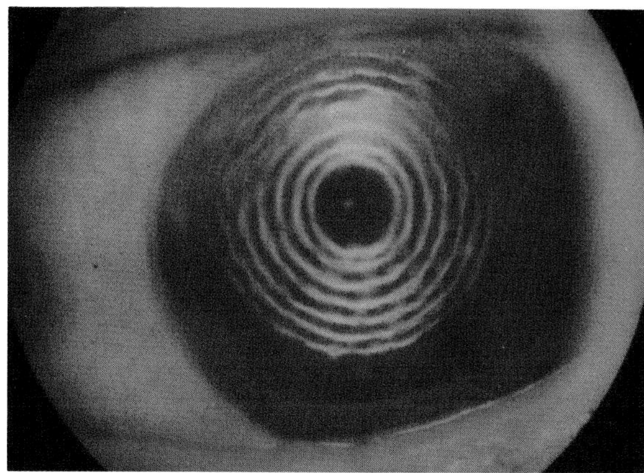

FIGURE 1–3 **Corneal topography.** Keratoscopy appearance of the reflection of the Placido disc from a patient with bullous keratopathy. The contour of the concentric ring reflection can be a useful qualitative tool to detect irregularities in the surface of the cornea.

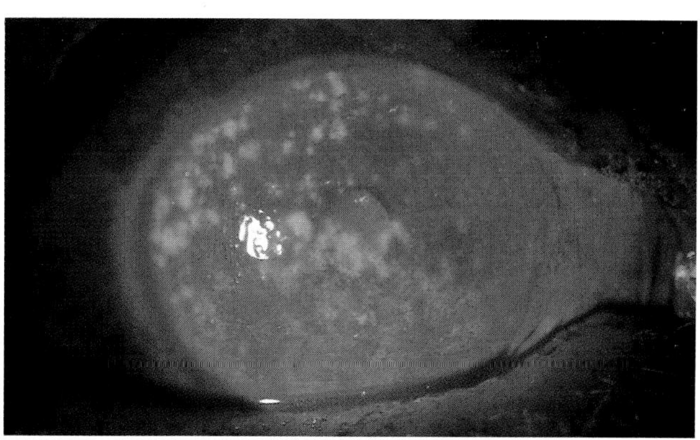

FIGURE 1–4 **Fluorescein staining.** Using cobalt blue illumination, fluorescein staining can be used to demonstrate superficial punctate keratopathy. (Courtesy of K. R. Kenyon, M.D.)

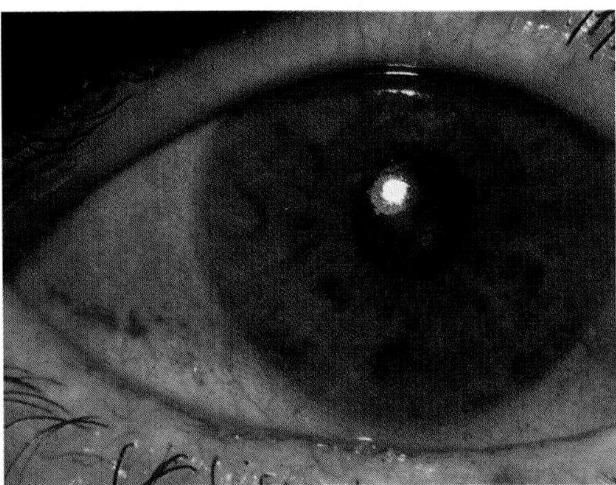

FIGURE 1–5 **Rose bengal staining.** Rose bengal staining demonstrates epithelial defects as well as degenerating or dead epithelial cells. In this case, note the rose bengal staining of the interpalpebral conjunctival epithelium, aiding in the diagnosis of keratoconjunctivitis sicca.

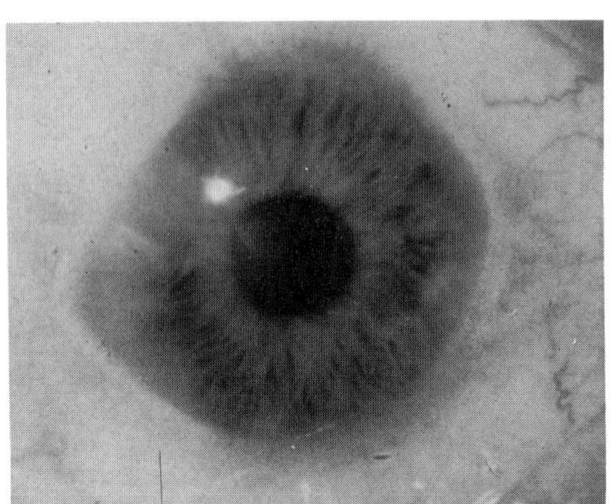

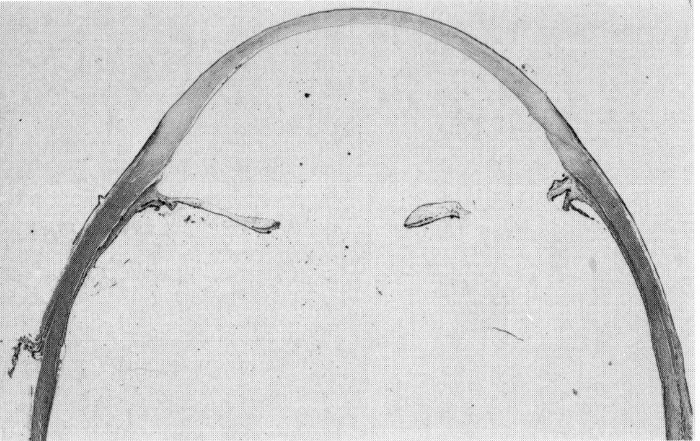

FIGURE 1–6 *Left,* Microcornea. A young child had a cornea of 9.5 mm diameter and subtle peripheral sclerocornea. *Right,* Megalocornea. Light microscopy of a 62-year-old man with corneal diameters of 13 mm. Note the anterior segment with no abnormalities (except beveled scar of cataract incision and surgical aphakia). H&E, ×3. (*Right,* From Wood WJ, Green WR, Marr WG: Megalocornea: A clinicopathologic case report. Md State Med J 23(7)57–60; 1974.)

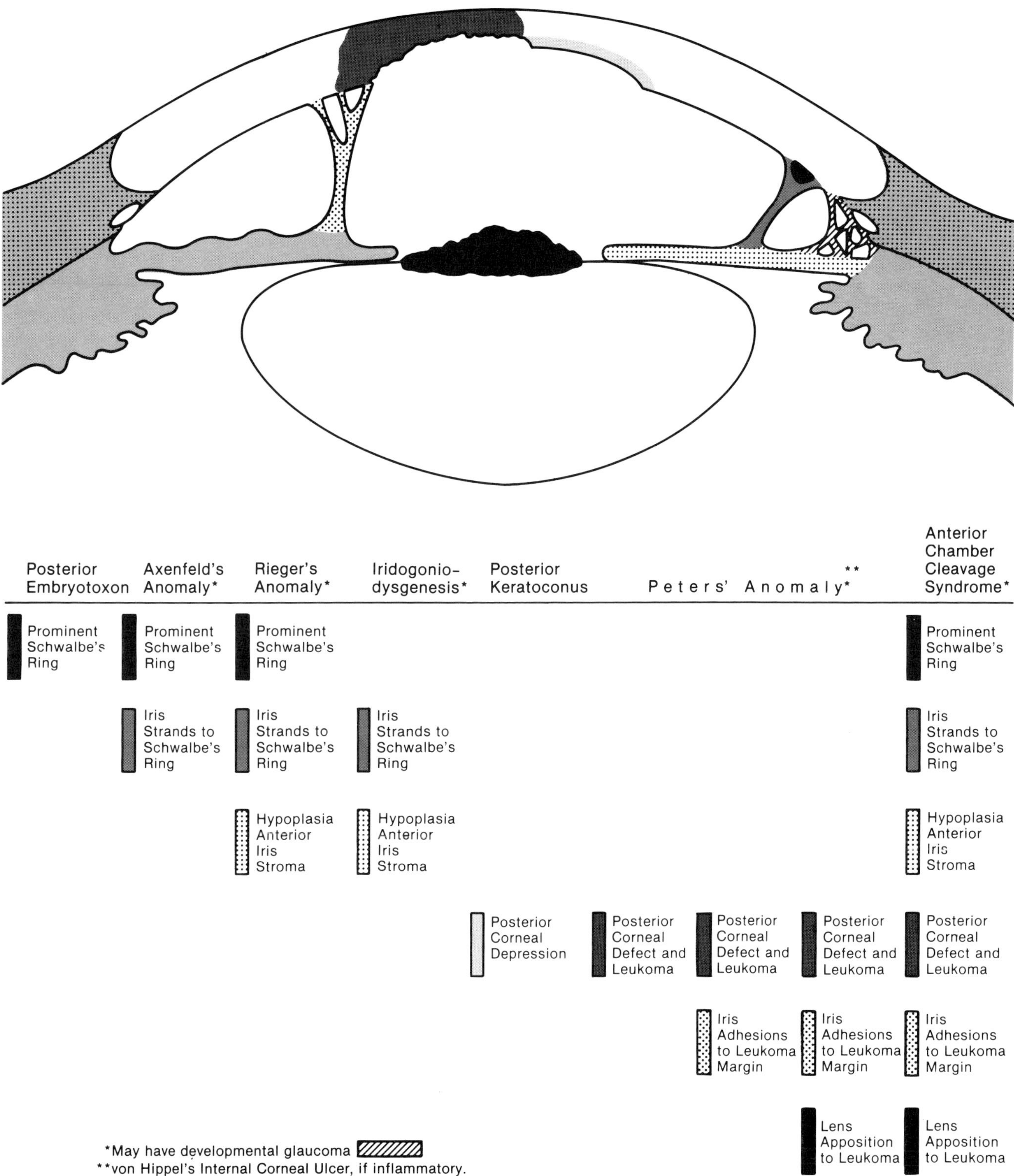

FIGURE 1-7 **Mesenchymal dysgenesis of the anterior segment.** The stepladder table demonstrates a spectrum of anatomic combinations of terms by which they are commonly known. The markers in the table indicate the corresponding anatomic component in the illustration. The central abnormalities occur because of the focal absence or attenuation of the endothelium. (From Waring GO III, Rodrigues MM, Laibson PR: Anterior chamber cleavage syndrome: A stepladder classification. Surv Ophthalmol 20:3, 1975.)

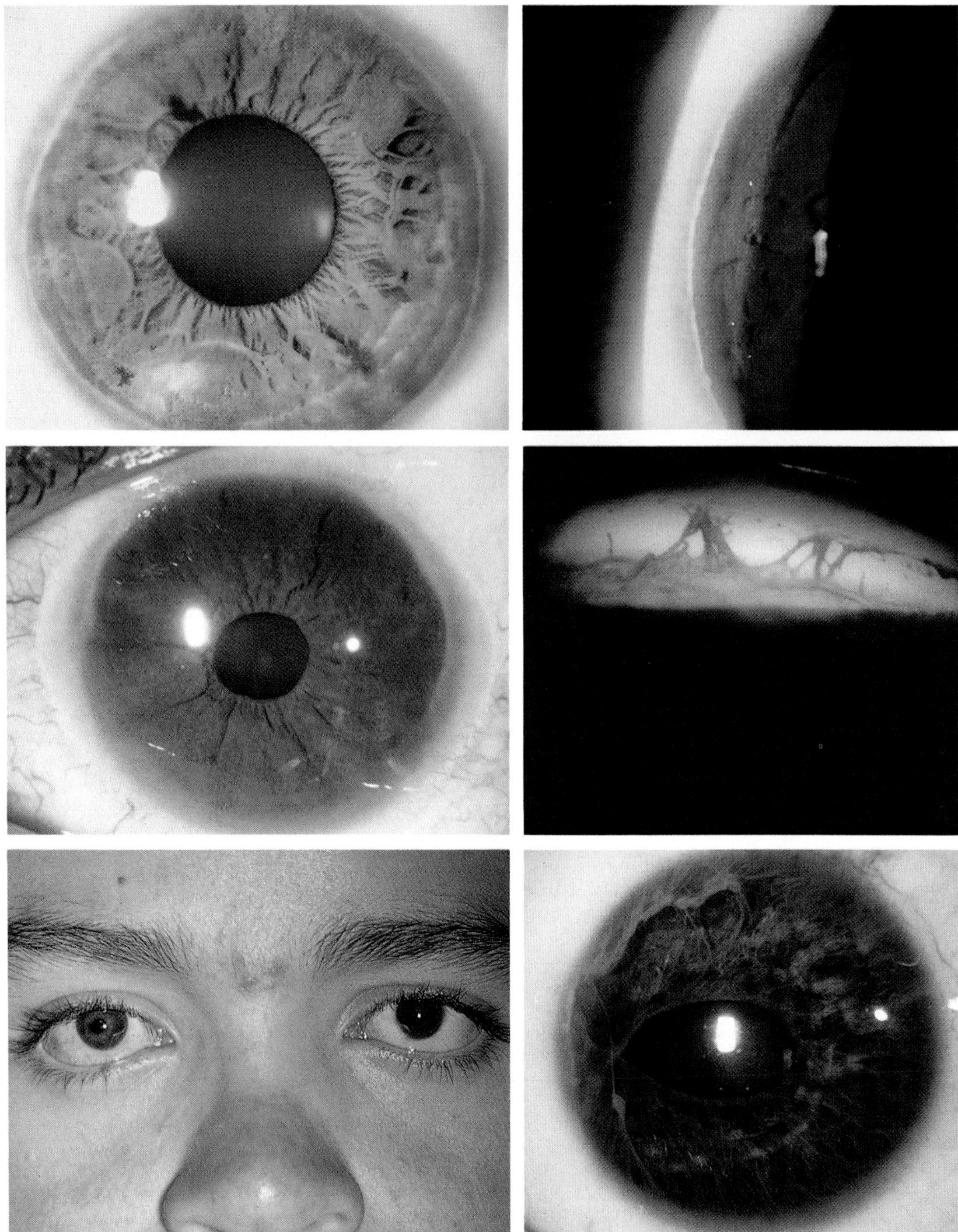

FIGURE 1–8 *Top left and right,* Posterior embryotoxon. Note the anteriorly and centrally displaced Schwalbe's line. *Middle,* Axenfeld's anomaly. Markedly dense and advanced Schwalbe's line *(left)* accompanied by adherent abnormal iris processes bridging the anterior chamber *(right)*. *Bottom,* Rieger's syndrome. *Left,* Multiple facial anomalies such as telecanthus, low nasal bridge, and maxillary hypoplasia. *Right,* This same patient exhibits posterior embryotoxon, hypoplasia of the anterior stroma, corectopia, and peripheral anterior synechiae.

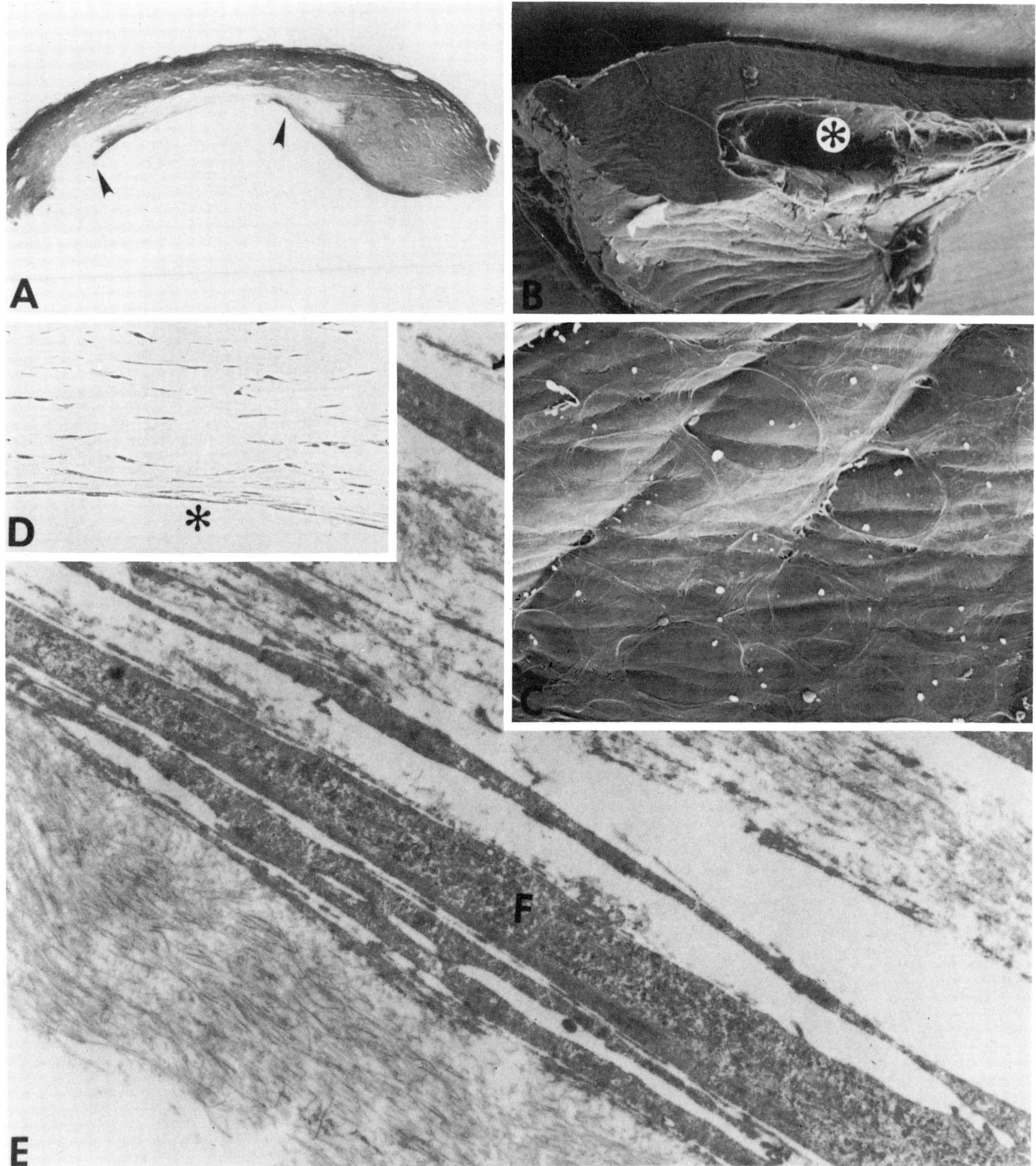

FIGURE 1–9 **Peters' anomaly.** *A,* Light micrograph of a keratoplasty specimen shows the posterior central stromal defect *(between the arrowheads)* devoid of Descemet's membrane and endothelium. H&E, ×15. *B,* By scanning electron microscopy the posterior central defect *(asterisk)* is prominently displayed and appears lined by fibrous tissue. ×31. *C,* Higher-power scanning electron microscopy of the posterior fibrous tissue shows the loose collagenous network of this layer. ×310. *D,* Phase-contrast microscopy of the posterior cornea discloses only attenuated fibroblastic cells *(asterisk)* covering the posterior stromal surface. PPDA, ×250. *E,* Transmission electron microscopy of the area in *D* shows loosely aggregated collagen fibrils of normal dimensions and thin fibroblasts (F). ×12,600.

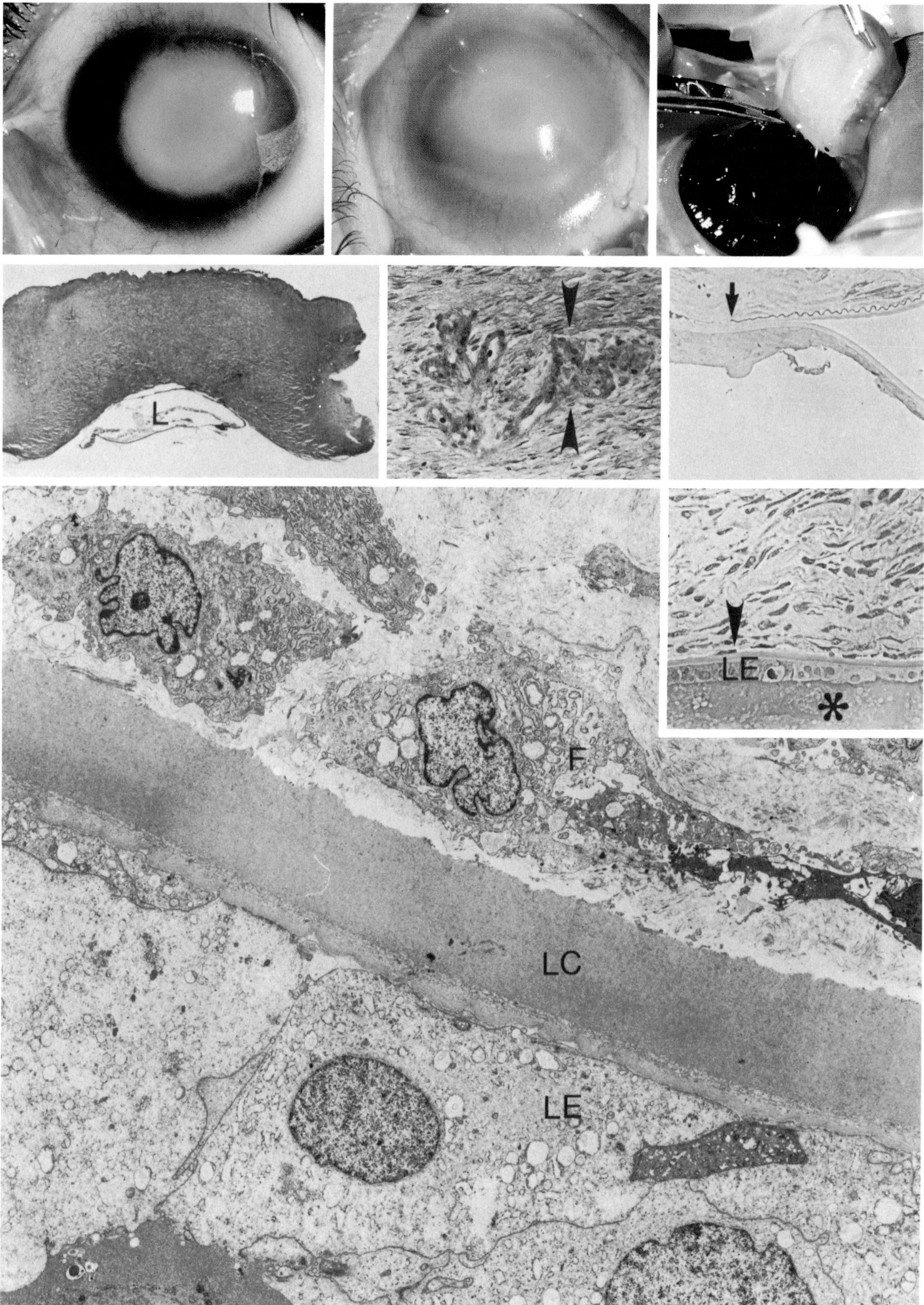

FIGURE 1–10 *See legend on opposite page*

◀ FIGURE 1–10 **Peters' anomaly.** *Top left,* Clinical photograph of a typical bilateral case with large leukomas that was successfully treated by penetrating keratoplasty with optical iridectomy of the fellow eye. *Top center,* A more diffuse corneal opacity in a 7-month-old baby. *Top right,* Intraoperative photograph demonstrates adhesion of the lens to the posterior cornea as a corneal button (grasped with forceps) is trephined. No iris could be identified. *Middle left,* Light micrograph of a corneal button showing a posterior central depression in which lodged the cataractous lens (L). H&E, ×10. *Middle center,* Higher magnification of light microscopy of the posterior cornea adjacent to the central stromal defect demonstrates fragments of presumed lens capsule and lens epithelium *(between arrowheads)* immersed in the stromal collagen. PAS, ×200. *Middle right,* Phase-contrast microscopy of the same cornea resolves the thin and undulating Descemet's membrane, which terminates *(arrow)* at the site of keratolenticular apposition. PPDA, ×250. *Bottom inset,* Phase-contrast micrograph of central area of the cornea devoid of Descemet's membrane and lined by lens capsule *(arrowhead),* lens epithelium *(LE),* and cataractous lens cortex *(asterisk).* PPDA, ×250. *Bottom,* Transmission electron micrograph of this same area discloses numerous fibroblastic cells (F) in the posterior stroma, lined by a uniform, 8-μm-thick lens capsule (LC) and lens epithelium (LE). ×4000.

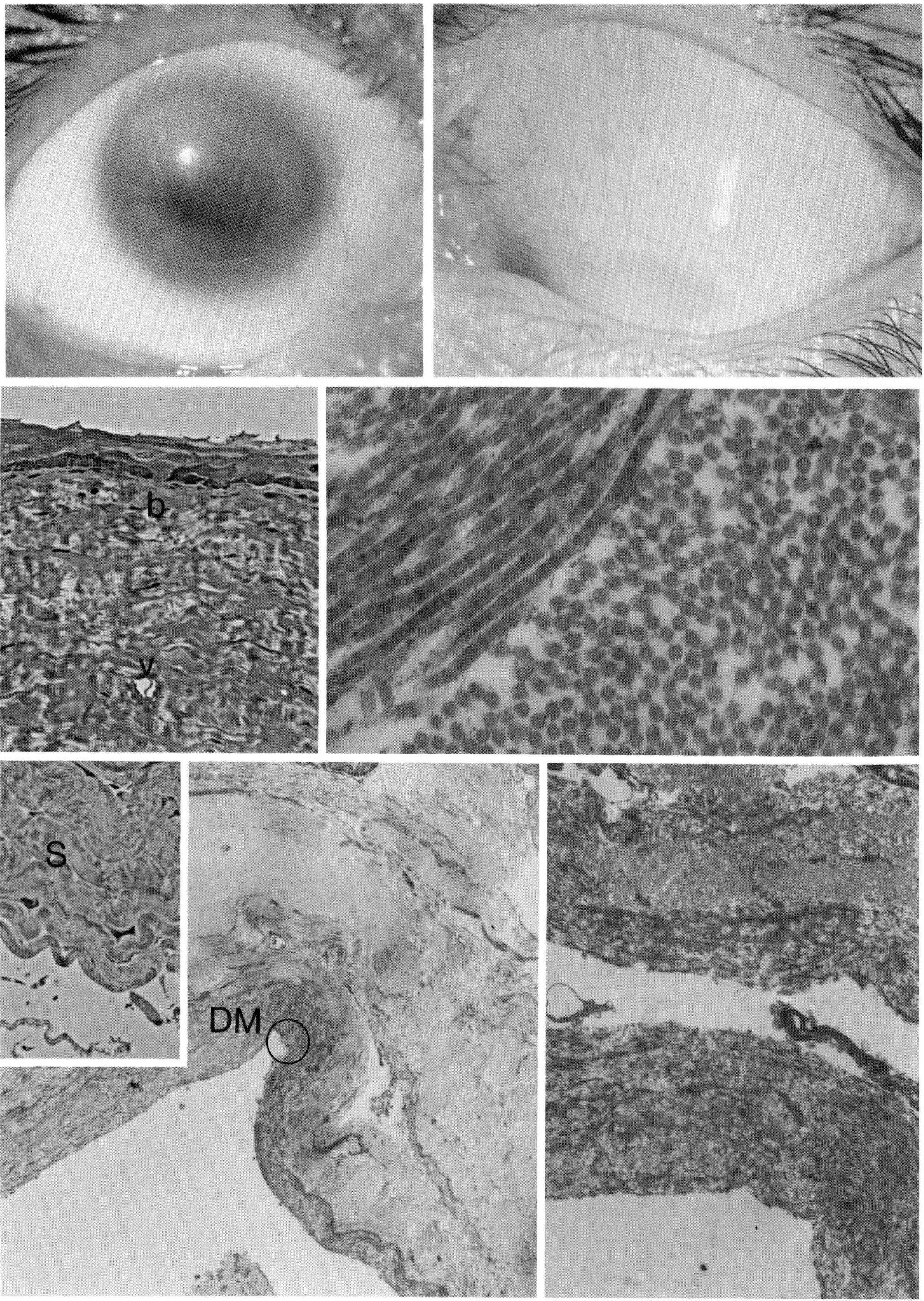

FIGURE 1–11 *See legend on opposite page*

◀ FIGURE 1–11 **Sclerocornea.** *Top left,* Moderate corneal haze in a partially affected patient. *Top right,* In this advanced bilateral case with multiple congenital abnormalities, the entire cornea is sclerified, and the fine vascular arcades extend centrally from the conjunctiva and sclera. *Middle left,* Light micrograph of anterior cornea shows disorganization of the epithelium, fragmentation of Bowman's layer (b), and interstitial vascularization (v). PPDA, ×350. *Middle right,* Transmission electron microscopy discloses a disorganized array of collagen fibrils that measure as much as three times normal diameter. ×52,500. *Bottom inset,* Light microscopy of the posterior cornea shows irregularly thick and wavy stromal lamellae (S). Descemet's membrane could not be easily identified. PPDA, ×350. *Bottom left,* Transmission electron micrograph of the same area discloses rudimentary Descemet's membrane (DM) with notable absence of endothelial cells. ×4,000. *Bottom right,* Higher-magnification electron micrograph of the area circled in *bottom left figure* reveals multilaminar basement membrane material interspersed with fine filaments. ×75,000.

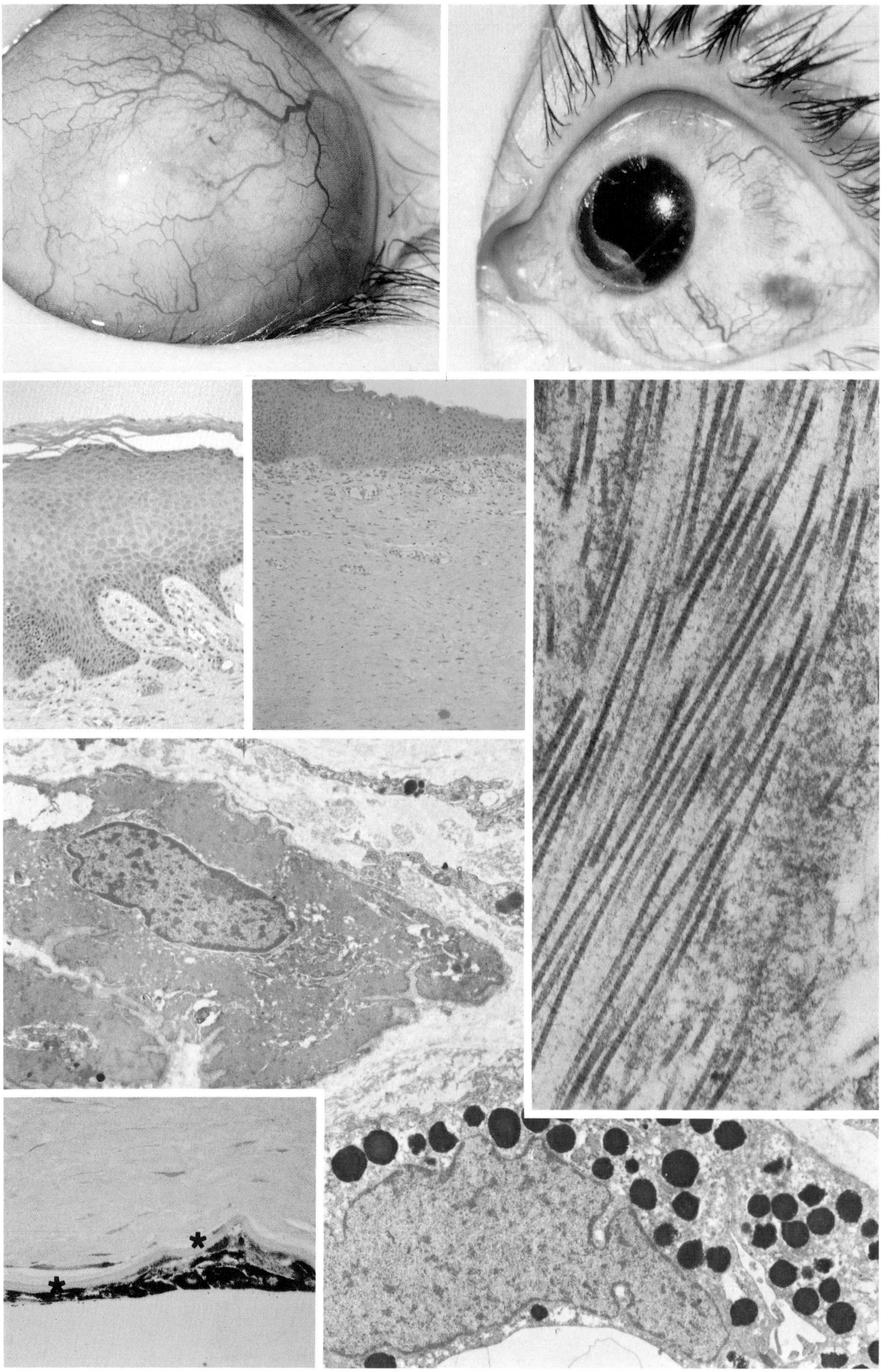

FIGURE 1–12 *See legend on opposite page*

◀ FIGURE 1–12 **Congenital anterior staphyloma.** *Top left,* A 1-year-old girl was born with anterior staphyloma of the right eye and anterior segment mesodermal dysgenesis of the left. The right eye showed enormous proptosis of the enlarged and scleralized cornea. The axial length is elongated to 24 mm owing to disproportionate enlargement of the anterior segment. *Top right,* The left eye immediately after penetrating keratoplasty and anterior segment reconstruction. *Middle left,* Light microscopy of keratoplasty specimen shows secondary epithelial metaplasia into keratinized stratified squamous epithelium. *Middle center,* Involved stroma of the same specimen assumes the morphologic features of scleral tissue with the presence of abundant blood vessels. H&E, ×75. *Middle right,* Transmission electron microscopy of the corneal stroma discloses abnormally thick (440 Å) collagen fibrils. ×43,400. *Bottom inset,* Light microscopy of posterior cornea demonstrates pigmented epithelium of the iris apposed to Descemet's membrane *(asterisk).* PAS, ×75. *Bottom,* Transmission electron microscopy of this same area discloses iris pigment epithelial cells and stromal tissue lining the posterior corneal surface. ×6400.

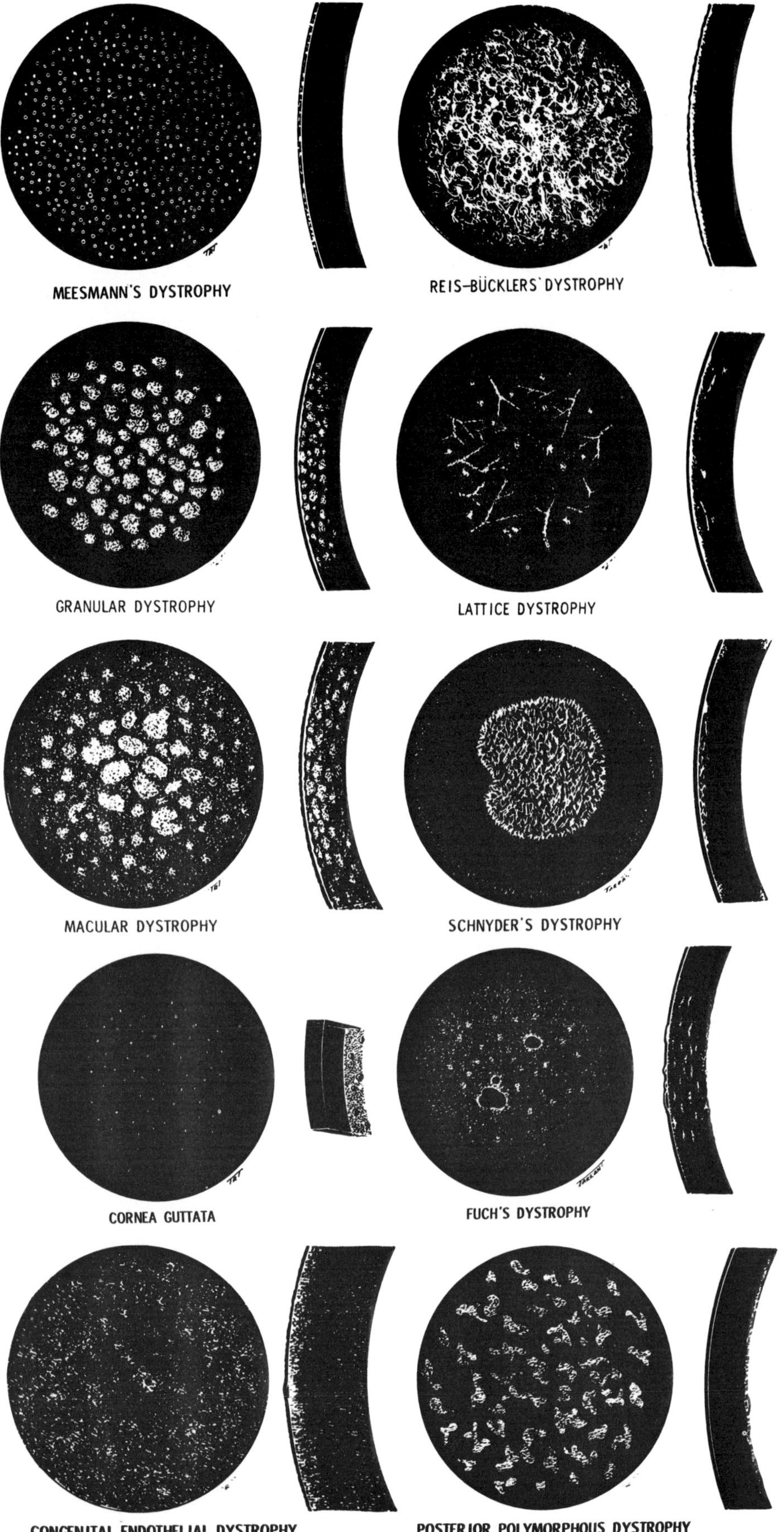

FIGURE 1–13 **Corneal stromal dystrophies.** The morphologic appearance of the more common corneal dystrophies. The sagittal corneal views depict the level of the affected corneal tissue. (Courtesy of Dr. A. Bron, From Coney A, Miller J, Krachmer JH: Corneal diseases. *In* Goldberg M: Genetic and Metabolic Eye Disease. Boston: Little, Brown, 1974, pp. 283–285.)

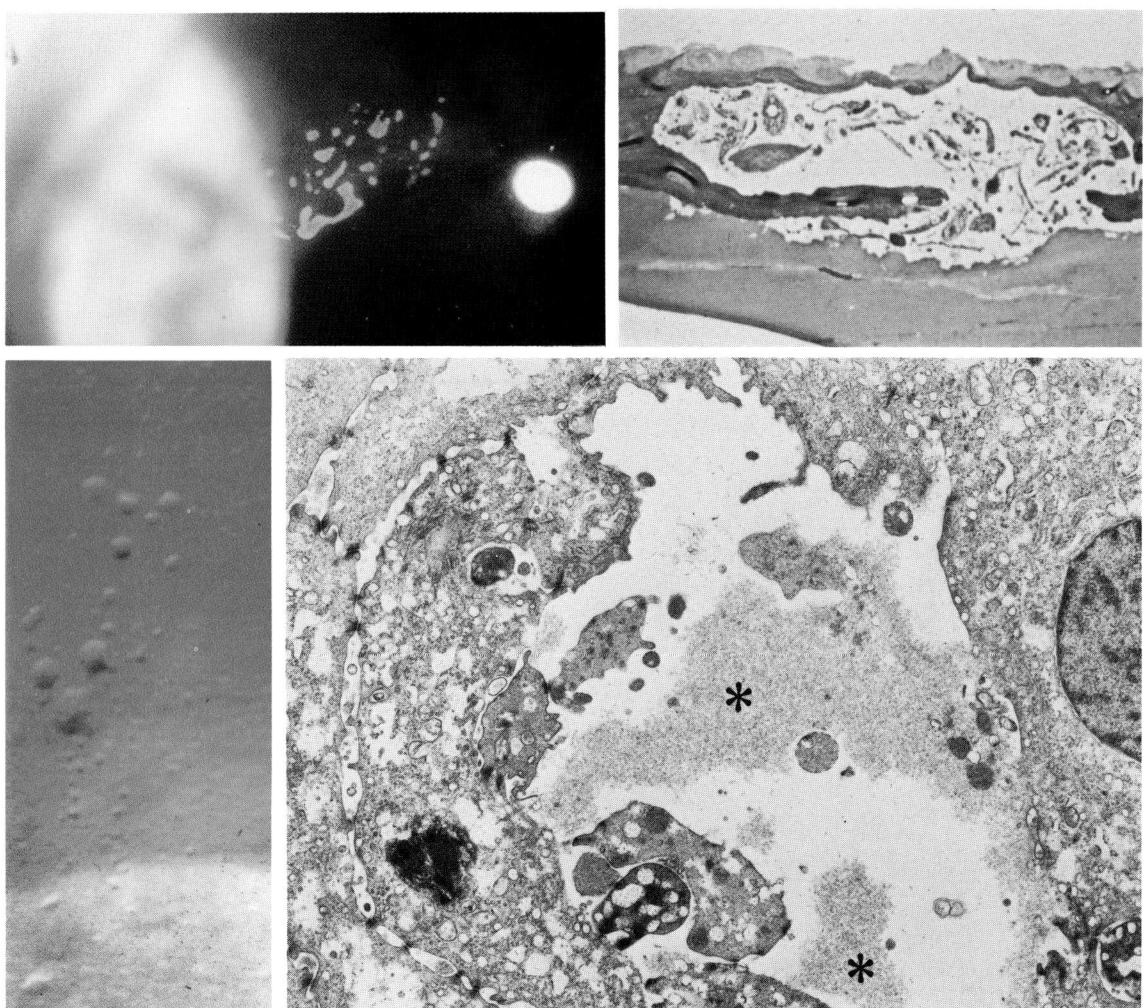

FIGURE 1–14 **Map-dot-fingerprint dystrophy.** *Top left,* Clinical photo of a 42-year-old woman with nontraumatic erosions shows characteristics of map dystrophy with superficial geographic haze interrupted by clear areas and few dots. *Top right,* Light microscopy of the clinical dot pattern reveals a large debris-containing intraepithelial cyst. PPDA, ×400. *Bottom left,* Enhanced transillumination view of the dot pattern. *Bottom right,* Transmission electron microscopy of the evolving cyst that results from cellular dissolution leaving residual nonspecific cytoplasmic granular debris *(asterisks).* ×8000.

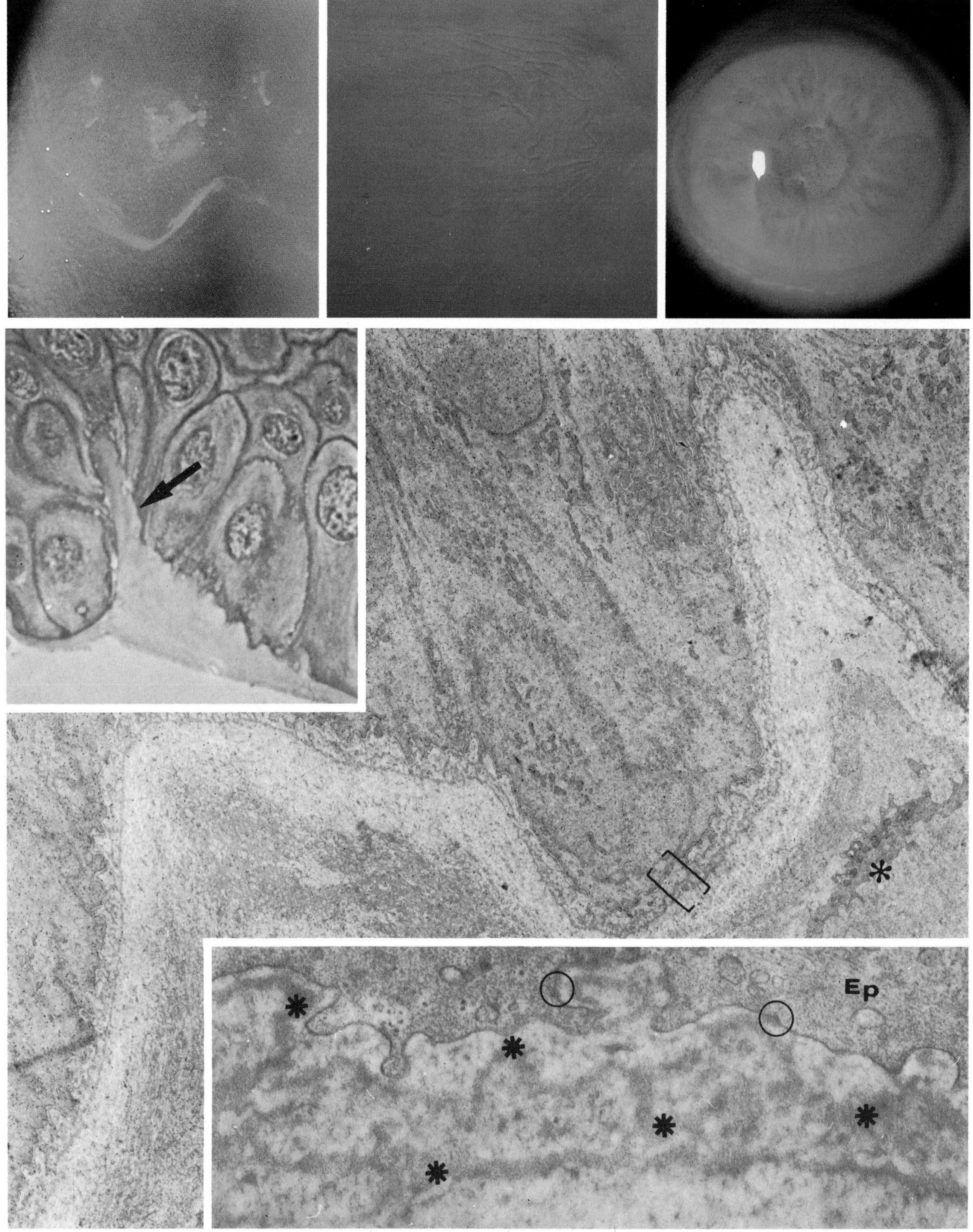

FIGURE 1–15 *See legend on opposite page*

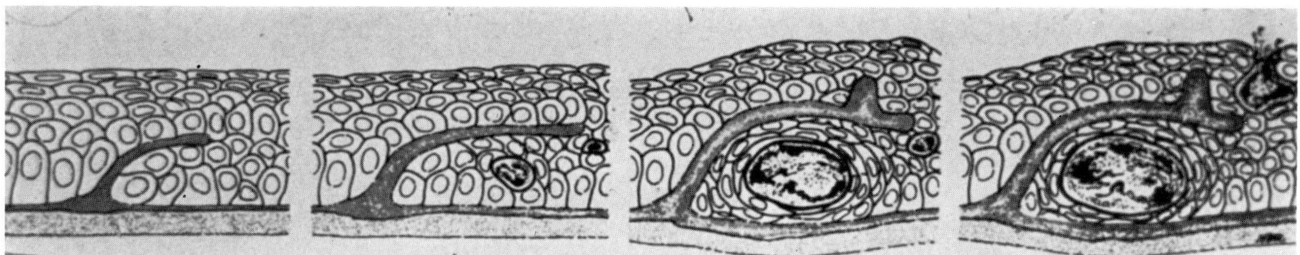

FIGURE 1-16 **Theorized pathogenesis of epithelial basement membrane dystrophy.** Epithelial cells produce abnormal multilaminar basement membrane, both in the normal location and intraepithelially. As the intraepithelial basement membrane thickens, it blocks a normal migration of epithelial cells toward the surface. Trapped epithelial cells degenerate to form intraepithelial microcysts that slowly migrate to the surface. The abnormal basement membrane produces map and fingerprint changes, and microcysts produce the dot pattern seen clinically. (From Waring GO III, Rodrigues MM, Laibson PR, et al: Corneal dystrophies. 1. Dystrophies of the epithelium, Bowman's layer and stroma. Surv Ophthal 23:71, 1978.)

◀ FIGURE 1-15 **Map-dot-fingerprint dystrophy.** *Top left and center,* Two variants of fingerprint dystrophy show subepithelial ridges and appear refractile against the red fundus reflection. (Courtesy of Dr. L. Hirst.) *Top right,* Under direct illumination, otherwise faintly visible fingerprint lines are enhanced with fluorescein staining and cobalt light. Irregular corneal tear film and abnormal tear breakup are evident. *Bottom, upper inset,* Phase-contrast photomicrograph illustrates a prominent intraepithelial "fingerprint" extension *(arrow)* from the subepithelial zone with marked rearrangement of the basal epithelium. PPDA, ×1200. *Bottom,* Transmission electron microscopy of the same area discloses collagenous and granular composition of the subepithelial material as well as cellular elements *(asterisk)* and an elaborate multilaminar basement membrane *(bracketed area)* loosely apposed to an undulating basal cell membrane. ×7000. *Bottom, lower inset,* Higher magnification of the bracketed area in *bottom figure* resolves typical redundant laminations of the basement membrane *(asterisks),* underdeveloped hemidesmosomes *(encircled areas),* and absence of anchoring fibrils; Ep indicates basal epithelium. ×40,000.

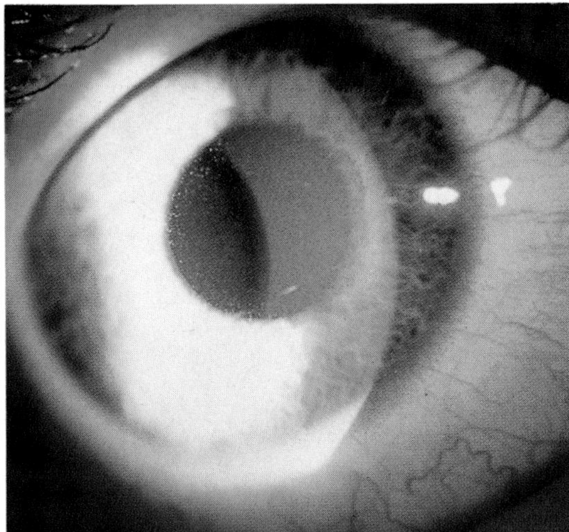

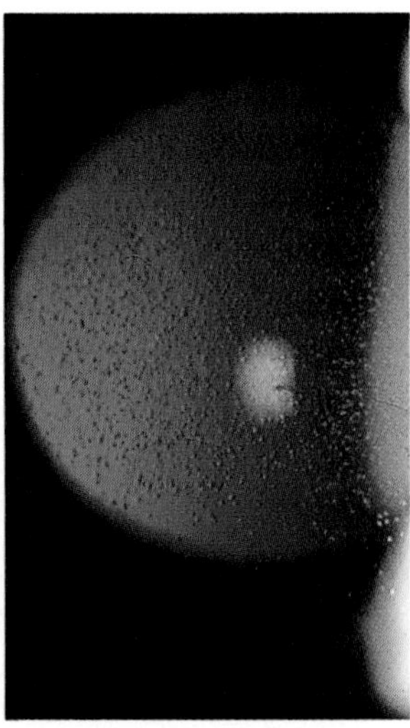

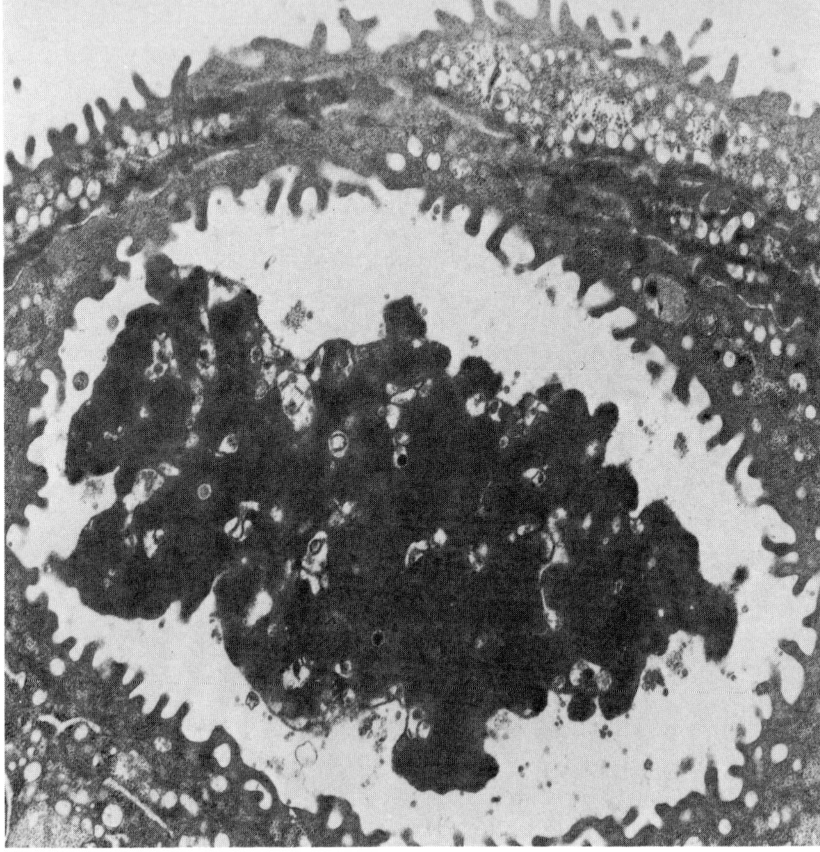

FIGURE 1–17 **Hereditary epithelial dystrophy (Meesmann; Stocker-Holt).** *Top left,* Photograph discloses myriad small, clear to gray-white punctate opacities in the interpalpebral zone. *Top right,* The intraepithelial vesicles stand out with retroillumination. *Bottom,* Transmission electron micrograph of the corneal epithelium shows an intraepithelial pseudocyst containing desquamated cellular debris. ×18,000.

FIGURE 1–18 **Reis-Bücklers dystrophy.** *Top left,* Clinical photograph of a 26-year-old woman with recurrent erosions exhibits a diffuse superficial corneal haze. *Top right,* Slit-lamp photograph shows a more typical reticular pattern of gray ringlike superficial opacities. *Middle left,* Light microscopy demonstrates the sawtooth configuration of accumulated subepithelial material with an irregular basal epithelial layer. H&E, ×220. *Middle right,* Phase-contrast microscopy reveals a prominent deposit of subepithelial fibrocellular tissue *(asterisk)* with a distorted Bowman's layer. PPDA, ×300. *Bottom inset,* Phase-contrast microscopy demonstrates degeneration of dark-staining basal cells and fragmentation of Bowman's layer *(asterisk)* by nodular fibrous pannus. PPDA, ×800. *Bottom left,* Transmission electron microscopy confirms thin remnants of a disarrayed Bowman's layer (B) and apparent continuity *(arrowheads)* between basal cell epithelium (Ep) and degenerate cellular debris (D) with Bowman's layer. Basement membrane complexes *(encircled area)* are discontinuous and lack anchoring fibrils. ×30,000. *Bottom right,* High-magnification electron micrograph of fibrillar deposits resolves as masses of irregular curled 6–8 nm diameter filaments. ×63,000. ▶

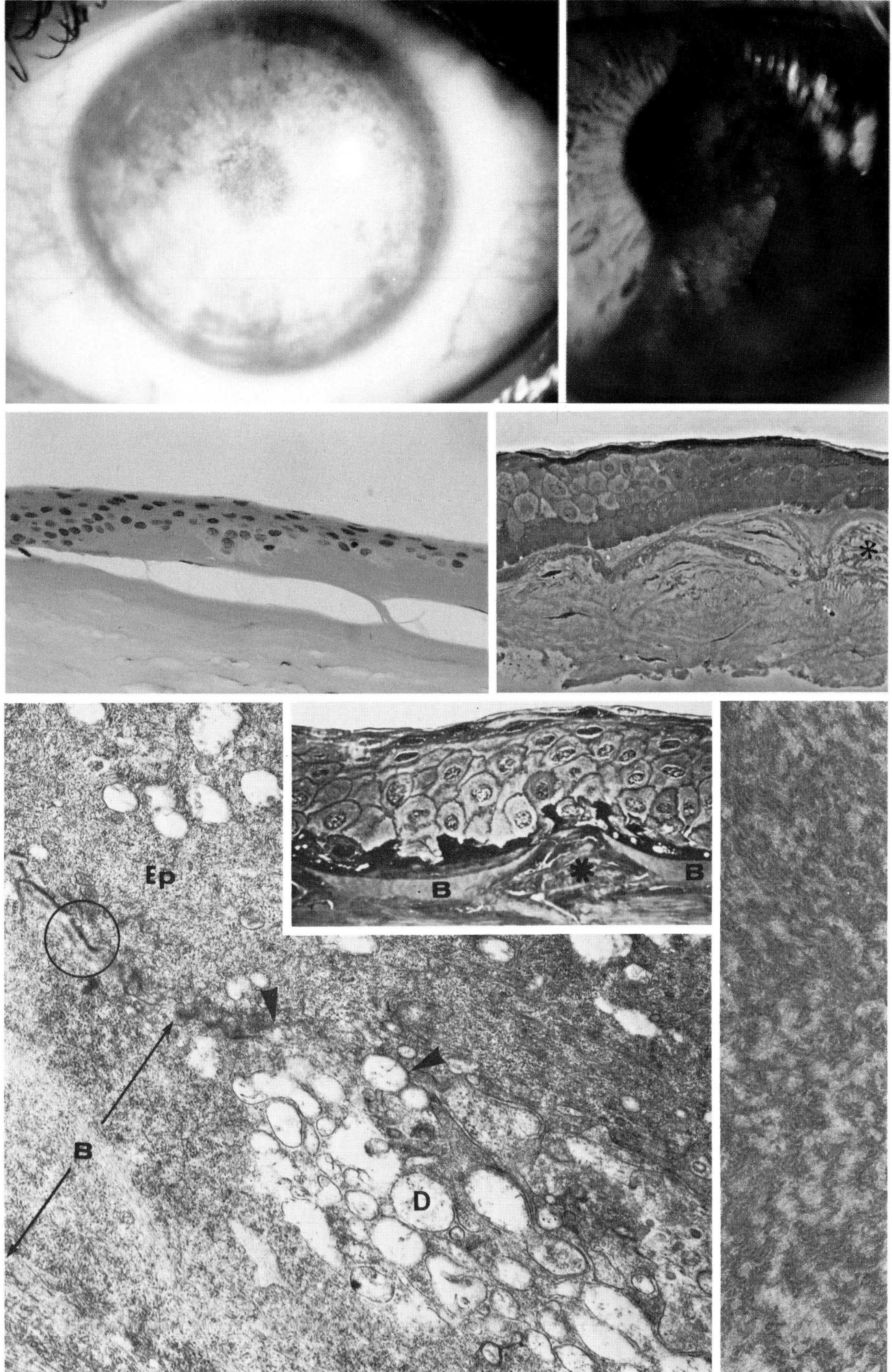

FIGURE 1–18 *See legend on opposite page*

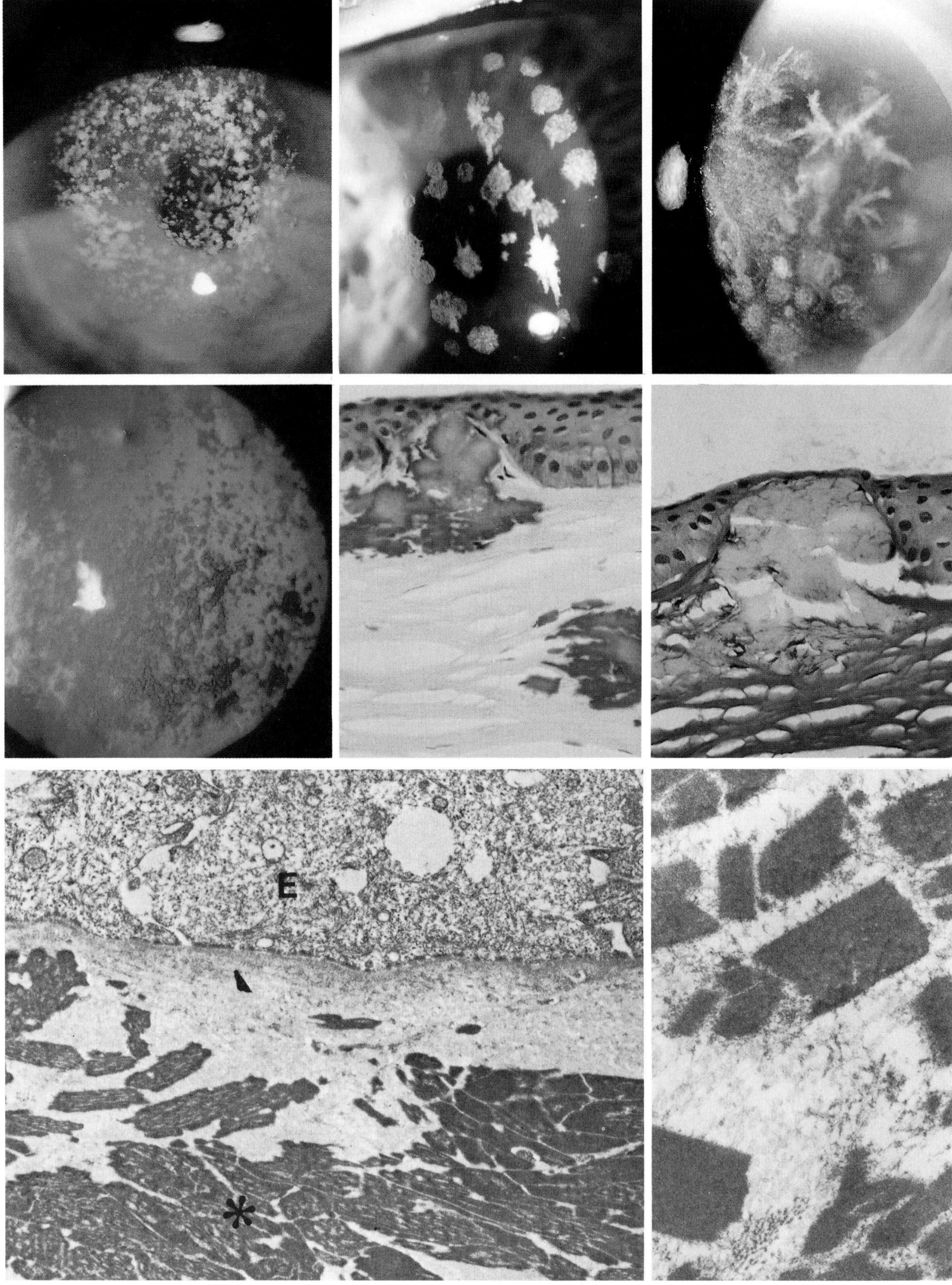

FIGURE 1–19 *See legend on opposite page*

◀ FIGURE 1-19 **Granular corneal dystrophy.** *Top,* Three different clinical configurations of granular dystrophy. *Top left,* Densely axial nontransluscent gray-white deposits simulating bread crumbs. *Top center,* More discrete and well-defined round and oval shapes with clear stroma between lesions. *Top right,* Christmas tree–like opacities with moderate anterior stromal scarring. *Middle left,* Retroillumination emphasizes the optical clarity of intervening stroma between the granular opacities. (Courtesy of Dr. Lawrence Hirst.) *Middle center,* Light microscopy of irregularly shaped hyaline deposits is accentuated with Masson's trichrome stain. ×220. *Middle right,* Light microscopy of a patient with severe recurrent erosion reveals a superficial deposit evolving to break the epithelial surface. PAS, ×220. *Bottom left,* Transmission electron microscopy shows relatively normal epithelium (E) and basement membrane *(arrowhead)* anterior to large electron-dense deposits *(asterisk)* within Bowman's layer and anterior stroma. ×15,000. *Bottom right,* Higher-magnification transmission electron microscopy of granular deposits shows the characteristic homogeneous rod-shaped paracrystalline structure. ×50,000.

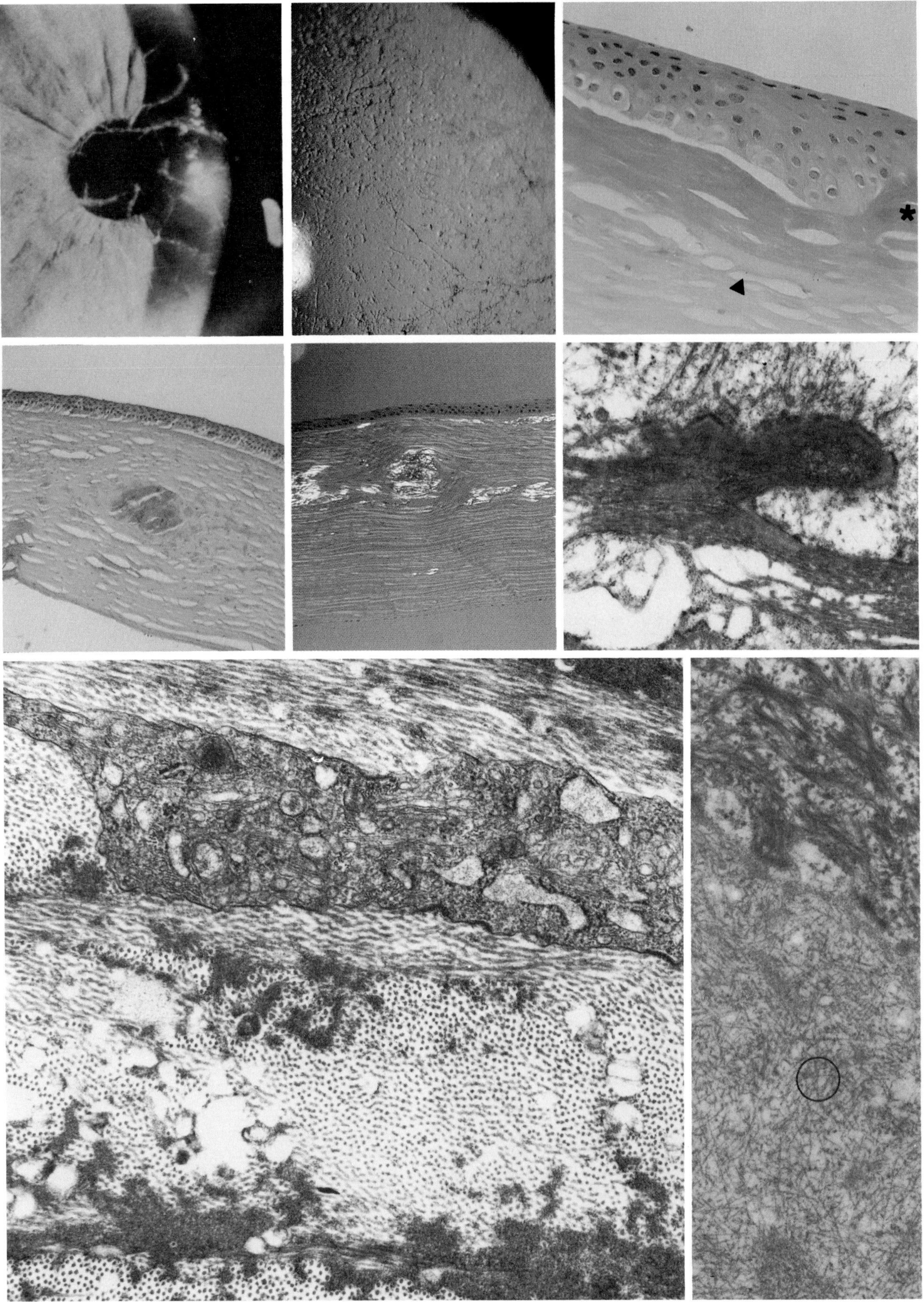

FIGURE 1–20 *See legend on opposite page*

◀ FIGURE 1-20 **Lattice corneal dystrophy.** *Top left and center,* Slit-lamp photography demonstrates pathognomonic branching lattice figures throughout the stroma. (*Top left,* Courtesy of Dr. W. J. Stark.) *Top right,* Light microscopy of a cornea in a patient with multiple episodes of recurrent erosions discloses an irregular epithelial layer, partial absence of Bowman's layer *(arrowhead),* and predominantly subepithelial amyloid deposits *(asterisk).* PAS, ×220. *Middle left,* Congo red stain of fusiform lesion that distorts the normal stromal lamellar architecture. Congo red, ×55. *Middle center,* Corneal amyloid shows birefringence and dichroism under the polarizing microscope. ×20. *Middle right,* Transmission electron microscopy of basement membrane complexes reveals basement membrane irregularity and discontinuity resulting from underlying amyloid fibrils. ×21,300. *Bottom left,* Transmission electron micrograph of the stroma shows normal collagen fibrils and keratocytes with electron-dense material abnormally dispersed extracellularly. ×16,000. *Bottom right,* High-magnification transmission electron micrograph resolves lattice material as masses of fine 80-100 Å diameter amyloid fibrils *(circled area).* ×43,400.

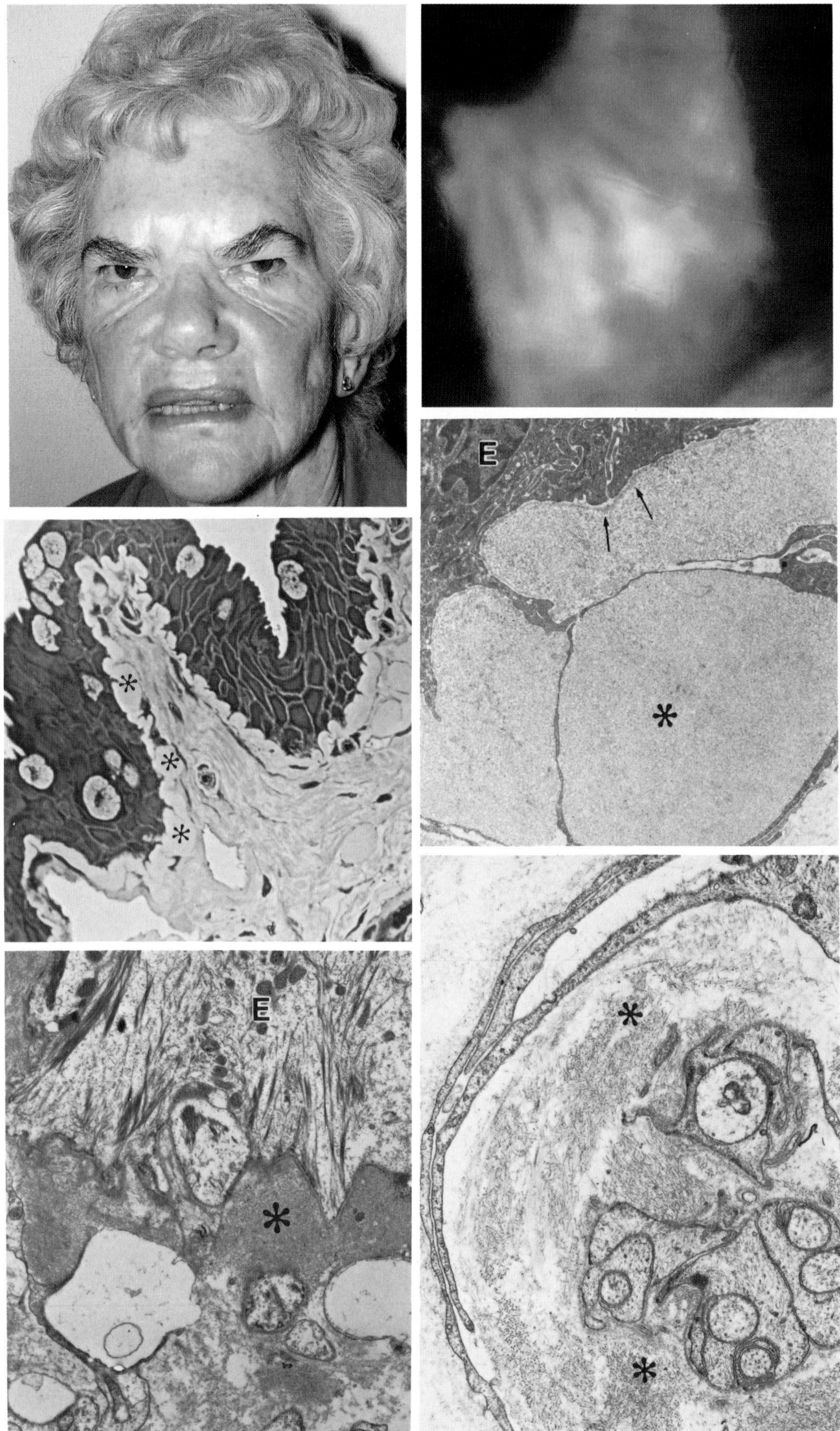

FIGURE 1–21 *See legend on opposite page*

◀ FIGURE 1–21 **Lattice corneal dystrophy and systemic amyloidosis (Meretoja syndrome).** *Top left,* A 73-year-old woman with typical "masklike" facies including skin thickening, prominent dermatochalasis, depressed eyebrows, and bilateral facial nerve palsies. *Top right,* Slit-lamp view of lattice lines beginning at the periphery and sparing the visual axis. *Middle left,* Light microscopy of conjunctival biopsy specimen shows continuous subepithelial layer *(asterisks)* of extracellular material. PPDA, ×300. *Middle right,* Transmission electron microscopy of this biopsy specimen demonstrates masses of fine amyloid fibrils *(asterisk)* beneath the epithelial membrane *(arrows).* (E, epithelium.) ×8700. *Bottom left,* Transmission electron microscopy of skin biopsy specimen reveals deposition of extracellular material *(asterisk)* immediately beneath the normal epithelial basement membrane. ×8100. *Bottom right,* Similar deposits *(asterisks)* are found associated with the perineurium and endoneurium of peripheral nerves. ×12,060.

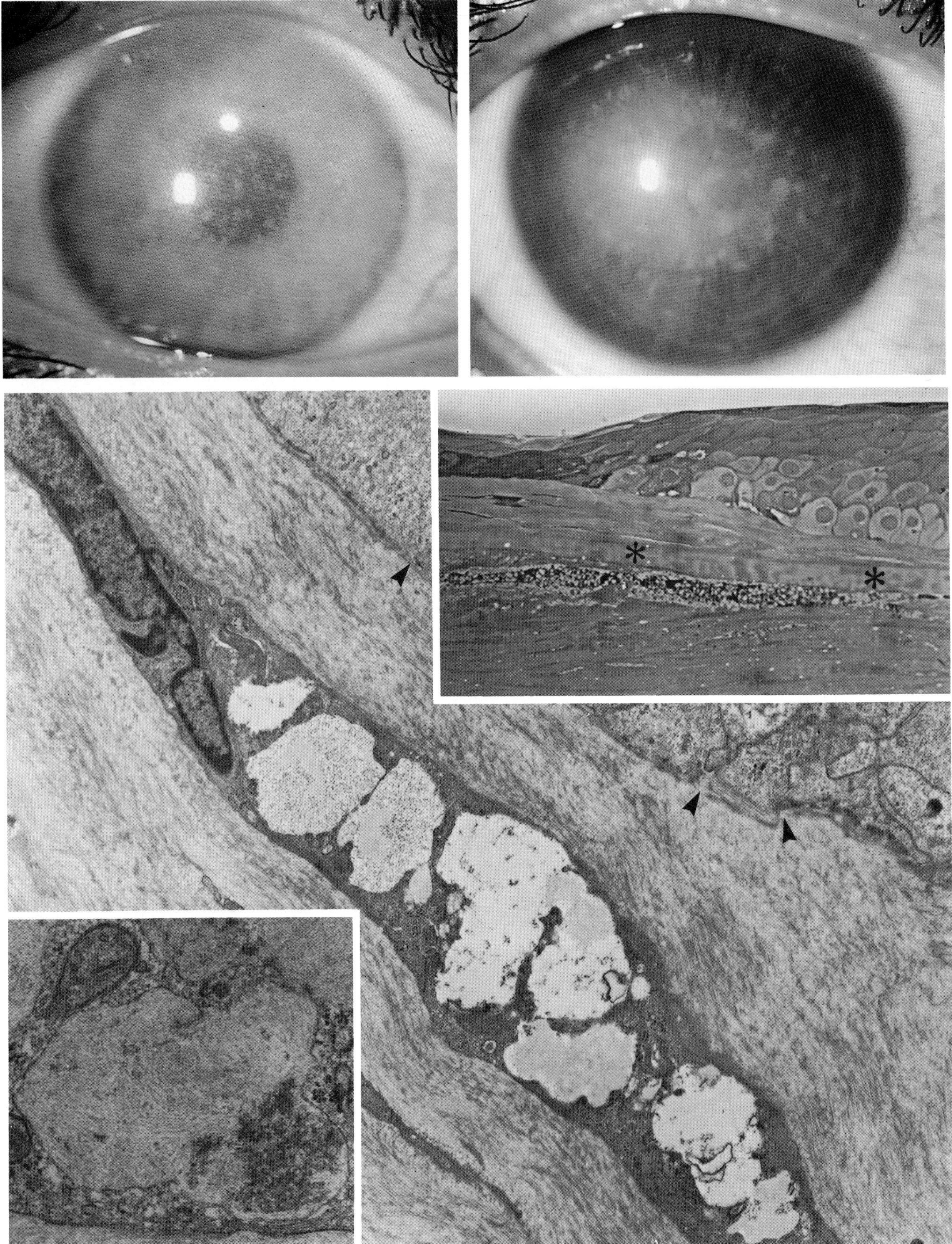

FIGURE 1–22 *See legend on opposite page*

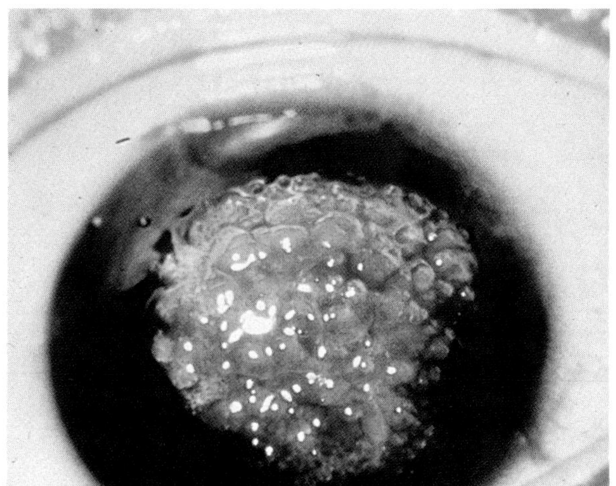

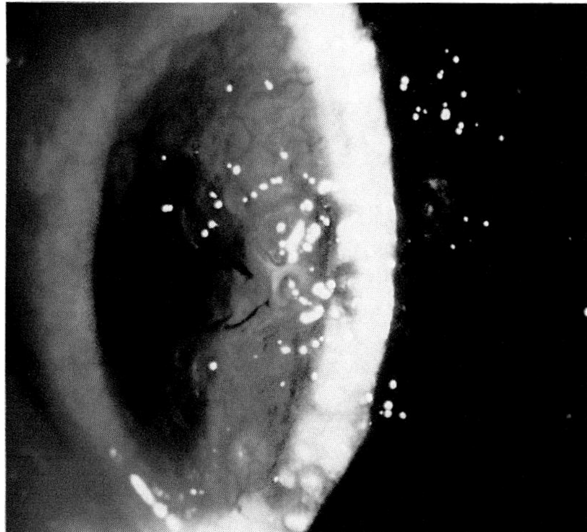

FIGURE 1–23 **Gelatinous droplike dystrophy.** Central "mulberry-like" opacity has protuberant subepithelial mounds that appear white on focal illumination *(left)* and semitransparent on retroillumination *(right).* Minor stromal neovascularization is present superonasally. This dystrophy is another clinical manifestation of primary, localized corneal amyloidosis.

◀ FIGURE 1–22 **Macular corneal dystropy.** *Top left,* Clinical appearance of cornea features diffuse stromal haze with a "ground-glass" appearance extending to the limbus. Centrally, superimposed gray-white spots with indistinct edges are observed. *Top right,* In a clinical variant, larger, amorphous lesions involve only the central cornea sparing the limbus. *Bottom, right inset,* By phase-contrast microscopy, the epithelium is seen to be irregular. Fibrocellular pannus intervenes between the epithelium and the unaffected Bowman's layer *(asterisks).* Several extensively vacuolated keratocytes are evident in the anterior stroma. PPDA, ×250. *Bottom, main figure,* Transmission electron microscopy demonstrates irregular thinning and breaks *(arrowheads)* of basement membrane. Within the fragmented Bowman's layer, subepithelial cells are distended by membrane-limited intracytoplasmic inclusions containing fine granular and reticular material. ×12,000. *Bottom, left inset,* Higher-magnification transmission electron microscopy resolves the reticular pattern of accumulated intracellular material. ×43,500.

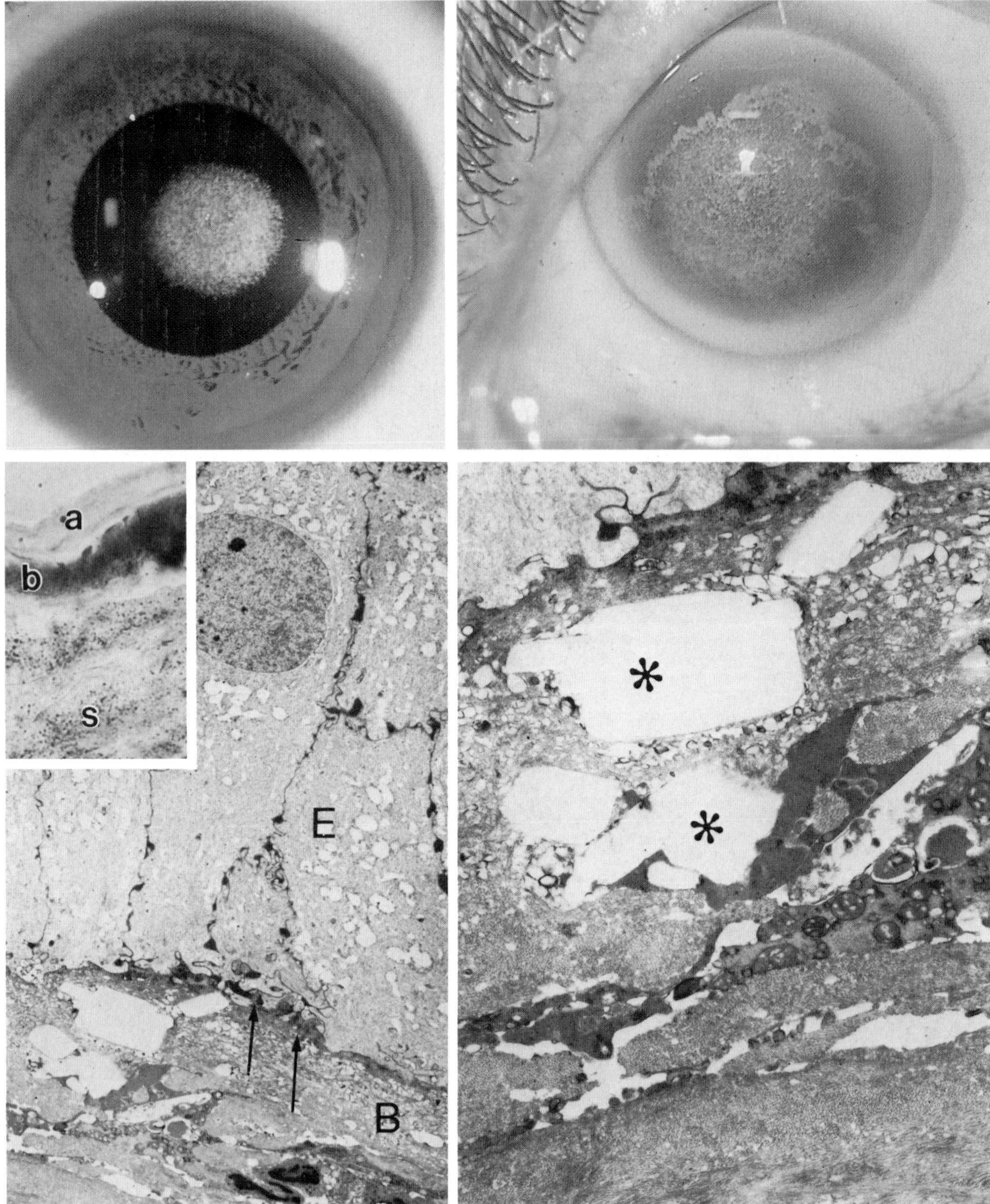

FIGURE 1–24 **Central crystalline dystrophy (Schnyder).** *Top left,* Clinical appearance of the eye of an 8-year-old boy includes an axial ring-shaped opacity formed by densely packed, fine, needle-shaped polychromatic crystals. Associated genu valgum was present in this pedigree. *Top right,* In a different variant, more extensive involvement of the central cornea and associated arcus senilis was present. *Bottom inset,* frozen section of keratoplasty specimen of superficial cornea reveals the epithelium (a) unstained, Bowman's layer (b) with intense lipid deposits, and stroma (s) with scattered lipid staining. Oil red O stain, ×350. *Bottom left,* Electron micrograph of basement epithelium in Bowman's layer reveals vacuolated corneal epithelium (E); thickened basement membrane *(arrows);* and distorted, vacuolated Bowman's zone (B) with polygonal profiles. ×10,000. *Bottom right,* High-magnification transmission electron microscopy of the same area discloses multiple polygonal spaces *(asterisks),* typical of cholesterol crystalline ghosts. ×25,000. (*Bottom,* From Burns RP, Connor W, Gipson I: Cholesterol turnover and hereditary crystalline corneal dystrophy of Schnyder. Trans Am Ophthalmol Soc 76:184, 1978.)

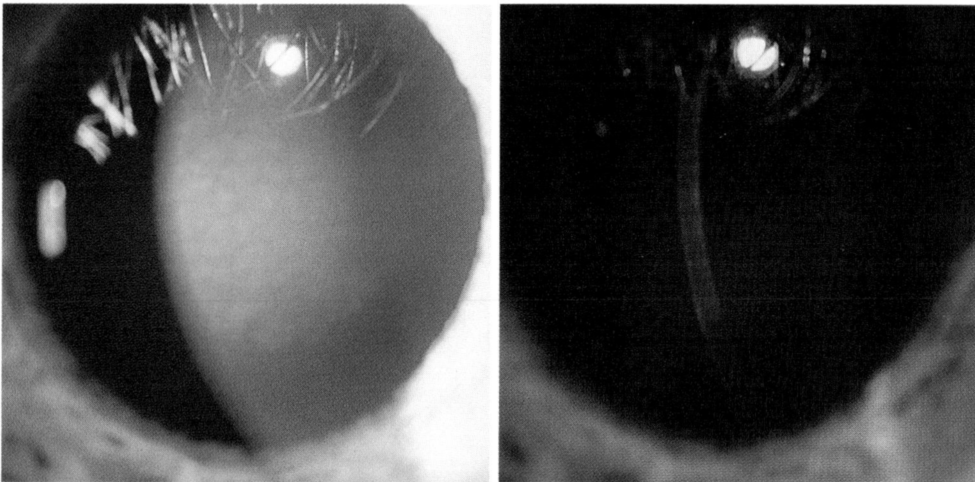

FIGURE 1–25 **Central cloudy dystrophy (François).** This 62-year-old man with visual acuity of 20/30 in both eyes demonstrates clouding of the central cornea into segmental areas of opacification with intervening clear tissue *(left)*. Similar view *(right)* features mainly posterior opacities extending forward but becoming much less dense. Vision is minimally affected, although the group of opacities are mainly axially. The patient is otherwise asymptomatic, and hence no therapy is required.

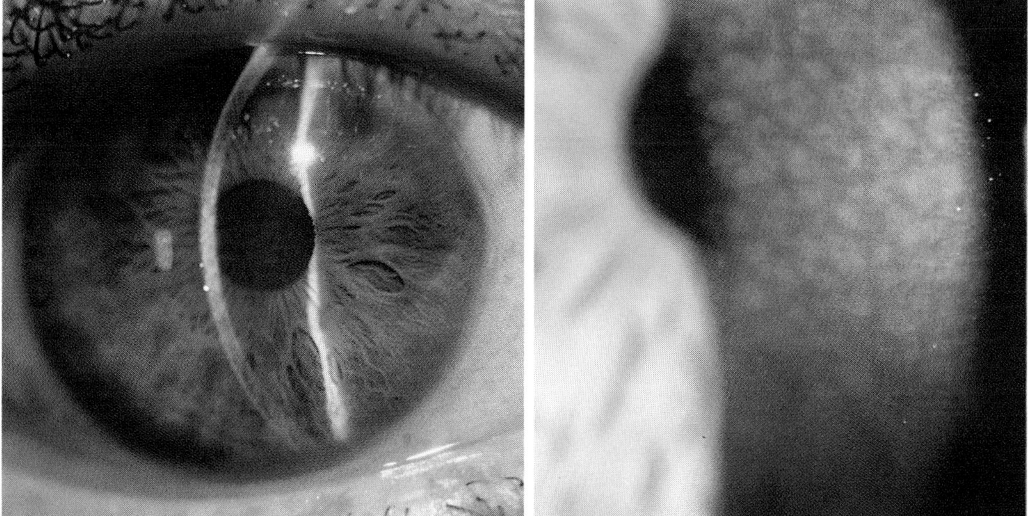

FIGURE 1–26 **Posterior mosaic crocodile shagreen (Vogt).** Clinical photography *(left)* of a 55-year-old asymptomatic woman demonstrates bilateral central opacification compromising the entire corneal thickness. Broad slit-lamp photography *(right)* discloses multiple small, fluffy, and indistinct grayish areas in a polygonal pattern separated by clear, cracklike zones. These regions are located at the level of Descemet's membrane. Transmission electron microscopy (not shown) reveals that the grayish opacities correspond to sawtooth-like configurations of the corneal collagen lamellae.

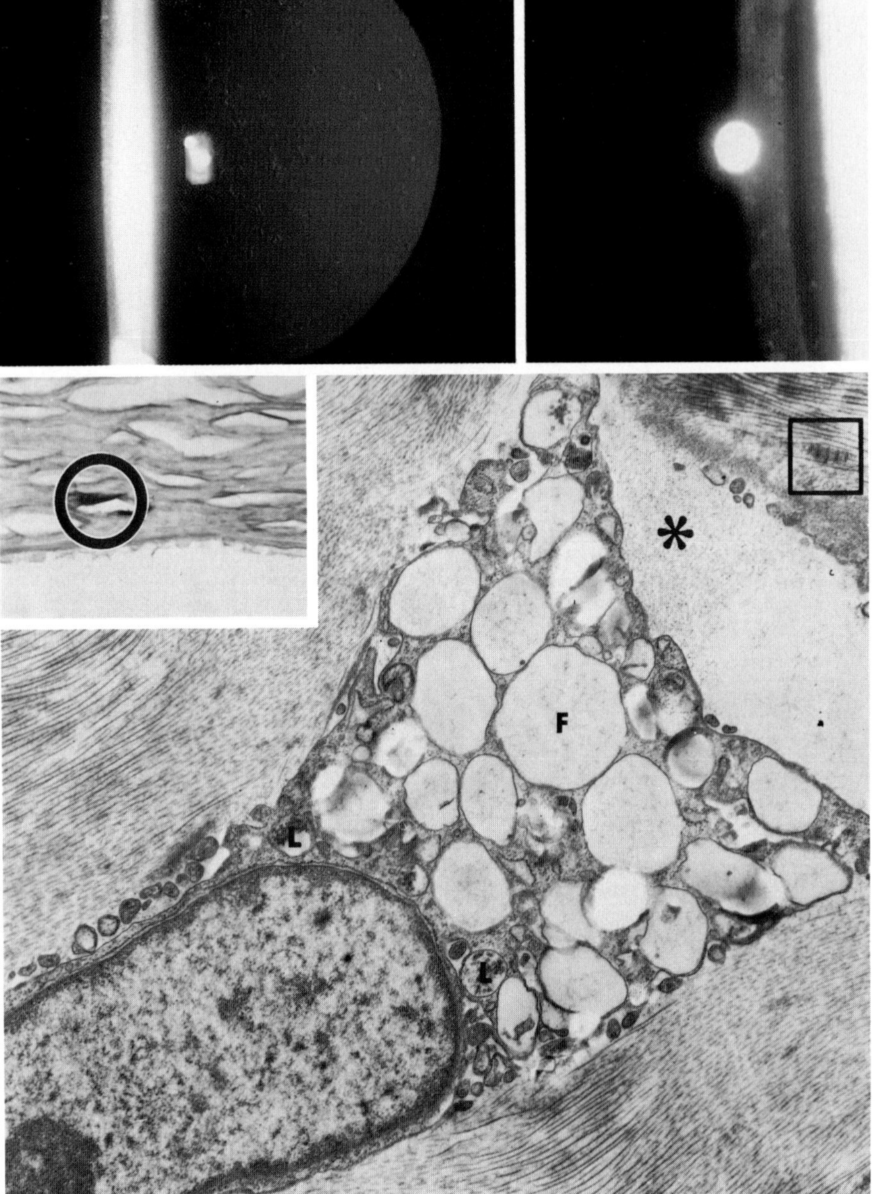

FIGURE 1-27 **Fleck dystrophy (François-Neetens).** *Top,* Retroillumination *(left)* and slit-lamp view *(right)* demonstrate discrete flattened white flecks with comma, wreath, or dot configuration present throughout the entire stroma. *Bottom inset,* Light microscopy of the posterior cornea illustrates positive staining for acid mucopolysaccharide limited to a swollen keratocyte *(circled area).* Colloidal iron, ×500. *Bottom,* Transmission electron microscopy of a markedly vacuolated keratocyte filled with fibrillogranular (F) or lipid (L) substances. There are no extracellular abnormalities except for accumulation of the fine granular material *(asterisk)* and occasional foci of long-spacing collagen *(square).* ×14,400. (*All,* From Nicholson DH, Green WR, Cross HE, et al: A clinical and histopathological study of François-Neeten's speckled corneal dystrophy. Am J Ophthalmol 83:554–560, 1977. Published with permission from the American Journal of Ophthalmology. Copyright by the Ophthalmic Publishing Company.)

FIGURE 1-28 **Congenital hereditary endothelial dystrophy.** *Top left,* Clinical photograph of an affected 20-year-old woman shows diffuse corneal haze and visual acuity of 20/200. *Top center,* On slit-lamp biomicroscopy, diffuse edematous thickening of the corneal stroma is evident in this same patient. *Top right,* Comparison of similarly prepared survey light micrographs of congenital hereditary endothelial dystrophy (a) and normal human corneas (b). Note the extraordinary increase in the thickness of the stroma in the former. H&E, ×60. *Bottom, upper right inset,* Light micrograph of the edematous stroma demonstrates vesicular water clefts *(asterisks).* PAS, ×200. *Bottom, upper middle inset,* Electron micrograph of the central stroma shows a cross section of collagen fibrils to have enlarged diameters (approximately 500 Å with some at 700 Å) *(arrowheads).* ×45,000. *Bottom, main figure,* Transmission electron micrographs of the posterior cornea. The anterior portion of Descemet's membrane (DM) appears to have banding of normal thickness, but the posterior collagenous layer is markedly thickened (8–15 μ). An additional abnormal posterior collagenous layer is present *(asterisk).* No endothelial cells are present. (S, stroma; AC, anterior chamber.) ×10,240. *Bottom, lower inset,* At higher magnification, the components of this posterior collagenous layer are visible as fine filaments (approximately 12 nm diameter) interspersed with basement membrane–like material *(asterisk).* (AC, anterior chamber.) ×50,000.

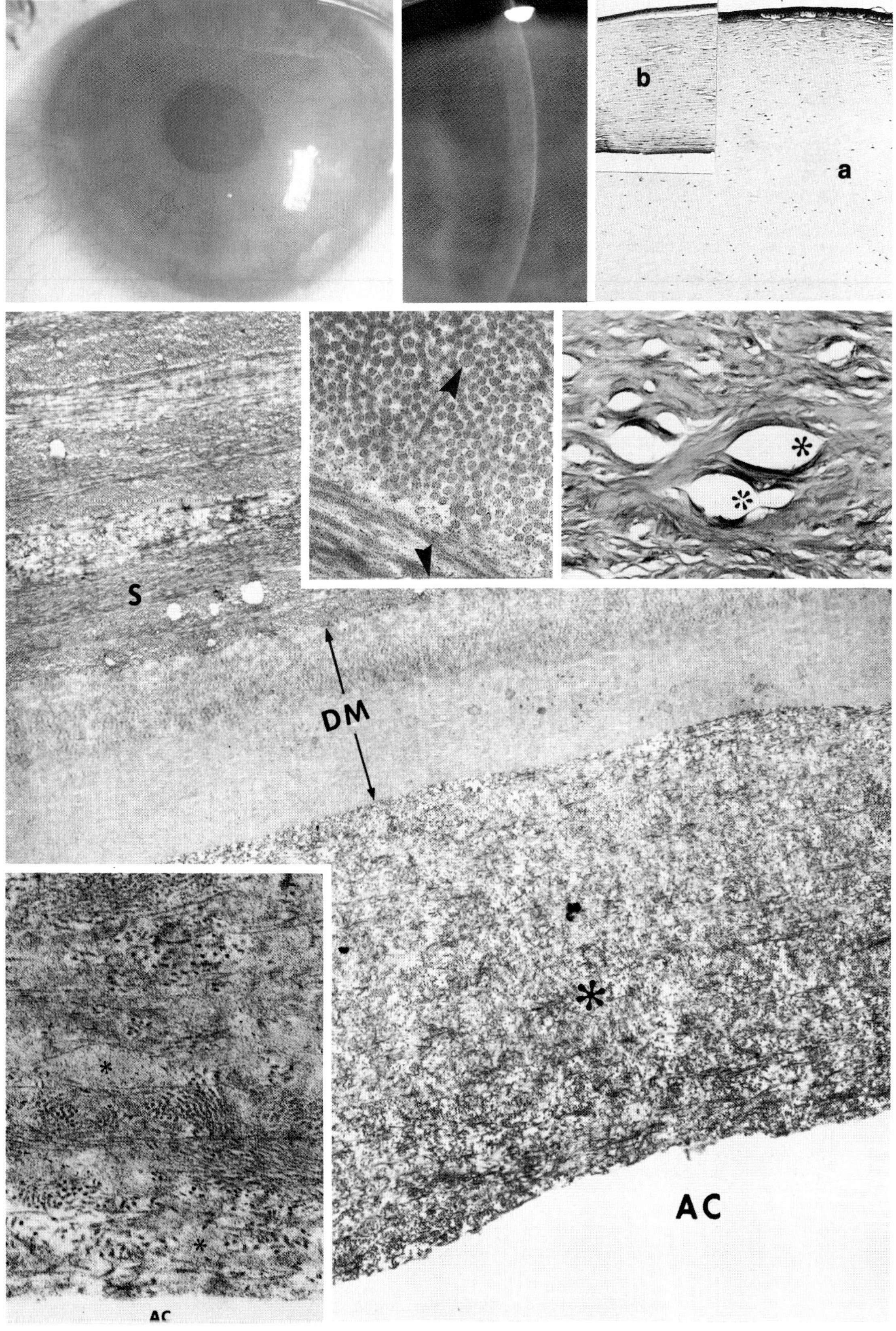

FIGURE 1–28 *See legend on opposite page*

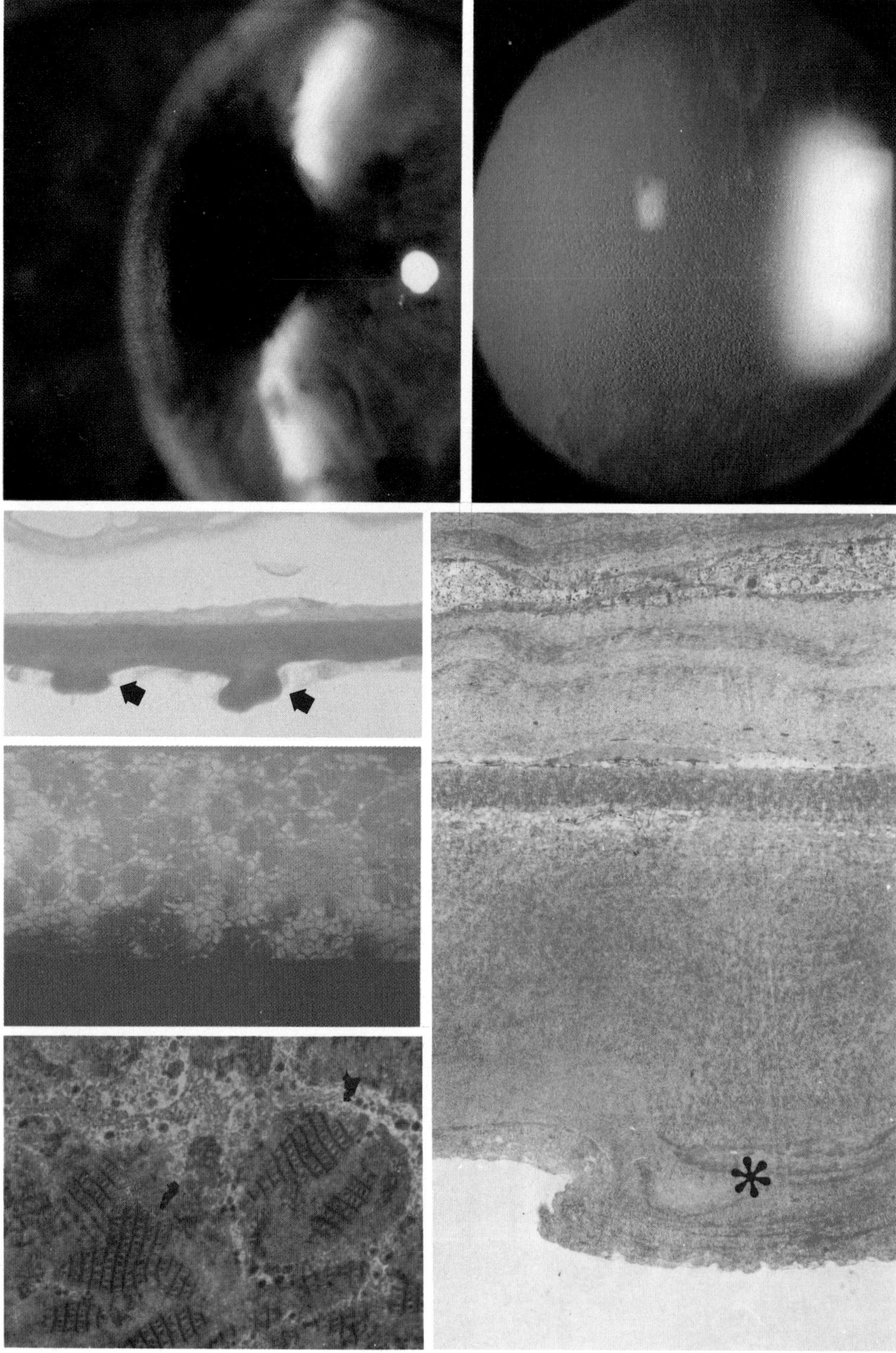

FIGURE 1–29 **Corneal guttata.** *Top left,* Slit-lamp photography shows stromal edema and folds in Descemet's membrane with metal-beaten appearance. *Top right,* Extensive endothelial guttae are demonstrated by retroillumination. *Left, upper inset,* By light microscopy, excresences *(arrows)* of Descemet's membrane are evident with loss of endothelial cells. PAS, ×100. *Left, middle inset,* Specular photomicrograph of the endothelial mosaic represents such guttae as dark holes. *Bottom right,* Transmission electron micrograph features a thickened Descemet's membrane with individual guttae *(asterisk).* ×3000. *Left, bottom inset,* At higher magnification, the guttata are resolved as fine filaments, multiple segments of basement membrane material, and collagen in long-spacing configuration *(arrowheads).* ×40,500.

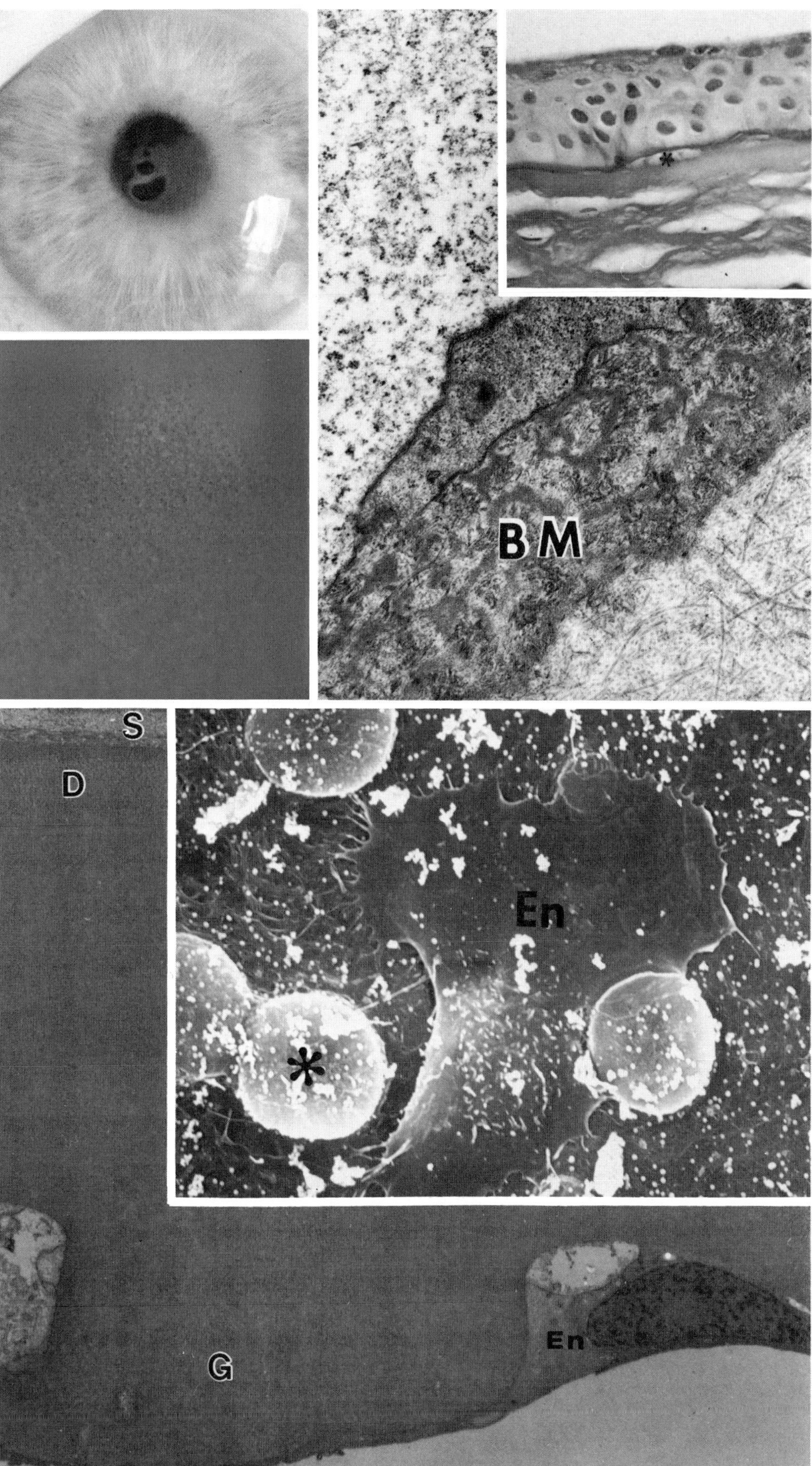

FIGURE 1–30 **Late hereditary endothelial dystrophy (Fuchs).** *Top left, upper and lower,* Clinical photographs of moderately advanced cases illustrate severe stromal edema and surface irregularities secondary to epithelial microcysts and coalescent bullae. *Top right, inset,* Light microscopy demonstrates intraepithelial edema, thickening of the basement membrane, subepithelial bullae *(asterisk),* and fibrocellular pannus with an adjacent break in Bowman's layer. H&E, ×350. *Top right,* Transmission electron micrograph of basal epithelial cells and Bowman's layer shows multilaminar basement membrane complexes (BM), the sequela of chromic epithelial edema. ×25,000. *Bottom, main figure,* Transmission electron micrograph of posterior corneal stroma shows unremarkable stroma (S) and anterior Descemet's membrane (D), but remarkable thickening of the posterior Descemet's membrane to 12 μ with additional superimposition of large guttae (G). The remaining endothelial cells (En) are severely degenerated and attenuated. ×5,000. *Bottom inset,* By scanning electron microscopy, the comparable picture shows disconnected and enormously attenuated endothelial cells (En) and numerous exposed mushroom-shaped excrescences *(asterisk)* projecting from the posterior collagenous layer. ×1600.

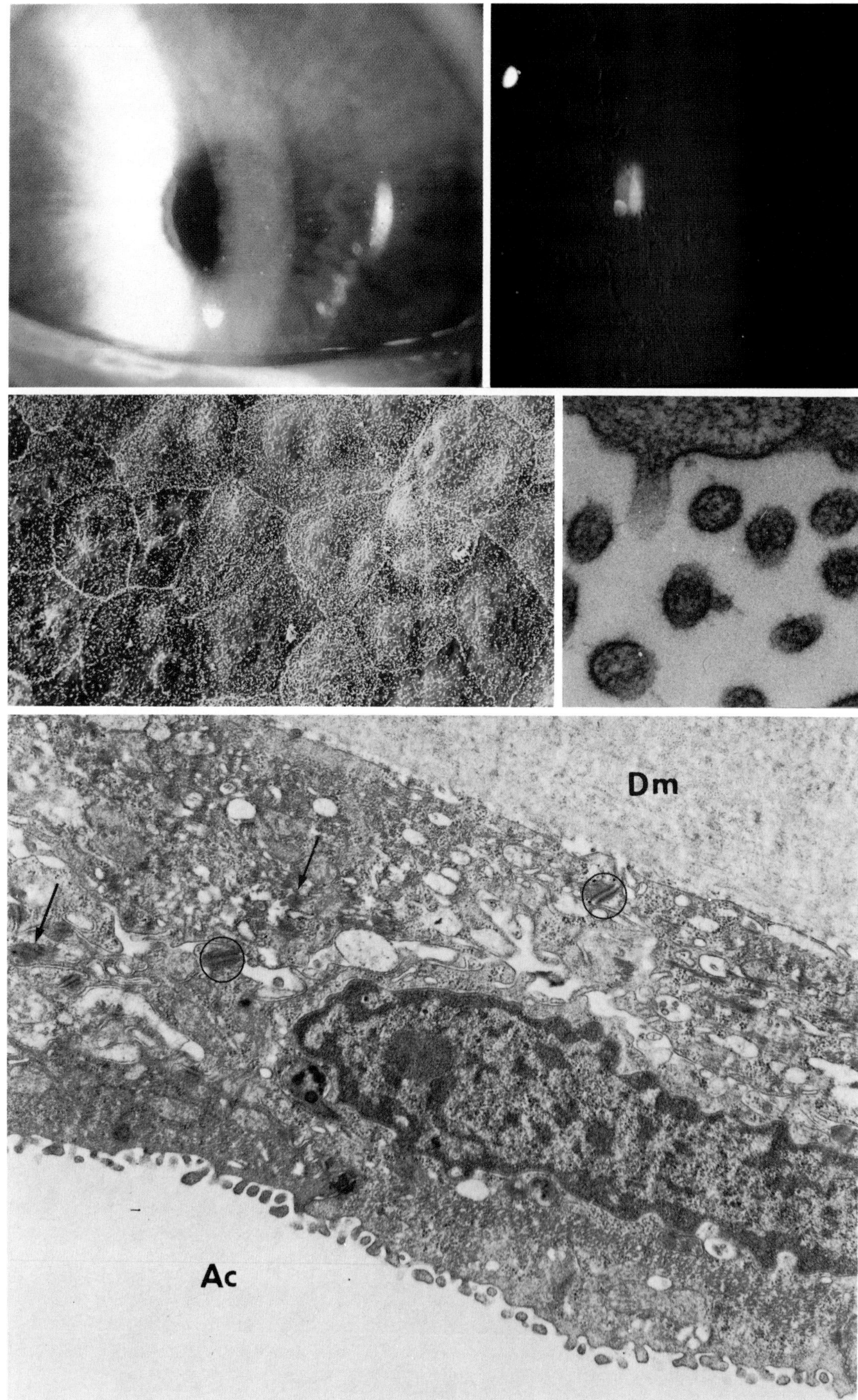

FIGURE 1–31 *See legend on opposite page*

◀ FIGURE 1–31 **Posterior polymorphous dystrophy.** *Top left,* Broad transillumination reveals multiple coalescent posterior vesicles with surrounding halos. *Top right,* In a similar case, retroillumination highlights bandlike and polymorphous configurations of the posterior cornea. *Middle left,* Scanning electron microscopy discloses an epithelial-like cell with characteristic myriad microvilli lining the posterior corneal surface. ×1000. *Bottom,* Transmission electron micrograph illustrates other features of these multilayered cells, such as desmosomal attachments *(circles)* and bundles of cytoplasmic filaments *(arrows).* (Dm, Descemet's membrane; Ac, anterior chamber.) ×19,000. *Middle right,* Higher-magnification transmission electron microscopy shows details of the microvilli as seen in transverse and longitudinal sections. Note resolution of the central filamentous core typical of cilia. ×87,500.

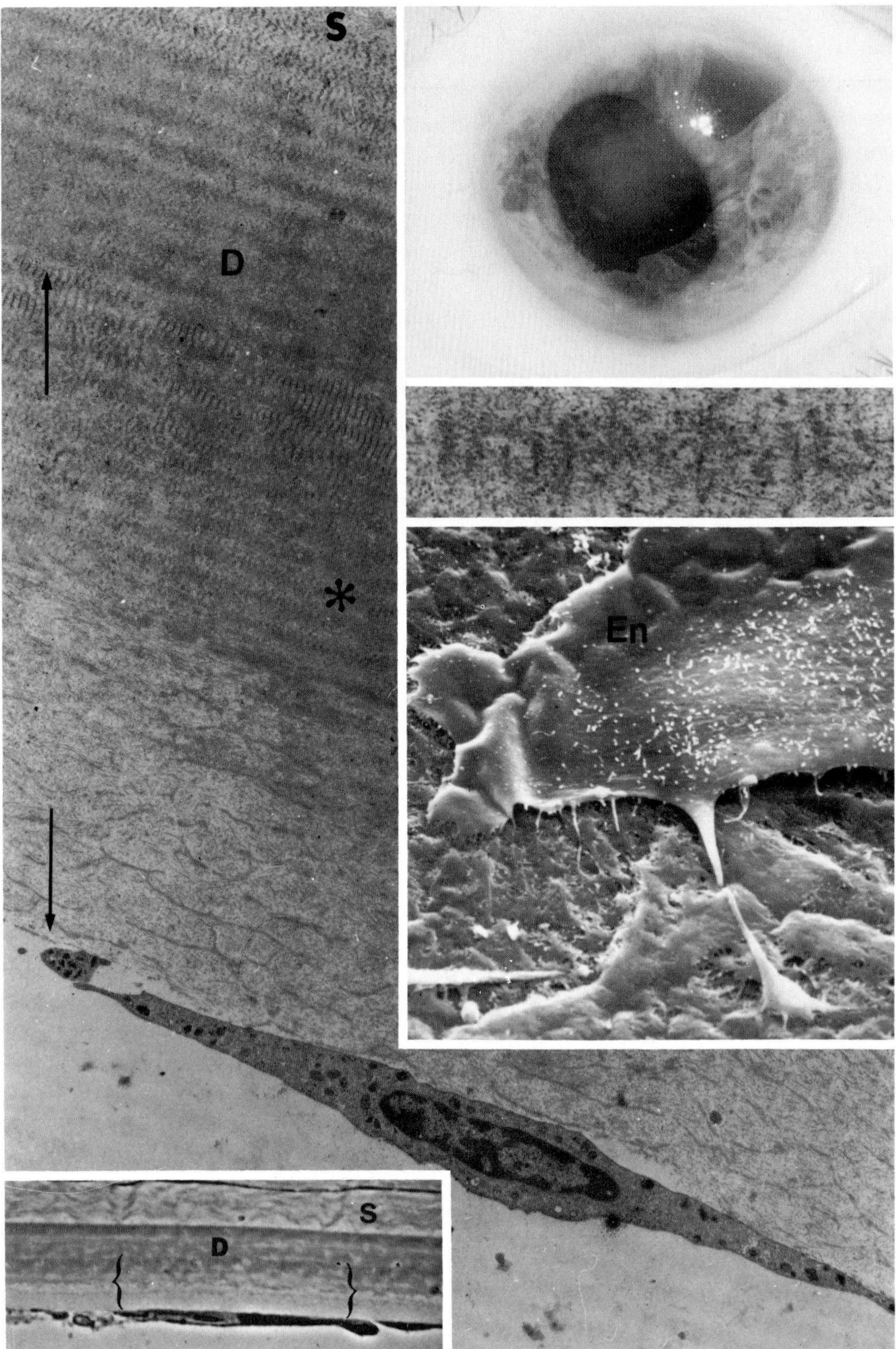

FIGURE 1–32 **Iridocorneal endothelial syndrome.** *Top right,* Clinical appearance in a 48-year-old woman with unilateral stromal edema, peripheral anterior synechia, iris atrophy, and glaucoma. *Bottom left,* Phase-contrast photomicrograph illustrates posterior stroma (S), anterior Descemet's membrane (D), and the approximately 10-μ-thick posterior collagen layer *(bracketed area).* The endothelial layer is irregular and discontinuous. PPDA, ×400. *Main figure,* Transmission electron micrograph shows a corresponding area with posterior stroma (S), ultrastructurally normal Descemet's membrane (D), thick posterior collagen layer *(between arrows),* and an attenuated epithelial cell. ×9000. *Middle right inset,* Higher magnification of area indicated by *asterisk in main figure* to resolve basement membrane–like material, fine filaments, and long-spaced banding patterns of the posterior collagen layer. ×50,000. *Lower right inset,* Scanning electron microscopy of keratoplasty specimen shows an attenuated endothelial cell (En) extending numerous cytoplasmic processes. ×2000.

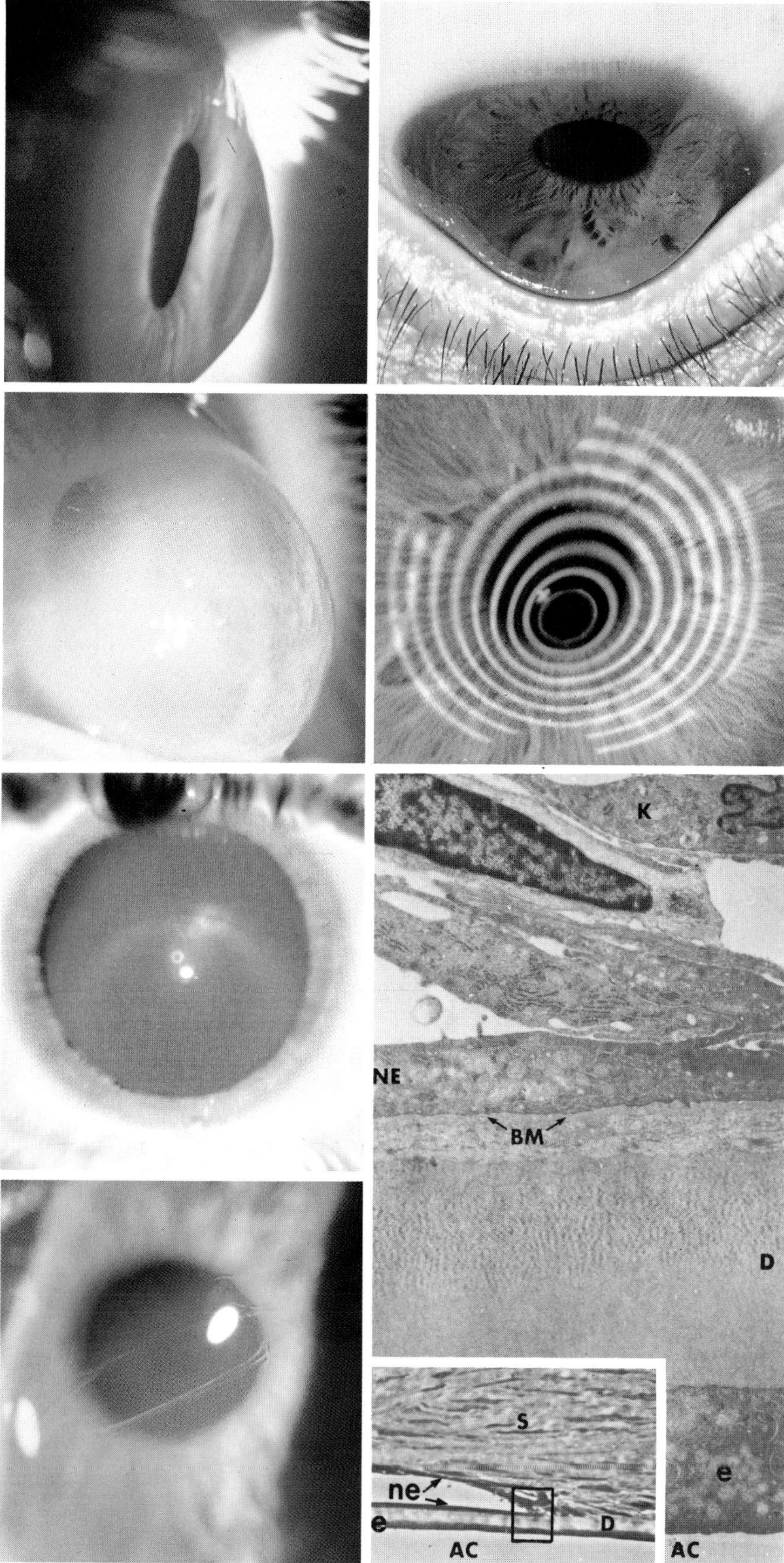

FIGURE 1–33 **Keratoconus.** *Top left,* Clinical photograph in lateral projection demonstrates extreme anterior protrusion of the markedly ectatic cornea. The apex of the cone is typically in the inferonasal position. *Top right,* Munson's sign. The V-shaped conformation on the lower lid is produced by the ectatic cornea when the patient is in downgaze. *Upper middle left,* Acute hydrops due to a break in Descemet's membrane is accompanied by extreme stromal and epithelial edema. Endothelium typically bridges the break in Descemet's membrane in 6 to 8 weeks, with resultant stromal deturgescence and residual stromal scarring of varying severity. *Upper middle right,* Keratoscopic view of typical "egg-shaped" appearance of the central corneal mires caused by inferotemporal steepening in this particular case. *Lower middle left,* Corneal retroillumination is a useful technique to identify the position and the extent of the cone. *Bottom left,* "Fish-mouth" break in Descemet's membrane remains following resolution of corneal hydrops. *Bottom right inset,* Light micrograph of a cornea with healed hydrops showed a ledge formed by detached Descemet's membrane (D) and endothelium (e). New regenerated endothelium (ne) lines the anterior surface of the ledge and posterior stroma (s). (AC, anterior chamber.) Phase contrast, PPDA, ×400. *Bottom right,* Electron micrograph of area indicated by *square in inset* demonstrates normal ultrastructure of endothelium (e) and Descemet's membrane (D). A thin basement membrane (BM) is subjacent to the new endothelium (NE). (K, keratocyte.) ×8100.

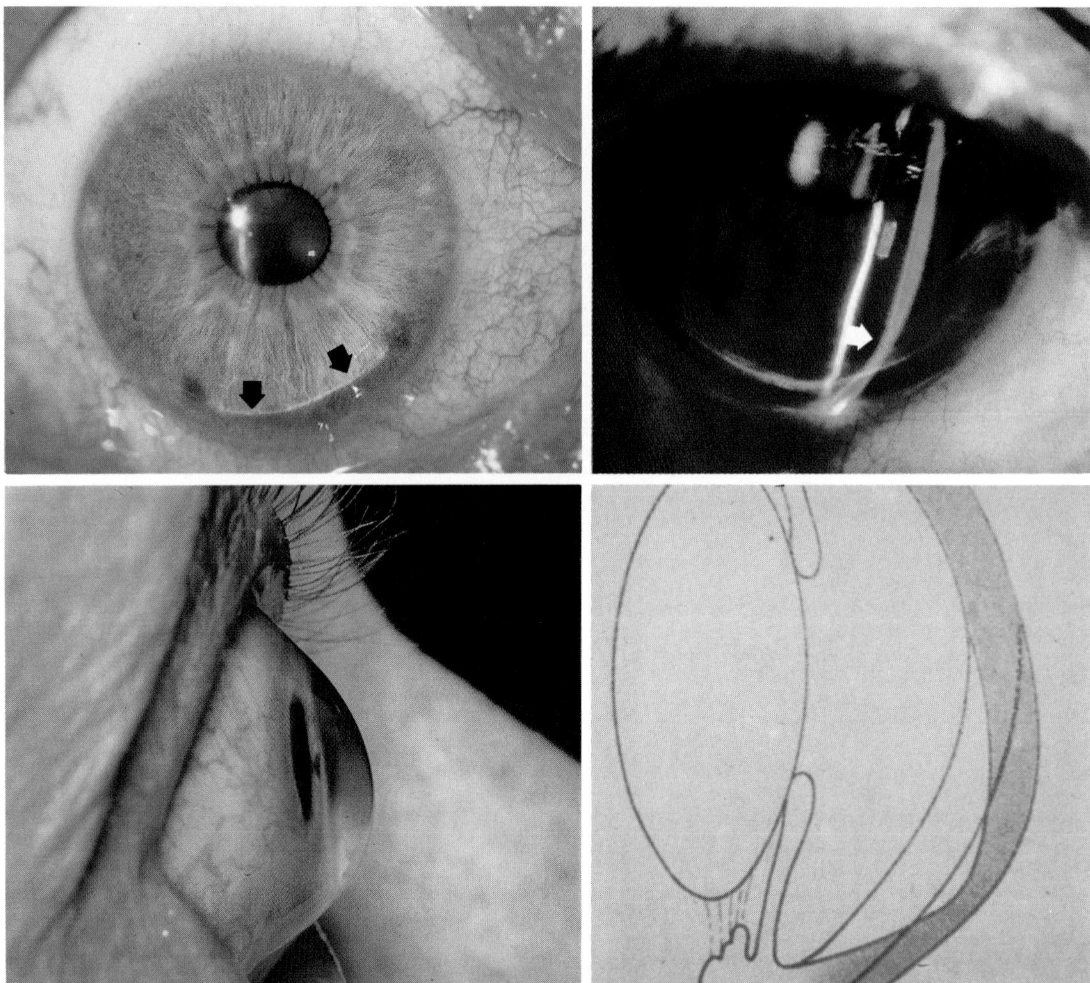

FIGURE 1–34 **Pellucid marginal degeneration.** *Left, top and bottom,* Clinical photographs feature corneal ectasia occurring above the narrow band of clear, thin, nonvascularized cornea that parallels the inferior limbus *(arrows)*. *Right, top and bottom,* Slit-lamp view and correspondent illustration show normal corneal thickness central and peripheral to the band of thinning *(arrow)*. (*Bottom right,* From Krachmer JH, Feder RS, Belin MW: Keratoconus and related noninflammatory corneal thinning disorders. Surv Ophthalmol 28:293, 1984.)

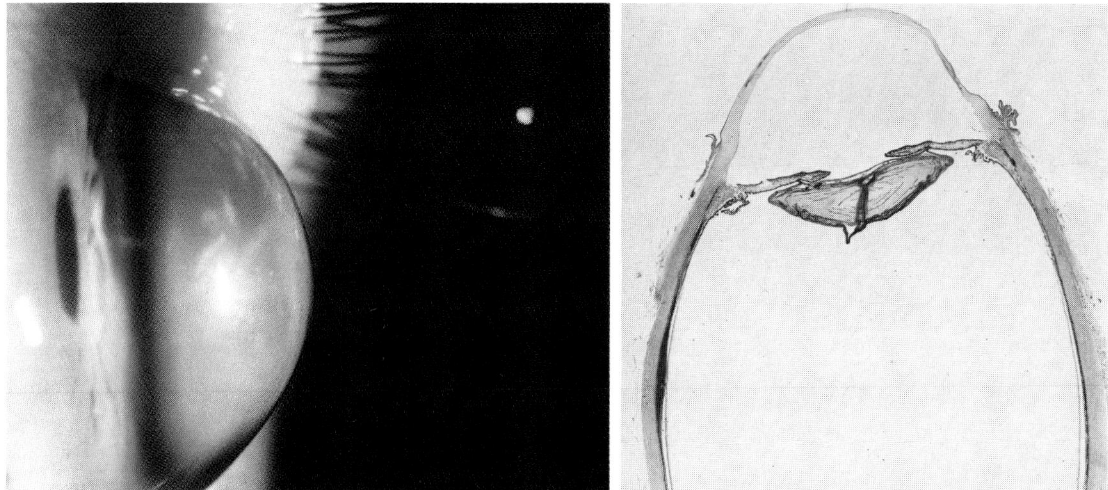

FIGURE 1–35 **Keratoglobus.** *Left,* Clinical photograph of acquired keratoglobus shows globoid protrusion of clear, diffusely thin cornea. Corneal thickness is one-third normal. *Right,* Horizontal pupil–optic nerve section of this eye reveals bulging cornea and deep anterior chamber. The entire cornea is approximately one-third normal thickness except in the extreme periphery nasally and temporally. H&E, ×4. (*Right,* From Jacobs DS, Green WR, Maumenee AE: Acquired keratoglobus. Am J Ophthalmol 77:393–399, 1974. Published with permission from the American Journal of Ophthalmology. Copyright by the Ophthalmic Publishing Company.)

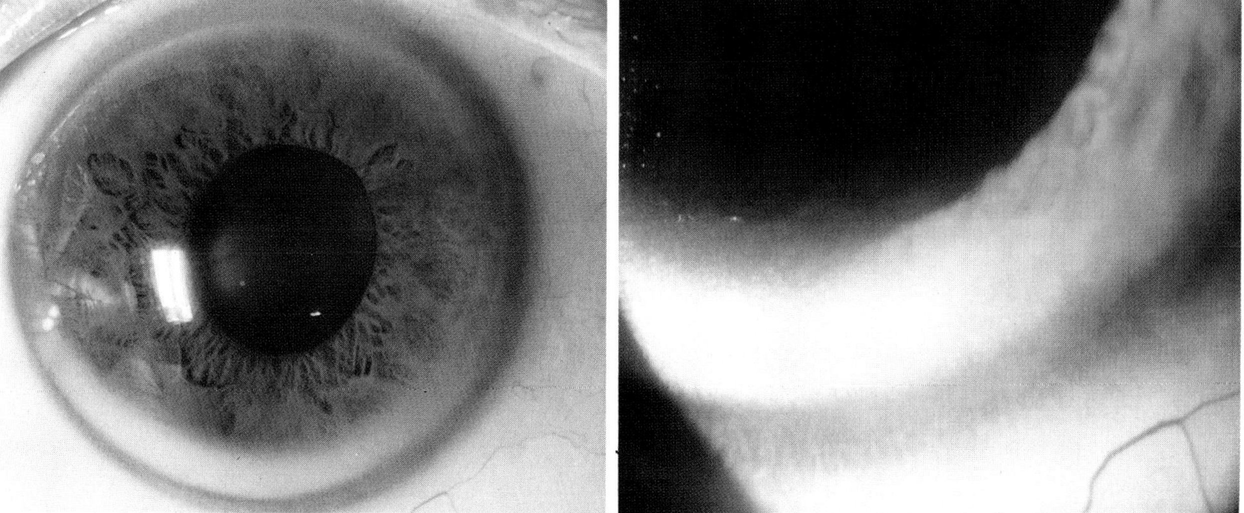

FIGURE 1–36 **Corneal arcus.** The arcus lipoides shows a dense white annular opacity of the peripheral stroma. *Right,* At higher magnification, an intervening zone of clear stroma separates lipid deposition from the limbus. The accumulations of cholesterol esters, triglycerides, and phospholipids are more prominent near Bowman's layer and deep at Descemet's membrane.

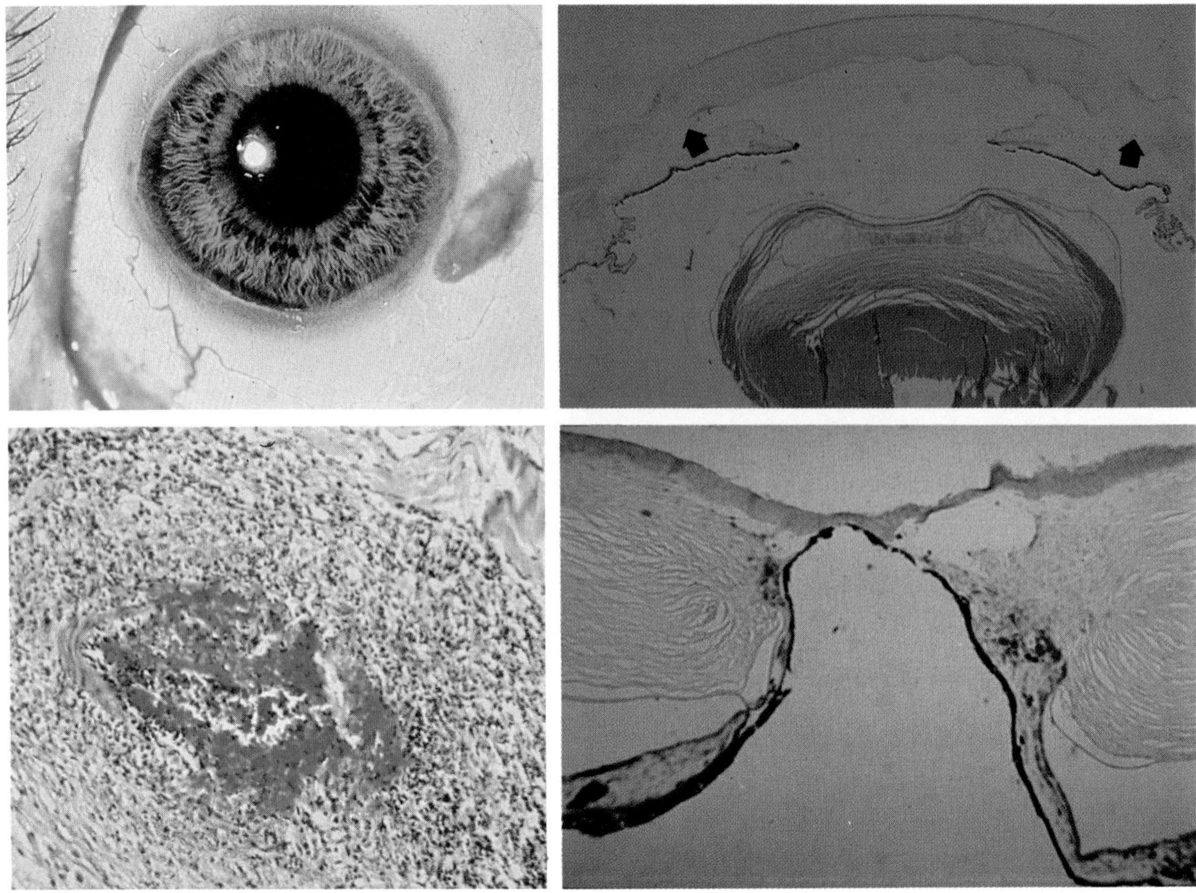

FIGURE 1–37 **Furrow degeneration associated with systemic disease.** *Top left,* Clinical photograph of patient with polyarteritis nodosa shows a full ring ulcer associated with lipid deposition near the limbus. *Top right,* Light microscopy of the same eye illustrates peripheral corneal thinning *(arrows)* corresponding to the area of clinical ulceration. H&E, ×3. *Bottom left,* Severe necrotizing vasculitis of medium-caliber artery confirms the diagnosis. H&E, ×100. *Bottom right,* Light microscopy of a 47-year-old woman with rheumatoid arthritis who developed a peripheral marginal corneal ulcer shows adjacent iris incorporated into a fibrous scar. PAS, ×32.

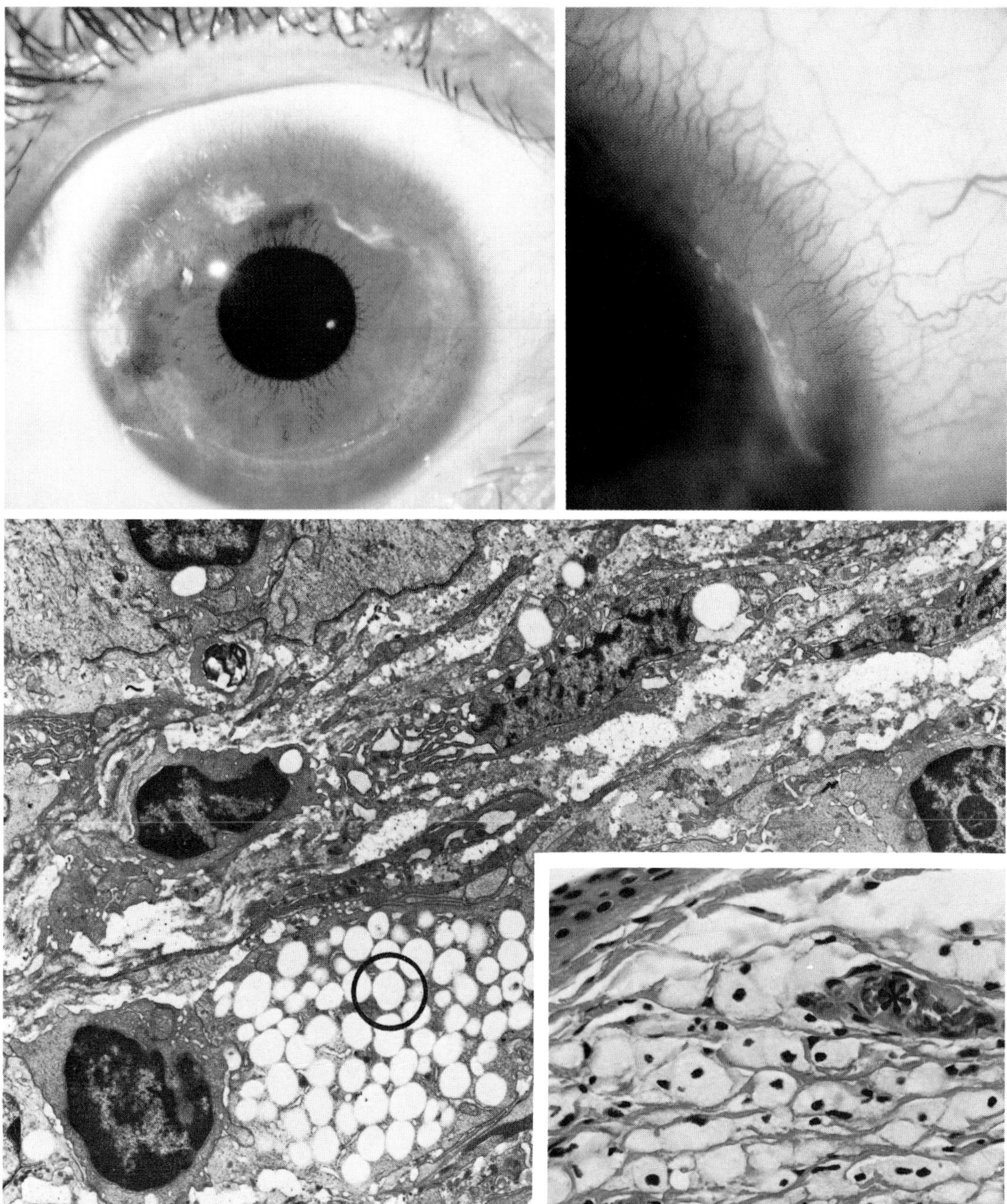

FIGURE 1–38 **Terrien's marginal degeneration.** *Top left,* Clinical photograph of a patient with extensive thinning of the peripheral stroma circumferentially from 9 o'clock to 2 o'clock. *Top right,* Higher magnification discloses vascularization of the involved stroma with lipid deposition at the advancing edge. *Bottom inset,* Light microscopy reveals numerous foamy histiocytic cells and blood vessels *(asterisk)* within the anterior stroma. H&E, ×300. *Bottom,* Transmission electron micrograph shows histiocytic cells laden with neutral lipid inclusions *(circled area).* Several reactive fibroblasts and chronic inflammatory cells are also seen. ×5000.

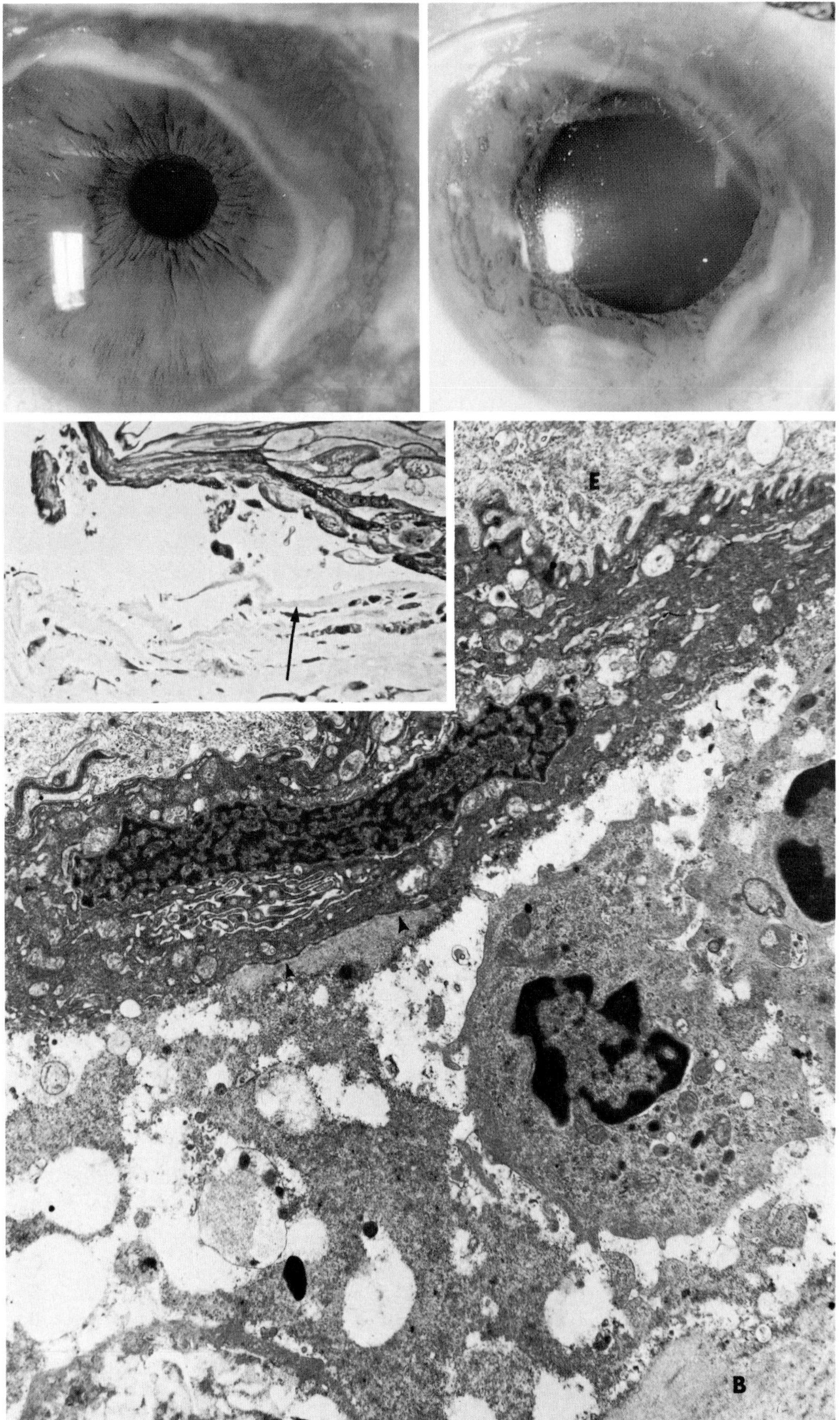

FIGURE 1–39 *See legend on opposite page*

◀ FIGURE 1–39 **Mooren's ulcer.** *Top left,* Clinical photograph of a 55-year-old man with painful, rapidly progressive ulcerative keratitis. *Top right,* Same patient 15 days after conjunctival resection reveals a marked improvement with decreased inflammatory response and arrest of ulceration. *Bottom inset,* Phase-contrast micrograph of the stroma at the margin of the ulcerating area includes abrupt termination of Bowman's layer *(arrow)* with numerous acute inflammatory cells. PDDA, ×800. *Bottom,* Transmission electron micrograph of the area in the figure, *bottom inset,* resolves multiple intrastromal inflammatory cells actively engaged in degranulation and phagocytosis. Note the remnants of the epithelial basement membrane *(arrowheads).* (E, epithelium; B, Bowman's layer.) ×7500. In contrast to typical degenerations of the peripheral cornea, Mooren's ulcer is characterized by a fulminating, centrally progressive, and painful inflammation occurring more often in males.

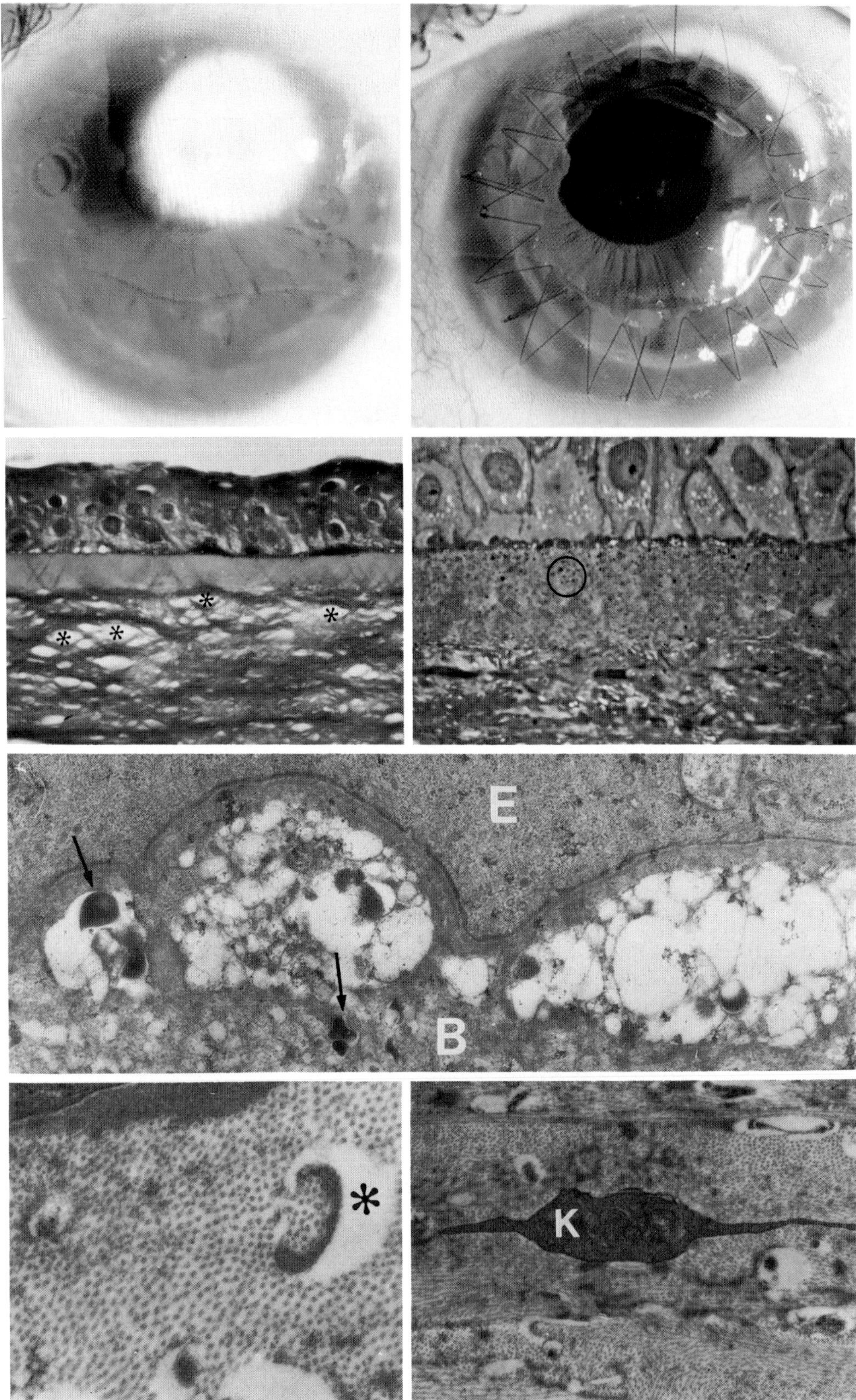

FIGURE 1–40 *See legend on opposite page*

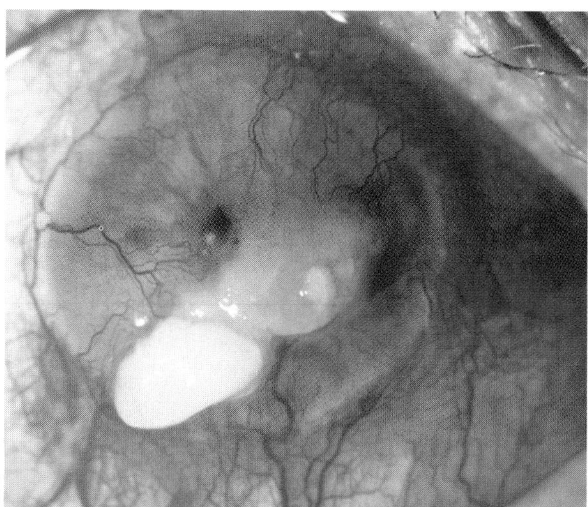

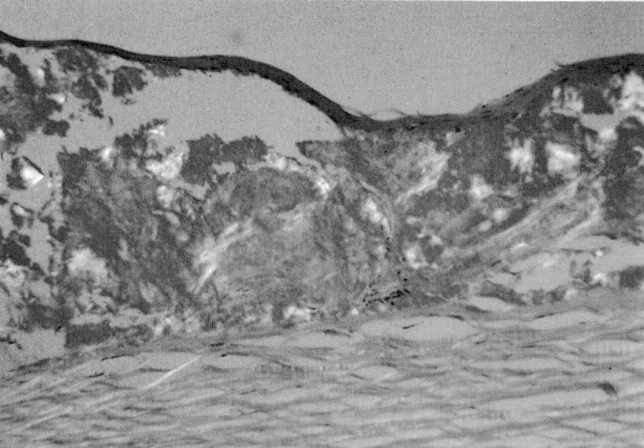

FIGURE 1–41 **Amyloid degeneration of cornea.** *Left,* In a patient with long-standing herpes keratitis and subsequent corneal scarring and vascularization, superficial irregular amyloid deposits developed. These corneal amyloid lesions consist of salmon-pink to yellow-white, raised, fleshy masses that create the nodular surface as depicted. Note that the cornea is also vascularized. *Right,* Light microscopy of corneal specimen discloses characteristic birefringent, Congo red–positive amyloid deposits. Note the location of the amyloid deposits in the epithelial layer. The amyloid itself contains protein, carbohydrate, and polysaccharide components as well as alpha-chain immunoglobulins. Congo red, ×100.

◀ FIGURE 1–40 **Lipid degeneration of the cornea.** *Top left,* Clinical photograph of a dense white deposit of lipid with feathery edges occurring in association with superior limbic pannus. Note this eye has previously undergone an intracapsular cataract extraction and secondary implantation of the anterior chamber lens. *Top right,* Same patient after keratoplasty shows a clear graft with residual opaque lipid deposition at the periphery superiorly. *Upper middle left,* Light microscopy shows an intact Bowman's layer with multiple clear vacuoles within the stroma *(asterisk)* ×400. *Upper middle right,* Phase-contrast microscopy includes numerous fine osmiophilic deposits *(circled area)* within Bowman's layer. PPDA, ×800. *Lower middle,* Transmission electron micrograph of the same area discloses confluent globular empty spaces below Bowman's layer (B) as well as some electron-dense complex lipid deposits *(arrows).* E, epithelium. ×40,000. *Bottom right,* Transmission electron micrograph of the anterior stroma illustrates the same type of deposits without disruption or other abnormality of the keratocytes (K). ×12,000. *Bottom left,* At higher magnification, lipid deposits of approximately 1 μ diameter have the characteristics of saturated neutral fats *(asterisk).* ×40,000.

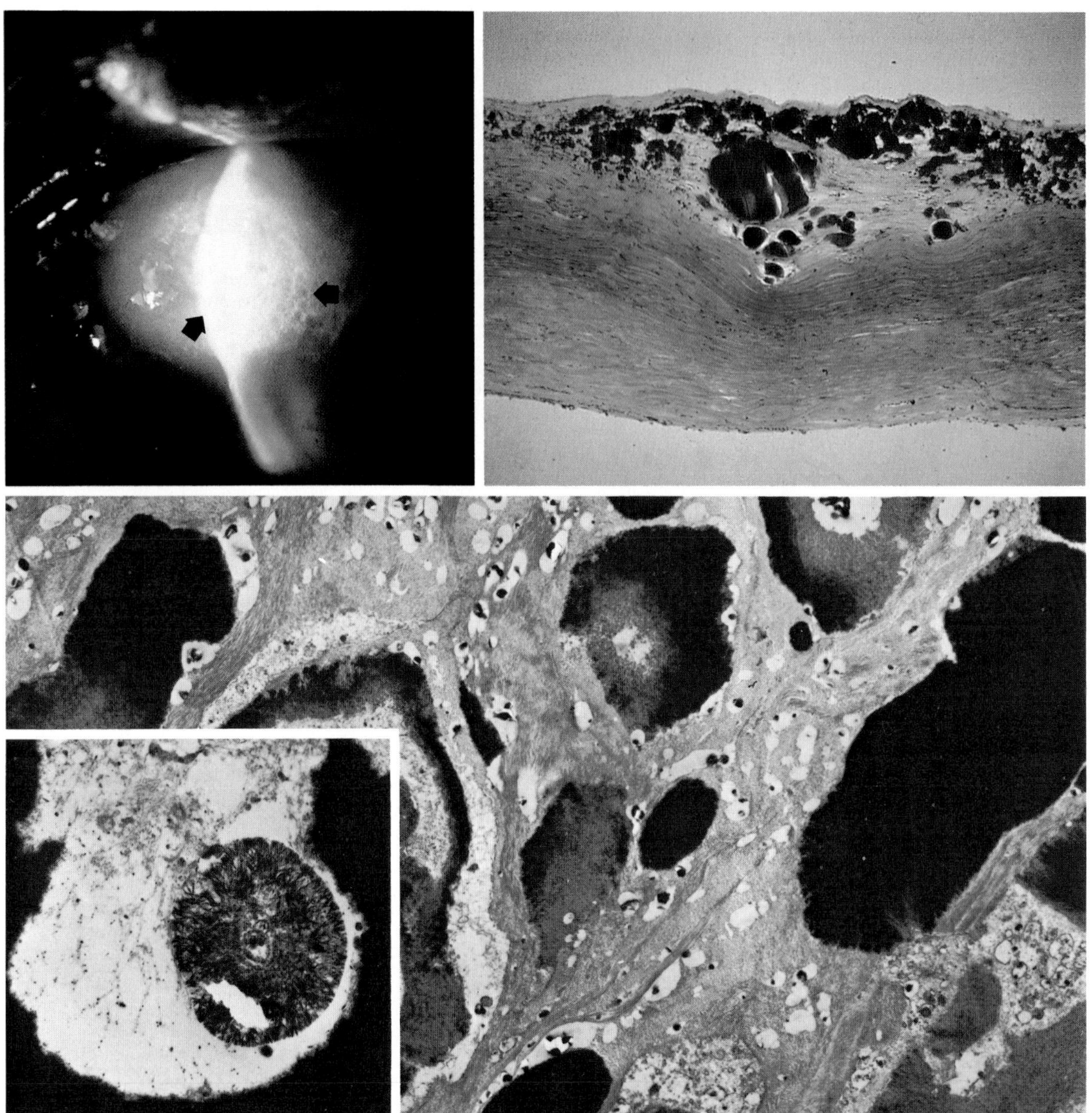

FIGURE 1–42 **Spheroid (keratinoid) degeneration of the cornea.** *Top left,* Clinically numerous spheroidal deposits appear over the anterior stroma *(arrows).* These yellow, oily-appearing subepithelial deposits characteristically are located within the interpalpebral fissure, generally beginning at the periphery. *Top right,* Histologic section reveals multiple densely staining spherules beneath the distorted epithelium and within the anterior stroma. H&E, ×20. *Bottom,* Survey transmission electron micrograph shows spheroidal deposits as extracellular accumulations of electron-dense material with variably crystalline structure. Lipid deposits and blood vessels are also seen. ×5000. *Bottom inset,* High-magnification transmission electron micrograph of these spheroidal deposits shows variable electron density with a crystalline fragment similar to calcium. ×40,000.

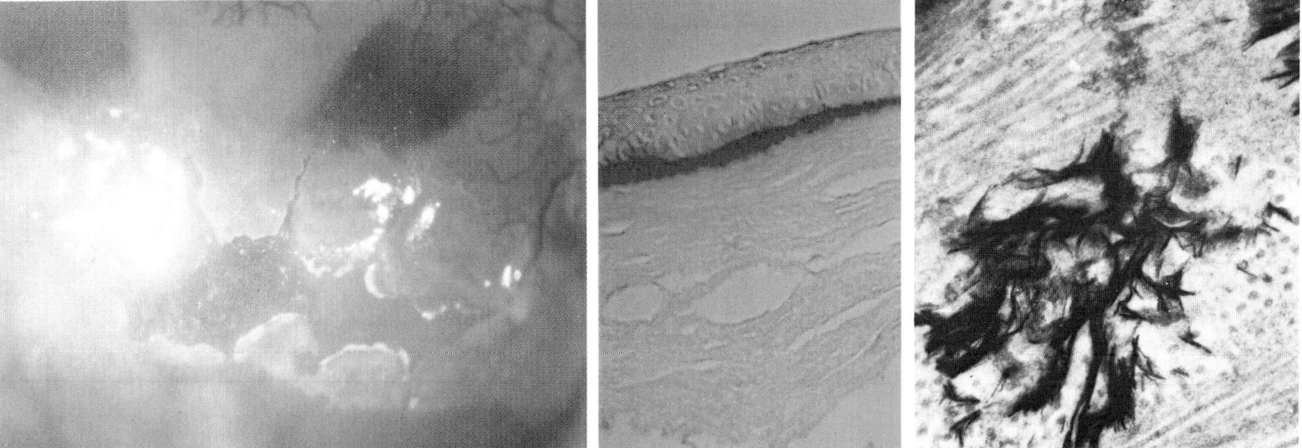

FIGURE 1–43 **Band keratopathy.** *Left,* In a 42-year-old woman with chronic uveitis, band keratopathy has resulted in epithelial erosion with a persistent central defect. Note that the band keratopathy is confined to the interpalpebral fissure area. A lucid interval generally separates the calcific band from the limbus. *Center,* Light microscopy discloses dense staining within Bowman's membrane. Histopathologically, the early changes consist of basophilic staining of the basement membrane of the epithelium. This staining is eventually followed by involvement of Bowman's layer with calcium deposition and eventual fragmentation. The calcium in this stain is red. Alizarin red, ×40. *Right,* Transmission electron micrograph resolves the fine crystalline characteristic and extreme electron density of calcium or hydroxyapatite particles. ×70,000.

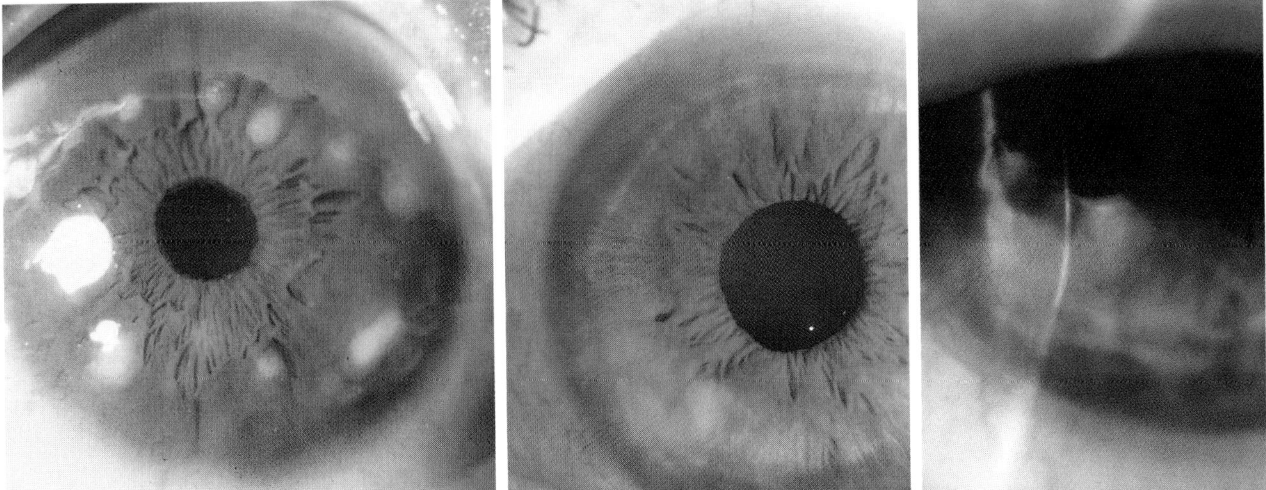

FIGURE 1–44 **Salzmann's nodular degeneration.** *Top left and center,* Clinical photographs of two patients with the classic bluish gray elevated paraaxial nodules with sparing of the remainder of the cornea. *Right,* Higher-magnification slit-lamp photograph emphasizes a minimal vascularization of the underlying stroma. These nodules represent focal areas of subepithelial fibrocellular, avascular pannus, replacing Bowman's layer and superimposed on a normal stroma.

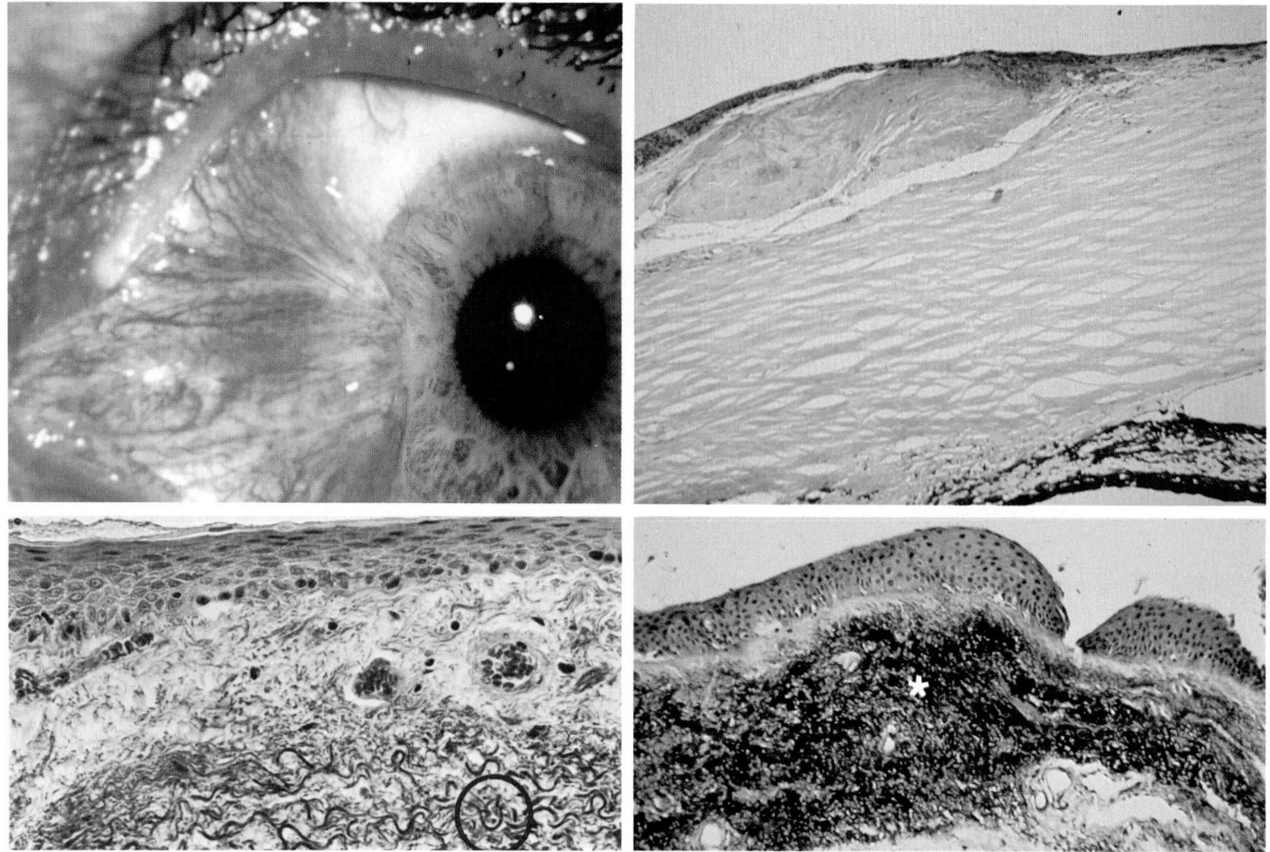

FIGURE 1–45 **Pterygium.** *Top left,* Clinical appearance of a typical interpalpebral pterygium shows extension of the fibrovascular conjunctival tissue onto clear cornea. True pterygia are found only in the interpalpebral fissure. *Top right,* Light microscopy of the limbus features a subepithelial mound of connective tissue invading the cornea. ×20. This subepithelial tissue exhibits newly synthesized (probably by fibroblasts from ultraviolet light stimulation) elastoid material rather than breakdown of the collagen. There is also an invasive destruction of Bowman's membrane. The subepithelial material stains positively for elastin but is not sensitive to elastase digestion. *Bottom,* Histologic sections show elastoid material *(circled area, left figure)* and positive stain for elastin *(asterisk, right figure).* Phosphotungstic acid–hematoxylin, ×375; elastin stain, ×40.

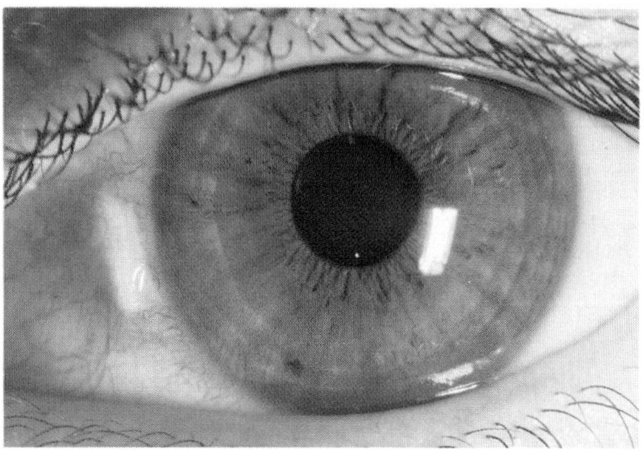

FIGURE 1–46 **Pinguecula.** Pingueculae appear as raised, cream-colored, white, or chalky subepithelial deposits of the conjunctiva adjacent to the limbus and within the palpebral fissure. These also represent elastoid material within the substantia propria of the conjunctiva, without corneal involvement, however.

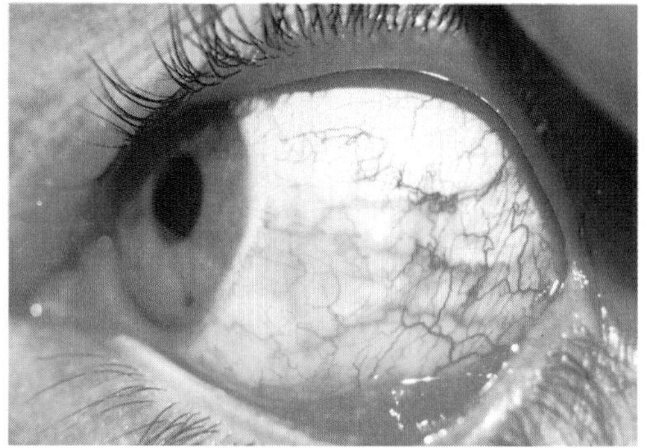

FIGURE 1–47 **Acute allergic conjunctivitis.** Conjunctival hyperemia is evident as is chemosis. Hyperemic swelling of the lids may or may not be present on examination, but patients often associate their exacerbation with knuckle rubbing. The hallmark symptom reported by patients is itching.

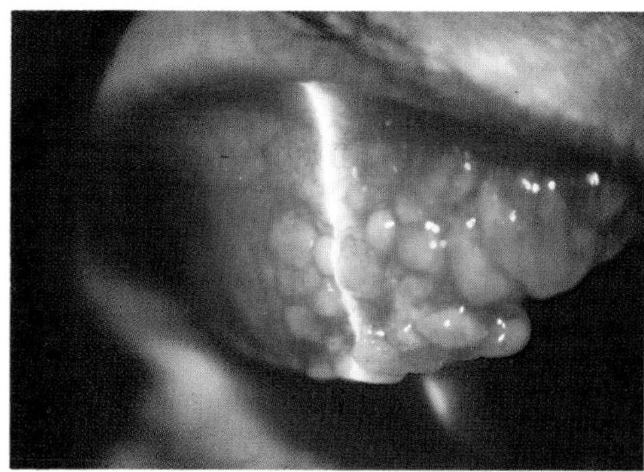

FIGURE 1–48 **Vernal conjunctivitis.** The palpebral form is characterized by enlarged papillae referred to as cobblestone papillae because of their shape and size, that are almost always confined to the upper tarsus. The conjunctiva is often pink.

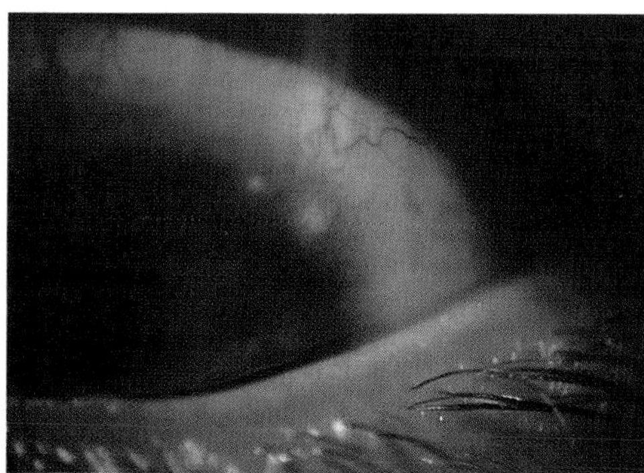

FIGURE 1–49 **Vernal conjunctivitis.** The limbal form exhibits Horner-Trantas dots, white infiltrates found at the limbus that can vary greatly in size and specific location or pattern. These Horner-Trantas dots are composed largely of eosinophils and degenerated cellular debris, but they may also contain polymorphonuclear cells and lymphocytes. In more severe cases, diffuse keratitis may be observed.

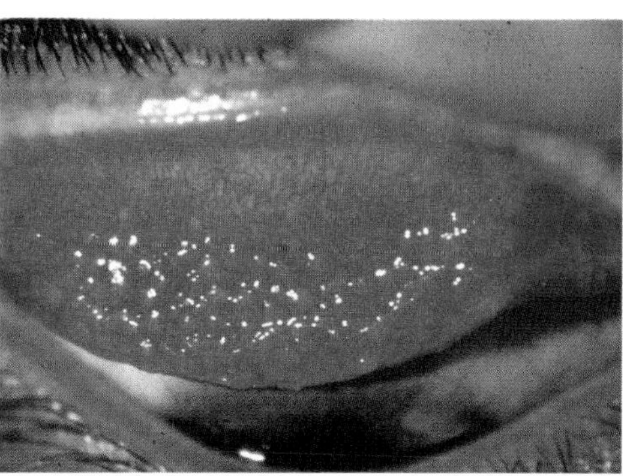

FIGURE 1–51 **Giant papillary conjunctivitis.** The papillae of giant papillary conjunctivitis, located on the upper tarsal conjunctiva, exceed 0.3 mm in diameter and may be somewhat translucent in the early stages of the disease but may become more opaque as the disease progresses. These papillae resolve with the removal of the foreign object, be it a contact lens, ocular prosthesis, or exposed suture, as opposed to the papillae resulting from vernal conjunctivitis.

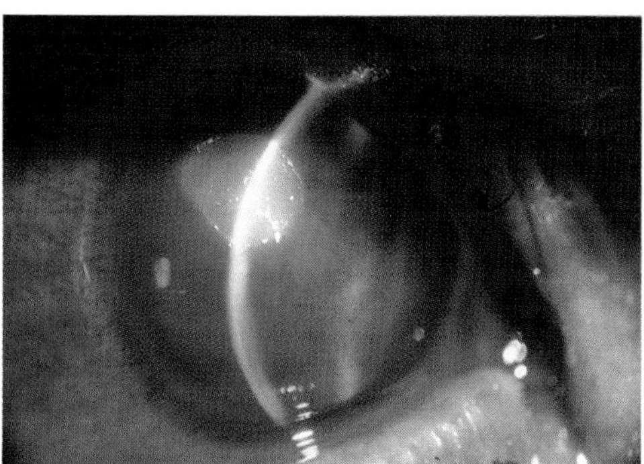

FIGURE 1–50 **Vernal conjunctivitis.** The shield ulcer is the most serious consequence of vernal conjunctivitis. It is a centrally located, white, fibrinous defect in the corneal epithelium. It lacks a surrounding haze often seen with other ulcer types and is rarely accompanied by iritis.

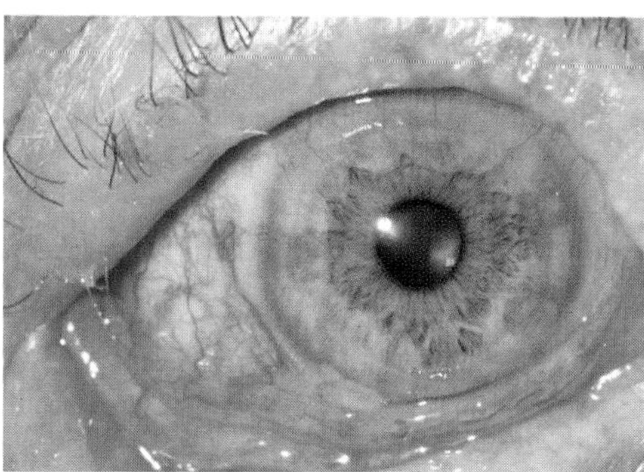

FIGURE 1–52 **Atopic keratoconjunctivitis.** Note the slight corneal haze, the conjunctival changes, and the accompanying blepharitis marked by structural changes at the lid margin and loss of lashes.

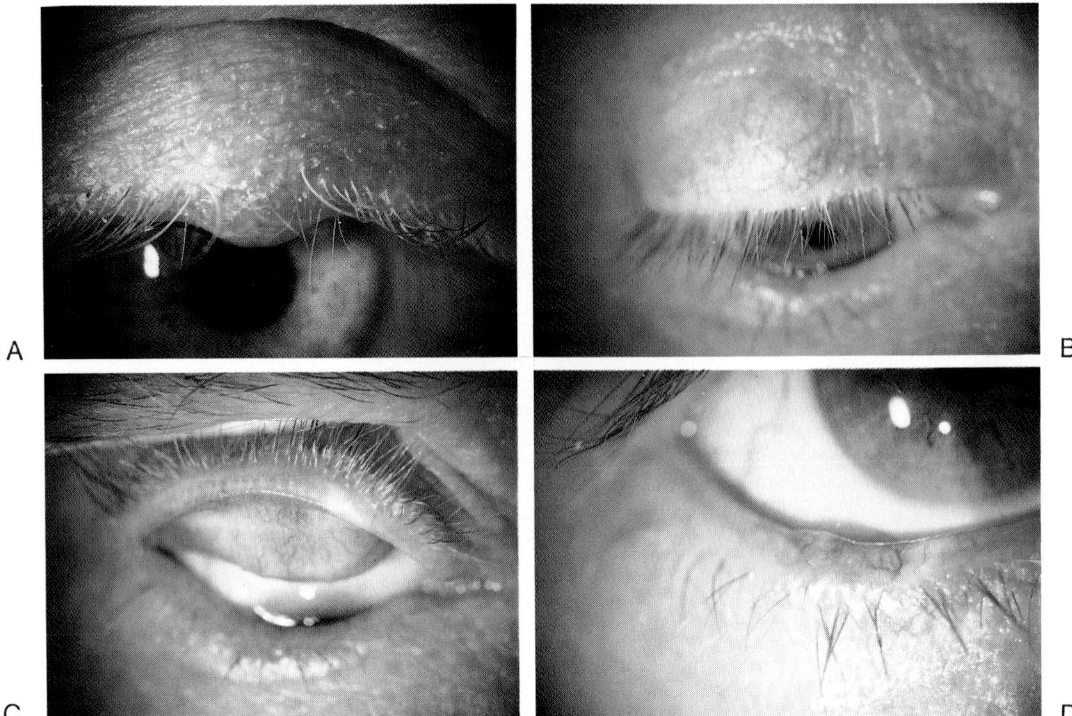

FIGURE 1–53 **Chalazion.** A chalazion is a granulomatous reaction to the inspissated secretions of the meibomian gland. It appears as a swollen tumor mass involving the eyelid. It may be associated with local inflammation around the mouth of a single gland *(A)*. It may show no external signs of inflammation *(B)*, with only a slight engorgement of vessels on the tarsal conjunctiva *(C)*. Chalazions may be small, presenting as only small granulomas at the posterior lid margin *(D)*. They may involve multiple glands and different lids *(B)*. They may cause blurring of vision owing to induced astigmatism from the pressure of the mass on the cornea. The patient in *B* and *C* complained of visual acuity that was reduced to 20/25; this returned to 20/15 when the chalazion was excised.

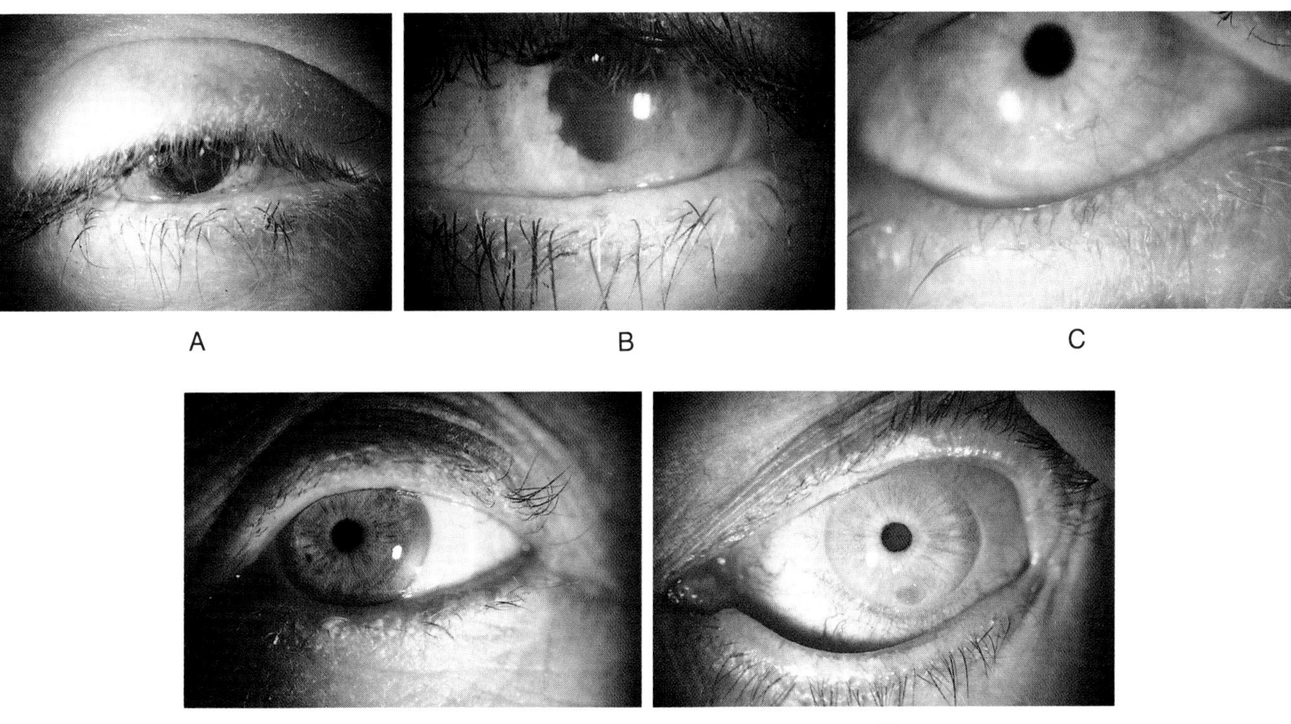

FIGURE 1–54 **Blepharitis.** *A*, This patient with chronic blepharitis shows the typical heavy crusting and scales along the bases of the eyelashes. There is a fairly uniform swelling to the lids with a chronic spotty redness to the lid margins. *B*, Patients with long-standing blepharitis demonstrate patchy loss of lashes (madarosis) and whitening or loss of pigmentation in lashes (poliosis) as well as chronic crusting and scale formation along the bases of their lashes. There may be patchy focal involvement with some portions of the lids affected more than others. *A* and *B* show the right and left eyes, respectively, of the same patient. *C*, Focal pouting of the individual meibomian glands may be seen, accompanied by telangiectasia of the lid margin. *D*, The upper and lower lids may be asymmetrically involved. *E*, Patients with chronic staphylococcal blepharitis frequently have a dry eye, as demonstrated here by rose bengal staining of the corneal and conjunctival epithelium. They are also susceptible to peripheral marginal ulcers of the cornea (*B* and *C*). It is postulated that hypersensitivity to components of the *Staphylococcus aureus* cell wall plays a role in the pathogenesis of staphylococcal blepharitis and peripheral corneal infiltrates.

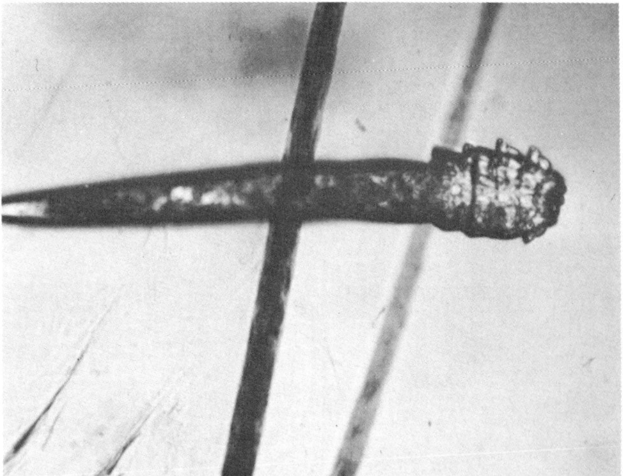

FIGURE 1–55 A *Demodex* mite is colorless and spindle-shaped. The anterior section of the body has four pairs of short legs, that limit their mobility. *Demodex* can be identified in normal-appearing eyelids by epilating lashes and observing the mites clinging to the lashes under a microscope. (From Smolin GR, Tabbara K, Whitcher J: Lids. *In* Infectious Disease of the Eye. Baltimore, Williams & Wilkins, 1984. Copyright 1984, The Williams & Wilkins Company, Baltimore.)

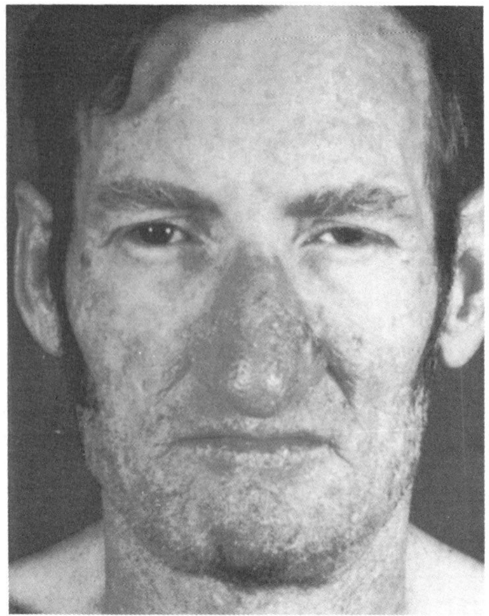

FIGURE 1–56 **Acne rosacea.** Severe rosacea results in facial disfigurement from rhinophyma and markedly dilated superficial telangiectatic blood vessels. Patients may exhibit a chronic low-grade conjunctivitis and tear film instability giving rise to ocular surface irritation and irregularity. In severe cases of rosacea, there may be peripheral corneal vascularization thinning, ulceration, and even perforation with serious visual and ocular morbidity. (From Browning DJ, Proia AD: Ocular rosacea. Surv Ophthalmol 31:145–158, 1986.)

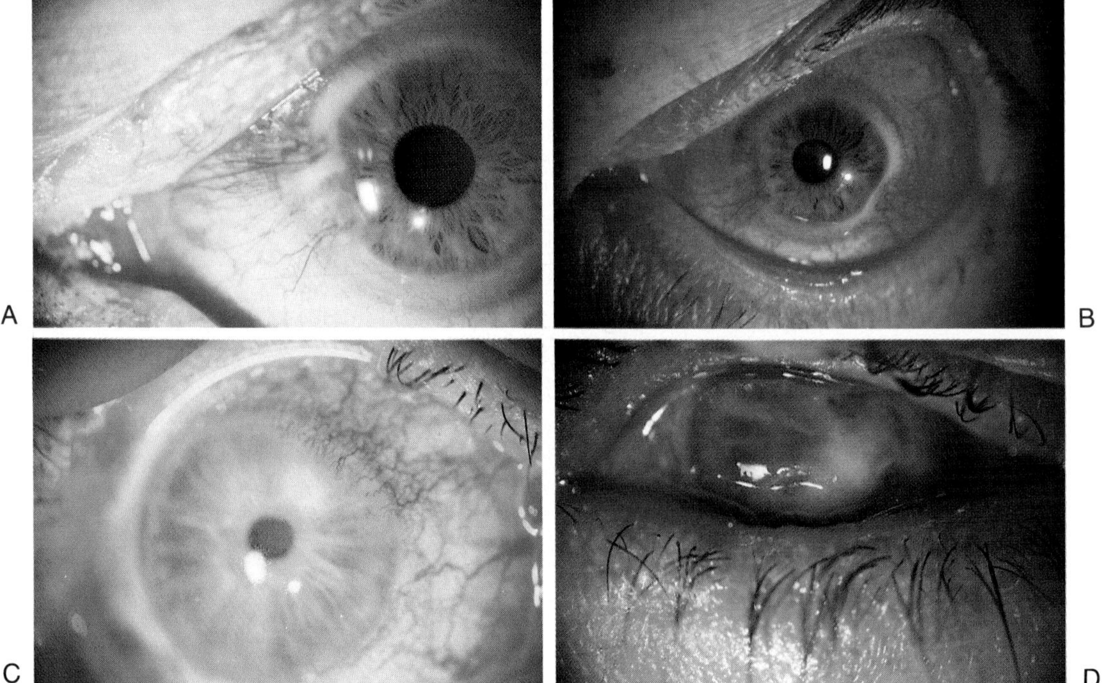

FIGURE 1–57 **Ocular rosacea.** Ocular involvement may be more severe than facial and lid involvement. Therapy tends to be chronic. *A*, A patient with rosacea after diagnosis and treatment with oral tetracycline and low-dose topical steroids shows quiet peripheral neovascularization. The patient had systemic hyperlipidemia with secondary deposition of lipid in the peripheral cornea. *B*, After cessation of therapy, the patient had a flare-up of his condition that responded to resumption of therapy with retention of excellent vision. *C*, Peripheral corneal ulceration may occur, leading to perforation *(D)*. Corneal transplantation may be necessary and has a good prognosis if the underlying disease can be controlled with topical and oral medication.

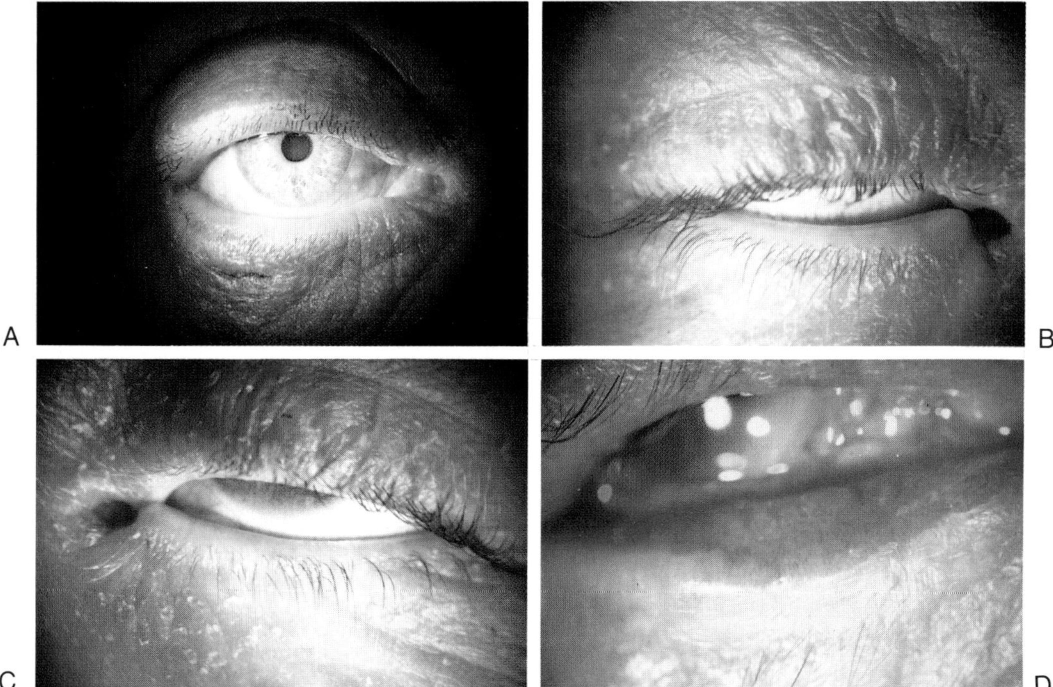

FIGURE 1–58 **Atopic dermatitis.** In atopic dermatitis, the skin may become thick and lichenified, resulting in cracking and fissuring with occasional bleeding as seen in the lower lid in *A*. The 6-year-old boy in *B* has ectropion of the right lower lid with lagophthalmos. *C*, His left eye has malposition of both upper and lower puncta as well as nocturnal lagophthalmos with corneal exposure. *D*, Frank ectropion may develop with keratinization of the tarsal conjunctiva and obliteration of the meibomian gland orifices by the lichenified epidermis. Patients with atopy are much more susceptible to chronic staphylococcal infections.

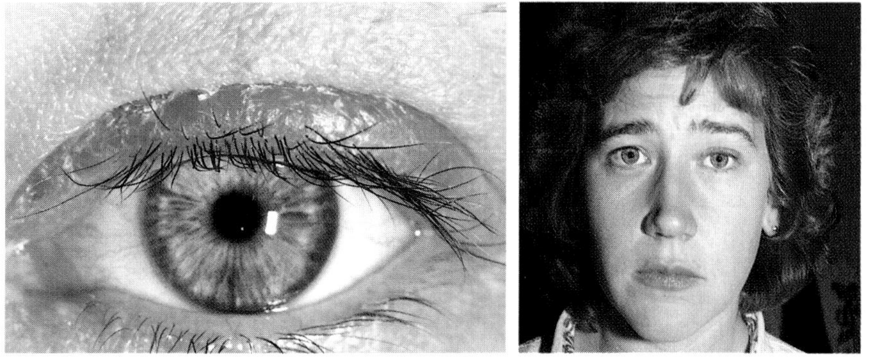

FIGURE 1–59 **Discoid lupus erythematosus.** A 28-year-old patient presented with chronic blepharitis that was resistant to the usual therapy, affecting the left upper lid. On careful questioning, a past history revealed pleurisy and chronic mouth ulcers of 8 years' duration. This led to the diagnosis of discoid lupus erythematosus presenting as chronic blepharitis.

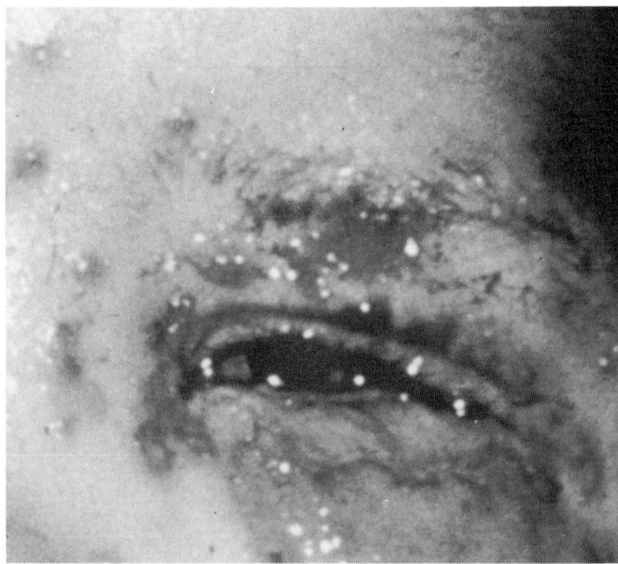

FIGURE 1-60 **Herpes simplex virus (HSV) blepharitis.** Acute HSV blepharitis with extensive vesicular eruption of the lids and periorbital area but no ocular involvement. Skin lesions healed within 3 weeks without scarring.

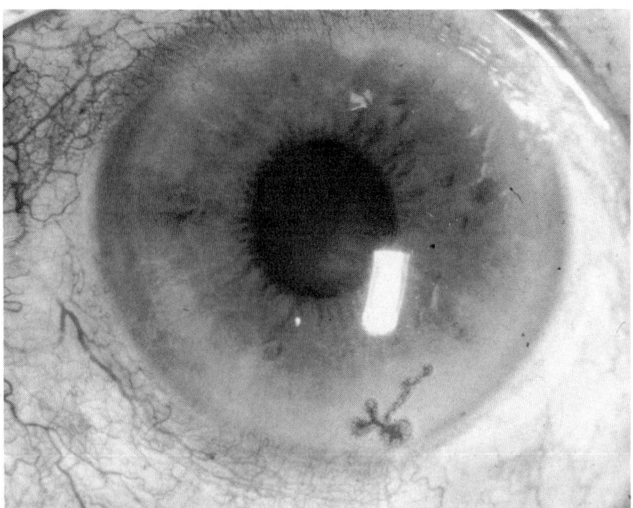

FIGURE 1-62 **HSV keratitis.** Recurrent HSV dendritic limbal ulceration. The ulcer shows the classic terminal bulbs not seen in herpes zoster dendrites. Under the dendrites, it is not uncommon to note a faint stromal infiltrate in the shape of the epithelial lesion. This infiltrate may represent diffusion of soluble antigen in the stroma, which ultimately leaves a dendritiform scar in the form of the previous dendrite.

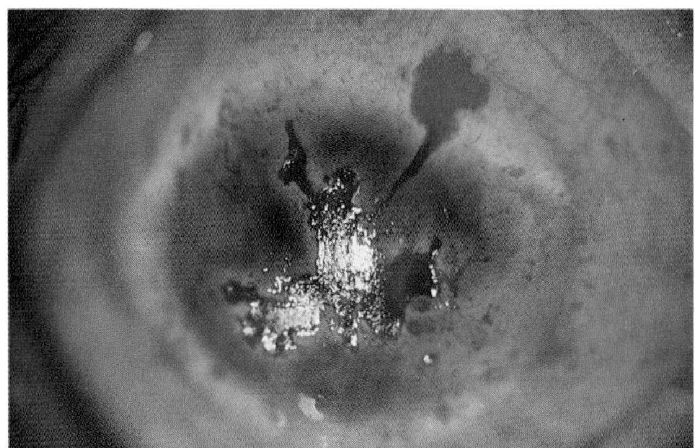

FIGURE 1-61 **HSV keratitis.** Acute HSV recurrent corneal dendrogeographic ulcer with extension onto the conjunctiva, as demonstrated by rose bengal staining.

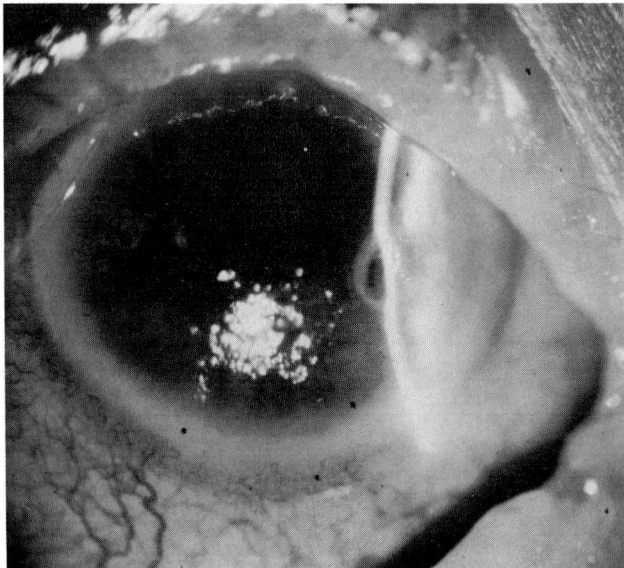

FIGURE 1-63 **HSV keratitis.** HSV postherpetic trophic ulceration with a 50% stromal melt.

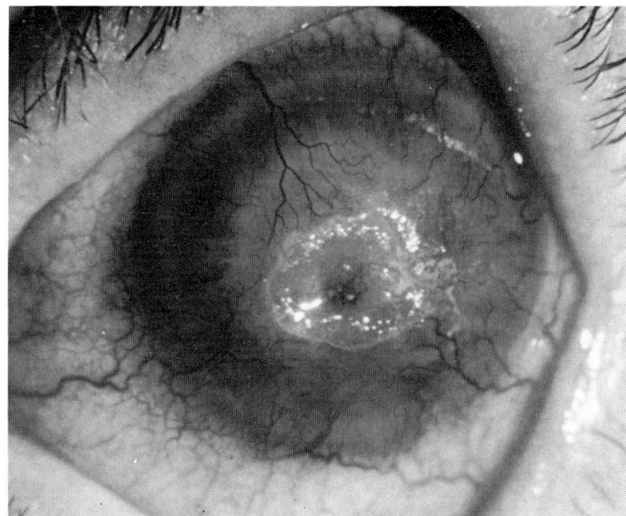

FIGURE 1-64 **HSV trophic ulcerative keratitis.** This vascularized cornea displays HSV trophic ulcerative keratitis with a deep periaxial melt filled with sterile tissue adhesive. The contact lens is placed over adhesive to prevent irritation of eyelids.

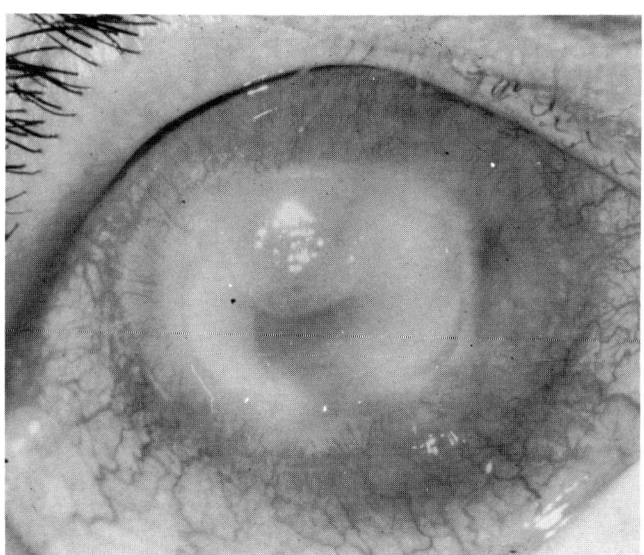

FIGURE 1-65 **HSV necrotizing interstitial keratitis.** Severe HSV necrotizing keratitis involving the entire cornea with deep neovascularization moving in 360 degrees. A conjunctival flap was placed to quiet the process.

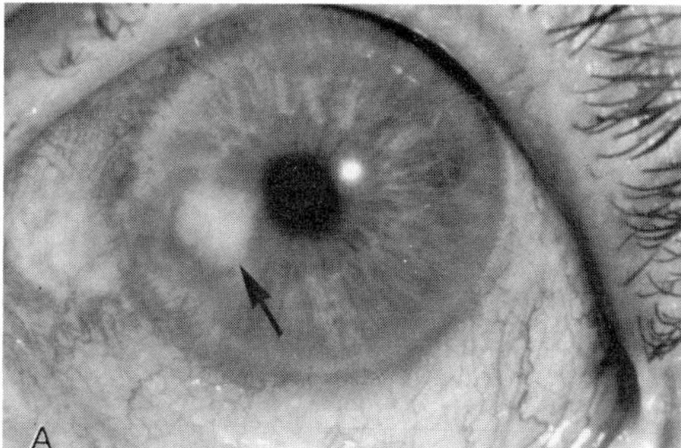

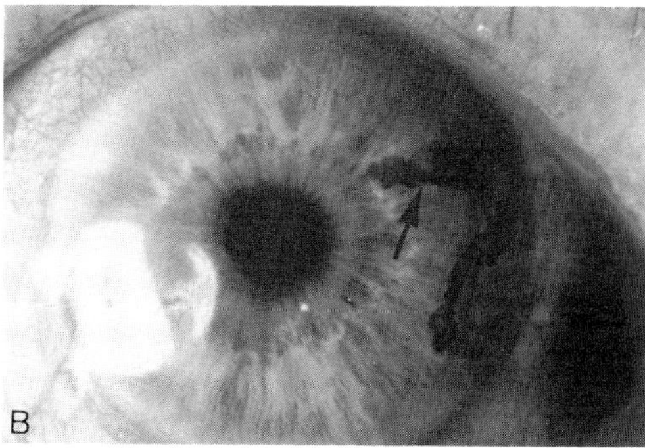

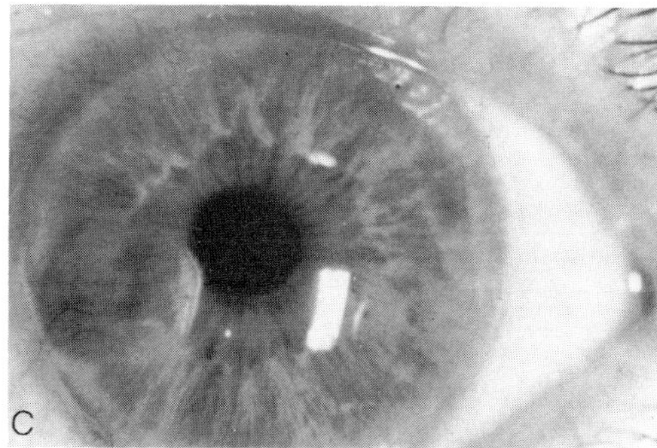

FIGURE 1-66 **HSV focal interstitial keratitis.** *A,* Acute HSV focal interstitial keratitis can resemble a bacterial infiltrate *(arrow). B,* Same eye 5 years later with acute recurrent limbal dendritic ulcer with typical terminal bulbs *(arrow). C,* Same eye 6 weeks later showing well-healed epithelium in the area of the previous dendritic ulcer and faceting with minimal scar in the area of the old herpes keratitis.

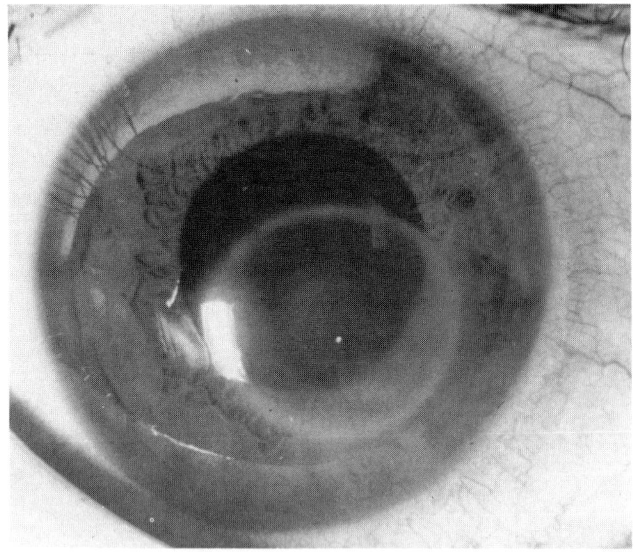

FIGURE 1–67 **Wessley ring.** HSV anterior stromal immune ring of Wessley under intact healthy epithelium. The ring is a manifestation of antigen-antibody-complement–mediated keratitis seen in HSV keratitis. These immune reactions may lie under ulcers or appear independently of them.

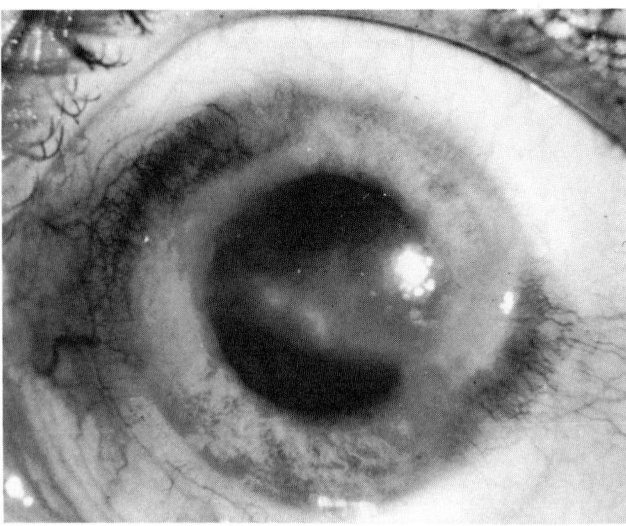

FIGURE 1–68 **HSV limbal vasculitis.** Acute HSV limbal vasculitis from 2:30 to 4:30 and 8:30 to 11 o'clock with central edematous stromal disciform edema in one eye with combined-mechanism immune disease (lymphocyte-mediated disciform keratitis and antigen-antibody-complement–mediated vasculitis).

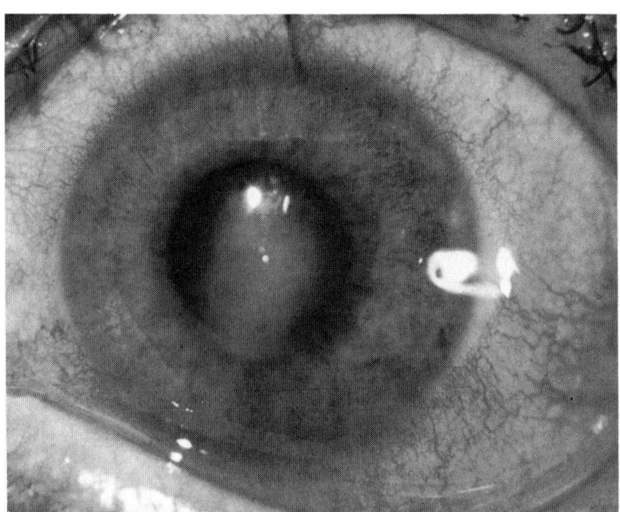

FIGURE 1–69 **HSV disciform keratitis.** Focal edematous acute HSV central disciform keratitis without necrosis or neovascularization. There may be focal keratic precipitates made up of plasma cells and lymphocytes clinging to the endothelium without anterior chamber reaction.

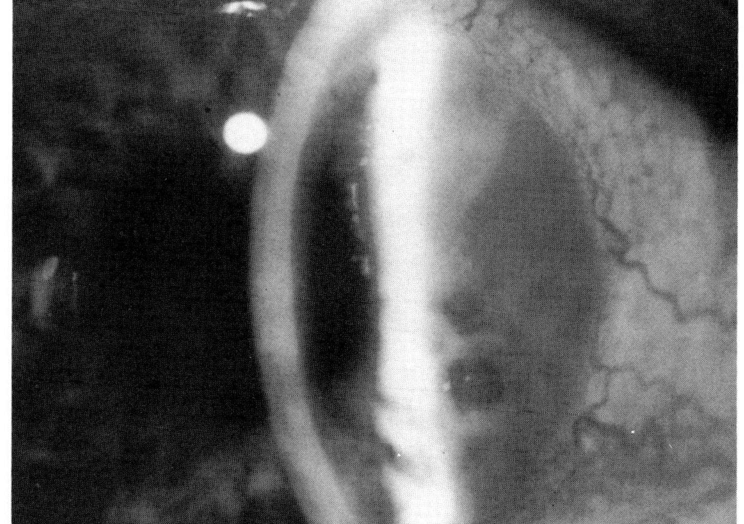

FIGURE 1-70 **HSV endotheliitis.** Acute HSV progressive endotheliitis similar to graft rejection with a lymphocyte line on the endothelium and focal full-thickness stromal edema medial to the lymphocyte line. These cases may be preceded by dendritic ulceration or marked elevation of intraocular pressure a few weeks before the onset of the demarcating keratic precipitate line. Anterior chamber reaction is usually minimal to nonexistent.

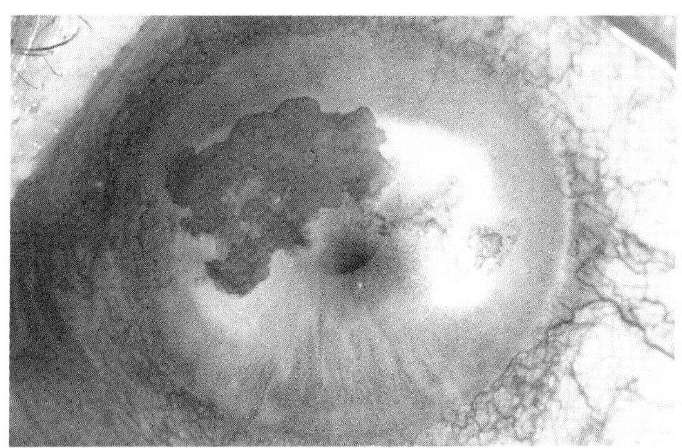

FIGURE 1-71 **HSV geographic ulcer.** Large HSV infectious geographic ulcer overlying necrotic stromal interstitial keratitis formed as a partial immune ring in an eye with combined-mechanism herpetic disease (infectious ulceration and antigen-antibody-complement–mediated interstitial keratitis and Wessley immune ring).

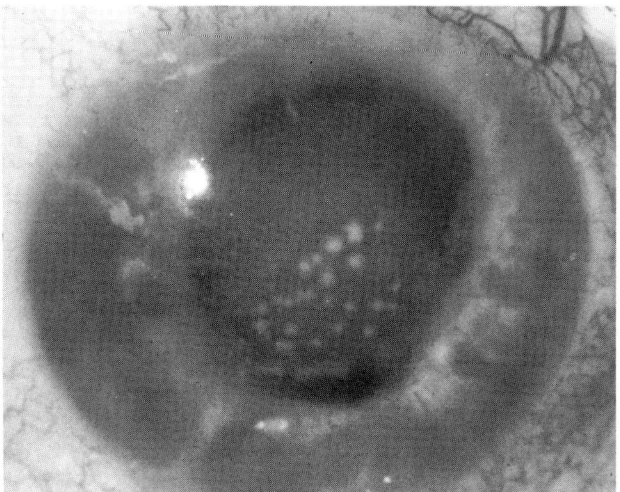

FIGURE 1-72 **HSV keratouveitis.** Acute HSV keratouveitis with mutton-fat keratic precipitates on the corneal endothelium and extensive anterior chamber cell and flare reaction. The cause of this entity is not well established, and it may occur before any known herpetic ocular disease or may be associated with active keratitis. Intraocular pressure is frequently elevated secondary to an associated trabeculitis.

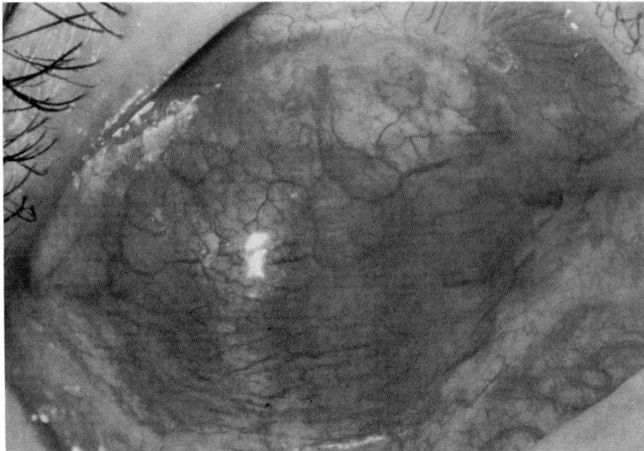

FIGURE 1–73 **Gunderson's conjunctival flap in HSV keratitis.** Complete Gunderson's conjunctival flap pulled down over a case of severe diffuse necrotic interstitial keratitis secondary to herpes simplex virus infection. The conjunctival flap is now largely reserved to resolve acute disease in inflamed, ulcerated, thinning corneas that cannot be controlled with medical or other therapeutic measures.

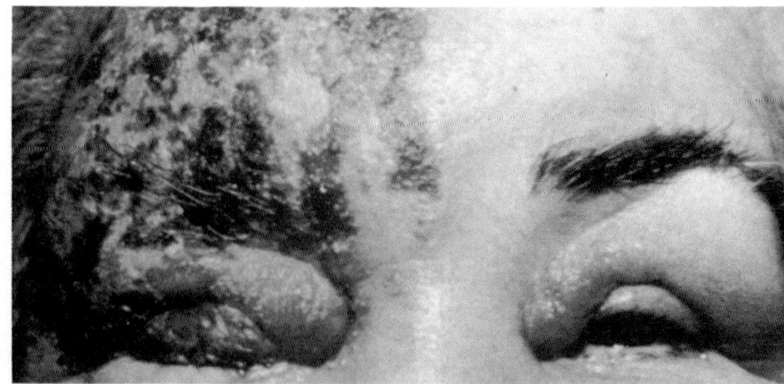

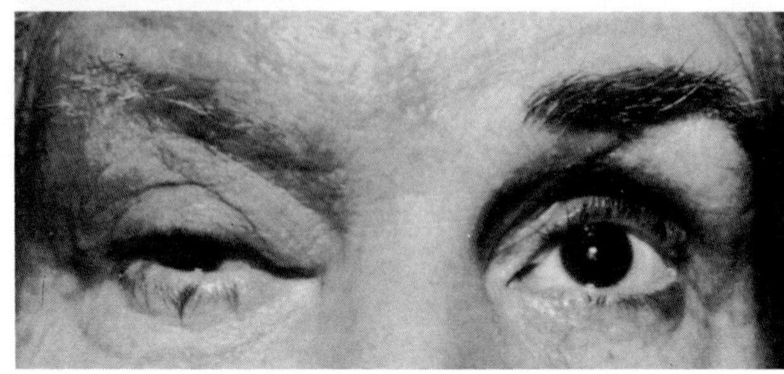

FIGURE 1–75 **Herpes zoster ophthalmicus (HZO).** *A,* Acute HZO of fresh and crusted vesicles at different stages of evolution in the V1 dermatomal distribution. *B,* Same patient 5 weeks later showing residual ptosis and partial third nerve palsy apparent on attempted upgaze. The palsy resolved completely over a 1-month period.

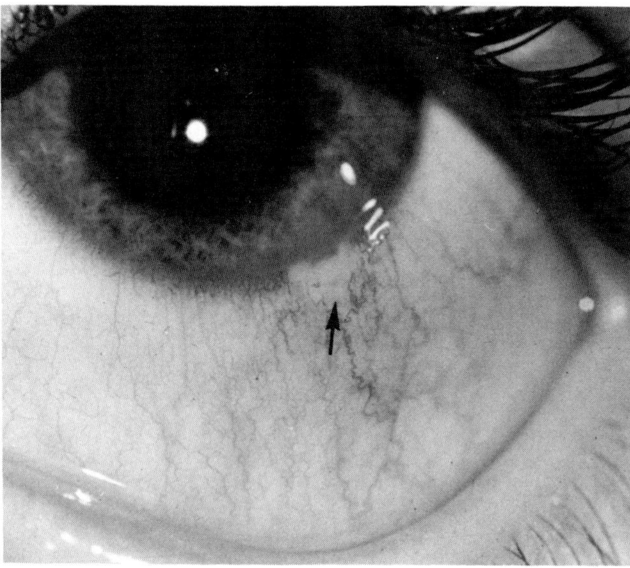

FIGURE 1–74 **Varicella phlyctenule.** Acute varicella limbal phlyctenule *(arrow)* appearing in the course of disseminated chickenpox. It is unclear whether these are due to live virus or an immune-like reaction or both.

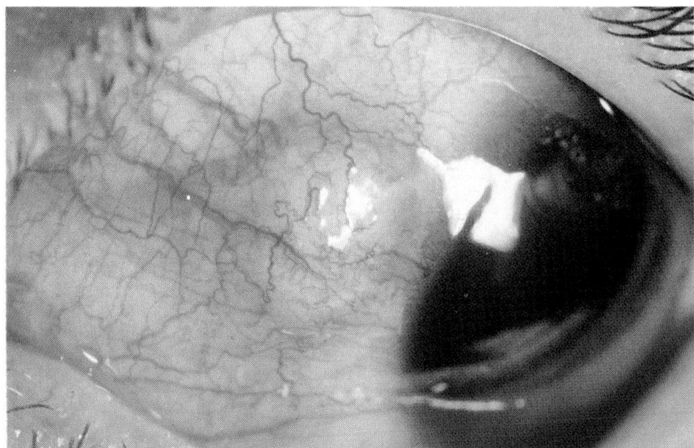

FIGURE 1–76 **HZO nodular scleritis.** Acute HZO nodular scleritis with onset several months after an acute attack of HZO. Scleritis responded to mild topical steroid and oral ibuprofen and resolved to a moderate focal scleral thinning. The scleritis may occur during the acute disease or several months after the cutaneous eruption has cleared.

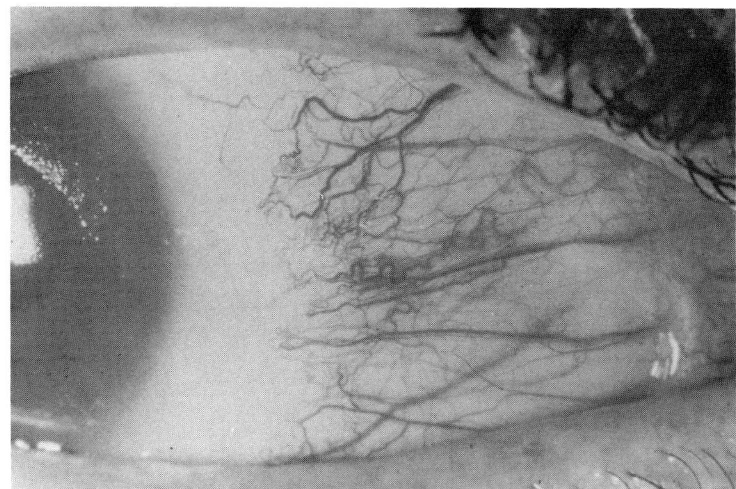

FIGURE 1–77 **HZO limbal vasculitis.** Acute severe HZO 360-degree occlusive limbal vasculitis manifests in this picture as loss of vasculature in the perilimbal region. Anterior ischemic necrosis resulted but responded to intensive topical and systemic steroids.

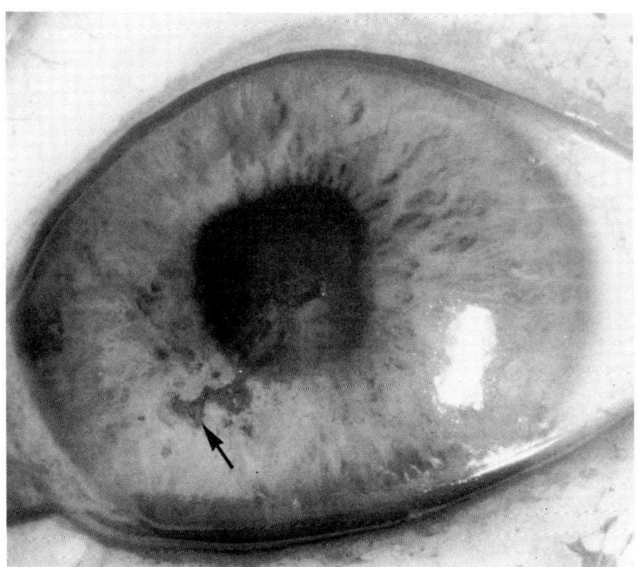

FIGURE 1–78 **HZO keratitis.** Acute HZO with zoster infectious viral dendritiform lesions appearing as transient, positive-staining, focally heaped-up areas of epithelium without terminal bulbs *(arrow)*. These vesicles may be differentiated from HSV dendrites in that HZV dendrites lack the rounded terminal bulbs at the end of the branches, and when they are wiped from the corneal epithelium, they tend to leave behind a layer of intact epithelium rather than the full-thickness ulcers noted with HSV. These HZV heaped-up lesions tend to resolve without therapy.

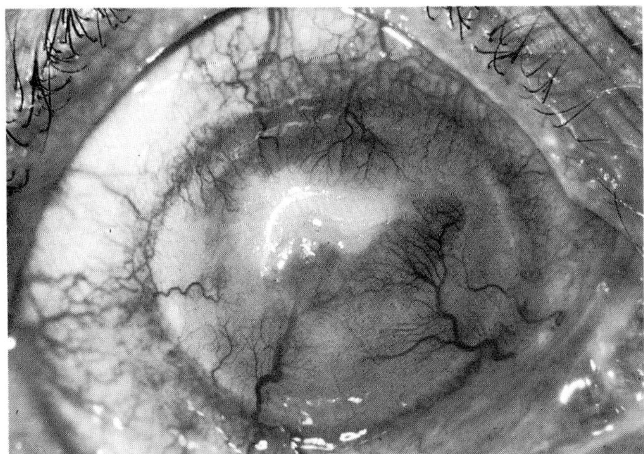

FIGURE 1–79 **HZO necrotizing interstitial keratitis.** Chronic HZO keratitis with active necrotic interstitial keratitis, soft neurotrophic ulceration, and superficial vascular pannus.

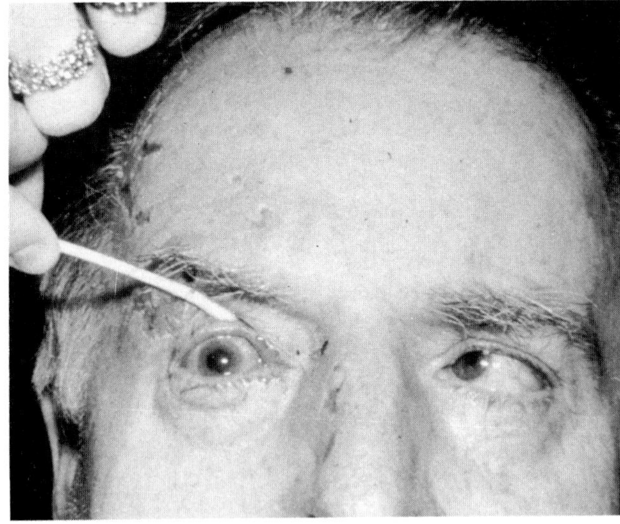

FIGURE 1–80 **HZV ocular motor palsy.** This man had a recent HZV infection with residual total third, fourth, and sixth palsies resulting in "frozen globe." The palsy resolved completely over an 18-month period.

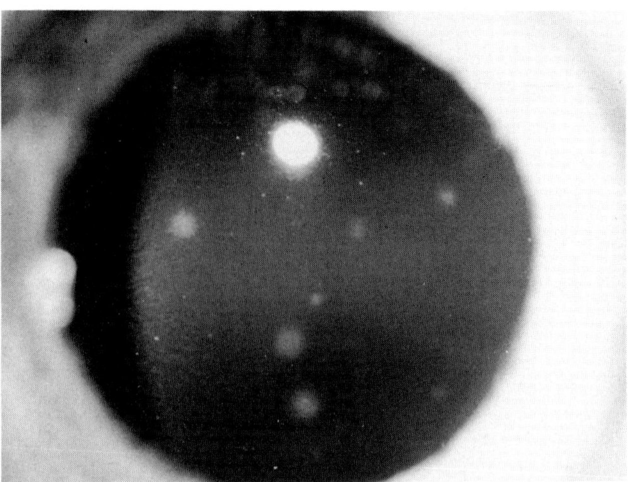

FIGURE 1–82 **Adenoviral keratoconjunctivitis.** Chronic adenoviral keratitis with anterior stromal whitish infiltrates. These may occasionally merge to form figures simulating focal HSV anterior stromal scars.

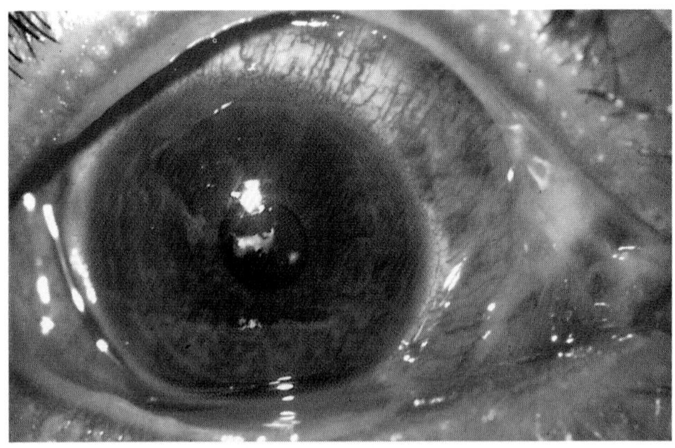

FIGURE 1–81 **Adenoviral keratoconjunctivitis.** Acute severe adenoviral conjunctivitis with true inflammatory membranes and symblepharon formations along with conjunctival chemosis and hyperemia.

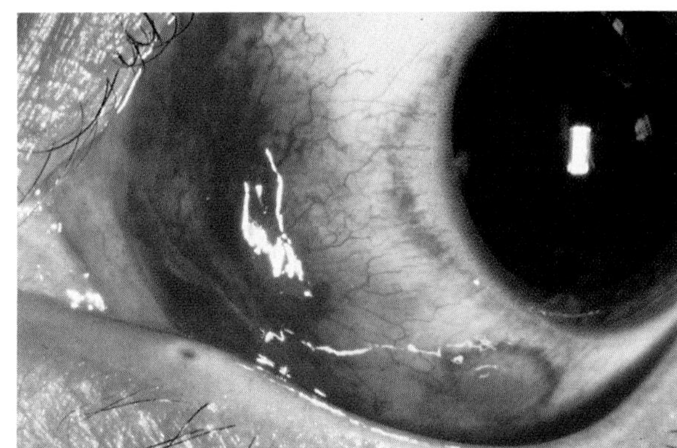

FIGURE 1–83 **Kaposi's sarcoma in an acquired immunodeficiency syndrome (AIDS) patient.** Such sarcomas appear typically in the lower or medial fornix and are soft and deep purple-red in color. Conjunctival involvement with Kaposi's sarcoma occurs in 10% of AIDS patients and may be focal nodules or diffuse infiltrative lesions.

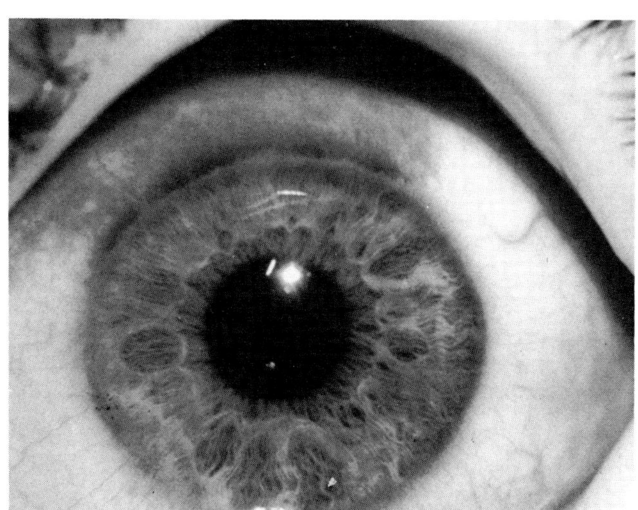

FIGURE 1–84 **Acute hemorrhagic conjunctivitis.** Acute hemorrhagic conjunctivitis showing a solid sheet of subconjunctival blood under the superior conjunctiva. Punctate keratitis developed 4 days later. This highly contagious ocular infection is caused by the enteroviruses, members of the picornavirus family.

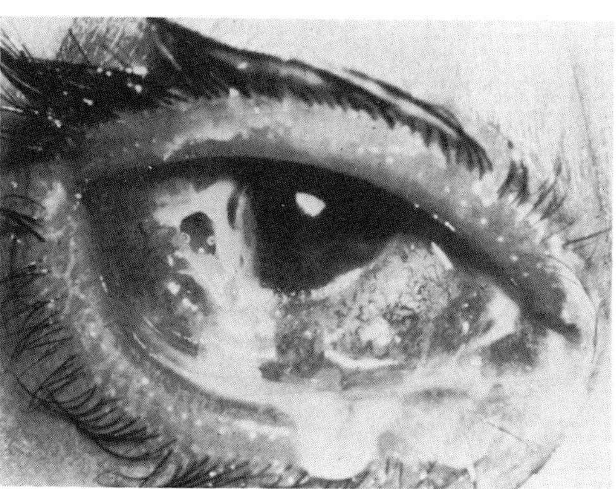

FIGURE 1–86 **Purulent gonococcal conjunctivitis (hyperacute).** Copious, thick, purulent discharge and marked conjunctival chemosis.

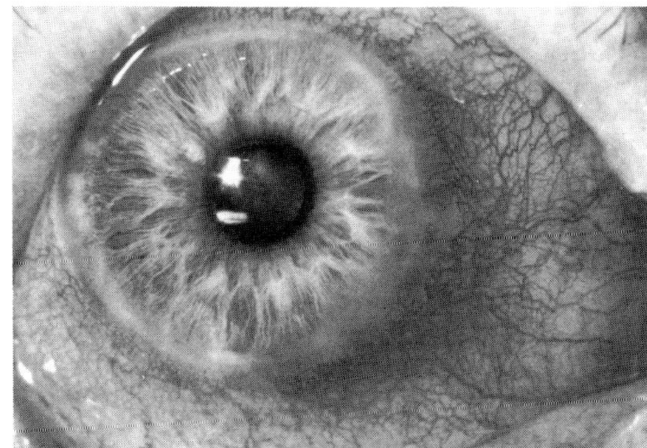

FIGURE 1–85 **Staphylococcal conjunctivitis.** Markedly hyperemic conjunctival vascular dilation with patchy anterior stromal infiltrates just inside the limbus.

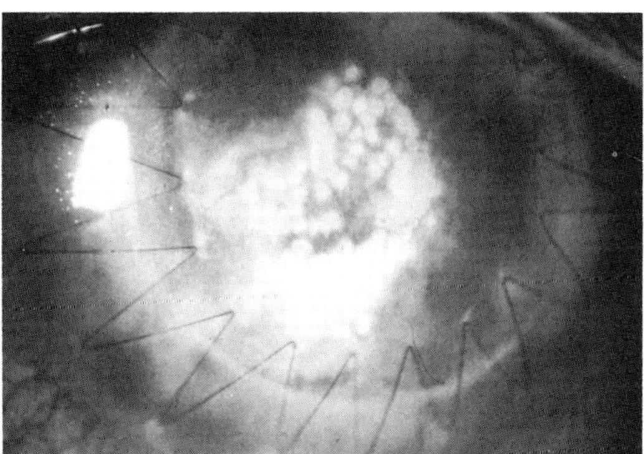

FIGURE 1–87 **Infectious crystalline keratopathy.** Scattered focal corneal lesions with crystalline pattern produced by a *Streptococcus viridans.* The distinct linear crystalline-appearing lesion is intrastromal in location and often occurs in corneas that have been treated with topical steroids. (Courtesy of L. Michael Cobo, M.D.)

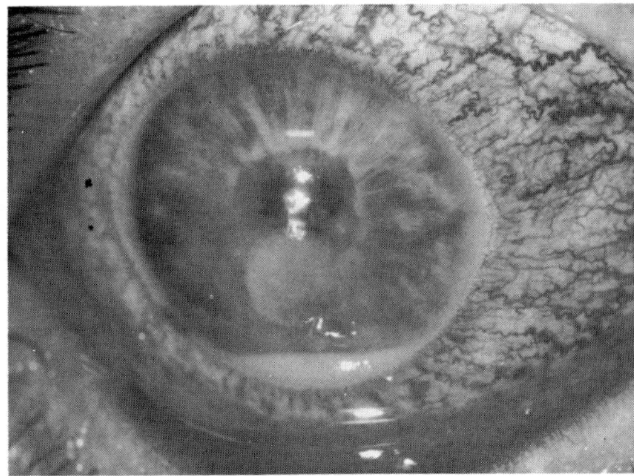

FIGURE 1–88 **Hypopyon corneal ulcer.** *Streptococcus pneumoniae* keratitis with stromal infiltration and anterior chamber hypopyon. This pathogen typically causes deep central ulceration with slightly undermined edges with a serpiginous contour but associated with deep, radiating striae in Descemet's membrane.

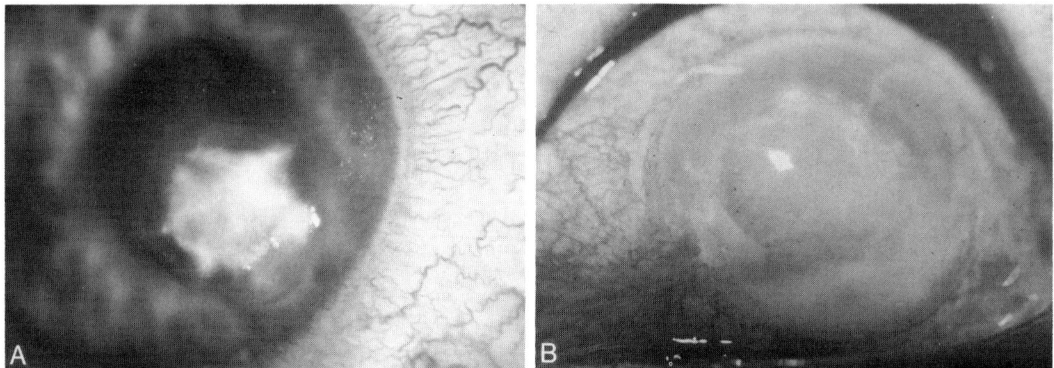

FIGURE 1–89 ***Pseudomonas aeruginosa* corneal ulcer.** *A*, Shaggy mucoid discharge adherent to cornea. The mucopurulent exudate is of a yellowish green hue, and ground-glass edema surrounding the ulcer may be present. *B*, Necrotic stromal infiltration with hypopyon. Rapid progression of a keratitis due to Pseudomonas is a real threat owing to a plethora of enzymes and toxins released by the organism.

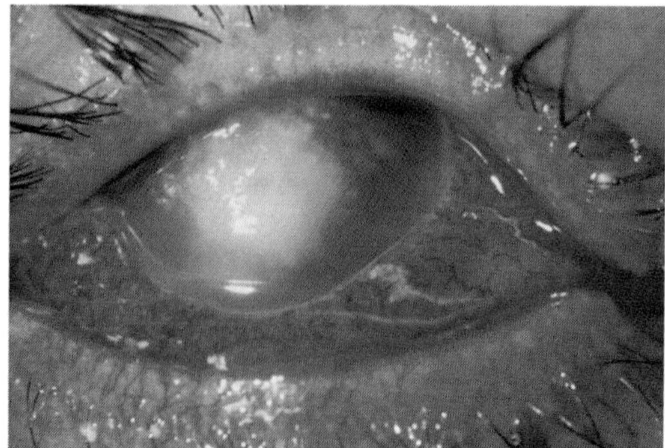

FIGURE 1–90 **Fungal keratitis.** Note the dense inflammatory infiltrate in the corneal stroma, with "satellite" lesions, and the feathery "hyphate" borders of the predominant lesion.

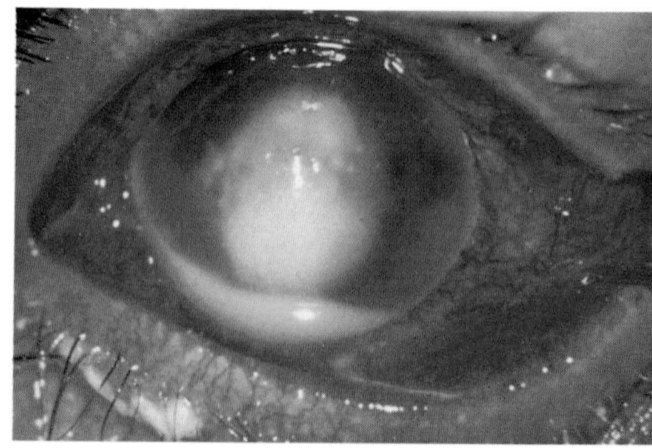

FIGURE 1–91 Same patient as in Figure 1–90. Worsening of the suppurative keratitis, with development of hypopyon.

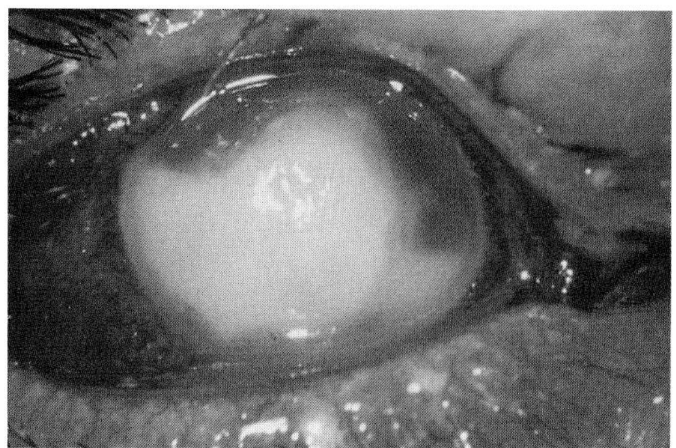

FIGURE 1–92 Same patient as in Figure 1–90. Increasing intraocular involvement from the inflammatory process.

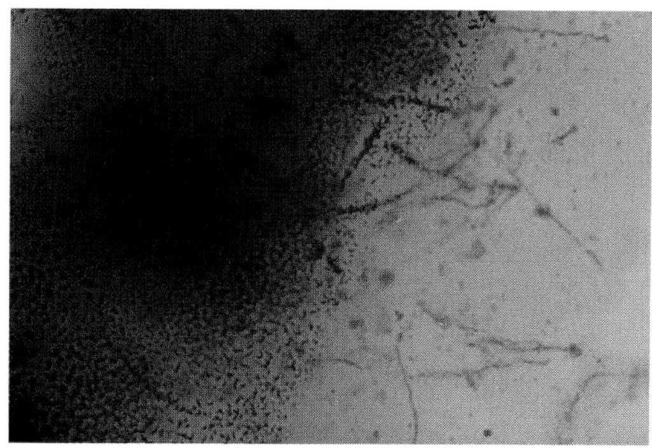

FIGURE 1–93 Same patient as in Figure 1–90. Histopathology slide of biopsied cornea, PAS stain. Note the filamentous fungal elements. These filamentous elements are septate in nature, and eventually the culture grew *Fusarium* species.

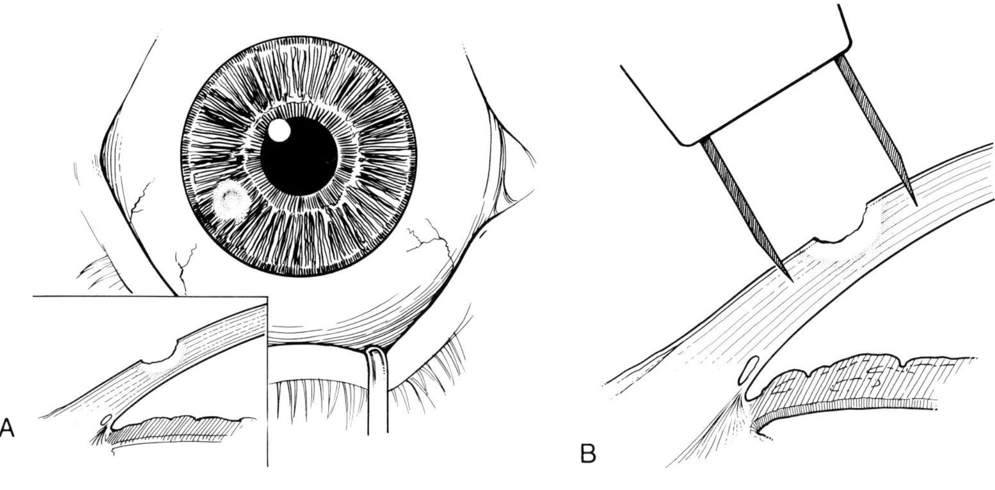

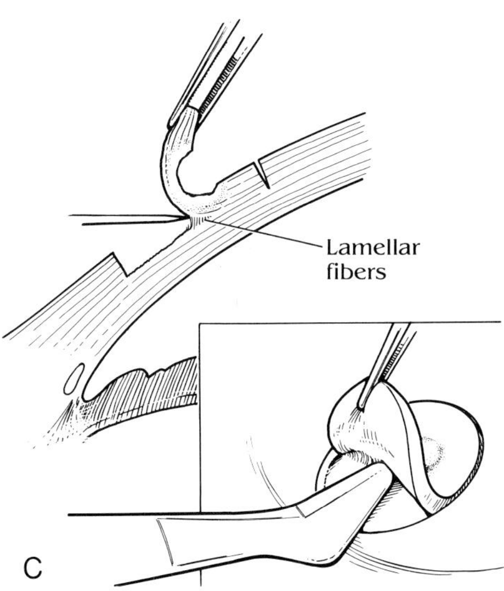

FIGURE 1–94 **Corneal biopsy technique.** *A,* Microbial corneal ulcer, 8 o'clock sector, midperiphery. The depth of the ulcer is approximately 25 percent and the depth of the infiltrate approximately 75 percent. *B,* Depth of trephination in the performance of a diagnostic corneal biopsy for this case of microbial keratitis. Note that the trephination is deep enough to ensure harvesting of material contained within the infiltrate below the deepest area of the ulcer itself. *C,* Dissection of the biopsy button after trephination illustrated in *B.* Note that the knife is dissecting the tissue in a lamellar plane, thereby avoiding an irregular or ever-deepening level of dissection. If keratomycosis is the primary clinical suspicion, but the smears are negative and the cultures are negative at 48 to 72 hours, and the patient is not improving on the broad-spectrum antibacterial therapy chosen, the recommendation is to proceed to corneal biopsy.

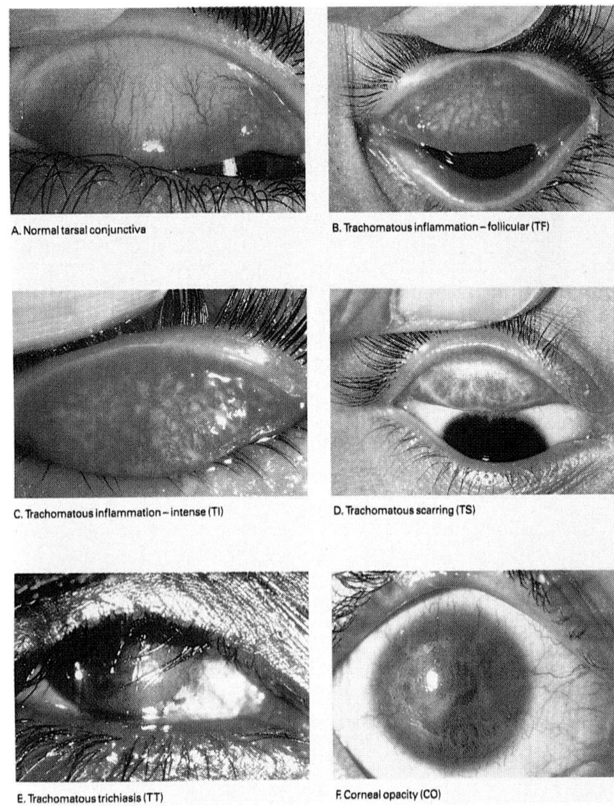

FIGURE 1–95 **Trachoma: World Health Organization classification scheme.** The inflammatory signs of the upper lid and cornea in trachoma are the basis for the classification. (From Thylefors B, Dawson ER, Jones BR, et al: A simple system for the assessment of trachoma and its complications. Bull WHO 65:481, 1987.)

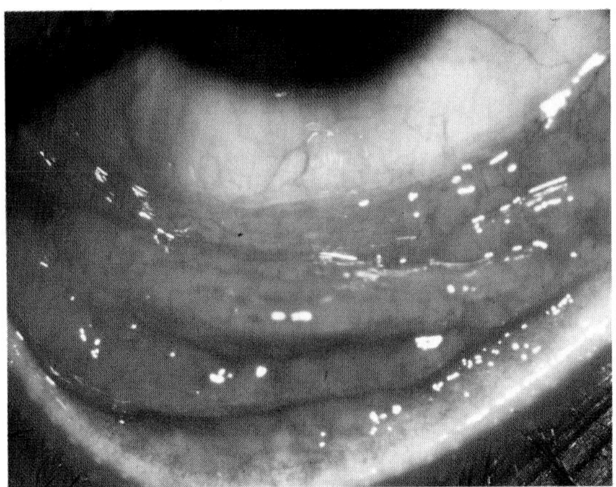

FIGURE 1–96 **Adult inclusion conjunctivitis.** Acute follicular conjunctivitis with a mucopurulent discharge involving the inferior tarsal conjunctiva is the primary feature of this disease.

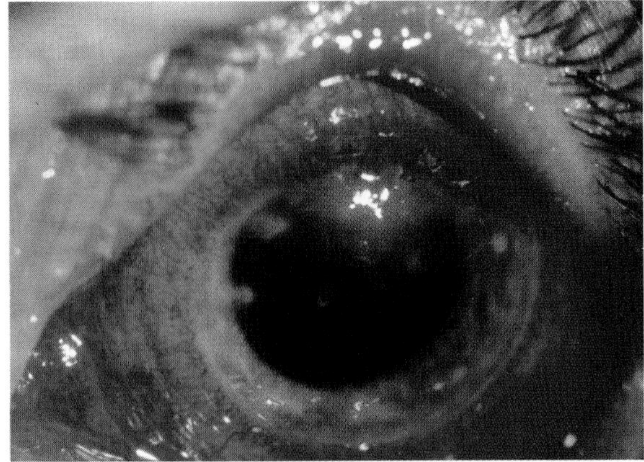

FIGURE 1–97 **Adult inclusion conjunctivitis.** Subepithelial corneal infiltrates and corneal neovascularization are present in this case of adult inclusion conjunctivitis.

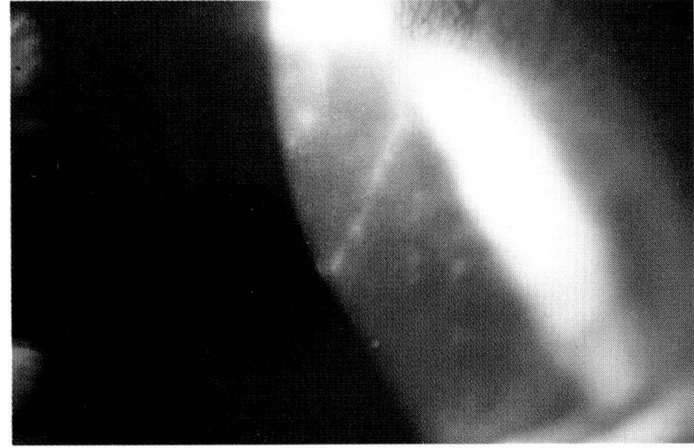

FIGURE 1–98 ***Acanthamoeba* radial keratoneuritis.** This broad slit-lamp beam view shows the inflammatory infiltrate along the radial course of a corneal nerve.

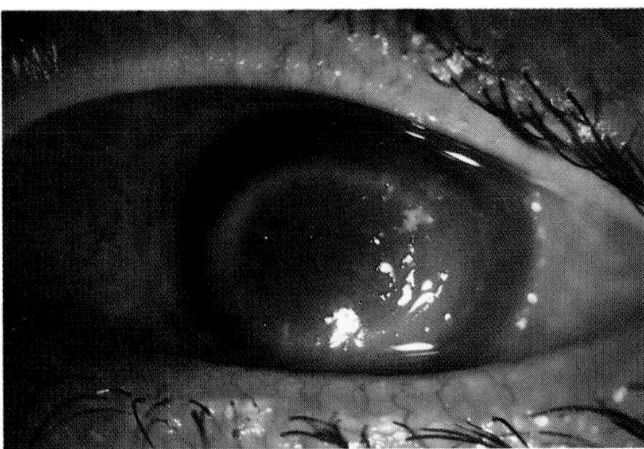

FIGURE 1–99 ***Acanthamoeba* ring infiltrate.** Characteristic ring infiltrate that formed 2 months after the onset of symptoms in a case of *Acanthamoeba* keratitis.

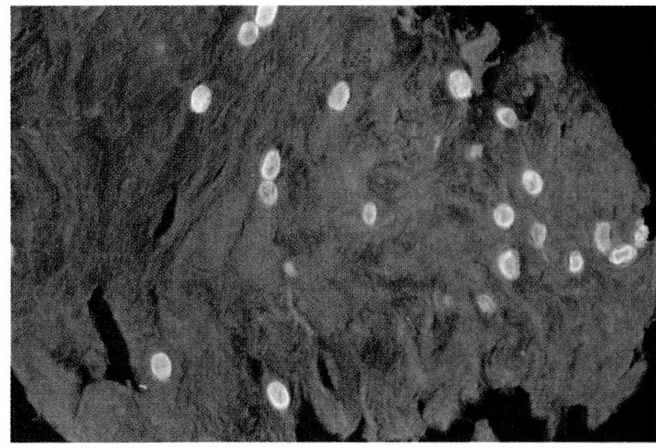

FIGURE 1-100 **Calcofluor white stain for *Acanthamoeba*.** A corneal biopsy specimen stained with Calcofluor white and viewed with ultraviolet light. These white cysts measure 10–25 μm in diameter. ×450. (From Wilhelmus KR, Osato MS, Font RL: Rapid diagnosis of *Acanthamoeba* keratitis using calcofluor white. Arch Ophthalmol 104:1309–1316, 1986. Copyright 1986, American Medical Association.)

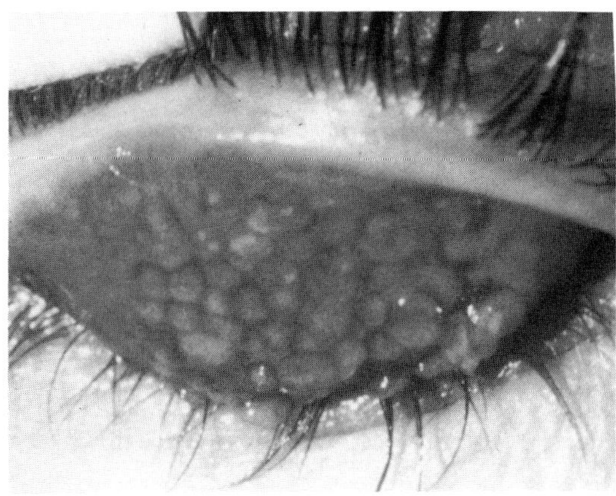

FIGURE 1-101 **Vernal keratoconjunctivitis (VKC).** Obvious giant papillae or cobblestones are present in the upper tarsal conjunctiva. These giant papillae are a classic sign of palpebral VKC.

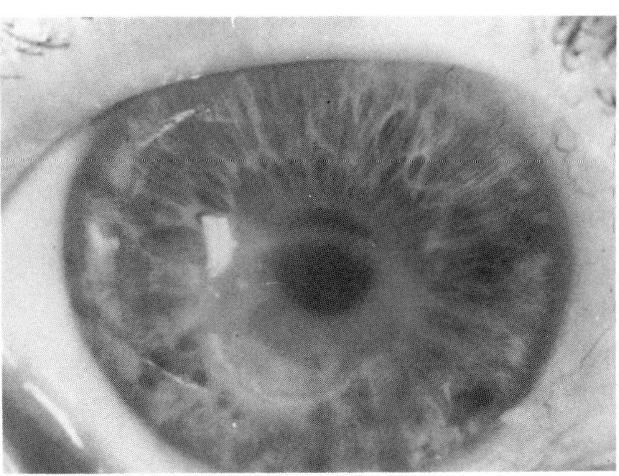

FIGURE 1-103 **VKC.** Shield ulcer in a patient with VKC. This ulcer had persisted for 4 months before referral. These epithelial defects are trophic, defining the therapeutic strategies that are usually successful in healing of corneal abrasions or epithelial defects.

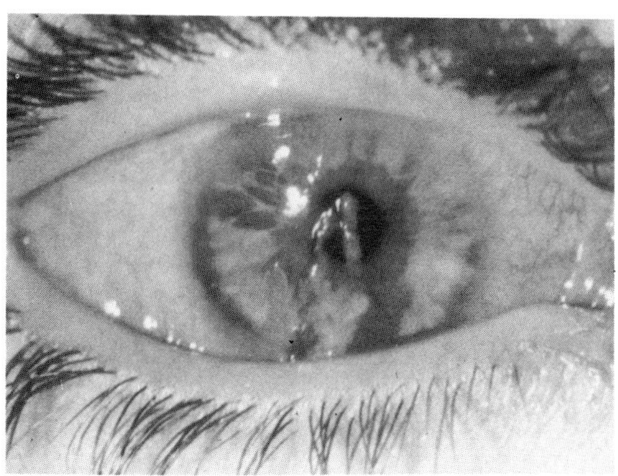

FIGURE 1-102 **VKC.** Note the bulbar conjunctival injection, the milky edema of the conjunctiva, and the characteristic ropy mucus thread on the corneal surface.

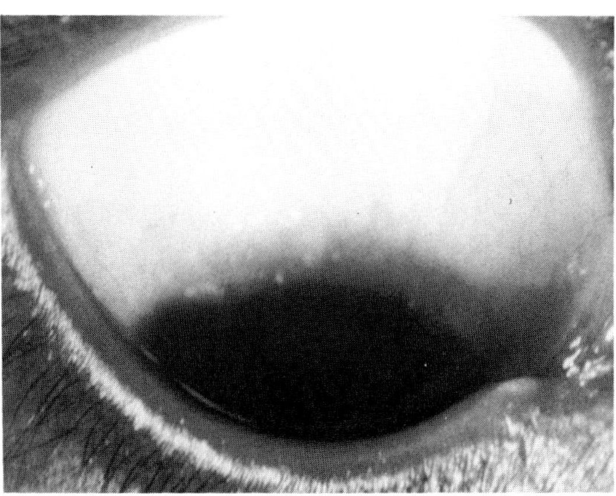

FIGURE 1-104 **Limbal VKC.** Note the limbal papillae with the white Horner-Trantas dots on the apices of the limbal papillae. These limbal papillae are rich in collections of inflammatory cells, especially eosinophils at the apices.

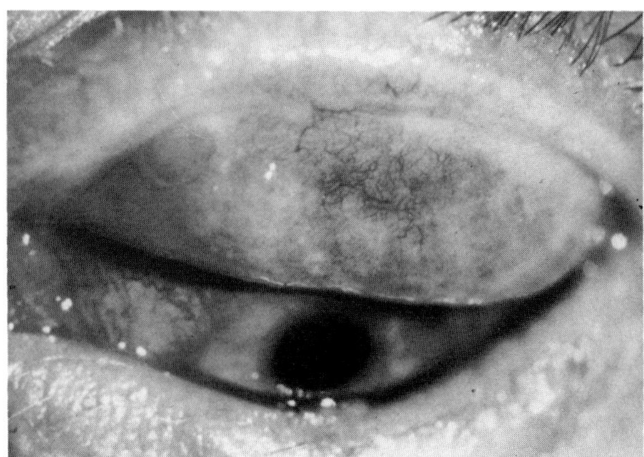

FIGURE 1-105 **Ocular cicatricial pemphigoid (OCP).** Everted upper lip demonstrating subepithelial fibrosis of the superior tarsal conjunctiva.

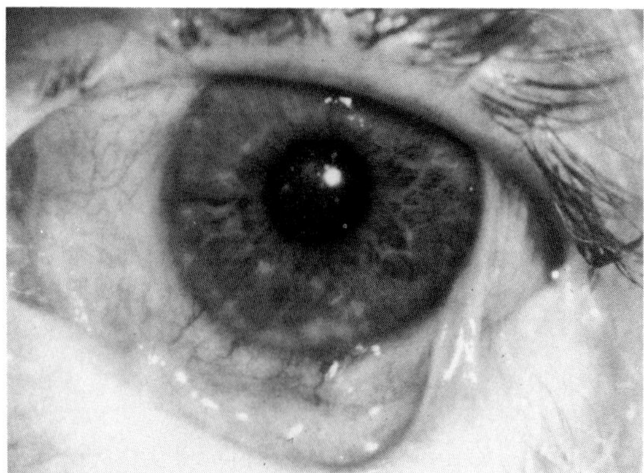

FIGURE 1-108 **OCP, stage 3.** The cicatrizing process has progressed to the point of formation of symblephara.

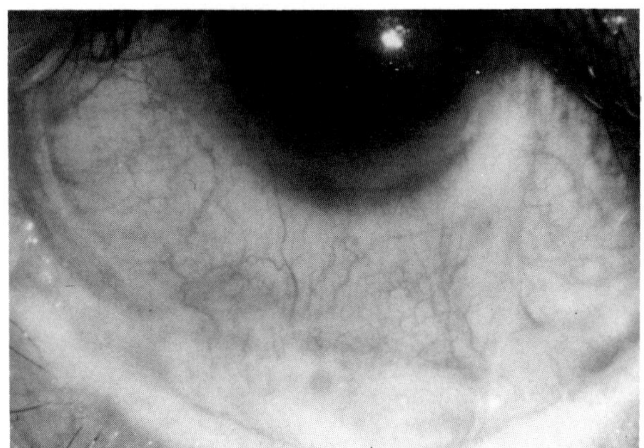

FIGURE 1-106 **OCP, stage 1.** Note the fibrotic striae under the inferior tarsal conjunctiva.

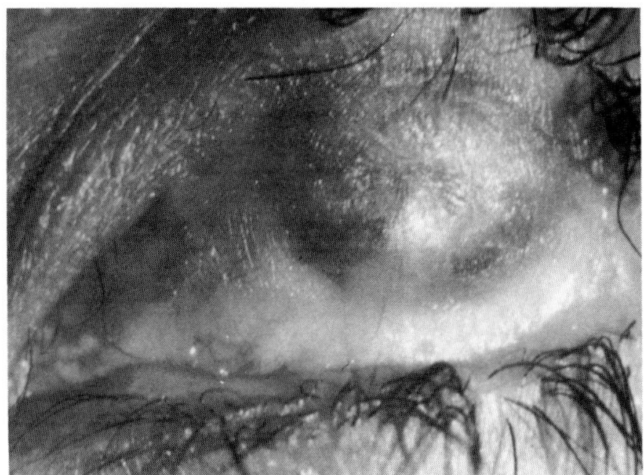

FIGURE 1-109 **OCP, stage 4.** Note the leatherization of the ocular surface and the adhesion of the lids to the globe. Note that the skin of the upper lid margin appears to blend imperceptibly into the epidermalization of the corneal surface.

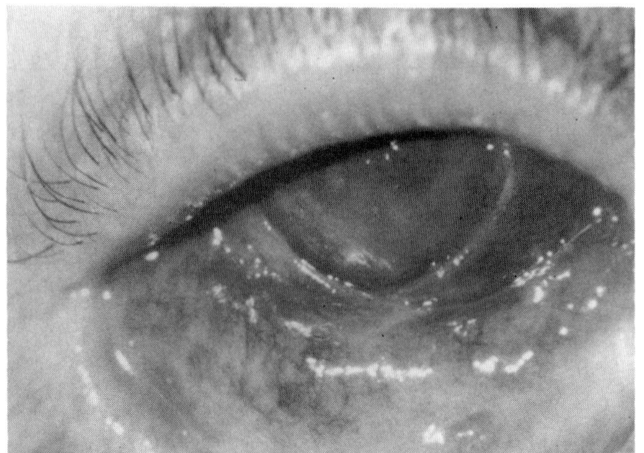

FIGURE 1-107 **OCP, stage 2.** Note the subepithelial fibrosis under the tarsal conjunctival epithelium, with formation of an extensive "feltwork" of the new collagen, and the loss of the normal depth of the inferior fornix, i.e., fornix foreshortening.

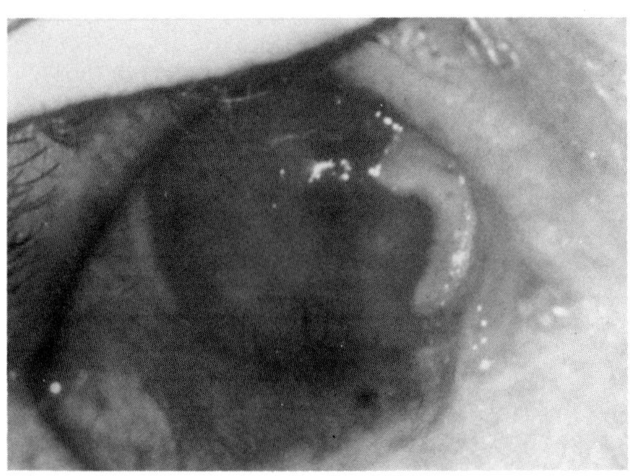

FIGURE 1-110 **OCP.** Extensive keratopathy, with corneal scarring and neovascularization, is present in this case.

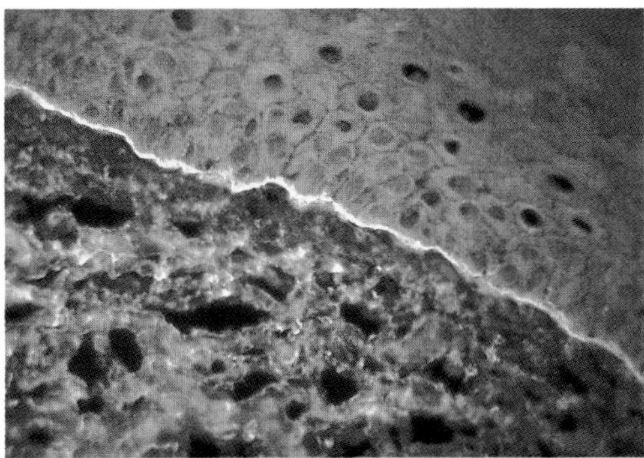

FIGURE 1–111 Conjunctival biopsy specimen of a patient with active OCP. This specimen is shown with immunofluorescent microscopy. The primary antibody used on this preparation has been anti-IgA. The bright apple-green, linear, continuous line of fluorescence of the epithelial basement zone shows that this patient has large amounts of IgA deposited at the epithelial basement membrane zone, an abnormal finding.

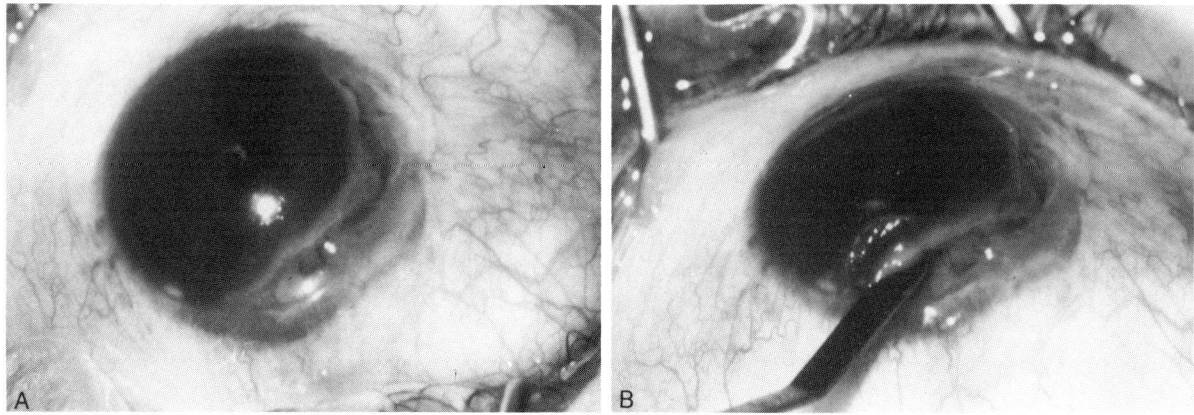

FIGURE 1–112 **Mooren's ulcer.** *A*, Note the peripheral ulcerative keratitis that has begun at 3 o'clock and has progressed clockwise to 6:30, counterclockwise to 1 o'clock, and centrally to involve 2.5 mm of the cornea. Note also the inflammatory infiltrates in advance of the edge of the ulcer. *B*, Probing of the edge of this ulcer demonstrates that the extent of the undermining and hence the destruction of the corneal stroma is astonishingly much greater than was apparent by slit-lamp biomicroscopy.

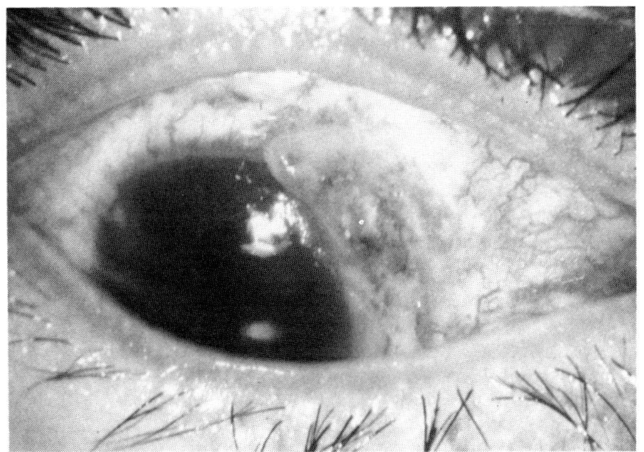

FIGURE 1–113 **Mooren's ulcer.** This cornea suffered perforation secondary to Mooren's ulcer. It displays status following conjunctival resections, ulcer débridement, and application of cyanoacrylate tissue adhesive at the perforation site at the 2 o'clock position at the limbus.

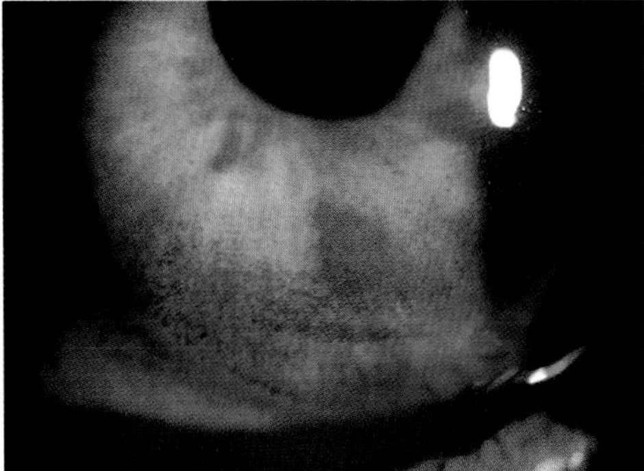

FIGURE 1–114 **Keratoconjunctivitis sicca.** This photograph has been taken with a red-free light source after instilling of 1 percent rose bengal dye. Note the punctate staining of the corneal epithelium in the interpalpebral fissure.

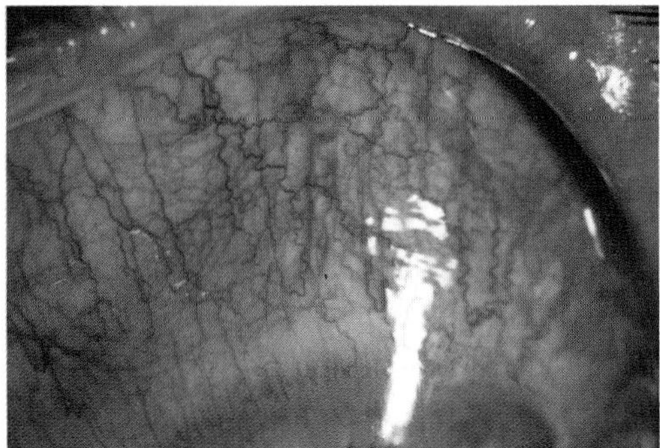

FIGURE 1-115 **Diffuse scleritis.** Note the slightly purple contribution to the reddened appearance of the eye. The presence of scleral edema is a sine qua non for establishing that a patient has scleritis.

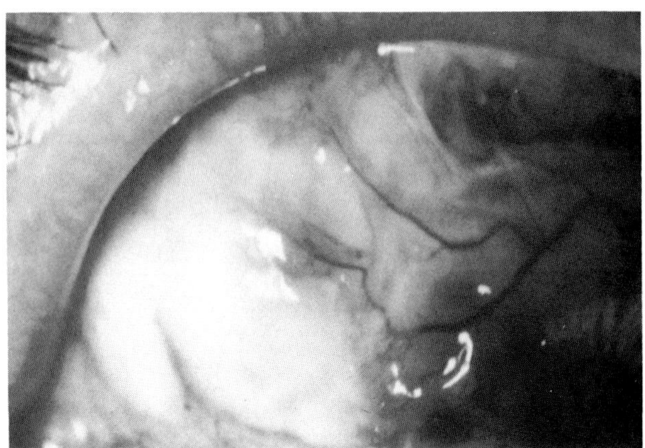

FIGURE 1-116 **Necrotizing scleritis.** Note the loss of sclera superiorly, down to choroid, and the associated extensive avascular area temporal to this area of near perforation.

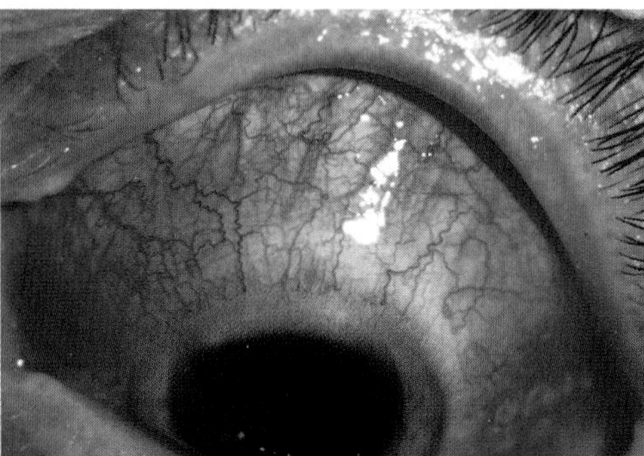

FIGURE 1-117 **Diffuse episcleritis.** Note the brilliant red characteristic of the conjunctival inflammation. In contrast to scleritis, there is no scleral edema seen in episcleritis.

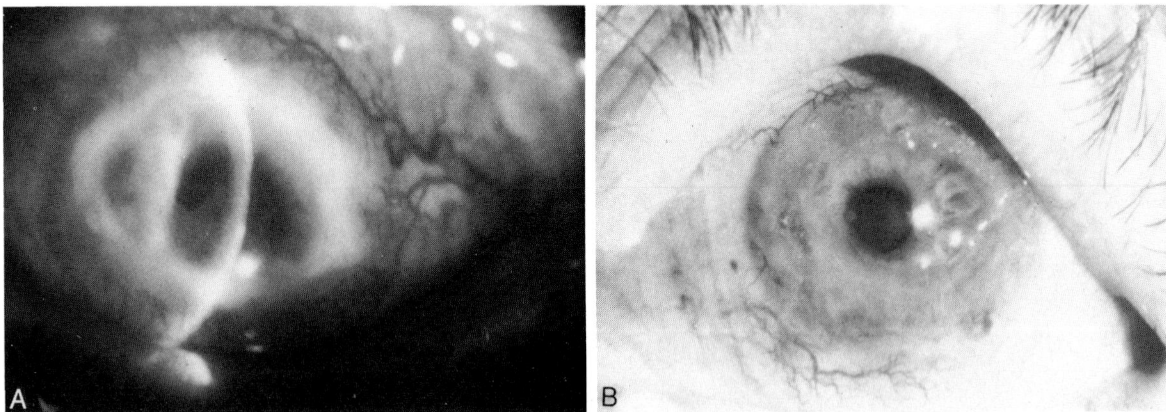

FIGURE 1-118 **Peripheral ulcerative keratitis.** *A*, Peripheral ulcerative keratitis in a patient with rheumatoid arthritis. Note the 360-degree ring infiltrate of the inflammatory cells with associated destruction of the peripheral cornea. *B*, Same eye as shown in *A*, following conjunctival resection, ulcer débridement, application of cyanoacrylate adhesive, and application of a soft contact lens.

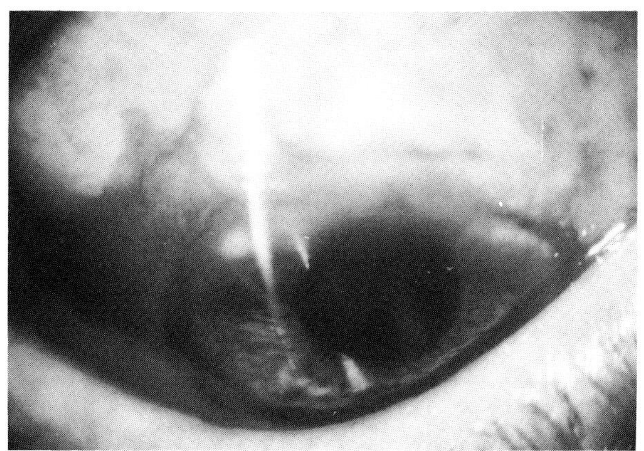

FIGURE 1-119 **Necrotizing scleritis in Wegener's granulomatosis.** Peripheral ulcerative keratitis and necrotizing scleritis are seen with increasing frequency as an initial significant manifestation of Wegener's granulomatosis. Here, one can see the areas of diffuse necrotizing scleritis along with peripheral ulcerative keratitis.

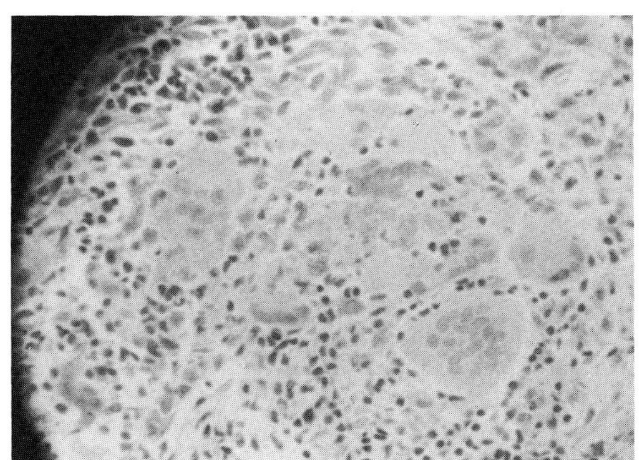

FIGURE 1-120 **Scleral biopsy specimen in Wegener's granulomatosis.** This H&E stain shows the histopathology of a scleral biopsy specimen in a patient with Wegener's granulomatosis. Note the extensive array of multinucleated giant cells.

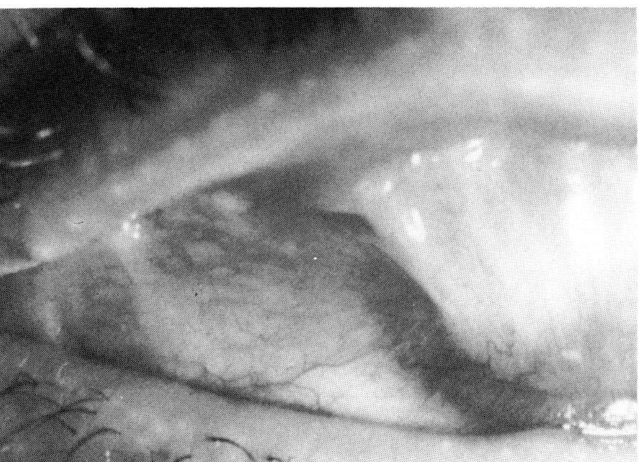

FIGURE 1-121 **Stevens-Johnson syndrome.** Ocular involvement in Stevens-Johnson syndrome with subepithelial fibrosis, fornix foreshortening, and dense symblepharon formation.

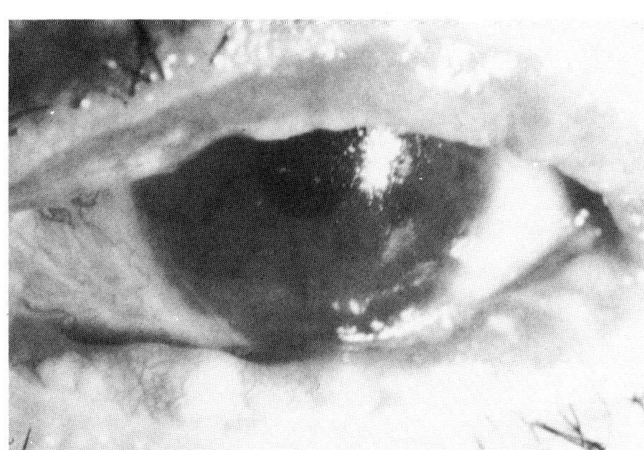

FIGURE 1-122 **Stevens-Johnson syndrome.** A patient with Stevens-Johnson syndrome had extensive keratinization of the tarsal conjunctiva, here shown following resection of that keratinization and performance of buccal mucosal membrane grafting to both upper and lower lids.

A. Normal

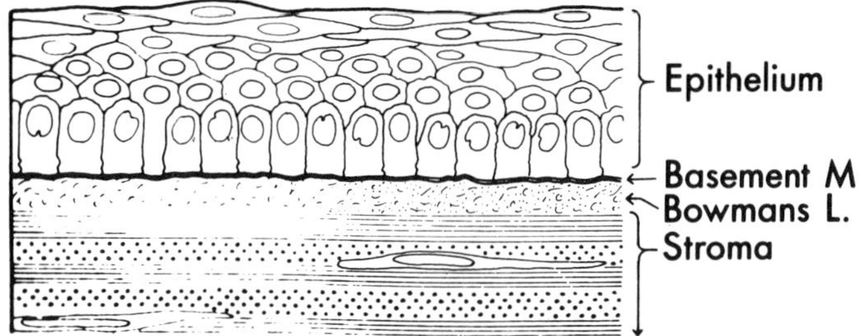

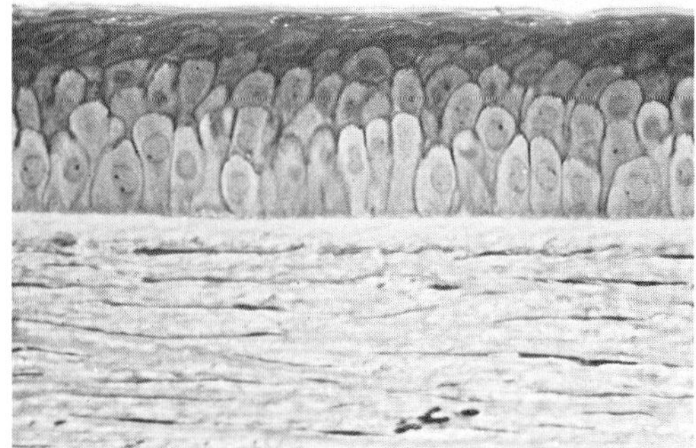

B. Recurrent erosion syndrome

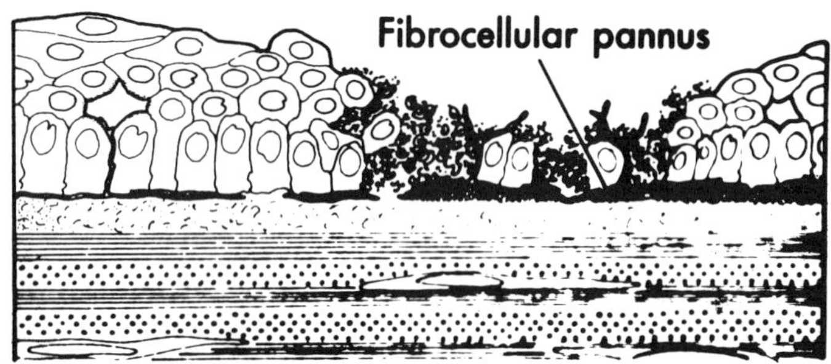

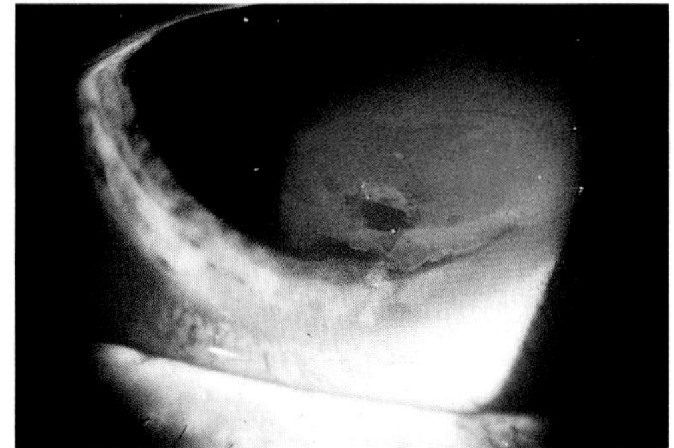

C. Persistent epithelial defect

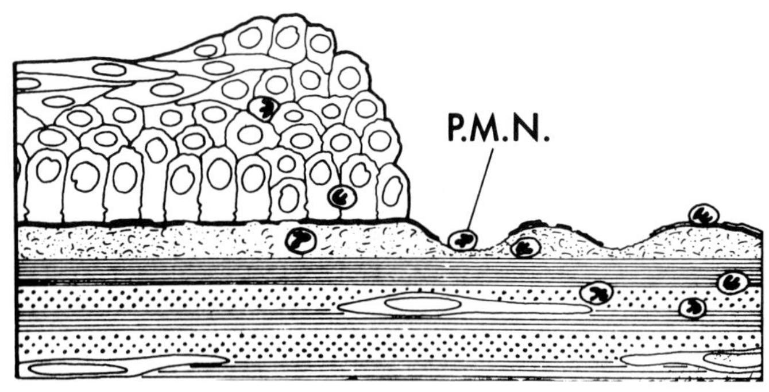

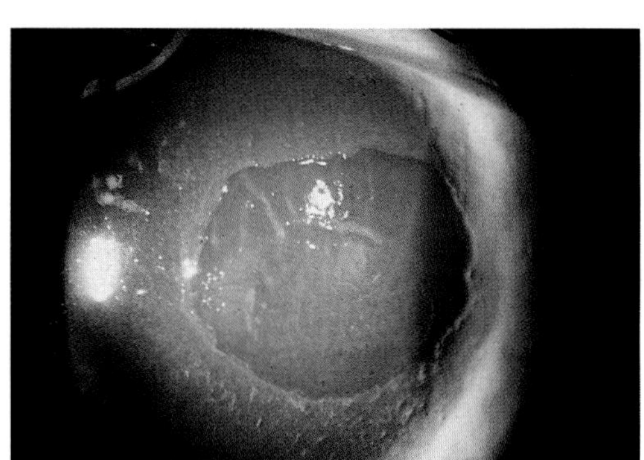

D. Sterile ulcer

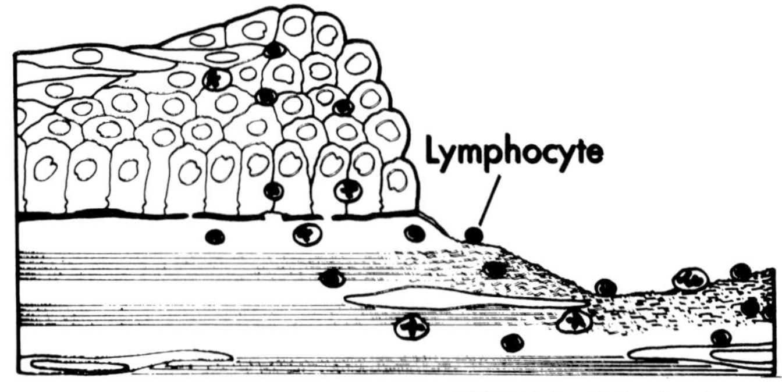

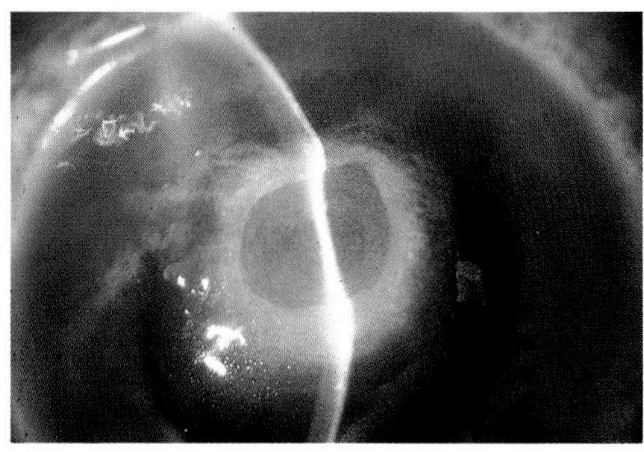

FIGURE 1–123 *See legend on opposite page*

◀ FIGURE 1–123 **Morphology and clinical appearance of normal cornea, corneal epithelial erosion, persistent defect, and ulceration.** *A, Left,* Normal cornea displays regular epithelial layers, a uniform continual basement membrane, and Bowman's membrane plus stroma devoid of inflammatory cells. *Right,* Phase-contrast biomicroscopy discloses these same features. Paraphenylenediamine, ×125. *B, Left,* Recurrent epithelial erosion involves epithelial defects associated with aberrant, discontinuous basement membrane plus subepithelial fibrocellular pannus but without Bowman's layer defect or inflammation. *Right,* Clinical features of posttraumatic recurrent epithelial erosion include extensive area of loose epithelial adhesion with devitalized threads of the epithelial sheet floating on the tear film. *C, Left,* Persistent epithelial defect is notable for thickened, nonmotile epithelial cell layer at defect edge, defects at basement membrane and Bowman's layer, and some inflammatory cells. (P.M.N., polymorphonuclear neutrophil.) *Right,* Neurotrophic keratitis in an anesthetic cornea displays typical persistent epithelial defect having gray, thickened margins of immobile epithelium overlying a somewhat edematous but structurally intact stroma. *D, Left,* Sterile ulceration involves enzymatically mediated degradation of Bowman's layer and stroma, usually in the presence of acute and chronic inflammatory cells. *Right,* Biomicroscopy of a sterile ulcer reveals features of persistent epithelial defect, plus stromal ulceration as evidenced in the thinning of the slit-lamp beam. (*A–D, Left,* From Conjunctival and corneal injuries. *In* Shingleton BJ, Hersh PS, Kenyon KR (eds): Eye Trauma. St. Louis, Mosby-Year Book, 1991.)

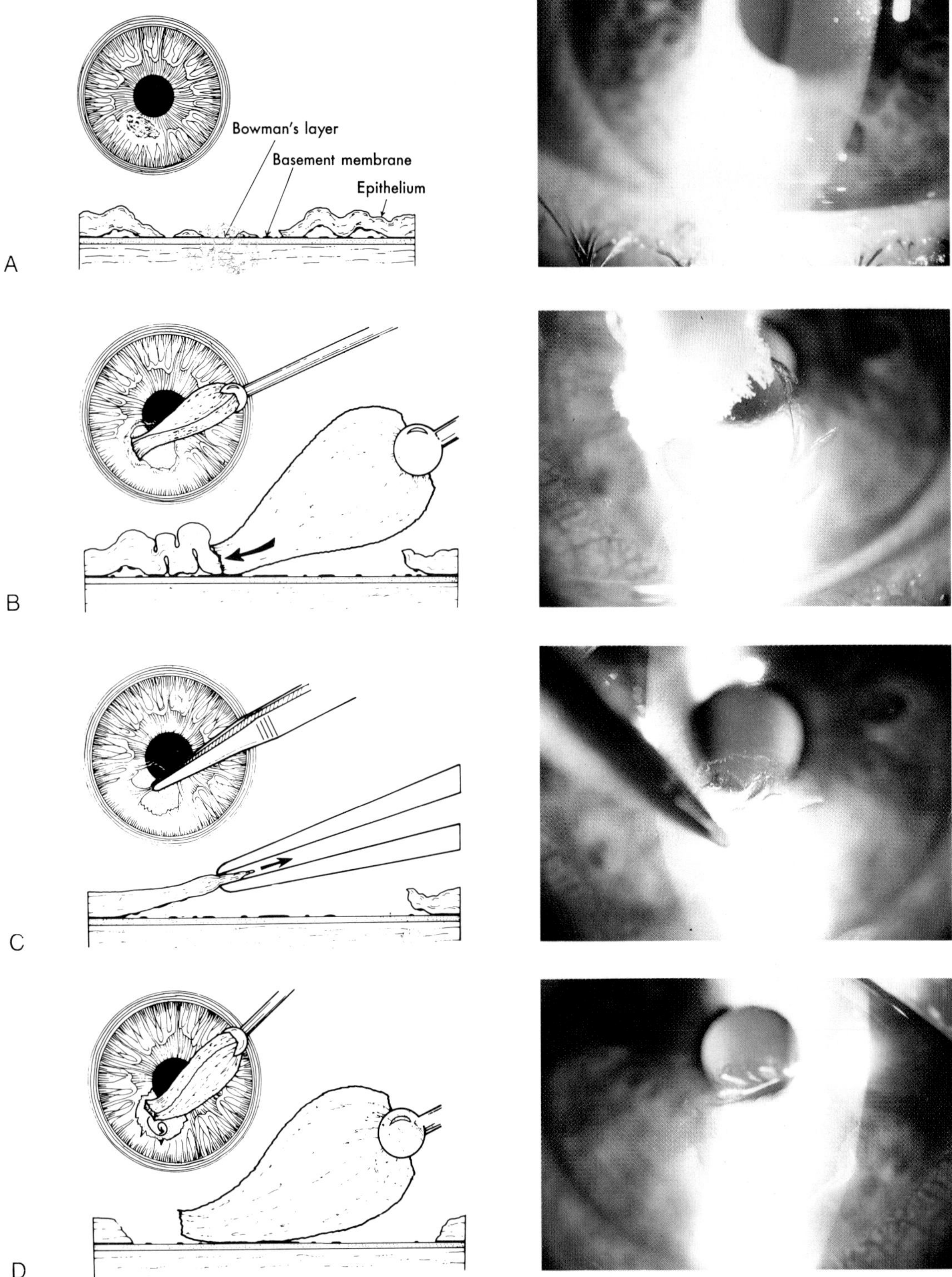

FIGURE 1–124 **Technique of epithelial débridement following recurrent erosion.** *A,* Devitalized epithelium and debris adherent to damaged basement membrane surface inhibit restoration of intact basement membrane and recovery of tight epithelial stromal adhesion. *B,* Following application of topical anesthetic, a dry cellulose sponge is used to sweep aside nonadherent epithelium and debris. *C,* Jeweler's forceps are used to remove loose shards of marginal epithelium. *D,* The surface of Bowman's layer is polished with a dry cellulose sponge. Topical antibiotic, steriod, and cycloplegic agents are applied followed by pressure pads. If epithelial defect persists beyond 72 hours, the patch is replaced by a bandage soft contact lens with continuation of the same medical therapy in decreasing doses for 6 to 8 weeks. (*A–D, Left,* From Conjunctival and corneal injuries. *In* Shingleton BJ, Hersh PS, Kenyon KR (eds): Eye Trauma. St. Louis, Mosby-Year Book, 1991.)

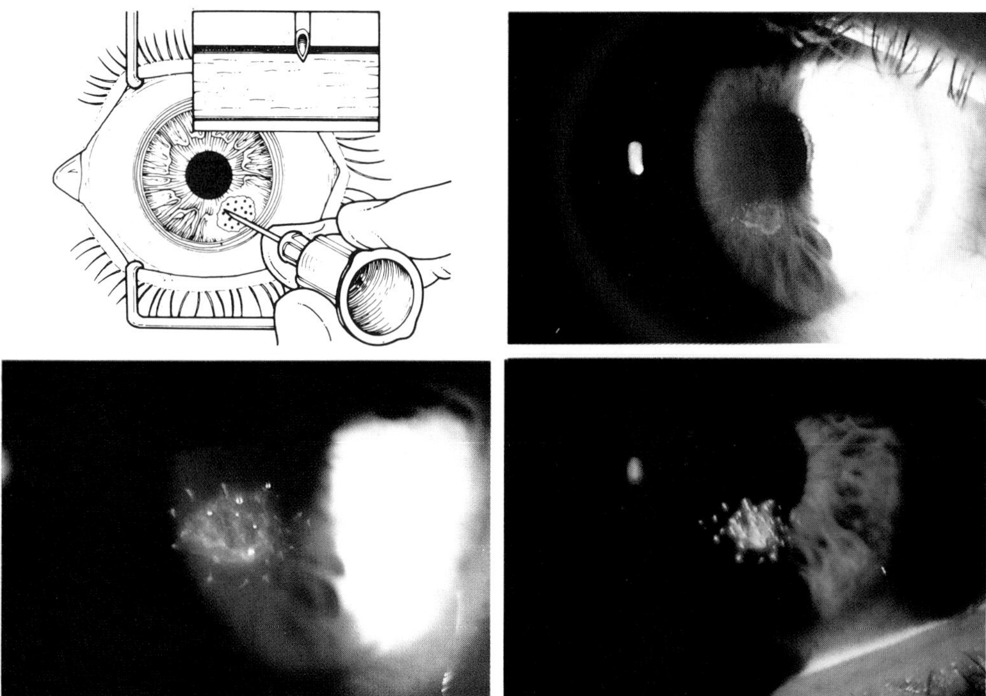

FIGURE 1–125 **Technique of anterior stromal puncture.** *Top left,* Multiple superficial punctures with a disposable No. 20 needle are used to stimulate microcicatrization between the epithelium, Bowman's layer, and the anterior stroma. *Top right,* Patient with recurrent erosion suitable for anterior stromal puncture displays an area of nonadherent epithelium. *Bottom left and right,* At completion of the procedure, multiple superficial punctures are evident within and around the area of defective epithelium. (*Top left,* From Conjunctival and corneal injuries. *In* Shingleton BJ, Hersh PS, Kenyon KR (eds): Eye Trauma. St. Louis, Mosby-Year Book, 1991. *Top right, bottom left and right,* Courtesy of Dr. S. M. MacRae.)

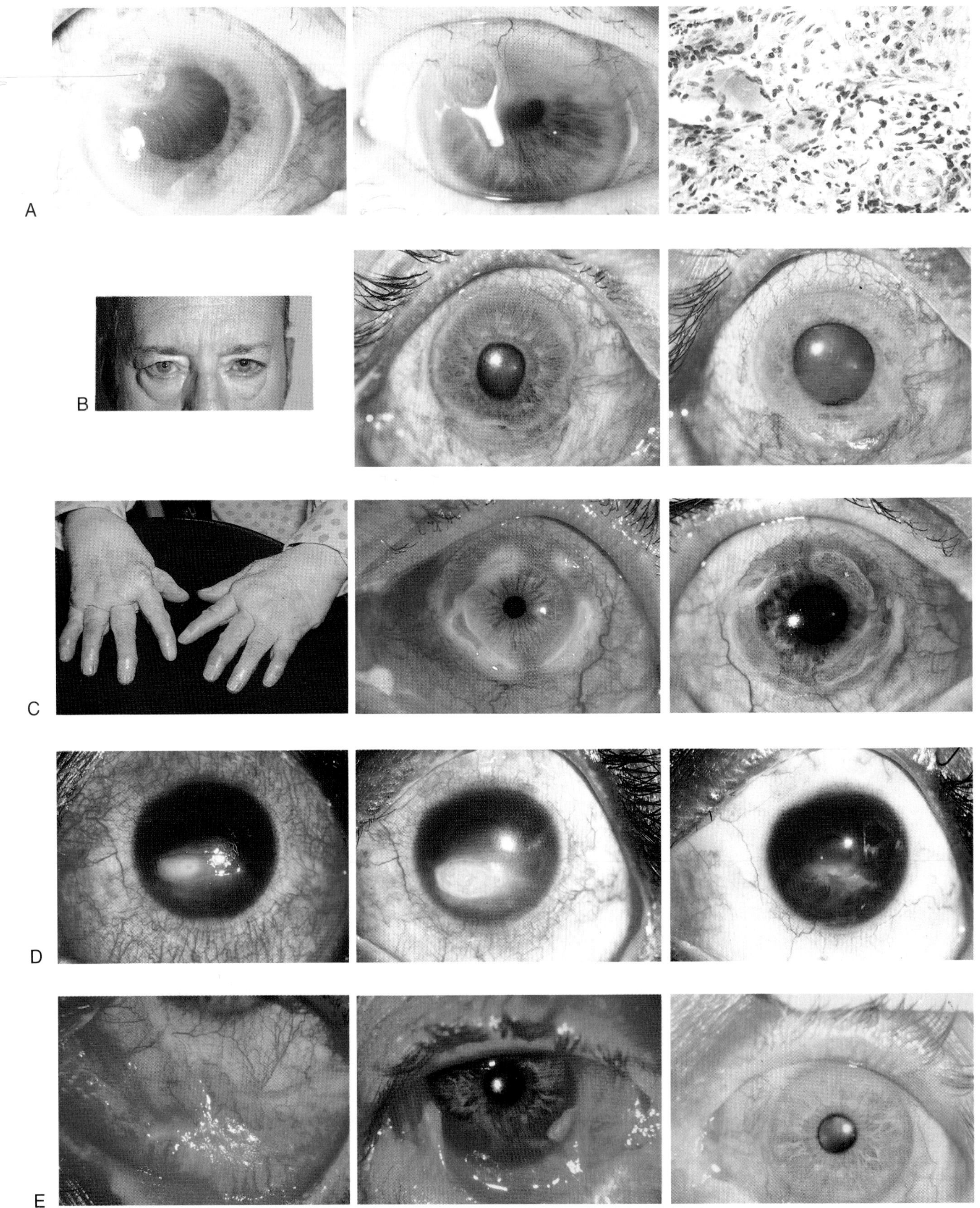

FIGURE 1–126 *See legend on opposite page*

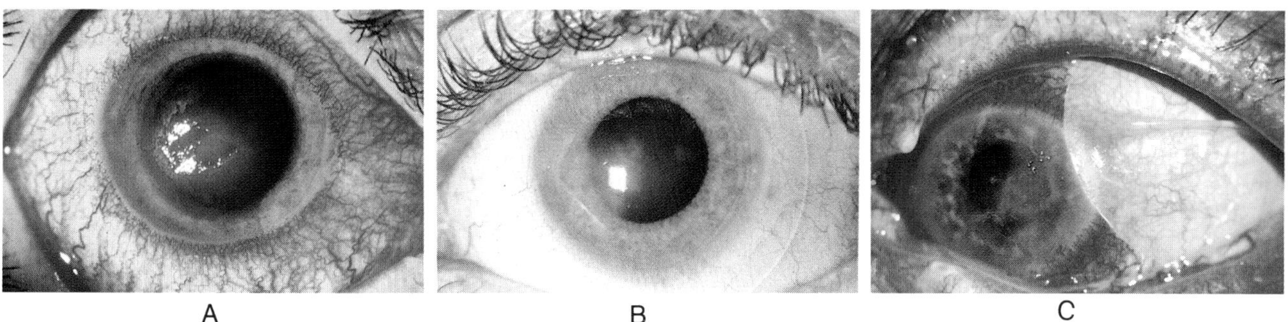

FIGURE 1-127 **Therapeutic soft contact lens.** *A,* In a patient with metaherpetic keratitis, a persistent defect, stromal haze, and conjunctival inflammation are evident. *B,* This same patient benefits from soft contact lens used to promote epithelial healing, improved stromal clarity, and reduced conjunctival inflammation. *C,* To assess corneal epithelial recovery in the presence of a bandage soft contact lens, topical anesthesia and fluorescein are instilled, the lens is slid to the side, the corneal surface is observed, and the contact lens is then repositioned. This technique is rapid and efficient, avoids corneal epithelial or contact lens damage from the manipulation of contact lens removal and replacement, and does not stain the contact lens. (*C,* From Conjunctival and corneal injuries. *In* Shingleton BJ, Hersh PS, Kenyon KR (eds): Eye Trauma. St. Louis, Mosby-Year Book, 1991.)

◀ FIGURE 1-126 **Noninfected stromal ulceration.** *A,* Peripheral ulcerative keratitis following cataract surgery. *Left,* In an elderly woman with keratitis sicca, uneventful cataract surgery was complicated by a 3-mm persistent epithelial defect with sterile stromal ulceration. *Middle,* This same patient was managed successfully with cyanoacrylate tissue adhesive and bandage soft contact lens. *Right,* In a similar clinical situation, peripheral ulceration occurred as a reaction to virgin silk suture used for cataract wound closure. Light microscopy reveals giant cell reaction in limbal episcleral tissue. H&E, ×100. *B,* Peripheral ulcerative keratitis associated with rosacea. *Left,* Patient displays subtle but typical skin changes of rosacea with concomitant chronic blepharitis and episodic conjunctivitis and scleritis. *Middle,* In the same patient, use of steriods to suppress conjunctival and scleral inflammation may have facilitated sterile stromal ulceration with perforation evident adjacent to inferior limbus. *Right,* This perforation was easily sealed with tissue adhesive. *C,* Peripheral ulcerative keratitis associated with rheumatoid arthritis. This woman exhibits hand deformities characteristic of rheumatoid arthritis. *Middle,* In the absence of keratitis sicca, multiple areas of rapidly progressive stromal ulceration developed with impending perforation. *Right,* Management of this patient included tissue adhesive and bandage soft contact lens, plus systemic immunosuppression with cyclophosphamide, resulting in preservation of 20/50 vision. *D,* Persistent epithelial defect and sterile stromal ulceration following herpes zoster keratitis. *Left,* Viral keratitis rendered the cornea anesthetic with resultant nonhealing epithelial defect and shallow stromal ulceration threatening the visual axis. *Middle,* Application of tissue adhesive arrested stromal ulceration until reepithelialization was completed. *Right,* Following removal of tissue adhesive, the epithelium remains stable while stromal scar and thinning are compatible with 20/25 vision. *E,* Ocular cicatricial pemphigoid. *Left,* In a patient complaining of chronic blepharoconjunctivitis, the presence of relatively minor conjunctival symblepharon establishes the clinical diagnosis. *Middle,* In a patient with advanced and active pemphigoid, systemic immunosuppressive therapy may be indicated. *Right,* This same patient displays remarkable resolution of inflammatory and ulcerative changes following immunosuppression. (*E, Middle and right,* From Mandel ER, Wagoner MD: Atlas of Clinical Disease. Philadelphia, WB Saunders, 1989.)

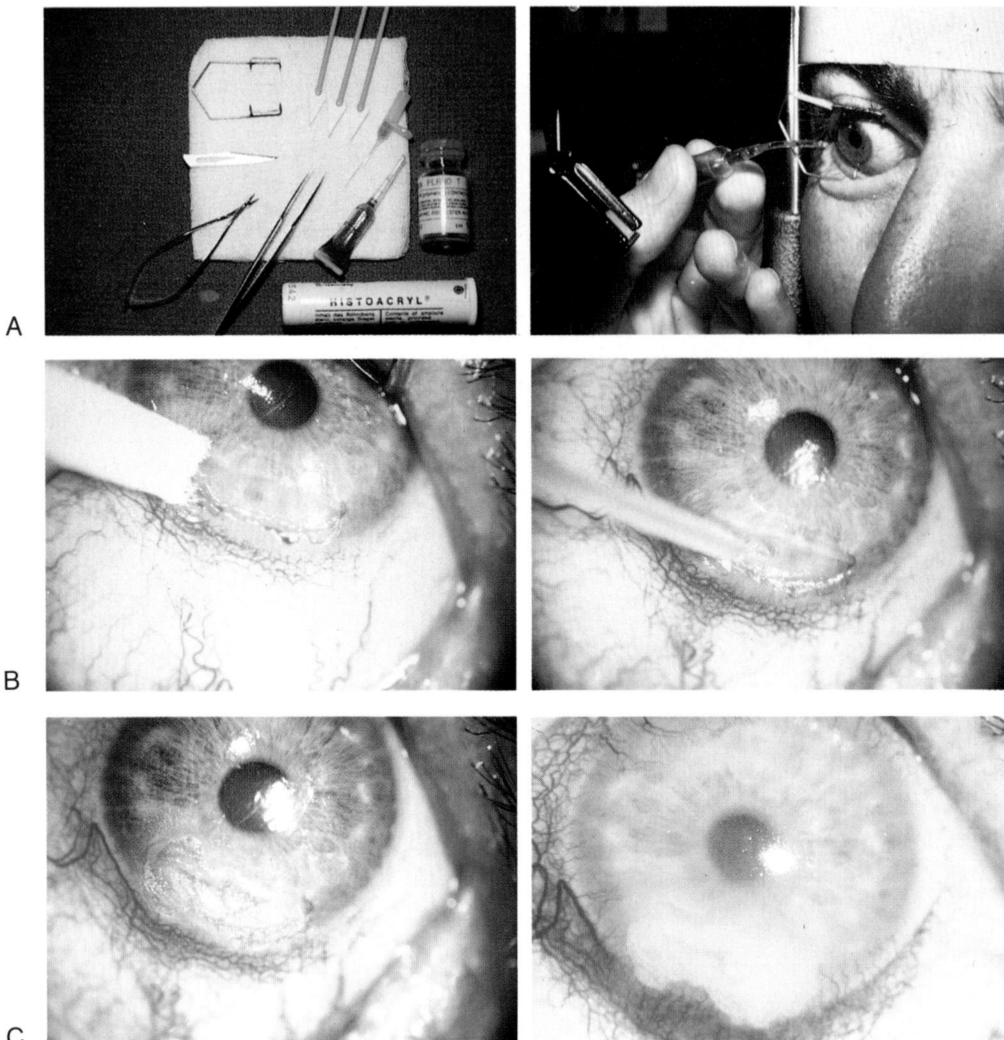

FIGURE 1–128 **Technique of cyanoacrylate tissue adhesive application.** *A, Left,* Materials required include isobutyl cyanoacrylate adhesive (Histoacryl, Braun, Melsungen, Germany) with capillary microapplicator or short, disposable No. 25 needle, wire lid speculum, cellulose sponges, and jeweler's forceps to dry and to débride corneal surface, scalpel blade to open adhesive ampule, and Vannas scissors to trim excessive adhesive before application of bandage soft contact lens. *Right,* The procedure can be performed at the slit lamp if perforation has not occurred or if perforation is minimal and without iris prolapse. *B, Left,* In a patient with peripheral ulcerative keratitis secondary to rheumatoid arthritis, a minute perforation is evident at the base of this 2-mm-by-4-mm sterile ulcer. A dry cellulose sponge is used to débride and to dry the ulcer base. *Right,* Minimal amounts of tissue adhesive are rapidly applied to coat thinly the ulcer base. *C, Left,* After the tissue adhesive has polymerized and a soft contact lens has been applied, the anterior chamber is observed to have spontaneously re-formed. *Right,* Three weeks after adhesive application, the eye remains tectonically stable and neovascularization is progressing to promote healing of the ulcerated stroma.

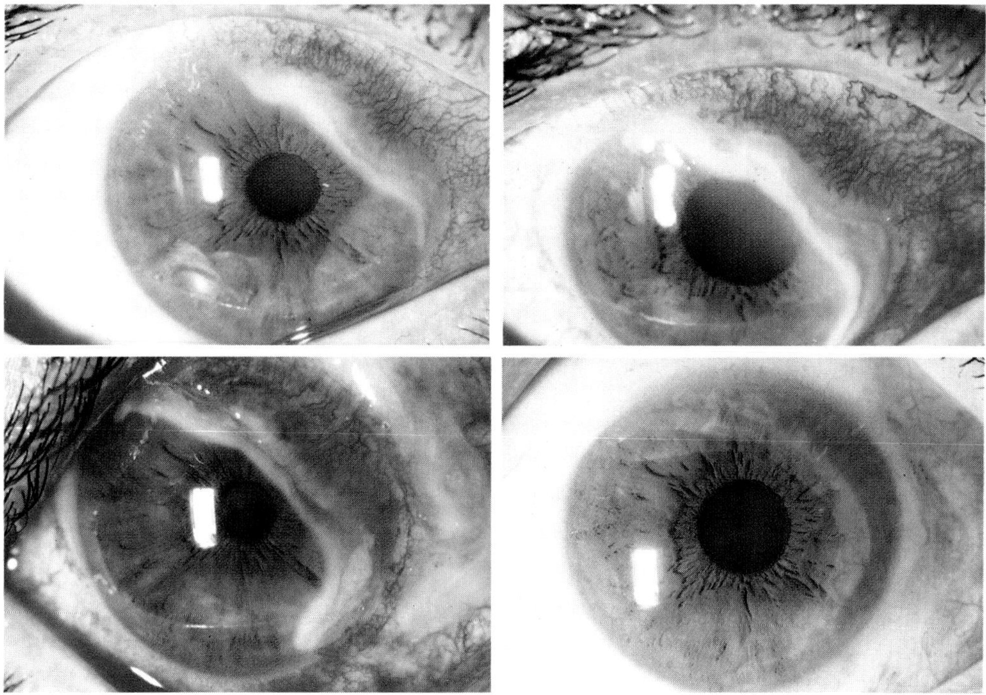

FIGURE 1–129 **Conjunctival resection for peripheral ulcerative keratitis.** *Top left,* In this 55-year-old white man with idiopathic Mooren's ulcer, the typical features of peripheral stromal ulceration followed by neovascularization and intense stromal inflammatory infiltrate at the advancing margin are evident. *Top right,* Within 3 days, despite intensive topical steroid therapy, inflammation, ulceration, and infiltration have markedly worsened. Resection of limbal conjunctiva from the 10 o'clock to the 4 o'clock meridians was performed at this time. *Bottom left,* Within 4 days after conjunctival resection and using only moderate steroid therapy, stromal ulceration has arrested and infiltration has subsided. *Bottom right,* One month later, vision has returned to 20/25, the eye is uninflamed, the corneal epithelium is intact, and the stroma is without infiltrate.

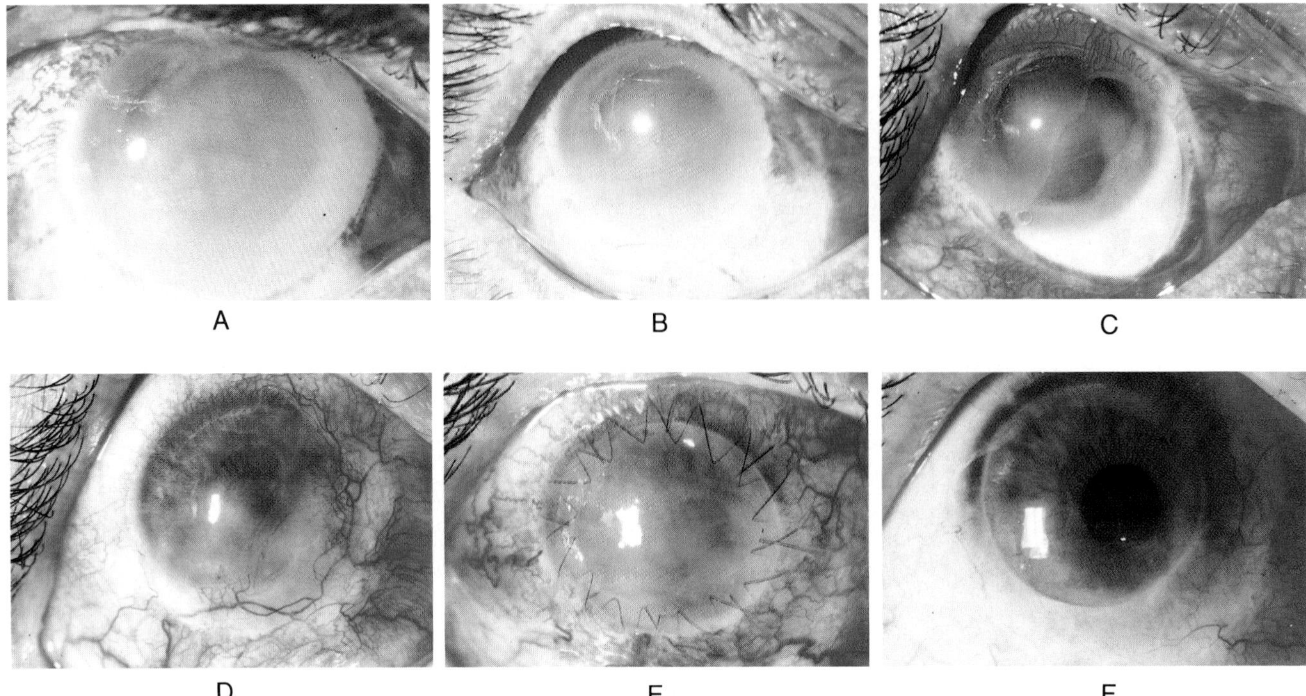

FIGURE 1–130 **Limbal autograft transplantation for persistent epithelial defect and stromal ulceration following chemical burn.** *A,* Severe acute chemical burn causes total destruction of ocular surface epithelium. *B,* One week following injury, an extensive persistent epithelial defect with limbal and scleral ischemia develops. *C,* One month later, despite conventional medical therapy, a nonhealing defect of corneal and conjunctival epithelium with necrosis of the totally ischemic sclera ensues. *D,* Within days after limbal autograft from the less severely burned fellow eye, plus advancement of the adjacent bulbar conjunctiva, the epithelial defects have healed completely. *E,* A deep keratoplasty is performed approximately 8 months later. *F,* Two years after lamellar keratoplasty, visual acuity is 20/60 with intact epithelial surface, clear stroma, and regression of neovascularization. (*A–F,* From Conjunctival and corneal injuries. *In* Shingleton BJ, Hersh PS, Kenyon KR (eds): Eye Trauma. St. Louis, Mosby-Year Book, 1990.)

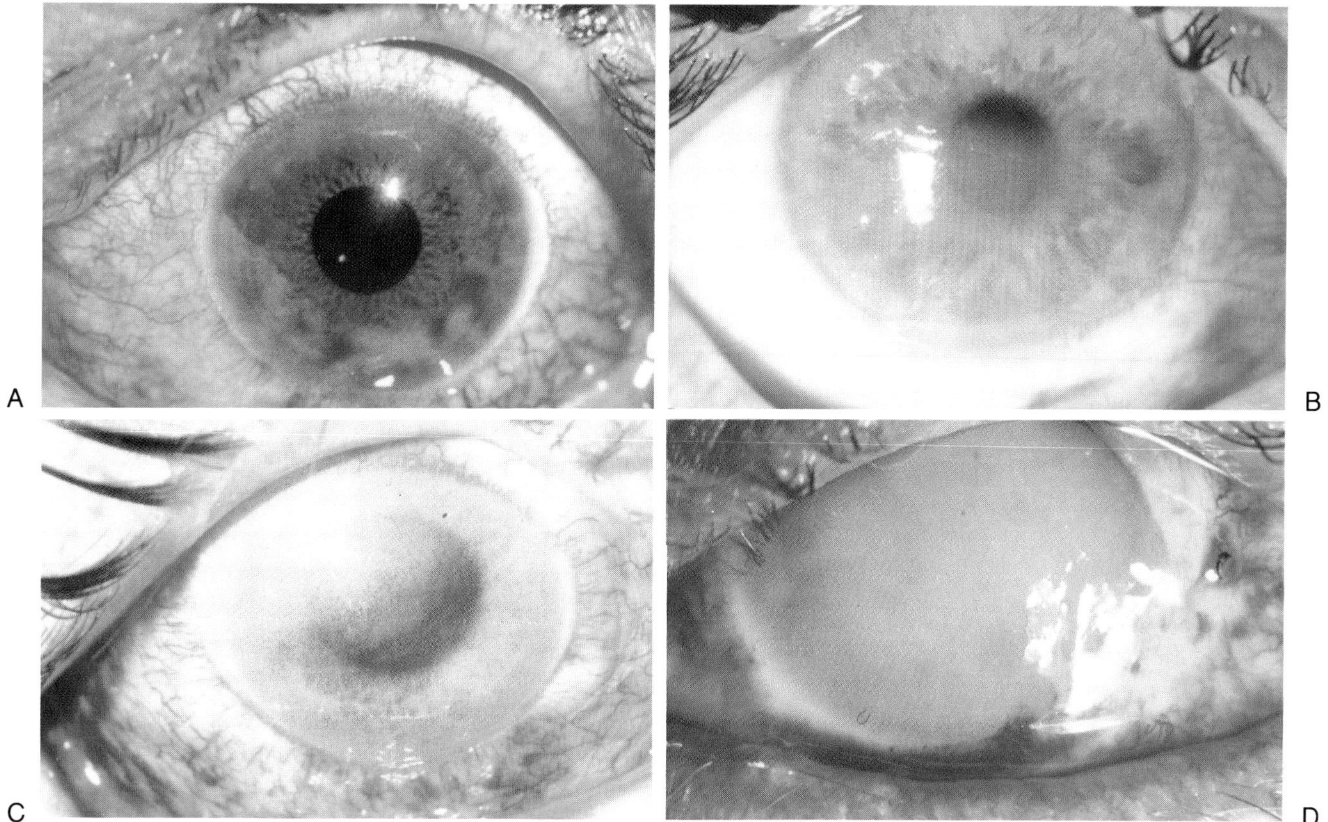

FIGURE 1–131 **Pictorial classification of chemical injury.** *A,* Thoft–stage 1. *B,* Thoft–stage 2. *C,* Thoft–stage 3. *D,* Thoft–stage 4. (*From* Wagoner MD, Kenyon KR: Chemical injuries. *In* Shingleton BJ, Hersh PS, Kenyon KR (eds): Eye Trauma. St. Louis, CV Mosby, 1990.)

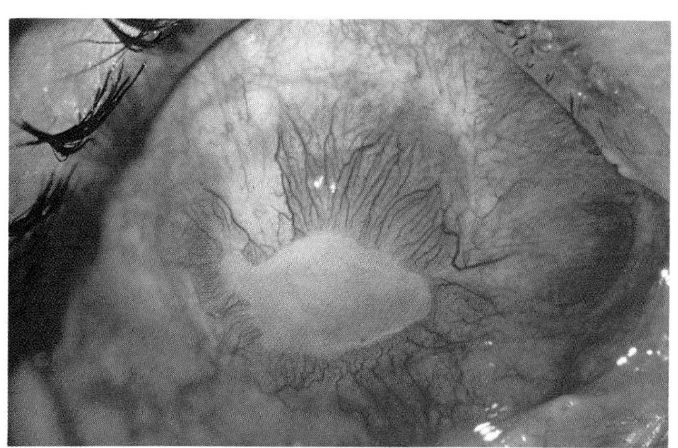

FIGURE 1–132 **Sequelae of failure of reepithelialization in alkali injury.** The peripheral cornea has developed severe vascular pannus, and the central 4-mm zone is undergoing stromal collagenolysis and progressive thinning, with impending perforation.

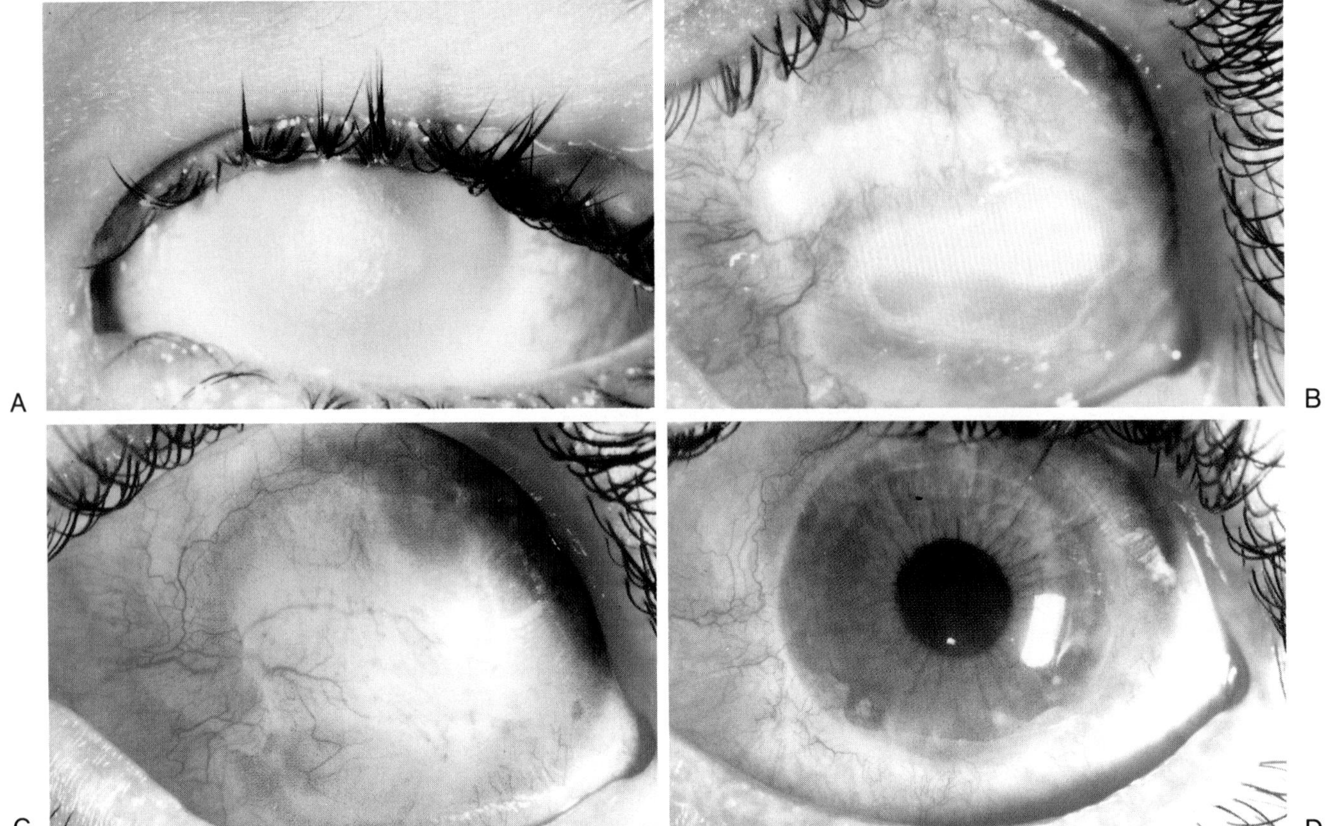

FIGURE 1–133 **Severe alkali injury with visual rehabilitation.** *A,* This 5-year-old boy sustained a severe alkali injury to the left eye with total ocular surface epithelial loss and extensive limbal and scleral ischemia. *B,* Despite maximum medical therapy, including corticosteroids and ascorbate, an extensive epithelial defect persisted. Limbal autograft transplantation was performed 4 weeks postinjury with slow resolution of the epithelial defect. *C,* The ocular surface epithelium is intact and stable 6 months after injury, and stromal neovascularization and edema have subsided, albeit with dense scarring. *D,* A deep lamellar keratoplasty was performed 1 year after injury. Visual acuity is 20/60 2 years later, and the cornea remains stable, uninflamed, and avascular without topical medications or lubricants. (From Wagoner MD, Kenyon KR: Chemical injuries. *In* Shingleton BJ, Hersh PS, Kenyon KR (eds): Eye Trauma. St. Louis, CV Mosby, 1990.)

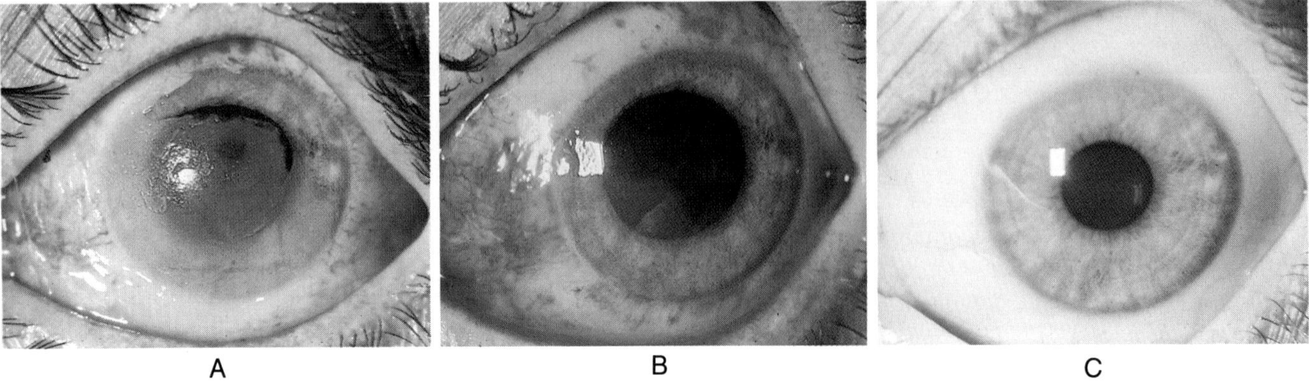

FIGURE 1–134 **Acid injury to ocular surface.** *A,* Epithelial necrosis following a severe acid injury. Only a scimitar-shaped area of epithelium remains superiorly. *B,* Prompt reepithelialization with intense topical corticosteroid use. *C,* One week after injury, epithelial recovery is complete, and inflammation has subsided.

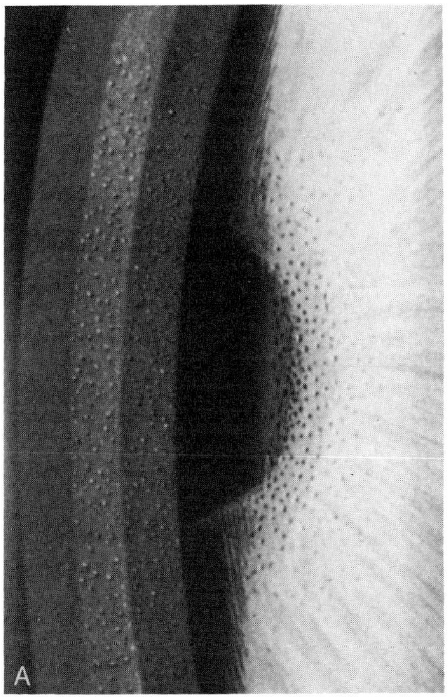

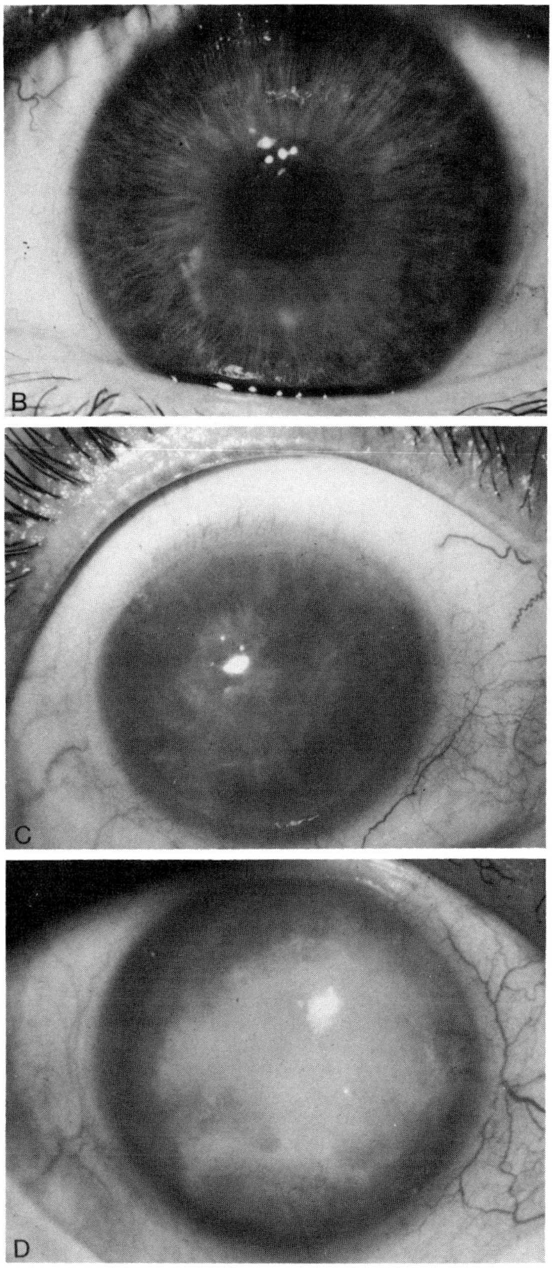

FIGURE 1-135 **Natural history of progressive corneal edema.** *A,* Corneal guttata of Fuchs' dystrophy often begins in young adulthood and progresses slowly over decades. Some edema gradually ensues for a long time without affecting vision. *B,* Epithelial edema begins in middle to late life, first as fine microcysts that early distort the surface and cause reduction of vision. *C,* Frank epithelial edema with visible blebs, opacity, and gross surface irregularities. *D,* End stage of chronic edema after many years of often painful bullous epithelium. A connective tissue pannus has formed between the epithelium and Bowman's layer. At this stage, the cornea is really opaque, but the epithelium has scarred down, and the pain is gone.

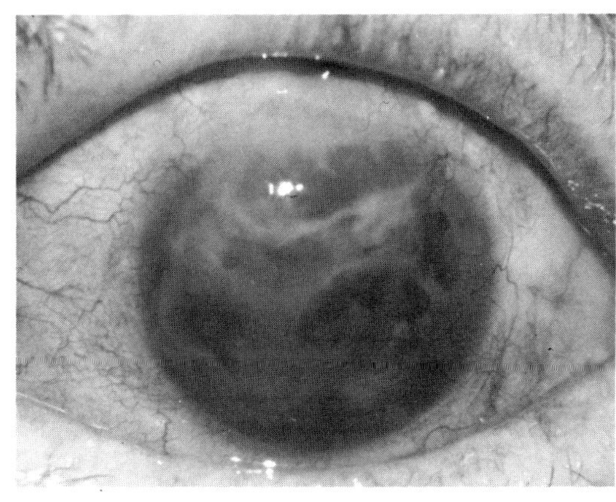

FIGURE 1-136 **Pseudophakic bullous keratopathy.** Mechanical trauma after intraocular lens implantation can damage the endothelial cells with future resultant development of a bullous keratopathy.

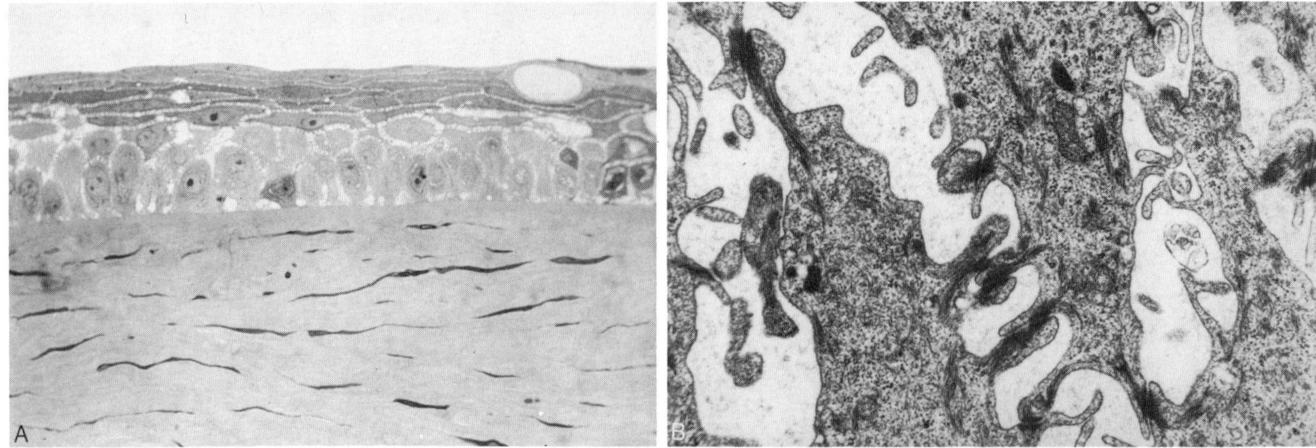

FIGURE 1–137 **Pathology of corneal epithelial edema.** *A,* Edema fluid is pushed into the epithelial cells and between the epithelial cells, resulting in intracellular and intercellular edema. *B,* Electron micrograph depicting intracellular edema. ×2000. (Courtesy of Toichi Kuwabara, M.D.)

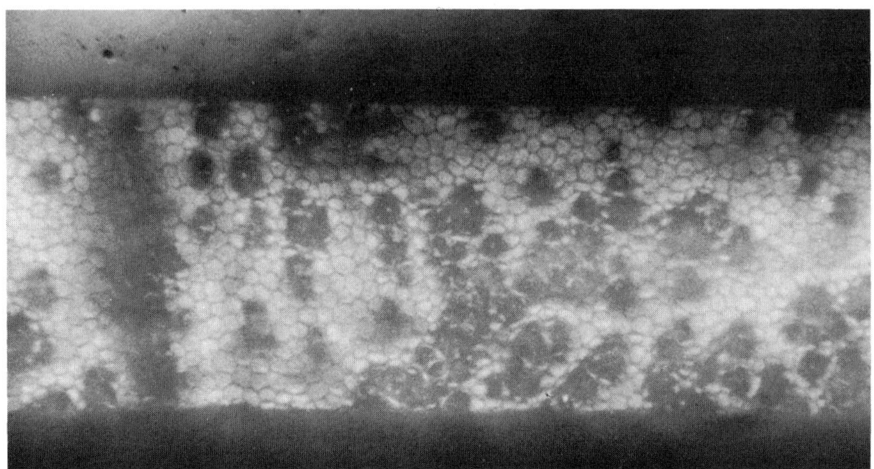

FIGURE 1–138 **Specular microscopy of corneal guttata.** The black dots indicate areas where the endothelium has been lifted posteriorly and out of focus by the excrescences on Descemet's membrane. Pathologically, these are areas of guttata formation.

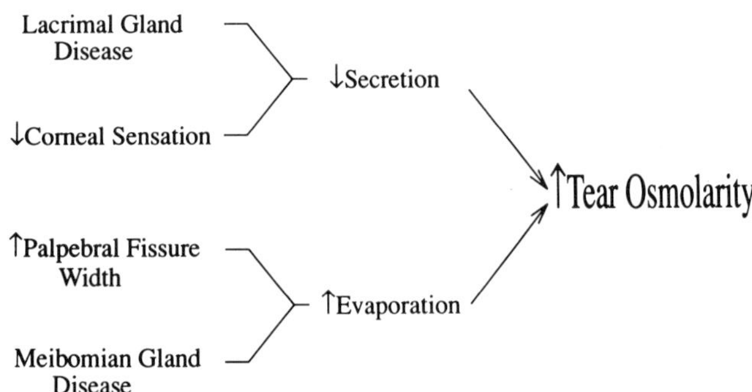

FIGURE 1–139 **Osmolarity.** Mechanisms for elevated tear film osmolarity. Conditions that increase osmolarity result in the surface disease of keratoconjunctivitis sicca.

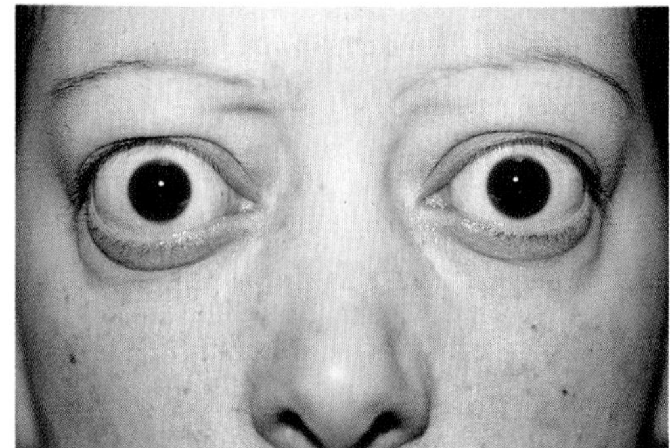

FIGURE 1–140 **Tear evaporation.** Increased surface area for evaporation is evident in this patient with thyroid eye disease. In such patients, it has been possible to correlate increased palpebral fissure with both elevated tear film osmolarity and ocular surface disease evidenced by rose bengal staining.

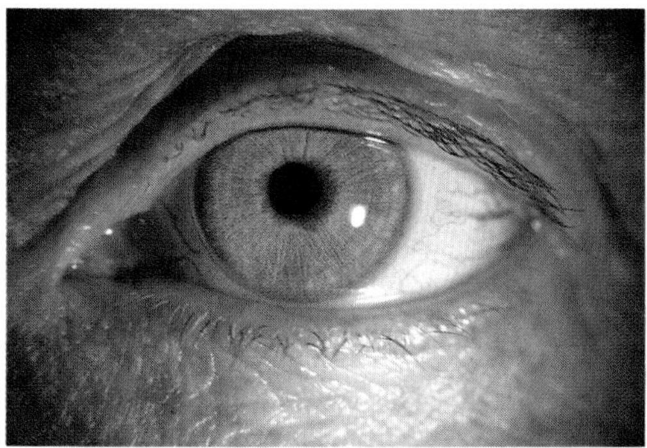

FIGURE 1–141 A patient with early keratoconjunctivitis sicca. The tear film appears normal before the instillation of dyes. The diagnosis of keratoconjunctivitis sicca was based on a sandy, gritty irritation that was worse toward the end of the day, rose bengal staining of the nasal bulbar conjunctiva within the exposure zone, and an elevated tear film osmolarity.

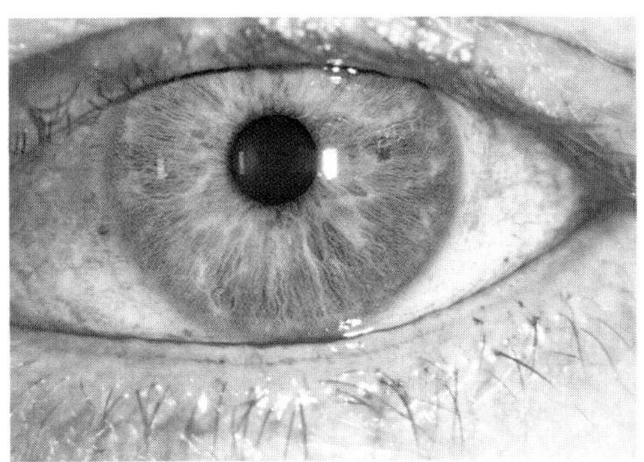

FIGURE 1–142 Rose bengal staining typical for moderate keratoconjunctivitis sicca. The conjunctiva stains more than the cornea, and the nasal conjunctiva stains more than the temporal conjunctiva.

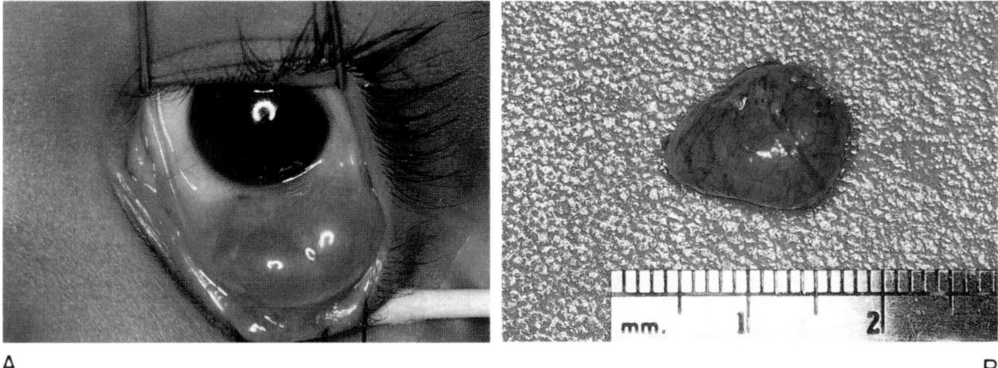

A B

FIGURE 1–143 **Dermoid of the conjunctiva.** *A,* Dermoid of the conjunctiva arising from the inferior fornix and protruding through the palpebral fissure. Characteristically these lesions tend to occur more temporally on the bulbar conjunctiva at the limbus. *B,* Macroscopic appearance of the lesion after excision.

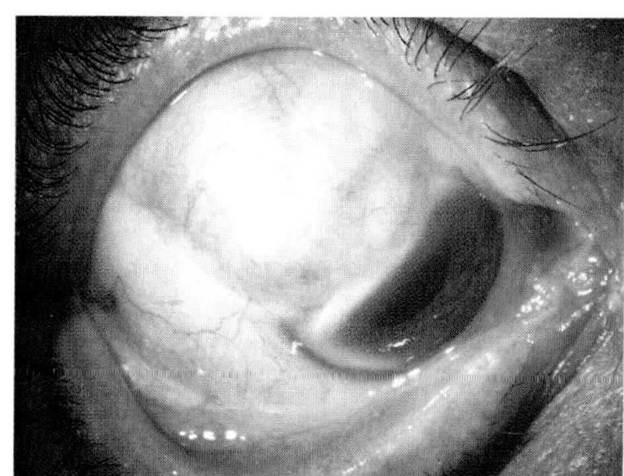

FIGURE 1–144 **Dermolipoma of the conjunctiva.** The lesion tends to arise from the superotemporal conjunctiva. The yellowish appearance is secondary to increased sebaceous material within the lesion, which distinguishes them histopathologically from dermoids. Often, fine hairs protrude from the surface; however, they are usually asymptomatic.

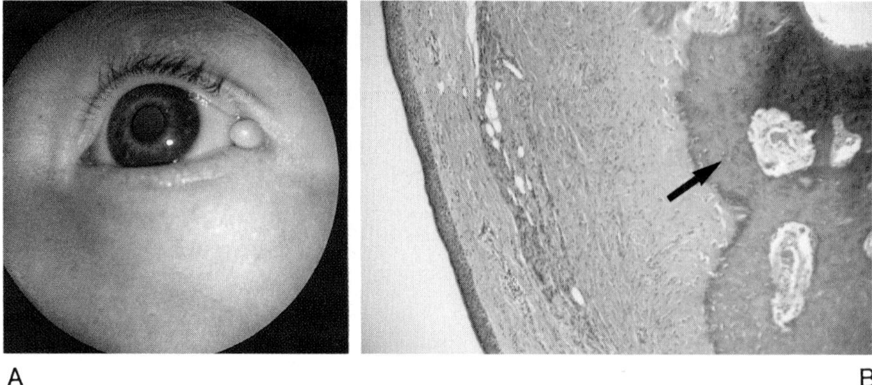

FIGURE 1–145 **Epibulbar osseous choristoma.** *A,* This osseous choristoma in a 1-year-old girl presented as a well-demarcated lesion on the lateral bulbar conjunctiva away from the cornea. This large lesion required surgical excision. *B,* A histologic section of the lesion shows mature compact bone *(arrow)* surrounded by dense connective tissue in pilosebaceous units. H&E, ×40.

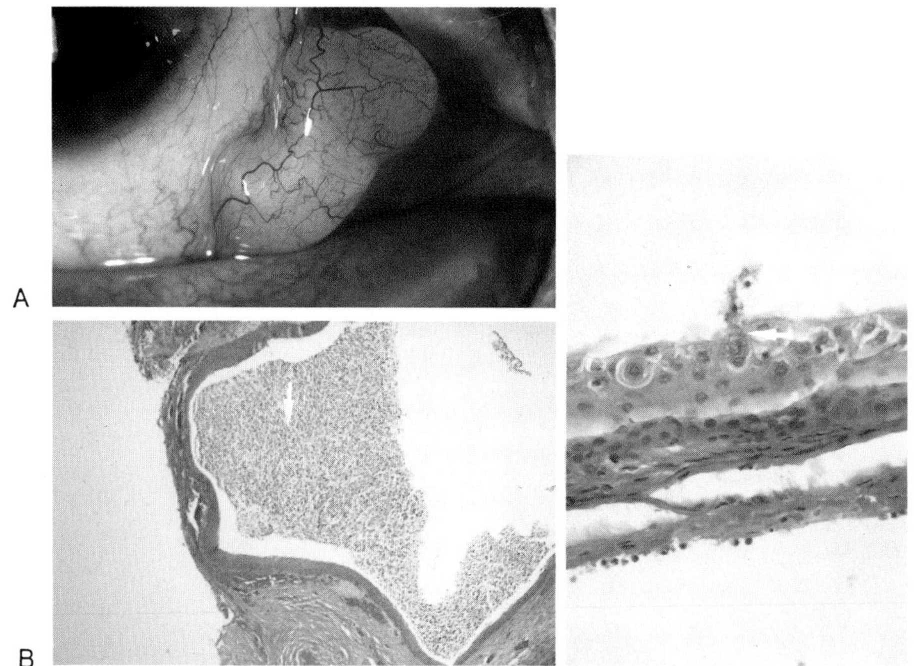

FIGURE 1–146 **Conjunctival inclusion cyst.** *A,* The lesion is usually well circumscribed and contains translucent fluid. Fine conjunctival vessels can be seen traversing the surface of the lesion. *B,* Histologic section of an inclusion cyst. The multiple layers of nonkeratinized epithelium forming the cyst wall distinguish the lesion from a ductal cyst, which is lined by a double layer of cuboidal epithelium. H&E, ×40. *C,* A high-power micrograph of the cyst walls showing a goblet cell discharging mucin into the lumen of the cyst. H&E, ×100.

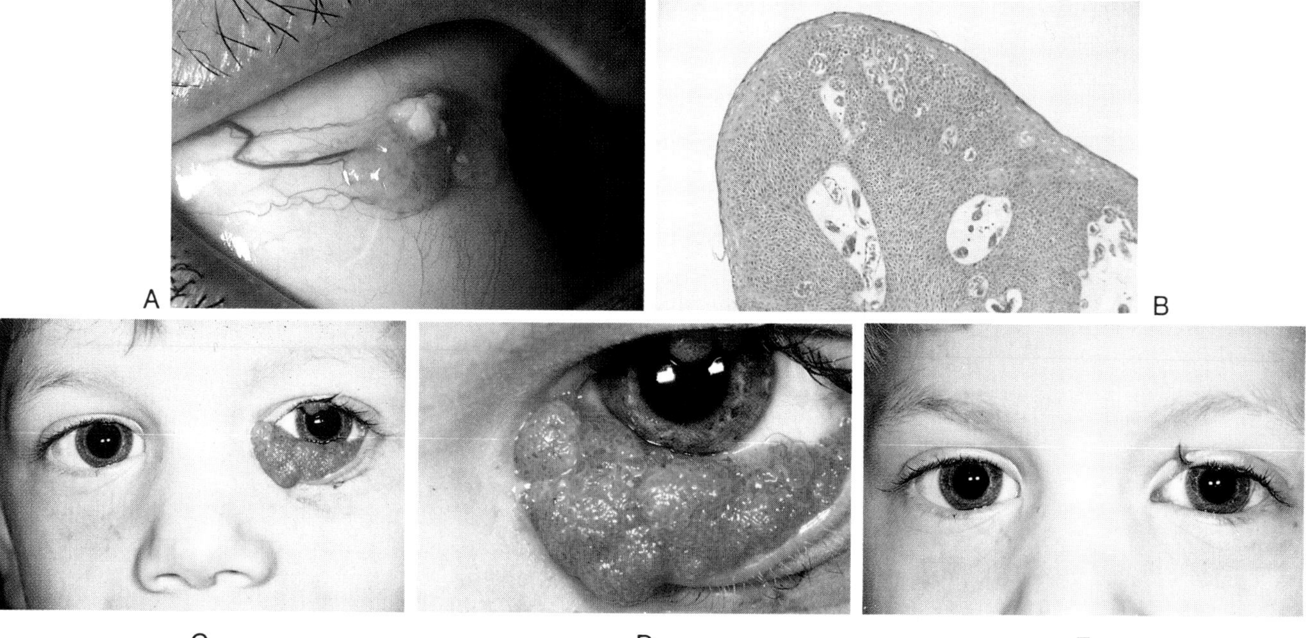

FIGURE 1-147 **Conjunctival papilloma.** *A,* Sessile papilloma of the conjunctiva. These are typically located 1 to 2 mm from the limbus as opposed to the juxtalimbal position of conjunctival intraepithelial neoplasia. The geometrically arranged red dots on the surface of the lesion are pathognomonic for papilloma and are secondary to central vasculature surrounded by thickened epithelium. Keratinization of the surface may be seen in both nondysplastic and dysplastic forms of this lesion. (Courtesy of Dr. A. Kaufman and Dr. Richard Darrell, New York, New York.) *B,* Microscopic appearance of a benign conjunctival papilloma sectioned transversely. Note the multiple well-vascularized lumens surrounded by acanthotic epithelium. The overlying epithelium contains normal polarity and has a low nucleus : cytoplasm ratio. H&E, ×40. *C,* An exuberant example of recurrence of conjunctival papillomas in a 4-year-old boy 1 month postexcision of the original lesion at its base. Note the multifocal growth pattern of this lesion. *D,* A closer view of the lesion from *B,* showing the geometrically arranged red dots present throughout the lesion. *E,* The appearance of the child following repeat excision and carbon dioxide laser treatment on the lesions. (*C–E,* Courtesy of James R. Patrinely, Houston, TX.)

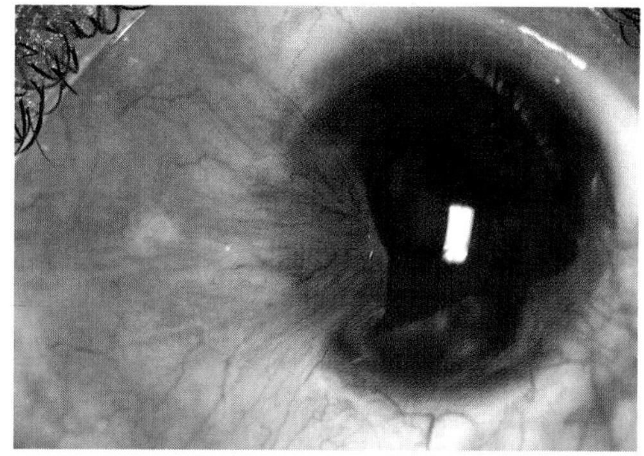

FIGURE 1-148 **Pterygium.** Typically these arise on the nasal bulbar conjunctiva and assume a triangular configuration with a base toward the nose. Growth occurs from the apex of the lesion toward the visual axis.

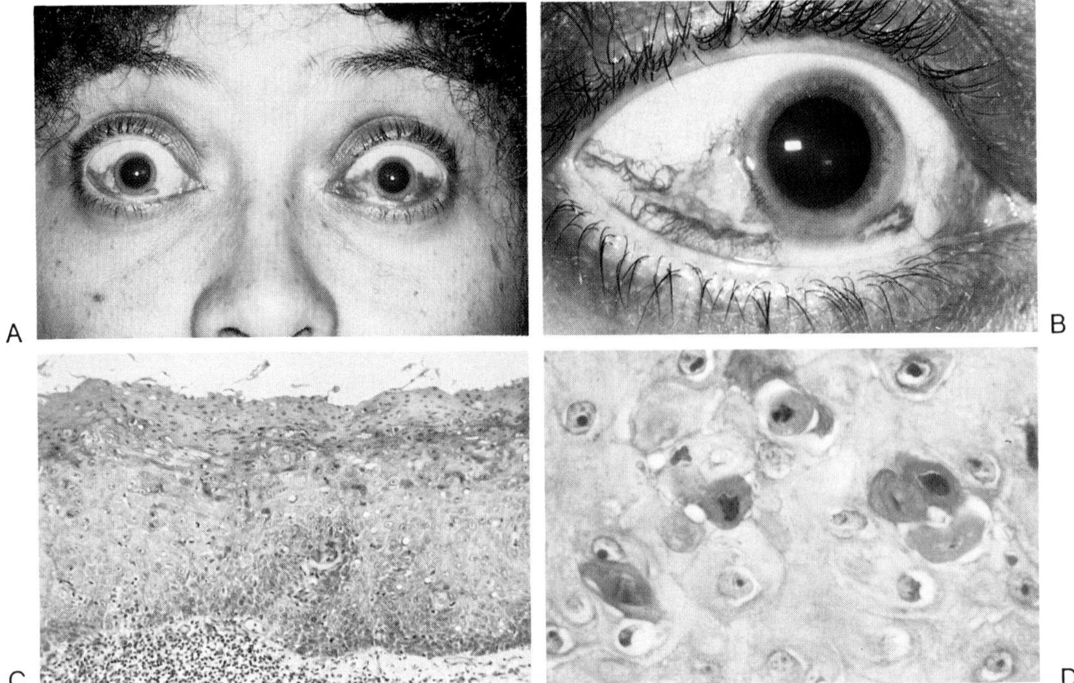

FIGURE 1-149 **Benign hereditary intraepithelial dyskeratosis.** *A,* Bilateral dilation of the conjunctival blood vessels associated with benign hereditary intraepithelial dyskeratosis. *B,* Closer view of the right eye showing white perilimbal plaque with adjacent hyperemia of the conjunctiva. *C,* Photomicrograph of the lesion demonstrating marked acanthosis, dyskeratosis, and parakeratosis of the conjunctival epithelium and an underlying inflammatory response in the substantia propria. H&E, ×25. *D,* Higher-power view demonstrating dyskeratotic cells typical of this condition. H&E, ×250. (*A–D,* From Shields CL, Shields JA, Eagle RA: Hereditary benign intraepithelial dyskeratosis. [Photo essay] Arch Ophthalmol 105:422–423, 1987. Copyright 1987, American Medical Association.)

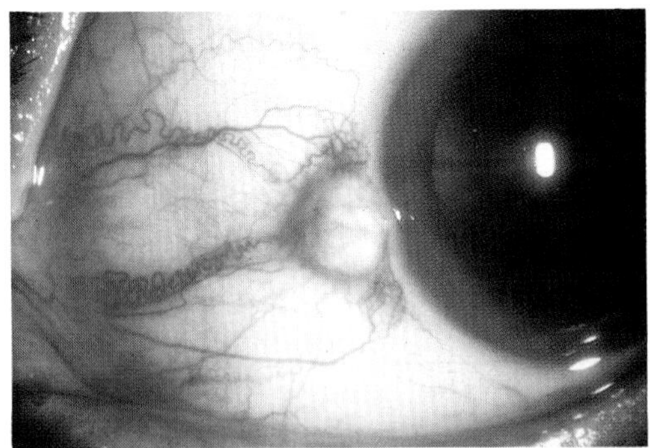

FIGURE 1-150 **Pseudoepitheliomatous hyperplasia of the conjunctiva.** Characteristically this lesion can be difficult to distinguish clinically from conjunctival intraepithelial neoplasia. The history of rapid onset points toward the diagnosis of pseudoepitheliomatous hyperplasia. Note the white component of the lesion, which corresponds to the presence of keratin.

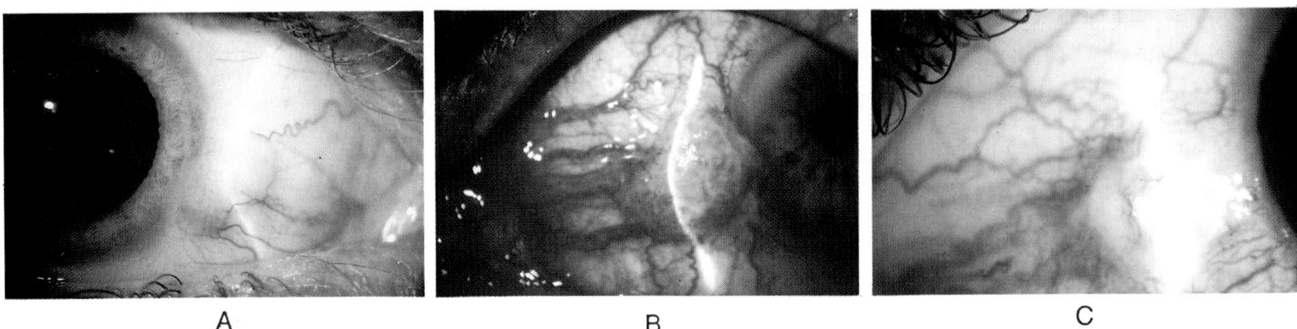

FIGURE 1-151 **Conjunctival intraepithelial neoplasia (CIN).** *A,* Typical gelatinous appearance of a mass arising at the limbus. *B,* This lesion typifies a papillomatous variety of this entity. The juxtalimbal location is more characteristic of CIN than of benign sessile papilloma, which tends to occur a few millimeters from the limbus. *C,* This photo of CIN displays the presence of keratin. This is also known as leukoplakia.

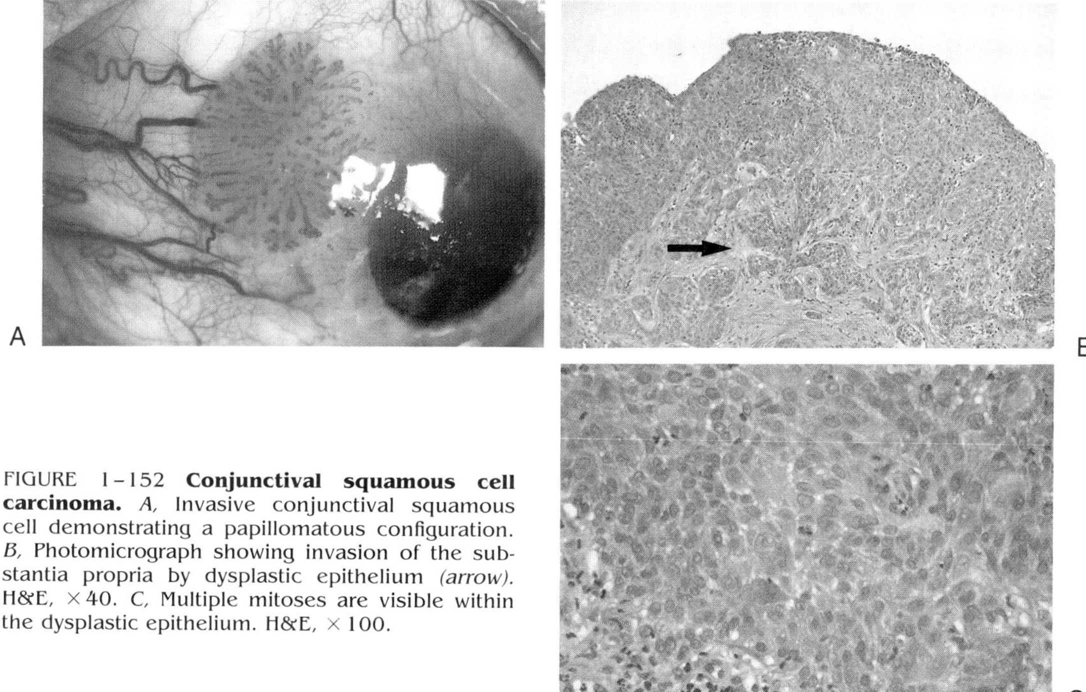

FIGURE 1-152 **Conjunctival squamous cell carcinoma.** *A,* Invasive conjunctival squamous cell demonstrating a papillomatous configuration. *B,* Photomicrograph showing invasion of the substantia propria by dysplastic epithelium *(arrow).* H&E, ×40. *C,* Multiple mitoses are visible within the dysplastic epithelium. H&E, × 100.

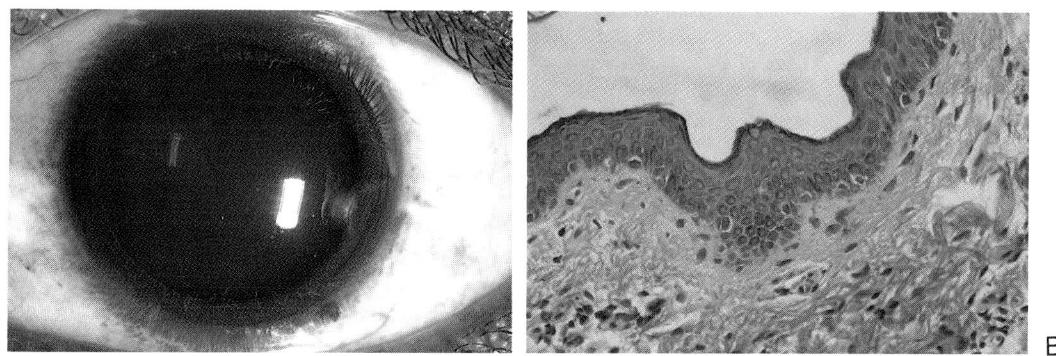

FIGURE 1-153 **Benign racial melanosis.** *A,* Circumlimbal distribution of golden brown pigmentation typically fades toward the fornices. This condition is seen primarily in darkly pigmented individuals and is bilateral. *B,* Histologic section of conjunctiva shows increased pigmentation of the basal and epithelium without proliferation in the number of melanocytes, consistent with benign racial melanosis.

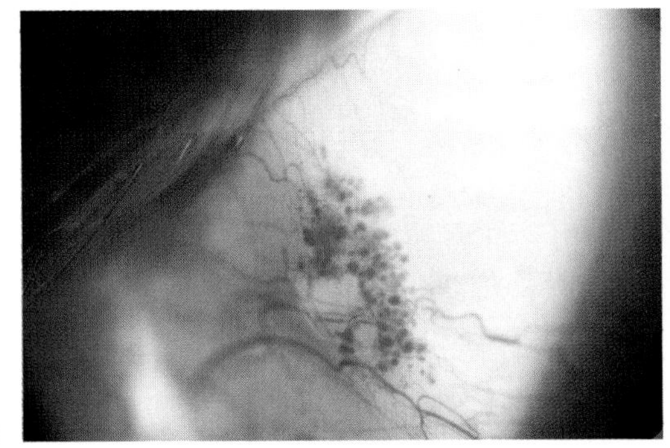

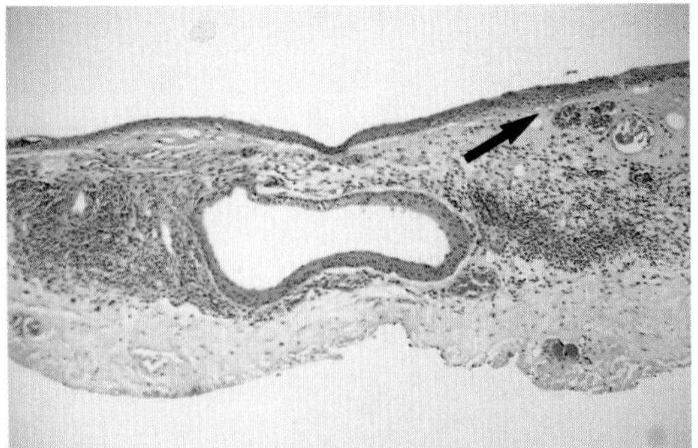

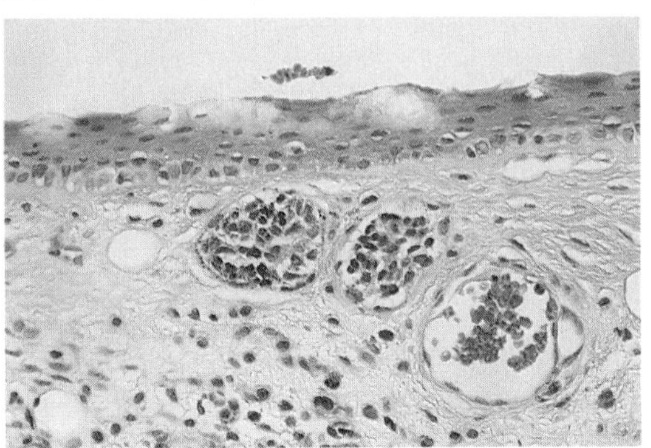

FIGURE 1-154 **Benign conjunctival nevus.** *A,* The presence of an epithelial cyst within the lesion is suggestive of a benign conjunctival nevus. These lesions are typically elevated. *B,* Microscopic picture of a conjunctival nevus showing a characteristic epithelial inclusion cyst. Also note the nesting pattern of the nevus cell *(arrow),* another feature that suggests a benign process. H&E, ×40. *C,* Higher-power view of the "nest" of nevus cells within the substantia propria. H&E, ×100.

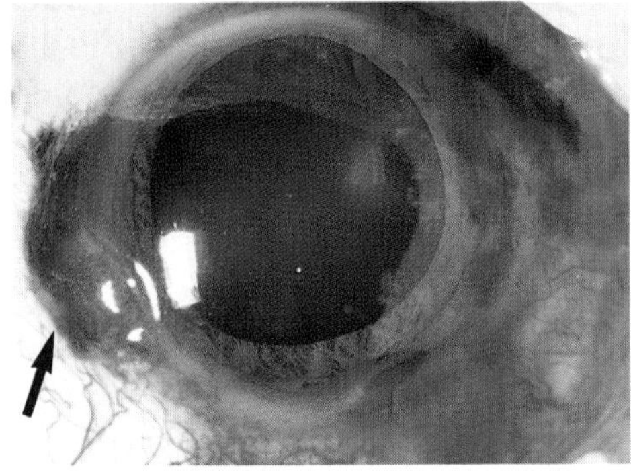

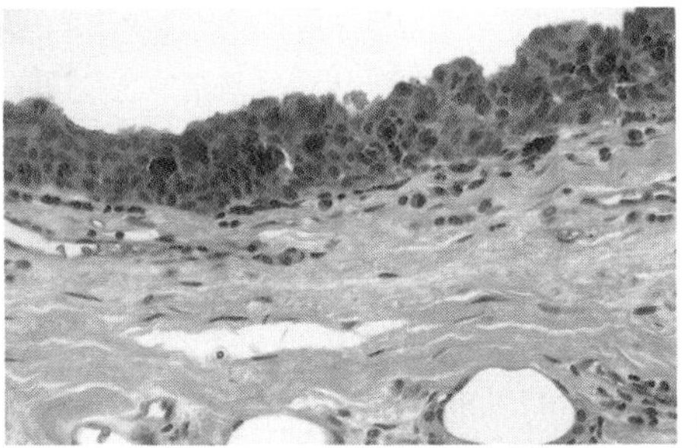

FIGURE 1-155 **Primary acquired melanosis (PAM).** *A,* PAM in a 50-year-old woman demonstrating extensive brown pigmentation of the bulbar conjunctiva and lid margins of the right eye. PAM is flat and overwhelmingly unilateral. (*A,* Courtesy of Frederick A. Jakobiec, Massachusetts Eye and Ear Infirmary, Boston, Massachusetts.) *B,* Histologic section of conjunctiva showing atypical melanocytes percolating throughout the epithelium with microinvasion of the underlying substantia propria. These features are consistent with the histologic diagnosis of PAM with atypia.

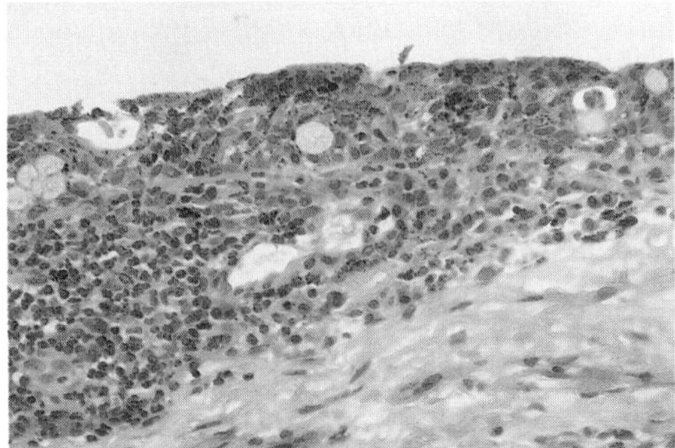

FIGURE 1-156 **Conjunctival malignant melanoma.** *A,* A nodule of malignant melanoma *(arrow)* of the conjunctiva arising in a patient with preexisting PAM. The incidence of eventual development of malignant melanoma from preexisting PAM with atypia approaches 90%. (Courtesy of Frederick A. Jakobiec, Massachusetts Eye and Ear Infirmary, Boston, Massachusetts.) *B,* Photomicrograph of malignant melanoma of the conjunctiva showing invasion of anaplastic cells into the underlying substantia propria. Note that the epithelium as well has full-thickness involvement with the melanoma process. H&E, ×100.

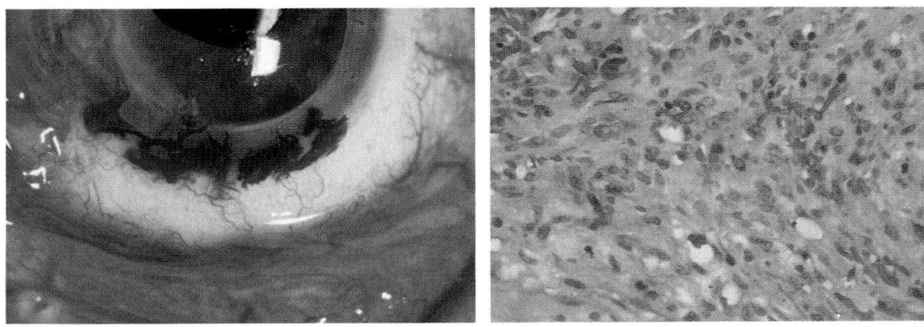

FIGURE 1–157 **Kaposi's sarcoma of the conjunctiva.** *A,* This conjunctival tumor shows invasion of adjacent cornea as well. This pathognomonic presentation is of a reddish vascular conjunctival lesion that may be diffuse or nodular in character. (Courtesy of Frederick A. Jakobiec and C. Stephen Foster, Massachusetts Eye and Ear Infirmary, Boston, Massachusetts.) *B,* Microscopic section showing plump endothelial cells with extravasation of red blood cells. × 100.

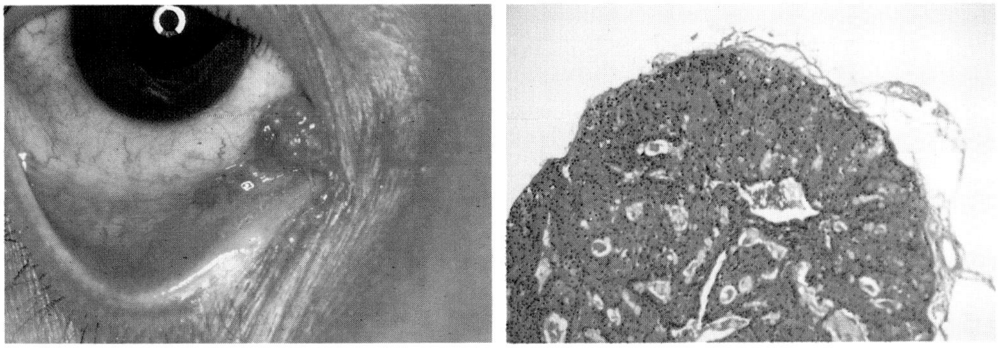

FIGURE 1–158 **Oncocytoma of the caruncle.** *A,* Typically this lesion arises in the caruncle; however, it may occur in the lacrimal gland, the conjunctiva, or the eyelid. Clinically, it appears as a small cystic mass and is characteristically yellow to red to tan in color. *B,* Histologic section shows eosinophilic tumor cells with a tendency toward lumen formation. H&E, ×40. *C,* Increased magnification shows eosinophilic granular cytoplasm *(arrow)* of the tumor cells that arise from ductal epithelium. Electron microscopy has shown these cells to be filled with abnormal mitochondria that contain fragmented cristae. H&E, × 100.

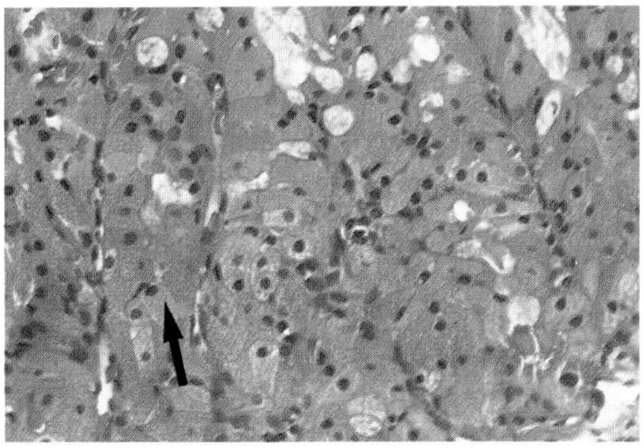

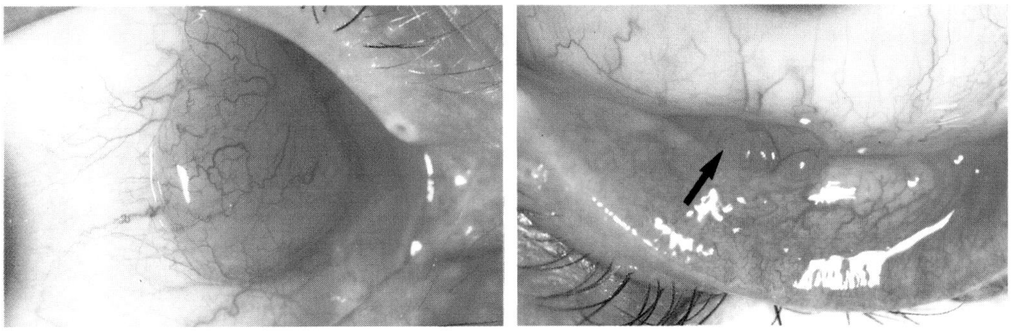

FIGURE 1–159 **Conjunctival lymphoma.** Bilateral conjunctival lymphoma arising superonasally in the right eye *(A)* and on the inferior tarsal conjunctiva *(arrow)* of the left eye *(B).* These lesions are typically a salmon-patch color and configuration. In this case, imaging failed to demonstrate orbital involvement, and systemic work-up was negative. Although a bilateral presentation is less common, it is not associated with a worse prognosis. The most accurate means of making this diagnosis and predicting the eventual clinical outcome is through a study of the cytomorphologic features of the lesion.

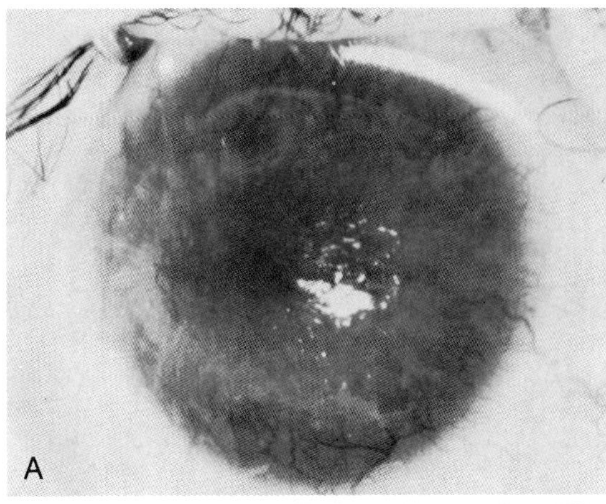

FIGURE 1-160 **Corneal changes in tyrosinemia, type II.** *A,* The left eye shows peripheral neovascularization, marked irregularity of the epithelium, patchy opacities, and loss of corneal transparency. *B,* The right eye shows even more extensive involvement. *C,* After 6 weeks of therapy, there is marked clearing of the lesions. (From Goldsmith LA: Cutaneous changes in errors of amino acid metabolism: Tyrosinemia, phenylketonuria, and argininosuccinic aciduria. *In* Fitzpatrick TB, Aisen AZ, Wolff K, et al (eds): Dermatology in General Medicine, 3rd ed. New York, McGraw-Hill, 1987, p. 1636. Copyright 1987 by McGraw-Hill, Inc. Used by permission of McGraw-Hill Book Company.)

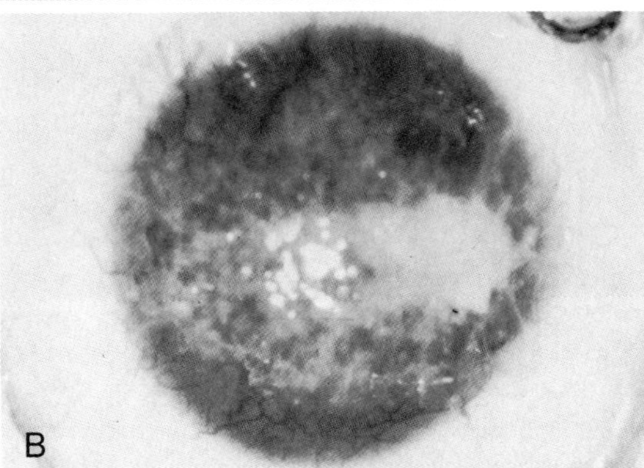

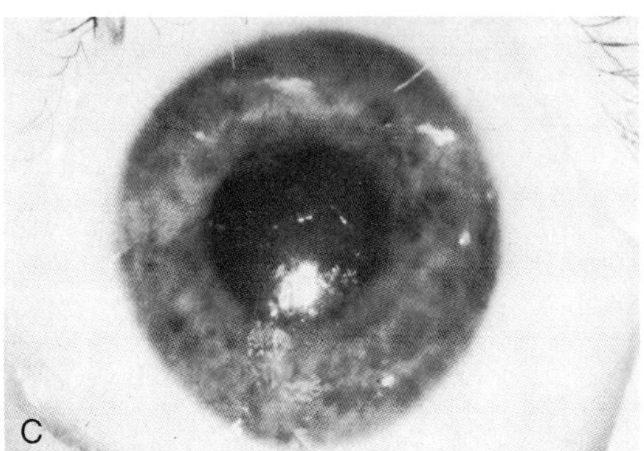

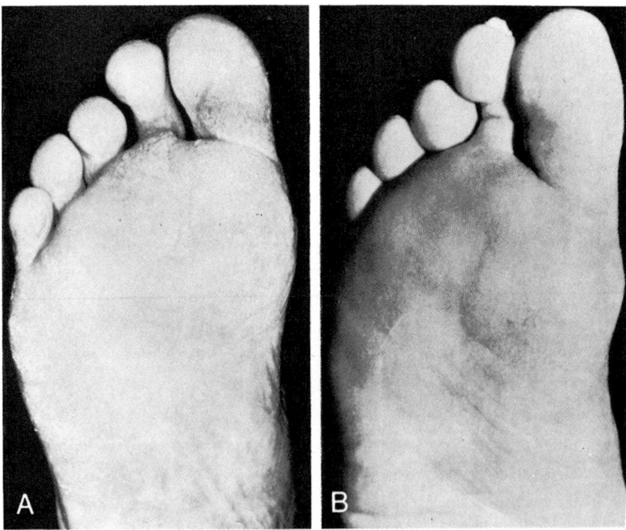

FIGURE 1-161 **Cutaneous changes in tyrosinemia.** *A,* Diffuse plantar hyperkeratosis in an adult with tyrosinemia. *B,* The hyperkeratosis cleared on a low-tyrosine, low-phenylalanine diet without topical treatment. (*A* and *B,* From Goldsmith LA: Cutaneous changes in errors of amino acid metabolism: Tyrosinemia, phenylketonuria, and argininosuccinic aciduria. *In* Fitzpatrick TB, Aisen AZ, Wolff K, et al (eds): Dermatology in General Medicine, 3rd ed. New York, McGraw-Hill, 1987, p. 1639. Copyright 1987 by McGraw-Hill, Inc. Used by permission of McGraw-Hill Book Company.)

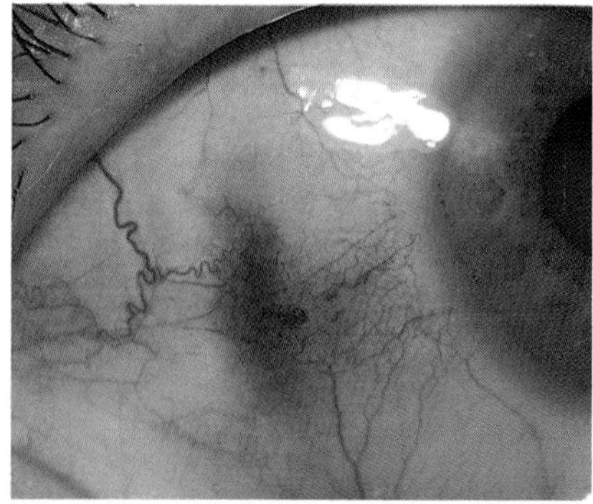

FIGURE 1-162 **Alkaptonuria.** Yellow-brown pigmentation in the paralimbal sclera with a predilection of deposition anterior to the insertion of the horizontal muscle tendons is characteristic. Over time the pigment deposition increases and takes on a darker, bluish black appearance that may be mistaken for melanoma. (From Donaldson DD: Atlas of External Diseases of the Eye, 2nd ed, vol. 3, Cornea and Sclera. St. Louis, CV Mosby, 1980, p. 65.)

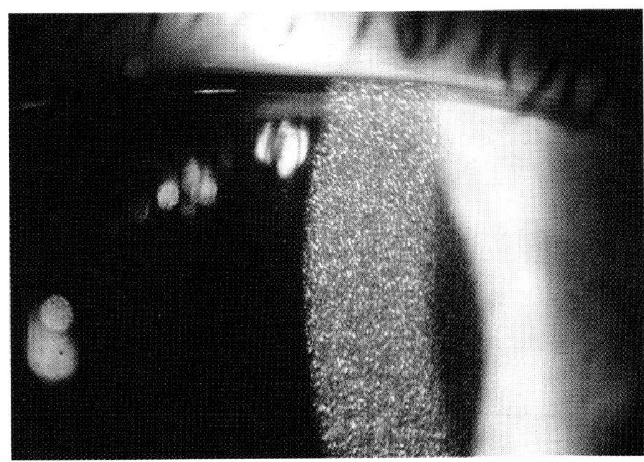

FIGURE 1-163 **Cystinosis.** Fine, needle-shaped refractile crystals can be seen within the corneal stroma. All forms of cystinosis show corneal changes. (From Mandel ER, Wagoner MD: Atlas of Corneal Disease. Philadelphia, WB Saunders, 1989, p. 47.)

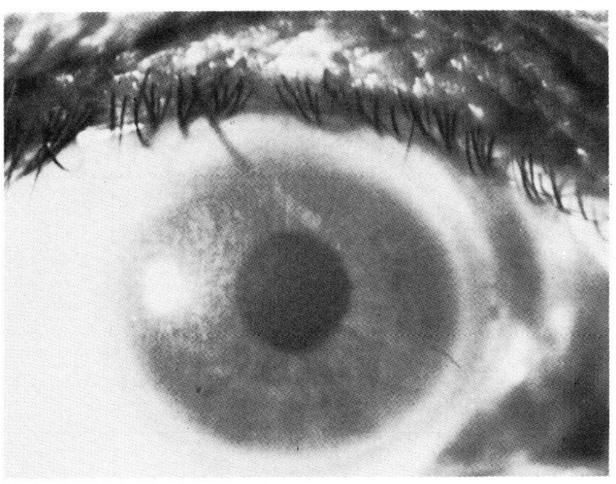

FIGURE 1-164 **Lecithin-cholesterol acyltransferase deficiency.** Dense peripheral arcus and diffuse stromal haze are present. Vision is relatively unaffected. Anterior and posterior crocodile shagreen is present in the midcorneal periphery. (From Puledo JS, Judisch GF, Vrabec NP: Hypolipoproteinemias. *In* Gold DH, Weingeist TA (eds): The Eye in Systemic Disease. Philadelphia, JB Lippincott, 1990, p. 337.)

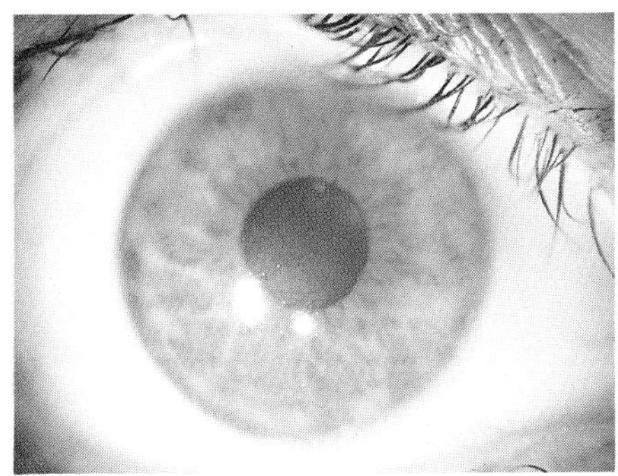

A

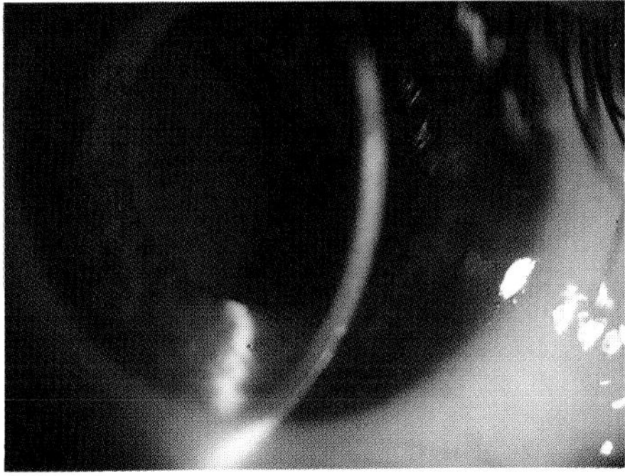

B

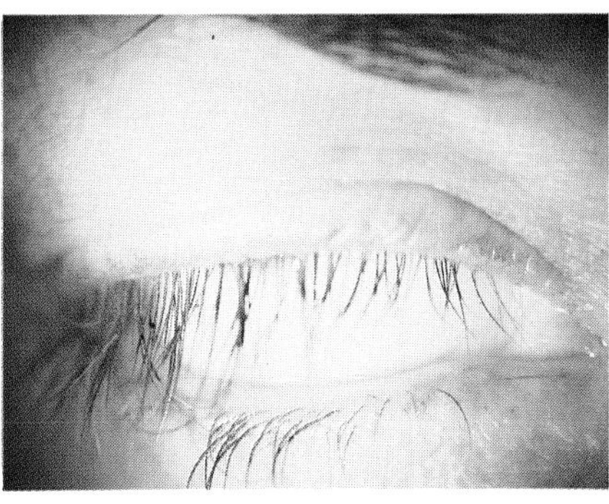

C

FIGURE 1-165 **Tangier disease.** *A,* The right eye of a 52-year-old woman shows subtle powdery stromal clouding. Vision is 20/15. The corneal clouding is subtle in the patient and must be astutely looked for despite the fact that she has had neuropathy for more than 20 years. *B,* The slit-beam photograph shows mild fluorescein staining of the epithelium of the junction of the mid and lower thirds of the cornea. *C,* Her major ocular problems are due to lagophthalmos from facial nerve palsy.

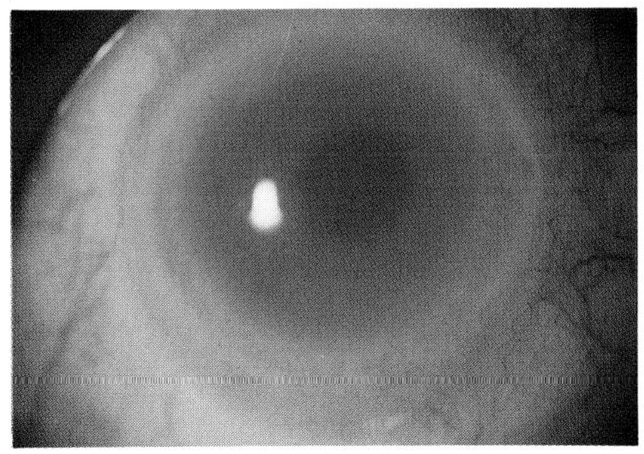

FIGURE 1-166 **Fish eye disease.** The cornea shows diffuse clouding with moderate reduction in vision owing to stromal opacification. There is denser, yellow-gray peripheral opacification. (Courtesy of Harry Koster, M.D., and Yves Pouliquen, M.D.)

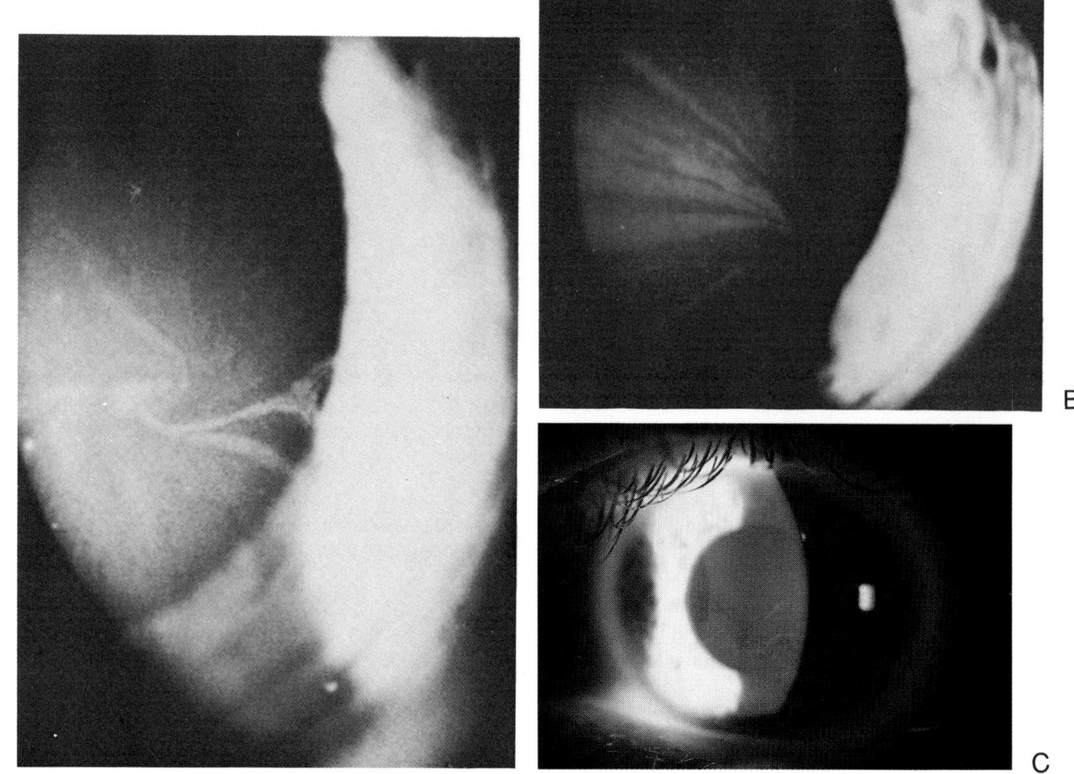

FIGURE 1-167 **Fabry's disease.** *A,* Subepithelial whorl pattern of corneal opacities in a man with Fabry's disease. *B,* Corneal involvement in his sister. (*A* and *B,* From Miller CA, Krachmer JH: Corneal Diseases. *In* Rene WA (ed): Goldberg's Genetic and Metabolic Eye Disease. Boston, Little, Brown, 1986, p. 350; reprinted with permission.) *C,* Fine whorls may give the appearance of force lines in a magnetic field. Similar corneal opacities may be seen in patients receiving chloroquine, amiodarone, and indomethacin.

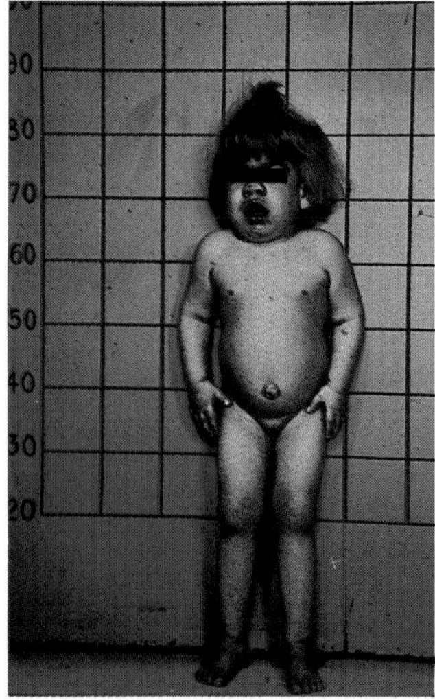

FIGURE 1-168 **Hurler's syndrome, mucopolysaccharoidosis (MPS) I-H.** Short stature and facial dysmorphism are characteristic of patients with MPS I-H. Facial features are coarse, the nares are anteverted, and the eyebrows are heavy and close, with wideset eyes. The abdomen is protuberant with an umbilical hernia. (Courtesy of Trexler M. Topping, M.D.)

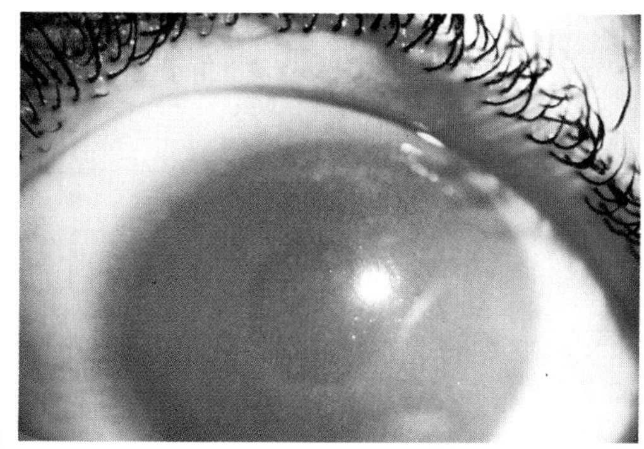
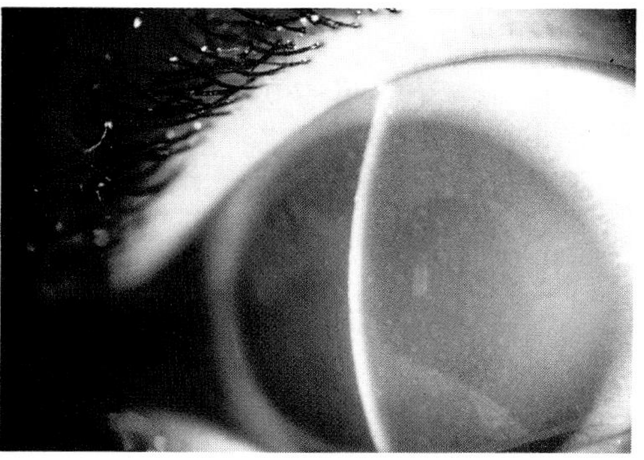

FIGURE 1–169 **Hurler's syndrome, MPS I-H.** Corneal clouding increases over time with punctate opacification of the stroma *(A)*, which can best be seen by slit-beam examination at the slit lamp *(B)*. (*A* and *B*, Courtesy of Roberto Pineda, M.D.)

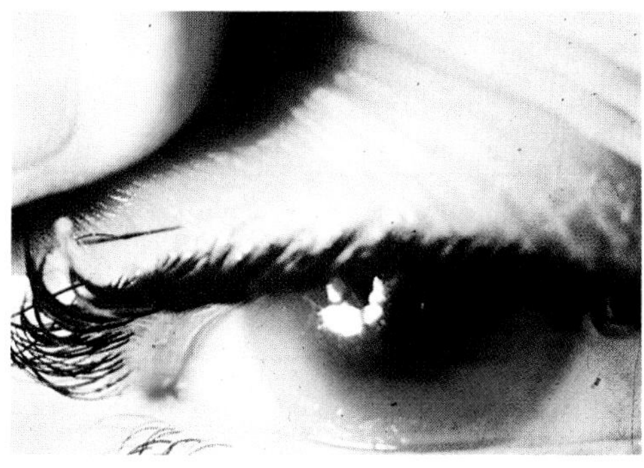

FIGURE 1–170 **Scheie's syndrome, MPS I-S.** Corneal clouding is fine, diffuse, and slightly more prominent in the peripheral stroma. (Courtesy of Trexler M. Topping, M.D.)

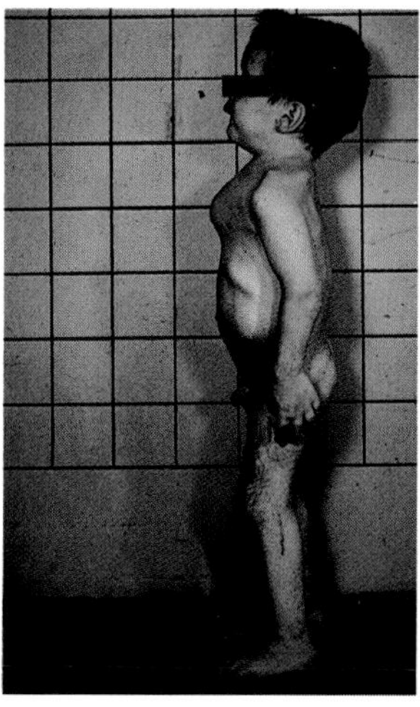

FIGURE 1–172 **Morquio's syndrome, MPS I-V.** Dwarfism, short neck, pectus carinatum, kyphoscoliosis, and other skeletal abnormalities characteristic of MPS I-V (Courtesy of Trexler M. Topping, M.D.)

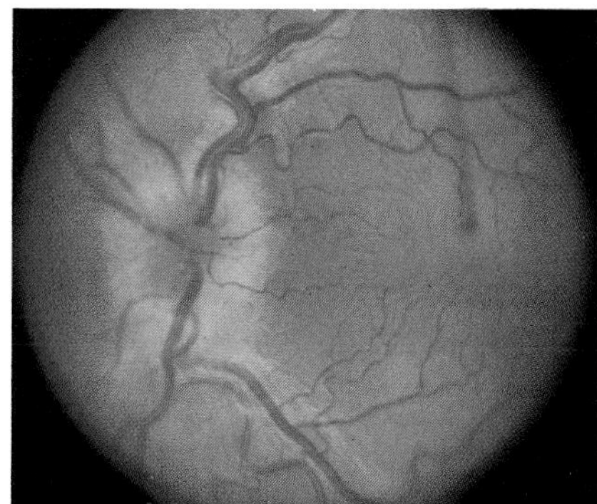

FIGURE 1–171 **Hunter's syndrome, MPS II.** A clinically clear cornea allows excellent visualization of disc edema in a 15 year-old boy with MPS II. (Courtesy of Trexler M. Topping, M.D.)

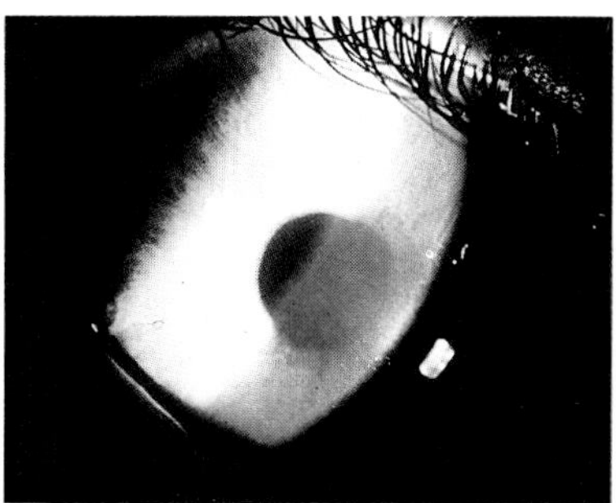

FIGURE 1–173 **Morquio's syndrome, MPS I-V.** Patchy dot-like and diffuse corneal clouding gives the cornea a ground-glass appearance. (Courtesy of Trexler M. Topping, M.D.)

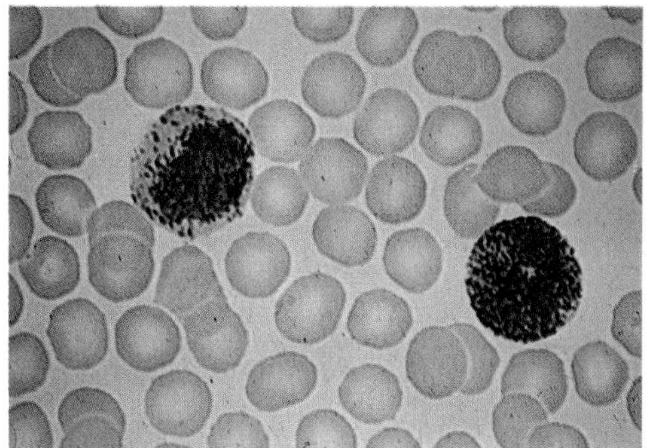

FIGURE 1–174 **Maroteaux-Lamy syndrome, MPS VI.** Circulating leukocytes often have prominent inclusion bodies. (Courtesy of Trexler M. Topping, M.D.)

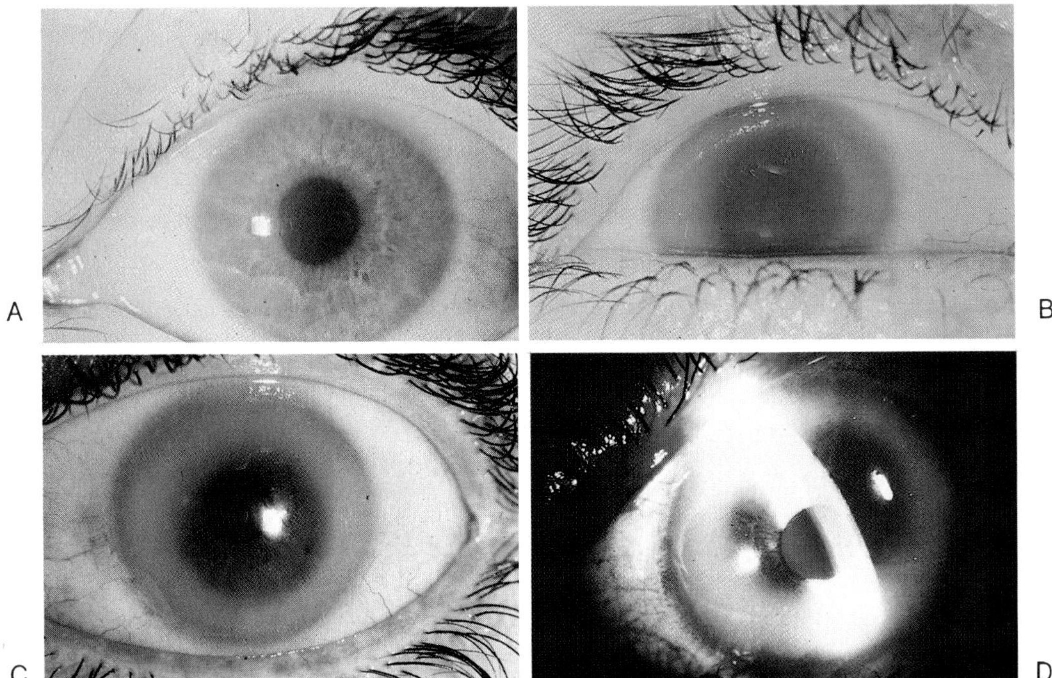

FIGURE 1–175 **Maroteaux-Lamy syndrome, MPS VI.** Corneal clouding varies from mild *(A)* to moderate *(B)* in type A. *C* and *D*, The peripheral corneal clouding is much more dense and visible to the unaided eye in type B disease. (Courtesy of Trexler M. Topping, M.D.)

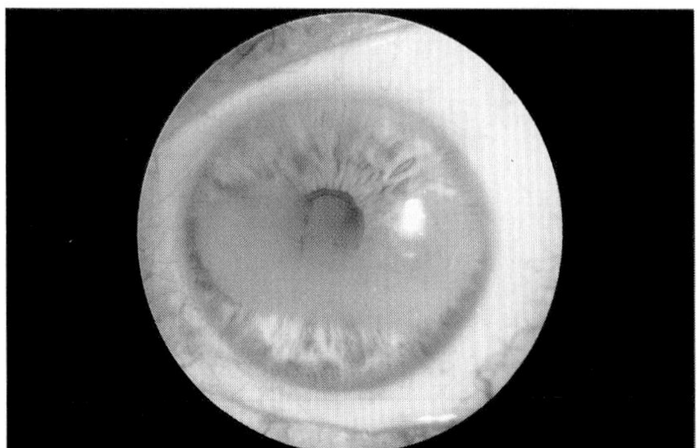

FIGURE 1–176 **Urate band keratopathy.** A 68-year-old man with gout presented with band keratopathy. The patient had dry eyes with a Schirmer test with anesthetic of 2-mm wetting. Vision was 20/50 and returned to 20/20 after the epithelium was scraped and subsequently reepithelialized.

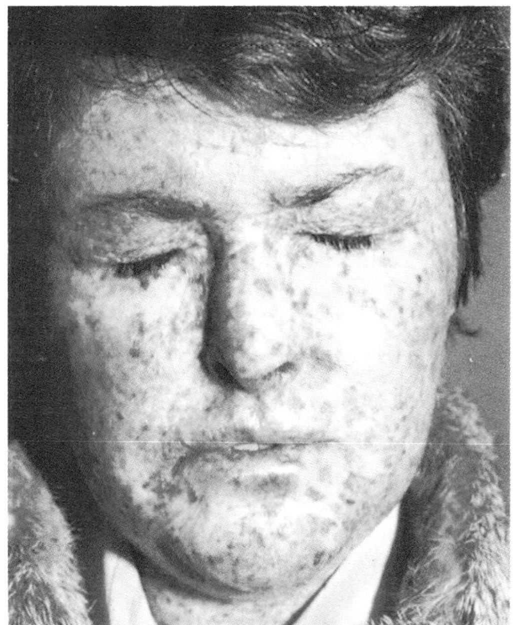

FIGURE 1–177 **Xeroderma pigmentosum.** Sun-exposed areas of skin showed hypopigmentation and hyperpigmentation with varying intensities of pigmentation. The deformity on the left part of the patient's nose is due to surgical excision of a tumor. (From Calonge M, Foster CS, Rice BA, et al: Management of corneal complications in xeroderma pigmentosum. Cornea 11:175, 1992.)

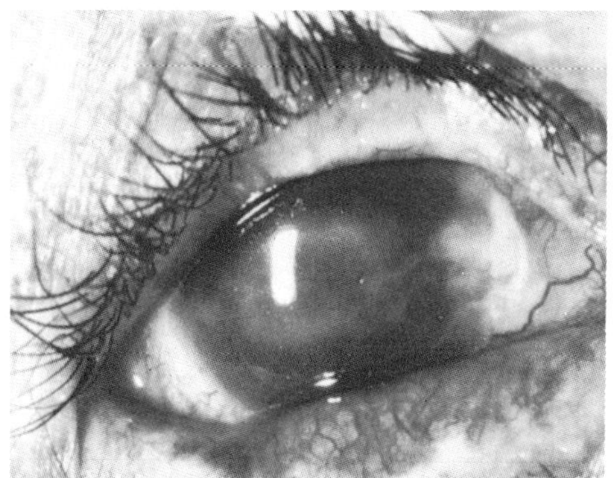

FIGURE 1–178 **Xeroderma pigmentosum.** The right eye of the patient in Figure 1–177 shows corneal stromal scarring with peripheral pannus and lipid deposition. The bulbar and tarsal conjunctiva are injected with notable telangiectasia of vessels. (From Calonge M, Foster CS, Rice BA, et al: Management of corneal complications in xeroderma pigmentosum. Cornea 11:175, 1992.)

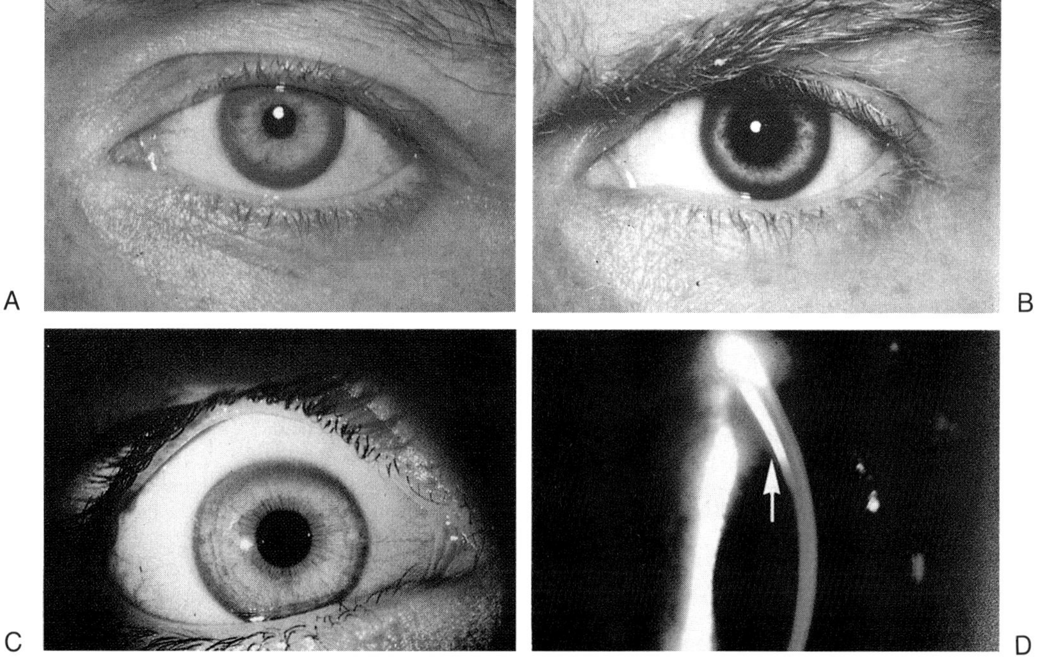

FIGURE 1–179 **Kayser-Fleischer ring in Wilson's disease.** *A* and *B,* These patients have full 360-degree copper deposits in Descemet's membrane of the cornea. *C,* This patient has involvement of only the upper cornea. *D,* The slit-lamp view of the patient in *C.* The *arrow* points to the Kayser-Fleischer ring at the level of Descemet's membrane. (*A–D,* From Wiebers DO, Hollenhorst RW, Goldstein NP: The ophthalmological manifestations of Wilson's disease. Mayo Clin Proc 52:414, 1977.)

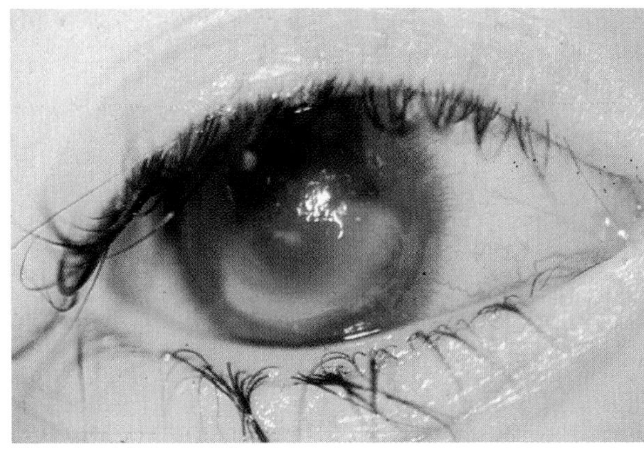

FIGURE 1–180 **Familial dysautonomia, Riley-Day syndrome.** The patient is a young girl with a neurotrophic corneal epithelial defect that resulted in sterile ulceration and stromal scarring. (From Mandel ER, Wagoner MD: Atlas of Corneal Disease. Philadelphia, WB Saunders, 1989, p. 48.)

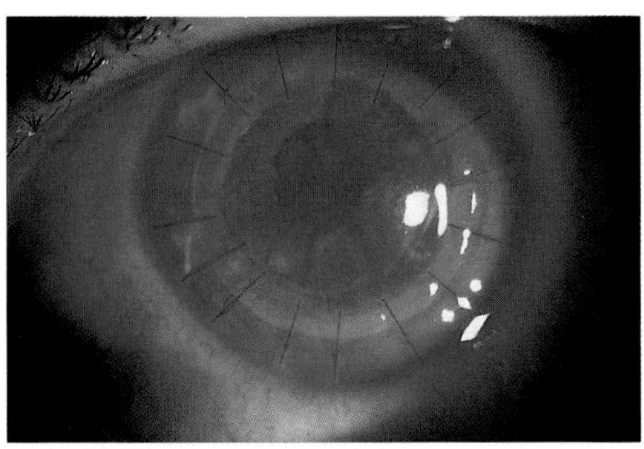

FIGURE 1–181 **Superficial punctate keratitis.** During the weeks after keratoplasty, the epithelium is fragile and especially subject to keratopathy from topical medications.

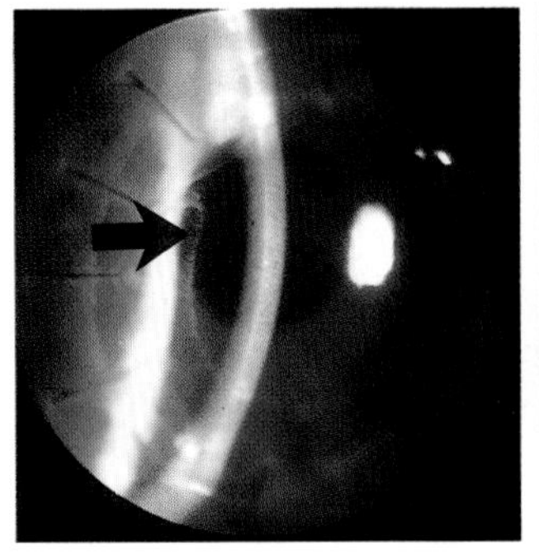

A

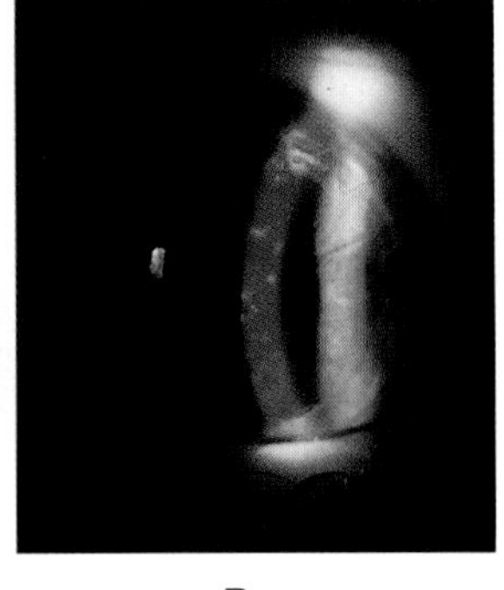

B

FIGURE 1–182 **Epithelial rejection after keratoplasty.** *A,* A linear opacity in the epithelium that migrates across the surface of the graft from one edge to the other over the course of several days is one of the first manifestations of epithelial rejection *(arrow). B,* The second major manifestation of epithelial rejection is the appearance of small, round, patchy infiltrates in the subepithelial zone.

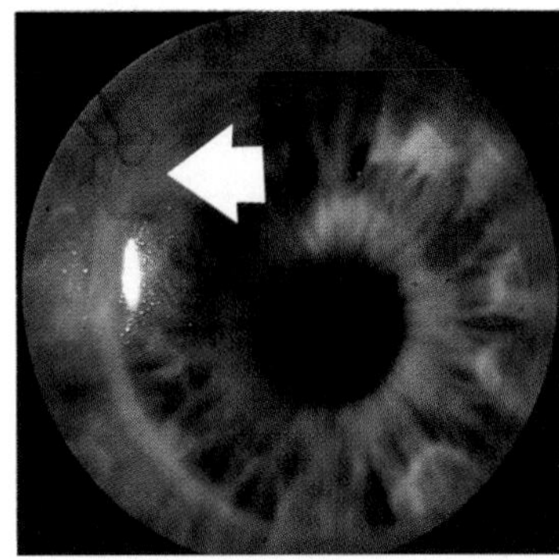

A

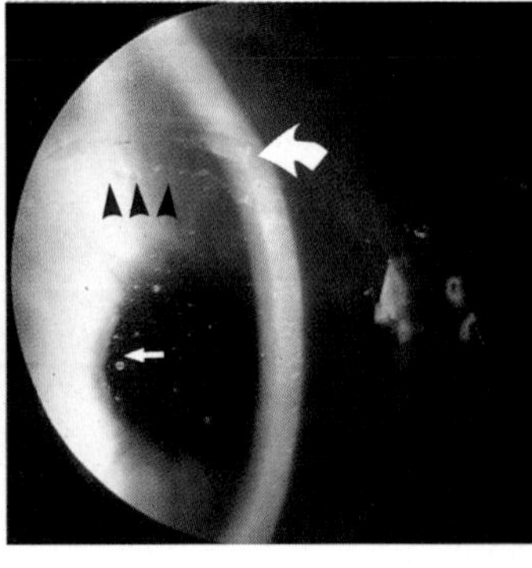

B

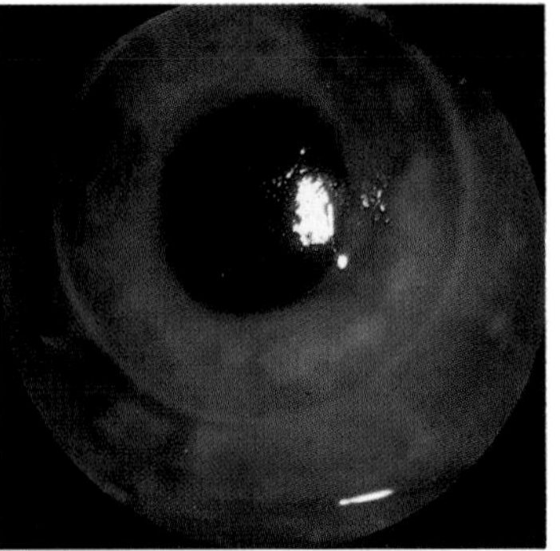

C

FIGURE 1–183 **Graft rejection.** *A,* At the junction of the graft and the host, there may be opening of previously dormant vessels with injection of the limbus in the affected area. Note the sectoral area of inflammation at the graft/host junction *(arrow). B,* Endothelial rejection: (1) edema at graft/host junction *(curved white arrow);* (2) Keratic precipitates *(white arrow);* (3) Khodadoust's line *(black arrowheads).* Khodadoust's line consists of endothelial precipitates in a linear arrangement that may progress in the affected area in the graft/host junction across the endothelium to the other side of the graft. *C,* Diffuse graft edema. This is the rejection manifestation having the poorest prognosis for improvement.

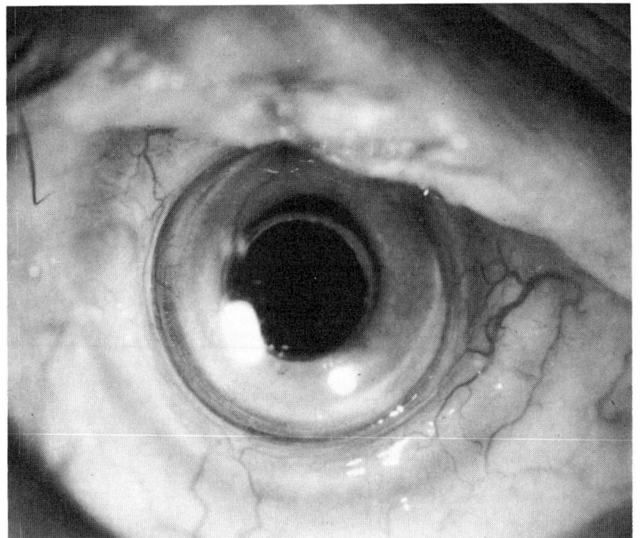

FIGURE 1-184 **Keratoprosthesis.** Collar button keratoprosthesis after severe herpes zoster. Vision is 20/40.

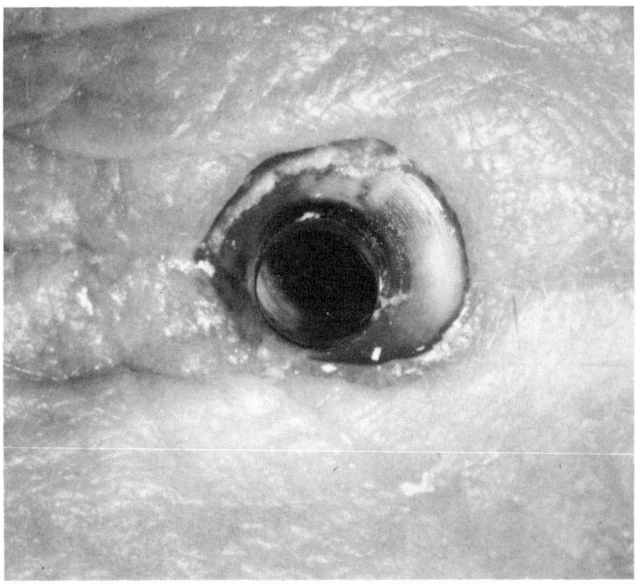

FIGURE 1-185 **Keratoprosthesis.** Through-the-lid prosthesis in end-stage pemphigoid. Vision is 20/25.

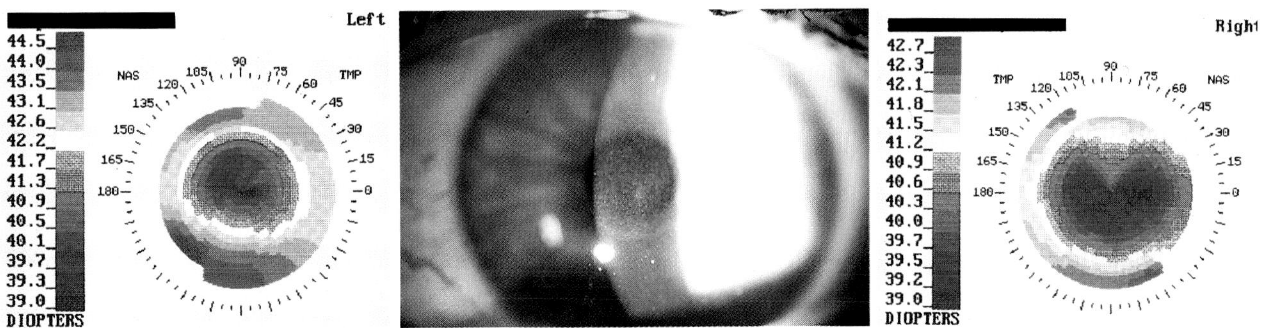

FIGURE 1-186 **Computer-assisted corneal topography.** *A,* Topographic analysis of patient's cornea 2 months after myopic excimer photorefractive keratectomy shows central flattening with reasonable centration on the optical zone. The overall optical zone is 4.5 mm. The intended and achieved correction was 3.5 D. *B,* Slit-lamp photograph of the patient shown in *A,* 2 months after excimer photorefractive keratectomy. A mild reticular haze can be seen with the broad slit beam in the anterior cornea, outlining the area of refractive keratectomy clearly. This haze was not visually apparent to the patient. It subsequently faded and was not detectable by the sixth month. *C,* Topographic analysis of patient's cornea after eight-incision radial keratotomy for 4 D of myopia. The optical zone can be seen as larger in diameter than that obtained with the excimer laser, with flattening extending out to 6 mm in some areas. Asymmetry of the correction is noted above. The clear corneal central optical zone in this case was 3.0 mm.

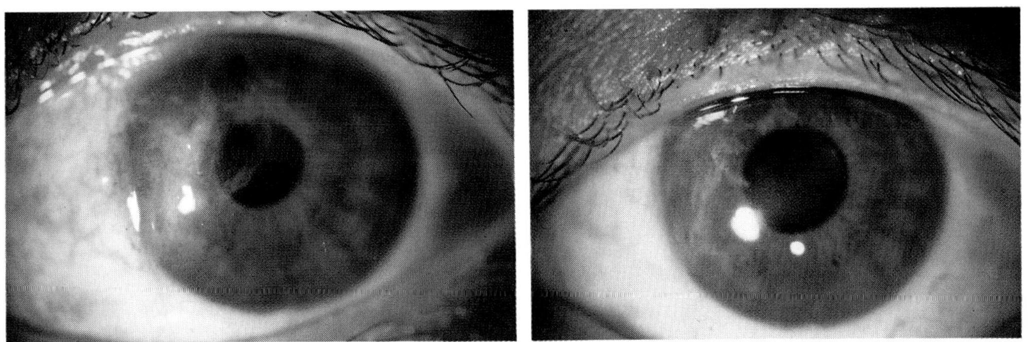

FIGURE 1-187 **Excimer laser treatment for corneal scarring.** Slit-lamp appearance before *(A)* and 1 month after *(B)* excimer laser phototherapeutic keratectomy performed to correct corneal scarring and irregular astigmatism in the visual axis following pterygium excision.

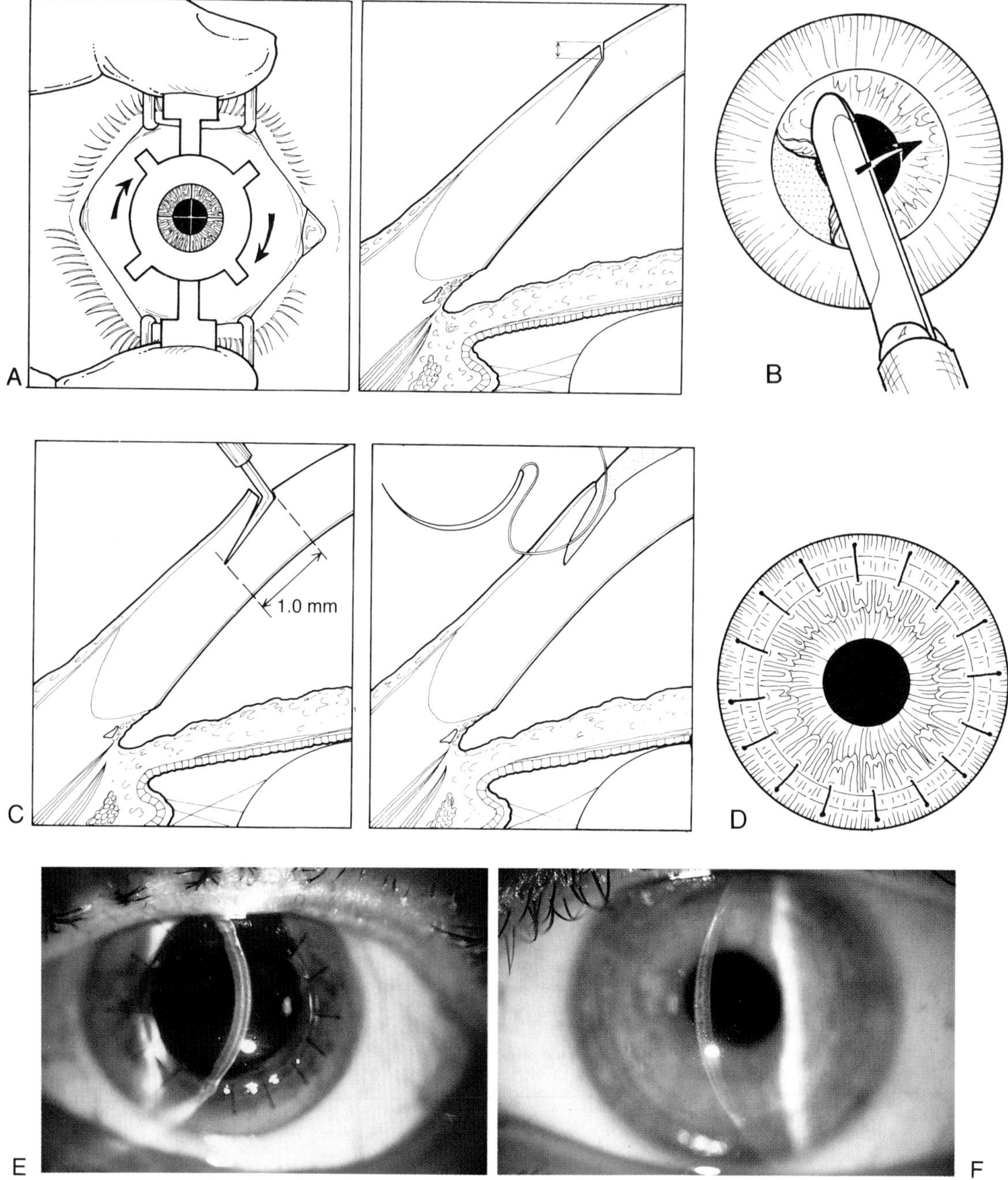

FIGURE 1–188 *See legend on opposite page*

◀ FIGURE 1–188 **Epikeratoplasty.** *A,* The Hessburg-Baron guarded suction trephine *(left)* is advanced to make an approximately 25 percent depth incision through Bowman's layer into the anterior stroma *(right). B,* The backside of a scarifier blade or similar instrument is used to deepithelialize the area within the trephination mechanically. Epithelium outside the trephination mark is left undisturbed. Care is taken to avoid the host's Bowman's layer. *C, Left,* A Suarez spreader or similar dissecting instrument then dissects a pocket from the depth of the trephination groove outward and downward toward the midstroma. The width of the lamellar bed should be 1.0 mm to accommodate the lenticule. *Right,* The lenticule is then placed into the stromal pocket. Suture with 10–0 nylon is performed meticulously so that the path of the suture passes through the tip of the wing. This anchors the edge of the lenticule within the stroma and prevents extrusion of the wing postoperatively. The suture is tied just tightly enough to lie down on the anterior surface of the cornea but not to place tension on the lenticule. *D,* At the completion of the suturing process, the lenticule is held securely within the dissected stromal bed but without tension. Qualitative astigmatism should be judged on the circular light reflex. Any tight or misplaced sutures should be replaced. Knots are rotated and buried just below the peripheral anterior cornea. Postoperative suture removal must not bring the knots through the lenticule to avoid displacing the edge of the lenticule. *E,* Aphakic epikeratoplasty 1 month postoperatively. Note that the host's Bowman's layer is visible in the thin slit beam, demarcating the interface between the epikeratoplasty lenticule and the patient's cornea. *F,* Appearance 1 year after aphakic epikeratoplasty in a 22-year-old man with spontaneous subluxation of the crystalline lens in Marfan's syndrome. The peripheral wound scar is beginning to fade. The epikeratoplasty lenticule is optically satisfactory, with normal visualization of the iris details through the lenticule on slit-lamp examination and a visual acuity of 20/20. Nevertheless, examination with a thin slit beam shows slightly more light scattering in the donor lenticule than in the underlying native host cornea.

SECTION 2

Uvea and Lens

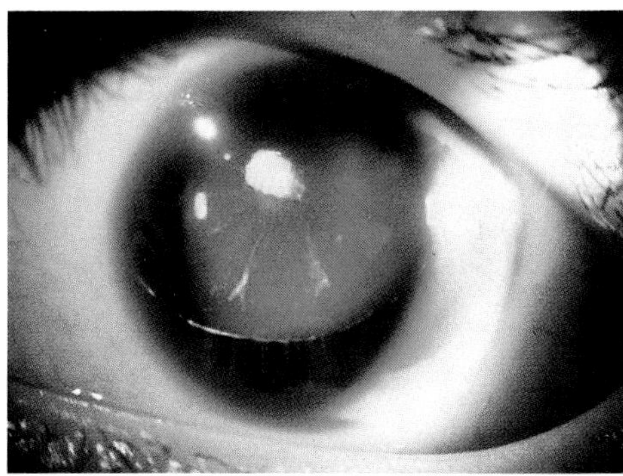

FIGURE 2-1 **Aniridia.** This patient has severe irideremia, superior dislocation of the lens, and a focal cataract. Zonular attachments of lens are clearly visible inferiorly.

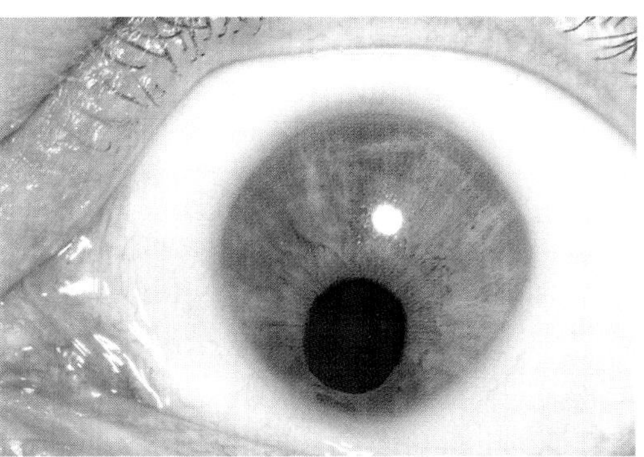

FIGURE 2-3 **Iris coloboma.** "Bridge" coloboma (fellow eye of Fig. 2-2). A bridge of mesectodermal tissue derived from the pupillary membrane stretched across the central portion of the defect. The choroidal coloboma was less extensive in this eye.

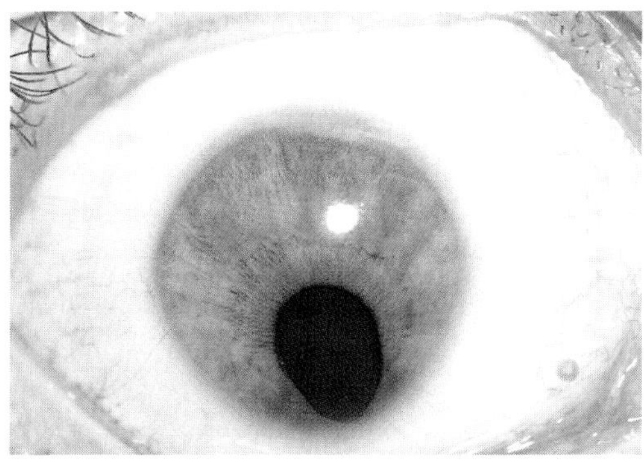

FIGURE 2-2 **Iris coloboma.** Typical iris coloboma is located inferonasally in the region of the embryonic fissure. The coloboma in this case also involved the ciliary body and the choroid.

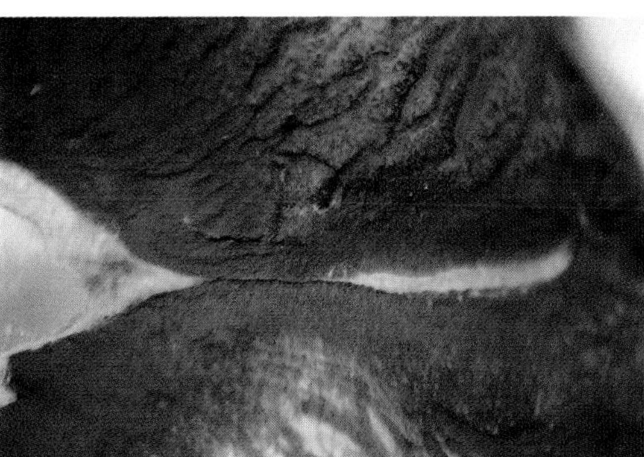

FIGURE 2-4 **Iridociliary coloboma.** Internal view of iridociliary coloboma in a fetal eye from a patient with 13q− syndrome. Anomalous ciliary processes flank the posterior extension of the colobomatous cleft into the pars plicata. Tan iris stroma fills the cleft and borders the pupil.

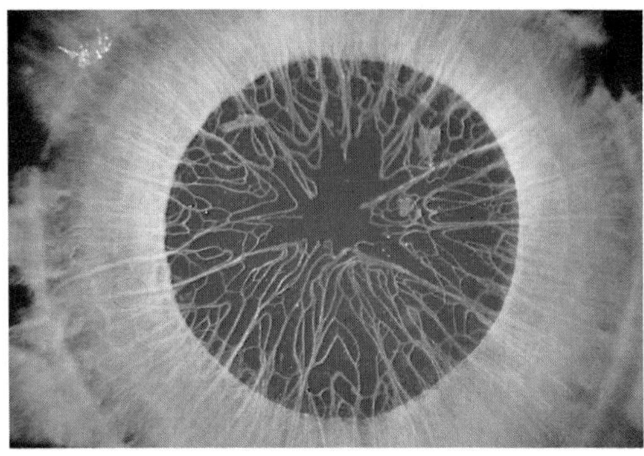

FIGURE 2–5 **Pupillary membrane, 6-month fetus.** Arcades of vessels nearly reach the center of the pupil.

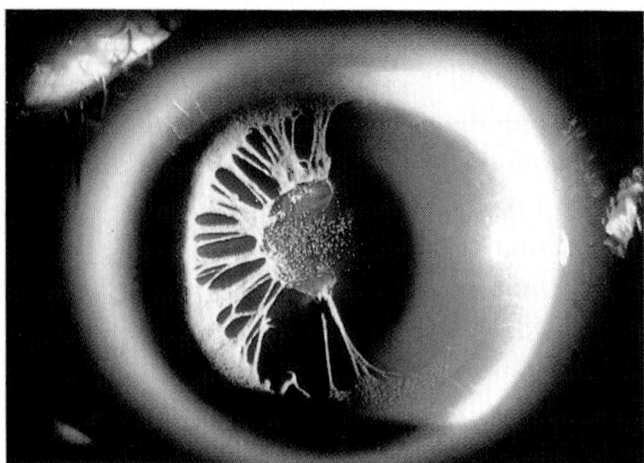

FIGURE 2–7 **Persistent pupillary membrane, type II.** Extensive iridolenticular adhesions are present in this patient. Iris stromal melanocytes form "pigment stars" on the anterior lens capsule.

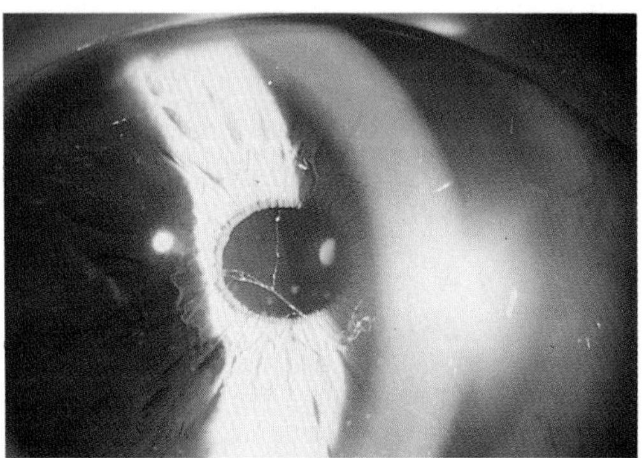

FIGURE 2–6 **Persistent pupillary membrane, type I.** Cobweb-like strands of tissue extend across the pupil from collarette to collarette.

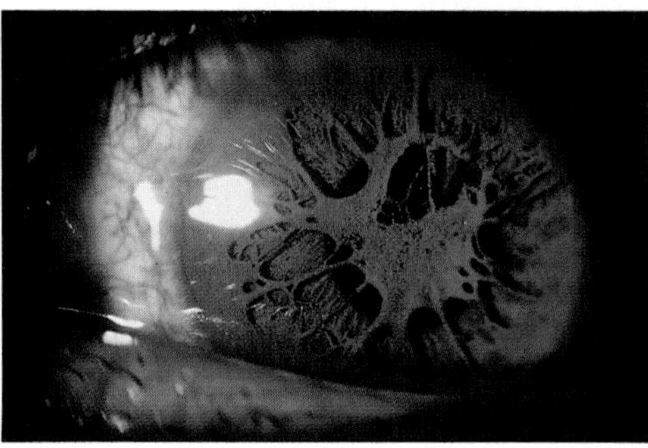

FIGURE 2–8 **Florid type I persistent pupillary membrane.** The patient has had yttrium-aluminum-garnet (YAG) laser photodisruption to clear a central opening through the visual axis. (Courtesy of Dr. Dario Savino, Caracas, Venezuela.)

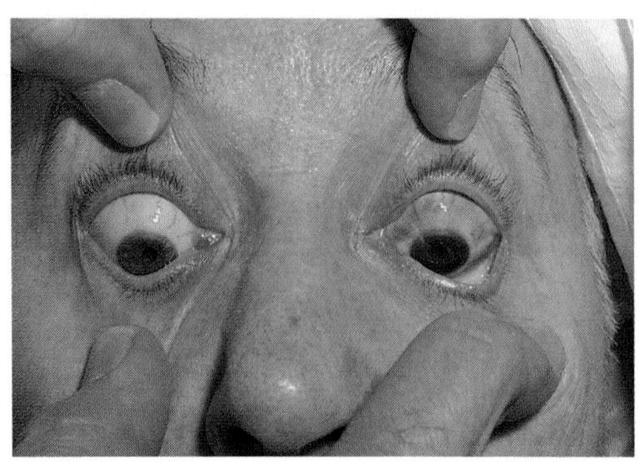

FIGURE 2–9 **Congenital oculodermal melanocytosis (nevus of Ota).** This patient with nevus of Ota displays heterochromia iridis secondary to the condition. This normal right eye has a light brown–colored iris. The affected left eye is deeply pigmented. Extensive slate-gray epibulbar pigmentation and subtle pigmentation on the periocular skin are present. Diffuse leptomeningeal melanosis was found post mortem after the patient developed primary central nervous system melanoma. (From Eagle RC Jr: Iris pigmentation and pigmented lesions: An ultrastructural study. Trans Am Ophthalmol Soc 86:581, 1988.)

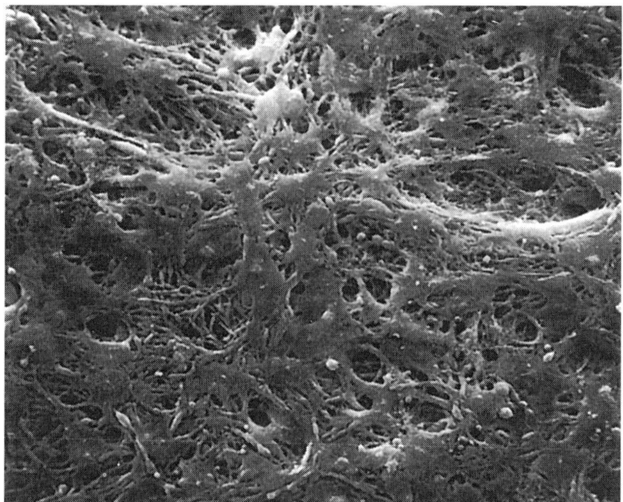

FIGURE 2–10 **Electron microscopy of nevus of Ota.** The normal light brown right iris of the patient seen in Figure 2–9. In contrast to the iris in the fellow eye with congenital melanocytosis (see Fig. 2–11), the anterior iris surface disclosed by scanning electron microscopy appears relatively smooth-surfaced and has delicate cellular processes. Scanning electron microscopy, ×640. (From Eagle RC Jr: Iris pigmentation and pigmented lesions: An ultrastructural study. Trans Am Ophthalmol Soc 86:581, 1988.)

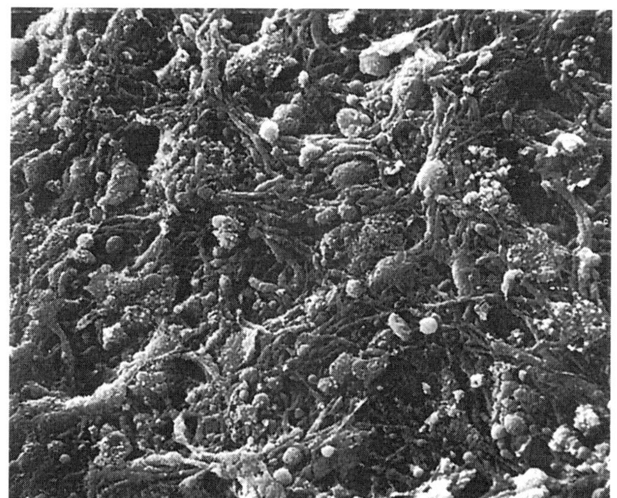

FIGURE 2–11 **Electron microscopy of nevus of Ota.** The anterior border layer of the iris with Ota's nevus has roughened texture and thickened processes engorged with pigment. Numerous round framboisiform processes project from the anterior surface. Scanning electron microscopy, ×640. (From Eagle RC Jr: Iris pigmentation and pigmented lesions: An ultrastructural study. Trans Am Ophthalmol Soc 86:581, 1988.)

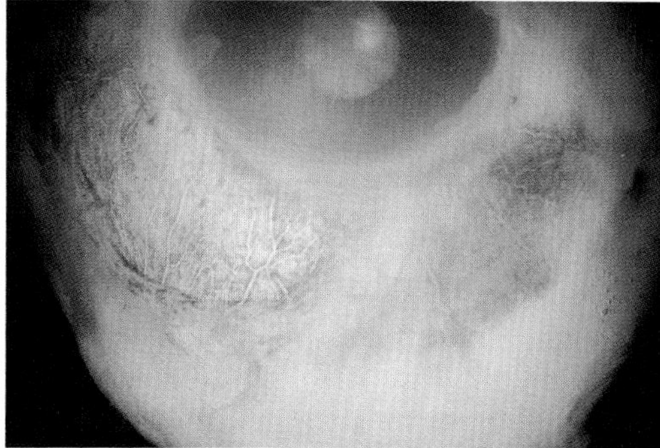

FIGURE 2–12 **Nevus of Ota.** The affected left eye was obtained post mortem from the patient seen in Figure 2–9. The conjunctiva was ripped during enucleation. The episcleral pigment exposed in the conjunctival defect at left appears brown. Pigmentation beneath the intact conjunctiva has the typical slate-gray color.

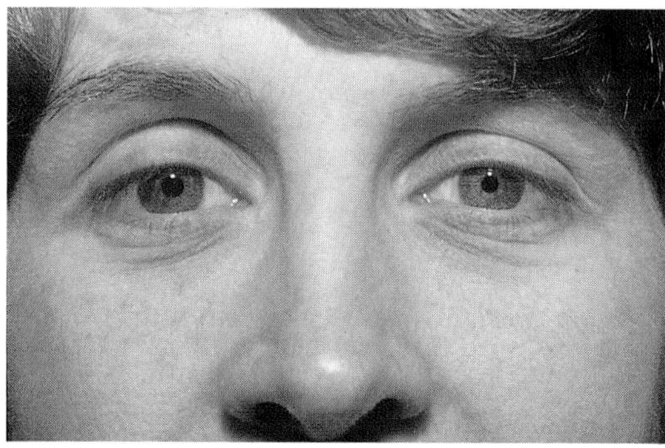

FIGURE 2–13 **Congenital Horner's syndrome with heterochromia iridis.** The involved left iris is subtly hypochromic. Pupillary miosis and minimal left ptosis are also evident.

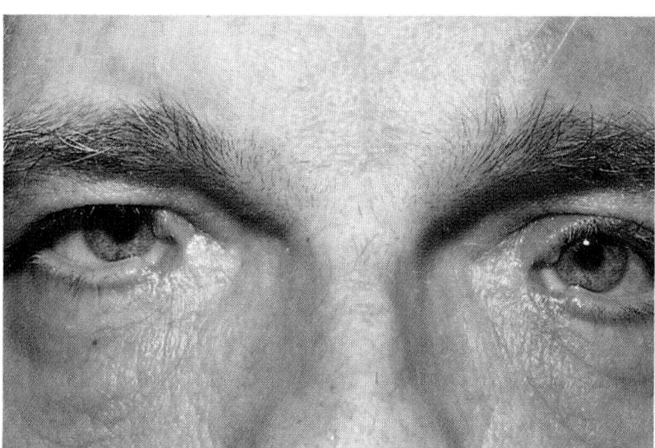

FIGURE 2–14 **Type I Waardenburg's syndrome with bilateral iris hypochromia.** The nasal bridge is broad, and the medial canthi and lacrimal puncta are displaced laterally (dystopia canthorum). The patient was also deaf and prematurely gray-haired.

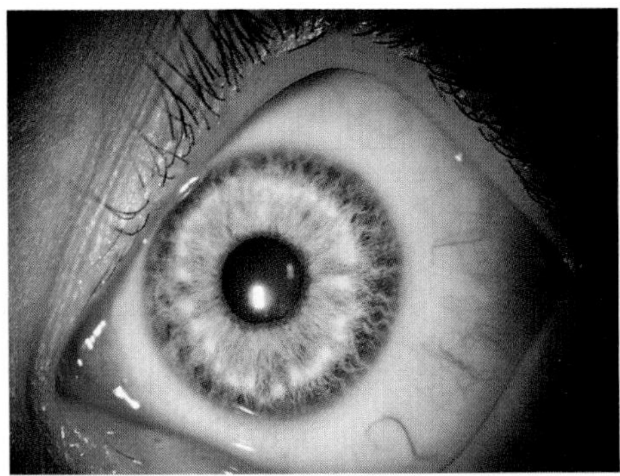

FIGURE 2-15 **Down's syndrome.** Brushfield's spots in a blue-eyed patient with trisomy 21. The ring of spots is located in the medial third of the iris stroma. These spots represent focal condensations of collagenous extracellular matrix material in the iris stroma. (Courtesy of Dr. Edward A. Jaeger.)

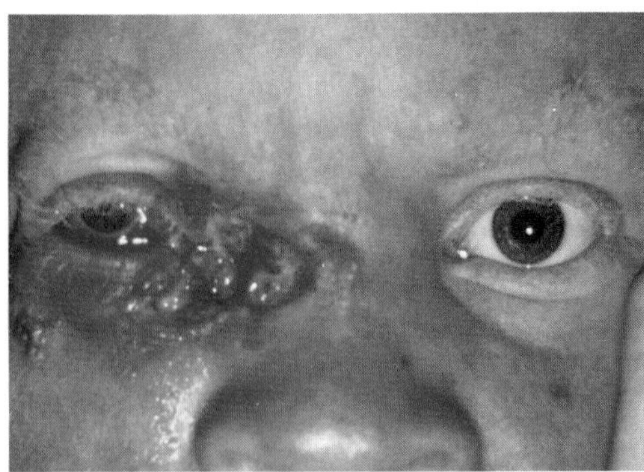

FIGURE 2-17 **Albinism.** A tyrosinase-positive albino black from Zaire. The patient, who has light skin and a light brown iris, has developed a large ulcerating invasive squamous cell carcinoma of the right medial canthus. The right orbit was exenterated. Albinos in the tropics frequently die from skin cancer.

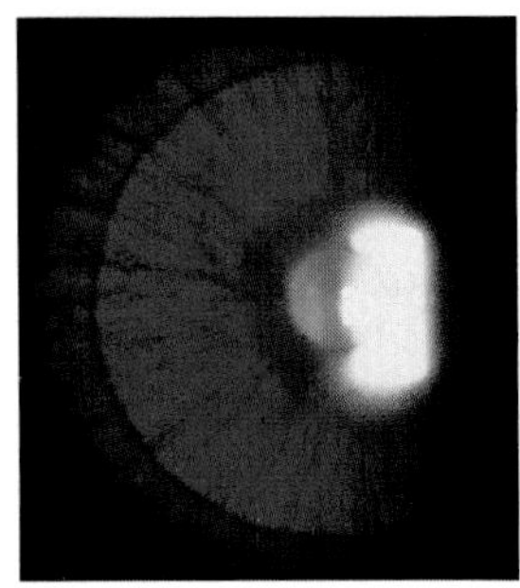

FIGURE 2-16 **Albinism.** A marked degree of iris transillumination in an albino patient. The equator of the lens and the ciliary processes are visible.

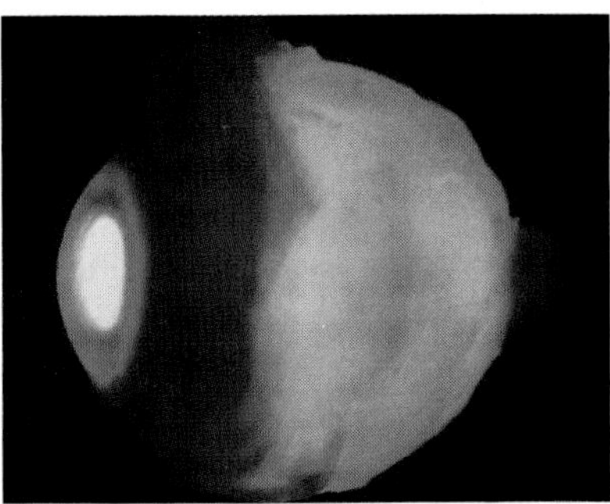

FIGURE 2-18 **Albinism.** The globe was enucleated from the African tyrosinase-positive albino patient shown in Figure 2-17. Both the iris and the choroid transilluminate vividly. Oddly, the pigment content on the ciliary body is relatively normal.

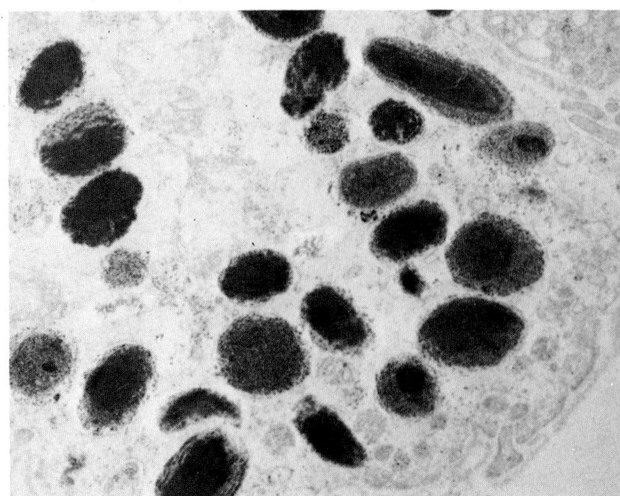

FIGURE 2-19 **Albinism.** Iris pigment epithelium from the African tyrosinase-positive albino patient seen in Figure 2-17 with iris transillumination. The melanosomes are immature and decreased in number. Transmission electron microscopy, ×9500.

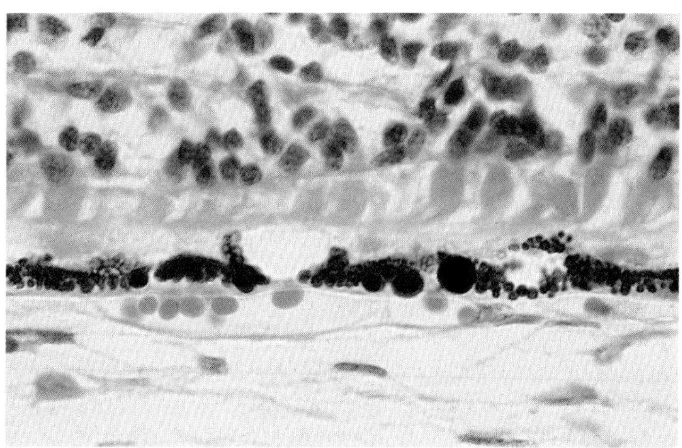

FIGURE 2–20 **X-linked ocular albinism.** Several retinal pigment epithelial cells contain giant pigment granules (macromelanosomes). These macromelanosomes are also found in the ciliary epithelium and in the keratinocytes and melanocytes of the skin. These are characteristic histologic markers in both affected male and female carriers with the Nettleship-Falls type of X-linked albinism. (From O'Donnell FE Jr, Hambrick GW Jr, Green WR, et al: X-linked ocular albinism: An oculocutaneous macromelanosomal disorder. Arch Ophthalmol 94:1883, 1976.)

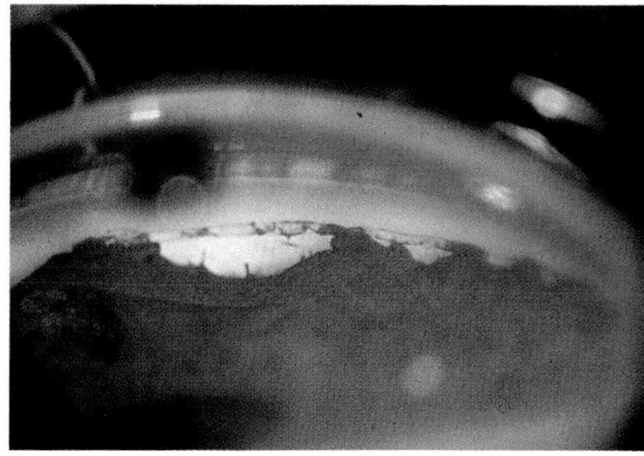

FIGURE 2–21 **Axenfeld's anomaly.** Gonioscopy discloses multiple broad iris processes bridging the angle to insert on the prominent anteriorly displaced Schwalbe's line. (Courtesy of Dr. Dario Savina, Caracas, Venezuela.)

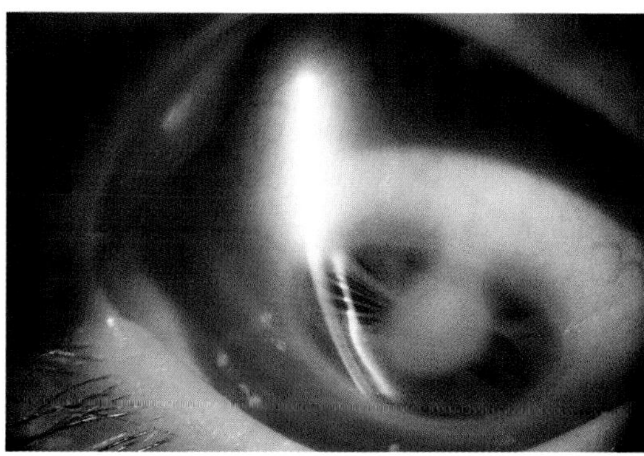

FIGURE 2–22 **Peters' anomaly with iridocorneal adhesions.** Cuneate strands of iris stroma insert into the periphery of the central corneal opacity. The lens is adherent to the posterior cornea centrally. (Courtesy of Irving Raber, M.D.)

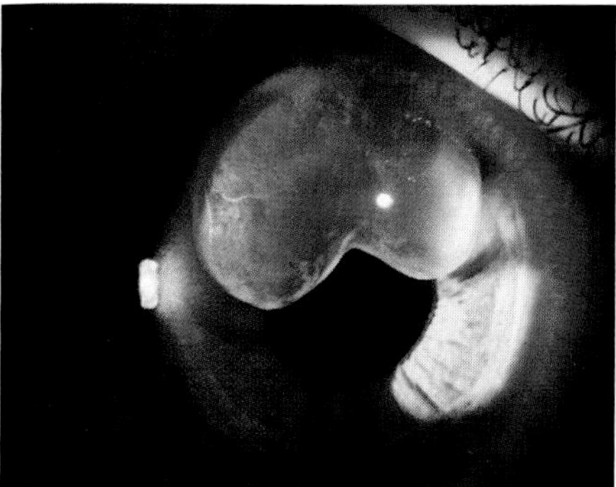

FIGURE 2–23 **Congenital epithelial cysts of the iris (congenital iris stromal cysts).** The patient had no history of surgery or trauma.

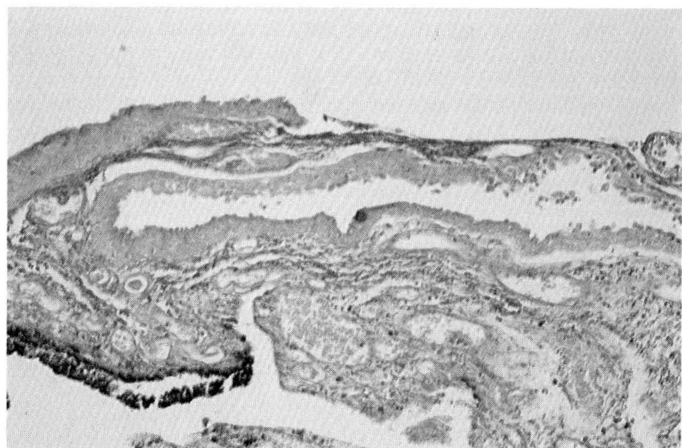

FIGURE 2–24 **Congenital iris stromal cyst.** Histopathology shows stratified squamous epithelium lining the cyst. The epithelium includes goblet cells in some cases, and the lumen contains clear fluid.

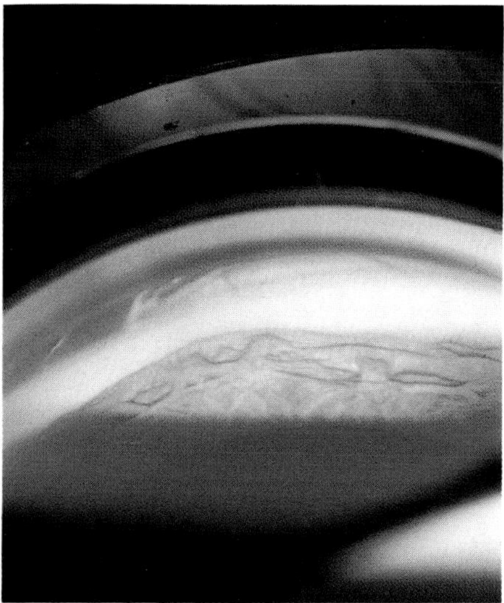

FIGURE 2–25 **Iris pigment epithelial cysts.** These cysts are important clinically because they are easily confused with uveal malignant melanomas. As in this case, the peripheral cysts are recognized on slit-lamp biomicroscopy as a subtle anterior displacement or "tenting up" of the peripheral iris whose appearance has been likened to "a ball thrown under a rug." (Courtesy of Jerry A. Shields, M.D.)

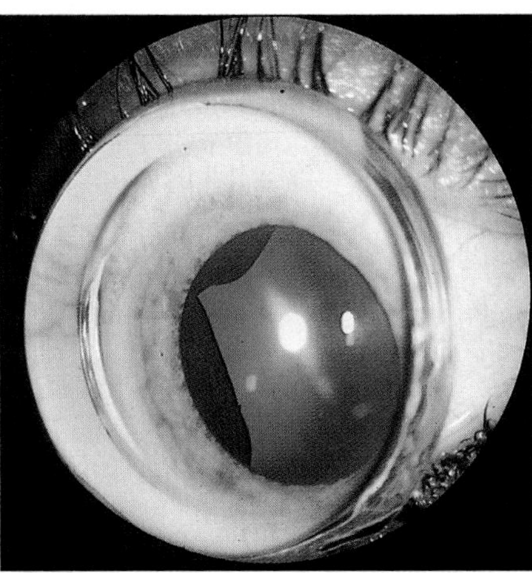

FIGURE 2–26 **Midzonal iris pigment epithelial cysts.** These pigment epithelial cysts are frequently multiple and bilateral. These are smooth, intensely pigmented masses that have an elongated or fusiform shape that can mimic a ciliary body melanoma. Slight undulations of the cyst wall caused by eye movements and focal transillumination defects are helpful differential features. The patient in this photograph was initially thought to have a malignant melanoma. (Courtesy of Jerry A. Shields, M.D.)

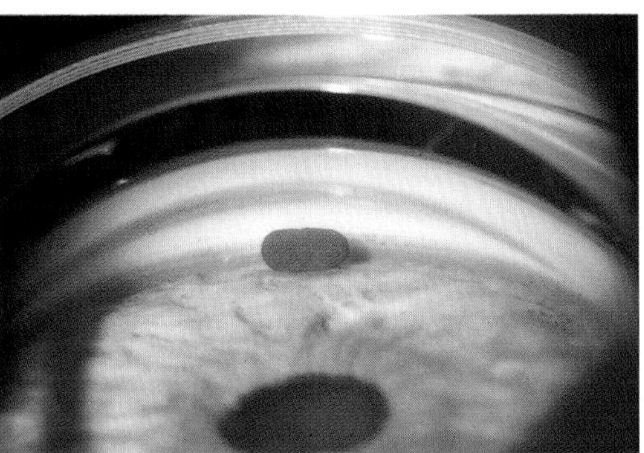

FIGURE 2–27 **Iris pigment epithelial cyst.** A gonioscopic view of a dislodged iris pigment epithelial cyst fixed to the anterior chamber angle. (Courtesy of Jerry A. Shields, M.D.)

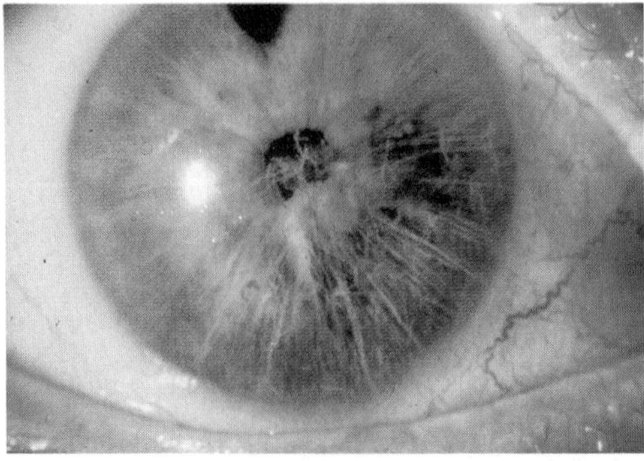

FIGURE 2–28 **Iridoschisis.** Ruptured anterior stromal fibers float freely in the anterior chamber. The posterior layer of stroma remains adherent to the neuroectodermal pigment epithelium and dilator muscle. Some of the anterior fibers rupture, and their distal ends float freely in the anterior chamber, occasionally damaging the corneal endothelium and causing frank corneal decompensation. (From Yanoff M, Fine BS: Ocular Pathology: A Text and Atlas, 3rd ed. Philadelphia, JB Lippincott, 1989, p. 606.)

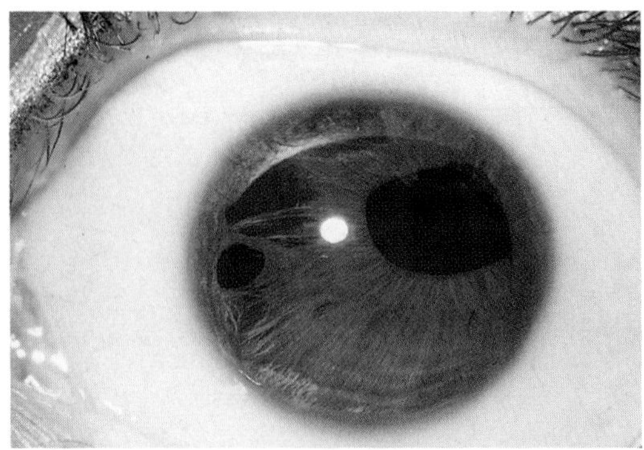

FIGURE 2–29 **Essential iris atrophy.** Full-thickness tractional holes have formed in the iris opposite the displaced pupil. The stretch holes initially form in the stroma and eventually involve the full thickness of the iris.

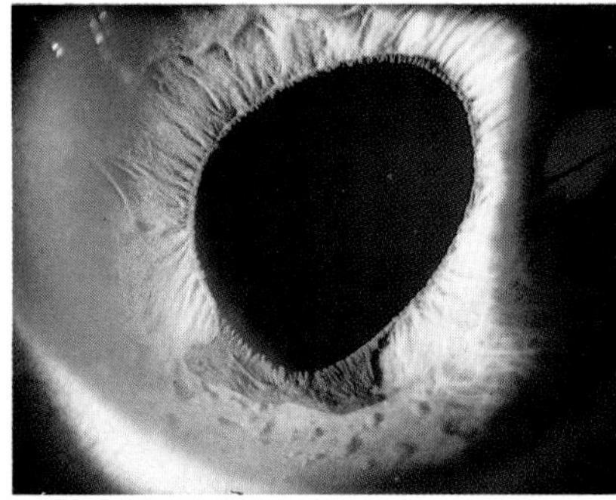

FIGURE 2–30 **Essential iris atrophy.** Multiple iris nodules are seen in a flattened, endothelialized area of the iris stroma adjacent to initial synechiae and ectropion iridis. As iris endothelialization progresses, islands of stromal melanocytes occasionally are encircled and pinched off by an advancing sheet of cells, forming the pigmented iris nodules. A full-thickness hole has developed at the right.

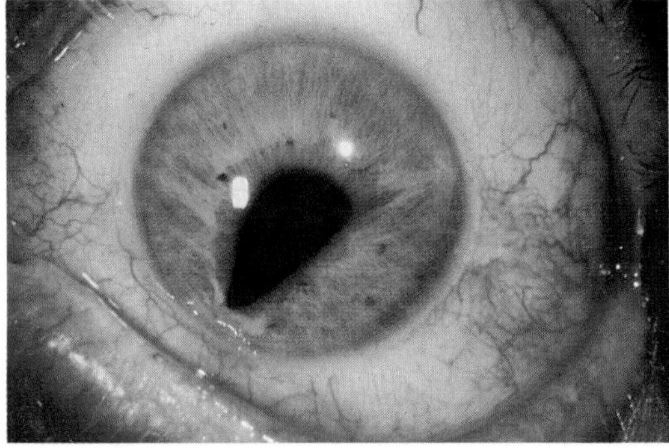

FIGURE 2–31 **Essential iris atrophy.** The pupil is peaked toward a synechia at 7 o'clock. These focal synechiae develop in an otherwise open angle. Studies indicate that the synechia forms consequent to endothelial migration across the trabecular meshwork onto the peripheral iris. A new synechia forming at 2:30 exerts traction on adjacent stroma and collarette. (From Eagle RC Jr, Shields JA: Iridocorneal endothelial syndrome with contralateral guttata endothelial dystrophy. Opthalmology 94:862, 1987.)

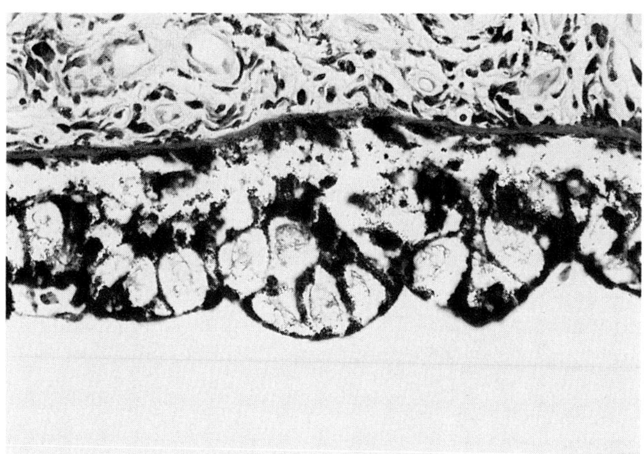

FIGURE 2–32 **Diabetic lacy vacuolization of the iris pigment epithelium.** Glycogen accumulates massively within the cytoplasm of the iris pigment epithelial cells, displacing the melanin granules and forming vacuoles or microcystoid spaces. In this histopathologic photograph, granular PAS-positive material is present. Diastase digestion confirmed that the material was glycogen. PAS, ×100.

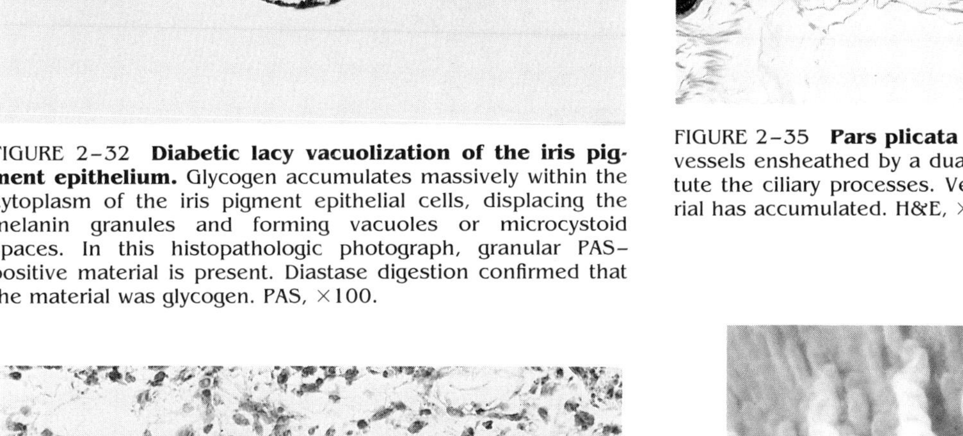

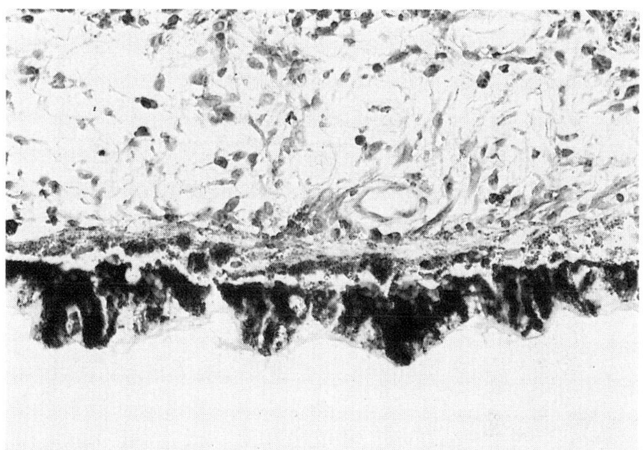

FIGURE 2–33 **"Sawtoothing" of the iris pigment epithelium in an eye with pseudoexfoliation syndrome.** Scanning electron microscopy would show that deposits of filamentary mucoprotein form strands or linear aggregates that radiate from the pupil and are oriented at right angles to a circumferential radius of the pigment epithelium, thus giving the pigment epithelium a "sawtooth" configuration. H&E, ×100.

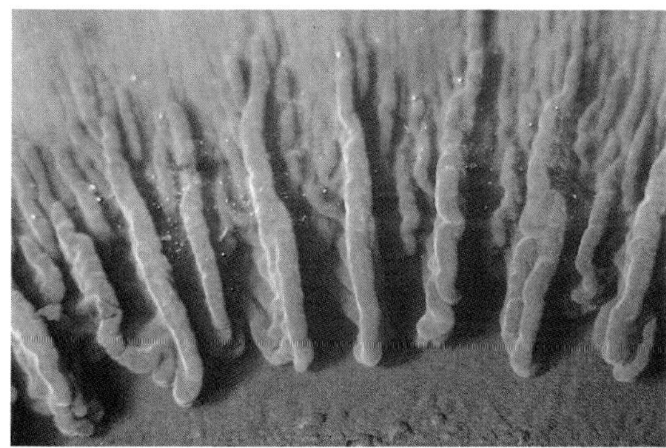

FIGURE 2–34 **Ciliary processes.** An eye from a 2-year-old child. The ciliary processes are pigmented, delicate, and relatively smooth in contour.

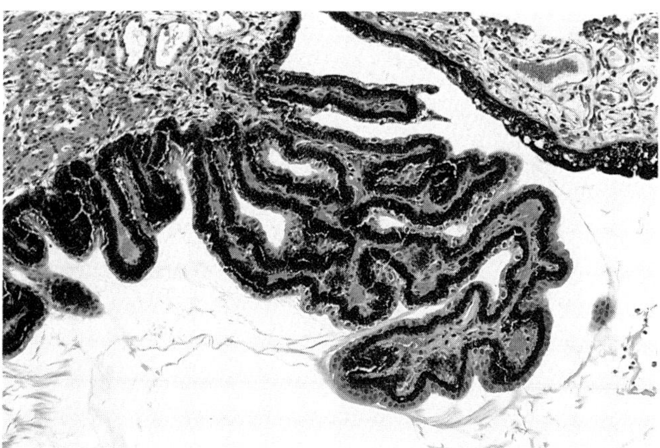

FIGURE 2–35 **Pars plicata in a 2-year-old child.** The central vessels ensheathed by a dual layer of ciliary epithelium constitute the ciliary processes. Very little extracellular matrix material has accumulated. H&E, ×100.

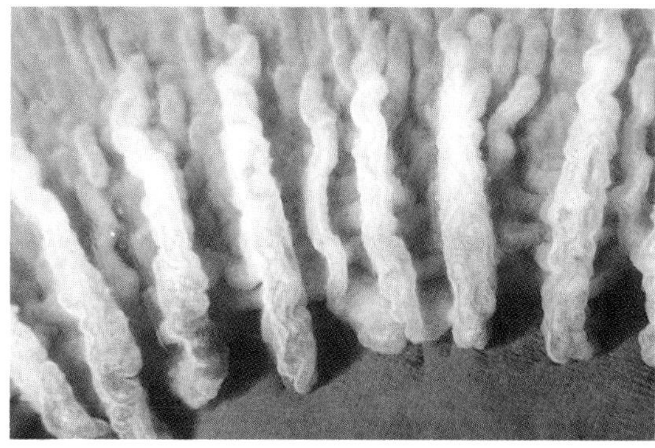

FIGURE 2–36 **Hyalinization of the ciliary processes in an elderly patient.** The processes are white, and they appear coarsely thickened when compared with the infant's processes shown at the same magnification in Figure 2–34.

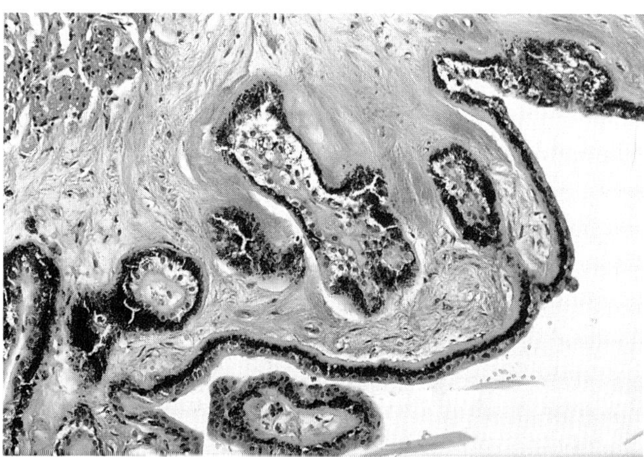

FIGURE 2–37 **Hyalinization of the pars plicata in an octogenarian patient.** The ciliary processes have a blunted configuration reflecting a lifelong accumulation of collagen. This process of increasing fibrosis may be responsible, in part, for the gradually decreasing production of aqueous humor in the elderly. H&E, ×100.

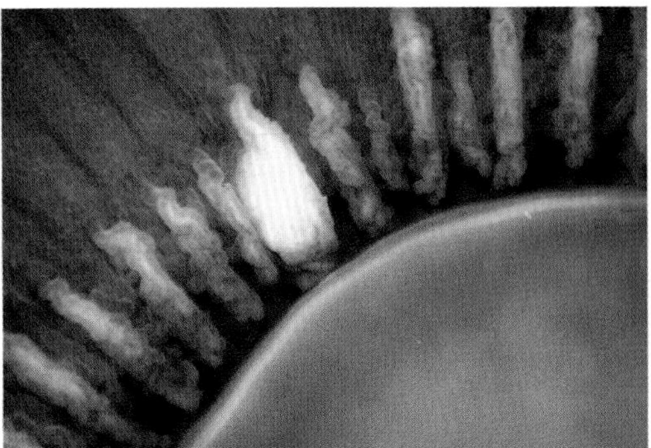

FIGURE 2–38 **Fuchs' adenoma of the pars plicata found incidentally in an elderly patient.** One study has shown that the observed incidence in vivo of this lesion was 18% in a group of older patients.

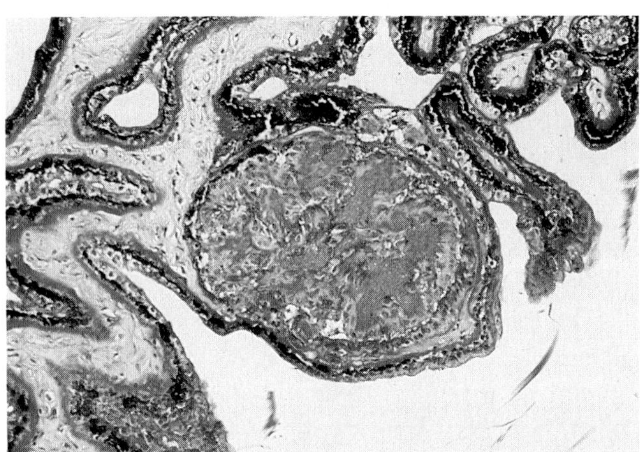

FIGURE 2–39 **Fuchs' adenoma.** Cords of benign, nonpigmented ciliary epithelium within hyperplastic nodule encompass pools of hyalinized PAS-positive extracellular matrix material. Thickening of the pigmented ciliary epithelial basement membrane suggests that the patient also had diabetes mellitus. PAS, ×100.

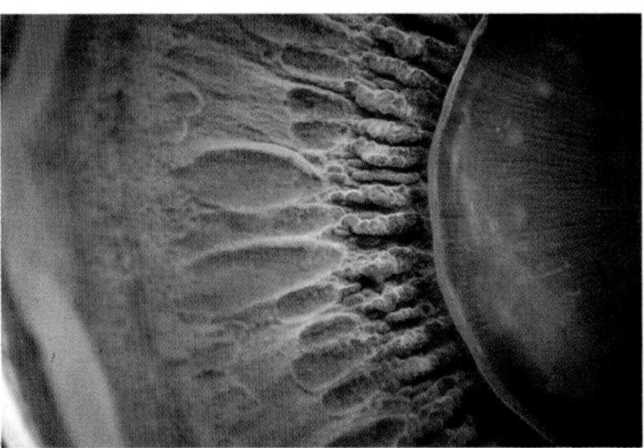

FIGURE 2–41 **Multiple pars plana cysts.** Multiple pars plana cysts in an unfixed postmortem eye from a patient with multiple myeloma. Myeloma cysts are clear before fixation. These cysts are filled with abnormal protein, which becomes precipitated by formaldehyde fixation, causing the cyst to appear milky-white.

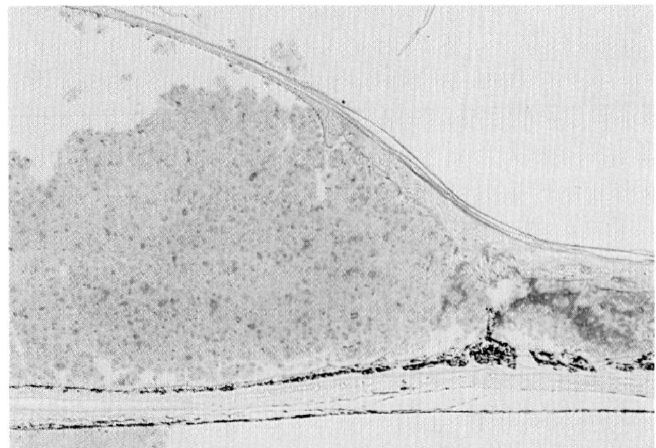

FIGURE 2–40 **Pars plana cyst, normal individual.** Blue-staining acid mucopolysaccharide material shows the lumen of the cyst bordered by pigmented and nonpigmented ciliary epithelium. Mucopolysaccharide staining was abolished by hyaluronidase digestion, indicating that the cyst contained hyaluronic acid. Hale's colloidal iron, ×25.

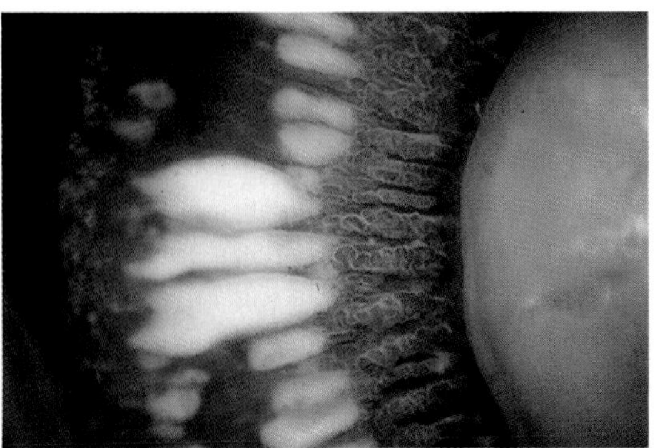

FIGURE 2–42 **Pars plana cyst.** Same region as in Figure 2–41 after fixation in 10% formaldehyde.

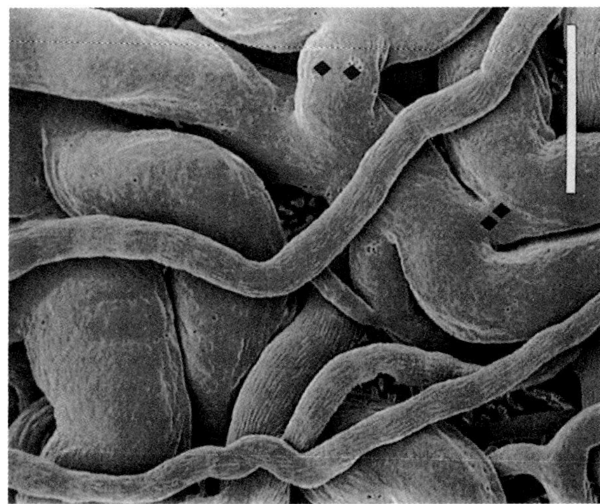

FIGURE 2–43 **Dense choroidal vasculature at the posterior pole close to the fovea.** Intervenous anastomoses are demonstrated *(diamonds).* Scleral surface of choriocapillaris is visible. B-R = 270 μm. (From Oliver JM: Functional anatomy of the choroidal circulation. Eye 4:262–273, 1990.)

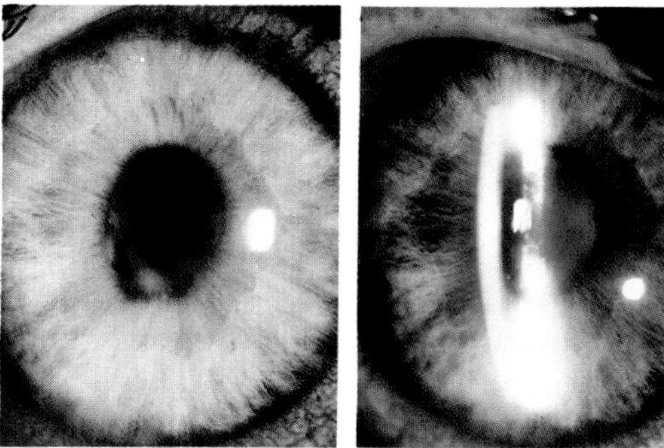

FIGURE 2–44 **Anterior segment inflammation and intermediate uveitis.** Slit-lamp photographs of the eye of a teenage girl with intermediate uveitis and anterior segment inflammation. Posterior synechiae have resulted in pupillary seclusion *(left).* Pupillary block in iris bombé with shallowing of the anterior chamber (demonstrated by the slit beam, *right*) resulted in secondary angle-closure glaucoma. Argon laser peripheral iridotomies did not remain patent. Pars plana vitrectomy and lensectomy were ultimately performed. The apparent heterochromia is an illumination artifact.

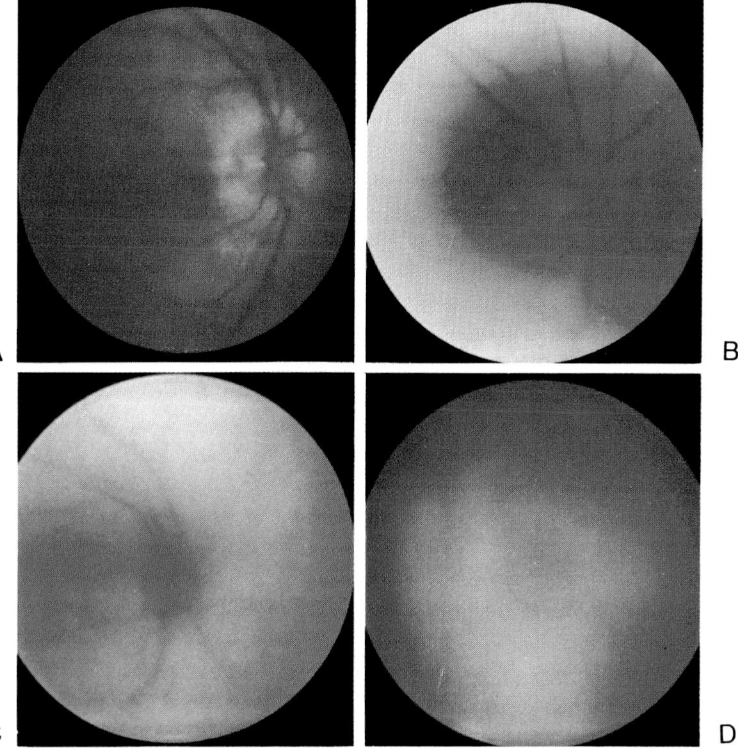

FIGURE 2–45 **Grading of vitritis.** A standardized system for the grading of vitreal inflammatory activity in intermediate uveitis based on the clarity of the optic nerve head, retinal vessels, and nerve fiber layer. *A,* 1+ vitreal haze. The nerve head topography and retinal vascular detail are discernible through the haze. *B,* 2+ vitreal haze. The optic nerve head margins and topography are moderately blurred, with retinal vessels well visualized. *C,* 3+ vitreal haze. The optic nerve head is markedly blurred yet discernible. *D,* 4+ vitreal haze. The view of the optic nerve head is obscured. (*A–D,* From Nussenblatt RB, Palestine AG, Chan C, Roberge F: Standardization of vitreous inflammatory activity in intermediate and posterior uveitis. Published courtesy of Ophthalmology [92:467–471, 1985].)

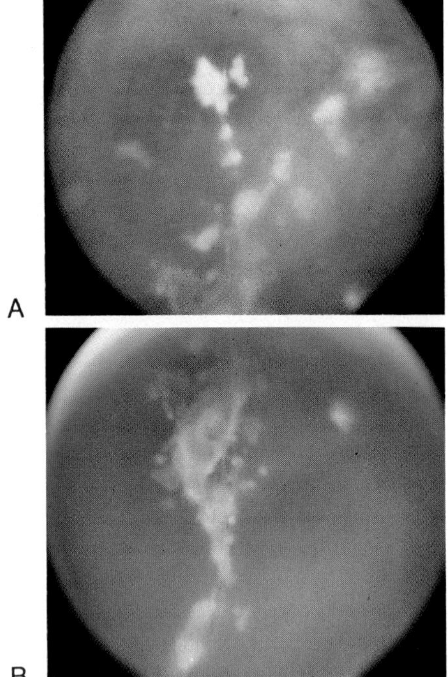

FIGURE 2–46 **Inflammatory vitreous debris.** The right *(A)* and left *(B)* eyes of a white man in his mid-20s who presented with a complaint of central floaters and decreased visual acuity. The aggregated mid-vitreous inflammatory debris pictured here interrupted the visual axis. There is 1+ vitreal haze. (The mid-vitreous plane of focus in these fundus photographs gives the false impression of 2+ vitreal haze.)

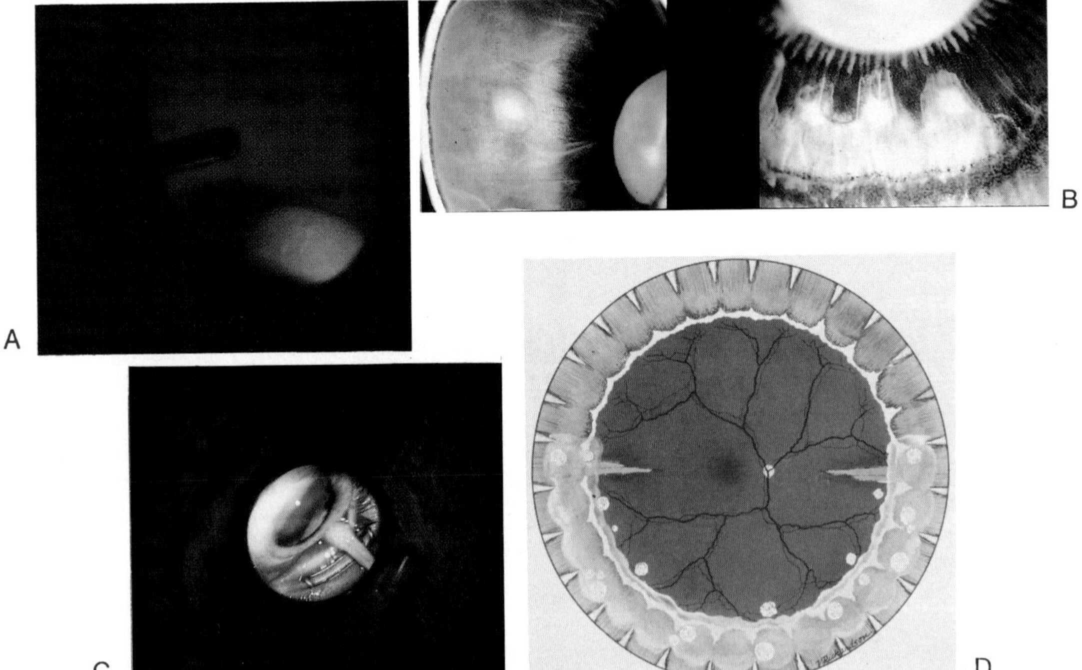

FIGURE 2–47 **"Snowbank" inflammatory aggregates.** *A,* Endoilluminated intraoperative photograph of "snowball" opacities overlying the peripheral inferior retina seen with scleral indentation. A vitrectomy instrument sits in the mid-vitreous. *B,* Gross histologic specimen of an eye demonstrating focal exudative accumulations *(left)* and "snowbank" inflammatory aggregates overlying the peripheral retina and posterior pars plana ciliaris *(right).* (Courtesy of J. D. M. Gass, M.D.) *C,* "Snowbank" exudate over the inferior vitreous base as seen by indirect ophthalmoscopy with scleral indentation. (Courtesy of Mano Swartz, M.D.) *D,* Schematic drawing depicting focal exudative accumulations and inferior "snowbank" inflammatory aggregates overlying the peripheral retina and posterior pars plana ciliaris. (From Aaberg TM, Cesarz TJ, Flickinger RR: Treatment of peripheral uveoretinitis by cryotherapy. Am J Ophthalmol 75:685–688, 1973. Published with permission from the American Journal of Ophthalmology. Copyright by the Ophthalmic Publishing Company.)

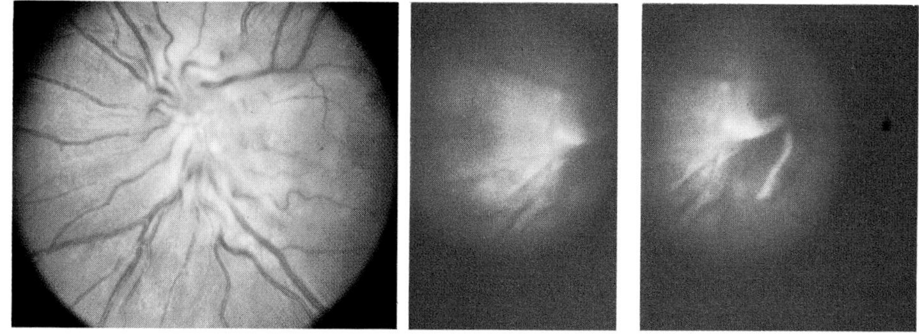

FIGURE 2–48 **Severe bilateral intermediate uveitis and neovascularization of the inferior vitreous base.** *A*, Fundus photograph of the right eye of a 7-year-old white boy who presented with bilateral intermediate uveitis and extensive neovascularization of the inferior vitreous base of both eyes. There is a tractional detachment of the macular and peripapillary retina. The gray-green area of discoloration along the temporal aspect of the disc is a localized subretinal hemorrhage. Note the loss of normal vascular tortuosity of vessels coming off the superior and inferior poles of the disc. *B*, Left eye of the same patient demonstrating a persistent hyaloid canal remnant that has become infected with neovascular tissue.

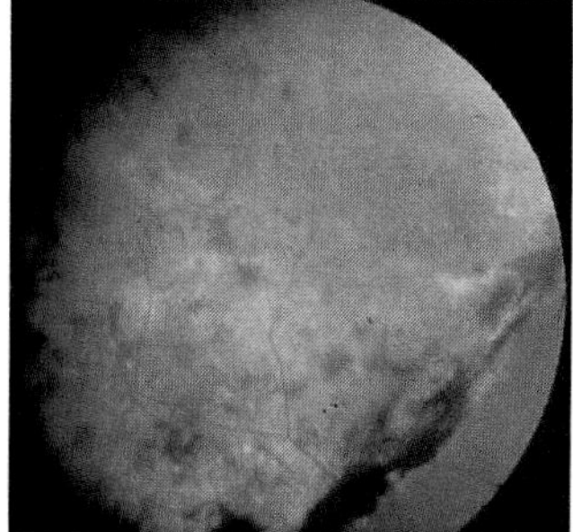

FIGURE 2–49 **Spontaneous reattachment of retinal detachment.** Demarcation line and clumped subretinal pigment indicate prior rhegmatogenous retinal detachment with spontaneous reattachment.

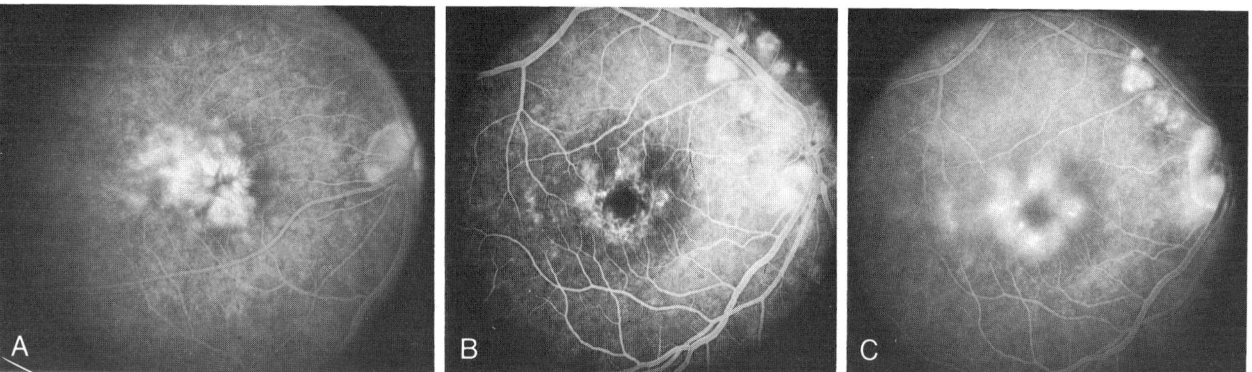

FIGURE 2–50 **Cystoid macular edema in intermediate uveitis.** *A*, Late-phase angiogram demonstrating florid classic cystoid macular edema (CME) in a patient with intermediate uveitis, the main cause of vision loss in these patients. *B*, Midvenous-phase angiogram from an eye with telangiectatic changes due to chronic posterior segment inflammation. Photocoagulation had been applied for retinal neovascularization. Treatment scars are present superotemporal to the disc. *C*, Late-phase angiogram in the same patient as in *B* demonstrating diffuse macular edema.

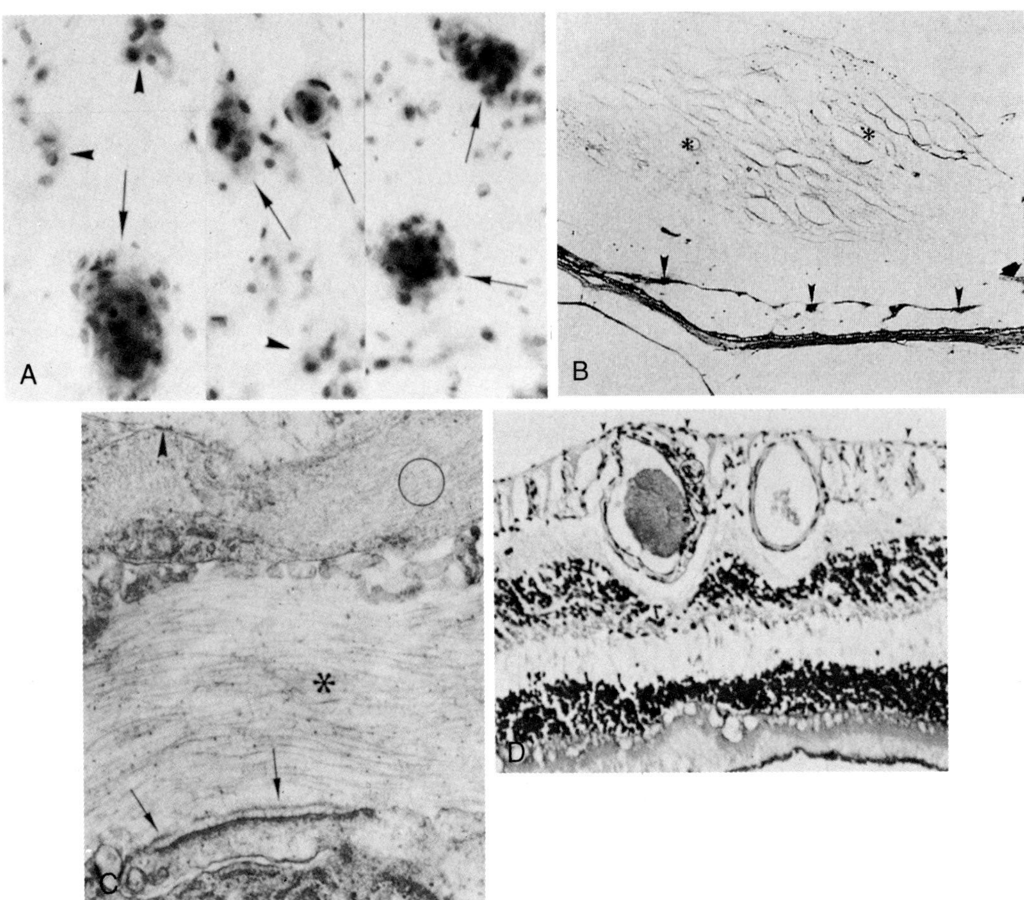

FIGURE 2–51 **Pars planitis.** *A,* Vitreous "snowballs" removed from the vitreous of a 9-year-old girl with intermediate uveitis, showing epithelioid cells *(arrowheads)* and multinucleated giant cells *(arrows).* Millipore filter, modified Papanicolaou's staining, ×500. (From Green WR, Kincaid MC, Michels RG, et al: Pars planitis. Trans Ophthalmol Soc UK 101:361, 1981.) *B,* Vitreous "snowbank" composed of collapsed, condensed vitreous; blood vessels *(asterisks);* scattered lymphocytes; spindle-shaped cells; and proliferated nonpigmented ciliary epithelium *(arrowheads).* The peripheral retina is shown by an *arrow.* H&E, ×100. *C,* Pars plana "snowbank" with cells containing 8 to 9 nm diameter intracytoplasmic filaments *(circled),* desmosome junctions *(arrowhead),* vitreous-like fibrillar collagen *(asterisk),* and segmented basement membrane 12 nm in diameter *(arrows).* ×42,000. *D,* This section from the posterior retina shows infiltration of the wall of the vein by lymphocytes *(circled).* The adjacent arteriole was not affected. A thin preretinal fibrous layer *(arrowheads)* overlies the internal limiting membrane. H&E, ×235. (From Pederson JE, Kenyon KR, Green WR, Maumenee AE: Pathology of pars planitis. Am J of Ophthalmol 86:762–774, 1978. Published with permission from the American Journal of Ophthalmology. Copyright by the Ophthalmic Publishing Company.)

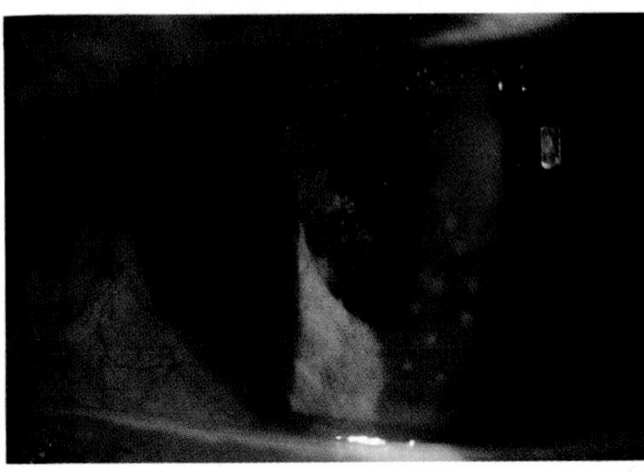

FIGURE 2–52 Granulomatous anterior uveitis in a patient with sarcoidosis.

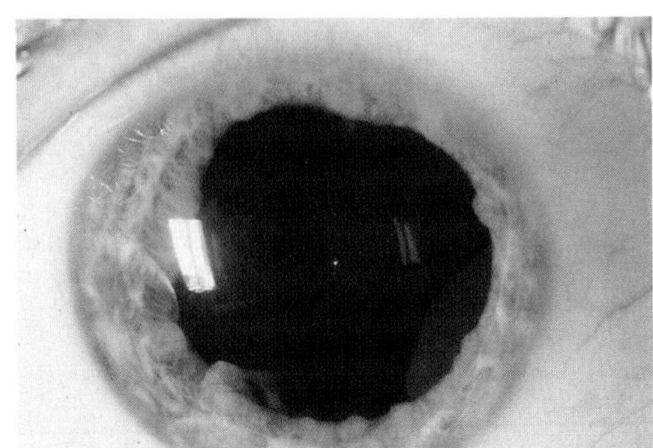

FIGURE 2–53 **Koeppe's nodules.** Nodules are present at the pupillary margin in the eye of a white woman with sarcoidosis. These nodules are precipitates of inflammatory debris. These are not true iris nodules, which consist of granulomatous inflammation within the iris substance.

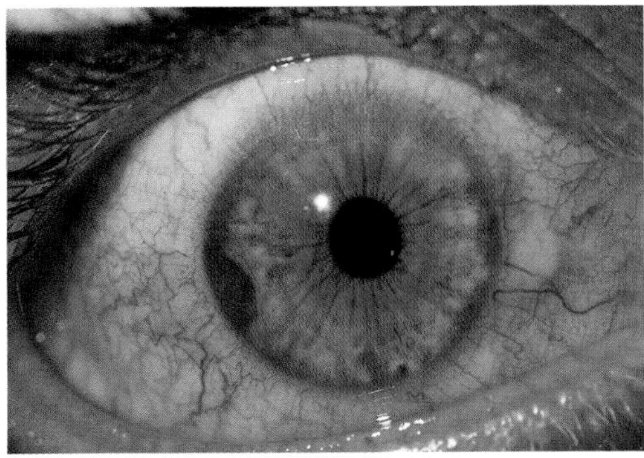

FIGURE 2–54 **True iris nodule in a sarcoidosis patient.** These true nodules can be massive, filling the anterior chamber and leading to phthisis bulbi.

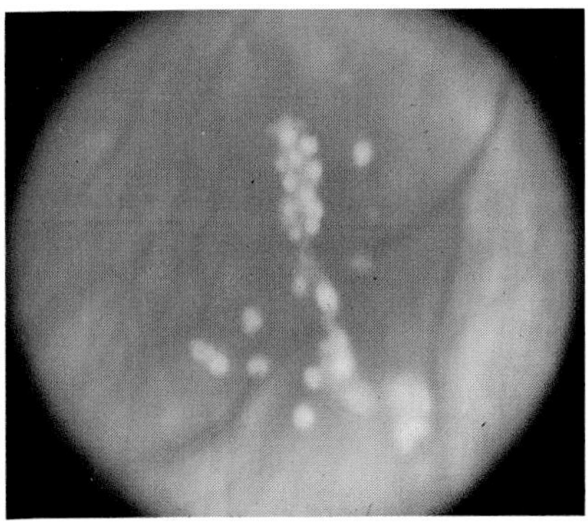

FIGURE 2–56 **Vitreous opacities in sarcoidosis.** These "snowballs" vary in size from small particles to one-third of a disc diameter, frequently occurring in chains ("string of pearls") and often casting a shadow from the examining light onto the retina.

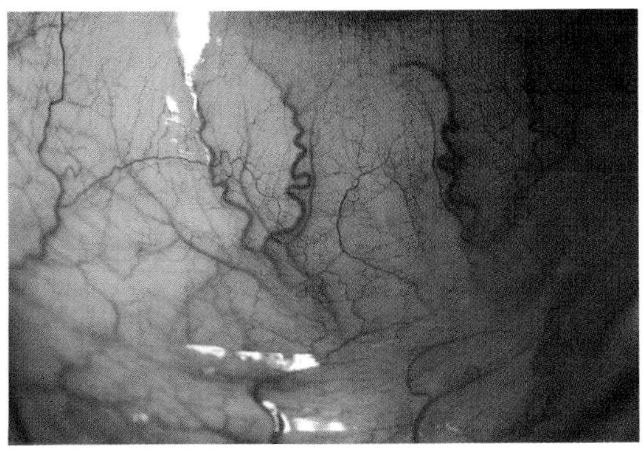

FIGURE 2–55 **Conjunctival nodules in sarcoidosis.** Nodule formation in the conjunctiva is the most common conjunctival lesion seen in this disorder.

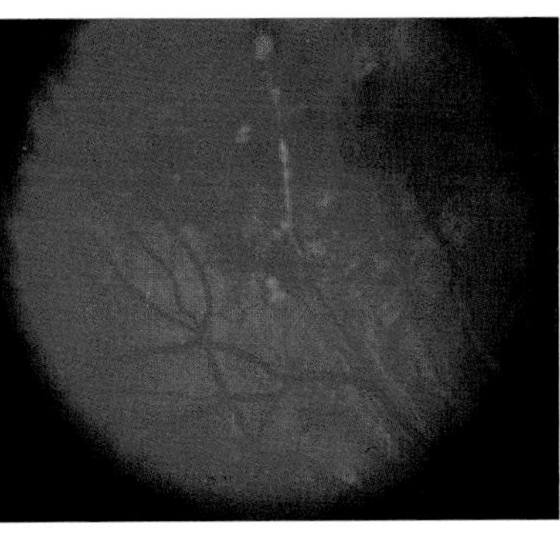

FIGURE 2–57 **"Candlewax drippings" in sarcoidosis.** These yellow waxy, discrete retinal infiltrates situated around the retinal veins are the most characteristic lesions of retinal sarcoidosis. These lesions are seen in 35 percent of patients with retinal manifestations of sarcoidosis.

FIGURE 2–58 **Optic nerve involvement with sarcoidosis.** Sarcoidosis involving the optic nerve in a 64-year-old white woman who presented to the Massachusetts Eye and Ear Infirmary with no light perception in her left eye. *A,* Before diagnosis and treatment. *B,* One week after initiation of systemic prednisone therapy, the nerve appeared less swollen. Vision was unchanged. As many as 40 percent of patients with posterior pole sarcoidosis may have optic disc changes.

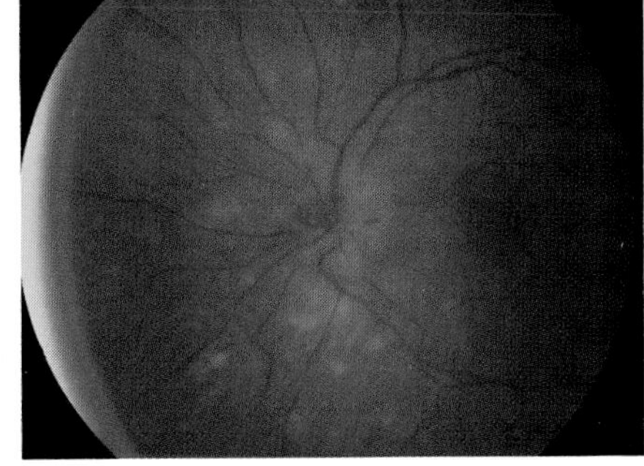

A

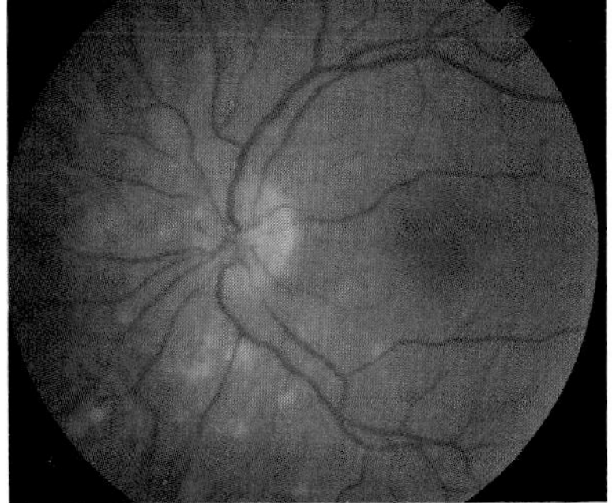

B

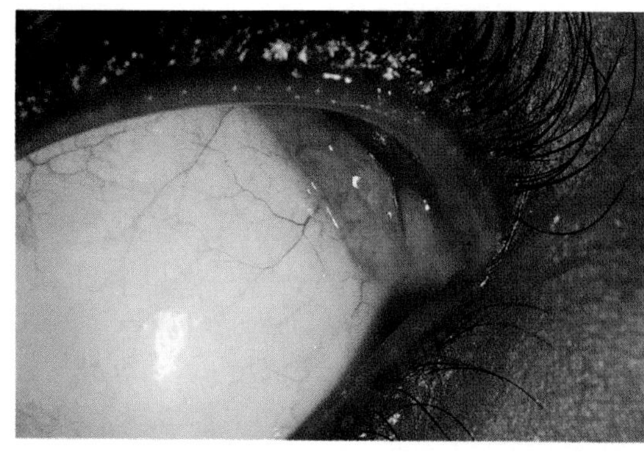

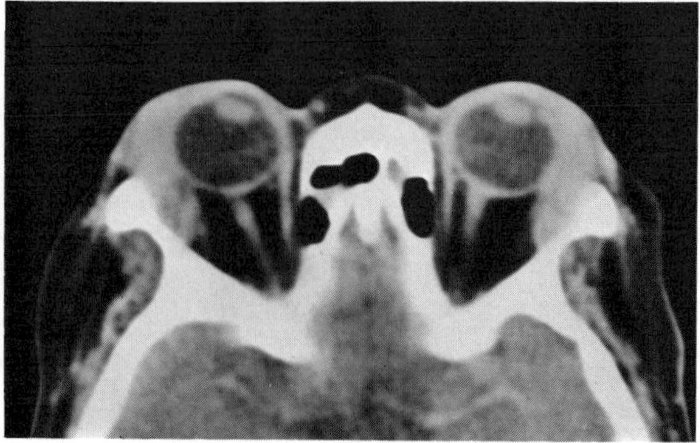

FIGURE 2-59 **Lacrimal gland enlargement in sarcoidosis.** This 30-year-old black woman has sarcoidosis. *A*, Clinical appearance of an enlarged lacrimal gland. Clinically apparent lacrimal gland enlargement is seen more frequently in patients under age 35 years. Gallium scans indicate that lacrimal gland involvement may occur in 60 to 75 percent of patients with sarcoidosis. *B*, Axial computed tomography of the orbits shows bilateral lacrimal gland enlargement. (*A* and *B*, Courtesy of Shizuo Mukai, M.D.)

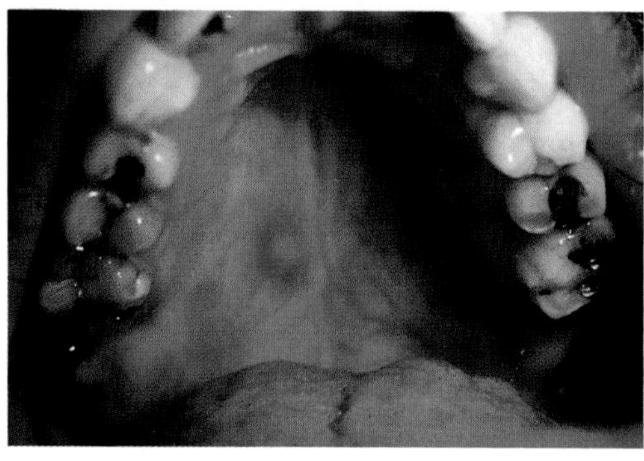

FIGURE 2-60 **Secondary syphilis.** A typical mucous membrane lesion in the mouth of a patient with secondary syphilis.

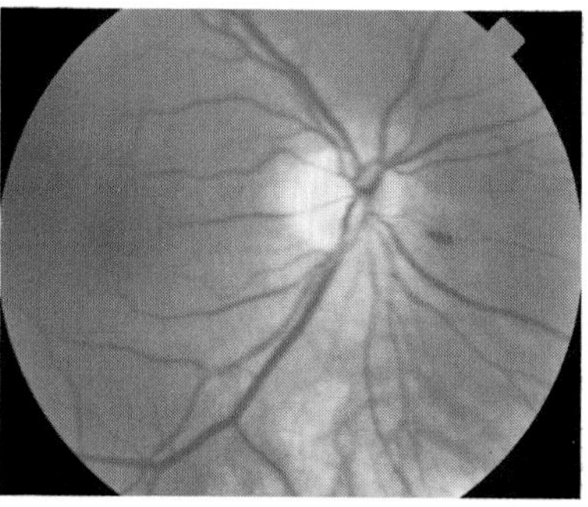

FIGURE 2-62 **Lyme disease.** The fundus photographs show a hemorrhage nasal to the disc. This retinal hemorrhage is only one of a multitude of ophthalmic manifestations caused by infection by the spirochete *Borrelia burgdorferi.*

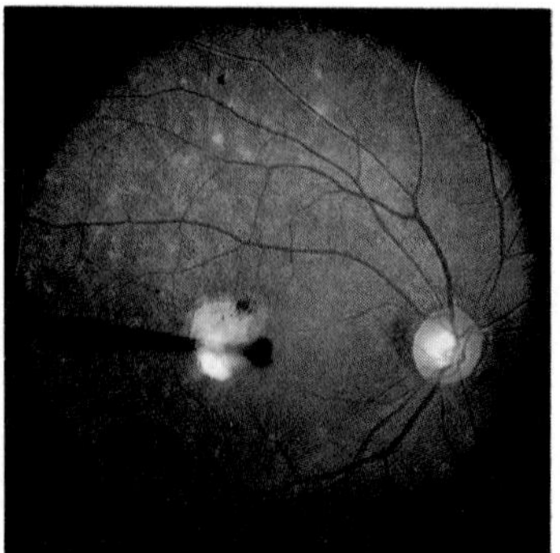

FIGURE 2-61 **Posterior segment manifestations of secondary syphilis.** This is the right eye of a patient with secondary syphilis. Note the focal and disseminated areas of lesions at the level of the choroid and retinal pigment epithelium. There are some areas of retinal pigment epithelial hyperplasia and depigmentation. Note also the area of subretinal neovascularization in the macula.

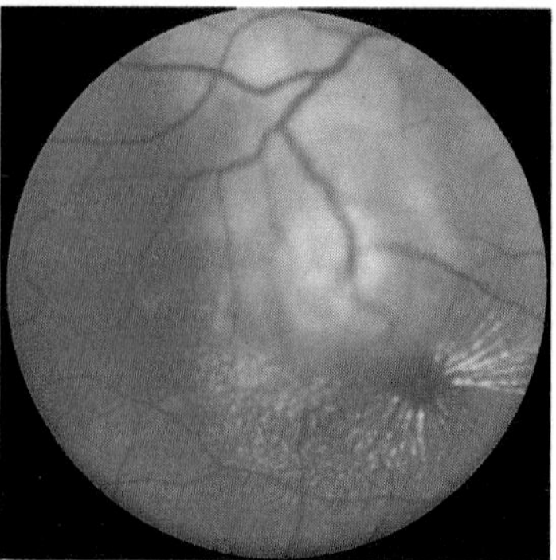

FIGURE 2-63 **Tuberculosis choroiditis.** Note the large tubercle superior to the macula. Note also the macular star of exudate accumulation.

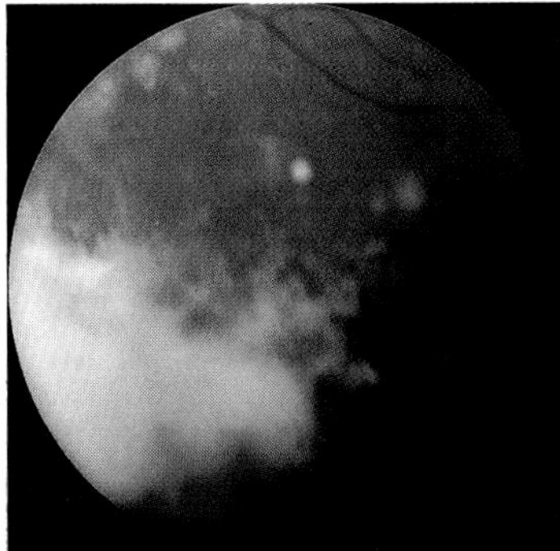

FIGURE 2–64 **Tuberculosis chorioretinitis.** A necrotizing chorioretinal lesion in a patient with tuberculosis. The most common posterior uveitis is a bilateral multifocal choroiditis, with or without overlying retinal necrosis, that may be seen with miliary or indolent tuberculosis.

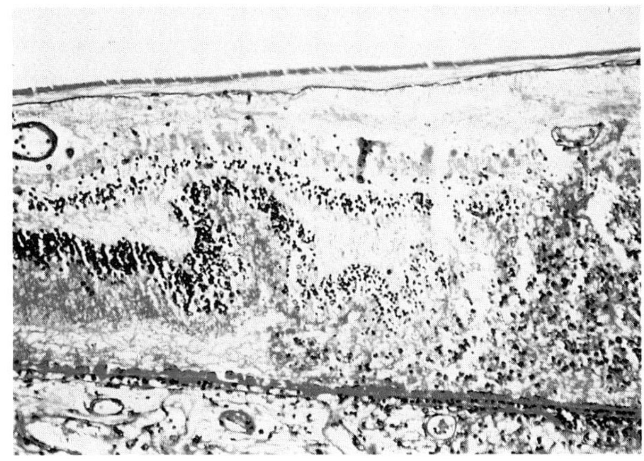

FIGURE 2–65 **Histopathology of chorioretinitis secondary to *Candida albicans*.** Note the full-thickness retinal necrosis and inflammation within the retinal layers.

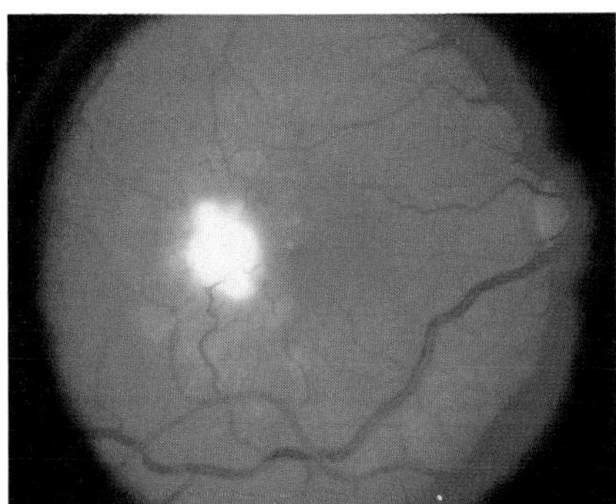

FIGURE 2–66 **Necrotizing *Candida* chorioretinitis.** A necrotizing lesion is seen adjacent to the fovea in an intravenous drug abuser with *Candida* chorioretinitis.

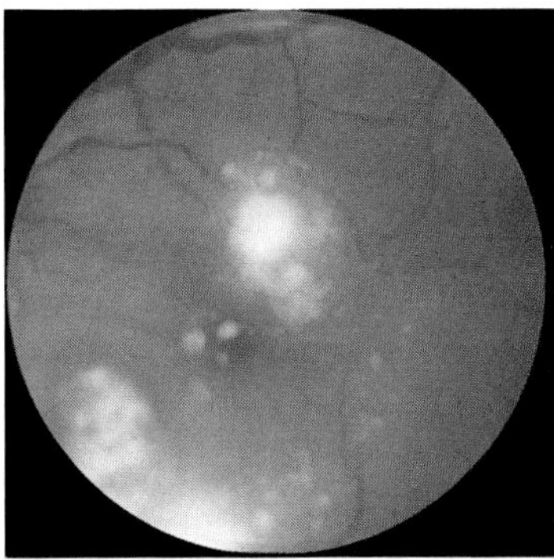

FIGURE 2–67 **Cryptococcosis necrotizing retinitis.** Fundus photograph of a renal transplant patient on immunosuppressive therapy who developed cryptococcosis of the eye and brain. Note the multifocal necrotizing lesions of the retina. In these severe cases, vascular sheathing, mutton-fat keratic precipitates, or endophthalmitis can be seen.

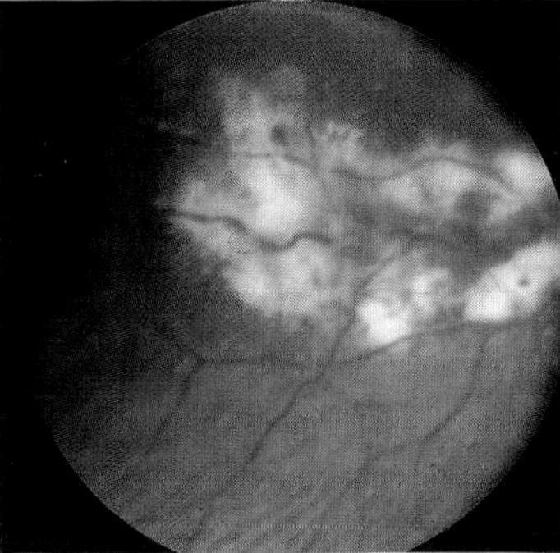

FIGURE 2–68 **Cytomegalovirus (CMV) retinitis.** Note the area of necrosis adjacent to an area of hemorrhage along a retinal vessel.

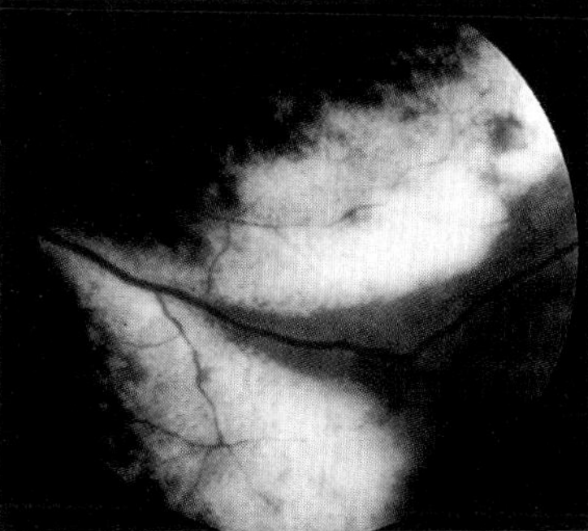

FIGURE 2–69 **CMV retinitis.** Fundus photograph showing necrotizing lesions superiorly and inferiorly in a patient with CMV retinitis. Among acquired immunodeficiency syndrome (AIDS) patients, there are two types of lesions: a slowly progressive, indolent infiltration of the retina that is usually restricted to the periphery, and a more progressive, white, necrotic lesion of the posterior pole with hemorrhage.

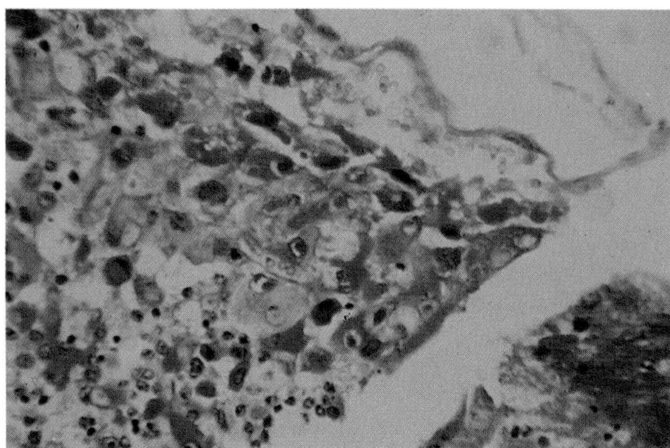

FIGURE 2–70 **Histopathology of CMV retinitis.** Photomicrograph of the retina of the patient seen in Figure 2–69 obtained after autopsy. Note the owl's eye appearance of the intracellular inclusion bodies in cells of the necrotic retina. These inclusion bodies along with multinucleated giant cells in a necrotic retina are pathognomonic for CMV retinitis.

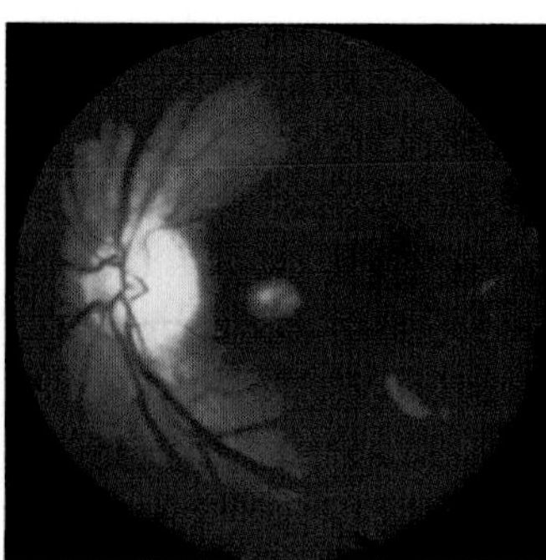

FIGURE 2–73 **Fundus photograph of a patient with subacute sclerosing panencephalitis (SSPE).** Note the areas of atrophy in and around the macula. In the early active phase of this disease, bilateral necrotizing retinitis with retinal hemorrhages and edema, cotton-wool spots, and disc edema may be seen. In the late phase, there is pigmented chorioretinal and optic nerve atrophy. (Courtesy of Gordon Klintworth, M.D.)

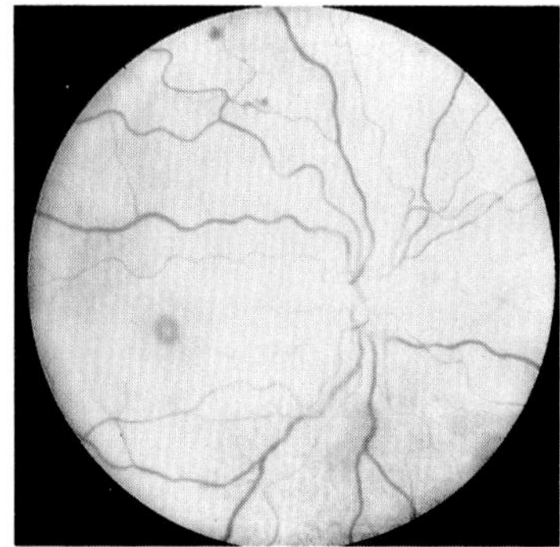

FIGURE 2–71 **Retinal necrosis with disseminated herpes simplex virus infection.** A widespread area of retinal necrosis is noted in this patient, along with overlying vitreous reaction.

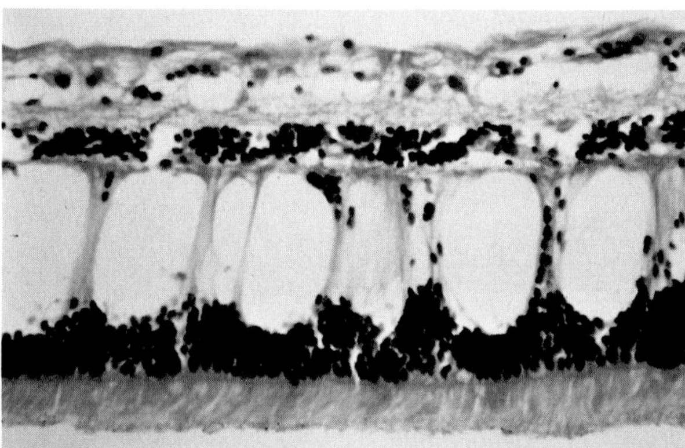

FIGURE 2–74 **Histopathology of necrotizing retinitis in SSPE.** This photomicrograph of the retina is from the patient in Figure 2–73 and shows atrophy of the inner retina along with cystoid changes in the outer plexiform layer. (Courtesy of Gordon Klintworth, M.D.)

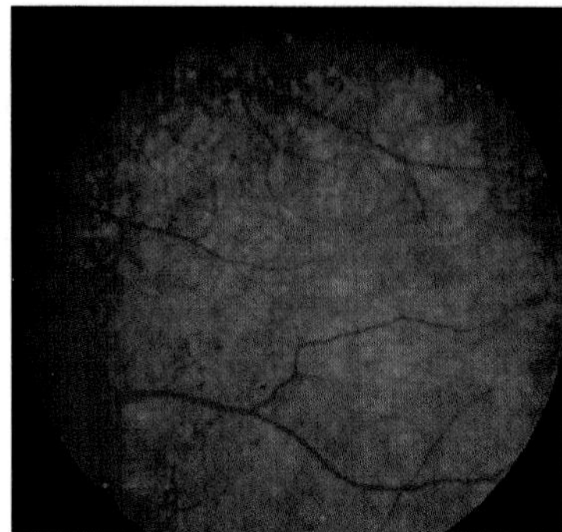

FIGURE 2–72 **"Salt-and-pepper" fundus in rubella.** Note the fine, granular, mottling of the pigment epithelium seen in this photograph of the fundus. Occasionally, pigment spicules and changes in the choroidal vasculature may be seen.

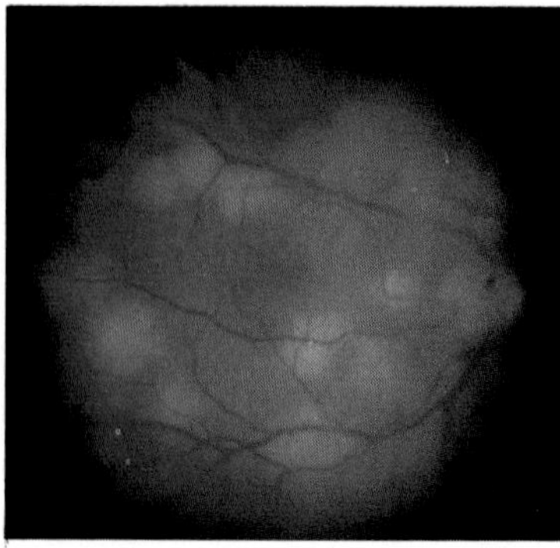

FIGURE 2–75 ***Pneumocystis carinii* choroiditis.** These choroidal lesions are in a patient with AIDS who went on pentamidine prophylactically. The association of multifocal yellow choroidal plaques in AIDS patients with disseminated *Pneumocystis carinii* infection has only recently been noted.

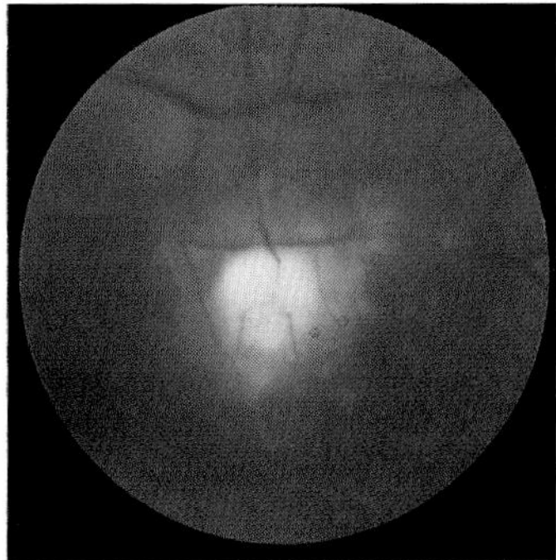

FIGURE 2-76 **Toxoplasmosis retinochoroiditis.** Clinical photograph of the necrotizing lesion in the retina of a patient with toxoplasmosis retinochoroiditis. In an immunocompetent patient with active retinochoroiditis, an isolated white fluffy focus of necrotizing retinitis is seen with associated retinal edema and vitritis. In contrast, in immunocompromised patients, the retinal lesions are multifocal and often seen bilaterally.

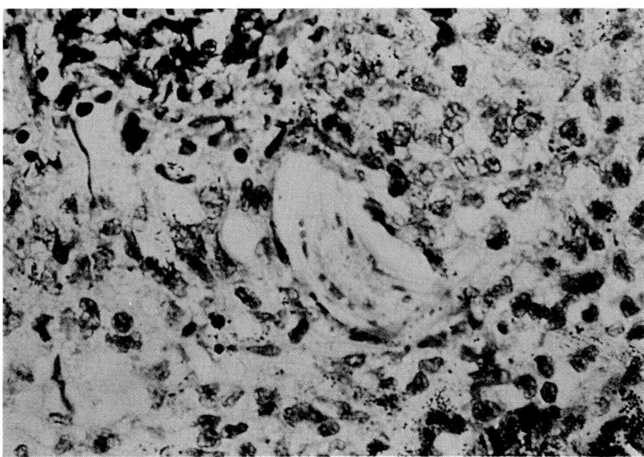

FIGURE 2-79 **Histopathology of the retina in a patient with toxocariasis.** Histologically, a focal granulomatous inflammation with prominent eosinophilic and lymphocytic infiltration is seen. Note the larva in the area of inflammation.

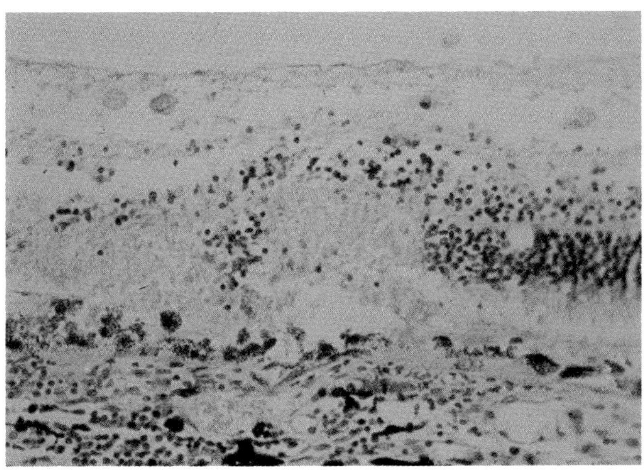

FIGURE 2-77 **Histopathology of toxoplasmosis retinochoroiditis.** Note the area of retinal necrosis on the left, whereas recognizable retinal architecture is seen on the right.

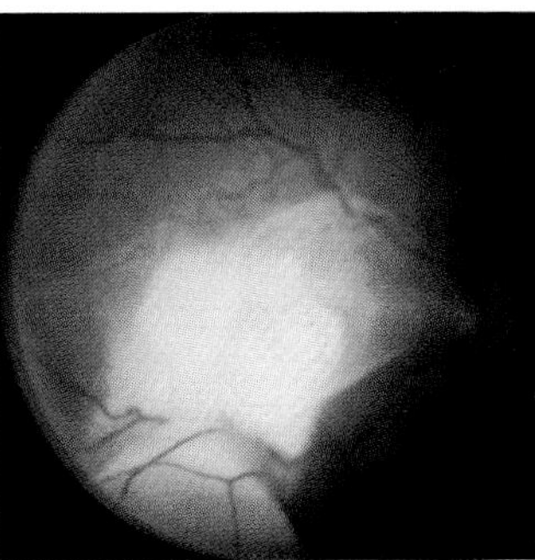

FIGURE 2-80 ***Cysticercus* larva in the subretinal space.** The most common ocular clinical manifestation is a unilateral subretinal whitish mass resulting from the larva entering the subretinal space via the posterior ciliary arteries. As the parasite grows and moves in the subretinal space, fibrous proliferation and inflammation can result.

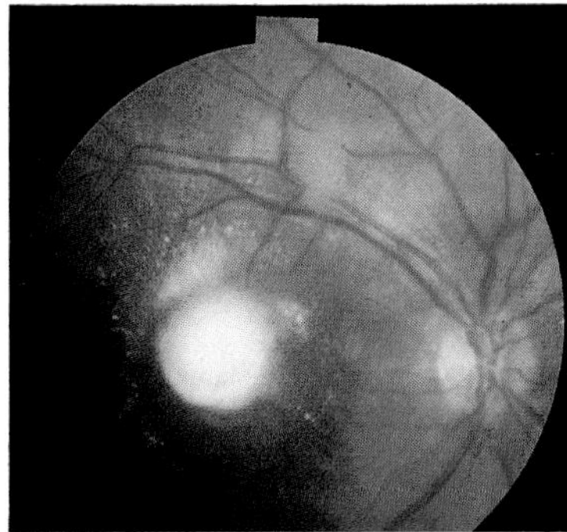

FIGURE 2-78 ***Toxocara canis* chorioretinal granuloma.** This lesion is located in the posterior pole of a patient with *Toxocara canis* infection. Along with a posterior pole granuloma, these patients can also present with a diffuse endophthalmitis or a peripheral localized granuloma.

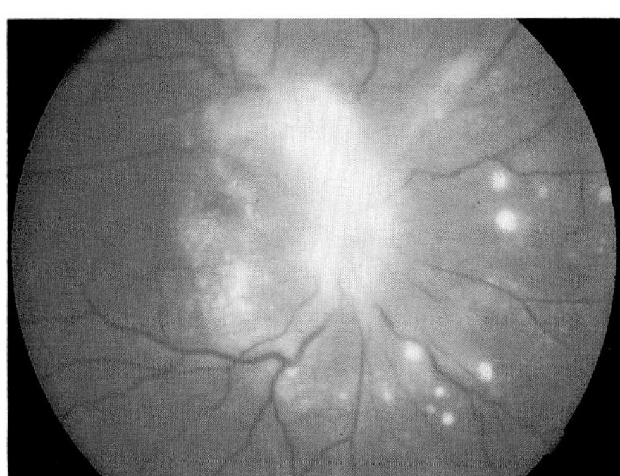

FIGURE 2-81 **Septic retinopapillitis.** A 23-year-old white woman with one abscessed necrotic tooth. Infected root canals or apical abscesses can extend into the paranasal sinuses and cause sinusitis or seed microorganisms into the circulation to cause a disseminated septic picture as depicted above.

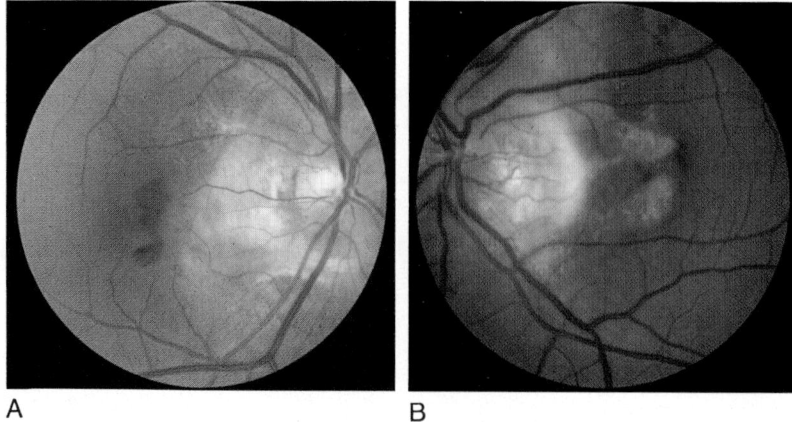

FIGURE 2–82 **Parasitic choroidosis *Entamoeba coli*.** *Entamoeba coli* was found in the stool of a 35-year-old white woman. This choroidosis is a peripapillary subretinal accumulation of opalescent fluid that may have associated hemorrhage and retinal edema. Persistence leads to a dense white subretinal exudate. *A*, Right fundus. *B*, Left fundus.

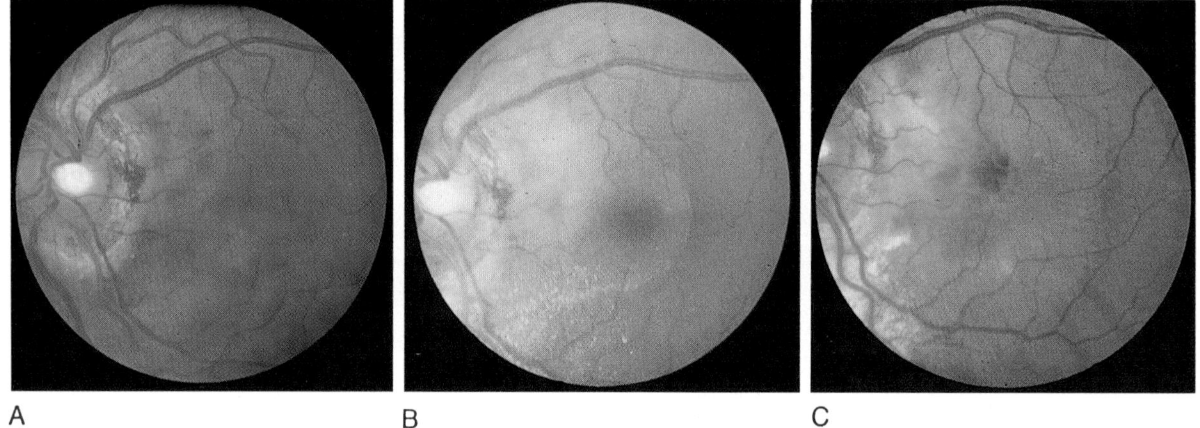

FIGURE 2–83 **Parasitic choroidosis.** *Endolimax nana* was found several times in the stools of a 35-year-old black man from Haiti. *A*, Left eye, August 15, 1977, reactivation. *B*, Left eye, November 4, 1967, extension. *C*, Left eye, June 4, 1968, less active.

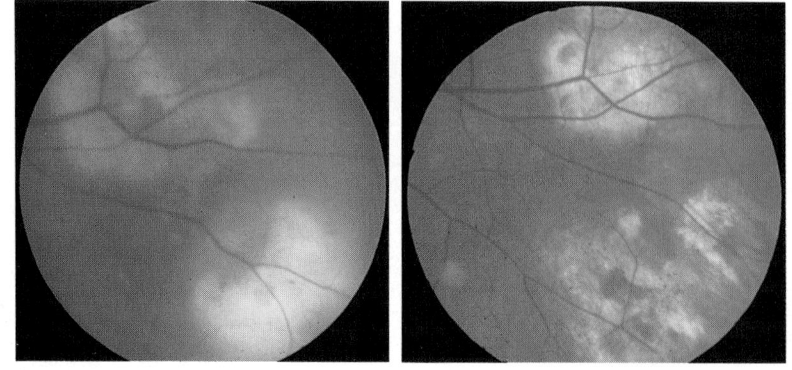

FIGURE 2–84 **Septic choroiditis.** Assumed abdominal abscess in a 25-year-old white woman. *A*, March 3, 1973, active lesion. *B*, July 10, 1973, inactive lesion after treatment with oral tetracycline.

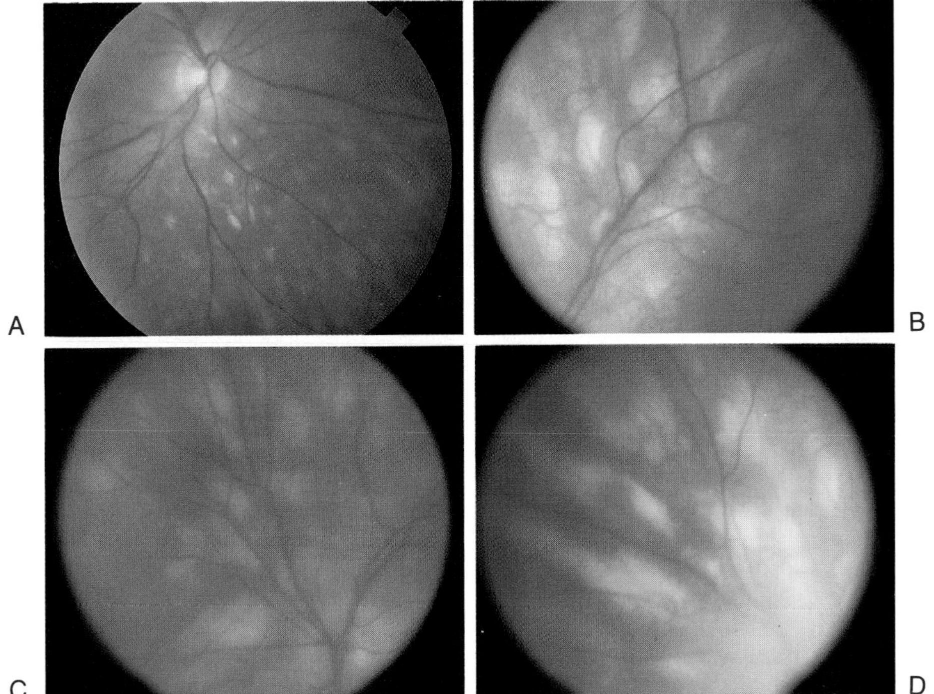

FIGURE 2–85 **Spectrum of retinochoroidal lesions in birdshot.** *A,* The small, ovoid, and depigmented nature of the lesions that lie deep to the retina. These lesions are typically located in the postequatorial fundus and often assume a radial orientation. *B,* Slightly larger, cream-colored lesions. *C* and *D,* Larger lesions with geographic involvement and lack of secondary pigmentation. The lesions still maintain a radial orientation and have "soft" borders. Vitreous haze is noted secondary to active vitritis. Cystoid macular edema is also common in birdshot retinochoroiditis.

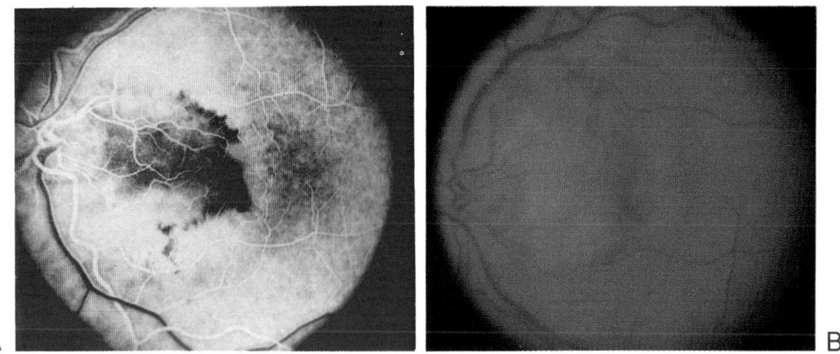

FIGURE 2–86 **Subretinal neovascular membrane formation in a patient with birdshot retinochoroiditis.** The visual acuity was 20/400 in this eye as a result of this process. *A,* Subretinal hemorrhage and fluid in the macula. *B,* A peripapillary juxtafoveal subretinal neovascular membrane extends to the fovea.

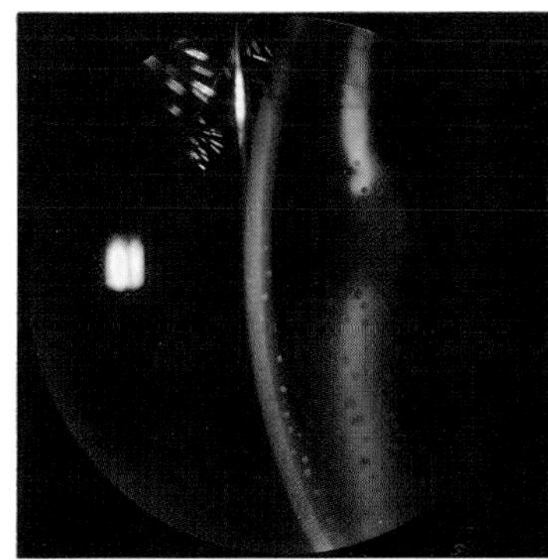

FIGURE 2–87 **Vogt-Koyanagi-Harada (VKH) disease.** Granulomatous, "mutton-fat" keratic precipitates on the corneal endothelium of a patient with VKH.

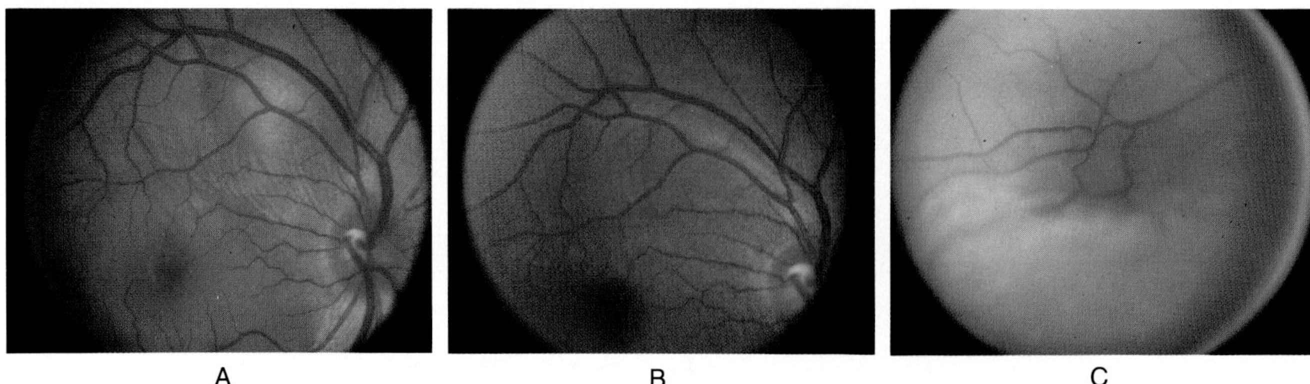

FIGURE 2–88 **Acute presentation of retinal exudation in VKH disease.** *A*, A retinal pigment epithelial detachment is seen along the superotemporal arcade, and a serous macular detachment is also present. Note the retinal striae. *B*, These largely resolved after 1 week of systemic steroid therapy. *C*, Serous retinal detachment in another patient with VKH disease. (*C*, Courtesy of the Armed Forces Institute of Pathology.)

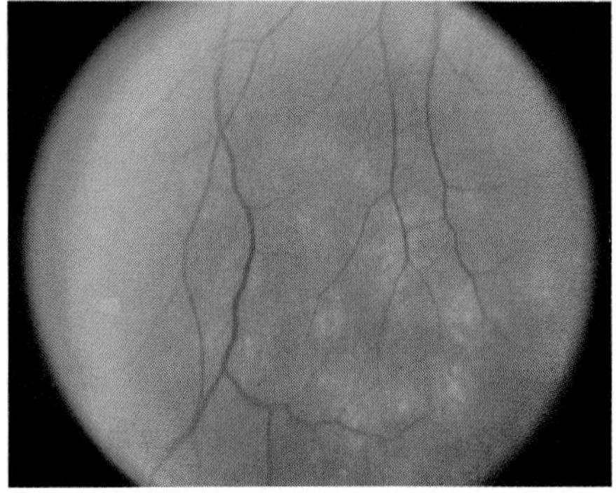

FIGURE 2–89 **Retinal pigment epithelium granulomas in VKH.** Numerous peripheral granulomatous lesions at the level of the retinal pigment epithelium, similar to Dalen-Fuchs nodules, were present in this patient.

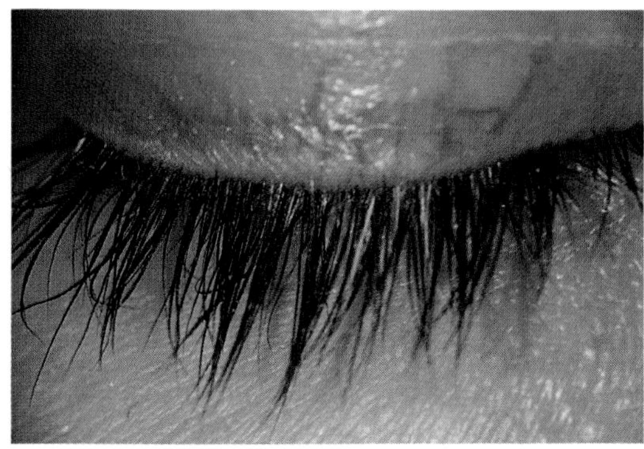

FIGURE 2–91 Lashes showing poliosis in a patient with VKH.

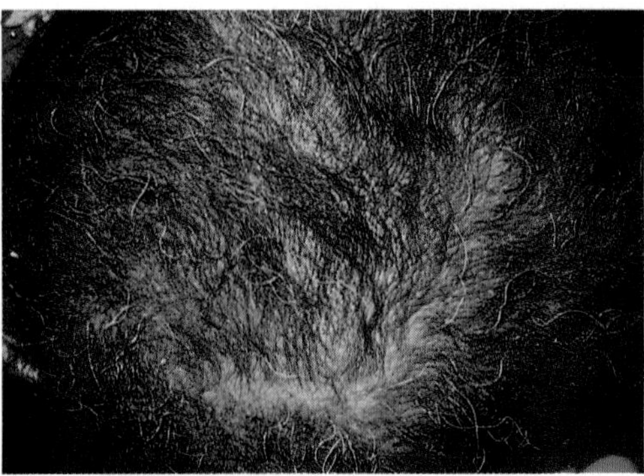

FIGURE 2–90 Alopecia in a patient with VKH.

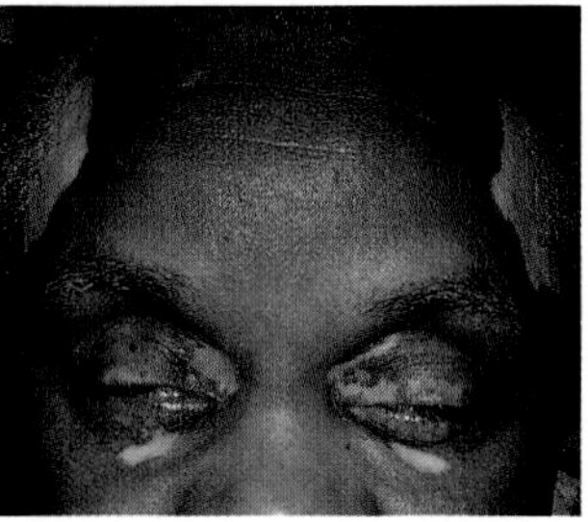

FIGURE 2–92 VKH disease showing a bilateral symmetric distribution of vitiligo.

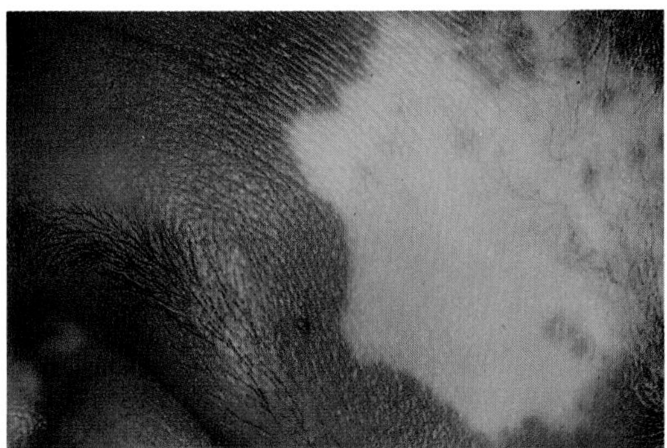

FIGURE 2–93 A prominent region of vitiligo in a black patient with VKH. (Courtesy of the Armed Forces Institute of Pathology.)

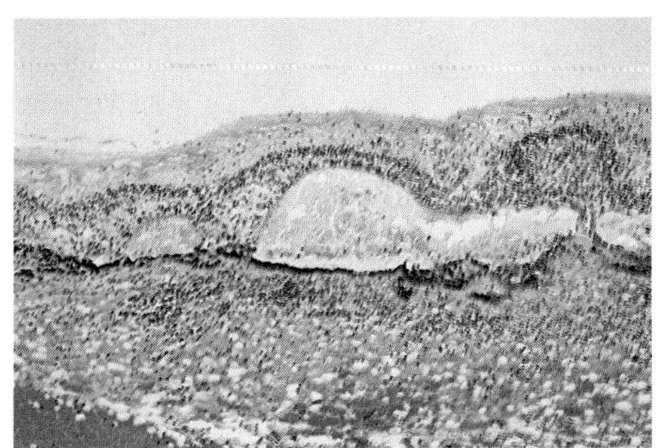

FIGURE 2–94 **Chorioretinal adhesions in VKH.** Areas of chorioretinal adhesion with focal proliferation of the retinal pigment epithelium. Lymphocytic infiltrates and edema are noted throughout the detached choroid. Blood fills the suprachoroidal space. These focal chorioretinal scars have been observed clinically to prevent a total bullous retinal detachment in the late stages of this disease. H&E, ×110. (Courtesy of Armed Forces Institute of Pathology.)

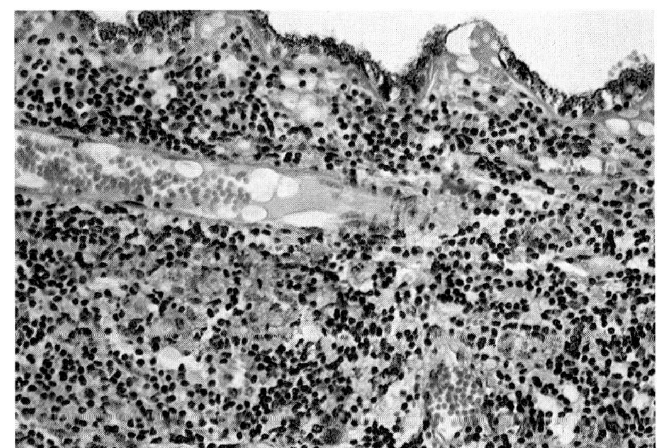

FIGURE 2–95 **Marked choroiditis in VKH.** Fully defined nests of epithelioid cells present throughout the thickened choroid with a moderate lymphocytic infiltrate in the eye of a patient with VKH. H&E, ×395. (Courtesy of Armed Forces Institute of Pathology.)

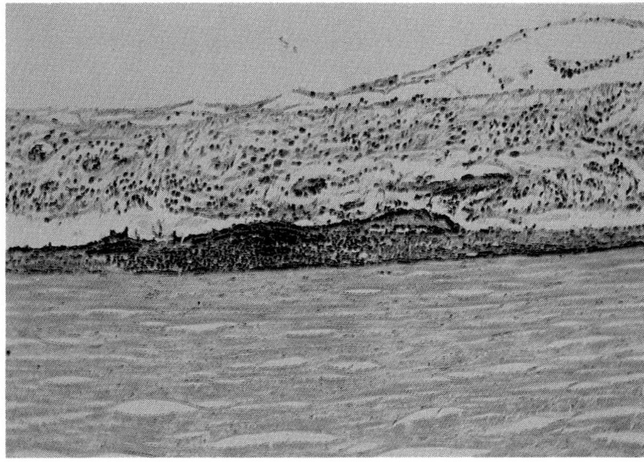

FIGURE 2–96 **Retinal gliosis in VKH.** Focal collections of lymphocytes in the choroid and proliferation of the retinal pigment epithelium with migration into the disorganized, gliosed retina are present. A thick, preretinal glial membrane is noted. H&E, ×115. (Courtesy of the Armed Forces Institute of Pathology.)

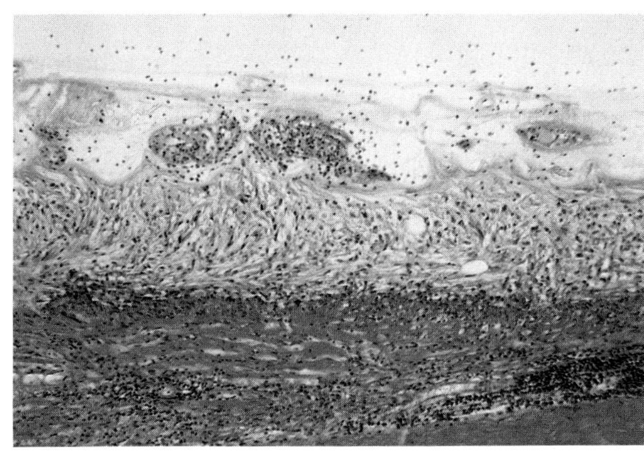

FIGURE 2–97 **Epiretinal membrane and gliosis of retina in VKH.** The markedly gliosed retina has wrinkling of the internal limiting membrane with neovascular nodules extending into the vitreous cavity, which contains a moderate number of chronic inflammatory cells. H&E, ×110. (Courtesy of the Armed Forces Institute of Pathology.)

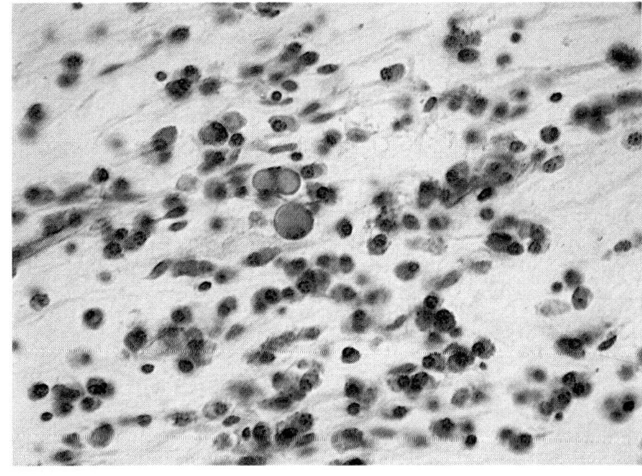

FIGURE 2–98 **Plasmacytic infiltrate in iris of patient with VKH.** Note the multitude of plasma cells and a few Russell bodies that are present within the iris of this patient with VKH. H&E, ×395. (Courtesy of the Armed Forces Institute of Pathology.)

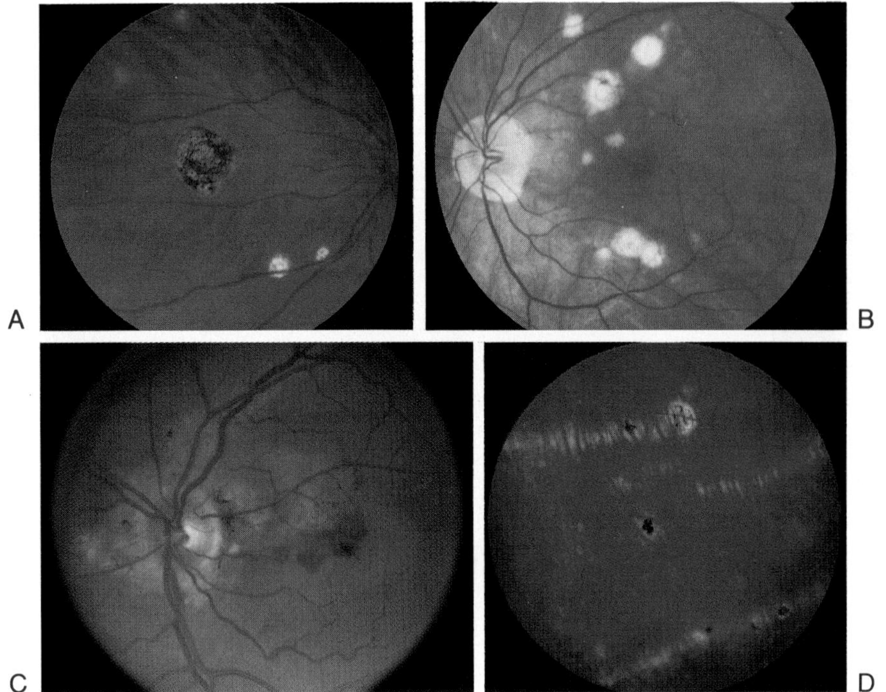

FIGURE 2–99 **Characteristic fundus lesions of the presumed ocular histoplasmosis syndrome (POHS).** *A,* Peripheral atrophic scars. Note the variable pigmentation among the scars. *B,* Peripapillary and macular atrophic scars. *C,* Peripapillary scars with associated choroidal neovascularization extending into the fovea. *D,* Linear peripheral streak lesions. The vitreous is quiet in patients with POHS.

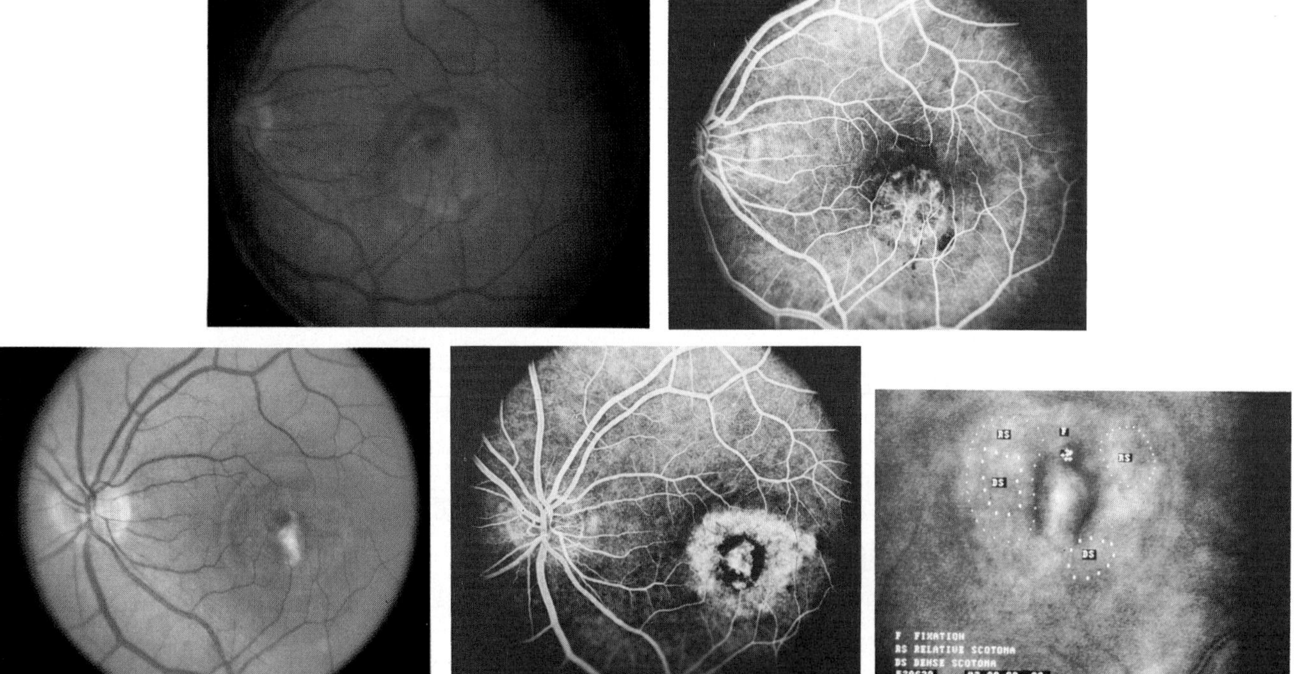

FIGURE 2–100 Glucocorticosteroid treatment for a choroidal neovascularization beneath the fovea in multifocal choroiditis. *A,* Color photograph showing a disciform lesion of the macula with subretinal hemorrhage and a serous detachment of the macula. *B,* Venous-phase fluorescein angiograms showing extensive choroidal neovascularization involving the fovea. Visual acuity was counting fingers at 3 feet. *C,* Color photograph 2 years later after periocular steroid injection showing a quiescent regressed choroidal neovascular membrane. *D,* Venous-phase fluorescein angiogram showing quiescent regressed choroidal neovascular membrane. *E,* Scanning laser ophthalmoscopic study showing preservation of foveal fixation. Visual acuity was 20/25.

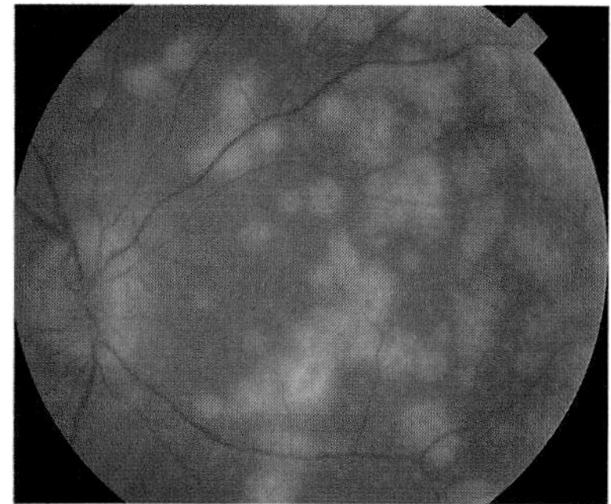

FIGURE 2–101 **Sympathetic ophthalmia post surgery.** A 40-year-old man had had multiple surgical procedures on his left eye by age 8 years for congenital cataract, glaucoma, and strabismus. When he was 39 years of age, his left eye was removed because of phthisis bulbi. Ocular inflammation occurred with visual decline to 20/40 in the right eye. Despite 1 year of intensive corticosteroid and cyclophosphamide (Cytoxan) systemic therapy, coupled with three plasmaphereses, the sympathetic ophthalmia in his right eye was not brought under control. At the time of referral, there were many yellowish confluent and nonconfluent choroidal infiltrates in the right eye, most pronounced, as depicted here, nasal to the optic disk. Note also the hyperemia of the optic nerve head. (Courtesy of Dr. Evangelos Gragoudas.)

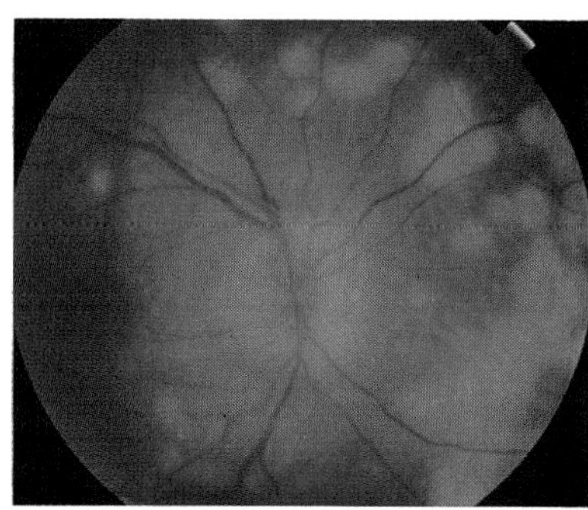

FIGURE 2–102 Same patient as in Figure 2–101, 1 month later, without a change in therapy. There is more swelling of the optic nerve head, enlargement of the choroidal infiltrates, and extension of the process in a circumpapillary fashion toward the temporal macular area. (Courtesy of Dr. Evangelos Gragoudas.)

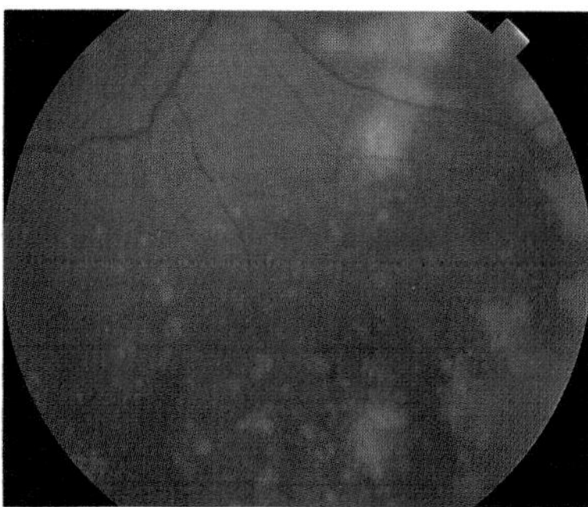

FIGURE 2–103 Same patient as in Figure 2–101. At the equatorial region, there are myriad small yellowish infiltrates at the level of the retinal pigment epithelium, corresponding to Dalen-Fuchs nodules. Cyclosporine (200 mg/day) was introduced along with prednisone, and a remarkable improvement in the condition was achieved. (Courtesy of Dr. Evangelos Gragoudas.)

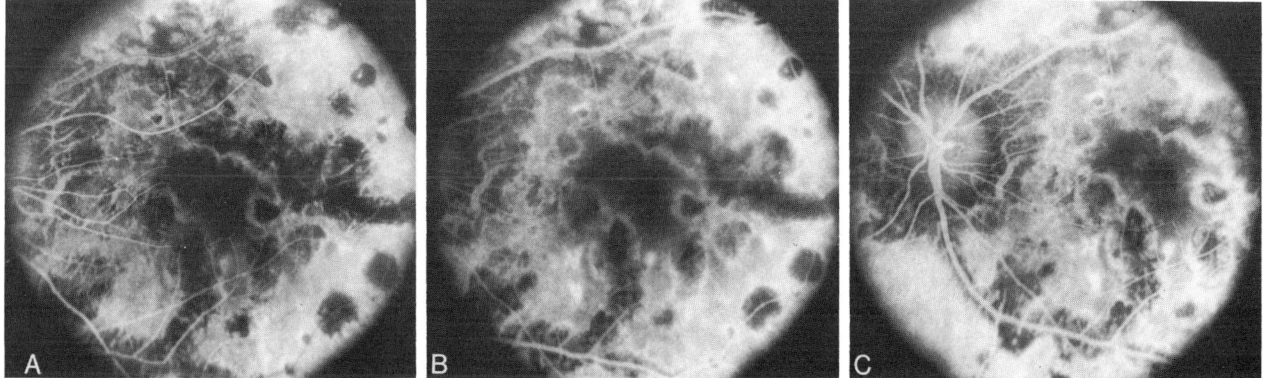

FIGURE 2–104 **Fluorescein angiogram of sympathetic ophthalmia.** *A*, Fluorescein angiogram reveals a large geographic zone and surrounding discrete round areas of nonperfusion of the choroidal infiltrates nasal to the nerve head shown in Figures 2–101 and 2–102. *B* and *C*, Later in the angiogram, dye begins to accumulate at the edges of the round nonperfused choroidal lesions, and the large geographic zone has somewhat diminished in size. Several minutes later (not shown here), there was leakage of dye into the centers of the lesions. (*A–C*, Courtesy of Dr. Evangelos Gragoudas.)

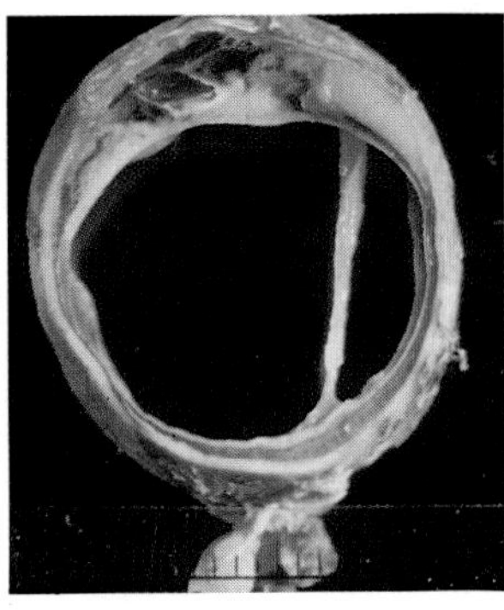

FIGURE 2-105 **Gross photograph of eye with sympathetic ophthalmia.** The pupillooptic section of a globe affected with sympathetic ophthalmia manifests anterior segment disorganization from antecedent trauma, retinal detachment, and marked inflammatory choroidal thickening.

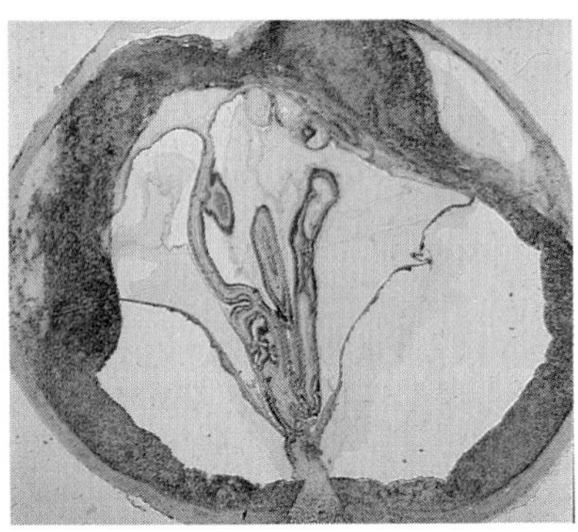

FIGURE 2-106 **Photomicrograph of a globe affected with sympathetic ophthalmia.** Note the dramatic uveal thickening from a panuveitis that extends throughout the choroid posteriorly and creates anterior ciliary body and iris masses. The retina is totally detached. The pale-staining areas in the uveal infiltrate are due to foci of granulomatous inflammation.

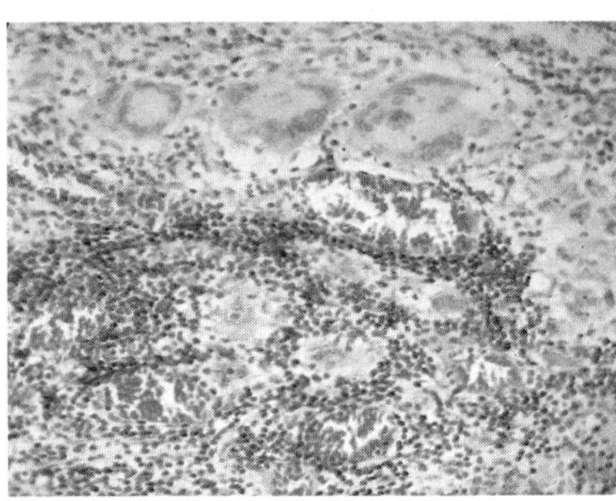

FIGURE 2-108 **Histopathology of sympathetic ophthalmia.** Pale-staining mononucleated epithelioid cells and multinucleated giant cells are intermixed with lymphocytes. Plasma cells are conspicuously absent, and the inflammation is nonnecrotizing.

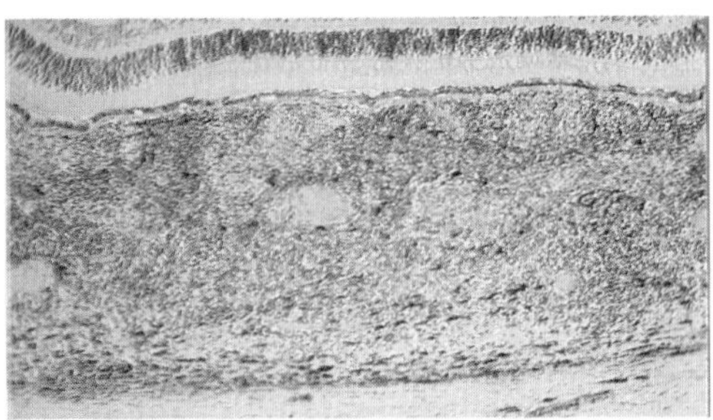

FIGURE 2-107 **Histopathology of sympathetic ophthalmia.** A moderately intense lymphocytic infiltrate in the posterior choroid contains interspersed and randomly organized granulomatous elements that are more pale-staining. Note that the choriocapillaris has been preserved as a thin layer immediately beneath the undisturbed pigment epithelium. The photoreceptors of the retina display remarkable preservation of their orientation in this case.

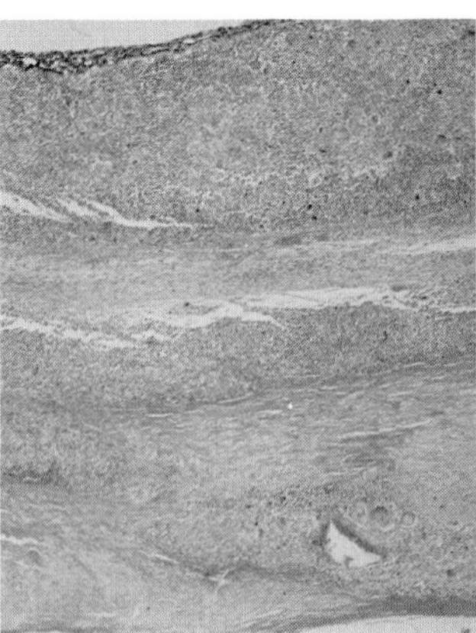

FIGURE 2-109 **Histopathology of sympathetic ophthalmia.** Marked granulomatous inflammation of the choroid in a case of sympathetic ophthalmia. Note extension of the process through the sclera at the site of an emissary vessel, shown clearly toward the bottom.

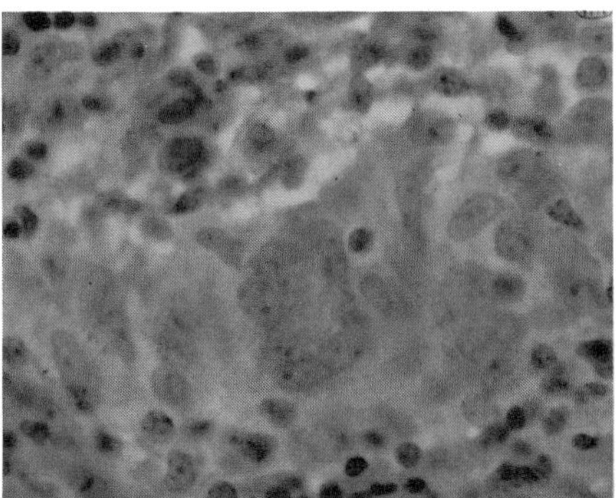

FIGURE 2–110 Multinucleated giant cells containing a white dispersion of monoparticulate melanin granules.

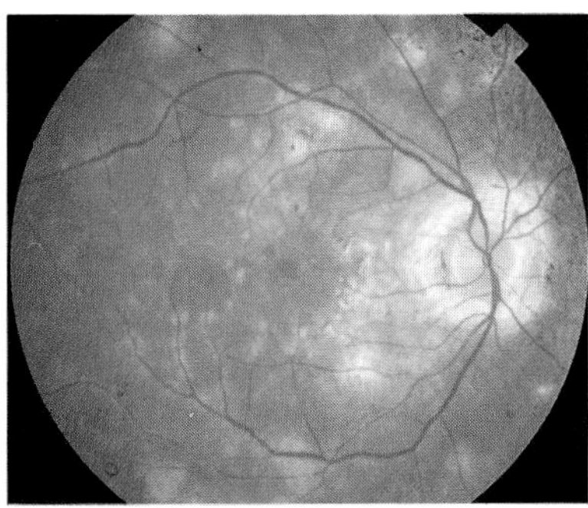

FIGURE 2–113 **Sympathetic ophthalmia post treatment.** Quiescent appearance of the fundus of the patient shown in Figures 2–101 and 2–102 after 2 years of therapy with cyclosporine and prednisone. Vision is 20/40 with multiple areas of chorioretinal atrophy and scarring, including pigment clumping with relative sparing of the macula. Note the circumpapillary atrophy and the venous perivascular sheathing in the perimacular region. Fluorescein angiography failed to disclose any dye leakage. (Courtesy of Dr. Evangelos Gragoudas.)

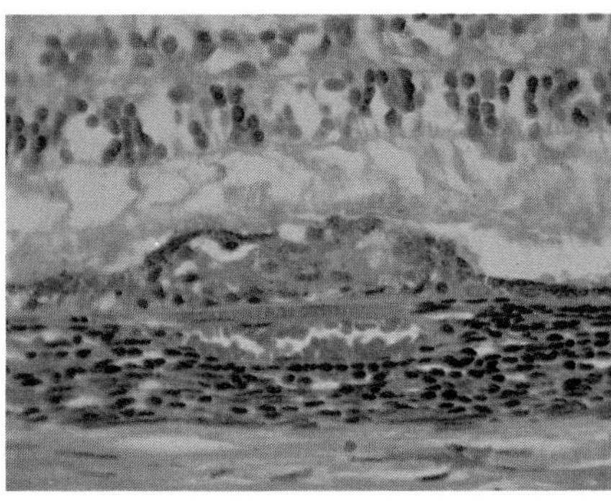

FIGURE 2–111 **Histopathology of sympathetic ophthalmia.** A placoid Dalen-Fuchs nodule, which is a collection of epithelioid cells situated above Bruch's membrane and covered by an intact or interrupted pigment epithelium. Note the misalignment and degeneration of the overlying photoreceptors. There is a nongranulomatous lymphocytic infiltrate in this segment of minimally thickened choroid.

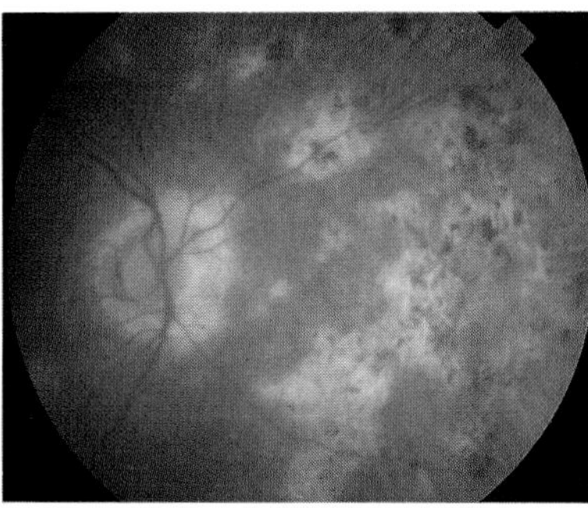

FIGURE 2–114 **Sympathetic ophthalmia post treatment.** Extensive chorioretinal atrophy with pigmentary disturbance nasal to the disc, corresponding to the resolution of the lesions shown in Figure 2–101. The patient is being maintained on low doses of cyclosporine (5 mg/day) and prednisone (10 mg/day). He has had a successful cataract extraction with posterior chamber lens implantation following the development of a subcapsular cataract from his sustained high doses of prednisone during the previous 2 years. (Courtesy of Dr. Evangelos Gragoudas.)

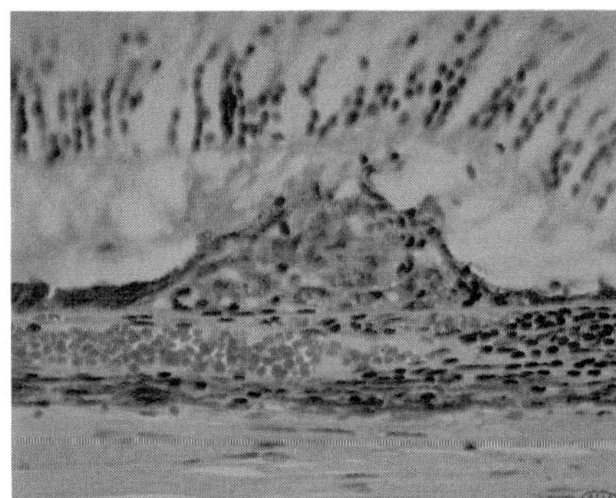

FIGURE 2–112 **Histopathology of sympathetic ophthalmia.** A more moundlike Dalen-Fuchs nodule reaching the outer limiting membrane of the retina has caused disruption of the surface covering of attenuated pigment epithelial cells. This leads to window defects during fluorescein angiography.

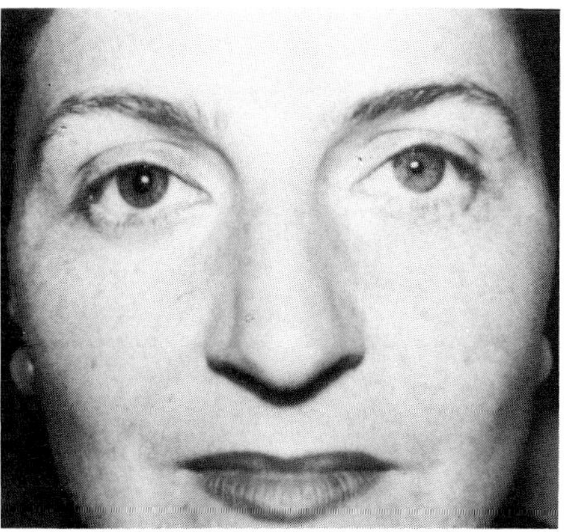

FIGURE 2–115 Full-face view of a patient with Fuchs' heterochromic iridocyclitis (FHI) affecting the right eye. The apparent hyperchromia of the right (affected) iris is due to the anterior border layer and stromal atrophy revealing the underlying iris pigment epithelium. (From O'Conner GR: Heterochromic iridocyclitis. Trans Ophthal Soc UK 104:221, 1985.)

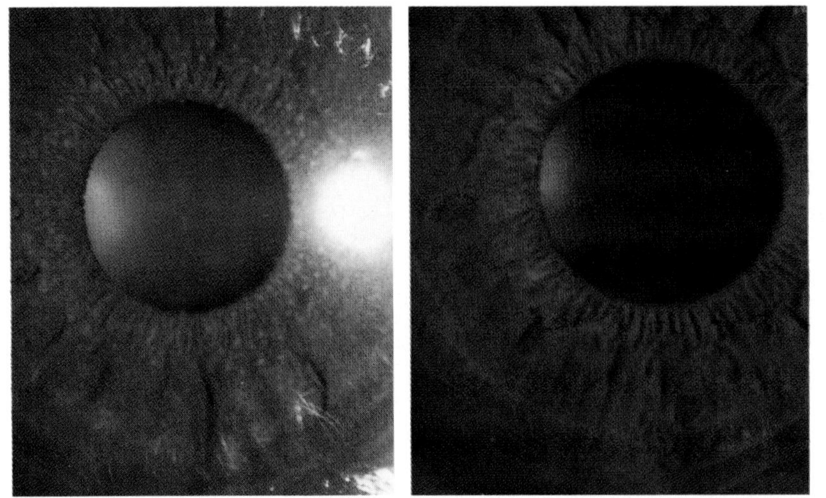

FIGURE 2–116 **FHI affecting the right eye *(A)*.** Heterochromia is subtle. Mild iris atrophy is detectable. Small peripupillary iris nodules are present. These nodules may be found in up to one-third of cases. (From Jones NP: Fuchs' heterochromic uveitis: A reappraisal of the clinical spectrum. Eye 5:653, 1991.)

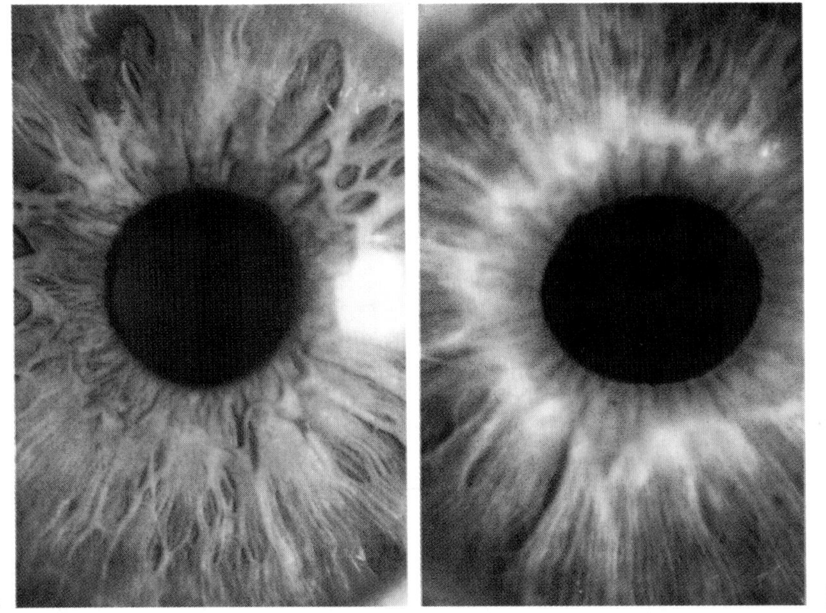

FIGURE 2–117 **FHI affecting the left eye *(B)*.** Heterochromia is due to depigmentation of the anterior border layer, resulting in a whitish, hazy appearance around the collarette. (From Jones NP: Fuchs' heterochromic uveitis: A reappraisal of the clinical spectrum. Eye 5:653, 1991.)

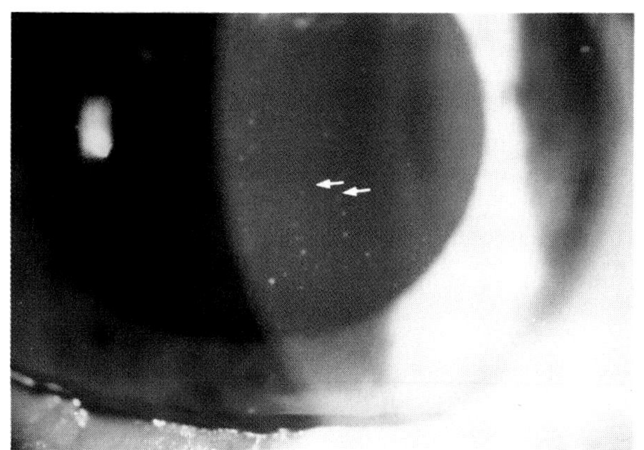

FIGURE 2–118 **Keratic precipitates in a patient with FHI.** The keratic precipitates are predominantly found on the inferior cornea but commonly extend superiorly. These keratic precipitates are stellate with interspersed wispy filaments *(arrows)*.

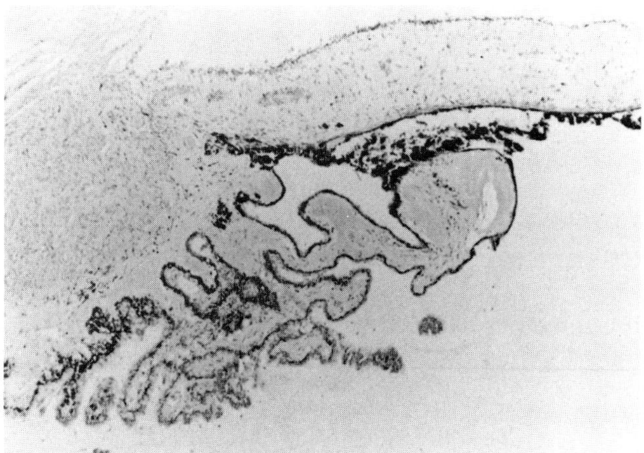

FIGURE 2–120 **Iris histology in FHI.** There is atrophy of the iris and ciliary body and hyalinization of the ciliary body stroma. Note the diffuse infiltration by plasma cells. H&E. (From O'Connor GR: Heterochromic iridocyclitis. Trans Ophthalmol Soc UK 104:225, 1985.)

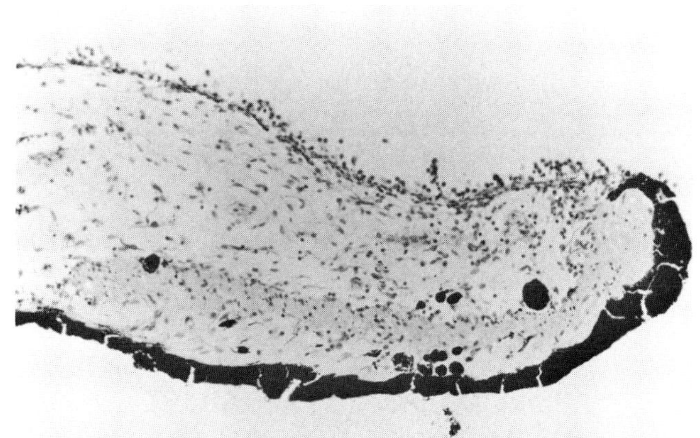

FIGURE 2–119 **Iris histology in FHI.** The anterior border layer of the iris is covered with plasma cells. H&E. (From O'Connor GR: Heterochromic unicycliastrae. Trans Ophthalmol Soc UK 104:225, 1985.)

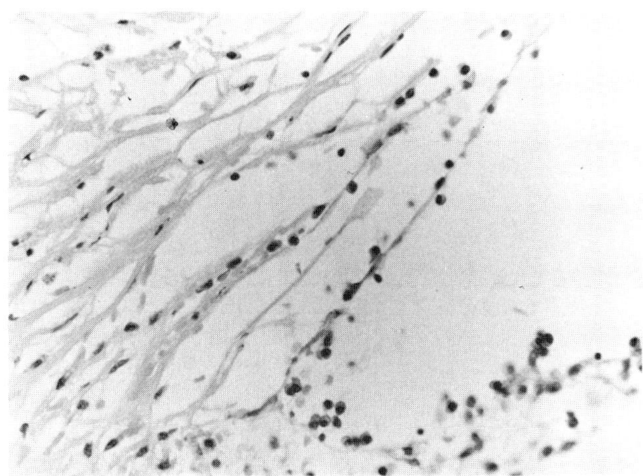

FIGURE 2–121 **Trabecular meshwork histology in FHI.** There is infiltration of the trabecular meshwork by plasma cells. H&E. (From O'Connor GR: Heterochromic iridocyclitis. Trans Ophthalmol Soc UK 104:225, 1985.)

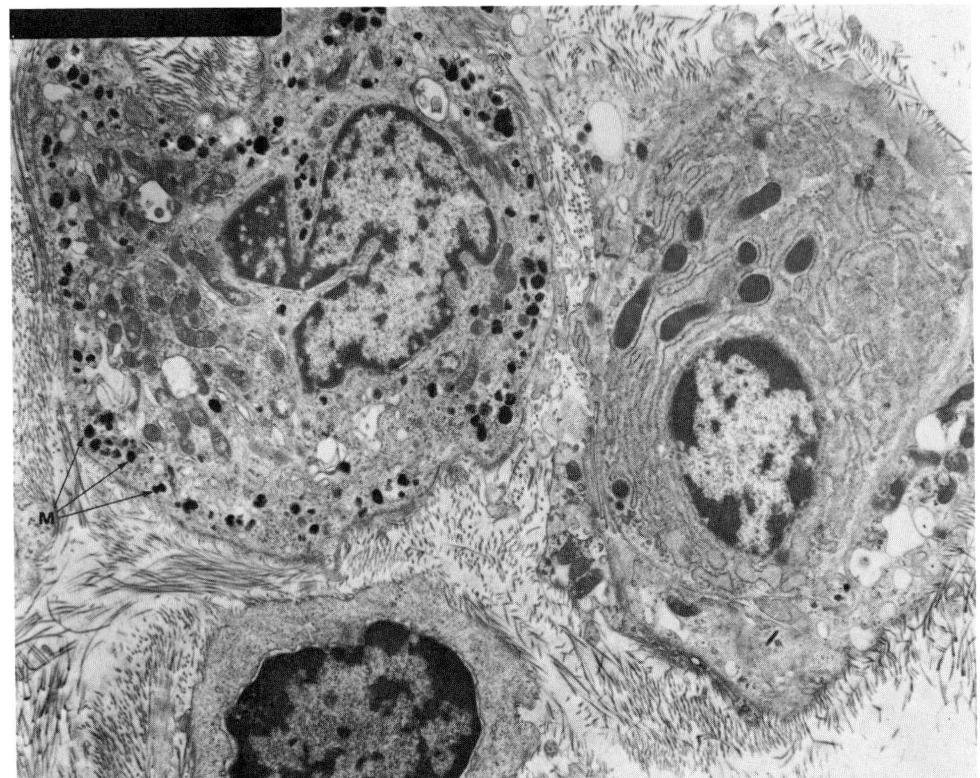

FIGURE 2–122 **FHI.** Electron micrograph showing an affected melanocyte with rare melanosomes (M). Note plasma cell at right and lymphocyte below. (From Melamed S, Lahav M, Sandbank U, et al: Fuchs' heterochromic iridocyclitis: An electron microscopic study of the iris. Invest Ophthalmol Vis Sci 17:1196, 1978.)

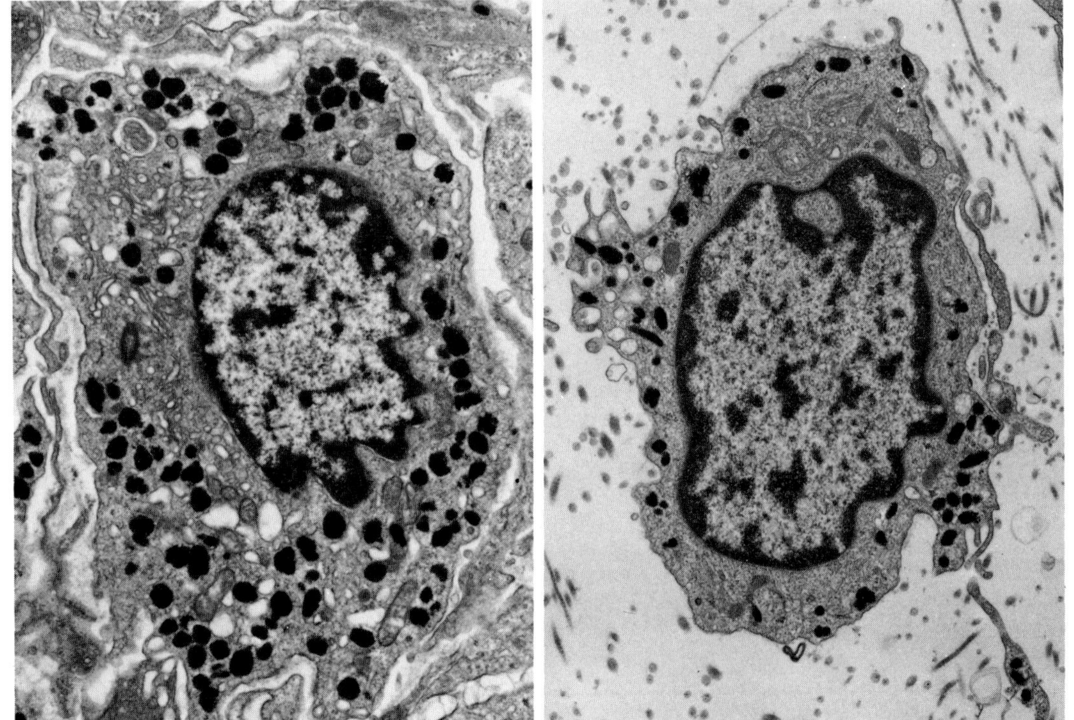

FIGURE 2–123 **FHI.** Electron micrograph of a normal melanocyte *(A)* and a melanocyte in FHI *(B)*. The affected melanocyte *(B)* is abnormally round and contains melanosomes that are markedly smaller than normal. (From McCartney ACE, Bull TB, Spaulton DJ: Fuchs' heterochromic iridocyclitis: An electron microscopic study. Trans Ophthalmol Soc UK 105:325, 1986.)

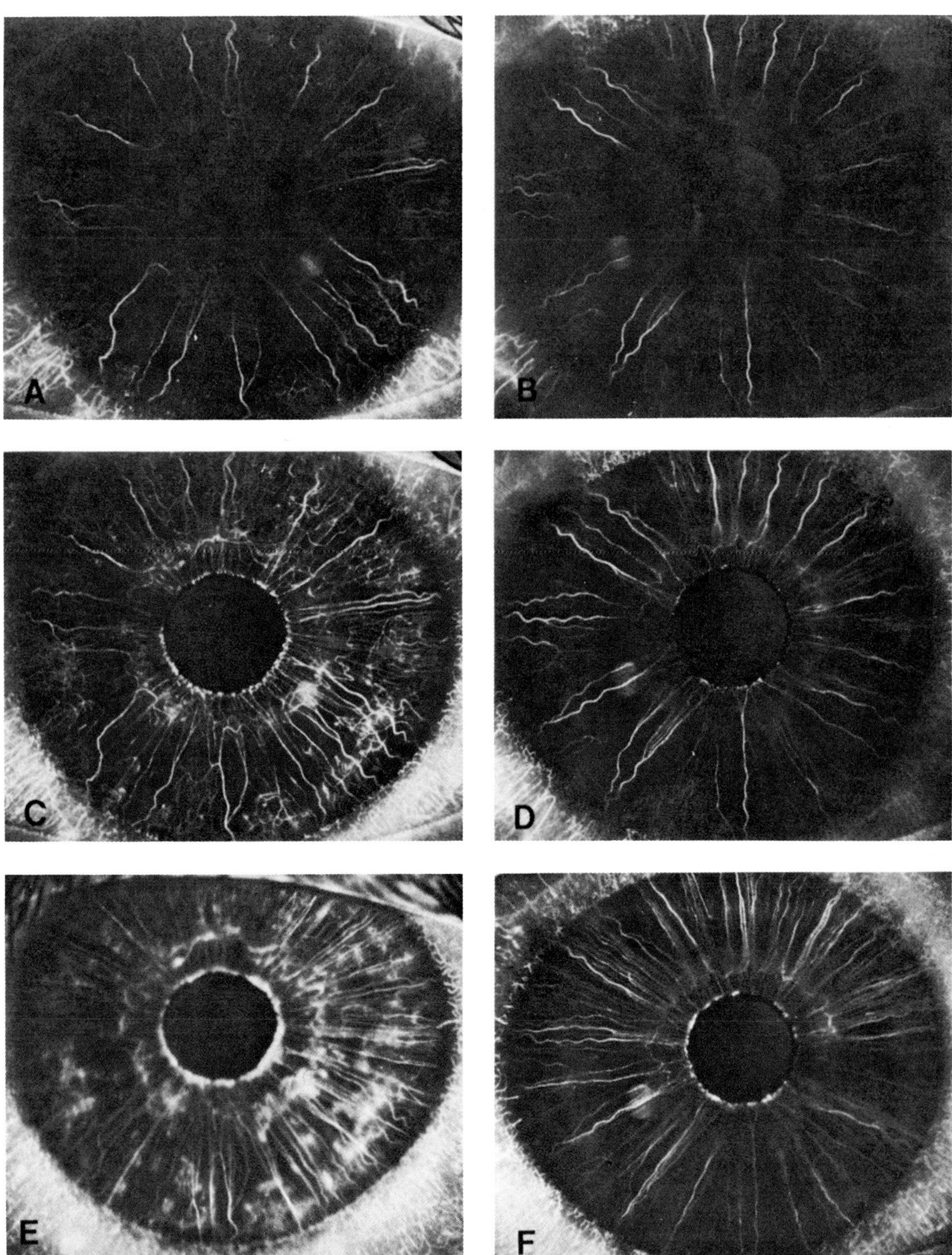

FIGURE 2–124 **FHI.** Simultaneous bilateral iris angiogram in FHI affecting the right eye. *A* and *B*, Arterial phase showing neovascularization of the iris in the affected iris *(A)* and a normal vascular pattern in the contralateral iris *(B)*. *C* and *D*, Arteriovenous phase showing increasingly prominent neovascularization in the affected iris *(C)* and a normal pattern in the contralateral iris *(D)*. *E* and *F*, Late venous phase showing fluorescein leakage from abnormal vessels in the affected iris *(E)* and a normal vascular pattern in the opposite iris *(F)*. (From Saari M, Vuorre I, Nieminen H: Fuchs' heterochromic cyclitis: A simultaneous bilateral fluorescein angiographic study of the iris. Br J Ophthalmol 62:719, 1978).

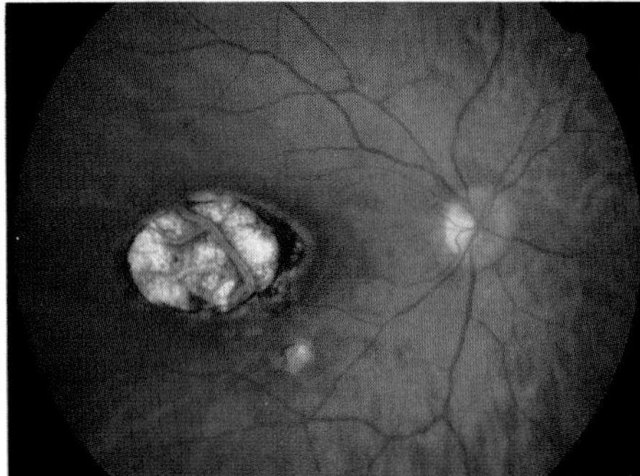

FIGURE 2–125 **FHI association with chorioretinitis.** A typical toxoplasmosis chorioretinal scar demonstrating a punched-out atrophic lesion surrounded by a well-defined pigment border. The association between FHI and ocular toxoplasmosis has been proposed by a number of authors, but the existence of conflicting studies highlights the need for further investigation. The incidence of all types of chorioretinal lesions in FHI ranges from 28 to 64 percent. (Courtesy of G. K. Asdourian; photography by H. Kachadoorian.)

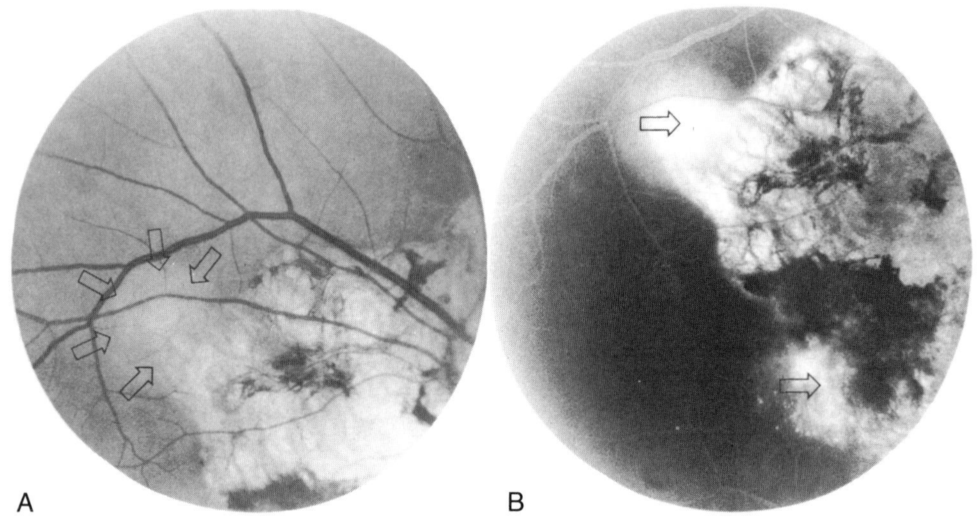

FIGURE 2–126 Fluorescein angiogram depicting active recurrent serpiginous choroiditis (SPC). *A*, Active focus of recurrent SPC *(arrows)*. *B*, Late-phase angiogram shows leakage from two foci of choroiditis. (*A* and *B*, From Jampol LM, Orth D, Daily MJ, Rabb MF: Subretinal neovascularization with geographic (serpiginous) choroiditis. Am J Ophthalmol 88:683–689, 1979. Published with permission from The American Journal of Ophthalmology. Copyright by the Ophthalmic Publishing Company.)

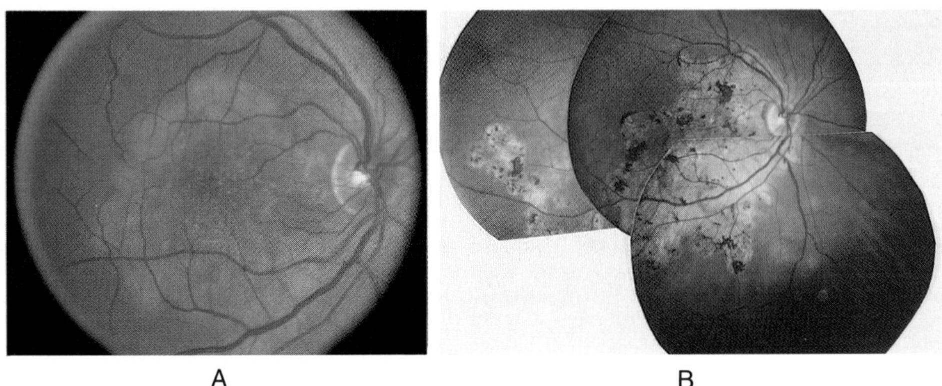

FIGURE 2–127 **Macular SPC.** *A*, Active initial lesion of macular SPC. *B*, Same patient 3 years and several recurrences later with serpentine extension. (*A* and *B*, From Mansour AM, Jampol LM, Packo KH, Hrisamalos NF: Macular serpiginous choroiditis. Retina 8:125, 1988.)

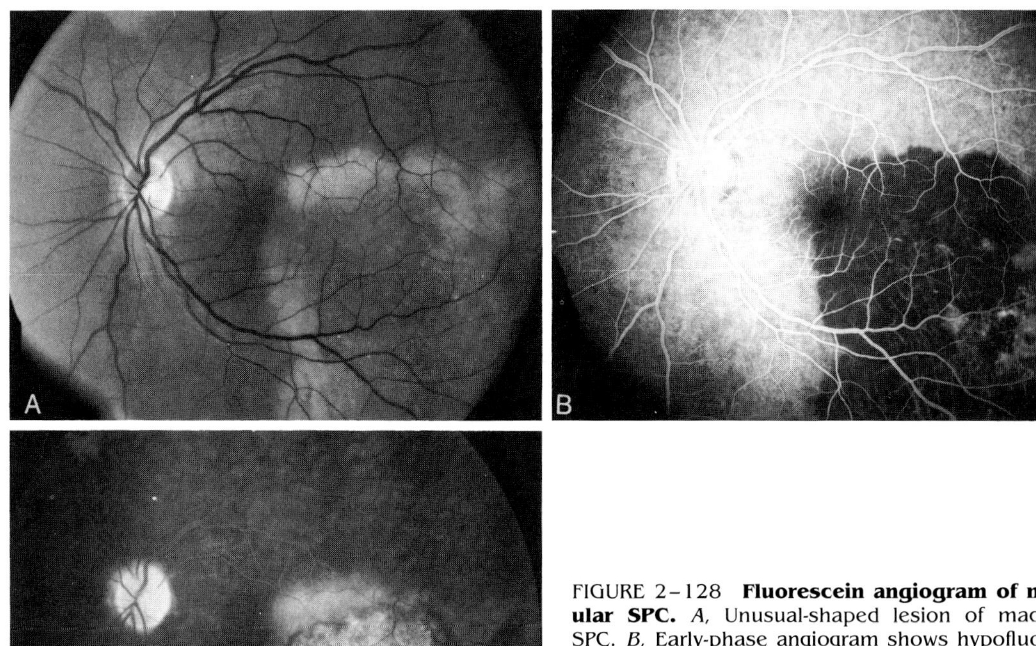

FIGURE 2-128 **Fluorescein angiogram of macular SPC.** *A*, Unusual-shaped lesion of macular SPC. *B*, Early-phase angiogram shows hypofluorescence. *C*, Late-phase angiogram shows staining of lesion. (*A–C*, Courtesy of Kirk Packo, M.D.)

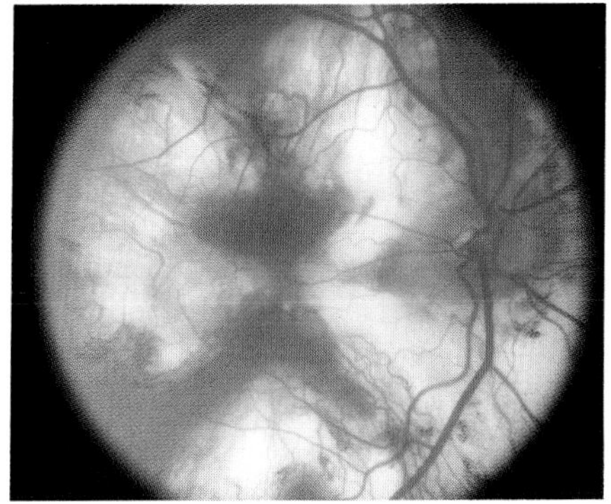

FIGURE 2-129 **End-stage scarring of inactive SPC.** Note the marked destruction of the choroid with variable pigmentary atrophy and clumping.

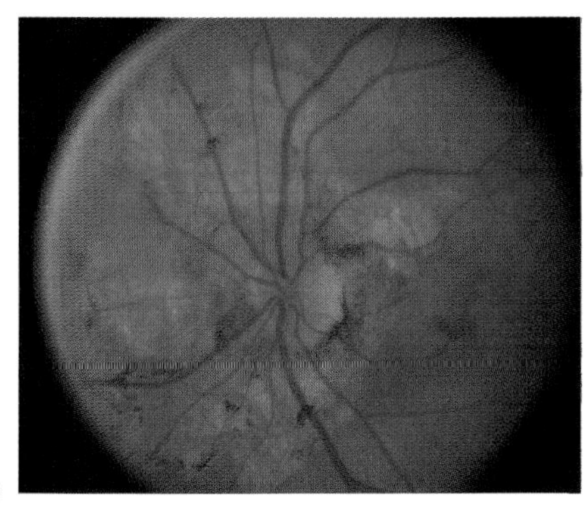

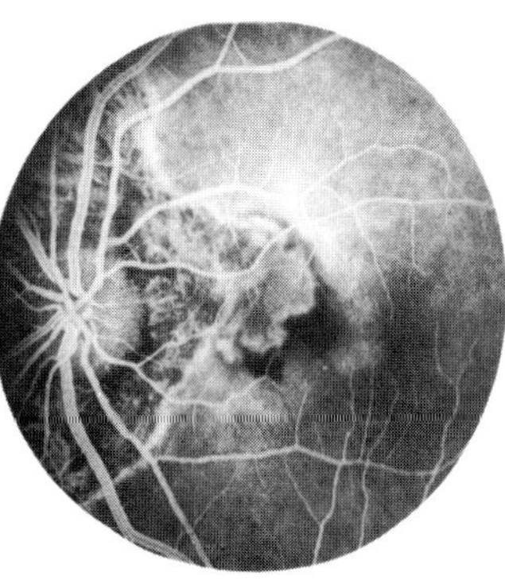

FIGURE 2-130 **Peripapillary SPC.** *A*, Peripapillary SPC with choroidal neovascularization at temporal margin. *B*, Angiography shows choroidal neovascular membrane that is well defined and extending from the papillomacular bundle into the fovea. (*A* and *B*, From Jampol LM, Orr D, Dailey MJ, Robb MF: Subretinal neovascularization with geographic (serpiginous) choroiditis. Am J Ophthalmol 88:683–689, 1979. Reprinted with permission from The American Journal of Ophthalmology. Copyright by The Ophthalmic Publishing Company.)

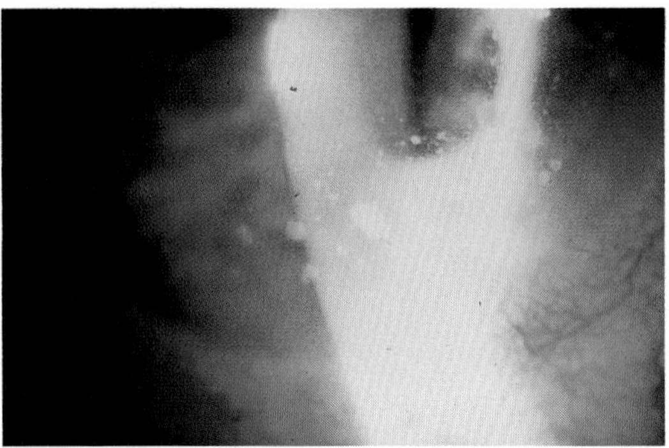

FIGURE 2–131 Primary intraocular and central nervous system (CNS) non-Hodgkin Lymphoma. There is a granulomatous anterior uveitis with keratic precipitates.

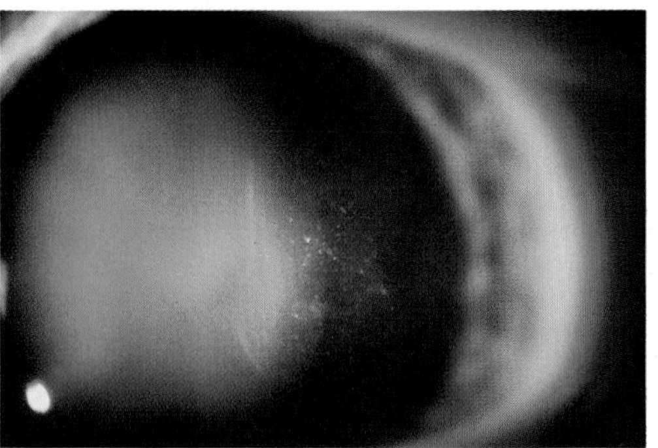

FIGURE 2–132 Retrolenticular and intravitreal cellular clusters in primary intraocular–CNS lymphoma.

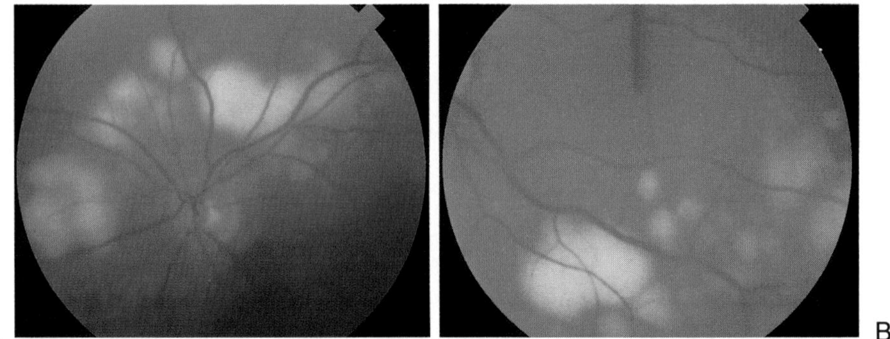

FIGURE 2–133 **Primary ocular and CNS lymphoma.** *A* and *B*, Multiple creamy to white deep retinal lesions, the smallest ones probably representing a subretinal pigment epithelial location. (*A* and *B*, Courtesy of Dr. Ronald Pruett.)

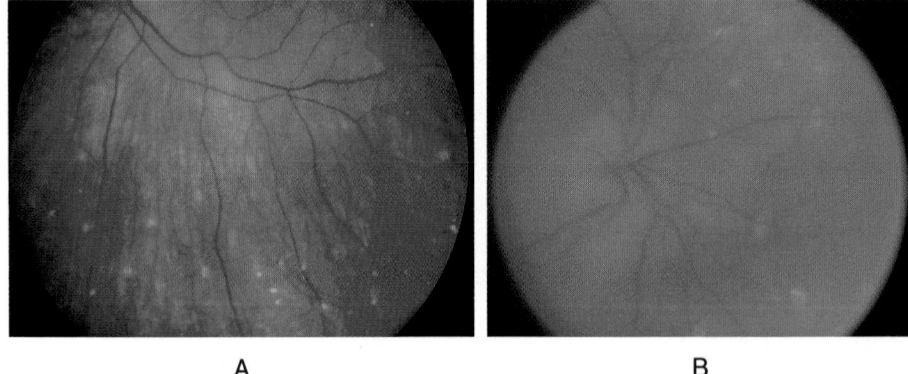

FIGURE 2–134 **Primary ocular and CNS lymphoma.** *A*, Small, white, deep retinal lesions, more likely to suggest a uveitis or an evanescent "white dot" syndrome. (Courtesy of Dr. William Mieler.) *B*, These small flecklike white lesions might invite the mistaken diagnosis of fundus flavimaculatus, but note the vitritis and the presence of optic nerve head swelling with the suggestion of a peripapillary mass.

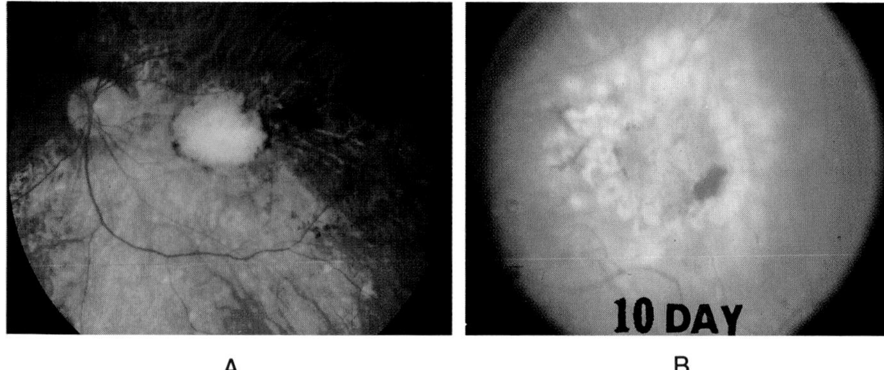

FIGURE 2-135 **Primary ocular and CNS lymphoma.** *A,* A white macular lesion simulating a disciform scar except that the lesion appears fluffy. There is clumping of the retinal pigment epithelium at the periphery of the lesion. (Courtesy of Dr. William Mieler.) *B,* Confluent macular lesions with a small associated hemorrhage resulting from a transvitreal biopsy. Note that several of the discrete foci at the periphery have an annular shape, shown particularly well at the left edge of the process. (Courtesy of Dr. Thomas Aaberg and Dr. Nancy Newman.)

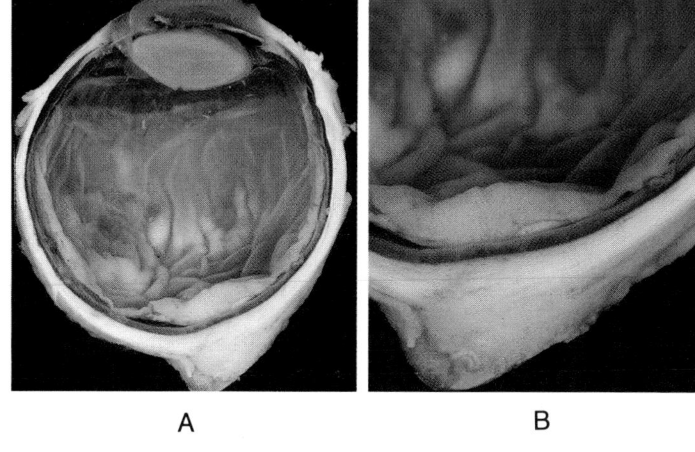

FIGURE 2-136 **Primary ocular and CNS lymphoma.** *A,* Pupillooptic section through an enucleated eyeball discloses fluffy white retinal lesions. *B,* At the posterior pole, there is a small lesion deep in the retina and just above Bruch's membrane, with a demarcating apical lamina of intact retinal pigment epithelium. Note that the choroid is minimally thickened by inflammation but not involved with the lymphomatous process. (*A* and *B,* Courtesy of Dr. Miguel Bernier.)

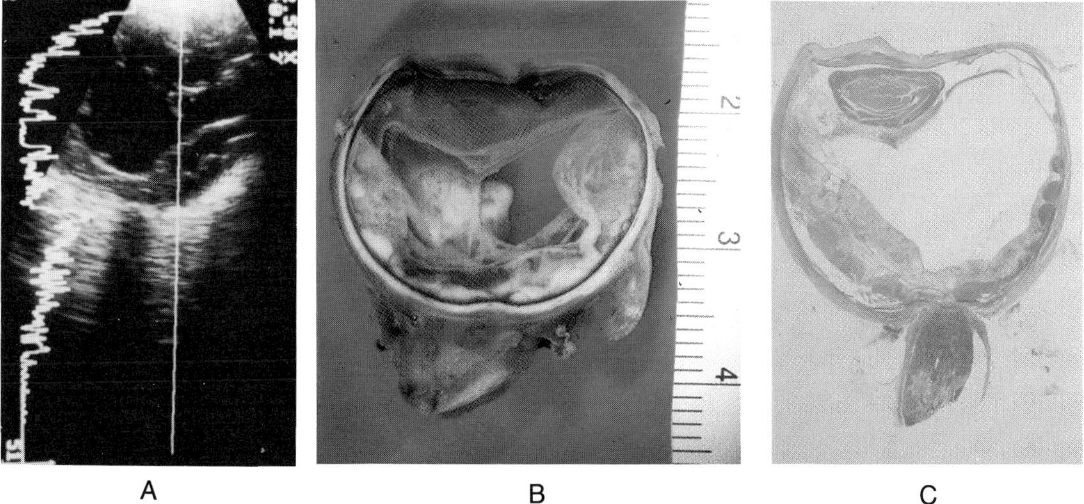

FIGURE 2-137 **Primary ocular and CNS lymphoma.** *A,* Ultrasonogram of an eye with a retinal detachment of clinically unknown origin. Beneath the retinal detachment shown toward the right are three small hillocks of thickening. The scan on the left running from top to bottom in the region of these hillocks shows minimal internal reflectivity. *B,* The enucleated globe contains many deep retinal moundlike masses corresponding to the hillocks displayed in the ultrasonogram. Note that the choroid remains pigmented and is only minimally thickened. *C,* Photomicrograph of the enucleated eyeball demonstrates multiple moundlike masses deep in the retina and sitting on Bruch's membrane. There is tumor involvement of the optic nerve.

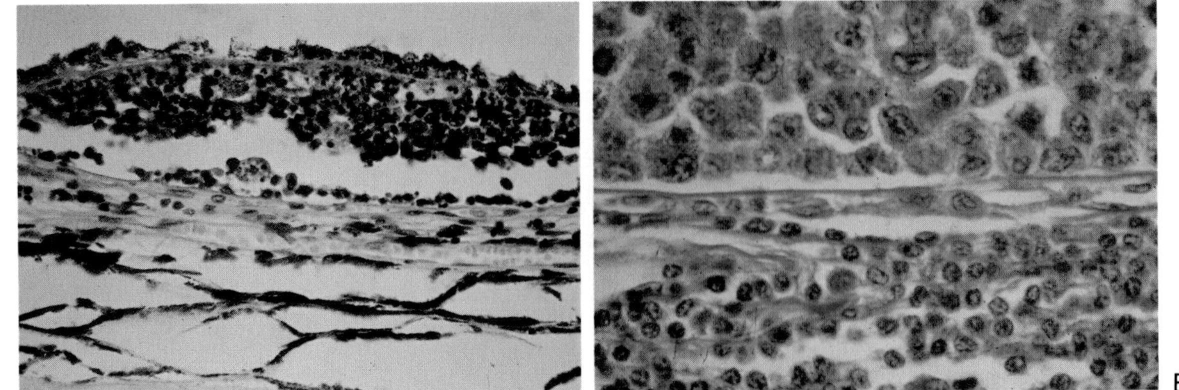

FIGURE 2–138 **Primary ocular and CNS lymphoma.** *A,* A collection of neoplastic lymphocytes that have detached the retinal pigment epithelium, shown above covering the lesion. The earliest lesions of primary ocular–CNS lymphoma probably commence above Bruch's membrane as neoplastic detachments of the pigment epithelium. *B,* The neoplastic lymphocytes are large and irregularly shaped and located exclusively above Bruch's membrane. There is an inflammatory lymphocytic infiltrate of the choroid below. The neoplastic lymphocytes are at least twice as large as the reactive lymphocytes in the choroid.

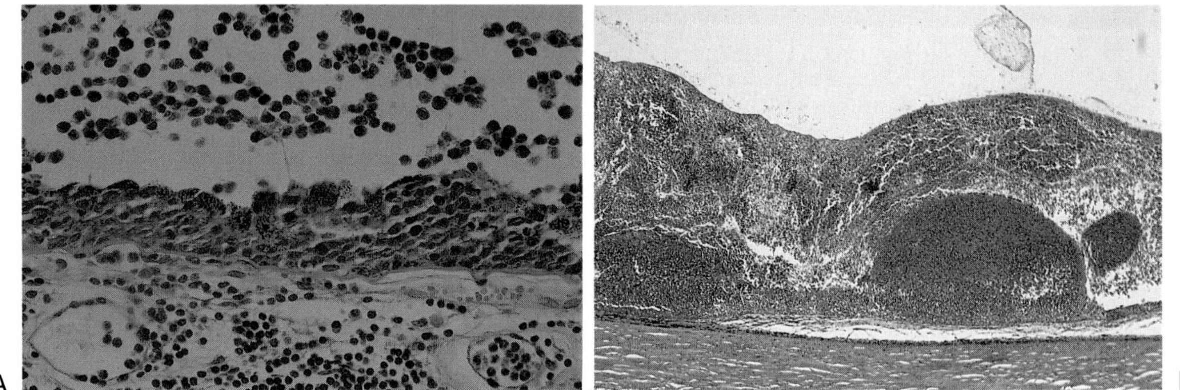

FIGURE 2–139 **Primary ocular and CNS lymphoma.** *A,* A cohesive layer of neoplastic lymphocytes is situated above Bruch's membrane, but dyscohesively sheds into the subretinal space. Again note the benign character of these small lymphocytes that have mounted a host response in the choroid. *B,* Mounds of what were probably initially subretinal pigment epithelial collections of neoplastic lymphocytes exhibit necrosis of their upper halves. The neoplastic cells have additionally infiltrated the retina. This process represents a more advanced stage of the incipient lesion shown in Figure 2–138*A*.

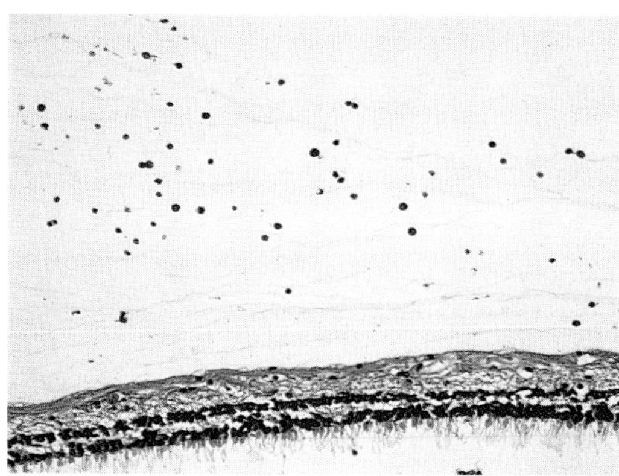

FIGURE 2–140 **Primary ocular and CNS lymphoma.** Hyperchromatic neoplastic lymphocytes in the vitreous of a most exceptional case that did not have any identifiable masses in the retina.

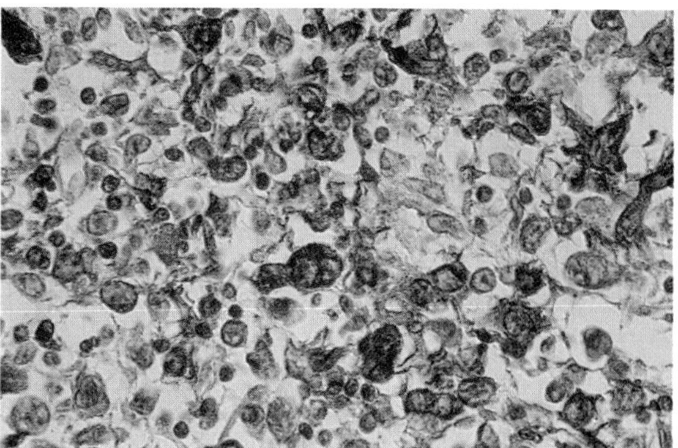

FIGURE 2–142 **Primary ocular and CNS lymphoma.** The vast majority of these lesions are of B-cell lymphocytic origin. These pleomorphic lymphocytes have been stained by the immunoperoxidase method for the presence of lambda light chain determinants. (Courtesy of Dr. Bruce Johnson.)

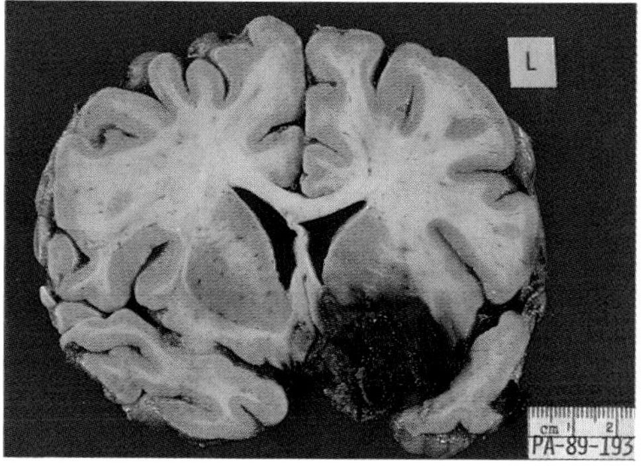

FIGURE 2–141 **Primary ocular and CNS lymphoma.** Hemorrhagic and partially necrotic brain lesion in a patient with ocular lymphoma. (Courtesy of Dr. Bruce Johnson.)

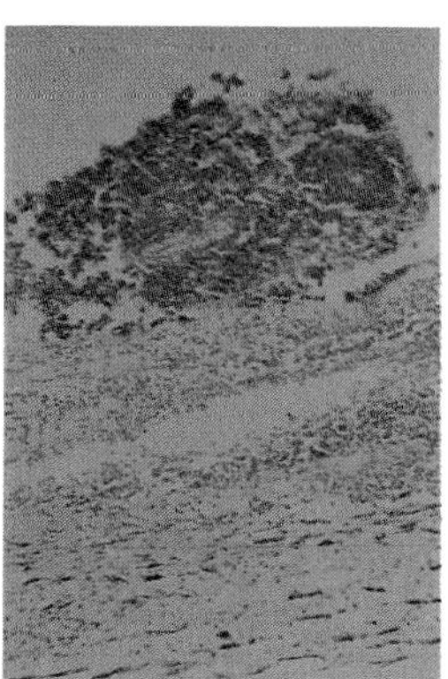

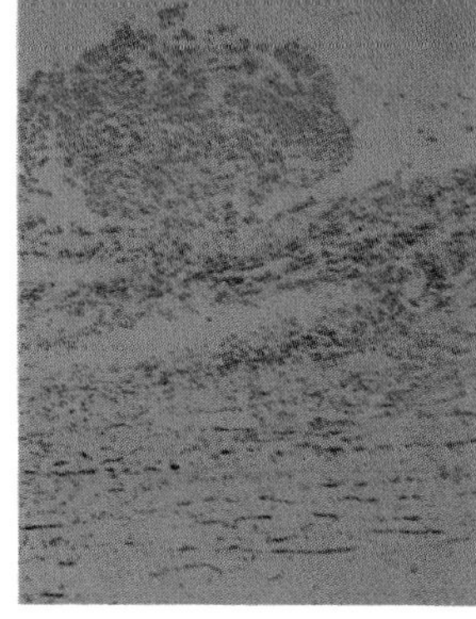

FIGURE 2–143 **Primary ocular and CNS lymphoma.** *Left,* The cluster of cells shown toward the top and above Bruch's membrane stains positively for a B-cell marker. Note that the majority of cells in the underlying choroid are not staining positively, although there is a light dispersion of some B cells. *Right,* A T-cell marker fails to react positively with the neoplastic cellular mass, but the majority of the cells in the choroid exhibit this lineage. Immunoperoxidase reaction. (Courtesy of Dr. Miguel Bernier.)

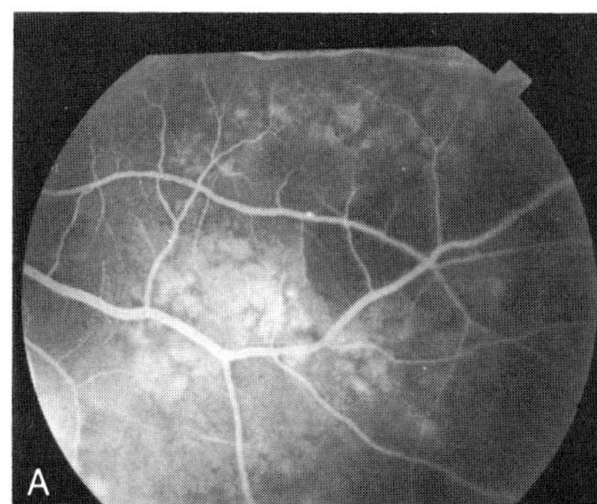

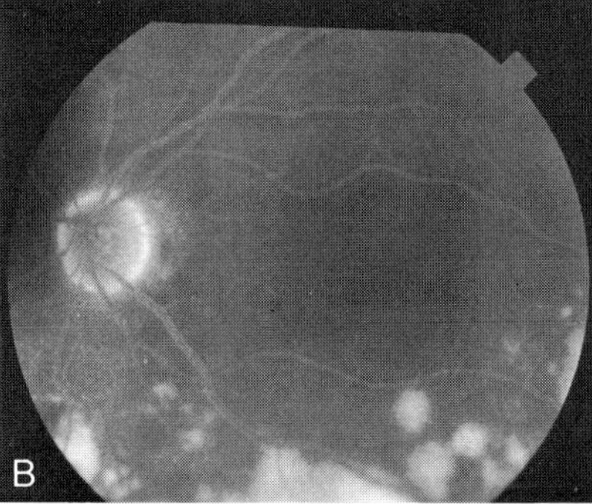

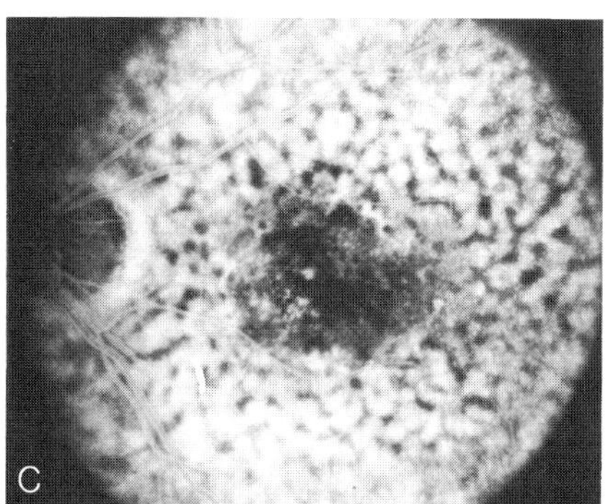

FIGURE 2–144 **Primary ocular and CNS lymphoma.** *A,* Arteriovenous-phase fluorescein angiogram displays early accumulation of dye within the deep retinal (mostly subpigment epithelial) lesions. *B,* Dye is retained late after most of the fluorescein has been recycled out of the fundus. (*A* and *B,* Courtesy of Dr. Ronald Pruett.) *C,* In another patient without deep retinal moundlike collections of tumor cells, there is a diffuse mottled blockage of dye in the choroid. (Courtesy of Dr. Thomas Aaberg.)

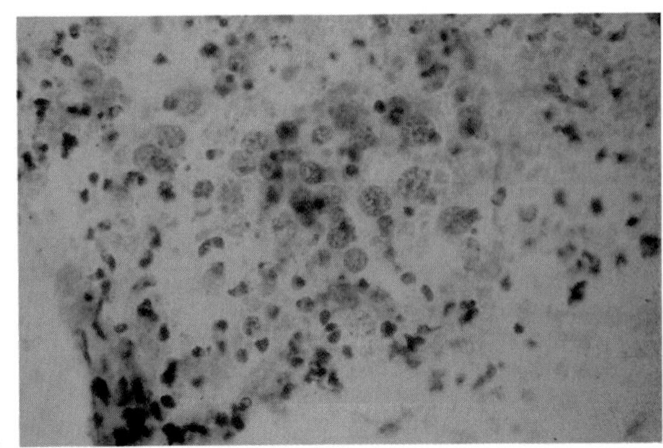

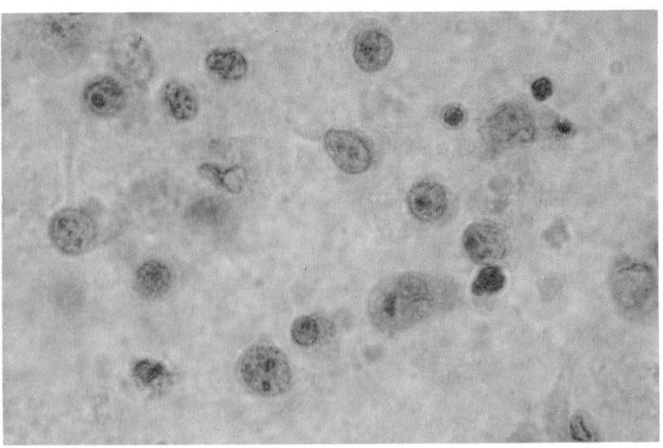

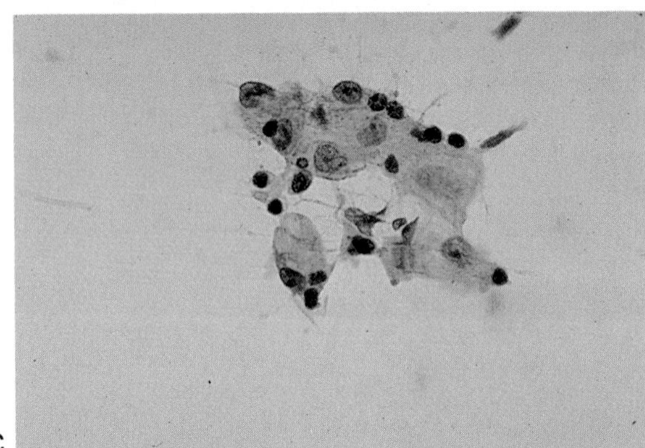

FIGURE 2–145 **Primary ocular and CNS lymphoma.** *A*, Cytologic preparation of a positive vitreous aspirate exhibits large pleomorphic lymphocytes. Many of the nuclei are pyknotic (not to be confused with polymorphonuclear leukocytes), and the background is "dirty" as a result of spontaneous cytolysis in the stagnant vitreous. *B*, The atypical large lymphocytes manifest coarse clumping of the nuclear chromatin. Note the amorphous cellular debris in the background. *C*, Benign macrophages shown here must be distinguished from atypical lymphocytes. The macrophages have delicate vesicular nucleoplasm without coarse clumping of the chromatinic material and more abundant and conspicuous cytoplasm. Note the association of small, dark, mature lymphocytes. Massive collections of histiocytes such as these may be seen in infectious endophthalmitis, including toxoplasmic retinochoroiditis. Papanicolaou stain.

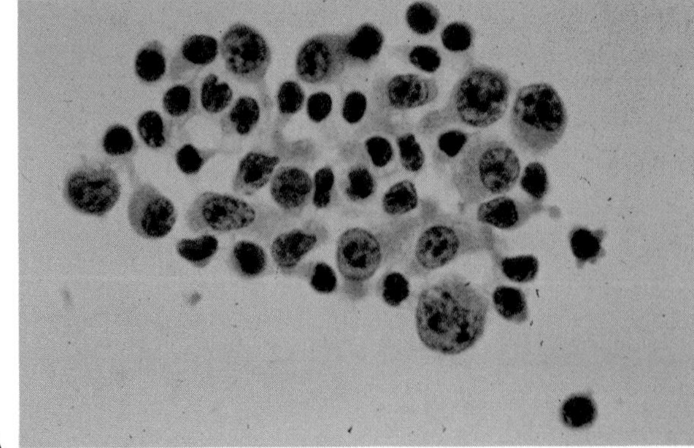

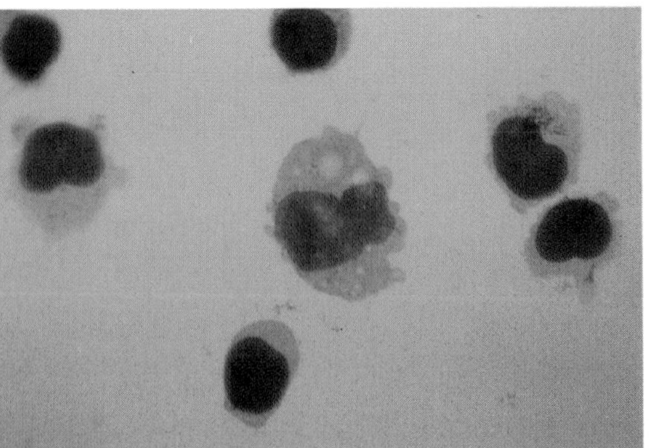

FIGURE 2–146 **Primary ocular and CNS lymphoma.** *A* and *B*, Atypical lymphocytes in the cerebrospinal fluid of patients with ocular and brain lymphoma. (*A*, Courtesy of Dr. Ramon L. Font; *B*, Courtesy of Dr. Nancy Newman.)

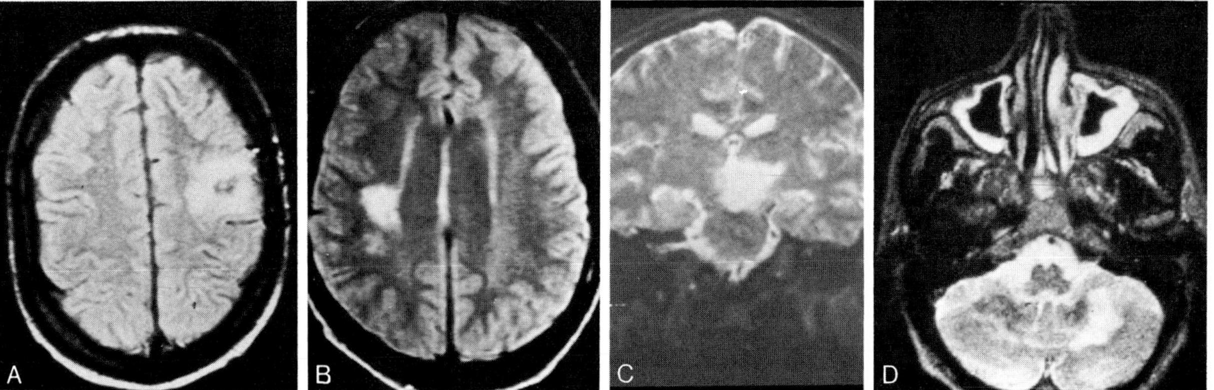

FIGURE 2–147 **Primary ocular and CNS lymphoma.** Magnetic resonance imaging after gadolinium injection is often more sensitive than computed tomography scanning in detecting hemispheric lesions. *A,* Frontoparietal mass in axial projection. *B,* Parietal mass. *C,* Coronal projection of deep white matter mass in the thalamic region. (*A–C,* Courtesy of Dr. Fred Hochberg.) *D,* Cerebellar hemispheric lesion in an AIDS patient. (Courtesy of Dr. Ramon L. Font.)

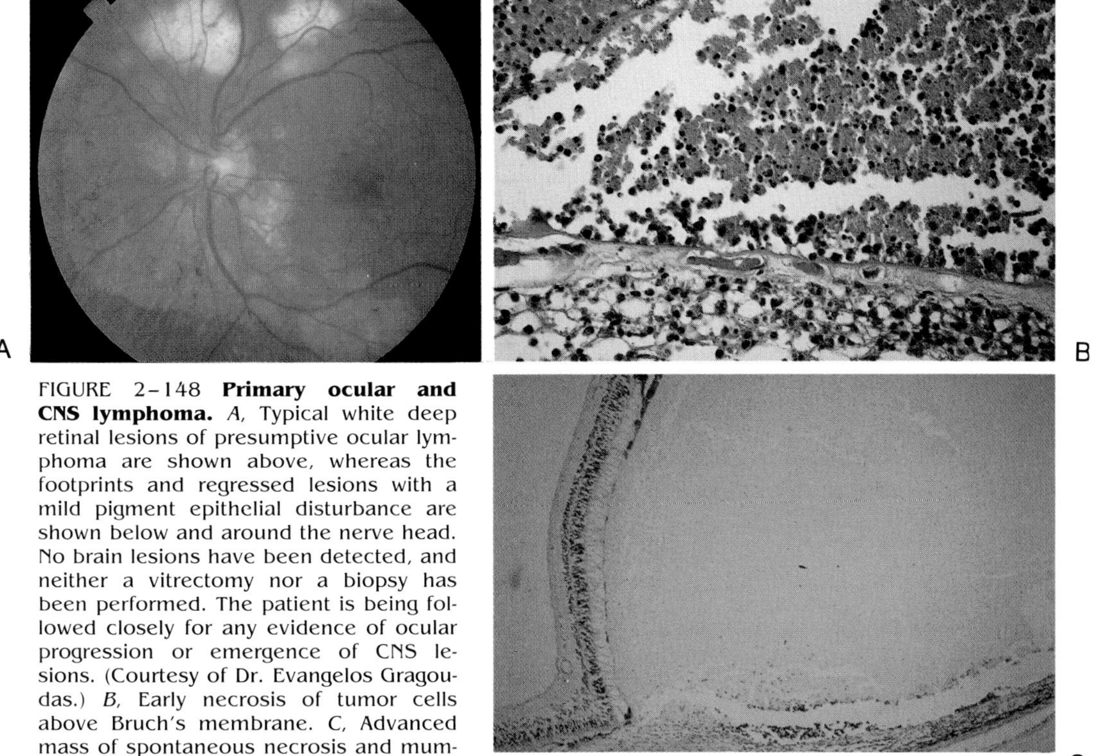

FIGURE 2–148 **Primary ocular and CNS lymphoma.** *A,* Typical white deep retinal lesions of presumptive ocular lymphoma are shown above, whereas the footprints and regressed lesions with a mild pigment epithelial disturbance are shown below and around the nerve head. No brain lesions have been detected, and neither a vitrectomy nor a biopsy has been performed. The patient is being followed closely for any evidence of ocular progression or emergence of CNS lesions. (Courtesy of Dr. Evangelos Gragoudas.) *B,* Early necrosis of tumor cells above Bruch's membrane. *C,* Advanced mass of spontaneous necrosis and mummification of a moundlike tumor with exudative detachment of the retina.

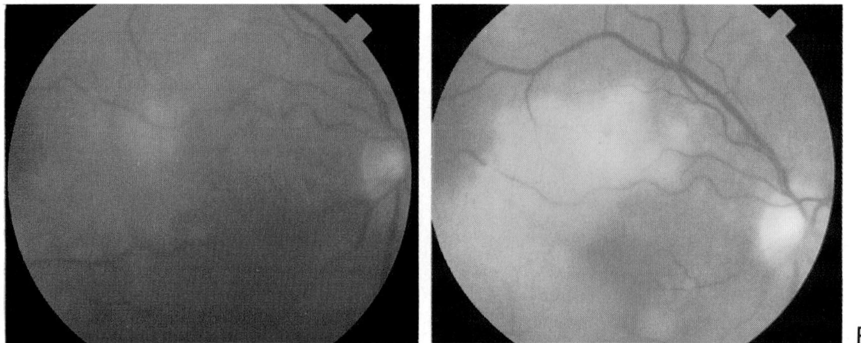

FIGURE 2-149 **Primary ocular and CNS lymphoma.** Progression of the lesion shown in *A* over a 6-week period into that shown in *B* resulted in threatening of the macula retinae and necessitated ocular radiotherapy. (Courtesy of Dr. Donald D'Amico.)

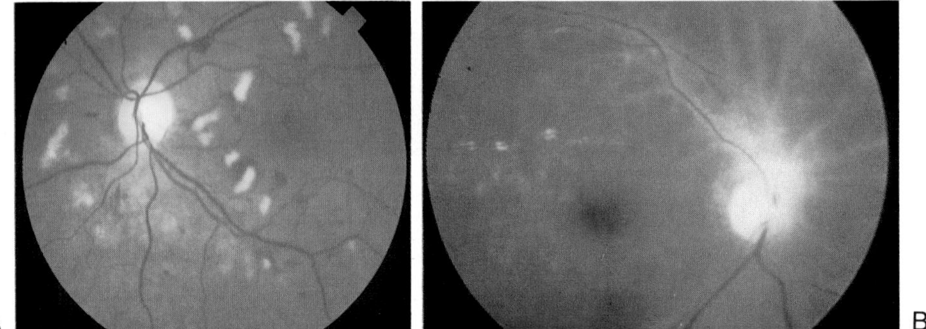

FIGURE 2-150 **Primary ocular and CNS lymphoma.** *A*, Eighteen months after the completion of ocular radiotherapy, there is evidence in this patient of a severe radiation-induced retinopathy, with cotton-wool spots, retinal hemorrhages, and optic nerve head pallor. (Courtesy of Dr. Donald D'Amico.) *B*, One month after the completion of radiotherapy, this patient with an AIDS-related ocular large cell lymphoma displayed almost complete resolution of the epipapillary lesion, which unfortunately has left advanced nerve head pallor in its wake. In this case, the tumor infiltrated the nerve head, and radiation therapy merely disclosed the underlying damage on disappearance of the lesional tissue. (Courtesy of Dr. Ramon L. Font.)

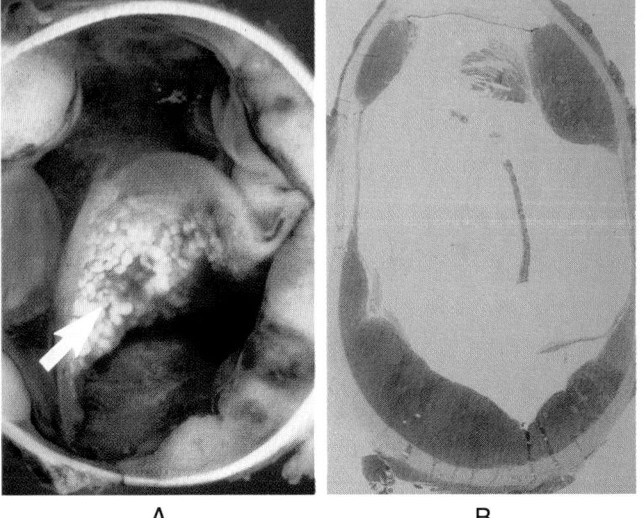

FIGURE 2-151 **Systemic lymphoma with secondary ocular involvement.** *A*, In contrast to primary ocular lymphoma in which the subretinal pigment epithelial space and the retina are sites of earliest involvement, in secondary ocular lymphoma from systemic spread, the uvea is the preferential site of localization and proliferation of the disseminating tumor cells. In this enucleated globe, note the massive thickening of the choroid posteriorly and the two bulbous expansions of the ciliary body shown above. The *arrow* points to a smaller fish egg component of the process that is located in the subretinal space. *B*, Photomicrograph of a globe with a diffuse proliferation of large anaplastic cells within the uvea, sparing the iris above. Note that both posteriorly and anteriorly there is episcleral extension of tumor cells. (*A* and *B*, Courtesy of Dr. William C. Lloyd III.)

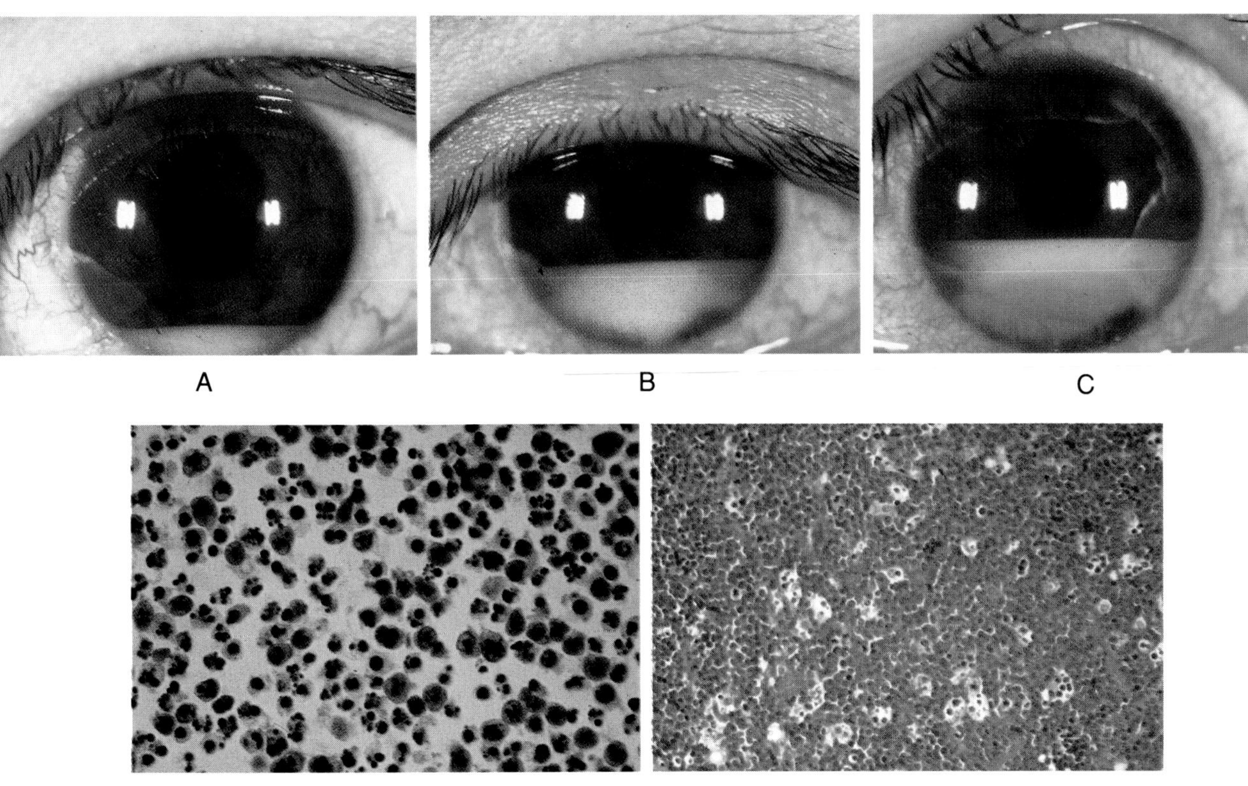

FIGURE 2-152 **Secondary lymphoma with ocular presentation.** *A–C*, A "neoplastic" hypopyon in a 32-year-old woman is shown developing over a 2-week period. Note that the eye is essentially quiet, belying the possibility that the condition is due to an infection. The small hyphema shown in *C* formed after a paracentesis was performed. Such an appearance is more often caused by leukemia. (A–C, Courtesy of Dr. Robert Ralph.) *D*, Anaplastic and dyscohesive tumor cells are present in the paracentesis specimen, suggesting a large cell lymphoma. The patient received 4000 rads of ocular radiotherapy, and the condition completely resolved. *E*, Although the initial work-up failed to reveal any evidence of a systemic lymphoproliferative disease, 4 months later the patient experienced a fracture of the femur and a pelvic mass was discovered. Biopsy revealed Burkitt's lymphoma with a starry-sky pattern caused by the dispersion of large pale-staining histiocytes among large round B lymphocytes. The patient died of disseminated disease. (*D* and *E*, Courtesy of Dr. Lorenz E. Zimmerman.)

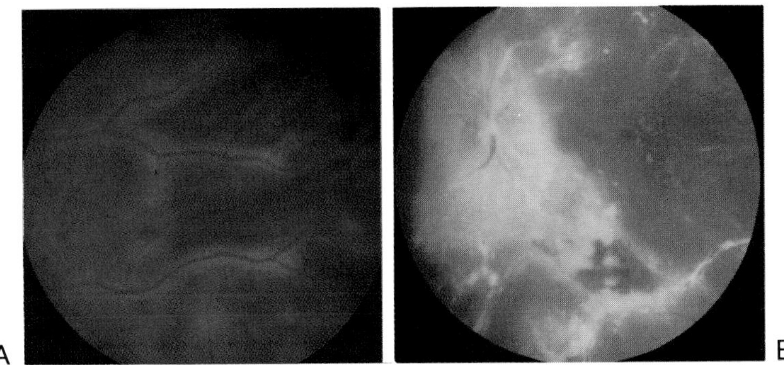

FIGURE 2-153 **Systemic leukemia involving the retina.** *A*, Initial perivascular infiltrates of the retinal arterioles with small hemorrhages. *B*, More massive extension of tumor cells out of the retinal arterioles obscures the optic nerve head and envelops the retinal vasculature. Note the associated hemorrhages. (*A* and *B*, Courtesy of Dr. John Flynn.)

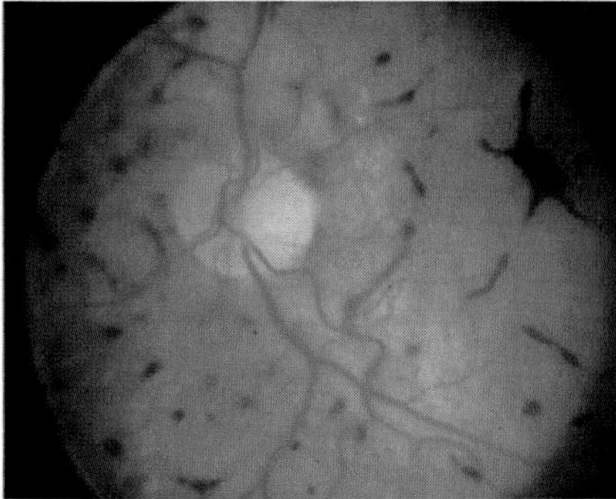

FIGURE 2–154 **Choroidal leukemic infiltration.** Leukemic infiltration of the choroid has caused a disturbance of the retinal pigment epithelium, which has assumed linear, stellate, and leopard pigment aggregations. (Courtesy of Dr. William Mieler.)

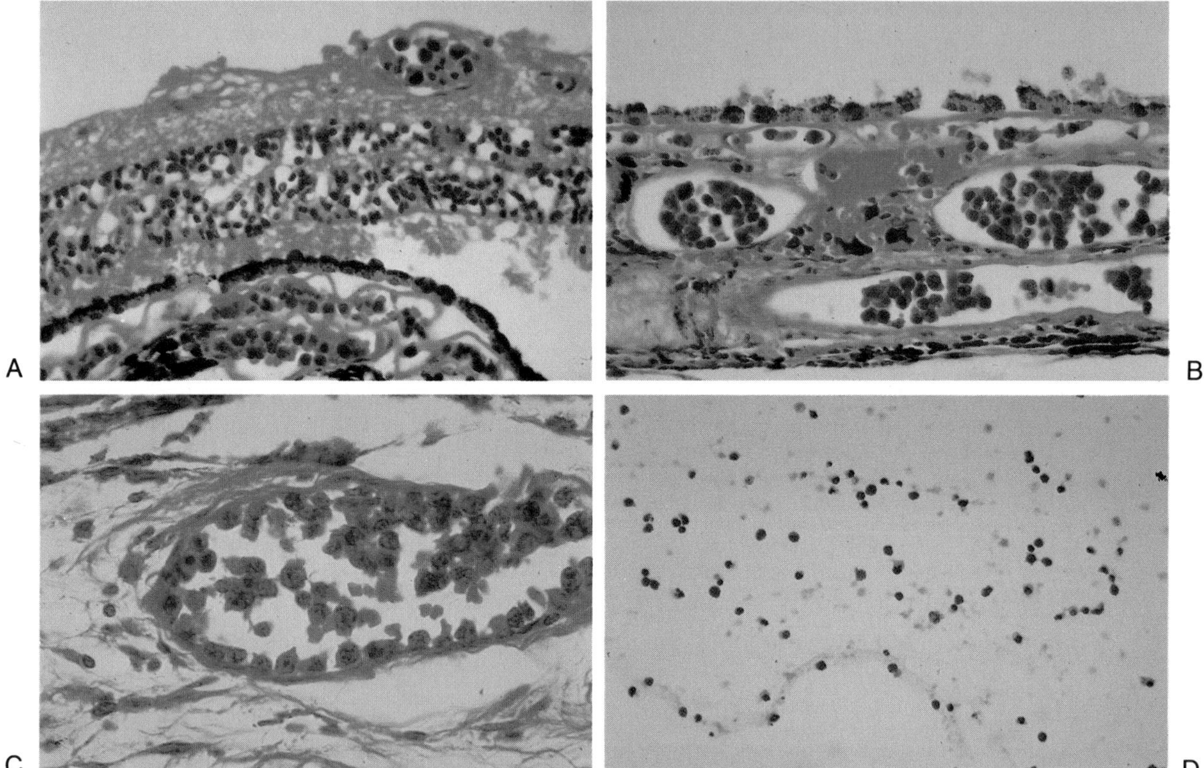

FIGURE 2–155 **Angiotrophic lymphoma (also called intravascular lymphomatosis and formerly referred to as malignant angioendotheliomatosis).** This proliferation of large atypical lymphocytes has a predilection for the lumina of small arteries, veins, and capillaries, typically in the absence of overt peripheral blood or bone marrow disease. Neurologic and cutaneous presentations are common, with a minority of patients having clinically significant eye lesions. *A,* A cluster of hyperchromatic lymphoma cells in the lumen of a retinal arteriole. *B,* Clusters of tumor cells in the choriocapillaris as well as in large choroidal vessels. *C,* Some of the tumor cells in this large choroidal vessel actually made contact with the endothelium, probably because of receptors on the cell surfaces of the neoplastic lymphocytes. *D,* Hyperchromatic cells in the vitreous.

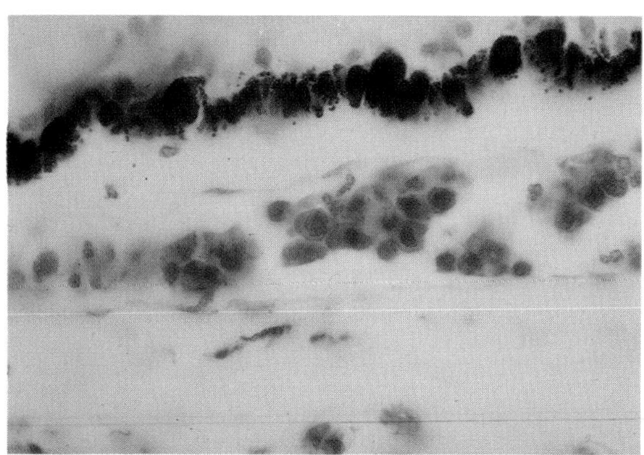

FIGURE 2-156 **Angiotrophic lymphoma.** Although "neoplastic angioendotheliomatosis" was initially believed to be a proliferation of neoplastic endothelial cells because of the pattern of intravascular dissemination, immunohistochemical studies have revealed that this condition is actually a lymphoma, as demonstrated here by positive staining of choroidal tumor cells with leukocyte common antigen. The new tumor cells in the majority of cases are of B-cell lineage, although a minority have been established to be of T-cell lineage.

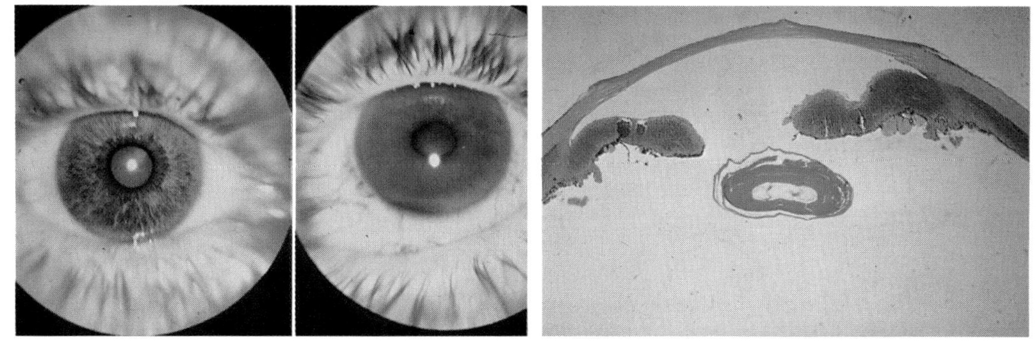

FIGURE 2-157 **Lymphoid hyperplasia of the uvea.** *A,* A brown heterochromia of the iris caused by massive lymphocytic infiltration *(right).* The normal contralateral iris is shown on the *left. B,* Histopathologic evaluation of the enucleated globe shows enormous thickening of the iris with extension toward the ciliary body on the right.

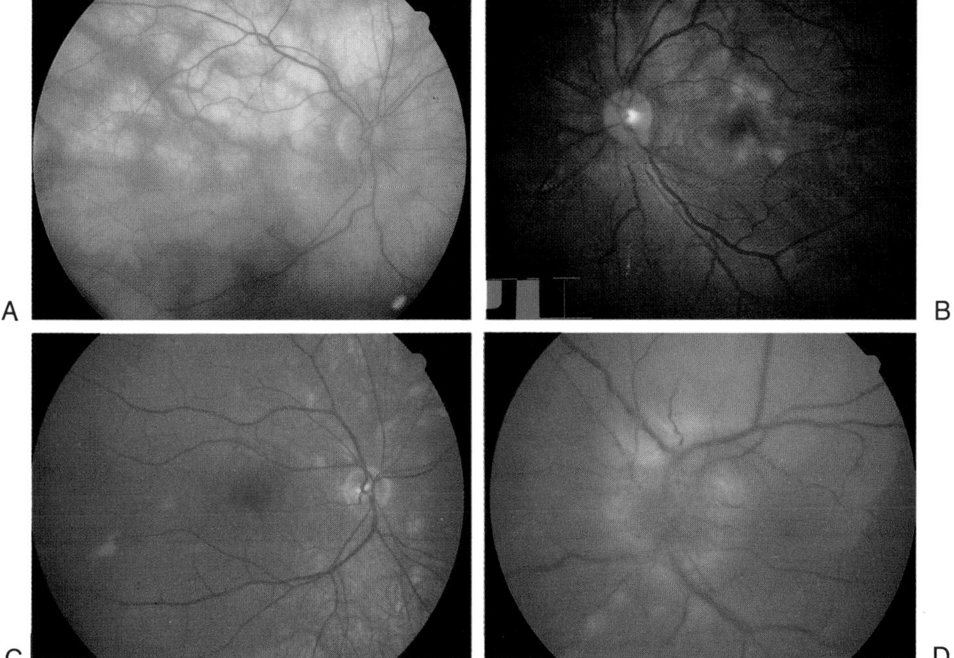

FIGURE 2-158 **Fundus appearance of lymphoid hyperplasia of the choroid.** *A,* Multifocal and confluent creamy infiltrates of the posterior pole. *B,* The creamy color of this peripapillary infiltrate is somewhat modified in this black patient by the hyperpigmented choroid. (Courtesy of Dr. Joseph Rizzo.) *C* and *D,* Bilateral infiltrates, with the lesions in the right eye *(C)* having irregular shapes and a small size, whereas in the left fundus *(D),* there is a prominent peripapillary mass with extension superiorly. Note also in *D* the presence of small lesions inferonasally. (*C* and *D,* Courtesy of Dr. John Gittinger.)

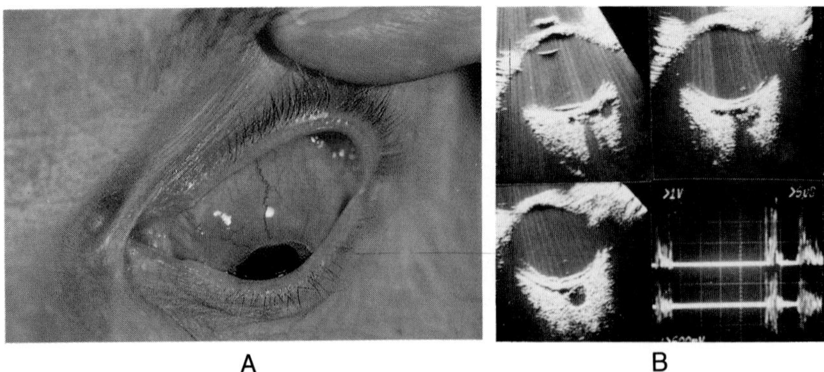

FIGURE 2-159 A painless epibulbar salmon-colored lesion of extraocular extension of uveal lymphoid hyperplasia. In contrast to most primary conjunctival lymphoid tumors, this mass was immovable on the sclera. In contrast, scleritis is typically painful and beefy-red. *B,* In addition to choroidal thickening in uveal lymphoid hyperplasia, the majority of patients also exhibit extraocular and episcleral extensions of the process, shown in this B-scan ultrasonogram as anechoic areas of epibulbar infiltrate on the posterior sclera as well as in a juxtapapillary location. (Courtesy of Dr. D. Jackson Coleman.)

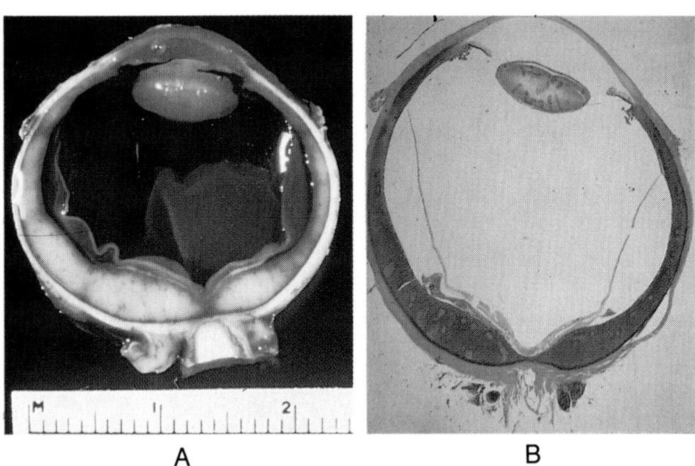

FIGURE 2-160 **Lymphoid hyperplasia of the uvea.** *A,* Note that the choroid is extensively thickened by a fish-flesh proliferation of lymphoid tissue, simulating the appearance of secondary ocular involvement with systemic lymphoma. In lymphoid hyperplasia of the uvea, however, the majority of patients do not have systemic disease, although the process may be mainly bilateral. *B,* Photomicrograph displays the intense cellularity of the uveal infiltrate, which is punctuated by pale-staining areas representing germinal centers. The iris has been spared in this case (as it frequently is), but there is a small amount of retrobulbar and episcleral lymphoid extension below. (*A* and *B,* Courtesy of Dr. Lorenz E. Zimmerman.)

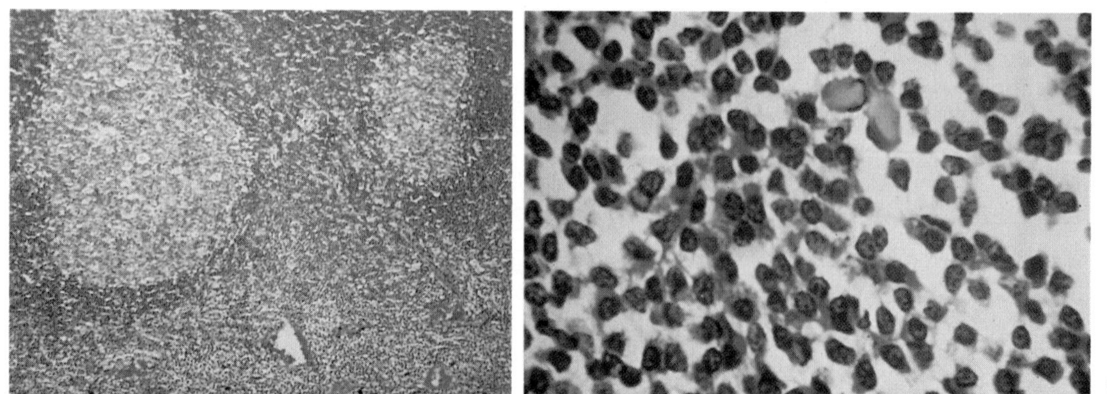

FIGURE 2-161 Lymphoid hyperplasia of the uvea. *A,* The hypercellular uveal infiltrate generally features small lymphocytes proliferating between variable-sized germinal centers. *B,* Often the tumor cells are plasmacytoid or lymphoplasmacytoid with evidence of intranuclear eosinophilic inclusions of immunoglobulin (Dutcher's bodies, one of which is *off-center left*) or similar eosinophilic inclusions in the cytoplasm (Russell's bodies, *upper right*). The tumor cells have more ample cytoplasm than lymphocytes, but they retain the small dark nuclei of lymphocytes and therefore are referred to as lymphoplasmacytoid cells. (*A* and *B,* Courtesy of Dr. Lorenz E. Zimmerman.)

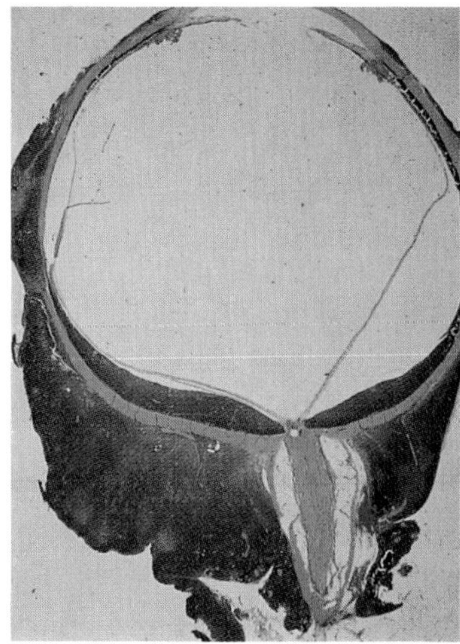

FIGURE 2–162 **Uveal lymphoid neoplasia.** The extraocular extensions of uveal lymphoid hyperplasia may sometimes overshadow the intraocular component and can lead to motility disturbances and proptosis. (Courtesy of Dr. Lorenz E. Zimmerman.)

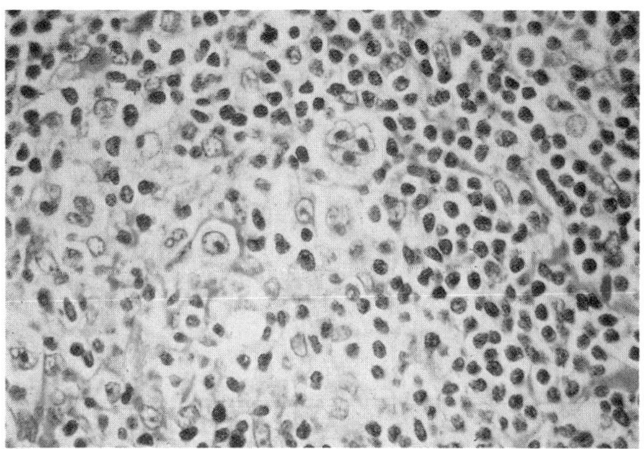

FIGURE 2–163 **Hodgkin's disease.** A Reed-Sternberg cell is shown slightly up and to the right of center in a biopsy specimen of a lymph node of a patient who had intraocular involvement with Hodgkin's disease. Note also the scattered atypical mononuclear cells toward the left. In the background, there are many mature lymphocytes and a scattering of eosinophilic leukocytes. (Courtesy of Dr. Lorenz E. Zimmerman.)

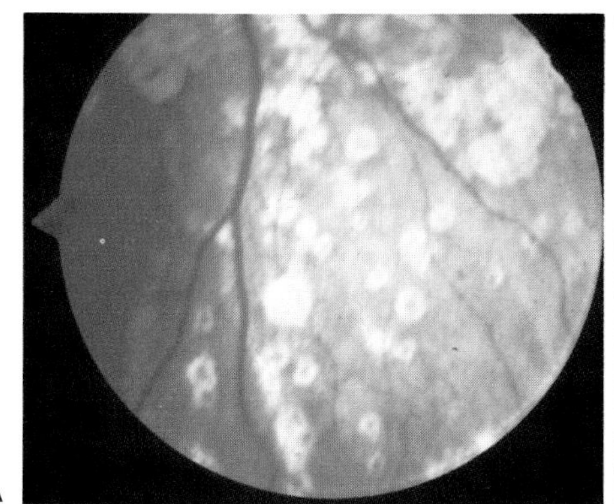

A

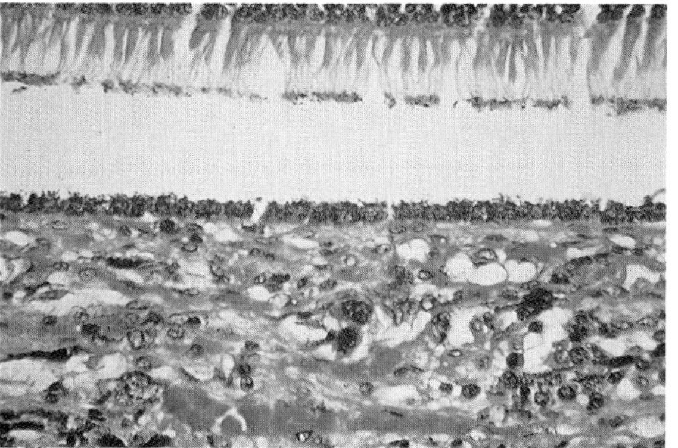

B

FIGURE 2–164 **Choroidal infiltration in systemic Hodgkin's disease.** *A*, The creamy choroidal infiltrates have a distinctive annular appearance. *B*, There are many large atypical mononuclear cells with hyperchromatic nuclei in the choroidal extravascular space, but no Reed-Sternberg cells are identifiable. These are sometimes difficult to find in extranodal tissues. (*A* and *B*, Courtesy of Dr. Lorenz E. Zimmerman.)

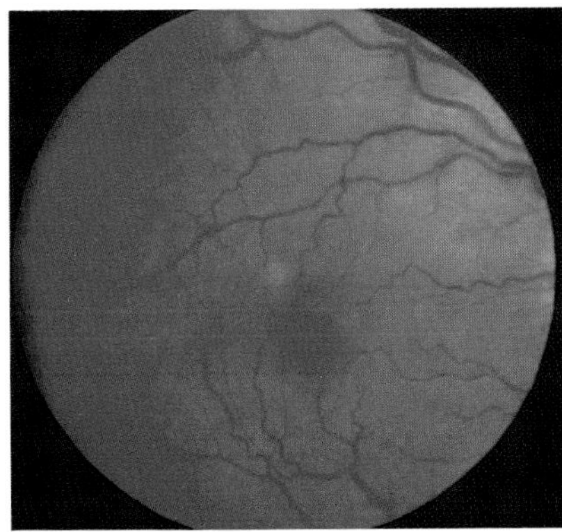

A

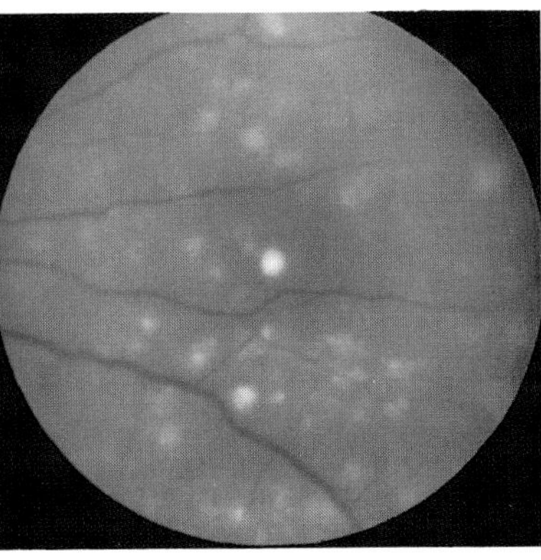

B

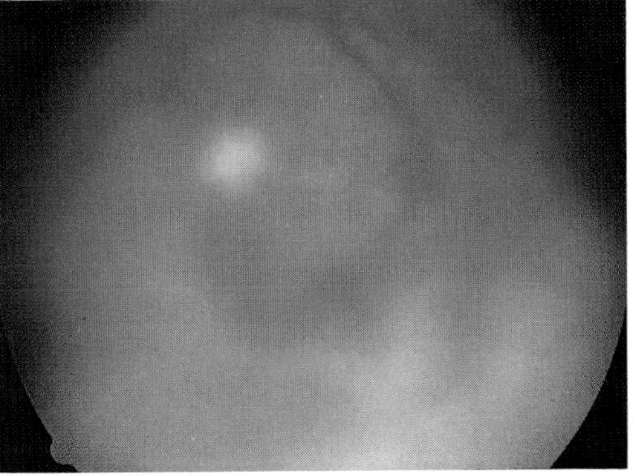

C

FIGURE 2–165 **Fundus involvement in mycosis fungoides, a T-cell cutaneous neoplasm.** *A*, In a patient with disseminated and end-stage mycosis fungoides, there is a small, round, creamy fundus lesion in the superotemporal perimacular region of the right eye. *B*, More peripherally in the left eye, there are myriad whitish lesions in the fundus. C, One month later, the lesions in *B* have achieved confluence and induced a retinal detachment. (*A–C*, Courtesy of Dr. B. C. Erny.)

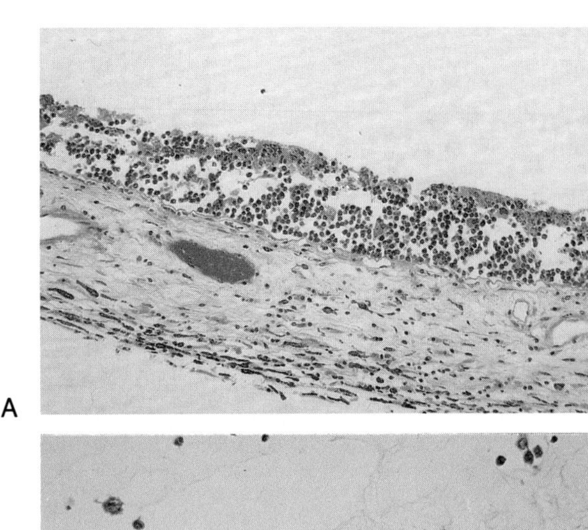

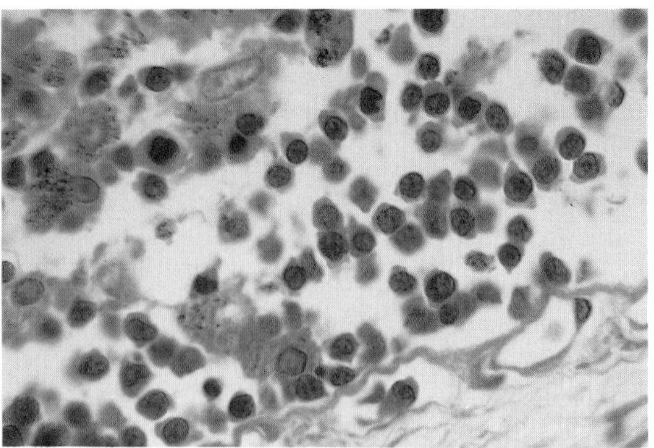

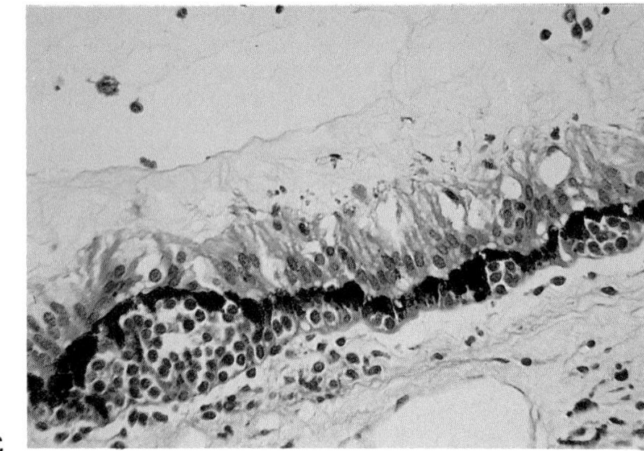

FIGURE 2–166 **Intraocular mycosis fungoides.** *A,* An extensive infiltrate of lymphocytes is situated beneath the pigment epithelium and above Bruch's membrane. Note the lack of neoplastic cells in the choroid. *B,* The neoplastic lymphocytes are hyperchromatic and occasionally show convoluted nuclear outlines. Bruch's membrane is shown toward the bottom right, and an atypical lymphocyte is found within a lumen of the choriocapillaris. *C,* Variable-sized collections of atypical T lymphocytes are found beneath the pigment epithelium of the pars plana region, above Bruch's membrane. There are also neoplastic cells in the vitreous. (*A–C,* Courtesy of Dr. Peter Egbert.)

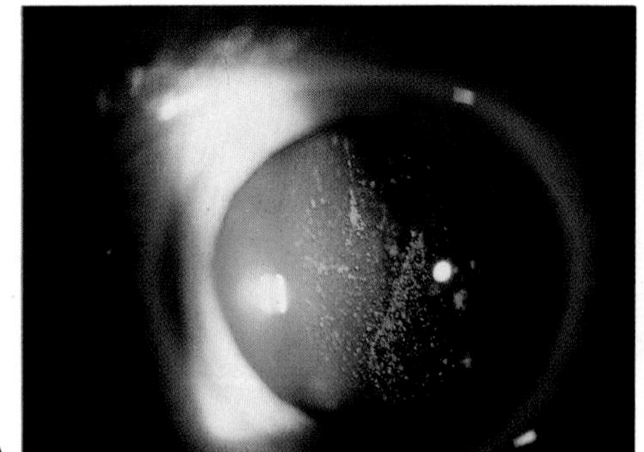

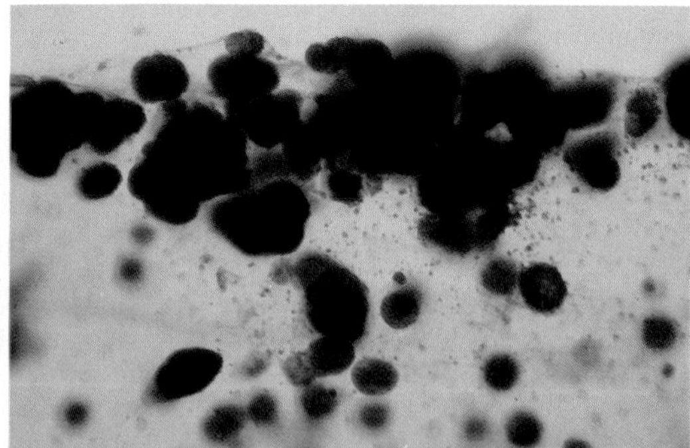

FIGURE 2–167 **Metastatic cutaneous melanoma to the eye.** *A,* A dispersion of pigment-laden tumor cells is present in the vitreous cavity. *B,* A cellular aspirate of the vitreous cavity shows clumps of tumor cells whose nuclear detail is obscured by the intense content of cytoplasmic melanin. (*A* and *B,* Courtesy of Dr. P. R. Sahel.)

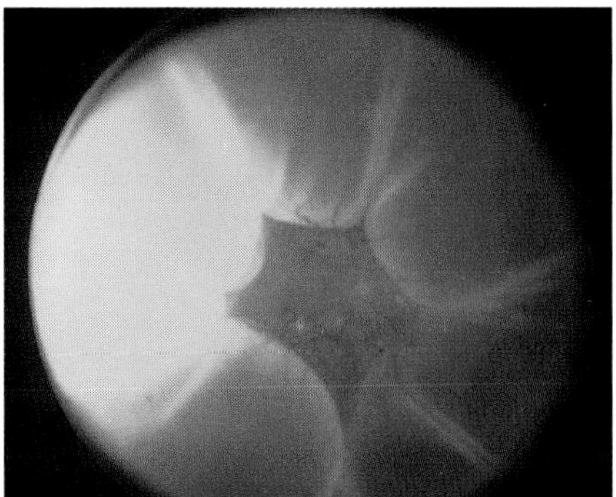

FIGURE 2–168 **Uveal effusion.** Fundus photograph (wide angle) shows a typical configuration of a nonrhegmatogenous retinal detachment. Note the absence of retinal breaks and fixed folds. The elevated retinal bullae are convex and show a smooth surface. (From Brockhurst RJ: Ciliochoroidal (uveal) effusion. *In* Ryan SJ, Ogden TE, Schachat AP (eds): Retina, vol. 2, St. Louis, CV Mosby, 1989; with permission.)

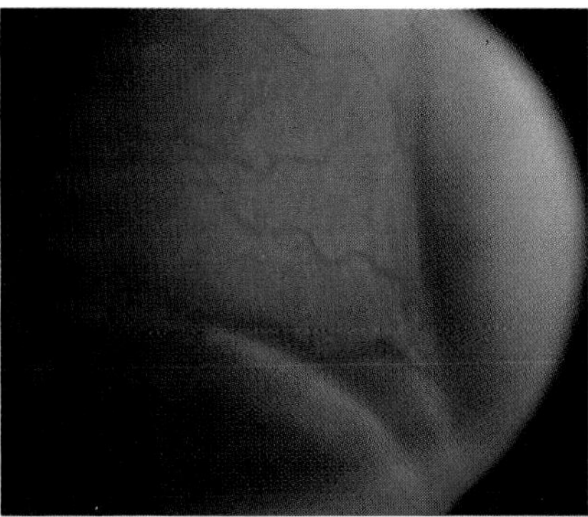

FIGURE 2–171 **Pseudomelanoma uveal effusion.** Fundus photograph of nanophthalmic uveal effusion shows choroidal detachment that resembles malignant melanoma.

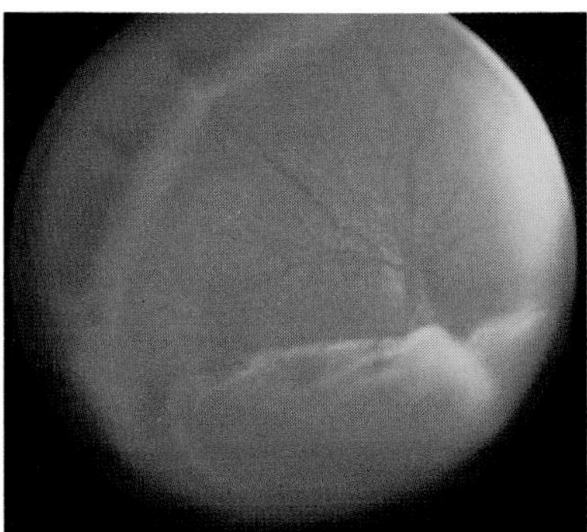

FIGURE 2–169 **Fundus photograph of nanophthalmic uveal effusion.** Note peripheral choroidal detachment in the upper temporal area and the absence of a choroidal pattern throughout the fundus (the vortex ampullae are not visible). In addition, the retina is detached in the dependent area below. Note that the retina is not detached in the periphery from the 7:30 to the 9 o'clock meridians.

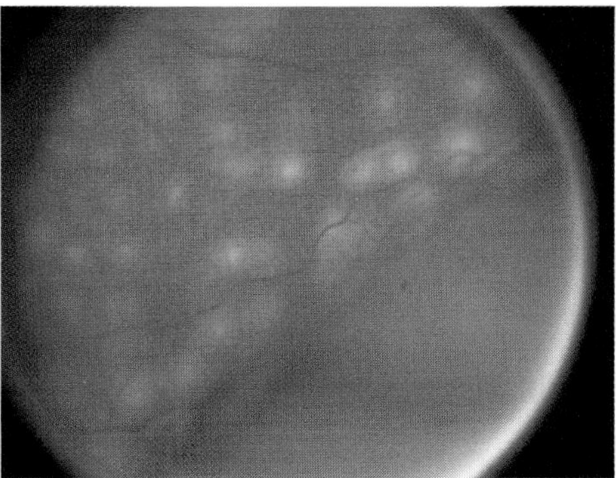

FIGURE 2–172 **Choroidal detachment after laser.** Fundus photograph shows a large choroidal detachment complicating panretinal argon laser photocoagulation. This generally occurs because an excessive amount of thermal energy was used during the therapeutic procedure.

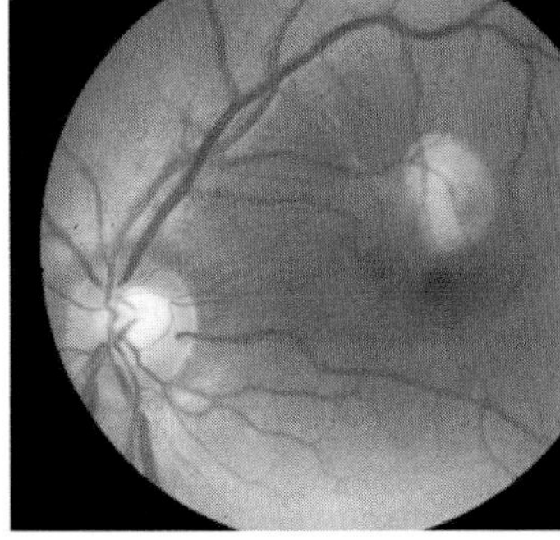

FIGURE 2–170 **Uveal effusion.** Fundus photograph shows yellowish subretinal exudate, seen as an early sign of uveal effusion. (From Brockhurst RJ, Lam KW: Uveal effusion II: Report of a case with analysis of subretinal fluid. Arch Ophthalmol 90:399, 1973. Copyright 1973, American Medical Association.)

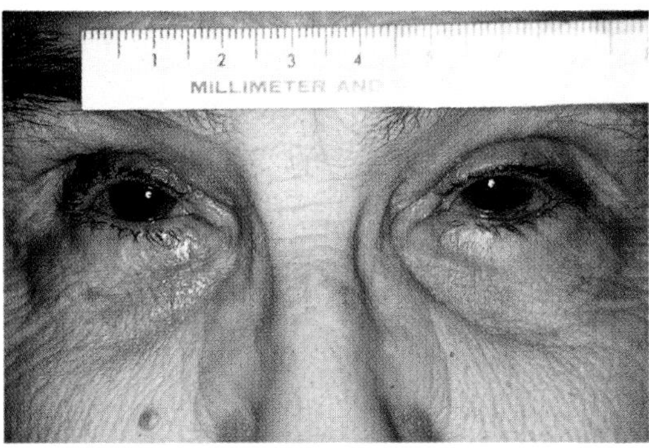

FIGURE 2–173 **Nanophthalmos.** The eyes of a patient with nanophthalmos. Note that the small eyes are deeply set in the eyelids. Nanophthalmos is always bilateral and is characterized by a diminutive eye, with one main exception: the crystalline lens, which has been reported to be of normal or slightly larger than normal size.

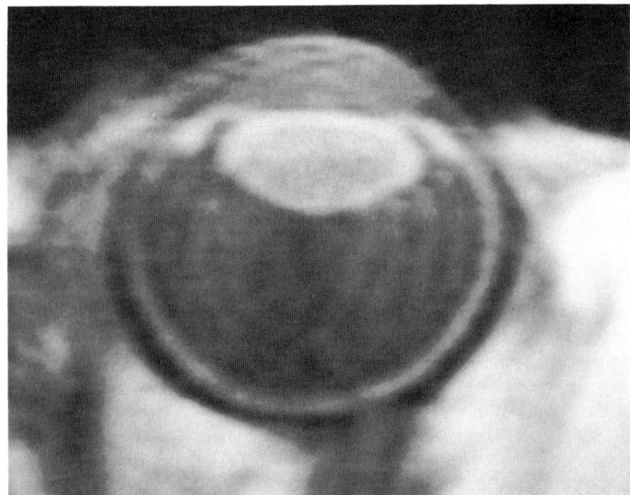

FIGURE 2–174 **Magnetic resonance imaging of a nanophthalmic eye.** The globe is small, measuring 17.5 mm in anteroposterior length, whereas the lens measures 4.5 × 9.0 mm. This technique clearly shows the thickened sclera *(black areas)* and the thickened choroid *(light areas).* (Courtesy of Hong-Ming Cheng, O.D., Ph.D., Massachusetts Eye and Ear Infirmary, who kindly provided this MRI, obtained using special coils that he developed.)

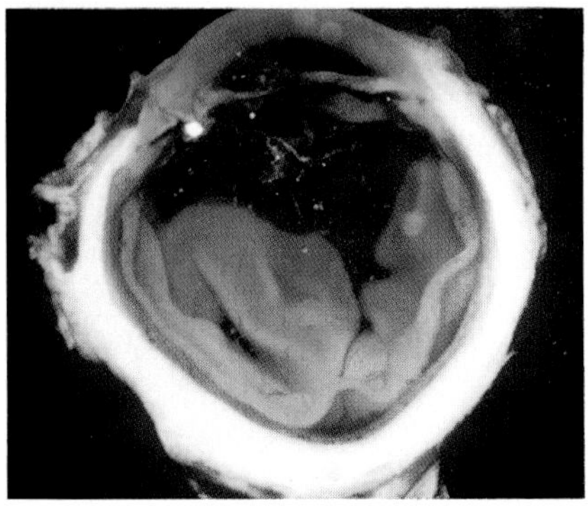

FIGURE 2–175 **Photograph of a nanophthalmic eye specimen.** Note the extremely thick sclera, thickened choroid, and nonrhegmatogenous retinal detachment.

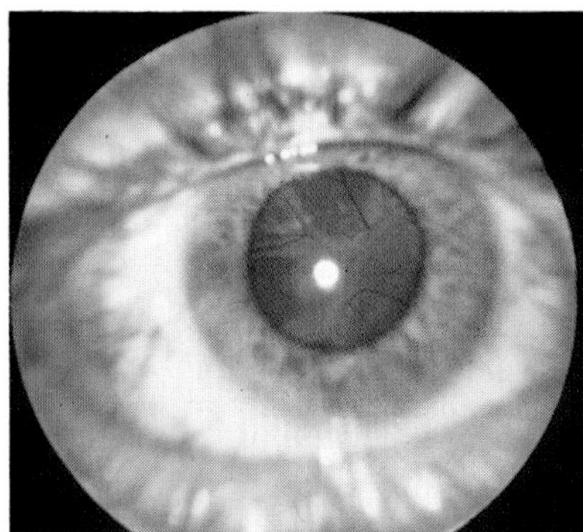

FIGURE 2–176 Anterior segment photograph of a nanophthalmic uveal effusion with the retina in contact with the crystalline lens.

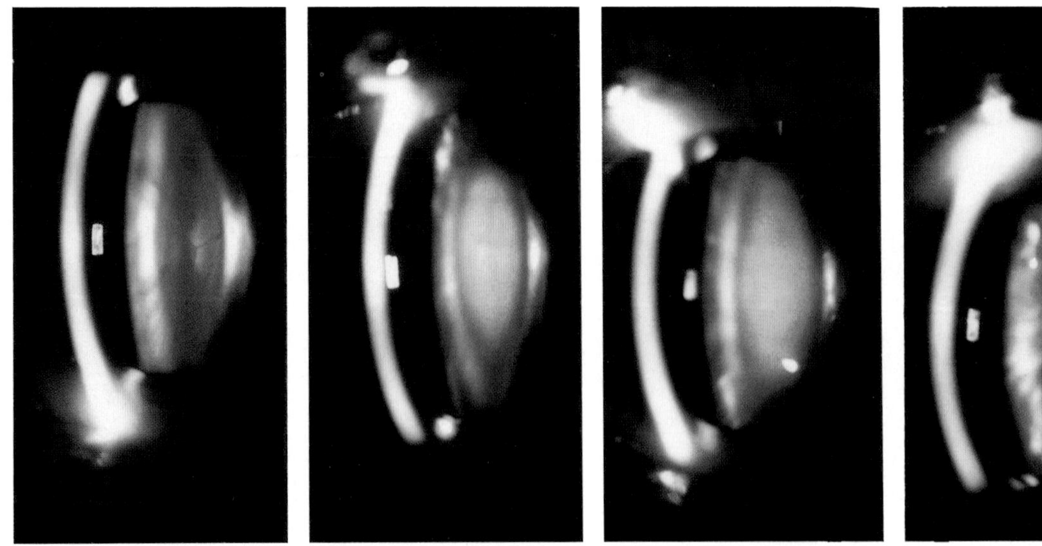

FIGURE 2–177 **Images of human lenses.** Direct, or transillumination, slit-lamp images of human lenses at different ages with various pathologies. *Left,* In a normal, noncataractous adult lens, these zones of discontinuity appear as partial, concentric shells of different color, density, and granularity. Note the Y suture within the fetal nucleus. *Left middle,* Nuclear cataracts have a central opacity that enlarges *(right middle)* as cataractogenesis proceeds. The nuclear opacities show varying degrees of discoloration ranging from white to yellow to brown as a function of the severity of the nuclear cataract. The nuclear opacity obscures the normally visible Y suture of the fetal nucleus. *Right,* Anterior subcapsular cataracts have a diffuse opacity consisting of metaplastic cells beneath the normal lens epithelium and above the normal fibrous cell mass. (Courtesy of L. T. Chylack, Jr.)

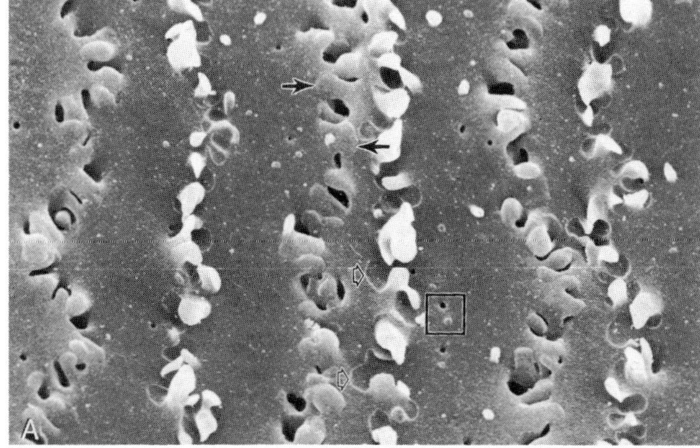

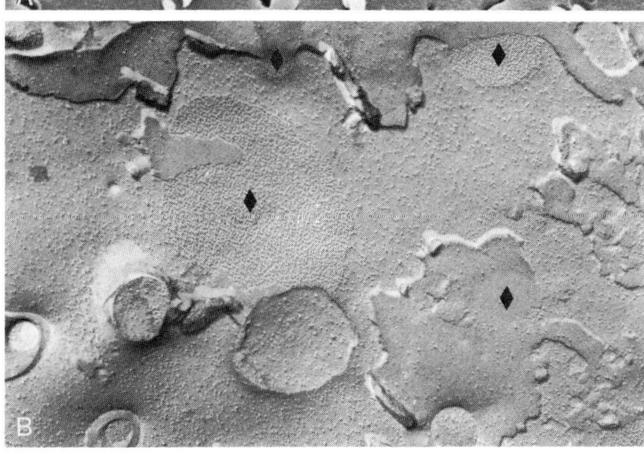

FIGURE 2–178 **Electron micrographs of normal lenses.** *A,* Scanning electron micrograph of superficial cortical fibrous cells of noncataractous lenses. The surface morphology of superficial cortical fibers of aged, noncataractous lens. Typical lateral interdigitations (flaps) *(solid arrows)* and the complementary imprints *(open arrows)* and balls and their complementary sockets *(square)* are arrayed along the length of superficial cortical fiber cells. *B,* Transmission electron micrograph of a freeze-etch replica showing the ultrastructure of the lateral membrane of these cells. Note the loose particle packing of the transmembrane proteins of fiber cell gap junctions *(diamonds)* and the relative lack of orthogonal arrays of particles.

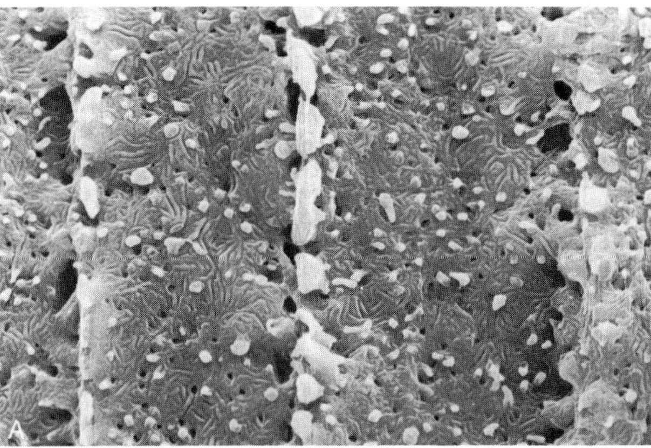

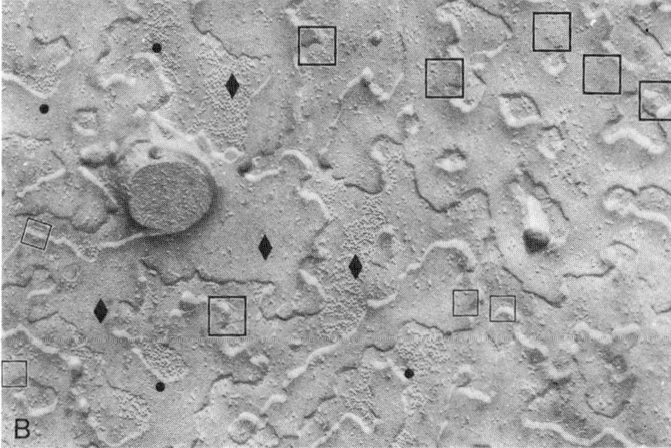

FIGURE 2–179 *A,* Scanning electron micrograph of intermediate cortical fibrous cells of noncataractous lens. The surface morphology of intermediate cortical fibers cells of aged, noncataractous lenses. The formerly planar apical, basal, and lateral membrane is progressively changed into polygonal domains of furrowed membrane. *B,* Transmission electron micrograph of a freeze-etch replica showing the lateral membrane ultrastructure of these cells. Loose aggregations of transmembrane proteins (*diamonds* and *circles*) and orthogonal rays of particles *(squares)* are common. Although many of the aggregations of transmembrane proteins *(diamonds)* meet the structural requirements of gap junctions (they bridge a narrowed, 2- to 4-nm extracellular gap), others *(circles)* have fracture shelves between the E and P faces of the membrane that are too far apart (derived from stereoscopic parallax measurements) to function as intercellular junctions. The size of the extracellular space at the sites of orthogonal arrays of particles (OAPs) is too large for these membrane-protein domains to function as intracellular junctions.

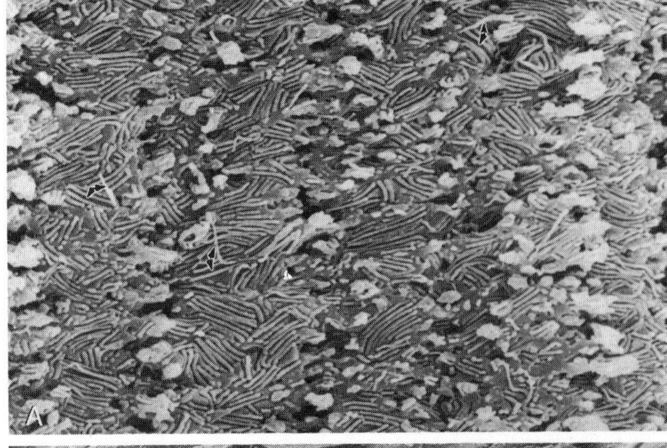

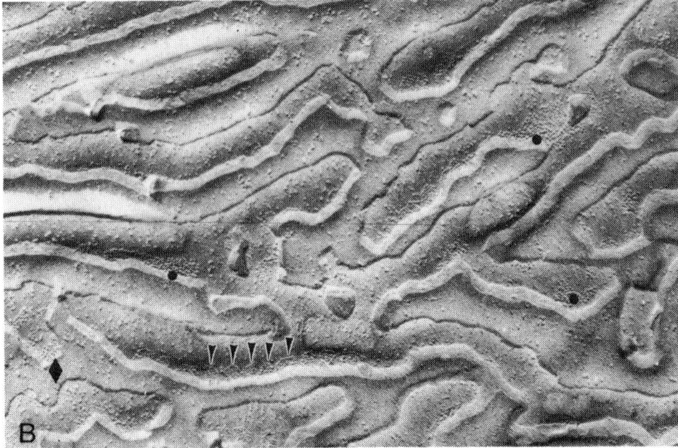

FIGURE 2–180 *A,* Electron micrograph of deep cortical fibers of noncataractous lens. The surface morphology of deep cortical fiber cells of middle-aged noncataractous lenses and adult nuclear fibers of senescent, noncataractous lenses. The lateral membrane of these cells has been transformed into polygonal domains of furrowed membrane with many of the ridges overlain by long microvilli *(arrows). B,* Transmission electron micrograph of a freeze-etch replica showing the ultrastructure of the lateral membrane of these cells. Many of the ridges are characterized by orthogonal arrays of particles (OAPs) *(arrowheads)* alternating with patches of protein-free membrane along their length. Occasionally, aggregations of larger transmembrane proteins *(circles)* are noted. Small gap junctions *(diamond)* are rare.

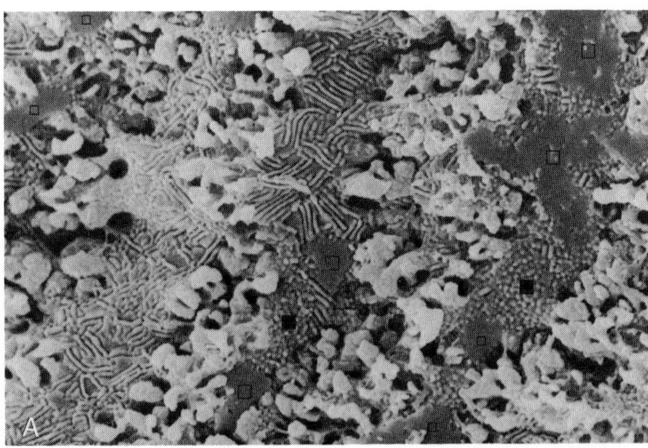

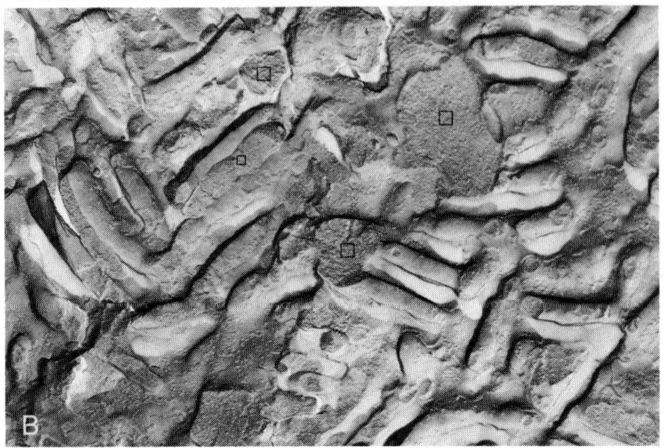

FIGURE 2–181 *A,* Electron micrograph of nuclear fibrous cells in a normal noncataractous lens. The surface morphology of nuclear fibrous cells in a normal, noncataractous senescent lens. Grossly, these cells have an inconstant, nonhexagonal shape and lateral interdigitations that are nonuniform and irregularly arrayed along the fibrous cell length. The polygonal domains of furrowed membrane are also less ordered and somewhat less numerous. Many are replaced by short microplicae *(solid squares)* and areas devoid of ridges, microvilli, and microplicae *(open squares). B,* Transmission electron micrograph of a freeze-fracture replica showing the ultrastructure of these cells. Both gap junctions and OAPs occur infrequently. Aggregation of membrane proteins, however, is common. Many areas devoid of ridges, microvilli, and microplicae are breaches in the plasma membrane *(squares).*

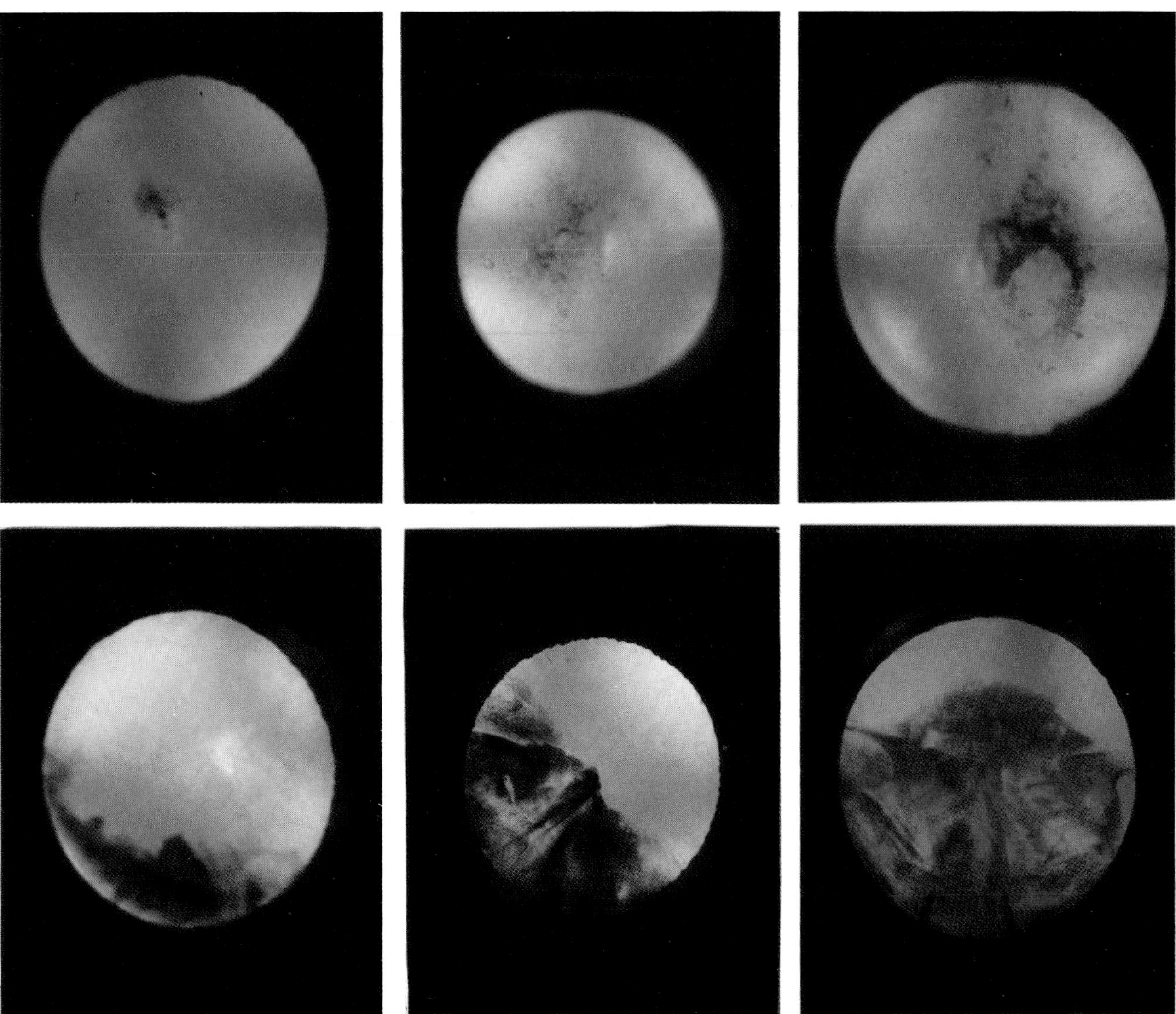

FIGURE 2–182 **Stages of cataract formation.** Retroillumination slit-lamp images of posterior subcapsular cataracts *(top row)* and cortical cataracts *(bottom row)* at different stages of cataract formation *(left to right)*. Posterior subcapsular cataracts are seen initially as dot opacities near the center of the visual axis. As the cataract forms, the opacities become larger and more diffuse. Cortical cataracts first appear as small spike-shaped and wedge-shaped opacities located at the lens periphery. As the cataract forms, the spikes and wedges enlarge toward the center of the visual axis. (Courtesy of L. T. Chylack, Jr.)

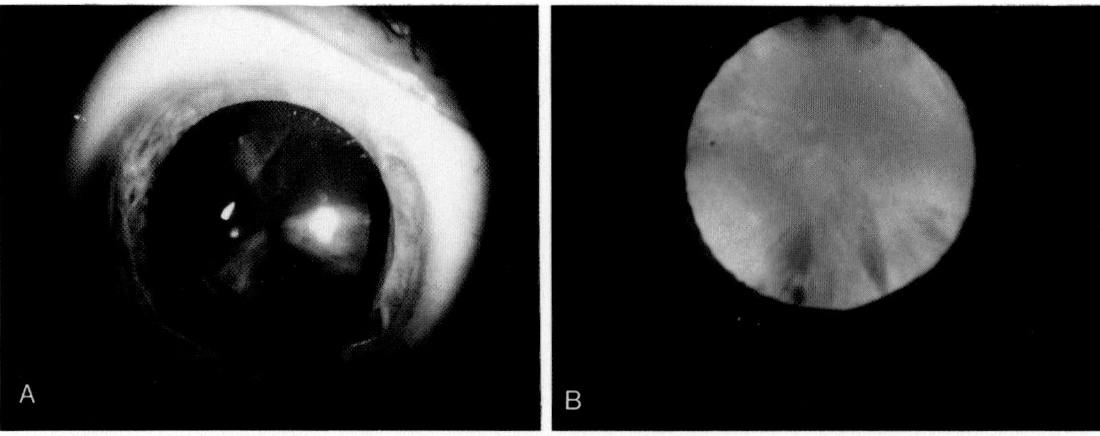

FIGURE 2–183 **Developmental cortical cataract.** *A,* Retroillumination slit-lamp images of an early developmental cortical cataract from a 35-year-old man. (Courtesy of M. S. Macsai-Kaplan.) *B,* A mixed cortical nuclear cataract. In a mixed cortical nuclear cataract, several spike-shaped and wedge-shaped cortical opacities can be seen in the lens periphery; a central darkening of the lens corresponds to a nuclear opacity that can be seen to greater advantage by direct illumination slit-lamp examination. (Courtesy of L. T. Chylack, Jr.)

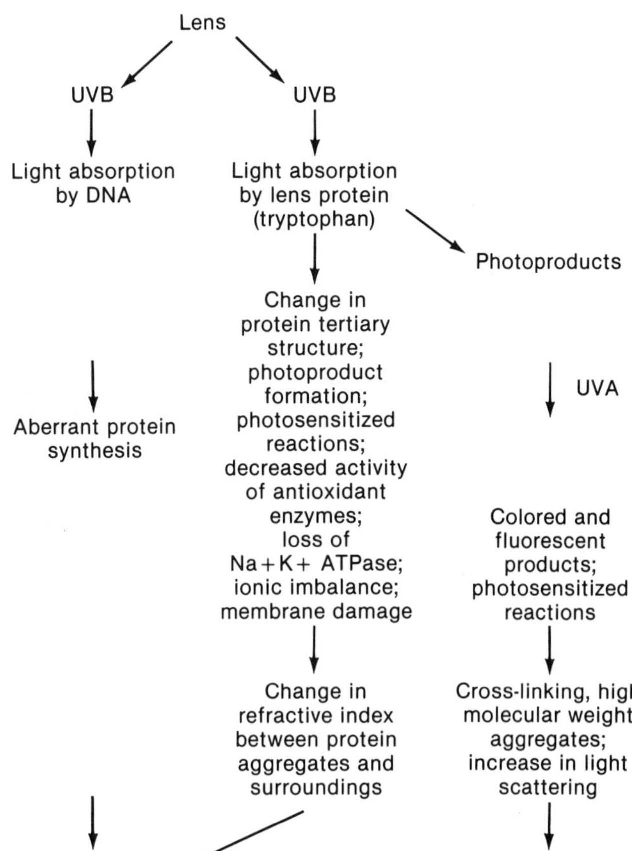

FIGURE 2–184 **A proposed scheme for cataractogenesis.** Light is absorbed by the chromophore (e.g., DNA bases and protein tryptophan). The absorption of electromagnetic energy of radiation produces an excited-state molecule, which undergoes a chemical change to form a photoproduct. The photoproduct may initiate complex biochemical changes, such as abnormal protein synthesis, altered protein structure, inactivation of enzymes, ionic imbalances, and generation of oxidants by photosensitized reactions. These processes culminate in a cellular response (e.g., abnormal fibrous cell formation and formation of high molecular weight protein aggregates). Multiple photochemical pathways may proceed simultaneously in the lens, resulting in the formation of cataracts.

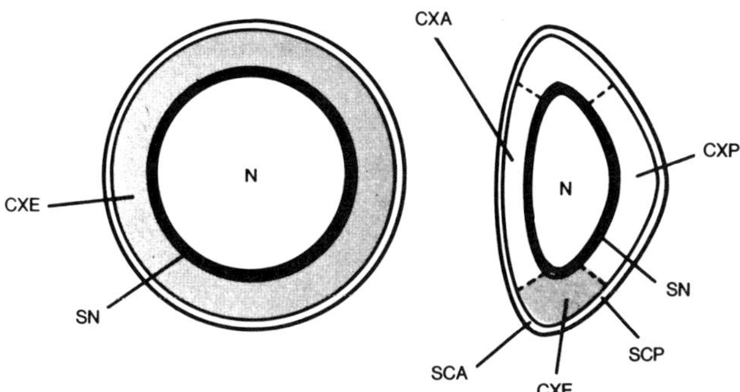

FIGURE 2–185 **Anatomic zones of crystalline lens.** Diagrammatic representation of anatomic zones of the human crystalline lens used in classifying cataractous change according to the American Cooperative Cataract Research Group method. (SCA, subcapsular anterior; SCP, subcapsular posterior; CXA, anterior cortical; CXE, equatorial cortical; CXP, posterior cortical; SN, supranuclear; N, nuclear. (From Chylack LT, Lee MR, Tung WH, Cheng HM: Classification of human senile cataractous change by the American Cooperative Cataract Research Group (CCRG) method. 1. Instrumentation and technique. Invest Ophthalmol Vis Sci 24:424, 1983.)

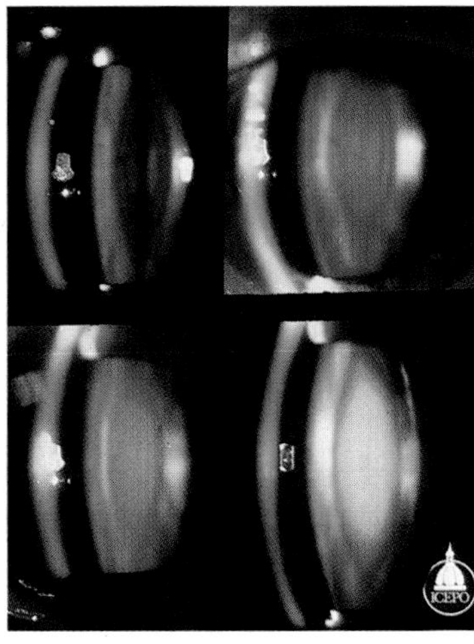

FIGURE 2–187 **"Wilmer" system: standard photographs for grading nuclear opacities.** *Upper left,* Nuclear standard 1; *upper right,* nuclear standard 2; *lower left,* nuclear standard 3; *lower right,* nuclear standard 4. (From Taylor HR, West SK: A simple system for the clinical grading of lens opacities. Lens Res 5(1 and 2):175, 1988; by courtesy of Marcel Dekker, Inc.)

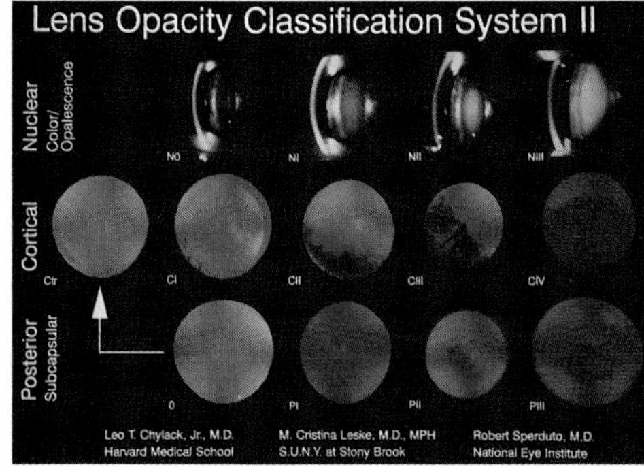

FIGURE 2–186 **Lens opacities classification system II (LOCS II).** This set of standard photographs is prepared as a 21.25- × 27.50-cm transparency for use at a slit lamp. It is placed on a light box near the patient and is used by the biomicroscopist to classify cataractous changes in vivo. (N0, nuclear standard 0; NI, nuclear standard I; NII, nuclear standard II; NIII, nuclear standard III; 0, cortical standard 0; Ctr, cortical standard trace; CI, CII, CIII, and CIV, cortical standards I through IV; 0, PI, PII, and PIII, posterior subcapsular standards 0 through III. 0 is the clear lens standard for both P and C grading.) (From Chylack LT Jr, Leske MC, McCarthy D, et al: Lens Opacities Classification System II (LOCS II). Arch Ophthalmol 107:991, 1989. Copyright 1989, American Medical Association.)

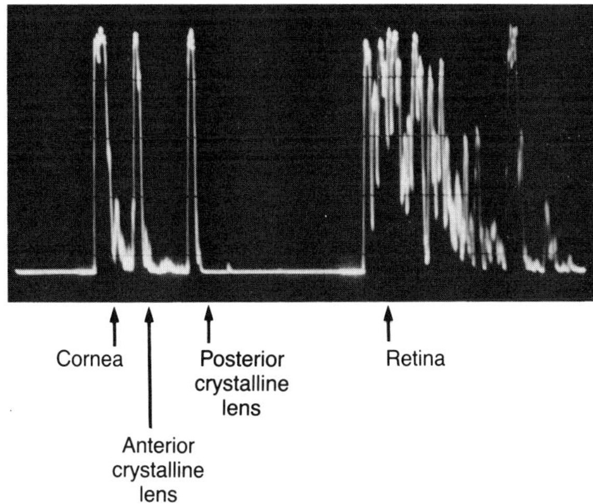

FIGURE 2–188 **A-scan biometry.** Axial length of a normal eye of 22.12 mm as measured by A-scan ultrasonography. (Courtesy of Lois Hart, R.D.M.S.)

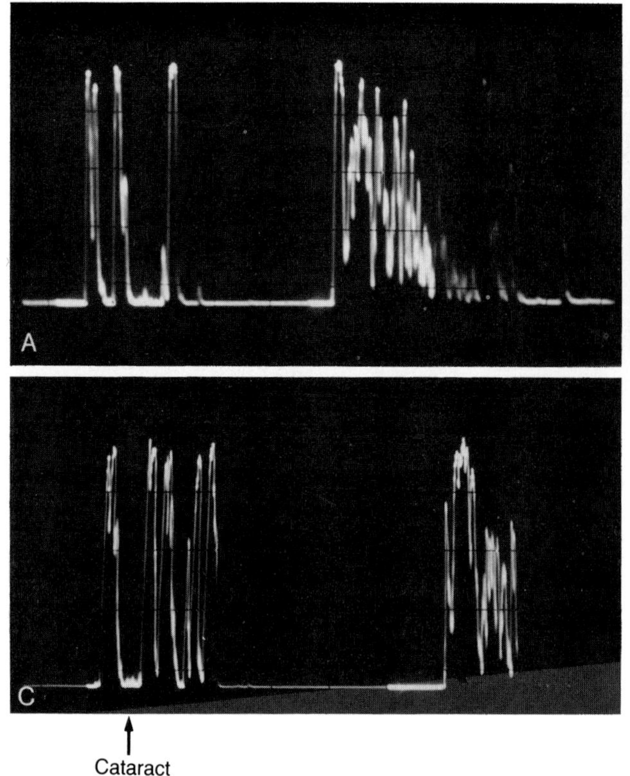

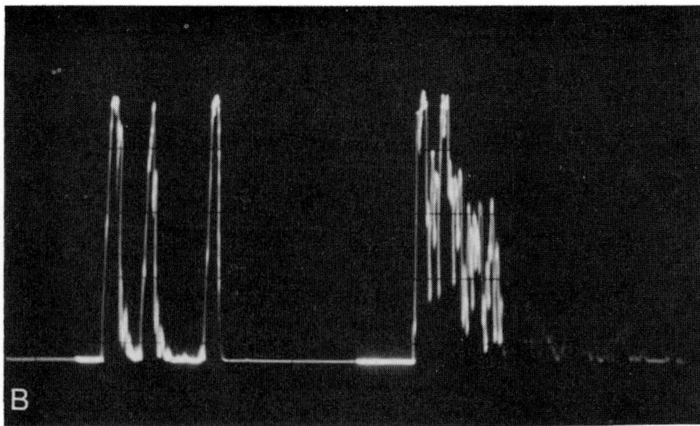

FIGURE 2–189 **A-scan biometry of hyperopic, emmetropic, and myopic eyes.** *A,* An A-scan of a "hyperopic" eye having a short axial length, measuring 20.20 mm. *B,* An A-scan of a normal-length eye with an overall length of 22.45 mm. Note the greater distance between the posterior lens echo and the retinal echo. *C,* Increasing distance between echoes as axial length increases is evident in this myopic eye with axial length of 22.45 mm. Note the increased echoes from within the crystalline lens, indicating the presence of a cataract. (*A–C,* Courtesy of Lois Hart, R.D.M.S.)

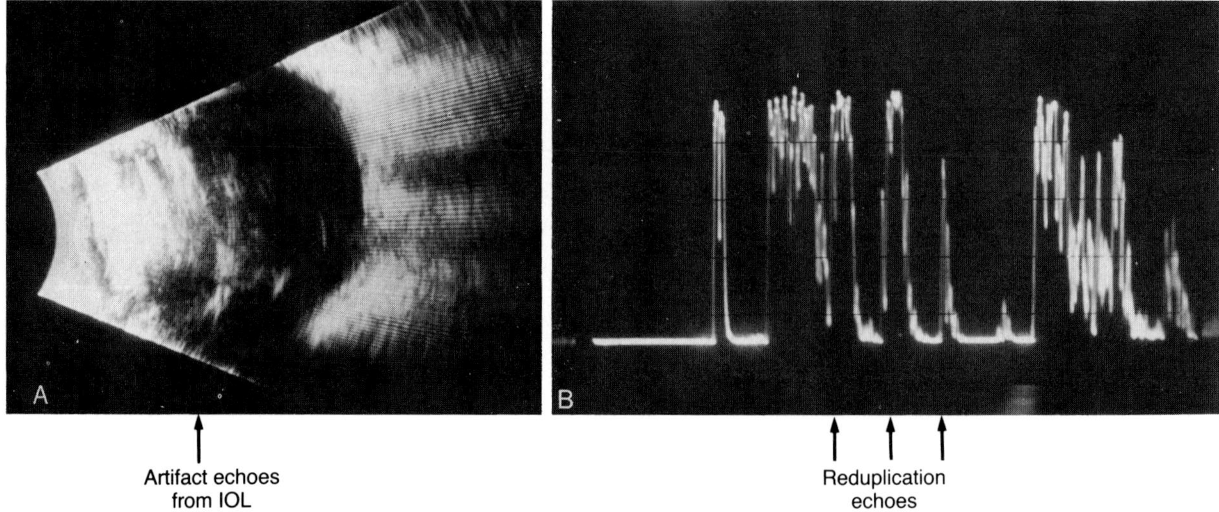

FIGURE 2–190 **Pseudophakic eye.** A B-scan *(A)* and an A-scan *(B)*. The intraocular lens (IOL) causes multiple "reduplication" echoes, obscuring the scans behind the lens. (*A* and *B,* Courtesy of Lois Hart, R.D.M.S.)

SECTION 3

Retina and Vitreous

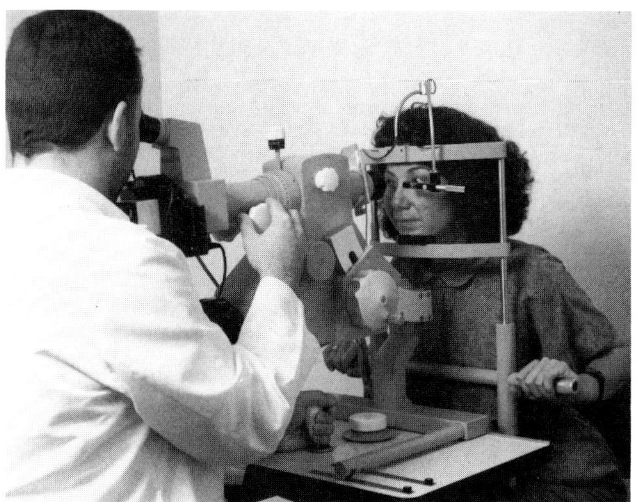

FIGURE 3–1 **Fundus camera used for fluorescein angiography.** Focusing is accomplished using a joystick (left hand) and is optimized via a focusing knob (right hand). Light from the strobe flash illuminates the fundus during the photographic exposure. Color transparencies are customarily obtained first, camera backs are changed, and the angiographic frames are recorded on black and white Kodak Tri-X film.

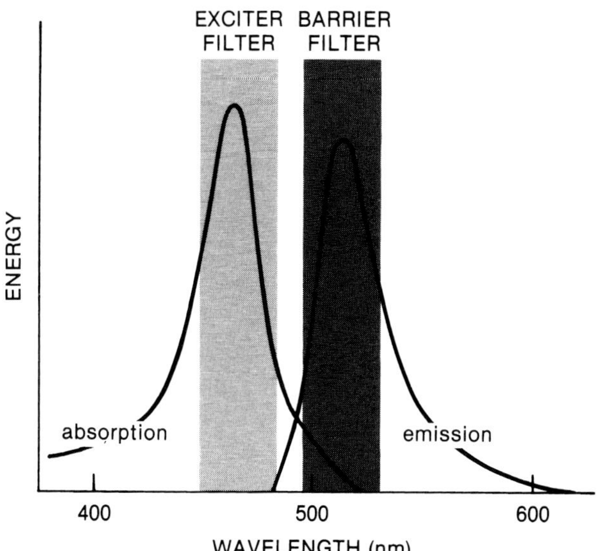

FIGURE 3–2 **Principles of fluorescence in fluorescein angiography.** Fluorescein dye absorbs visible light in the blue spectrum as indicated by its absorption curve. It then fluoresces, producing green light with an emission spectrum shown on the right-hand curve. In the fundus camera, white light passes through an excitation filter to produce the excitation wavelengths, while a barrier filter, interposed in front of the film pack, only transmits light of longer wavelengths, so light simply reflected off the fundus is not detected.

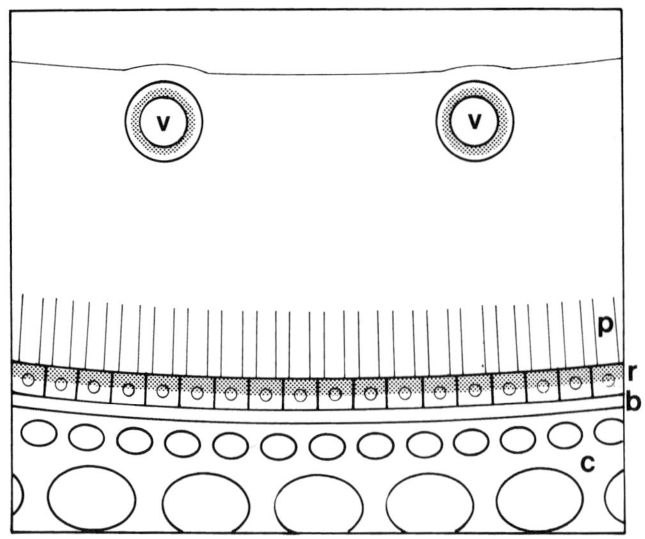

FIGURE 3–3 **Cross section of the eye wall.** The sensory retina contains vessels (v) located within its superficial layers, whereas the photoreceptors (p) are found in the deepest layer. The retinal pigment epithelial cells (r) lie directly adjacent to the photoreceptors and just above Bruch's membrane (b). The choroid (c), located beneath Bruch's membrane, provides nutrition to the outer layers of the sensory retina. Normal barriers to fluorescein leakage are the tight junctions of both the retinal vasculature and the retinal pigment epithelium, as indicated by the shaded zones.

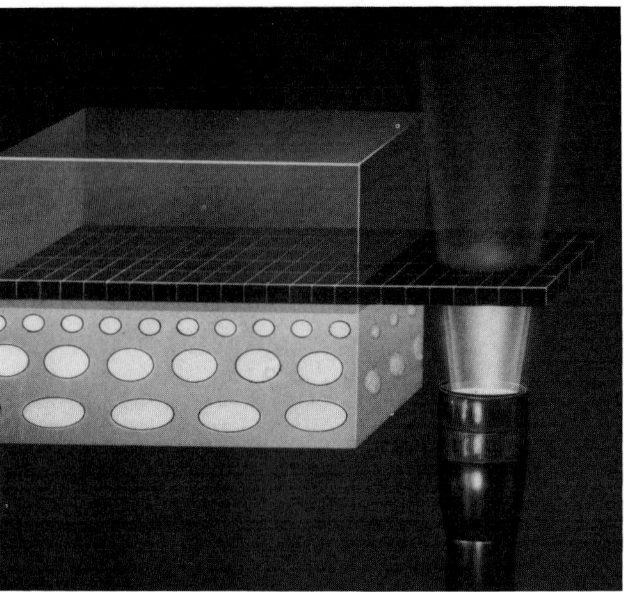

FIGURE 3–4 **Blocking of fluorescence by the retinal pigment epithelium.** The melanin granules of the retinal pigment epithelium act like an optical filter, attenuating the intensity of the underlying choroidal fluorescence, depicted here by the beam of a flashlight. Xanthophyll in the macula also blocks background choroidal fluorescence, contributing to the darker angiographic appearance of the fovea.

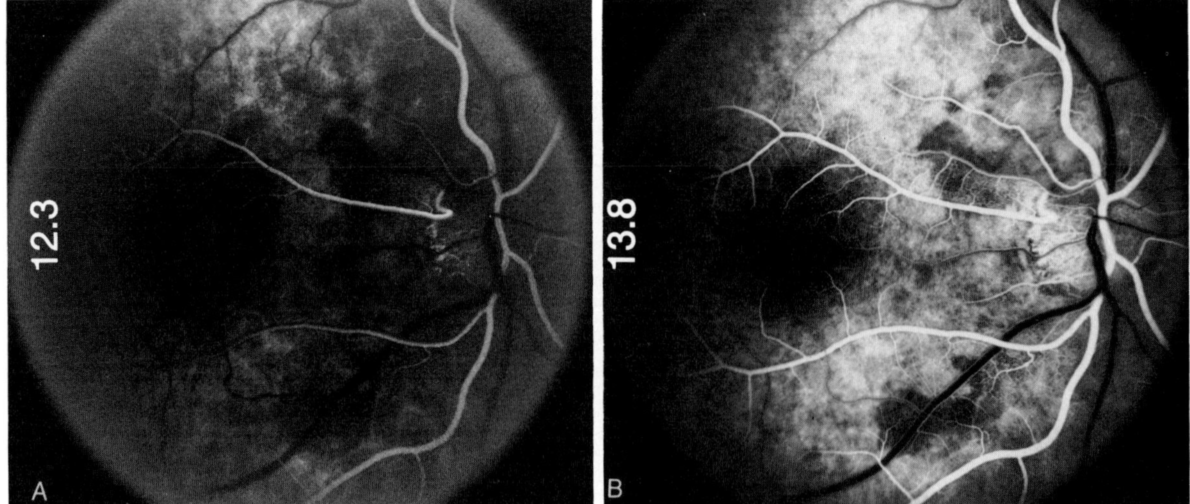

FIGURE 3–5 **Normal fluorescein angiogram.** The time after intravenous injection of fluorescein dye into an antecubital vein is indicated on each frame. Approximately 10 to 15 seconds later, the choroid exhibits patchy filling of its lobules via the short posterior ciliary arteries, and within seconds thereafter, the retinal arteries begin to fill quickly in the period known as the arterial phase *(A)*. Pathologic processes that interfere with the arterial supply of the choroid and retina, such as carotid occlusive disease or giant cell arteritis, may lead to substantial delays in the filling of the choroidal lobules and the retinal arterioles. The end of the arterial phase is characterized by complete filling of the arterioles with fluorescein dye *(B)*.

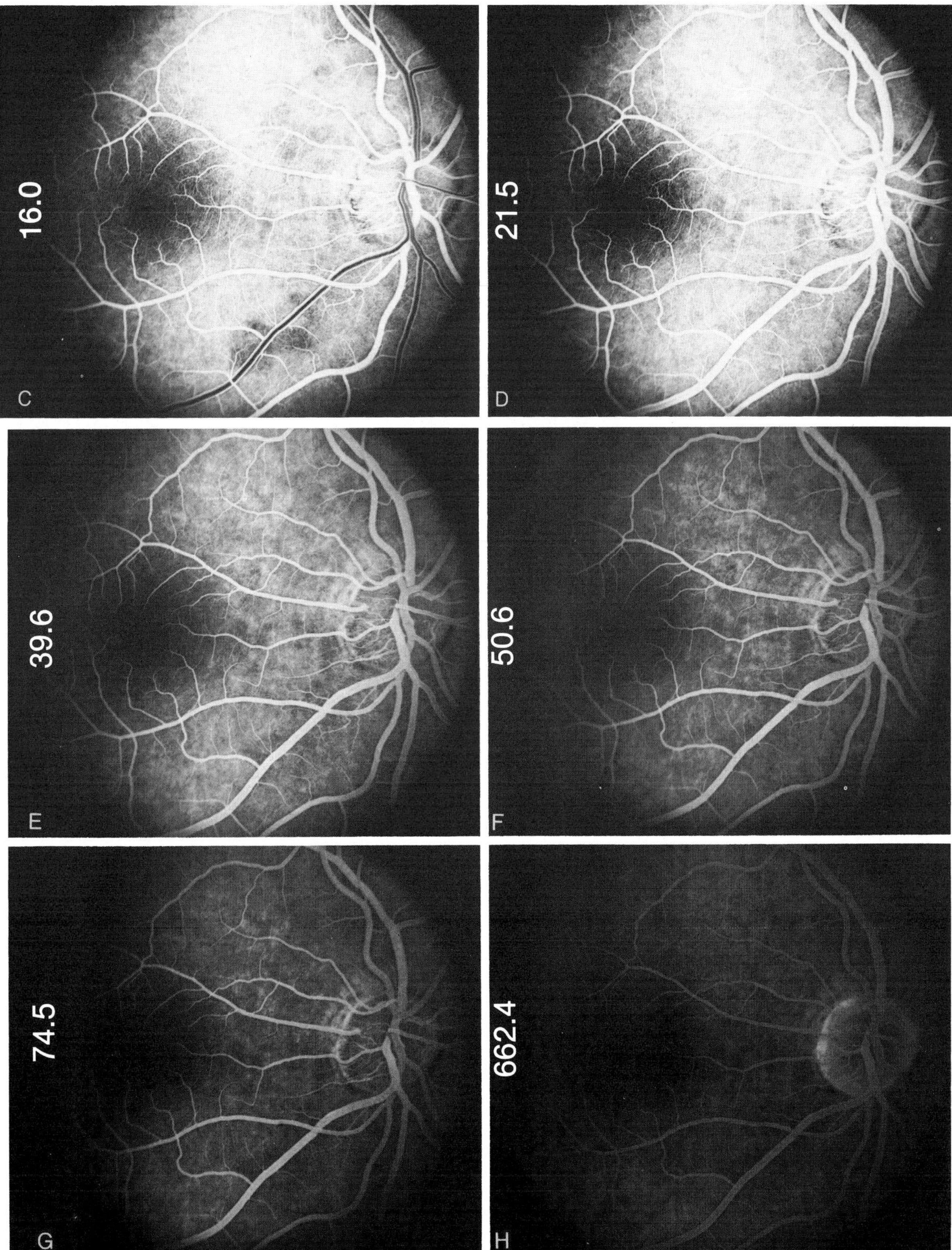

FIGURE 3–5 *Continued* Shortly thereafter, dye begins to accumulate near the walls of the larger veins, marking the laminar flow or early arteriovenous phase *(C)*. Gradually the concentration of dye in all vessels increases until it is maximal, indicating peak phase *(D)*. During this phase, the foveal avascular zone is most apparent. By 30 seconds after injection, the dye has begun to recirculate in the blood stream, decreasing its intensity in the eye. The study thus enters the late arteriovenous phases *(E–G)*. Ten minutes after injection and beyond, little fluorescein remains in the normal eye *(H)*. These late-phase films are important, however, when evaluating an eye for macular edema and neovascularization. (*A–H,* Courtesy of Constantine Balouris, M.D.)

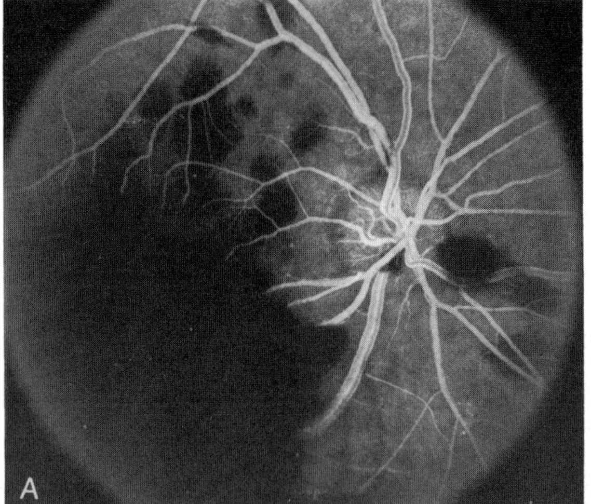

FIGURE 3–6 **Blockage of fluorescence.** Pigments such as hemoglobin in blood or excess melanin in the choroid or retinal pigment epithelium absorb some of the blue excitation wavelengths and attenuate the fluorescence of the deeper choroidal layers. *A,* Large areas of hypofluorescence secondary to preretinal and intraretinal hemorrhage are seen in a patient with Valsalva retinopathy. *B,* Hypofluorescence secondary to blocked choroidal fluorescence is shown in the area of the choroidal nevus just inferonasal to the fovea. A few window defects (see Fig. 3–8) within the nevus exhibit hyperfluorescence. *C,* The mechanism of hypofluorescence is shown in cross section demonstrating how the presence of excess pigment may attenuate deep choroidal fluorescence.

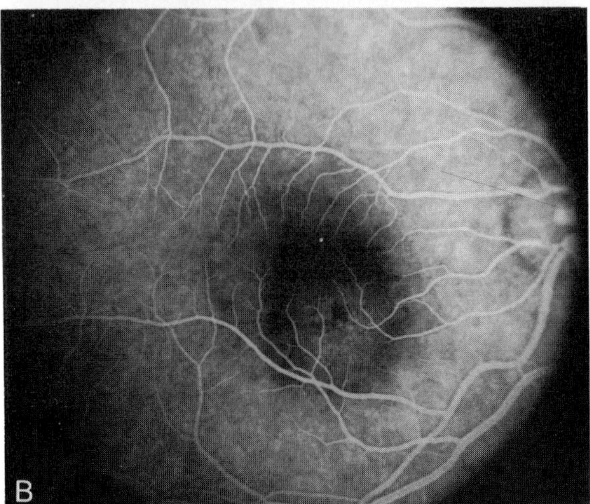

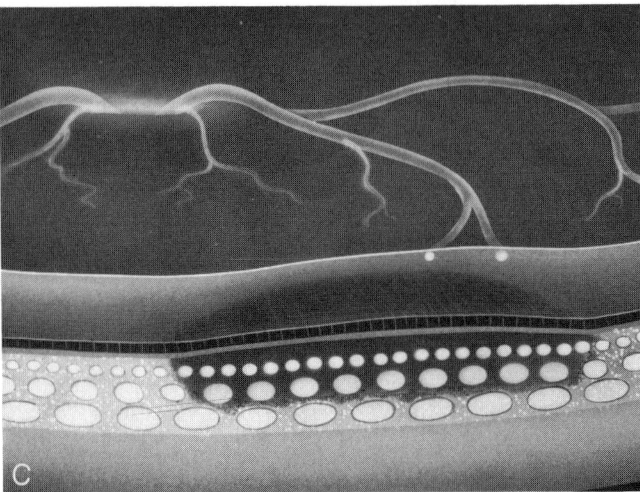

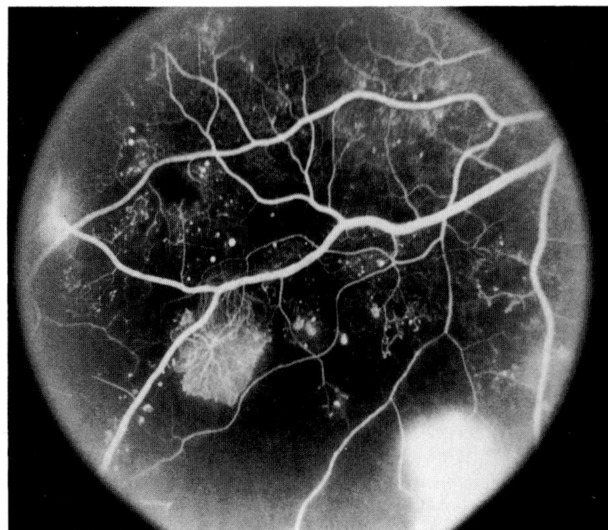

FIGURE 3–7 **Hypoperfusion.** Hypoperfusion from retinal ischemia (in this case secondary to diabetes mellitus) causes hypofluorescence. The retinal capillary bed has been occluded, decreasing the concentration of intraretinal fluorescein that normally would be seen in this arteriovenous phase of the angiogram. The bright regions of hyperfluorescence are areas of retinal neovascularization that are typically found at the border between ischemic and nonischemic retina.

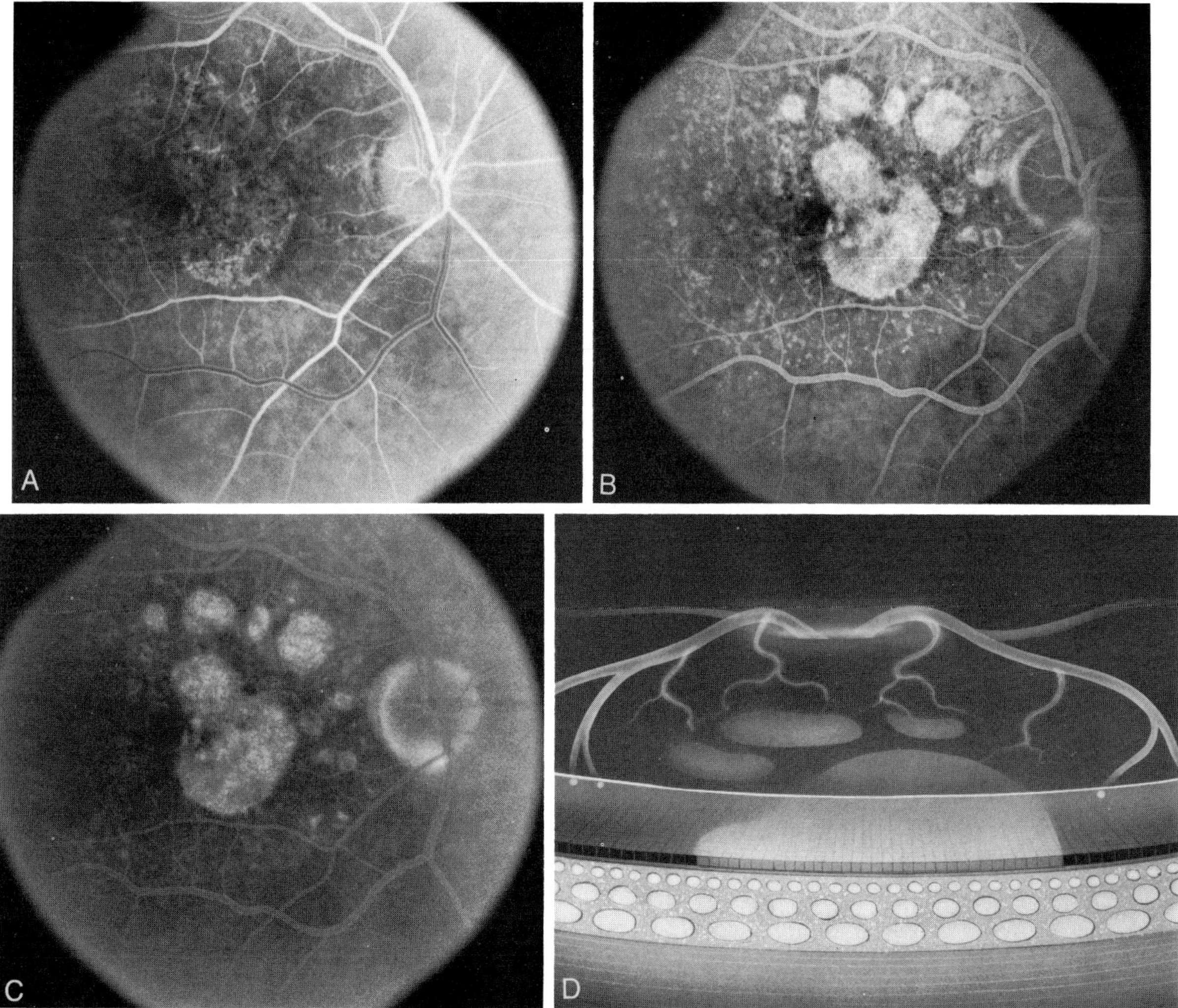

FIGURE 3–8 **Window defects.** Loss of the normal attenuation effect of the retinal pigment epithelium creates a footprint-like pattern of hyperfluorescent window defects surrounding the fovea in this patient with age-related macular degeneration. Although the retinal pigment epithelium contains little pigment, its tight junctions are intact and prevent leakage of dye into the subretinal space. The defects increase in brightness through the peak phase (*A* and *B*) and slowly fade as fluorescein leaves the eye in the late phase (*C*). These defects do not change in size through the course of the study. *D*, The cause of hyperfluorescent patches of window defects is shown schematically, demonstrating areas of depigmented retinal pigment epithelium.

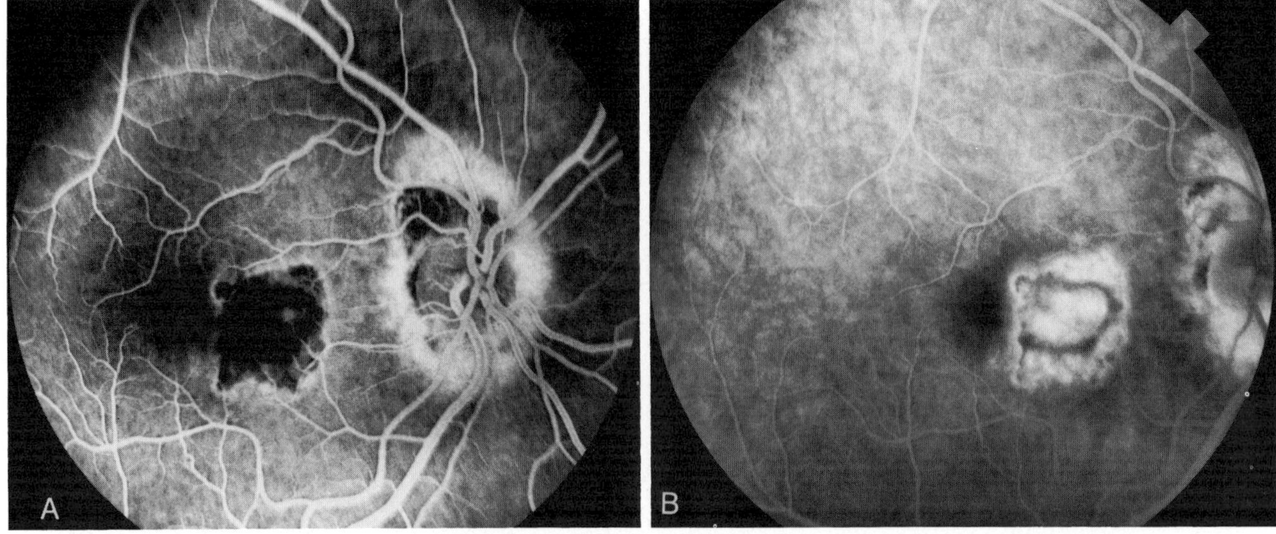

FIGURE 3–9 **Staining.** An atrophic chorioretinal scar (in this case secondary to laser photocoagulation) demonstrates staining of the sclera. This staining is not present early *(A)*, as there is no overlying choroid, so accumulation of fluorescein in the sclera occurs slowly from the intact choroid surrounding the scar. *B*, Later phases show hyperfluorescence from scleral staining.

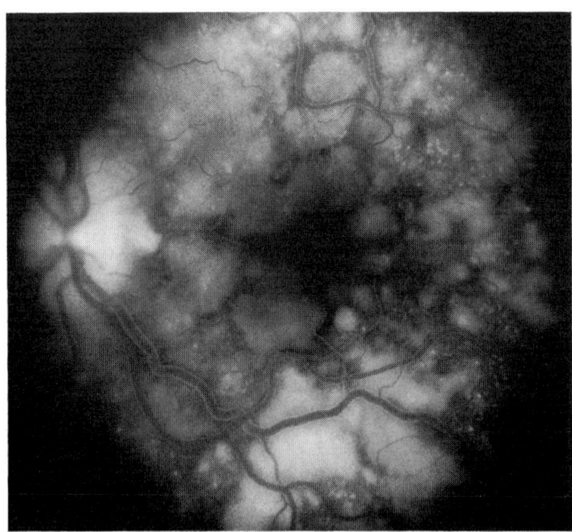

FIGURE 3–10 **Pooling.** Fluorescein accumulating within a potential space is said to pool, and the high concentration of fluorescein molecules within this pool produced hyperfluorescence. In this patient with Harada's disease, considerable dye has leaked into several regions within the subretinal space, producing scattered pools of hyperfluorescence.

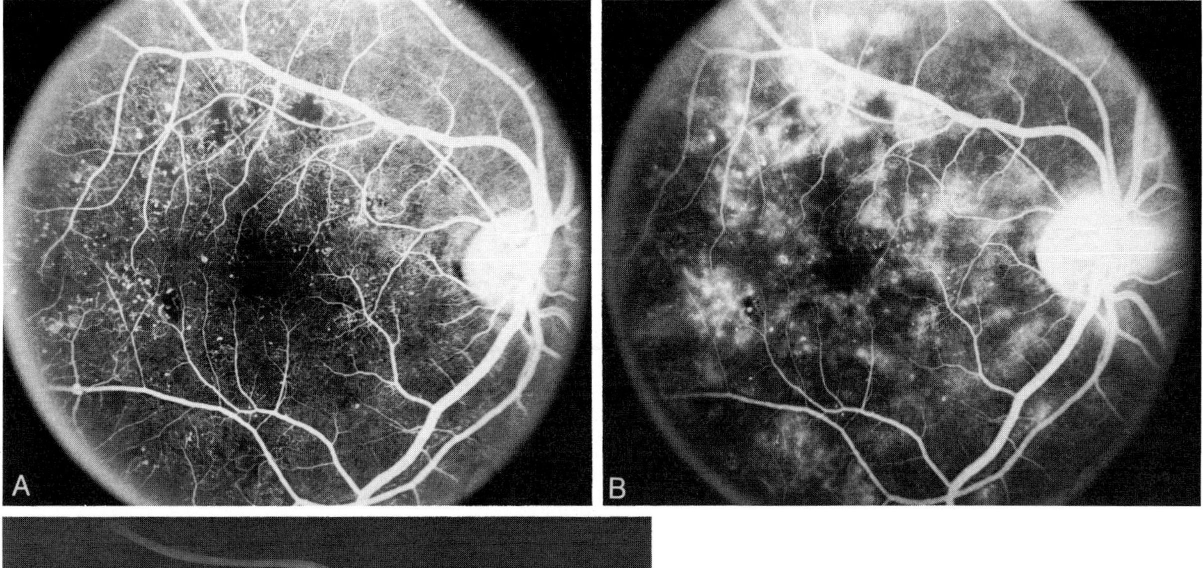

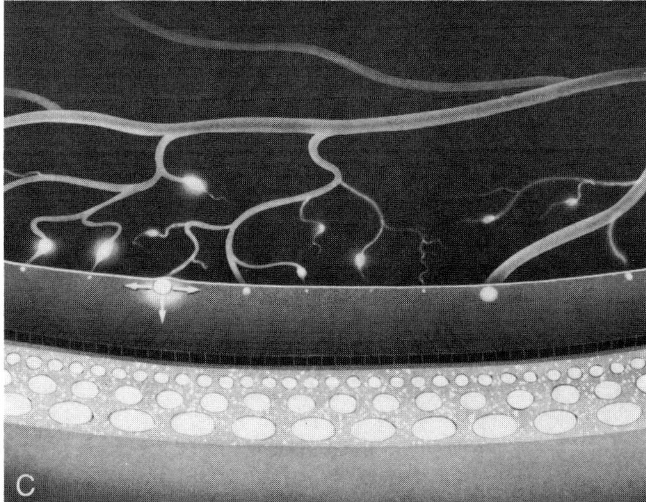

FIGURE 3–11 **Leakage.** Intraretinal fluorescein leakage is caused by defects in the tight junctions of the retinal vasculature, in this case secondary to diabetes mellitus. Intravascular fluid leaks out from areas of microaneurysms into the surrounding retina, producing retinal edema. Fluorescein dye shows the location of this leakage as the dye accumulates within the sensory retina, producing intraretinal hyperfluorescence (*A* and *B*). *C*, Leakage of fluorescein is shown schematically in cross section.

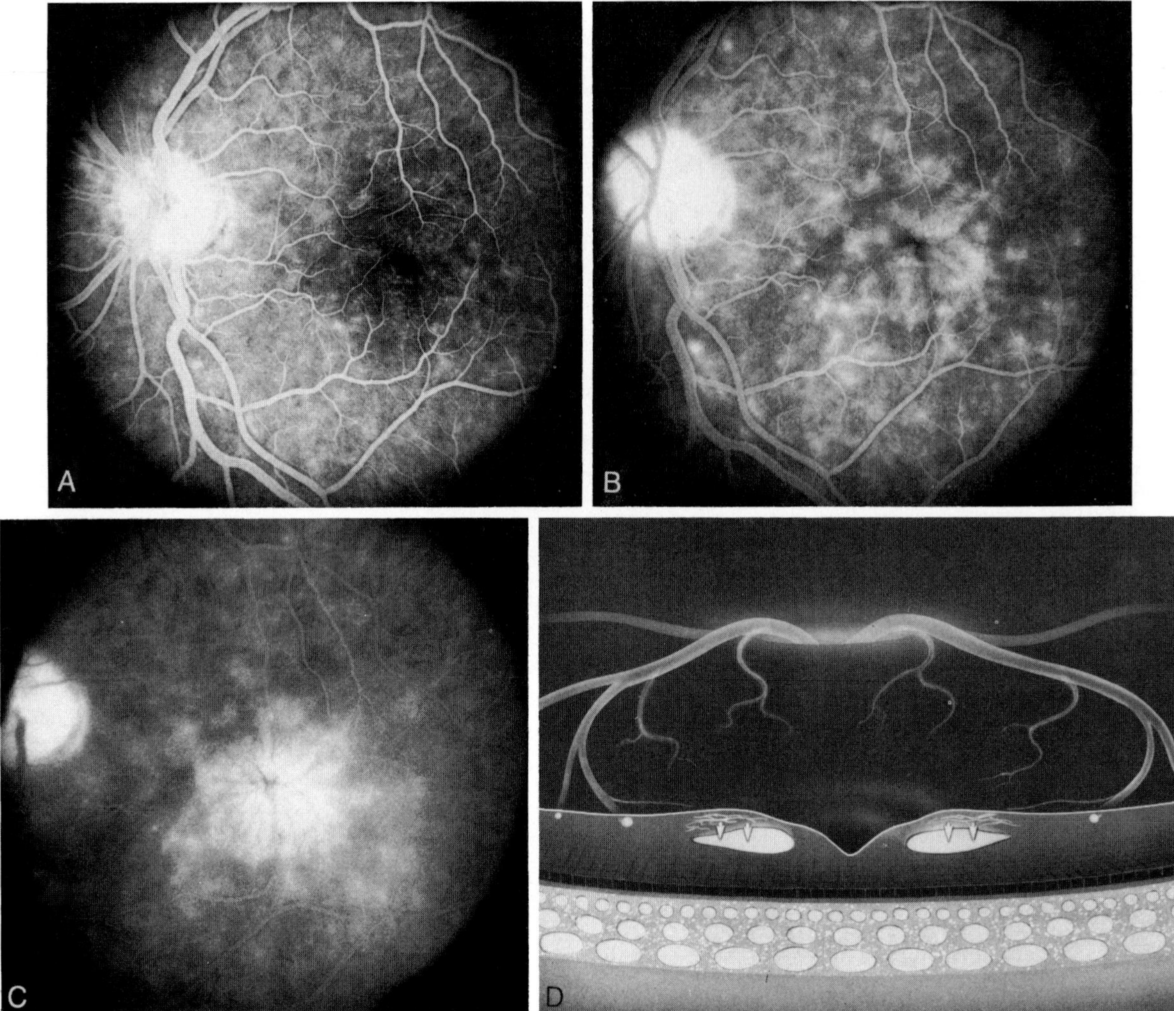

FIGURE 3–12 **Fluorescein angiography of cystoid macular edema.** In an eye with aphakic cystoid macular edema, dye from the perifoveal retinal capillaries leaks into the outer plexiform layer and pools in cystic spaces (*A* and *B*). The petalloid pattern of fluorescence, which becomes most prominent in the late-phase films *(C)*, is diagnostic of cystoid macular edema. *D*, This schematic cross section depicts the source of the edema and the location of the cystic spaces in the perifoveal area.

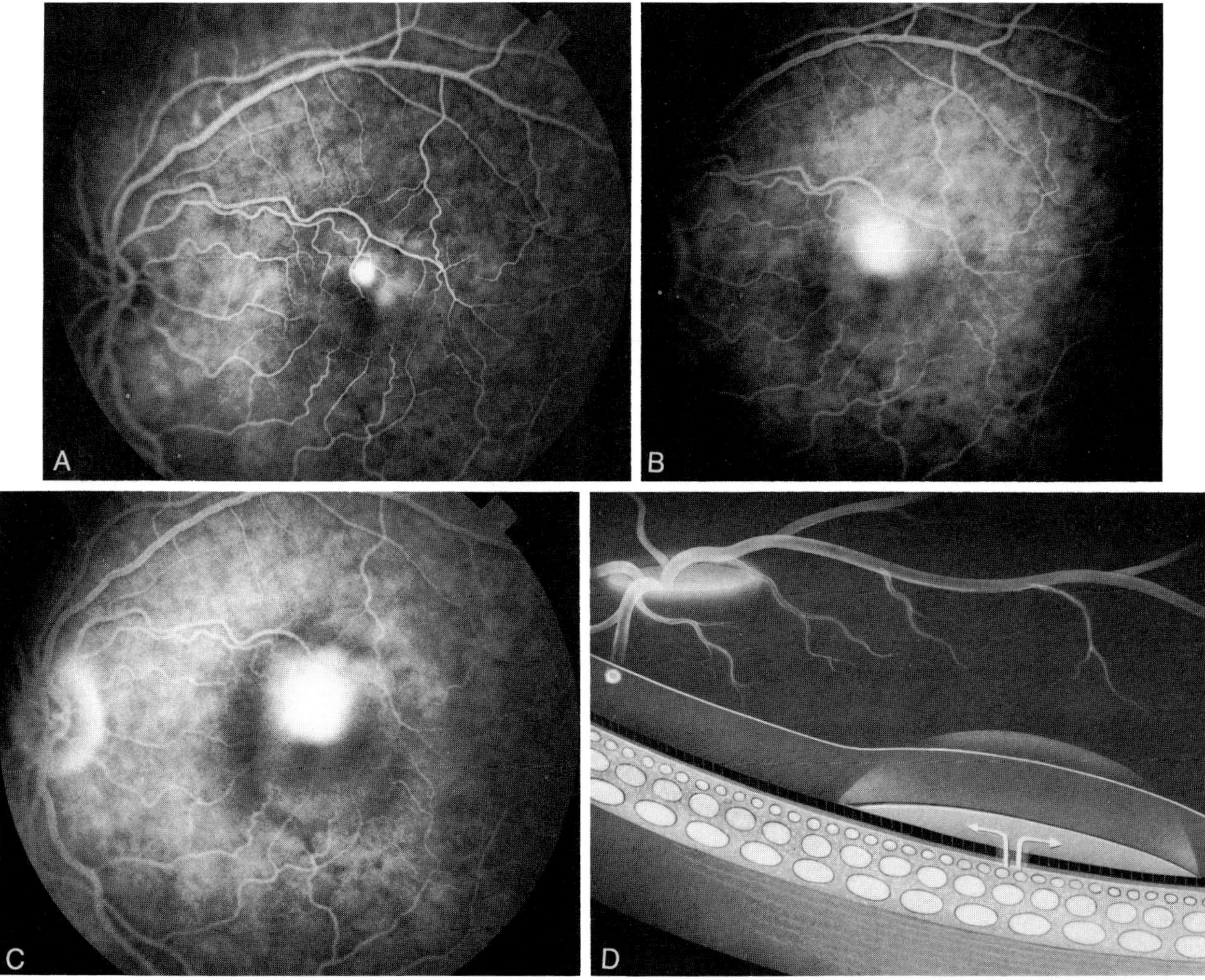

FIGURE 3-13 **Fluorescein angiography of central serous chorioretinopathy.** *A,* In this case of central serous chorioretinopathy, fluid from the choroid has leaked across defective tight junctions in the retinal pigment epithelium and accumulates in the subretinal space. On fluorescein angiography, a small round area of hyperfluorescence is seen in the early phase films and expands progressively as the dye is trapped (pools) within the subretinal space (*B* and *C*). *D,* The schematic representation demonstrates the fluorescein findings of central serous chorioretinopathy.

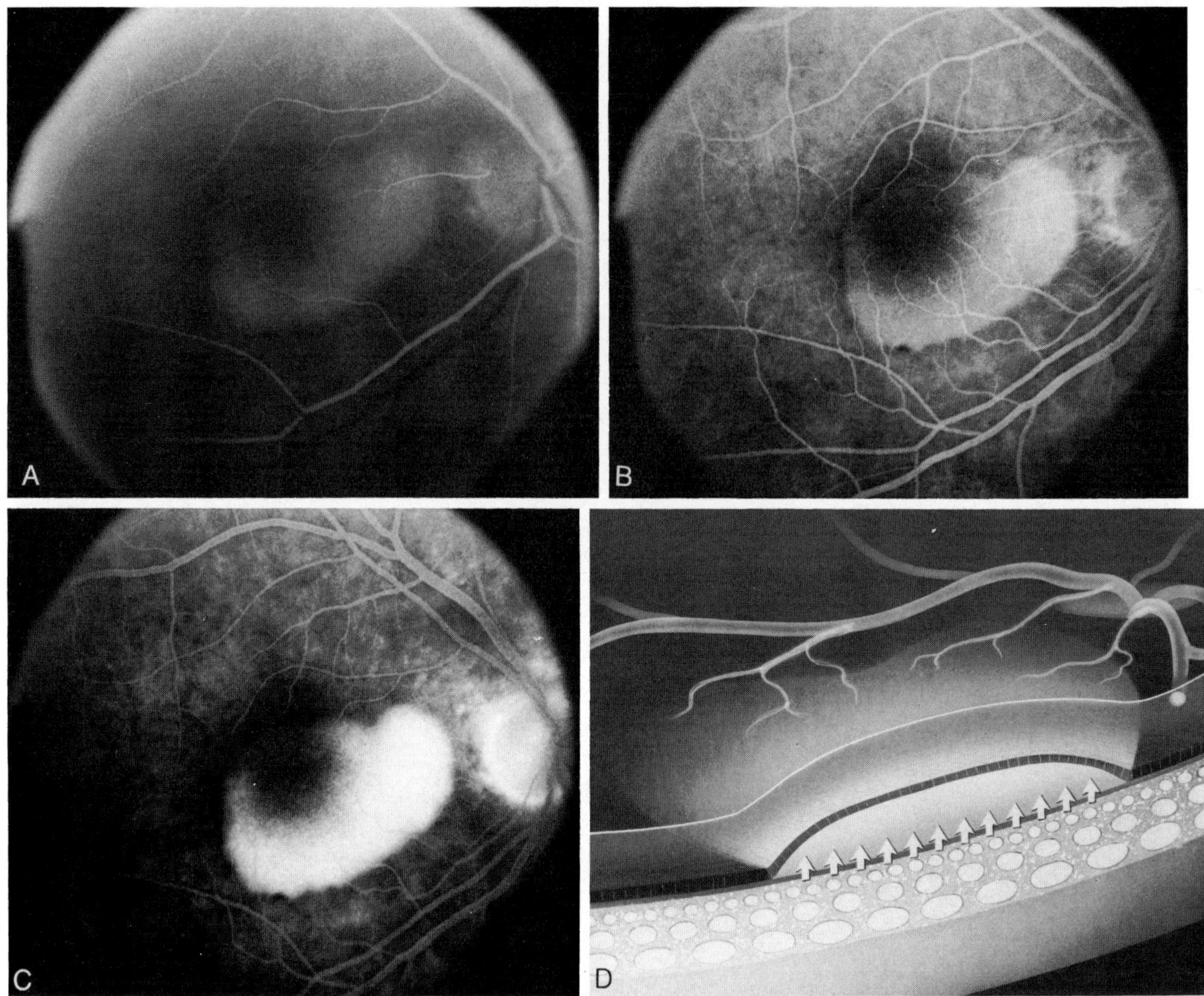

FIGURE 3-14 **Fluorescein angiography of a retinal pigment epithelial detachment.** Fluorescein dye leaks across Bruch's membrane and pools beneath a retinal pigment epithelial detachment, at which point it is confined. Angiographically, progressive pooling is seen, but the extent of the hyperfluorescent area remains constant *(A–C)*. *D,* Cross-sectional illustration depicts this course of events after fluorescein injection.

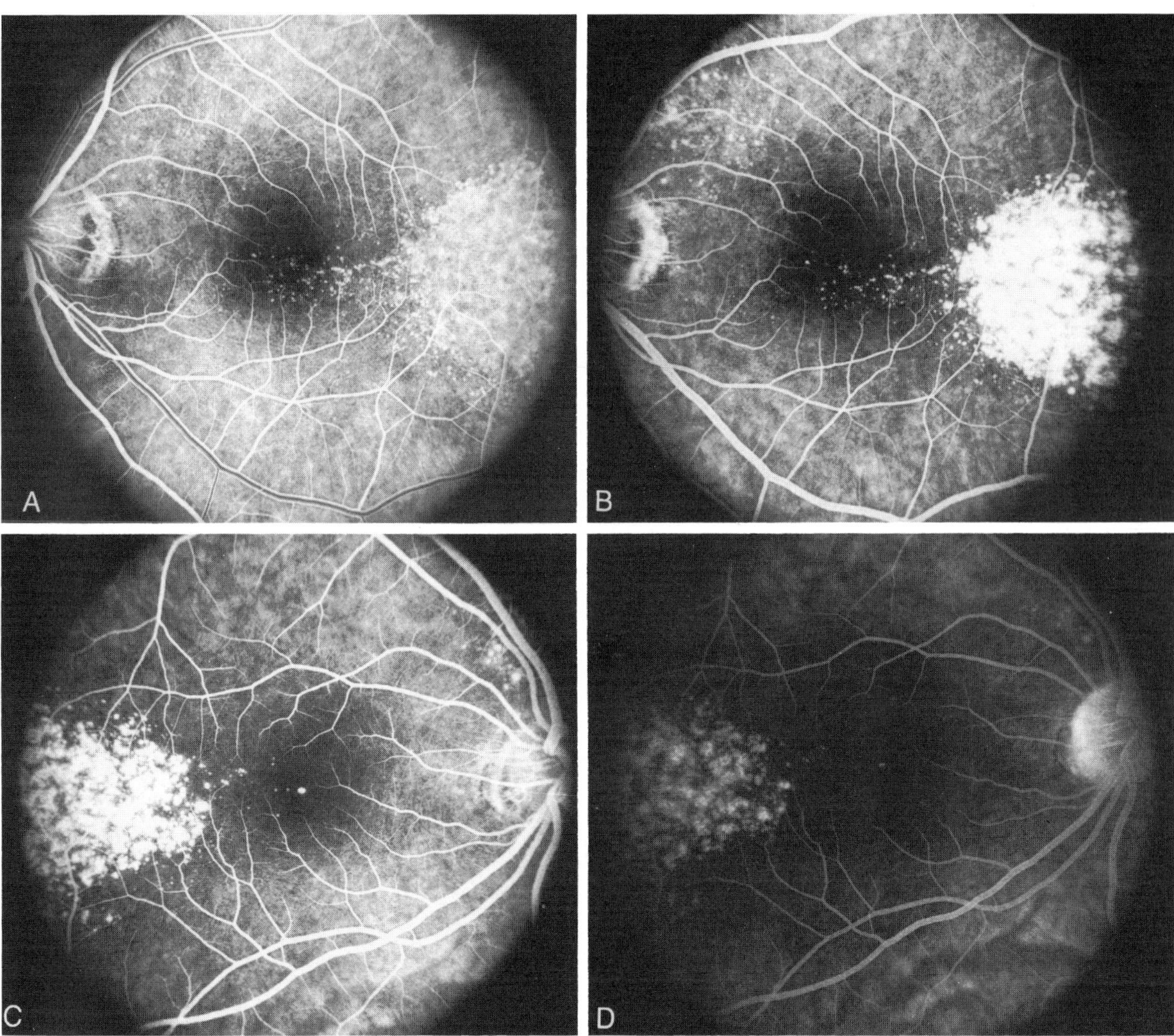

FIGURE 3–15 **Fluorescein angiography of drusen.** Drusen look similar to window defects on fluorescein angiography *(A)*. Later in the study, however, the borders of the drusen may become fuzzy (*B* and *C*). *D*, Arteriovenous late-phase photograph shows staining of the drusen. (*A–D*, Courtesy of Roberta Wilson.)

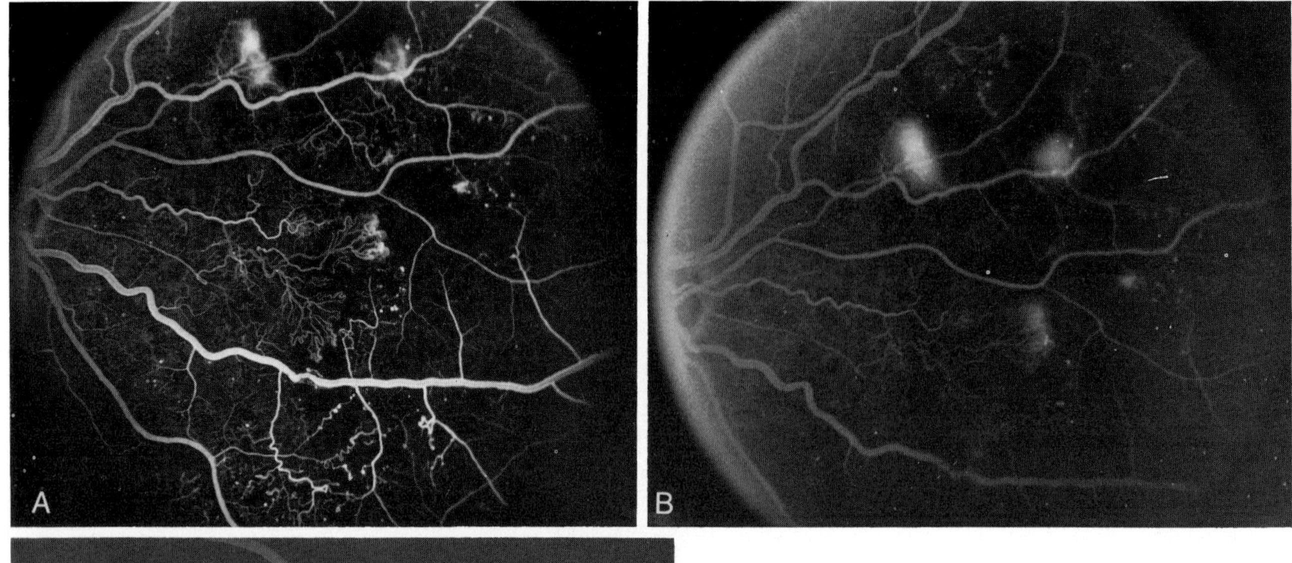

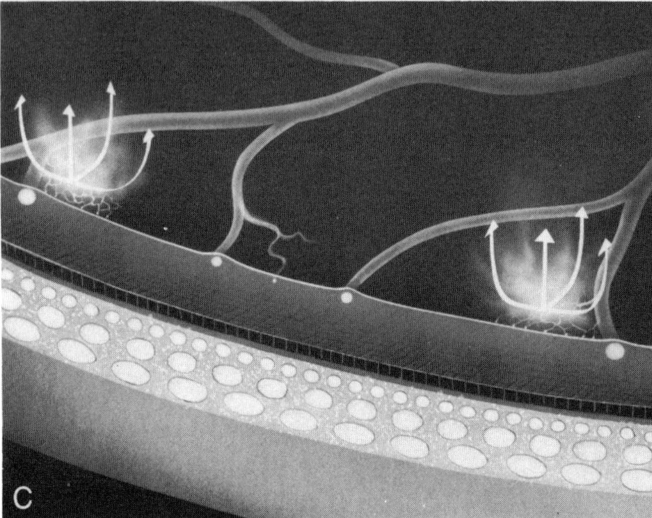

FIGURE 3–16 **Fluorescein angiography of retinal neovascularization.** The hyperfluorescence shown here is caused by retinal neovascularization, in this case secondary to sickle cell retinopathy. Because the new vessels lack tight junctions, dye continuously leaks out of the lumina *(A)*, staining the retina and vitreous more intensely in the later phases *(B)*. *C*, This schematic illustration summarizes these events.

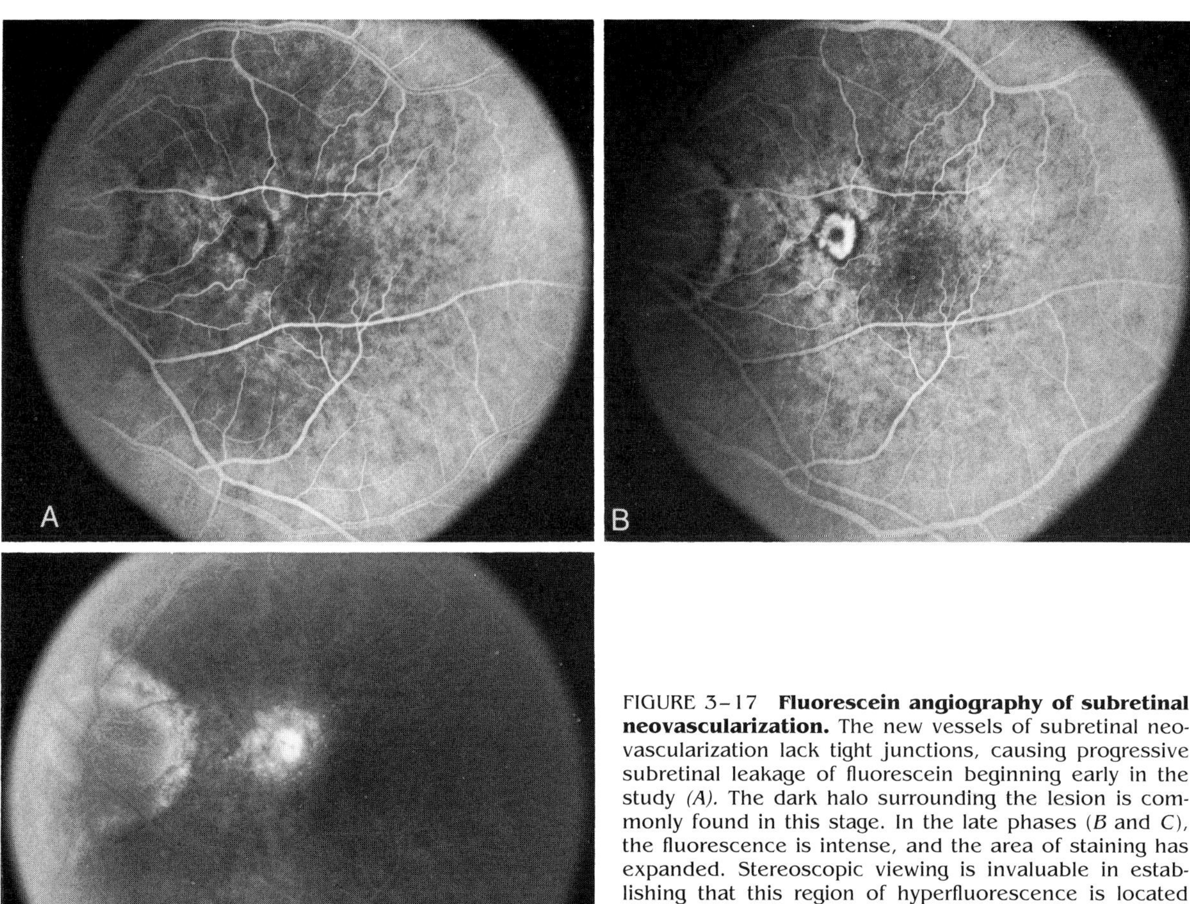

FIGURE 3–17 **Fluorescein angiography of subretinal neovascularization.** The new vessels of subretinal neovascularization lack tight junctions, causing progressive subretinal leakage of fluorescein beginning early in the study *(A)*. The dark halo surrounding the lesion is commonly found in this stage. In the late phases (*B* and *C*), the fluorescence is intense, and the area of staining has expanded. Stereoscopic viewing is invaluable in establishing that this region of hyperfluorescence is located beneath the retina.

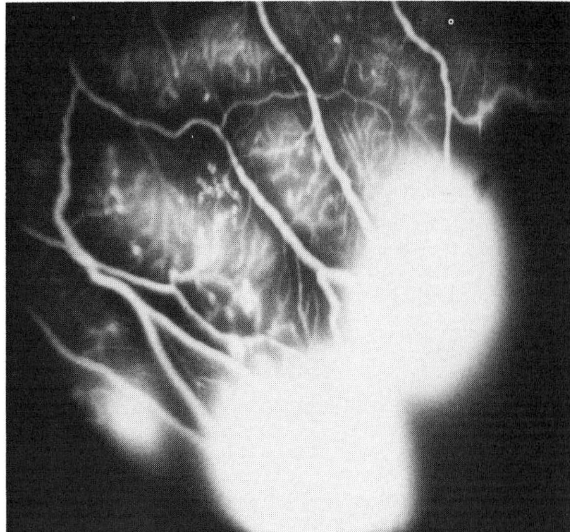

FIGURE 3–18 **Fluorescein angiography of Coats' disease.** The telangiectatic retinal vessels in a patient with Coats' disease lack normal tight junctions, allowing fluorescein to leak out and progressively stain the adjacent vitreous.

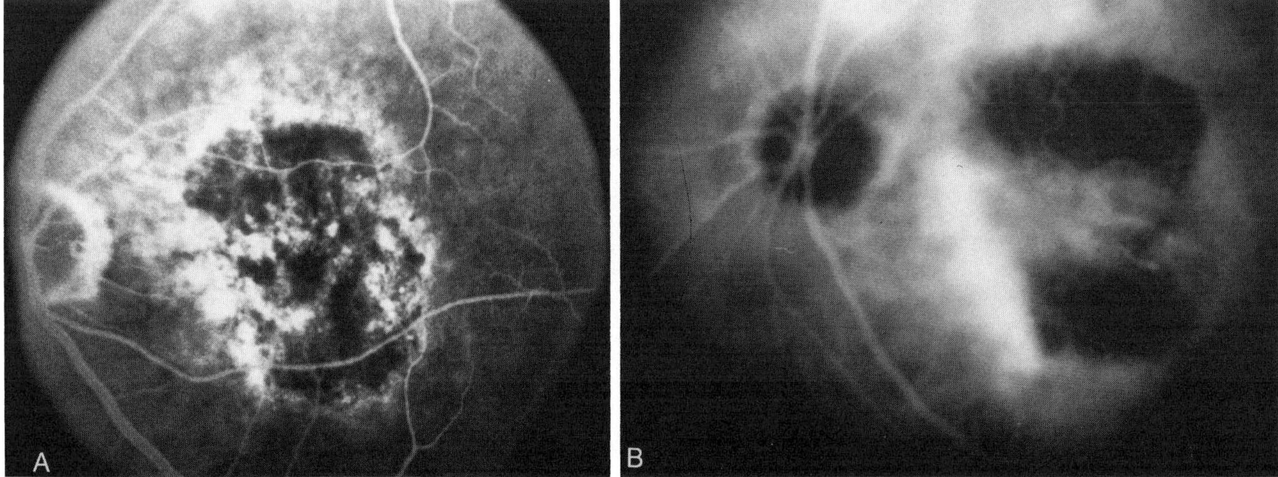

FIGURE 3–19 **Angiography of exudative macular degeneration.** *A,* This fluorescein angiogram (arteriovenous phase) demonstrates a large disciform area of chorioretinal atrophy centered at the fovea. A well-defined neovascular membrane cannot be discerned. *B,* Indocyanine green (ICG) videoangiographic frame of the same eye shows the presence of a large subretinal neovascular membrane beneath the fovea. In regions of chorioretinal scarring, subretinal neovascularization is often more easily detectable when ICG, rather than fluorescein angiography, is used. This is due in part to the fact that chorioretinal scars, which are hyperfluorescent on fluorescein angiography, are hypofluorescent on an ICG study. (*A* and *B,* Courtesy of Maryanna Destro, M.D.)

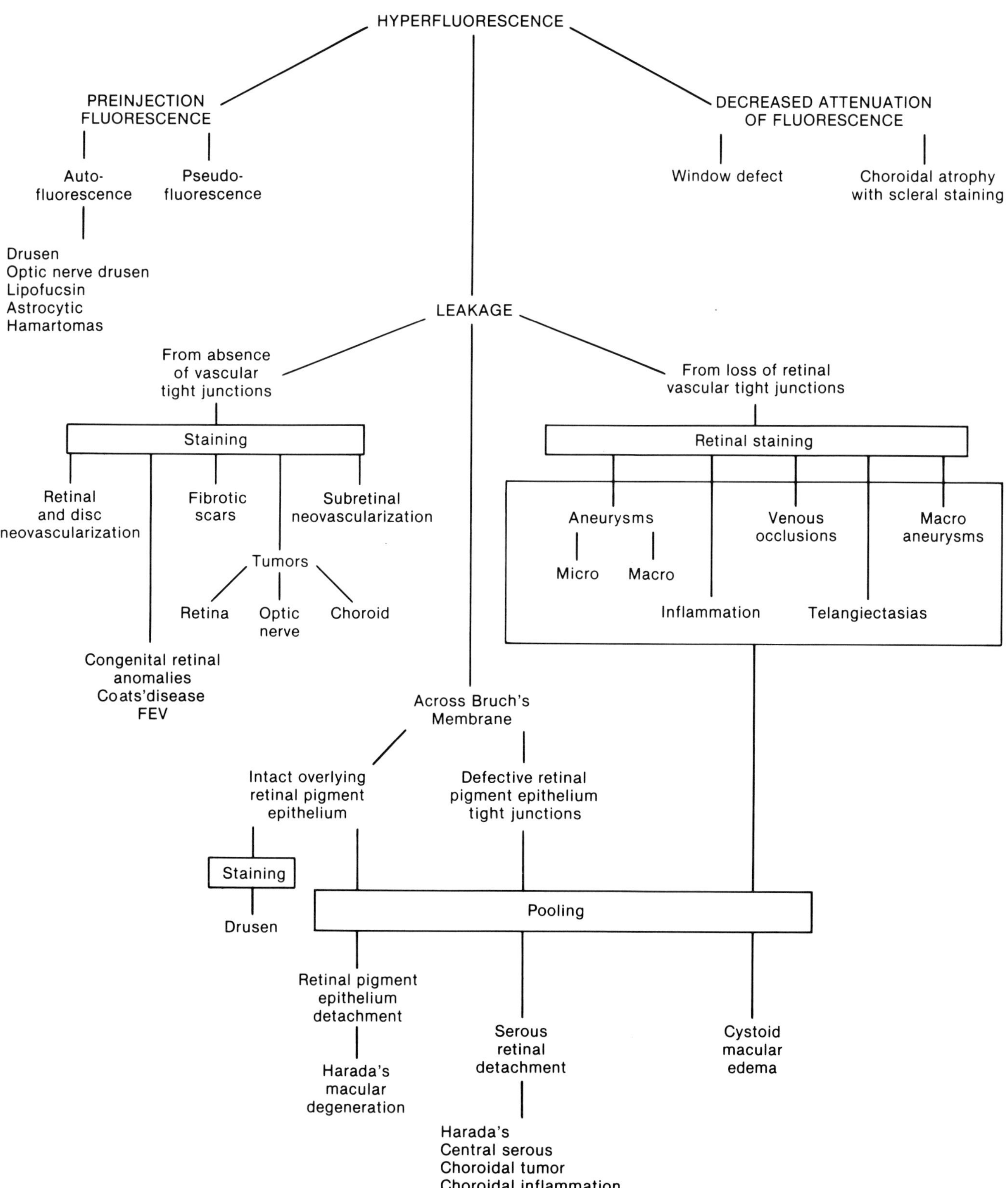

FIGURE 3–20 **Flow chart for hyperfluorescence in fluorescein angiography.** Preinjection fluorescence has been placed on this chart for convenience. (FEV, familial exudative vitreoretinopathy.)

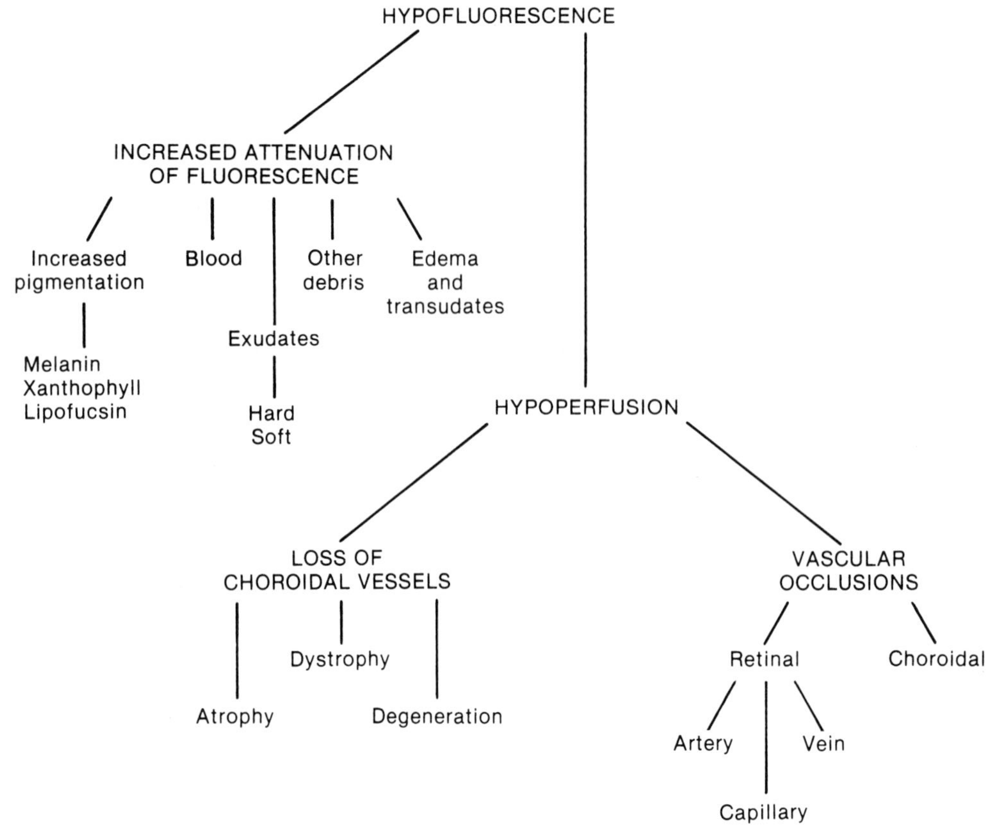

FIGURE 3–21 Flow chart for hypofluorescence in fluorescein angiography.

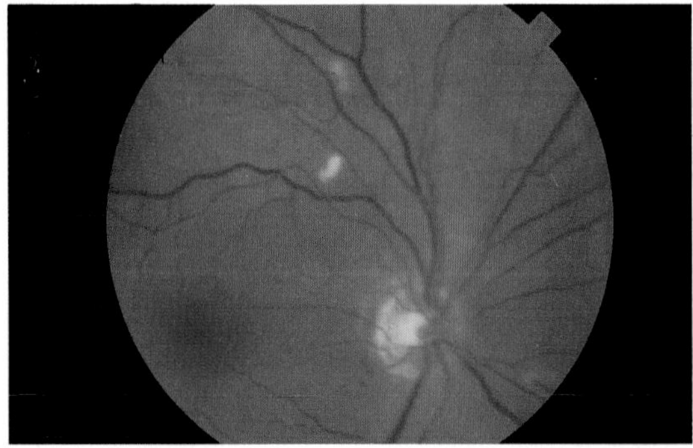

FIGURE 3–22 **Cotton-wool spots.** Cotton-wool spots in this fundus photograph from a patient with acquired immunodeficiency syndrome (AIDS) are transient, small, whitish opacities with feathery edges located within the superficial retina that represent microinfarctions of small retinal arterioles and the resultant disruption of neuronal axoplasmic flow. The presence and number of cotton-wool spots in patients with AIDS have been noted to indicate a poor systemic prognosis and may be useful in monitoring the severity of systemic disease.

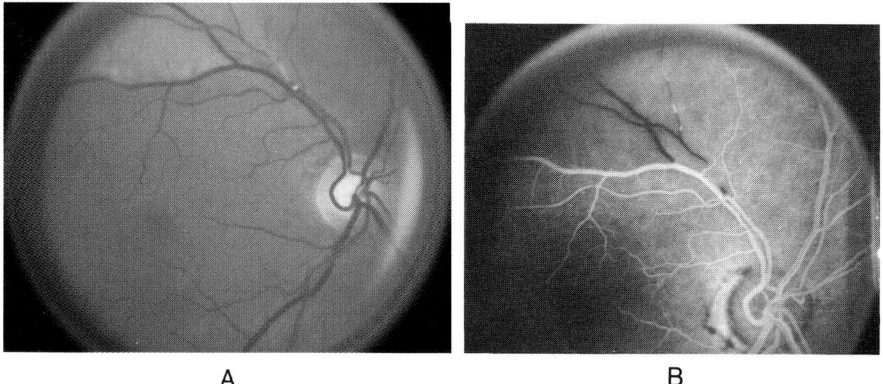

FIGURE 3–23 **Branch retinal artery occlusions.** In this superotemporal branch retinal artery occlusion, note the acute retinal whitening from edema in the distribution of the occluded arteriole distal to the embolus *(A)*, with lack of fluorescein filling on the corresponding angiogram *(B)*.

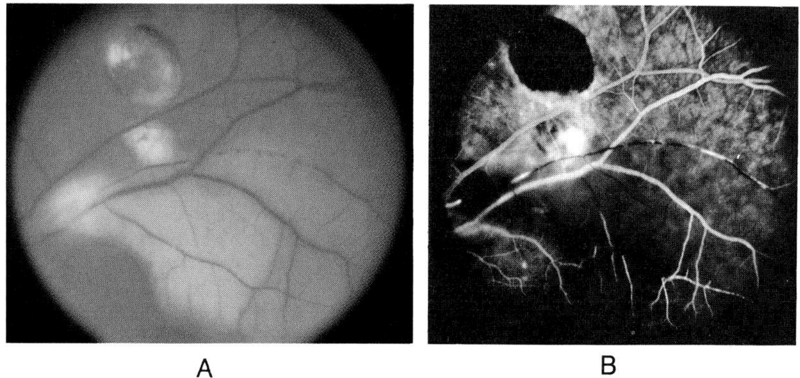

FIGURE 3–24 **Branch retinal artery occlusions.** Acute retinal whitening is associated with this superotemporal branch retinal artery occlusion distal to a focus of active toxoplasmic retinochoroiditis *(A)*. *B,* The fluorescein angiogram shows staining of portions of the wall of the occluded vessel consistent with vasculitis.

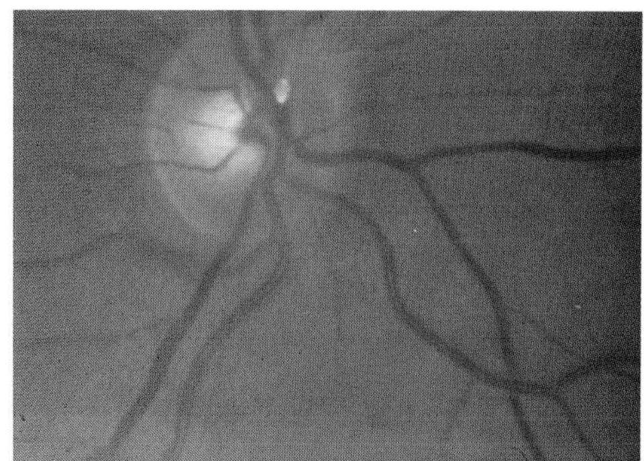

FIGURE 3–25 **Calcific emboli.** A calcific embolus overlies the optic disc in a patient with cardiac valvular disease. Although less common than either platelet-fibrin or cholesterol emboli, calcific emboli are still a frequent cause of branch arterial occlusions of the retina.

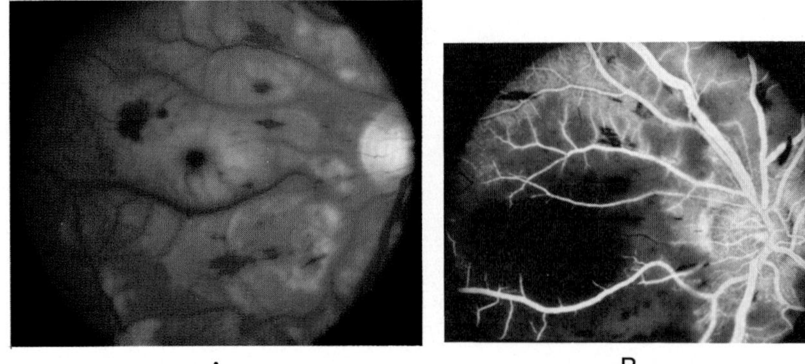

FIGURE 3–26 **Purtscher's retinopathy.** Fundus photograph *(A)* and fluorescein angiogram *(B)* from a patient with presumed Purtscher's retinopathy following a severe chest compression injury. The multiple arterial occlusions, evidenced by the numerous cotton-wool spots and the cherry-red spot in the macula, are thought to be due to leukoemboli.

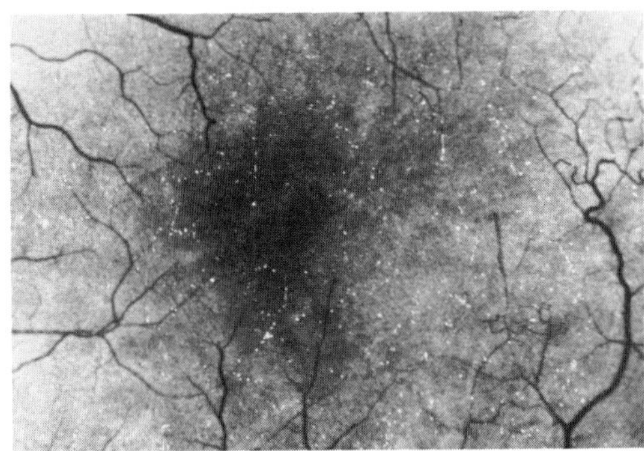

FIGURE 3–27 **Talc retinopathy.** Multiple talc emboli are present in this red-free photograph of the macula of an intravenous drug-abuser (From Friberg TR, Gragoudas ES, Regan CDJ: Talc emboli and macular ischemia in intravenous drug abuse. Arch Ophthalmol 97:1089–1091, 1979. Copyright 1979, American Medical Association.)

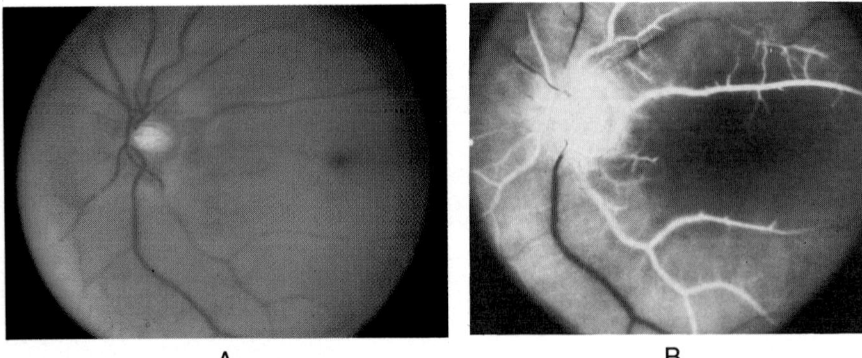

FIGURE 3–28 **Central retinal artery occlusions.** An acute central retinal artery occlusion typically causes a foveal cherry-red spot *(A)* because the retina in the foveal area is thin, allowing visibility of the underlying patent choroidal circulation that is obscured elsewhere by retinal edema. Note the delayed retinal arteriole filling with prolonged arteriole venous circulation time on the corresponding fluorescein angiogram *(B)*.

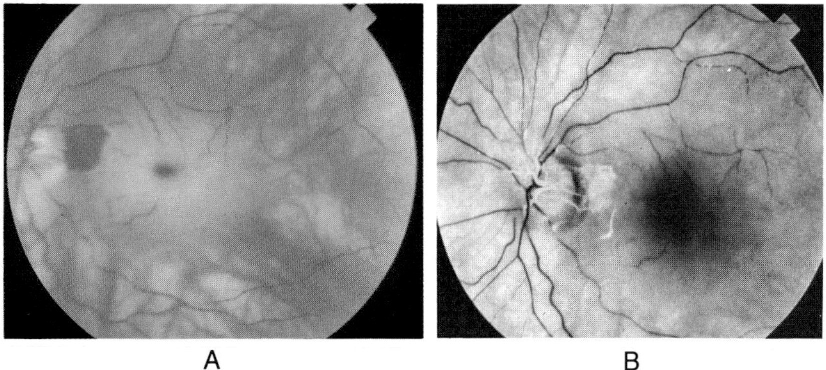

FIGURE 3-29 **Central retinal artery occlusions.** This patient with a central retinal artery occlusion has a patent cilioretinal artery perfusing a small portion of his retina near the optic disc *(A)*. Up to one tenth of patients with central retinal artery occlusions are more fortunate than this patient because they may retain central vision owing to the presence of a patent cilioretinal artery that perfuses the fovea. Note the filling of the cilioretinal artery and the lack of filling of the retinal arterioles on the corresponding fluorescein angiogram *(B)*.

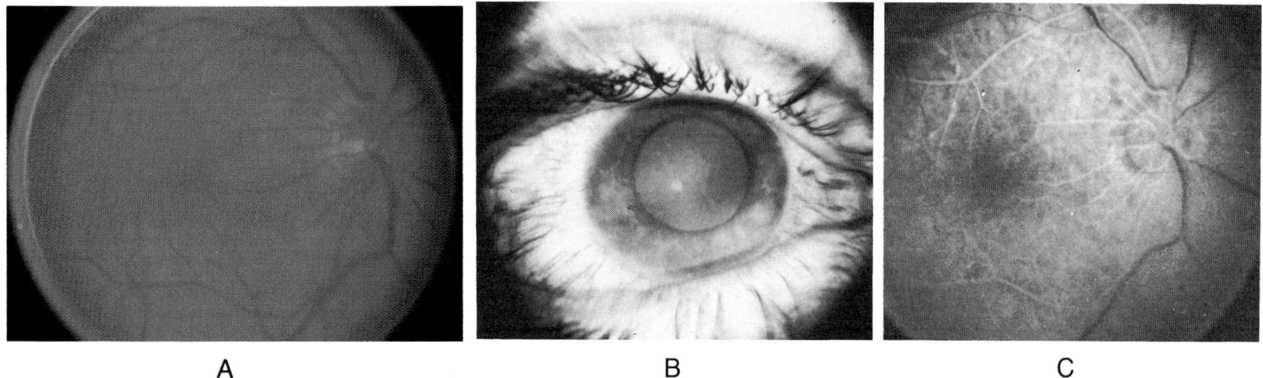

FIGURE 3-30 **Ocular ischemic syndrome.** This patient had ocular ischemia secondary to carotid occlusive disease. Note the retinal arteriolar narrowing and retinal venous dilatation without tortuosity *(A)*, fluorescein leakage from associated iris neovascularization *(B)*, and delayed retinal perfusion on fluorescein angiography *(C)*. Despite treatment with panretinal laser photocoagulation or carotid endarterectomy, visual prognosis usually remains poor.

FIGURE 3-31 **Central retinal vein occlusions.** This fundus photograph demonstrates the typical appearance of a fresh central retinal vein occlusion, with disc edema, venous dilatation and tortuosity, cotton-wool spots, and retinal hemorrhages in all quadrants.

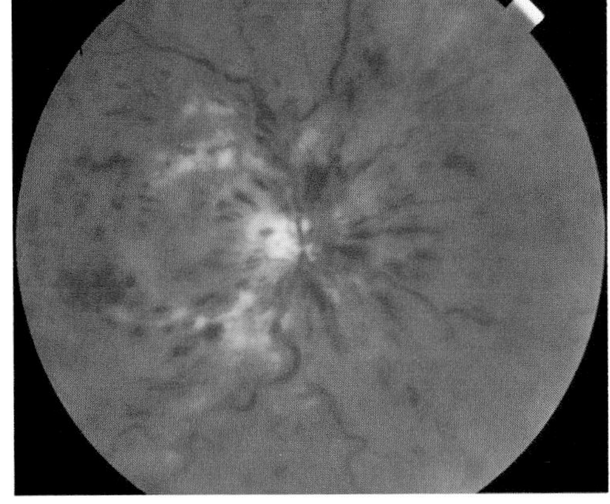

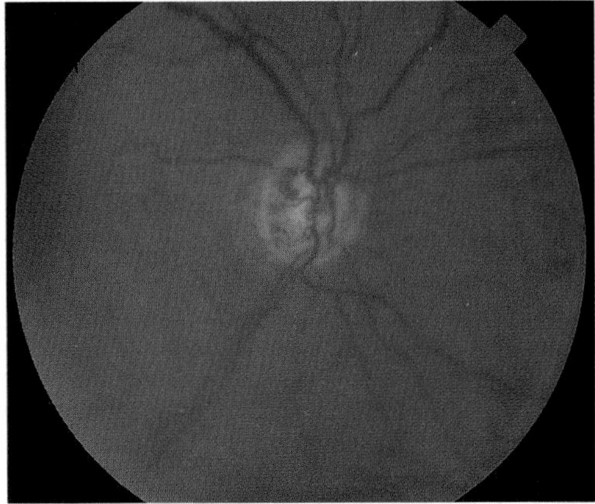

FIGURE 3–32 **Venous collaterals caused by central retinal vein occlusion.** As a central retinal vein occlusion resolves, tortuous collateral vessels connecting the retinal and choroidal circulations may appear at the optic disc. These collateral vessels, in contrast to neovascularization of the disc, do not leak on fluorescein angiography.

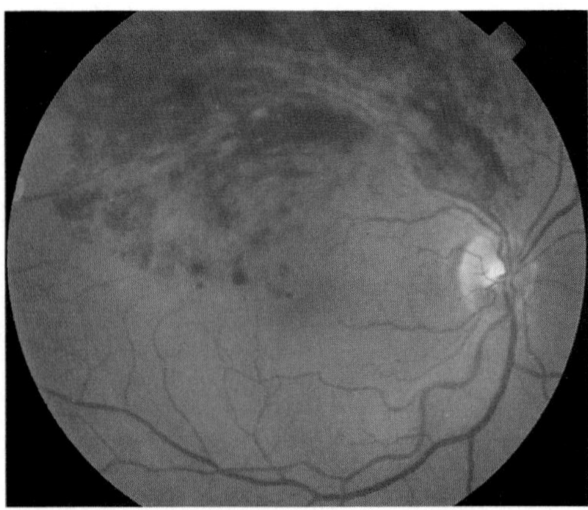

FIGURE 3–33 **Branch retinal vein occlusions.** Branch retinal vein occlusions occur almost exclusively at arteriovenous intersections such as the one shown here near the superior margin of the disc. The area of retina drained by the vein typically shows variable degrees of venous dilatation and tortuosity, superficial and deep hemorrhages, cotton-wool spots, and retinal edema.

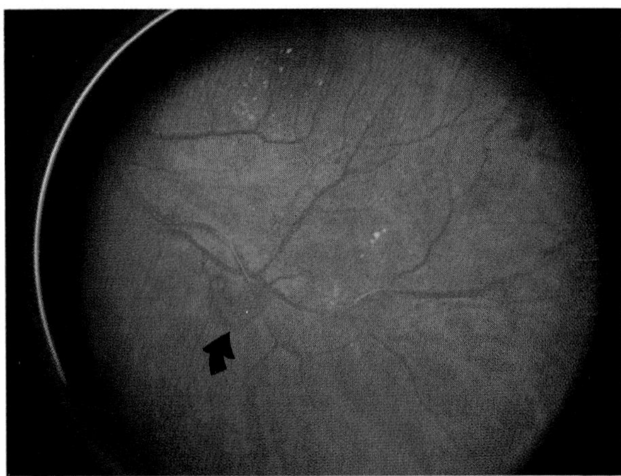

FIGURE 3–34 **Neovascularization caused by branch retinal vein occlusion.** After a branch retinal vein occlusion, retinal neovascularization *(arrow)* occurs most commonly at the border of perfused and unperfused retina, whereas neovascularization of the disc or iris are rare events. The Branch Retinal Vein Occlusion Study found that patients who develop neovascularization following a branch retinal vein occlusion should be treated with scatter laser photocoagulation to the ischemic area in an effort to prevent vitreous hemorrhage and further neovascular complications.

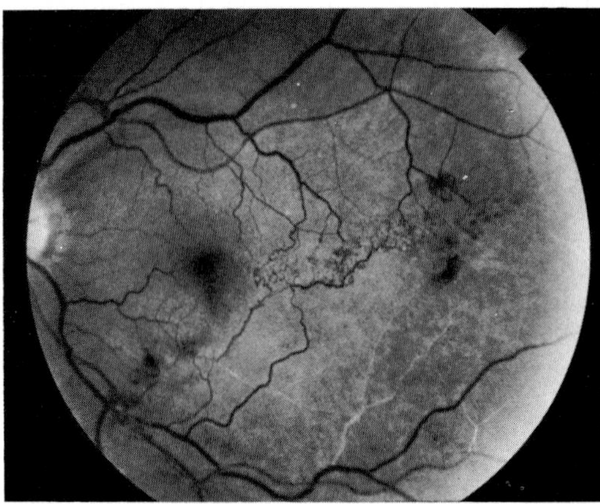

FIGURE 3–35 **Venous collaterals caused by branch retinal vein occlusion.** Venous collaterals may form after a branch retinal vein occlusion to drain the venous circulation in the affected retina into an unaffected area. The most characteristic type of collaterals shown here are small, tortuous venous channels that cross the horizontal raphe temporal to the fovea and drain into the venous circulation of the uninvolved quadrant.

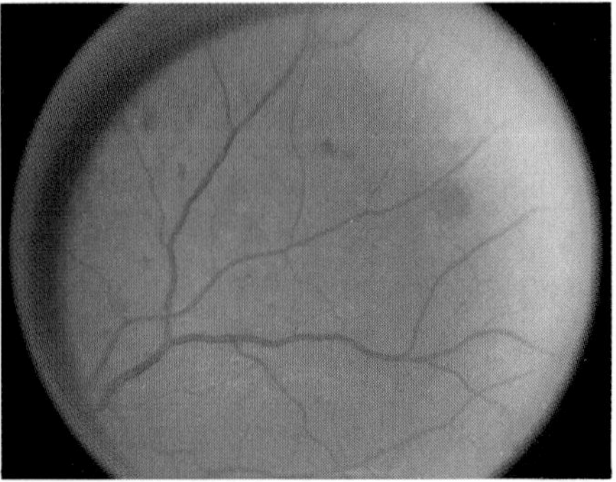

FIGURE 3–36 **Nonproliferative diabetic retinopathy.** Microaneurysms and intraretinal hemorrhages, typically the first clinical signs of diabetic retinopathy, are due to a selective and progressive loss of the capillary pericytes. (Standard photograph No. 2A of the Modified Airlee House Classification of Diabetic Retinopathy; courtesy of the Early Treatment Diabetic Retinopathy Study [ETDRS].)

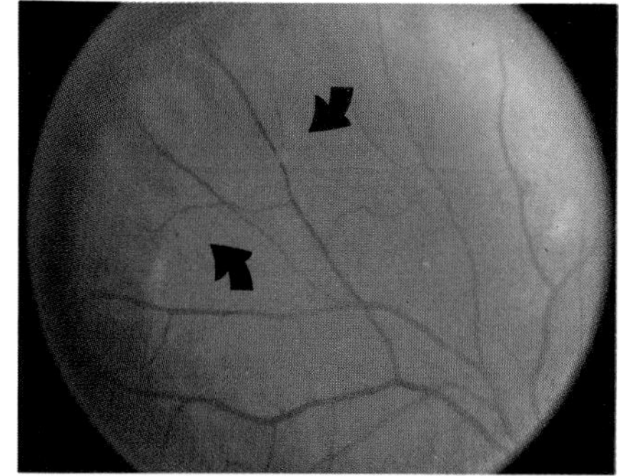

FIGURE 3-37 **Nonproliferative diabetic retinopathy.** Intraretinal microvascular abnormalities (IRMAs) *(arrows)* represent either new vessel growth within the retina or preexisting vessels with endothelial proliferation that become "shunts" through areas of nonperfusion. Multiple IRMAs mark a severe stage of nonproliferative diabetic retinopathy with a high risk of proceeding to frank neovascularization in the near future. (Standard photograph No. 8A of the Modified Airlee House Classification of Diabetic Retinopathy; courtesy of the ETDRS.)

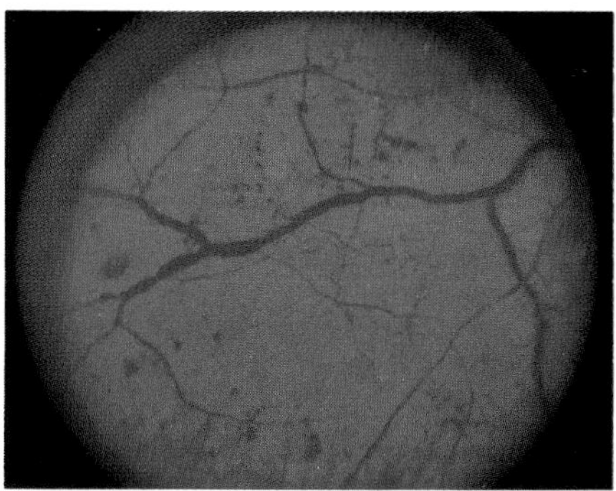

FIGURE 3-38 **Nonproliferative diabetic retinopathy.** The venous dilatation and beading shown here are indicators of severe retinal hypoxia in the diabetic retina. Treatment with scatter (panretinal) photocoagulation may cause these abnormal veins to become less dilated and more regular. (Standard photograph No. 6B of the Modified Airlee House Classification of Diabetic Retinopathy; courtesy of the ETDRS.)

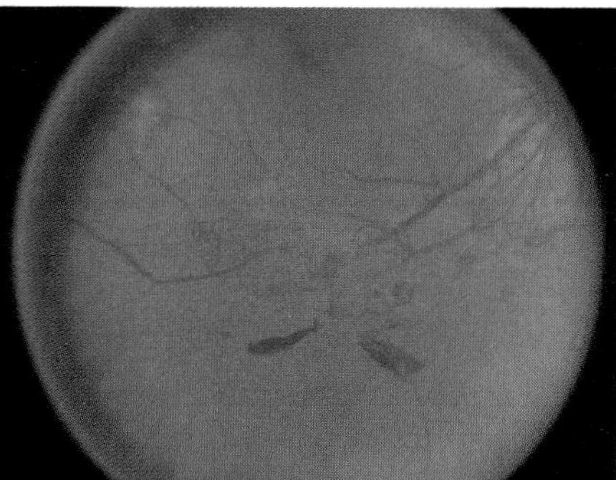

FIGURE 3-40 **Proliferative diabetic retinopathy.** Neovascularization elsewhere (NVE) in the retina greater than or equal to one half disc area when associated with fresh vitreous or preretinal hemorrhage fulfills a minimum criterion for high-risk proliferative diabetic retinopathy and requires immediate scatter laser photocoagulation. (Standard photograph No. 7 of the Modified Airlee House Classification of Diabetic Retinopathy; courtesy of the ETDRS.)

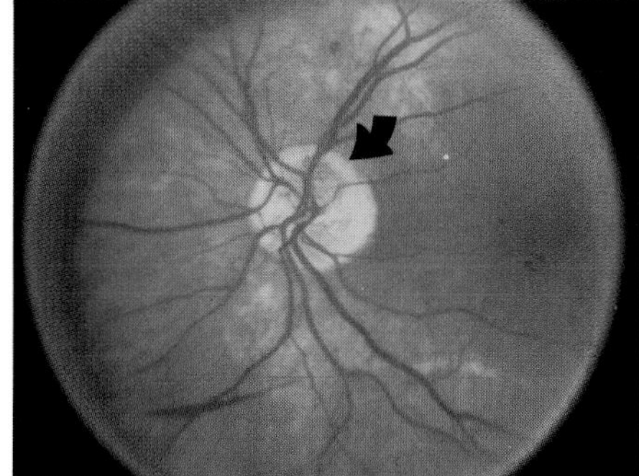

FIGURE 3-39 **Proliferative diabetic retinopathy.** Neovascularization of the optic disc (NVD) covering approximately one quarter to one third of the optic disc *(arrow)* fulfills a minimum criterion for high-risk proliferative diabetic retinopathy and requires immediate scatter laser photocoagulation. (Standard photograph No. 10A of the Modified Airlee House Classification of Diabetic Retinopathy; courtesy of the ETDRS.)

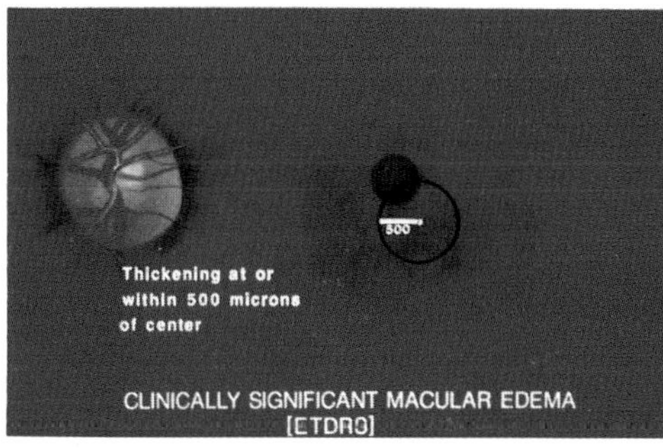

FIGURE 3-41 **Clinically significant macular edema (CSME).** Thickening of the macula at or within 500 μ of the center of the macula is CSME according to the ETDRS, and focal laser photocoagulation is recommended. (Courtesy of Robert Murphy, M.D.)

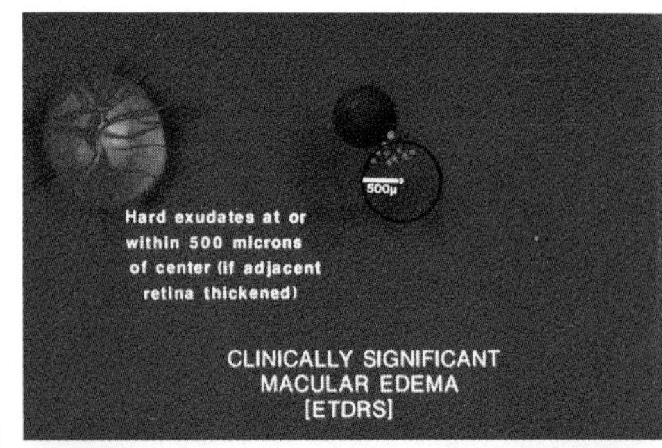

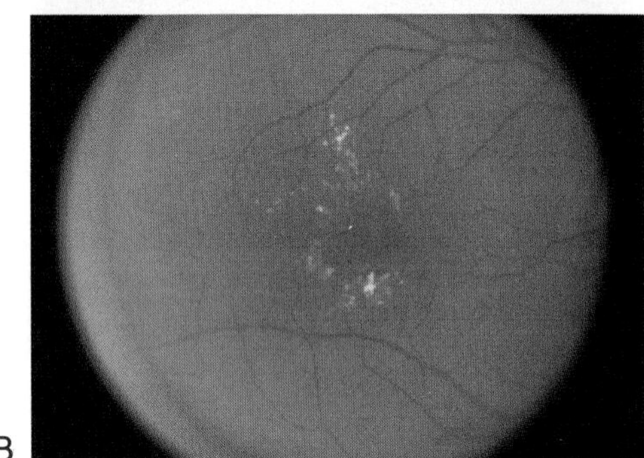

FIGURE 3–42 **CSME.** *A,* CSME is also denoted by hard exudates at or within 500 μ of the center of the macula, with thickening of the retina adjacent to the exudates. (Courtesy of Robert Murphy, M.D.) *B,* Clinical photograph demonstrates the appearance of hard exudates less than 500 μ from the center of the macula. There is thickening of the adjacent retina, which is not appreciated without stereoscopic observation. (Courtesy of the ETDRS.)

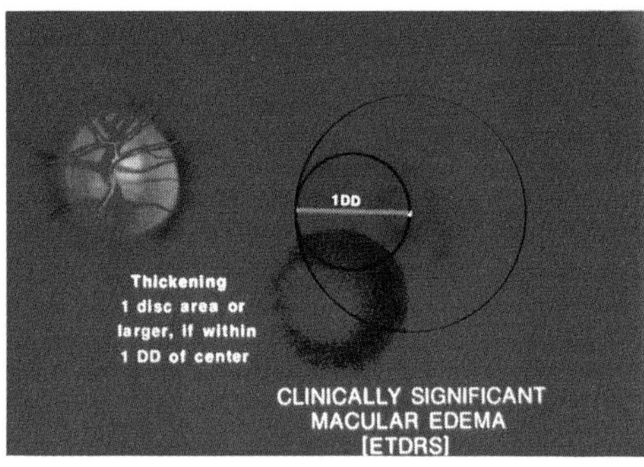

FIGURE 3–43 **CSME.** A third criterion for CSME is an area of retinal thickening, 1 disc diameter in size, part of which is within 1 disc diameter of the center of the macula. (Courtesy of Robert Murphy, M.D.)

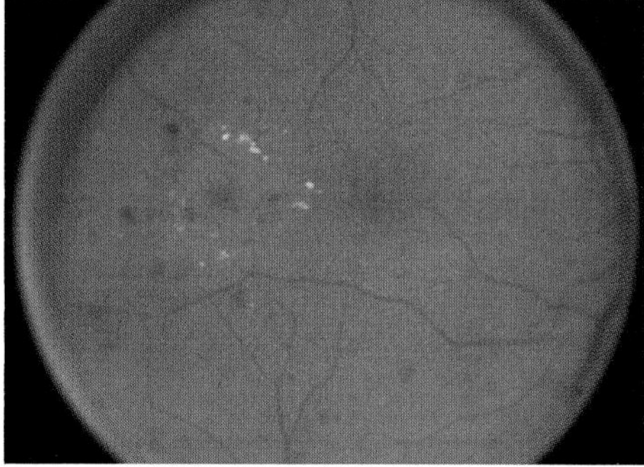

FIGURE 3–44 **CSME.** Clinical stereoscopic examination of the fundus shown in this photograph demonstrated greater than 1 disc diameter of thickening, part of which was within 1 disc diameter of the center of the macula. Focal laser treatment would be indicated to treat this clinically significant macular edema. (Courtesy of the ETDRS.)

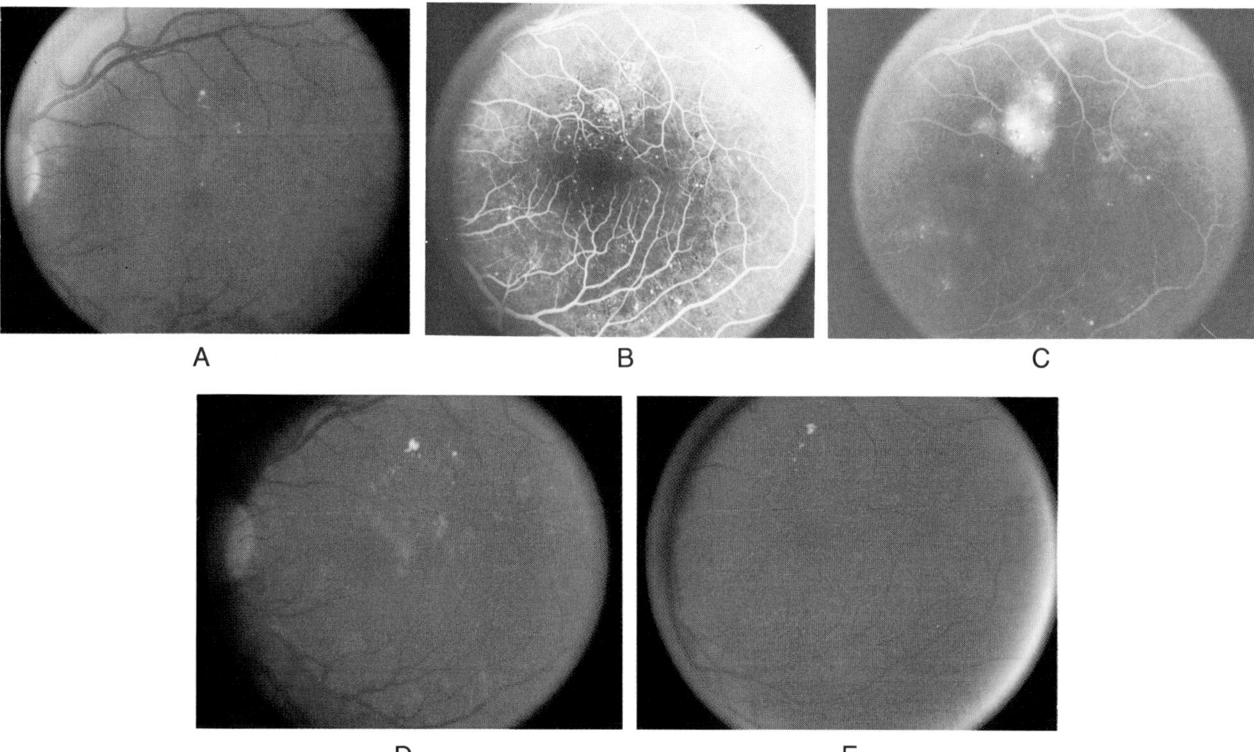

FIGURE 3–45 **CSME.** This series of photographs illustrates the diagnosis and treatment of CSME. *A,* In this patient with 20/15 vision, thickening is present just above the center of the macula (best appreciated with stereopsis). Because the thickening is within 500 μ of the center of the macula and there is associated exudate almost in the center of the macula, this macular edema is clinically significant. *B,* In the 17- to 18-second phase of the fluorescein angiogram, microaneurysms and slightly dilated capillaries are visible in the area of thickening. *C,* The 7-minute phase of the angiogram shows leakage into the retina from the two groups of microaneurysms noted in *B. D,* Focal laser photocoagulation has been applied to most of the microaneurysms. *E,* Four months later, the CSME has resolved. The center of the macula is flat, and most of the thickening noted before treatment has disappeared. Visual acuity remains at 20/15. (*A–E,* Courtesy of the ETDRS.)

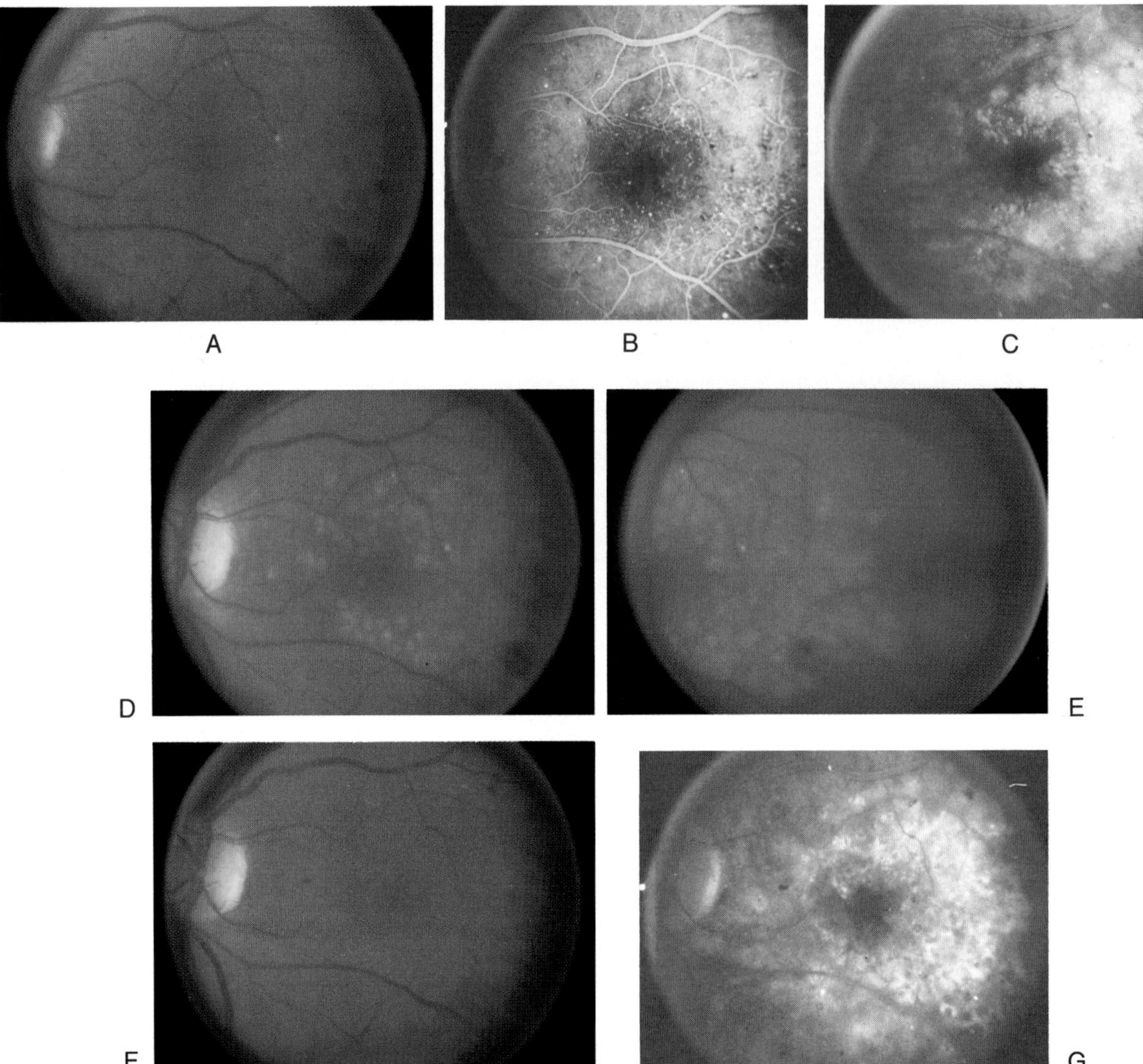

FIGURE 3–46 **CSME.** This series of clinical photographs depicts the diagnosis and treatment of a large area of CSME with cystoid changes of the macula. *A,* Clinical examination of the fundus in this photograph reveals retinal thickening temporal to the center of the macula extending just to the center. Visual acuity is 20/40 + 3. *B,* Early phase of the angiogram shows capillary loss adjacent to the foveal avascular zone, capillary dilatation, and scattered microaneurysms. *C,* The 7-minute phase of the angiogram shows extensive small cystoid spaces temporal to the center of the macula and above and below it, while the center appears uninvolved. *D,* The microaneurysms have been treated with focal laser photocoagulation. In addition, laser burns have been applied in a grid pattern to the areas of diffuse leakage between 500 and 3000 μ of the center of the macula. *E,* The temporal extent of the grid laser treatment is shown. *F,* Four months later, hemorrhages and hard exudates have decreased, and the retinal thickening can no longer be detected. Visual acuity is 20/25. *G,* The 7-minute phase of the angiogram demonstrates resolution of most of the cystoid spaces visible in *C.* (*A–G,* Courtesy of the ETDRS.)

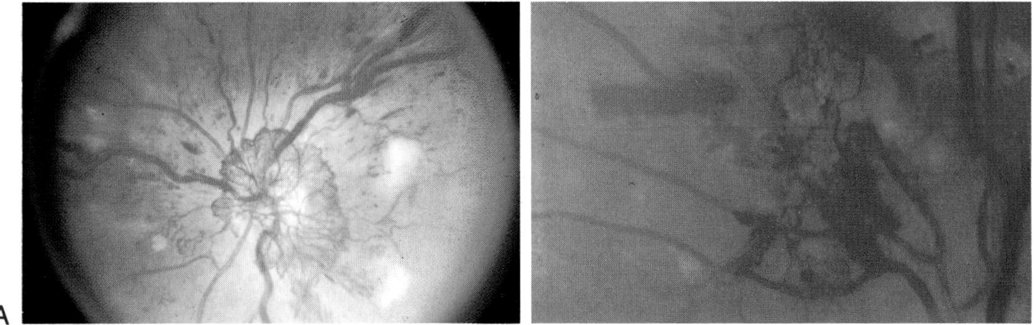

FIGURE 3-47 **Proliferative diabetic retinopathy.** *A,* NVD is thought to be stimulated by a diffusable angiogenic factor or factors released by ischemia retina, usually in the midperiphery. Typically, these vessels form in a cartwheel configuration with vessels radiating out from the center to a circumferential peripheral vessel. *B,* NVE develops from retinal vessels and tends to appear adjacent to regions of nonperfusion. Proliferative diabetic retinopathy also includes new vessels on the surface of the iris (rubeosis iridis) or in the anterior chamber angle.

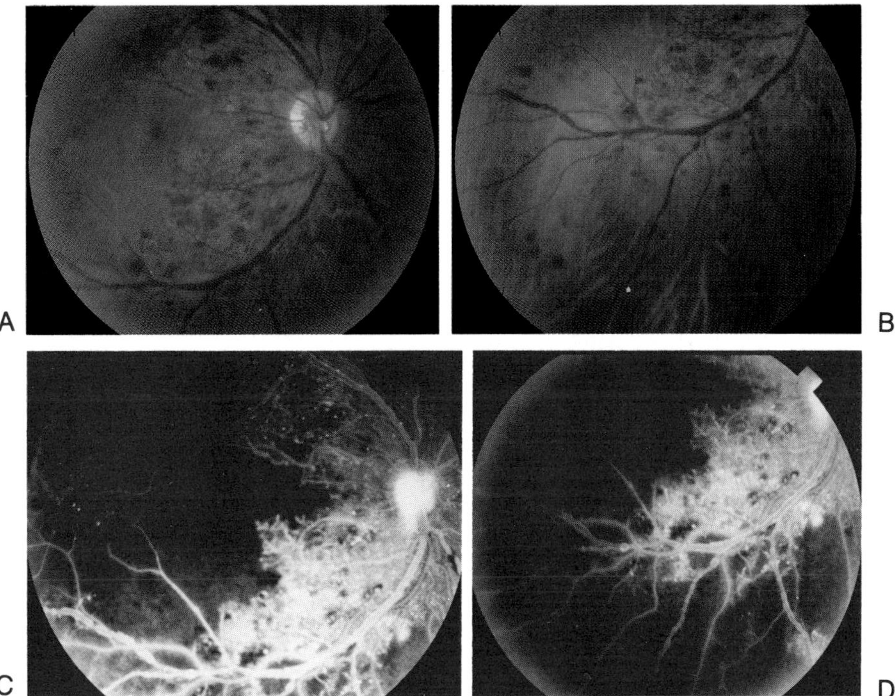

FIGURE 3-48 **Proliferative diabetic retinopathy.** *A,* A 27-year-old diabetic man presented with rubeosis and neovascular glaucoma in each eye. NVD was present, and visual acuity was 20/200. *B,* This view of the inferotemporal arcade demonstrates numerous intraretinal hemorrhages and a subtle intraretinal whitening indicative of retinal ischemia. *C,* A fluorescein angiogram documents severe capillary nonperfusion of the entire temporal macula and beyond; there is also hyperfluorescence of the disc denoting NVD. *D,* This inferior view shows nearly complete lack of capillary perfusion outside of the peripapillary area.

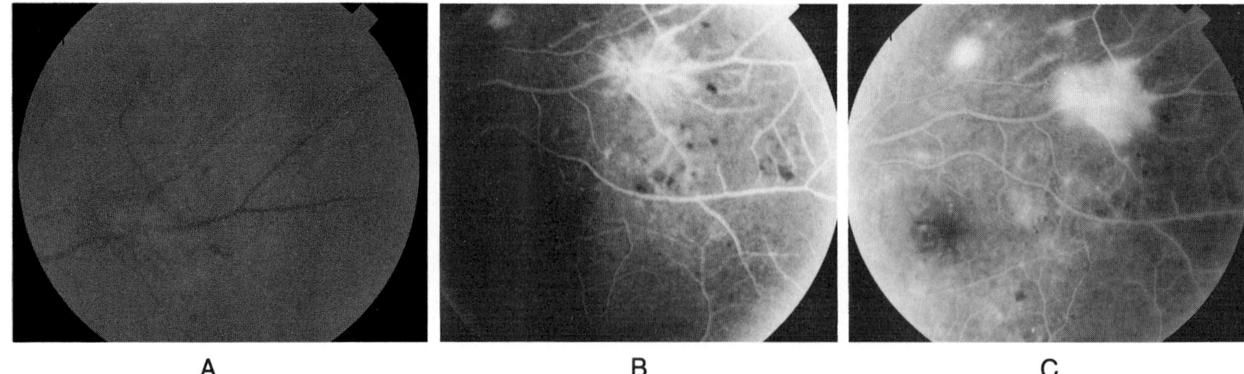

FIGURE 3–49 **Proliferative diabetic retinopathy.** *A,* NVE typically occurs adjacent to areas of capillary closure, marked by cotton-wool spots and hemorrhagic microaneurysms. *B,* An early transit fluorescein angiogram photograph shows hyperfluorescence of the same area of NVE. *C,* A late transit phase view demonstrates continued leakage of fluorescein from the NVE. IRMA may be difficult to differentiate from NVE; however, IRMAs usually do not leak as profusely as do new vessels.

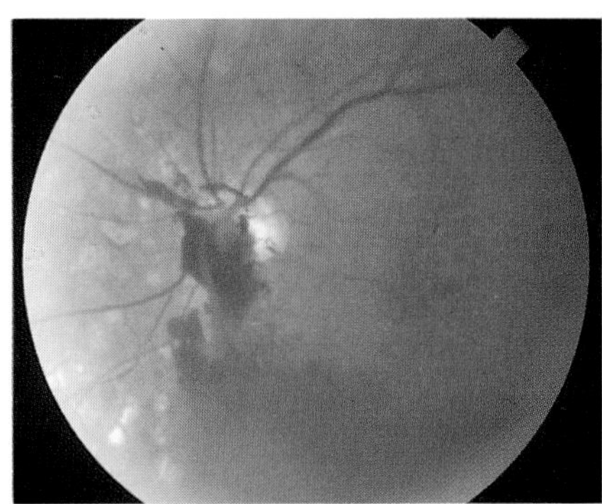

FIGURE 3–50 **Vitreous hemorrhage in proliferative diabetic retinopathy.** Vitreous hemorrhage from NVD may occur as the posterior hyaloid face of the vitreous begins to detach and exerts traction on friable neovascular tissue.

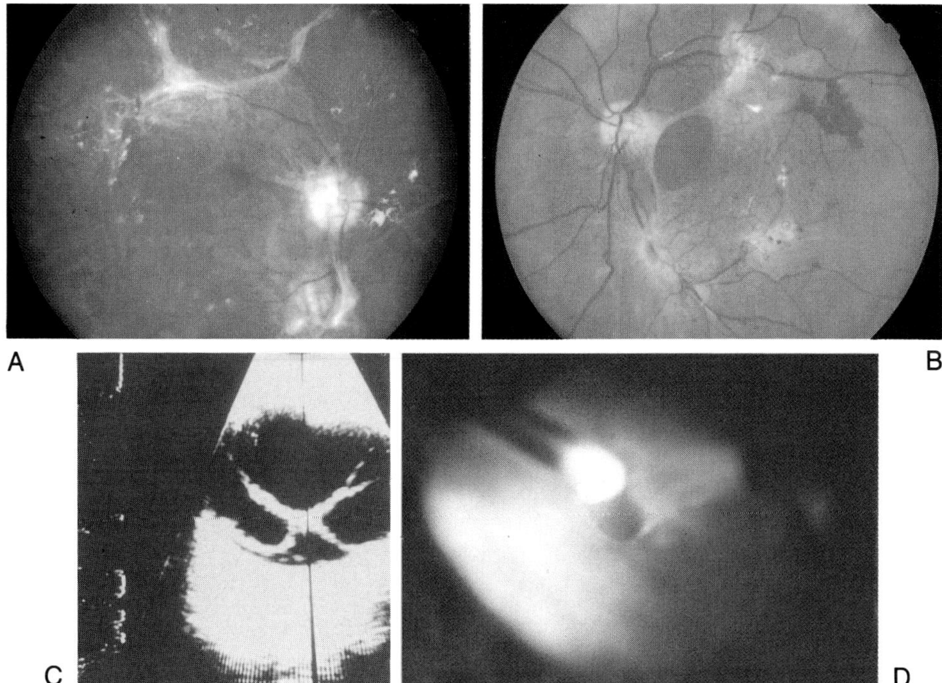

FIGURE 3-51 **Vitreous traction in proliferative diabetic retinopathy.** The posterior hyaloid (posterior vitreous face) may have a variety of complex configurations in proliferative diabetic retinopathy. *A,* In this fundus photograph, the posterior hyaloid is attached across the macula, at the disc, and just beyond each arcade; outside of these areas, the vitreous is detached. In this eye, the posterior hyaloid is fibrotic and slightly separated from the surface of the macula, rendering it visible. The underlying retina is totally attached, and the visual acuity is 20/30. *B,* The posterior hyaloid of this fundus has a large hole centrally, simulating an epiretinal membrane with hole. The residual attachment points of the posterior hyaloid at the disc in the superior, inferior, and inferotemporal locations may be seen. The retina is attached, and visual acuity is 20/30. *C,* An ultrasound scan may be useful to define vitreoretinal relationships in proliferative diabetic retinopathy, especially if there are media opacities present. This ultrasound scan demonstrates a traction retinal detachment and vitreous attachments (vitreous cone). *D,* This intraoperative view of vitreous surgery shows the creation of an opening in the detached peripheral vitreous with the vitrectomy instrument; the membranous character of the tissue is shown.

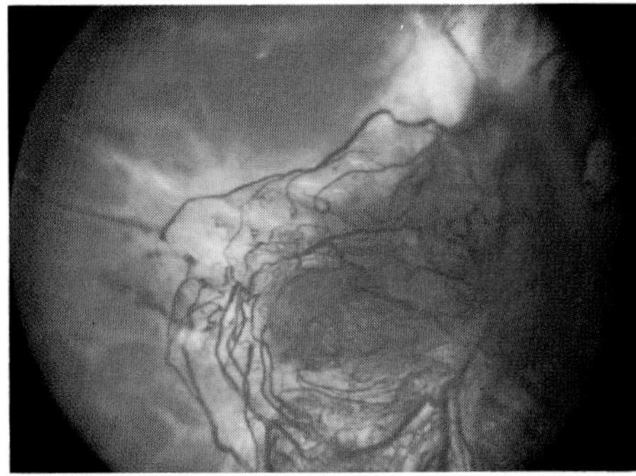

FIGURE 3–52 **Fibrous proliferation in proliferative diabetic retinopathy.** Severe neovascularization with vascular overgrowth may obscure the retina, and contraction of the associated fibrous tissue may lead to distortion of the normal retinal architecture and traction retinal detachment.

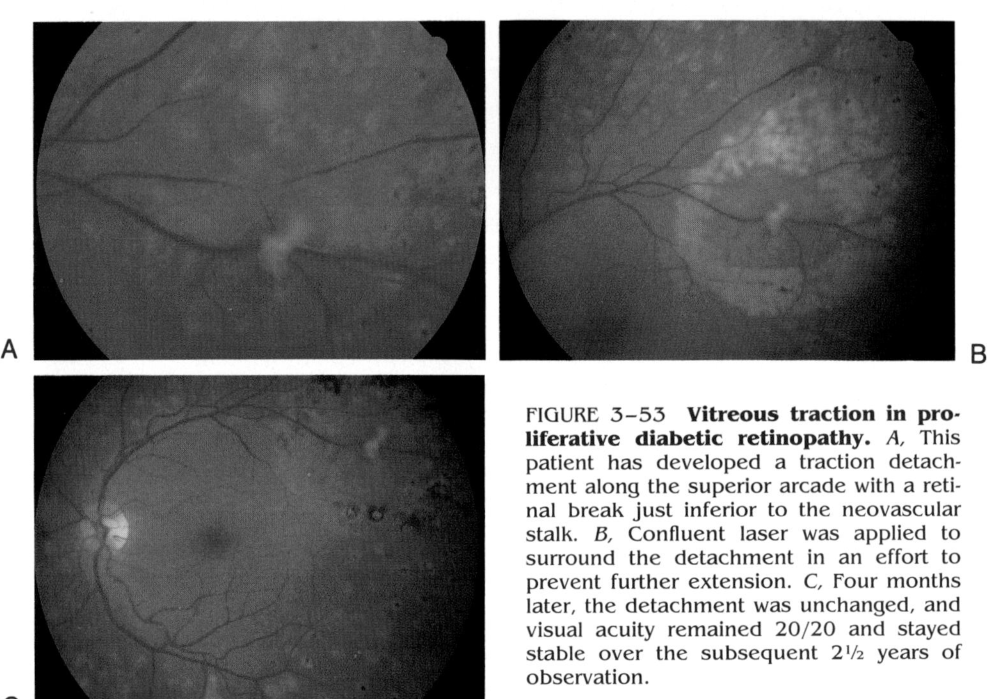

FIGURE 3–53 **Vitreous traction in proliferative diabetic retinopathy.** *A,* This patient has developed a traction detachment along the superior arcade with a retinal break just inferior to the neovascular stalk. *B,* Confluent laser was applied to surround the detachment in an effort to prevent further extension. *C,* Four months later, the detachment was unchanged, and visual acuity remained 20/20 and stayed stable over the subsequent 2½ years of observation.

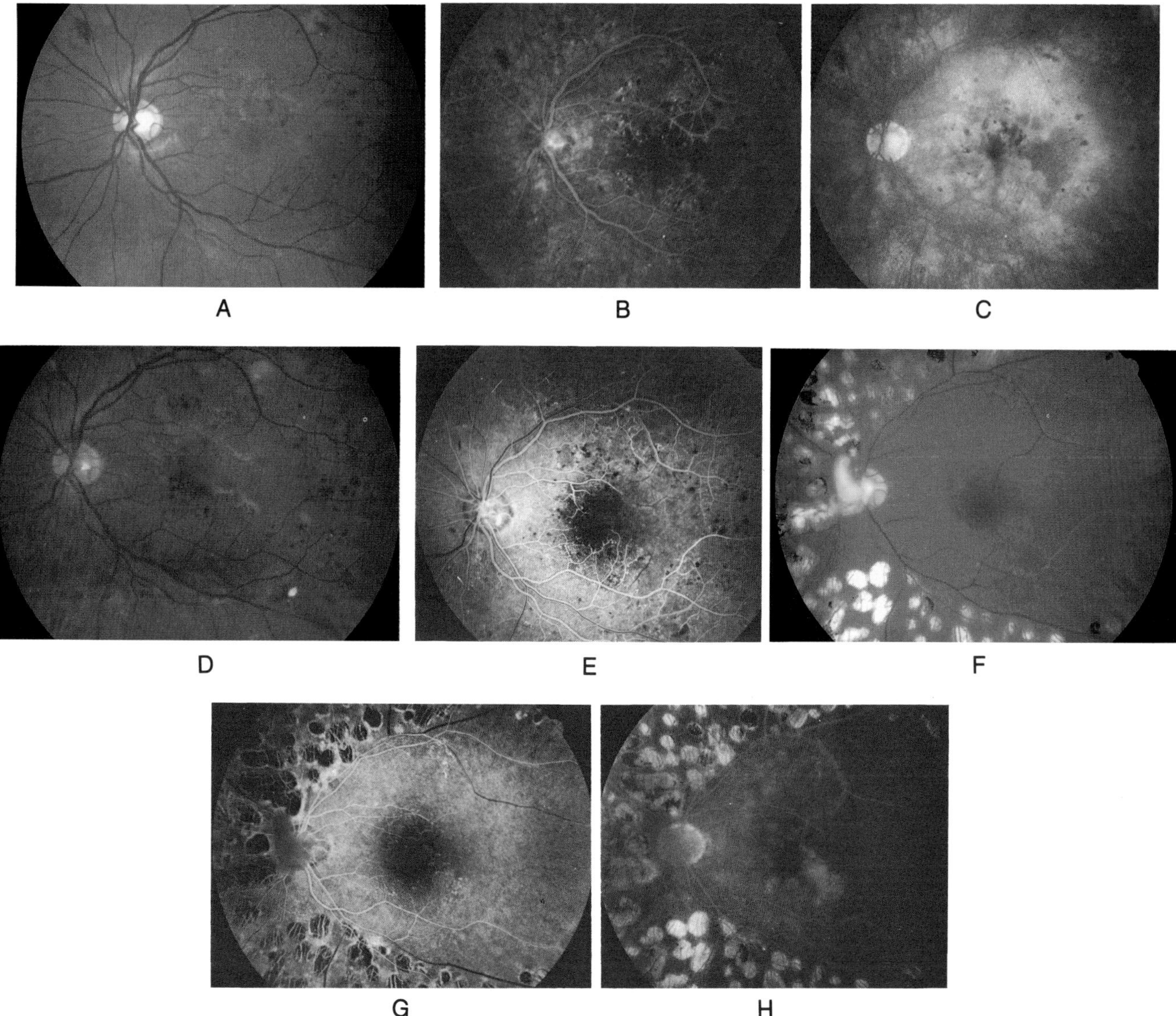

FIGURE 3-54 **Progression of proliferative diabetic retinopathy.** This series of photographs depicts the long-term progression of ocular disease in a 21-year-old man with diabetic retinopathy. *A,* Initially, the patient has intraretinal hemorrhages and cotton-wool spots with a visual acuity of 20/30. *B,* The transit phase of the fluorescein angiogram demonstrates macular capillary nonperfusion and early disc neovascularization. *C,* Late phase of the angiogram shows continued ischemia with diffuse leakage in the macula. *D,* Six months later, cotton-wool spots have increased, and visual acuity has dropped to 20/50. *E,* The fluorescein angiogram now displays NVD and extensive capillary nonperfusion, most prominent in the temporal macula. *F,* Eight years later, after extensive panretinal photocoagulation as well as a vitrectomy for vitreous hemorrhage, regressed proliferative changes are noted. Sclerotic vessels are present temporally with 20/80 visual acuity. *G,* A fluorescein angiogram shows delayed filling of the temporal vessels and a greatly increased foveal avascular zone. *H,* The late phase of the angiogram reveals continued ischemia, vascular wall leakage in the temporal vessels, and macular edema resulting from intraretinal vascular abnormalities.

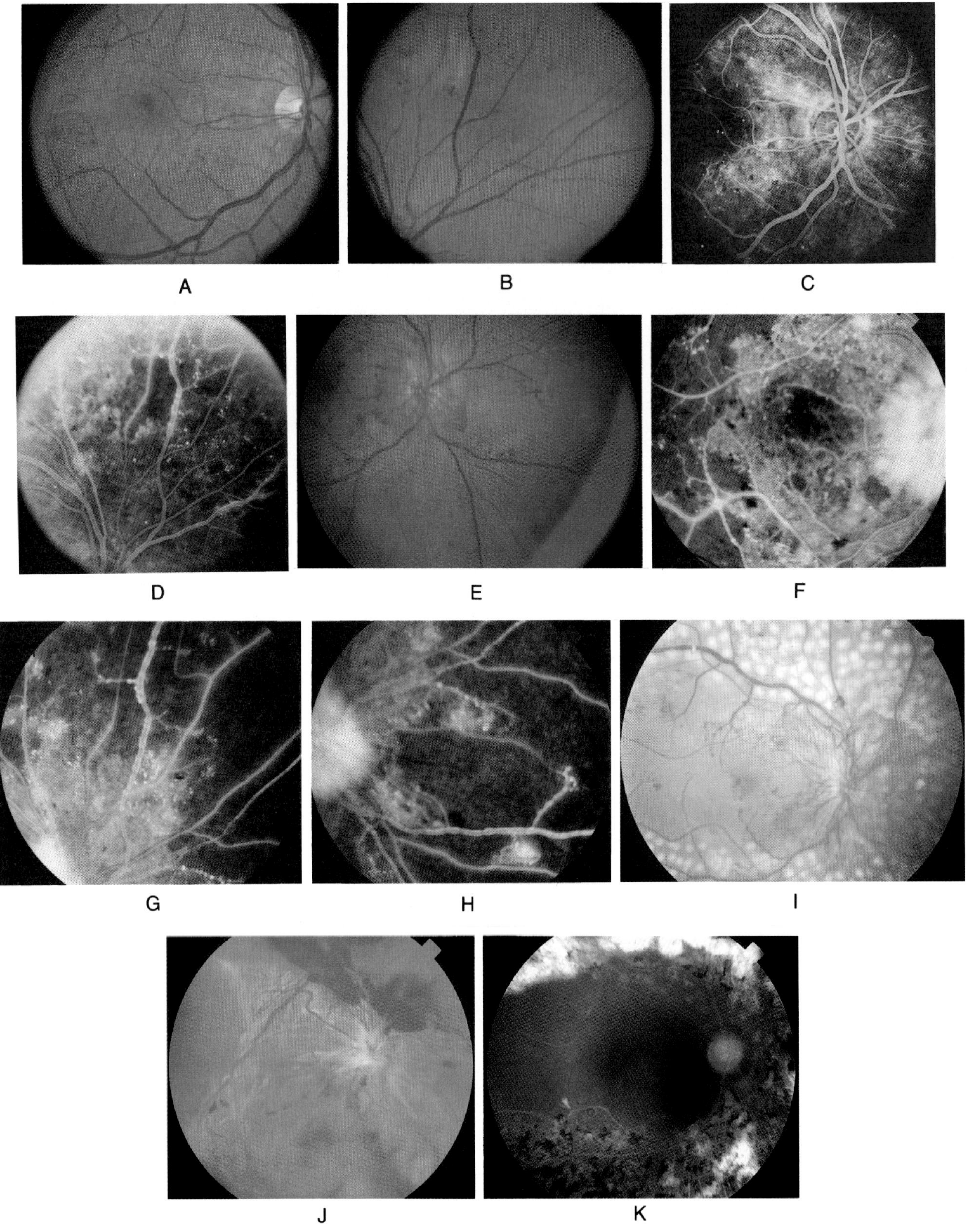

FIGURE 3–55 *See legend on opposite page*

◀ FIGURE 3–55 **Progression of proliferative diabetic retinopathy.** In some patients, proliferative diabetic retinopathy progresses despite panretinal photocoagulation. *A,* A 29-year-old man initially presented with 20/25 vision and preproliferative changes in his right eye. Vascular dilatation, cotton-wool spots, and intraretinal hemorrhages are seen. *B,* The superior retina shows similar preproliferative changes. *C,* A fluorescein angiogram is remarkable for numerous microaneurysms with leakage and an enlarged foveal avascular zone. *D,* The superior retina also has capillary nonperfusion and leakage into the vascular walls. *E,* The patient was lost to follow-up for 1½ years and returned with severe NVD; visual acuity was still 20/25. *F,* The fluorescein angiogram demonstrates marked progression of ischemic changes in association with prominent leakage from NVD. *G,* An angiogram of the superior retina shows greatly increased ischemia compared with the previous angiogram. *H,* In the nasal retina, the angiogram documents almost total closure of the capillary bed in association with areas of neovascularization. *I,* Six months later, NVD progresses despite extensive and repeated panretinal photocoagulation. *J,* After an additional 10 months, a traction retinal detachment involving the fovea developed. The retina is obscured by neovascular tissue, and the visual acuity had dropped to the counting fingers level at 1 foot. *K,* One year after vitrectomy and endolaser treatment, the retina is attached but displays optic atrophy. The final visual acuity is 20/200.

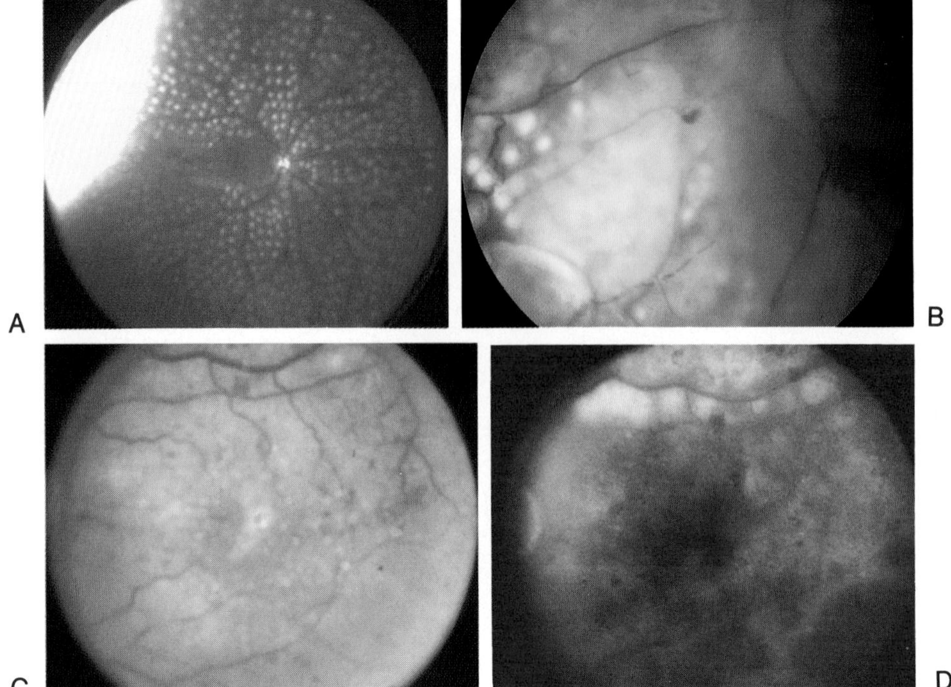

FIGURE 3–56 **Laser treatment of proliferative diabetic retinopathy.** Panretinal photocoagulation for proliferative diabetic retinopathy can lead to a variety of complications, especially after heavy treatment. *A,* This wide-angle photograph demonstrates a typical panretinal photocoagulation pattern, as recommended by the Diabetic Retinopathy Study. *B,* Extensive photocoagulation, as shown here for rubeosis, may lead to a choroidal and exudative retinal detachment, which usually resolves spontaneously. *C,* Macular edema can be exacerbated by panretinal photocoagulation. A loss of visual acuity of one to three lines can occur and is more common in patients with perifoveal capillary nonperfusion. *D,* A fluorescein angiogram documents cystoid edema; the edema resolved in 1 month with visual recovery.

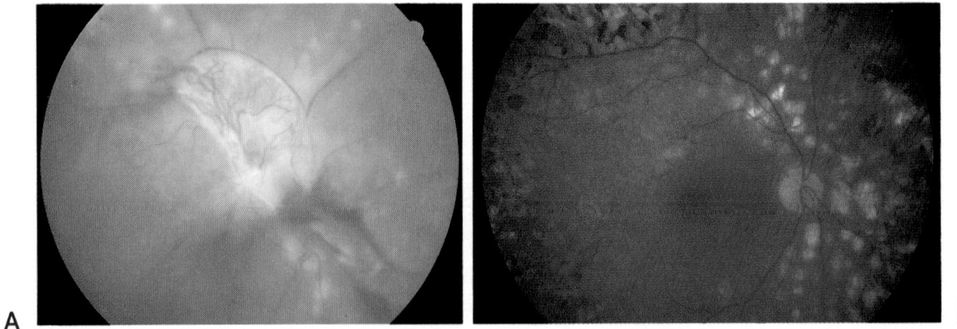

FIGURE 3–57 **Vitrectomy for proliferative diabetic retinopathy.** A traction retinal detachment involving the fovea is an indication for a prompt pars plana vitrectomy in an effort to preserve central vision. *A,* This preoperative photograph of a patient with 20/400 vision illustrates extensive neovascularization emanating from the disc with a traction retinal detachment. *B,* The postoperative photograph after vitrectomy shows retinal reattachment and removal of neovascular tissue. Visual acuity had improved to 20/40.

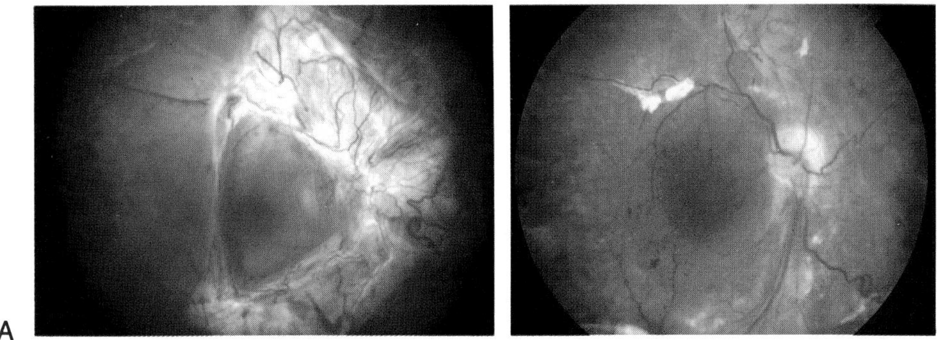

FIGURE 3-58 **Vitrectomy for proliferative diabetic retinopathy.** The majority of patients with a traction retinal detachment involving the fovea can expect to have improved vision after a pars plana vitrectomy. *A*, This preoperative photograph shows severe neovascularization with detachment of the fovea in a patient with 20/400 vision. *B*, After a vitrectomy, the retina was reattached; however, visual improvement was limited to 20/200, in part as a result of continued distortion of the inferior macula.

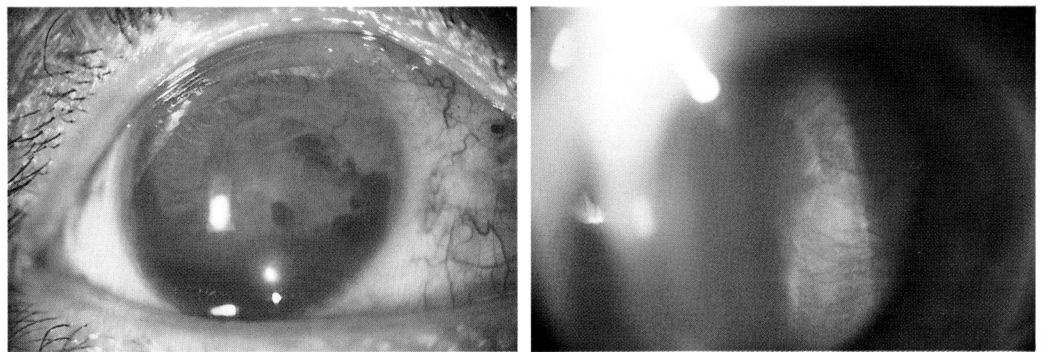

FIGURE 3-59 **Complications of vitrectomy for proliferative diabetic retinopathy.** *A*, After a failed vitrectomy, rubeosis, hyphema, and neovascular glaucoma may arise secondary to recurrent detachment and persistent retinal ischemia. Visual acuity was at the no-light perception level. *B*, Anterior hyaloid fibrovascular proliferation is a serious complication most commonly observed in juvenile diabetics undergoing vitrectomy without lens removal. Unless surgical intervention, including lensectomy and extensive peripheral retinal ablation, is performed promptly, these eyes are invariably lost.

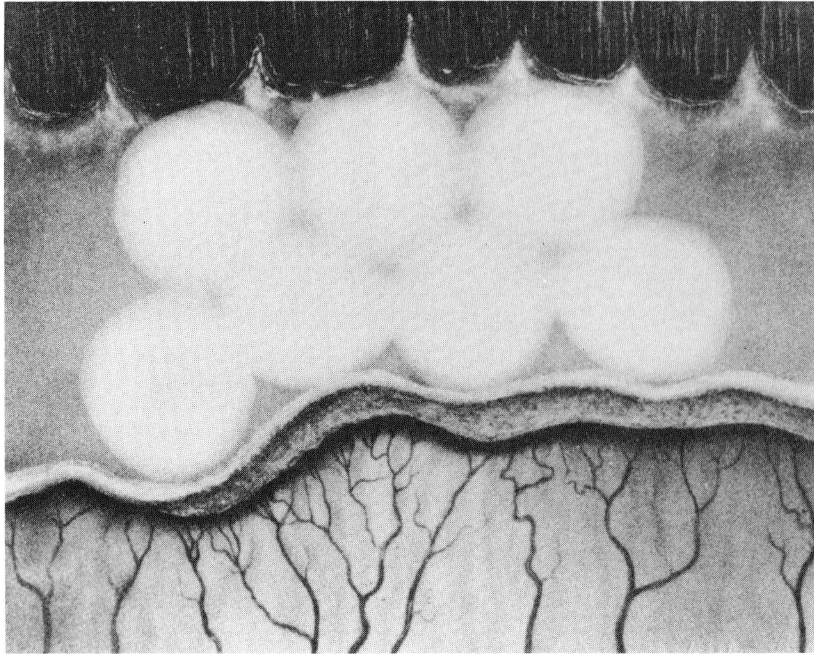

FIGURE 3-60 **Cryotherapy for retinopathy of prematurity.** When treating retinopathy of prematurity, the entire avascular retina peripheral to the ridge of neovascular tissue is ablated. Shown here is a fundus drawing of the avascular retina immediately after seven spots of cryoapplications anterior to the fibrovascular ridge. (From Cryotherapy for Retinopathy of Prematurity Cooperative Group: Multicenter trial of cryotherapy for retinopathy of prematurity: Preliminary results. Arch Ophthalmol 106:471–479, 1988. Copyright 1988, American Medical Association.)

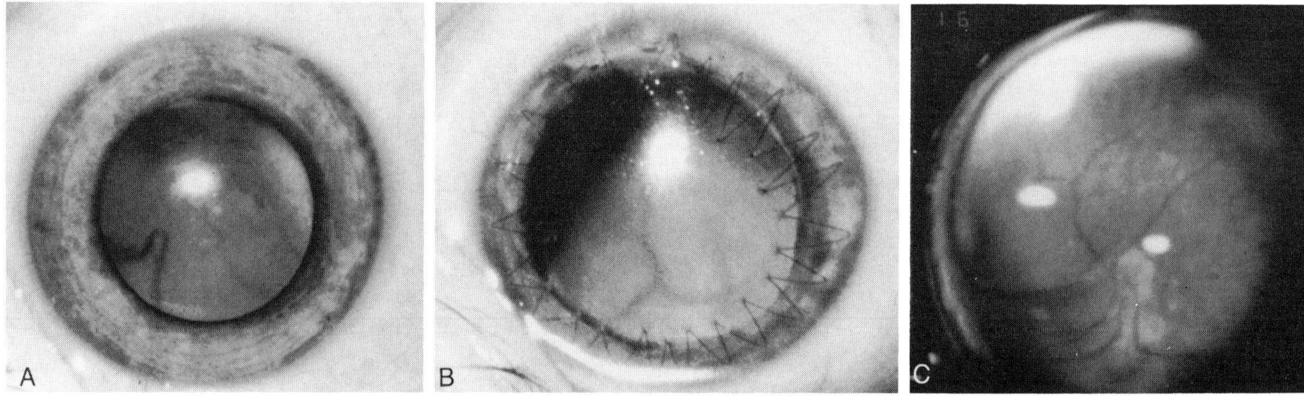

FIGURE 3-61 **Vitrectomy for retinopathy of prematurity.** *A,* This eye of a 16-month-old boy has stage 5 retinopathy of prematurity with a totally detached retina pulled forward toward the lens. The vessels of the detached retina are seen through the thin retrolental fibrous membrane. *B,* A postoperative photograph shows the same eye 1½ months after open-sky vitrectomy. *C,* The postoperative fundus photograph demonstrates an attached retina with the retinal vessels drawn into the broad dry fold inferiorly.

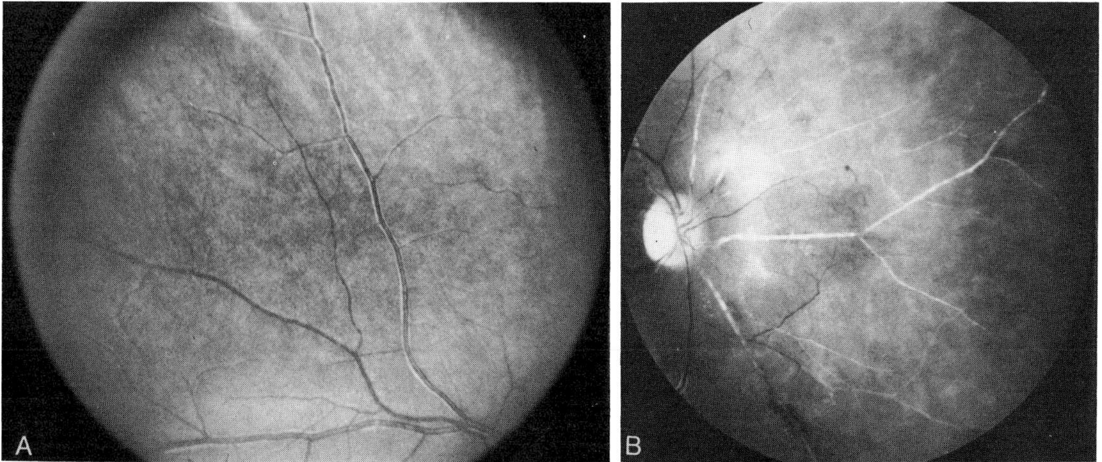

FIGURE 3–62 **Vasculitis in Eales' disease.** *A,* Vascular sheathing, as evidenced by the thin white lines surrounding this retinal venule, is a common clinical sign of ocular inflammation encountered in the idiopathic peripheral retinal vasculitis of Eales' disease. (From Gieser SC, Murphy RP; Eales' disease. *In* Ryan S (ed): Retina. St Louis, CV Mosby, 1989.) *B,* This photograph of the retina of a patient with Eales' disease demonstrates extensive arteriolar sheathing with retinal vascular nonperfusion nasal to the disc.

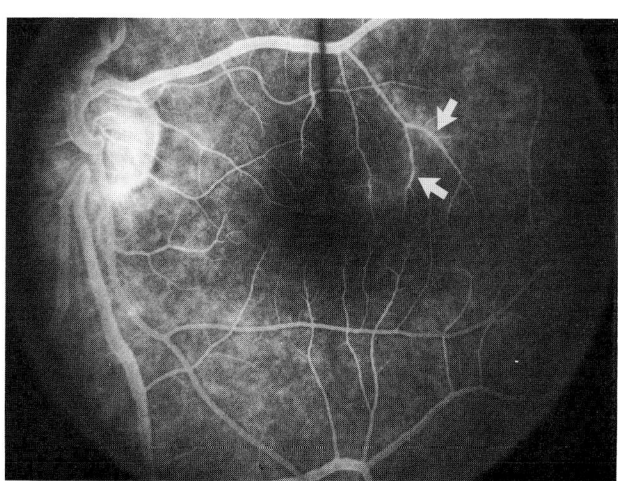

FIGURE 3–63 **Vasculitis in Eales' disease.** Fluorescein angiography in patients with Eales' disease often demonstrate abnormal staining in areas of vascular sheathing *(arrows);* however, the intensity of hyperfluorescence seen on fluorescein angiography does not necessarily correlate with the intensity of inflammation on clinical examination.

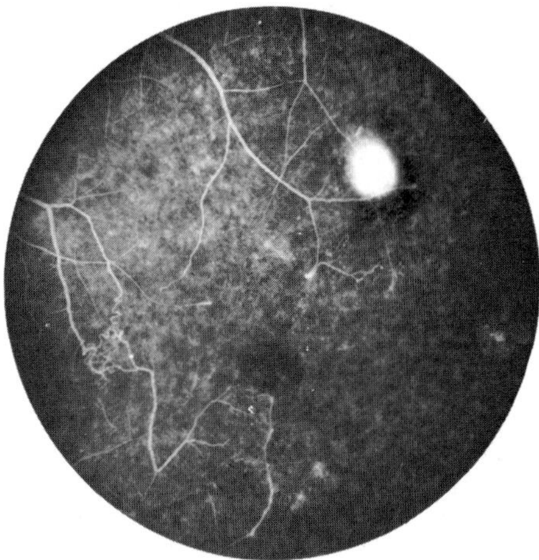

FIGURE 3-64 **Peripheral retinal nonperfusion in Eales' disease.** Peripheral retinal nonperfusion is invariably present in patients with Eales' disease, particularly in the temporal retina. Note the vascular abnormalities and the small area of neovascularization at the junctional zone between perfused and nonperfused retina in this fluorescein angiogram.

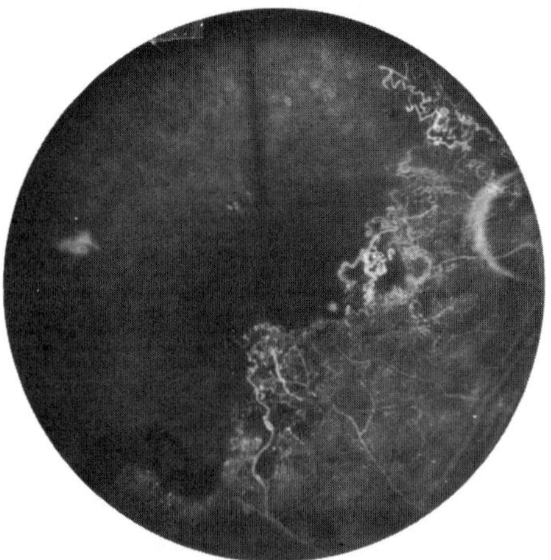

FIGURE 3-65 **Peripheral retinal nonperfusion in Eales' disease.** This fluorescein angiogram demonstrates that peripheral nonperfusion may expand massively and ultimately involve a substantial portion of the macula. Note the microaneurysms, arteriovenous shunts, and staining of the stumps of the obliterated vessels at the junction between perfused and nonperfused retina.

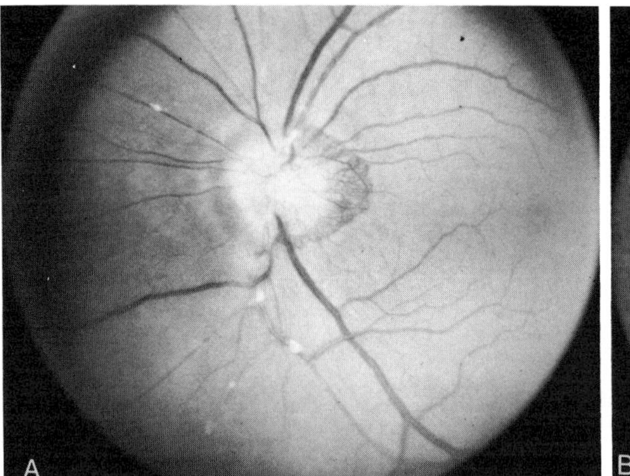

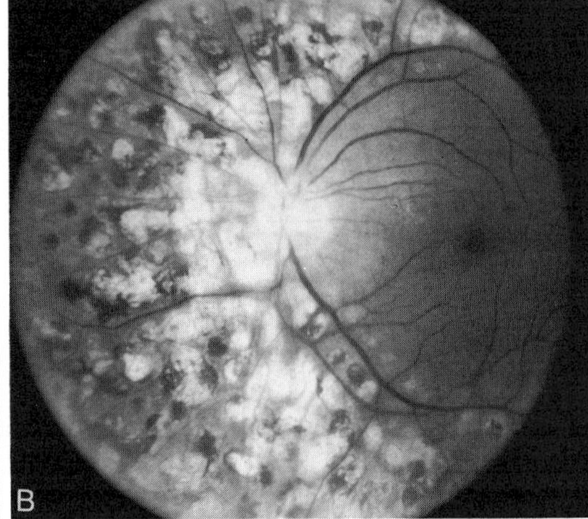

FIGURE 3-66 **Laser treatment of Eales' disease.** *A,* This patient with Eales' disease manifests neovascularization of the disc and segmental arteriolar sheathing. *B,* The patient was treated with scatter photocoagulation to all areas of nonperfused retina. Two and a half years later, note that the neovascularization has regressed, and the areas of arteriolar sheathing have resolved. (*A* and *B,* From Gieser SC, Murphy RP: Eales' disease. *In* Ryan S (ed): Retina. St Louis, CV Mosby, 1989.)

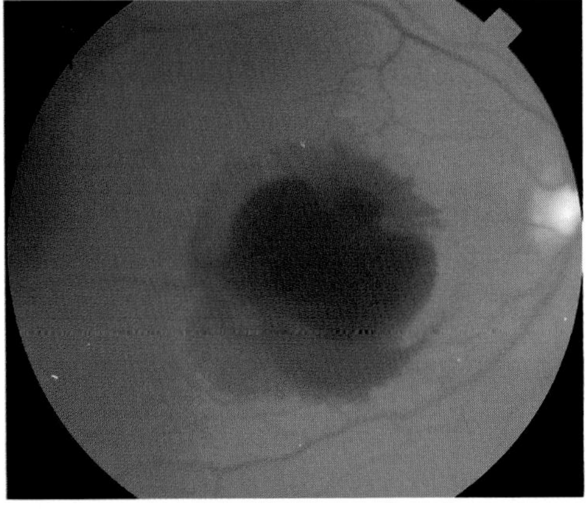

FIGURE 3-67 **Rupture of a retinal arterial macroaneurysm.** It is thought that chronic vascular wall damage owing to hypertension and associated arteriosclerotic changes predisposes the retinal arteries to focal dilatation in the presence of increased intraluminal pressure. Progressive weakening of the arterial wall may result in a rupture of the macroaneurysm as shown in this patient. Note that the hemorrhage has gained access to the subretinal, intraretinal, and retrohyaloidal spaces obscuring the macroaneurysm.

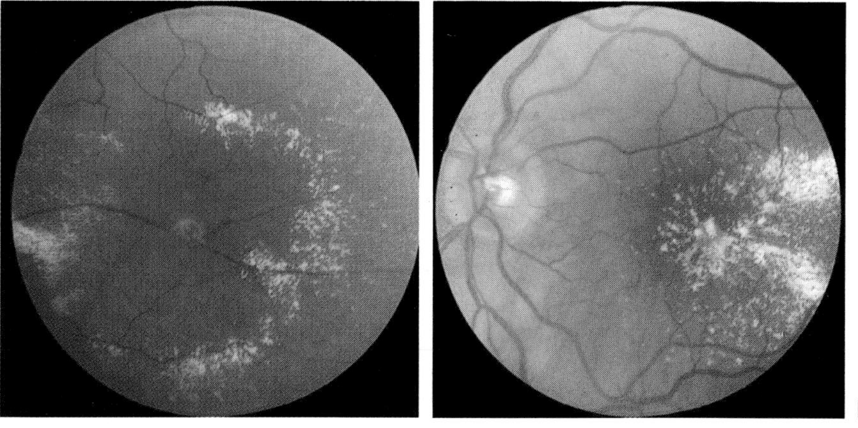

FIGURE 3-68 **Exudative retinopathy secondary to a retinal arterial macroaneurysm.** *A,* A large macroaneurysm is located in the temporal retinal periphery. Note the circinate pattern of intraretinal lipid deposition resulting from the altered permeability of the arterial wall. *B,* The exudate extends to involve the fovea producing macular edema and reduced visual acuity.

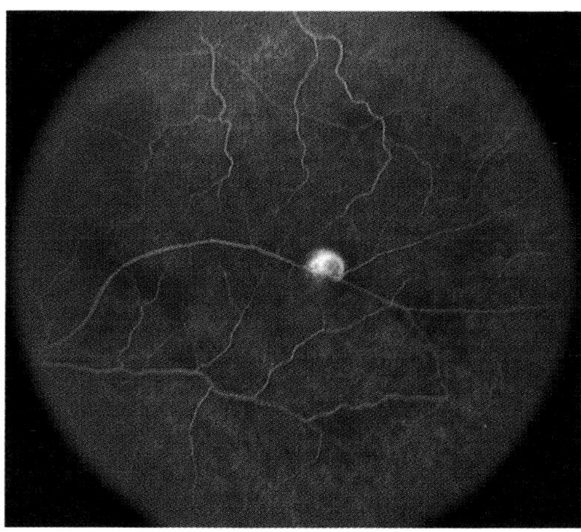

FIGURE 3-69 **Fluorescein angiographic features of a retinal arterial macroaneurysm.** The fluorescein angiogram demonstrates rapid, incomplete filling of the macroaneurysm, which is consistent with partial thrombosis. Although it is not evident in this figure, macroaneurysms are often surrounded by capillary microaneurysms with capillary nonperfusion, intraretinal microvascular abnormalities, telangiectasis, and fluorescein dye leakage.

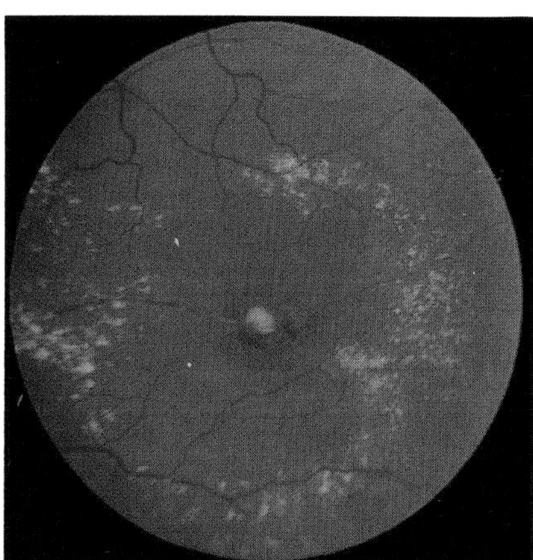

FIGURE 3-70 **Retinal arterial macroaneurysm following laser photocoagulation.** Three months after argon-green photocoagulation, the lesion appears to be fibrotic with partial closure of the vessel, resolution of the surrounding macular edema, and residual retinal exudate. Reduced arterial blood flow and a corresponding reduction in hydrostatic pressure following photocoagulation of the surrounding retina result in diminished vascular leakage and a lesser risk of spontaneous rupture.

FIGURE 3-71 **Exudative retinal detachment in Coats' disease.** Coats' disease exists on a spectrum. Mild forms may be characterized by one or more foci of retinal telangiectasis with altered vascular permeability leading to localized retinal edema and lipid exudate. Severe forms, as shown here, often present in early childhood with leukocoria secondary to total exudative retinal detachment. In addition to telangiectasis, microaneurysms, areas of capillary nonperfusion, and saccular outpouchings of retinal venules may be seen.

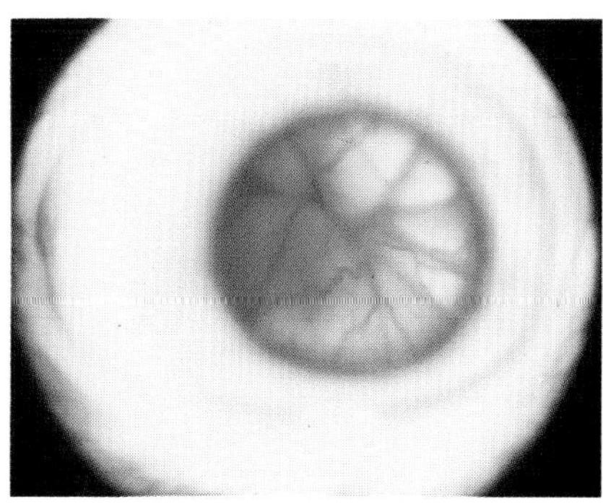

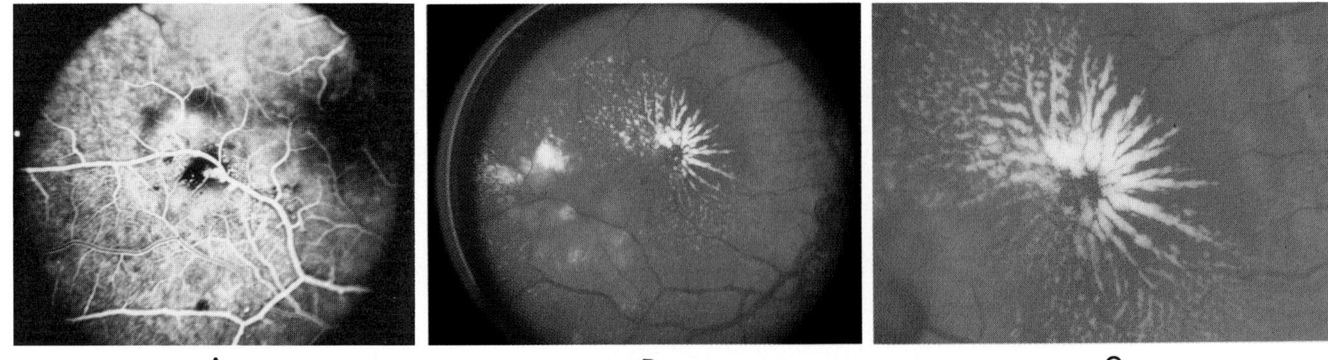

FIGURE 3-72 **Macular edema and lipid exudation in Coats' disease.** Retinal telangiectasis in a patient with Coats' disease resulting in decreased visual acuity secondary to macular edema and lipid exudation. Note the area of retinal telangiectasis temporal to the fovea on fluorescein angiography (A) as well as macular star formation secondary to lipid exudation (*B* and *C*). *B* depicts the abnormal blood vessels following recent laser photocoagulation to the region of telangiectasis.

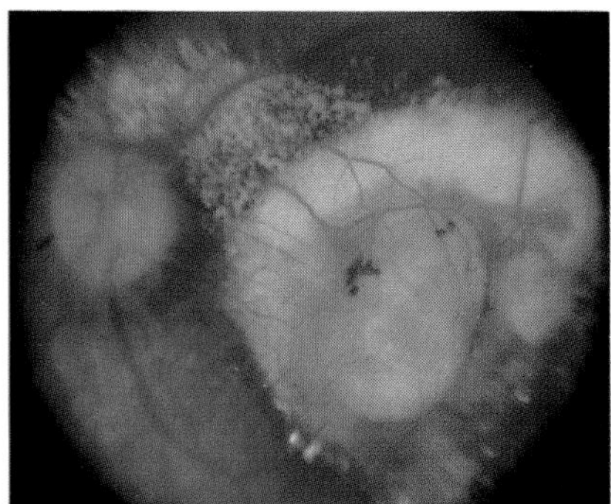

FIGURE 3-73 **Massive subretinal exudate in Coats' disease.** A subretinal mass with an overlying exudative retinal detachment secondary to progressive accumulation of subretinal lipid exudate in a patient with Coats' disease. The source of vascular leakage is typically located in the temporal retinal periphery; however, migration of fluid and exudate when the patient is supine may involve the dependent posterior pole.

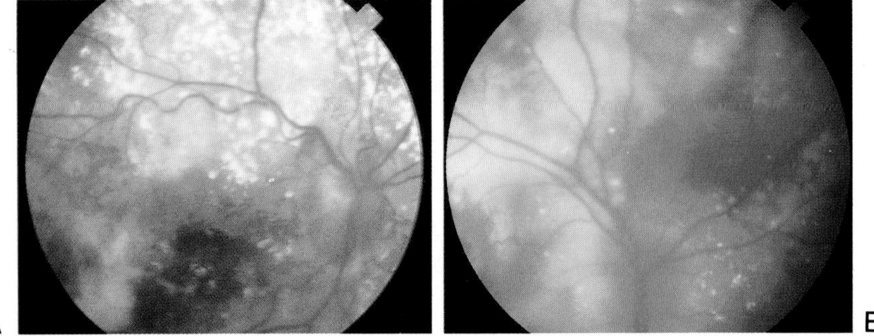

FIGURE 3-74 **Proliferative retinopathy in Coats' disease.** *A* and *B*, Subretinal cholesterol-rich "crystalline bodies" and associated hemorrhage in a patient with Coats' disease. Iris, retinal, and optic disc neovascularization may also occur, often resulting in neovascular glaucoma and retinal and vitreous hemorrhage.

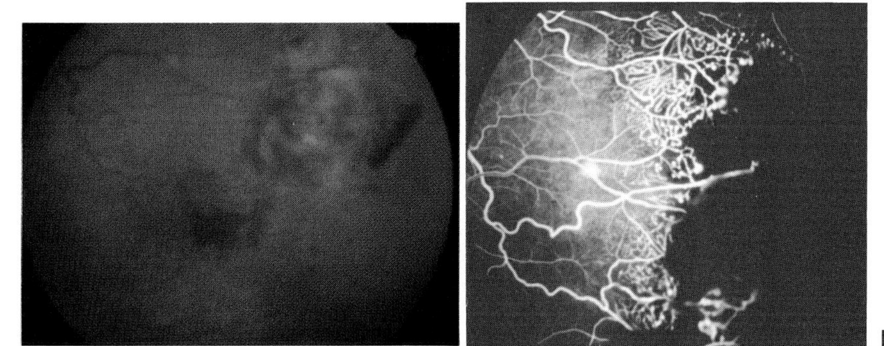

FIGURE 3–75 **Fluorescein angiographic features of Coats' disease.** *A* and *B*, A peripheral angiomatous mass in a patient with Coats' disease. Fluorescein angiography aids in distinguishing this lesion from angiomatosis retinae. Note the typical retinal vascular changes of Coats' disease, including capillary nonperfusion, saccular and beadlike "light bulb" dilatations of the retinal vessels, and associated dilatation of the adjacent capillary bed.

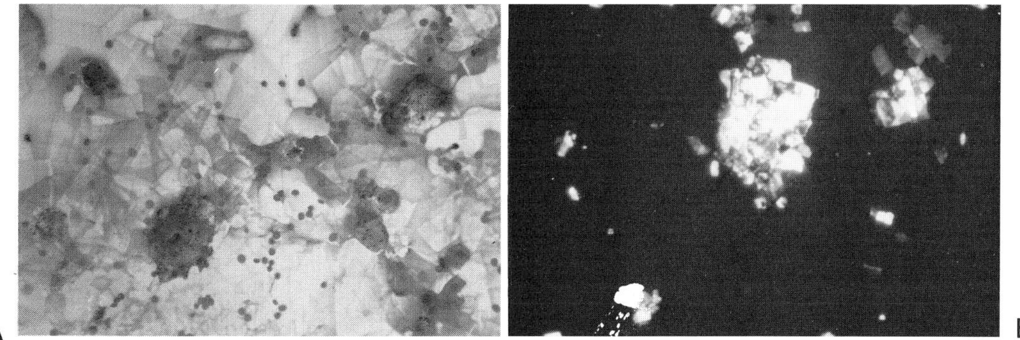

FIGURE 3–76 **Histopathologic features of Coats' disease.** Cholesterol crystals of a subretinal fluid aspirate in a patient with Coats' disease as visualized with H&E staining *(A)* and polarized microscopy *(B)*.

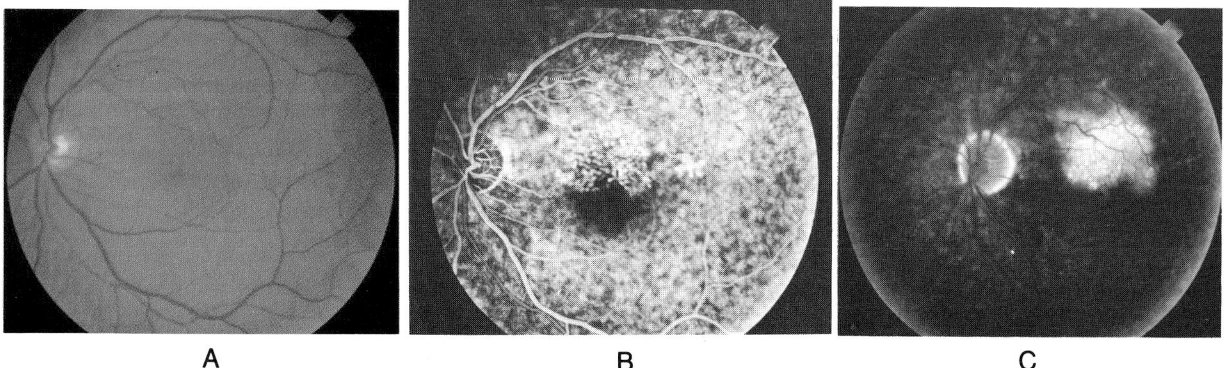

FIGURE 3–77 **Unilateral congenital parafoveal telangiectasia.** *A–C*, This patient has group IA: unilateral congenital parafoveal telangiectasia that most likely represents a mild form of Coats' disease. *A*, Telangiectatic vessels are present within 2 disc diameters of the center of the fovea. *B* and *C*, Fluorescein angiography demonstrates telangiectatic vessels in the superior parafoveal region in the early phase *(B)* and leakage of fluorescein dye in the late phases *(C)*. Unilateral, idiopathic parafoveal telangiectasis (group IB) is typically associated with less prominent vascular incompetence and a better visual prognosis.

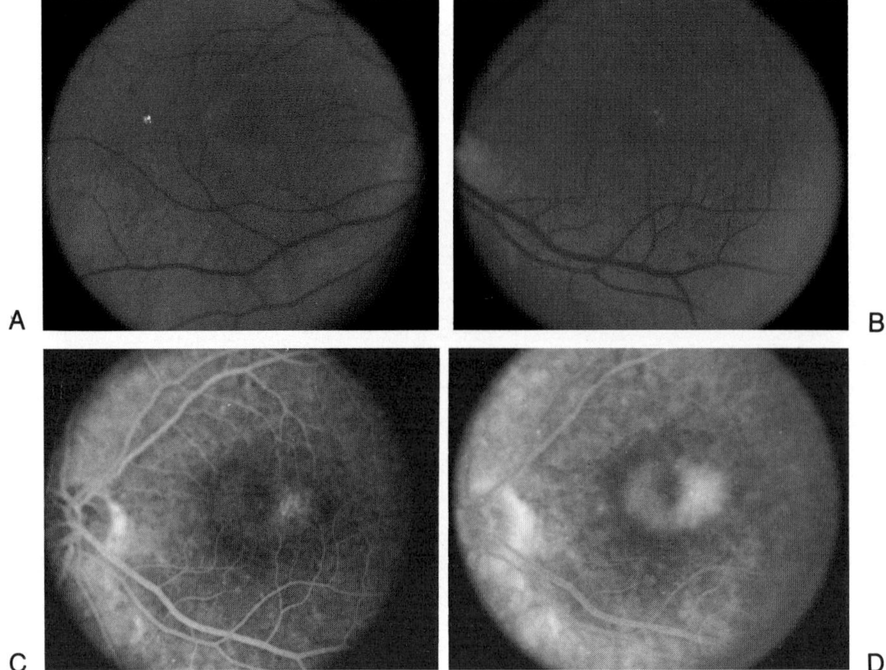

FIGURE 3–78 **Bilateral idiopathic acquired parafoveolar telangiectasia.** Bilateral idiopathic acquired parafoveal telangiectasia (group II) is the most common form of juxtafoveal telangiectasis. It occurs in both sexes, typically in the fifth and sixth decades, and there may be a familial component to the disease. *A–D,* Note the bilateral grayish parafoveal appearance, the yellow superficial retinal dots on the color photographs, and the parafoveal leakage on fluorescein angiography.

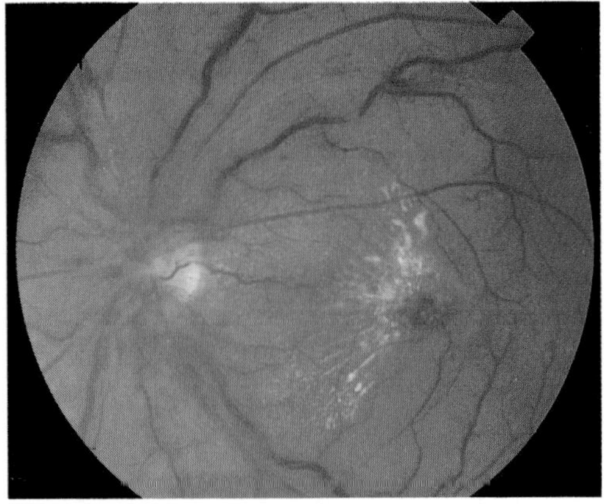

FIGURE 3–79 **Leber's idiopathic stellate neuroretinitis (LISN).** Ophthalmoscopic appearance of LISN with optic disc edema and macular star exudate. The patient was a 25-year-old woman with a 1-month history of scotoma and decreased vision in the left eye. The patient had numerous cats at home and was otherwise healthy. The visual acuity was 20/40; serologic test results for syphilis were negative, and the neurologic examination was otherwise normal. Recent reports have identified *Rochalimaea (Bartonella) henselae* in the serum of patients with cat scratch-related LISN.

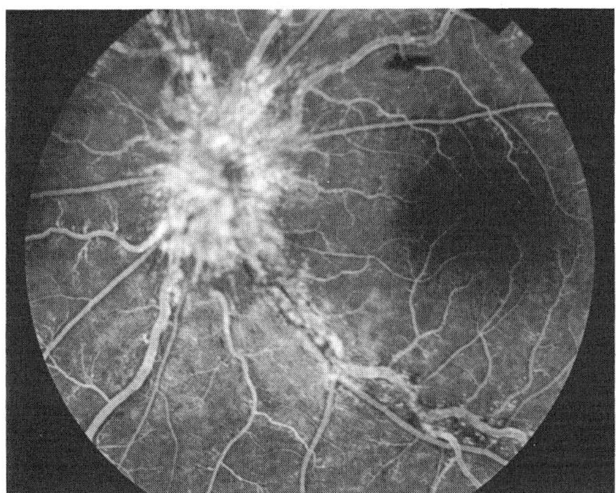

FIGURE 3–80 **LISN.** The fluorescein angiogram demonstrates diffuse fluorescence of the optic disc secondary to leakage from peripapillary capillaries and venous engorgement. Note that there is no leakage from the perifoveal capillaries.

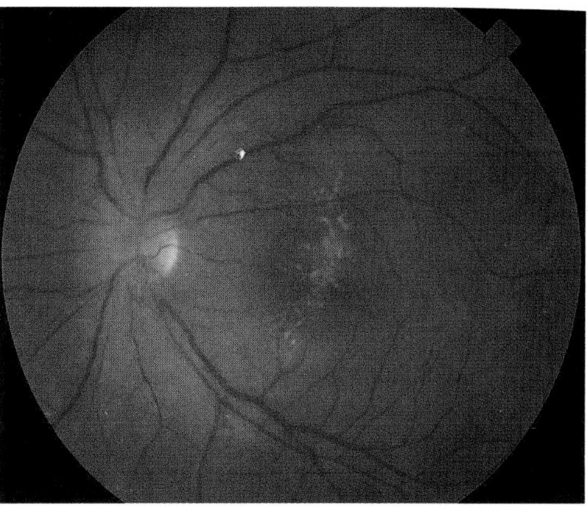

FIGURE 3–81 **LISN.** The same patient as in Figures 3–79 and 3–80. Seven weeks later, the visual acuity has improved to 20/30 + 2, with partial resolution of the optic disc edema and macular exudates.

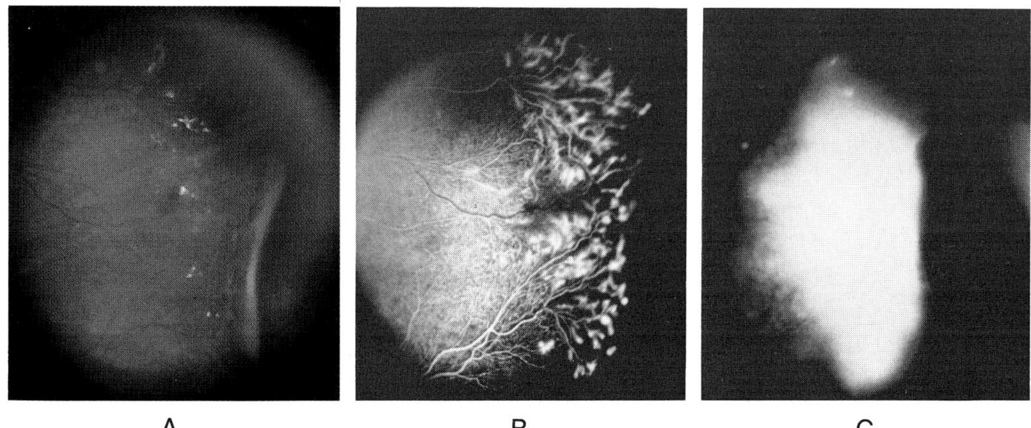

FIGURE 3–82 **Proliferative retinopathy in familial exudative vitreoretinopathy (FEVR).** Stage 1 represents a mild form of FEVR characterized by peripheral vitreoretinal abnormalities, such as white without pressure, cystoid degeneration, and vitreous bands. Vascular proliferation and exudation are not features of stage 1 disease. Stage 2, depicted above, shows the characteristic fibrovascular ridge in the temporal periphery *(A)*, and corresponding fluorescein angiography shows neovascularization at the vascular-avascular border *(B)* with late leakage *(C)*. *(A–C,* Courtesy of Tatsuo Hirose, M.D.)

FIGURE 3–83 **Macular traction in FEVR.** A patient with stage 2 FEVR with dragged disc and ectopic macula owing to contraction of the fibrovascular lesion in the temporal periphery. In stage 3 FEVR, the cicatricial lesion in the temporal periphery causes traction retinal detachments, falciform retinal folds, and rhegmatogenous retinal detachment.

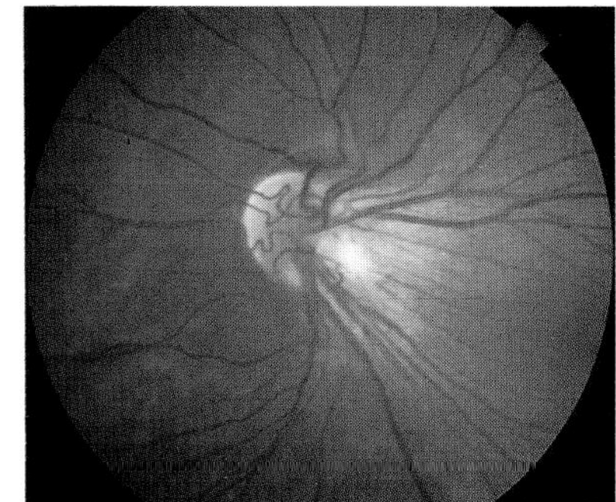

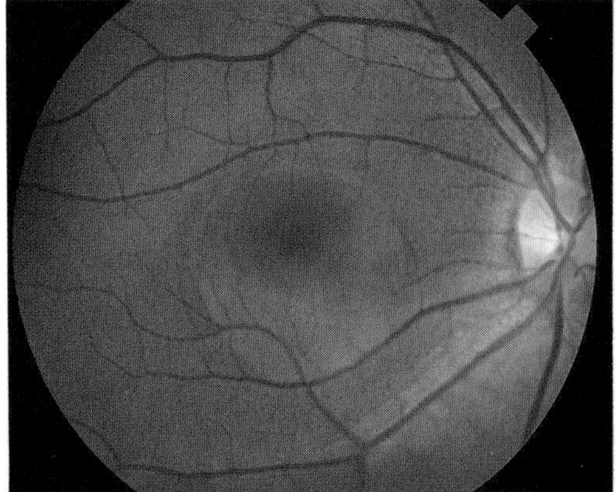

A

FIGURE 3–84 **Central serous chorioretinopathy.** There is considerable controversy regarding the pathogenesis of central serous chorioretinopathy. Fluorescein angiography typically reveals a focal disturbance of the outer blood retinal barrier, suggesting a defect at the level of the retinal pigment epithelium. *A,* A serous macular detachment consistent with central serous chorioretinopathy. *B,* Fluorescein angiography reveals early focal hyperfluorescence at the level of the retinal pigment epithelium in the early phase. *C,* Expansion of fluorescence into the subretinal space forms a classic smokestack configuration.

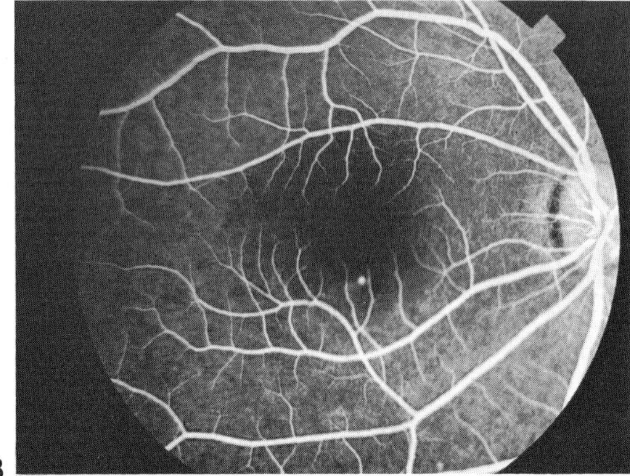

B

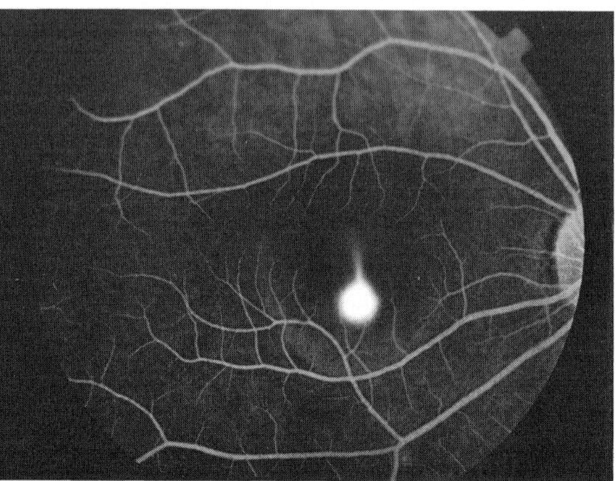

C

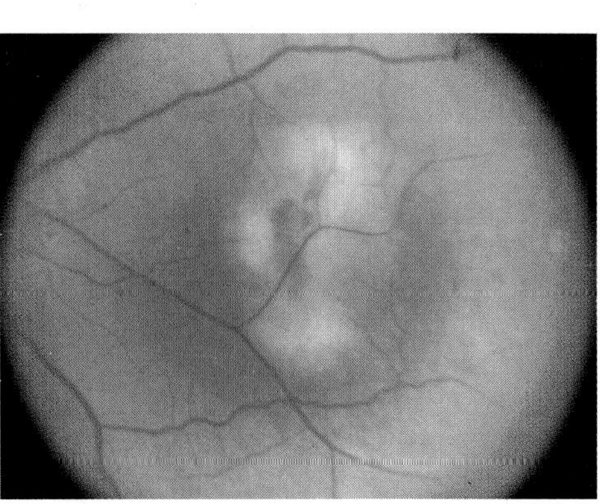

FIGURE 3–85 **Central serous chorioretinopathy with subretinal precipitates.** Patients may develop subretinal precipitates in association with serous neurosensory detachments in central serous chorioretinopathy. This figure depicts fibrin deposition, which probably represents a coalescence of these deposits.

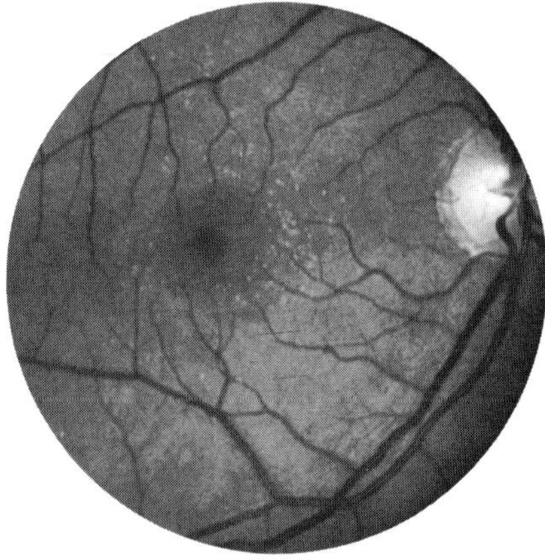

FIGURE 3–86 **Hard drusen in age-related macular degeneration.** Hard drusen usually appear clinically as small yellow punctate lesions at the level of the retinal pigment epithelium with sharp discrete borders. These changes have been shown to correspond to lipoid degeneration of a few discrete retinal pigment epithelial cells without evidence of diffuse thickening of the inner aspect of Bruch's membrane throughout the macula.

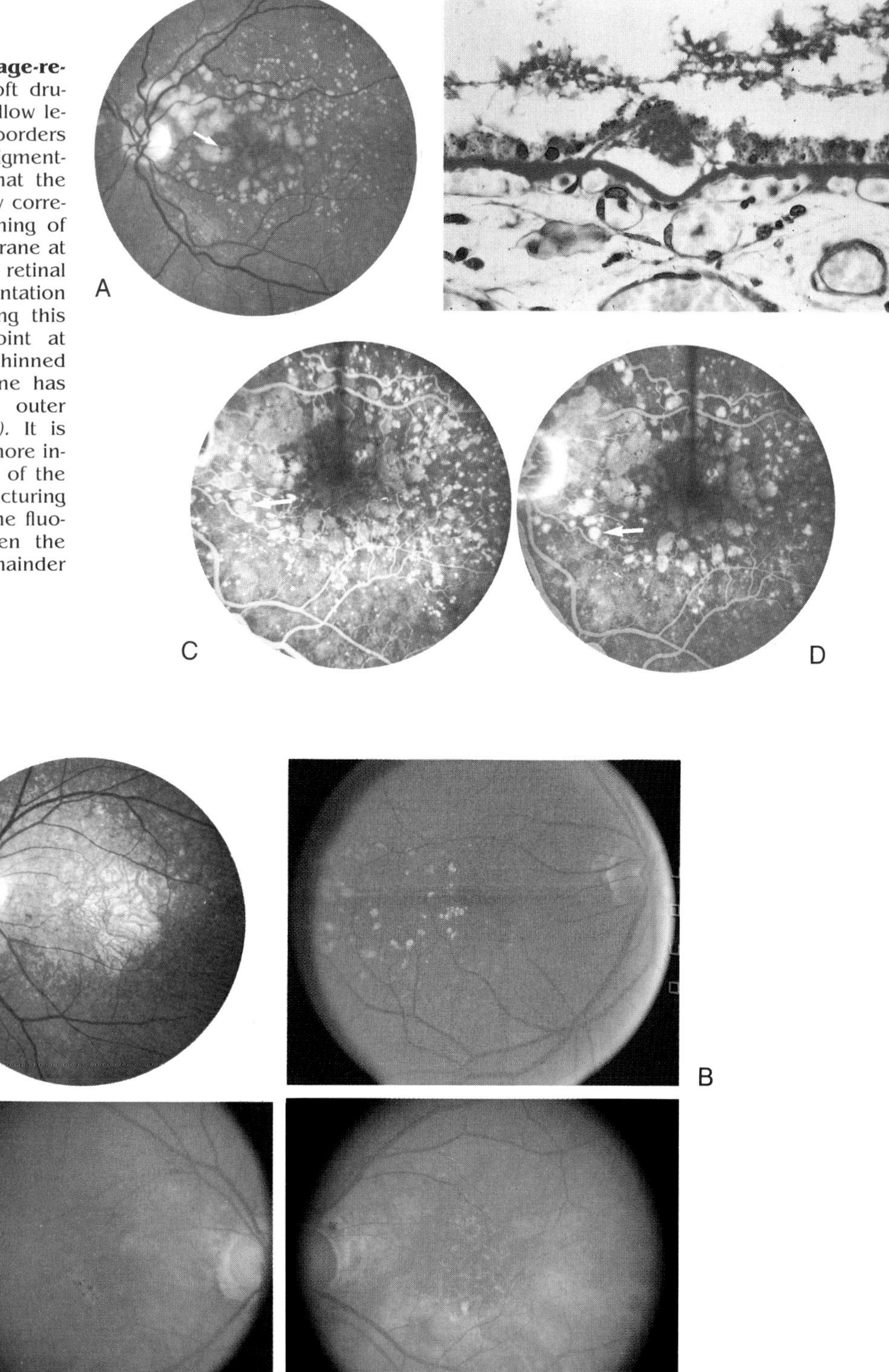

FIGURE 3–87 **Soft drusen in age-related macular degeneration.** Soft drusen are seen clinically as large yellow lesions with amorphous, ill-defined borders *(arrow)* at the level of the retinal pigment-epithelium *(A)*. It is suspected that the soft drusen noted clinically usually correspond to areas of diffuse thickening of the inner aspect of Bruch's membrane at the point at which focal areas of retinal pigment epithelium hypopigmentation have developed in areas overlying this diffuse thickening or at the point at which fracturing of the diffusely thinned inner aspect of Bruch's membrane has separated from the remaining outer aspect of Bruch's membrane *(B)*. It is suspected that drusen may stain more intensely *(arrow)* in the late phases of the angiogram (*C* and *D*) when this fracturing is present, presumably because the fluorescein molecules collect between the detached inner aspect and the remainder of Bruch's membrane.

FIGURE 3–88 **Geographic atrophy in age-related macular degeneration.** Abnormalities of the retinal pigment epithelium secondary to age-related macular degeneration. *A,* An area of geographic atrophy, with well-demarcated loss of pigmentation of the retinal pigment epithelium and overlying thinning of the neurosensory retina with more apparent underlying choroidal vasculature. *B,* Calcified drusen correspond histologically to dystrophic calcification at the level of the outer retina. *C,* Focal hyperpigmentation or pigment clumps correspond to clumps of pigment at the level of the retinal pigment epithelium or within the outer aspects of the sensory retina. *D,* Nongeographic atrophy refers to a finding of tiny mottled areas of hypopigmentation and hyperpigmentation that may show some thinning of the overlying sensory retina.

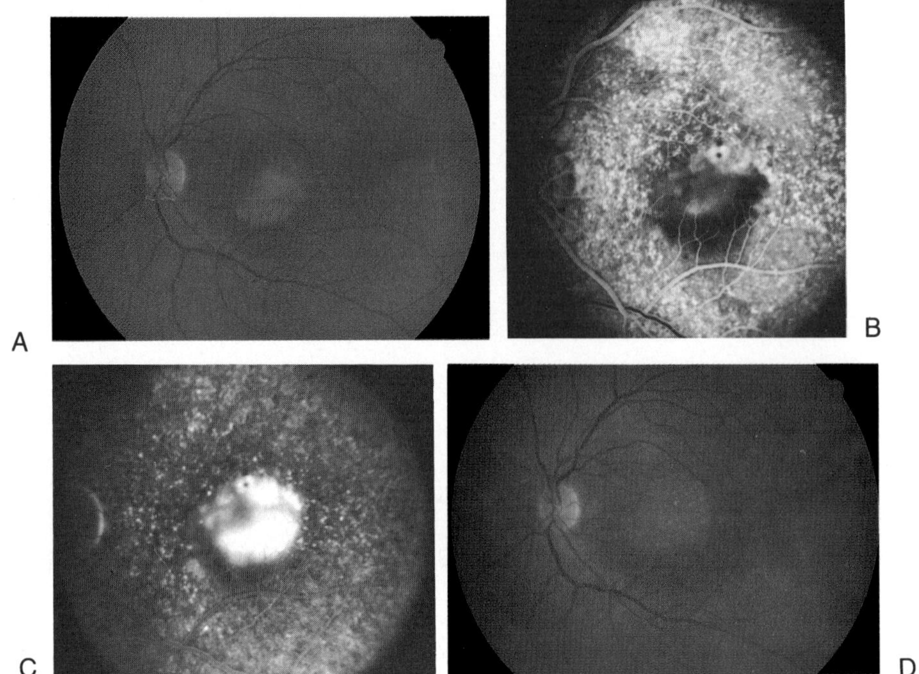

FIGURE 3–89 **Basal laminar or cuticular drusen.** *A,* Color photography showing innumerable small, uniformly sized, discretely round, and slightly raised yellow subretinal lesions and dull yellow material in the central macula referred to as *pseudovitelliform detachment. B,* The angiogram helps to highlight basal laminar drusen. In addition, hypofluorescence, from the associated pseudovitelliform lesion, blocks the underlying fluorescence of the choriocapillaris. *C,* Progressive staining of the pseudovitelliform material becomes apparent in the middle and late transit phases of the angiogram. *D,* With time, the pseudovitelliform detachment can clear spontaneously. Geographic atrophy sometimes develops with clearing.

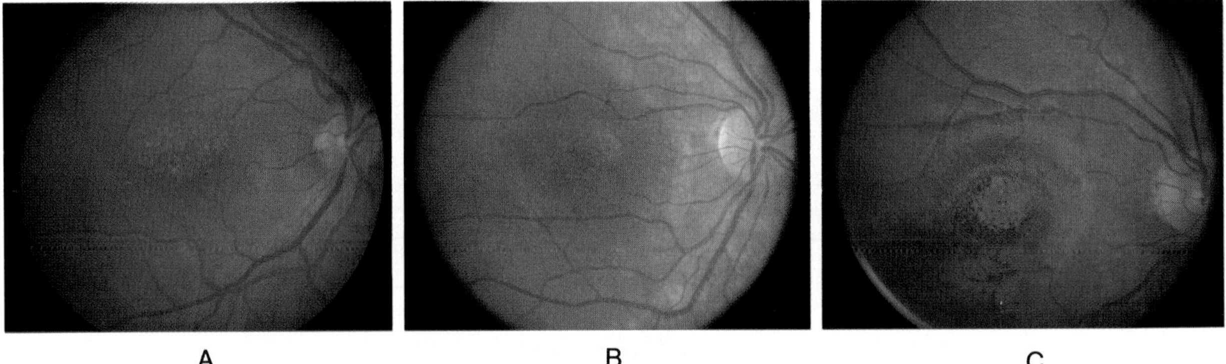

FIGURE 3–90 **Dominant drusen.** *A,* A woman in her 20s demonstrates typical large drusen, some of which have discrete boundaries. Similar findings are noted in her 9-year-old son *(B)* and her 6-year-old son *(C).*

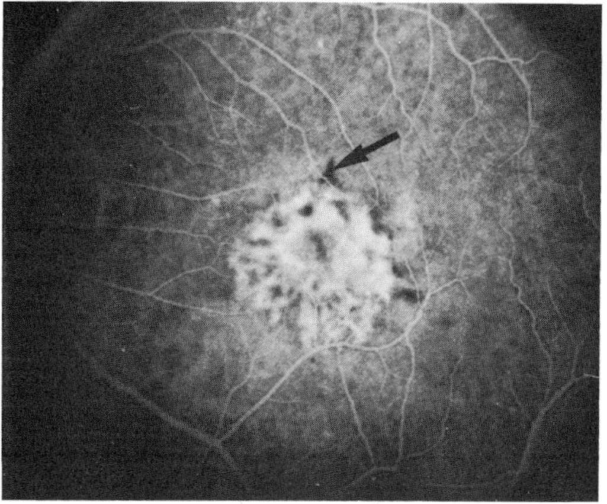

FIGURE 3–91 **Age-related macular degeneration: subfoveal choriodal neovascularization (CNV).** Fluorescein angiogram depicting subfoveal CNV with contiguous blood *(arrow).* The boundaries are well demarcated; the entire lesion is less than 3.5 disc areas: The lesion would meet the criteria for the Macular Photocoagulation Study. (From Macular Photocoagulation Study Group: Laser photocoagulation of subfoveal neovascular lesions in age-related macular degeneration. Results of a randomized clinical trial. Arch Ophthalmol 109:1220–1231, 1991. Copyright 1991, American Medical Association.)

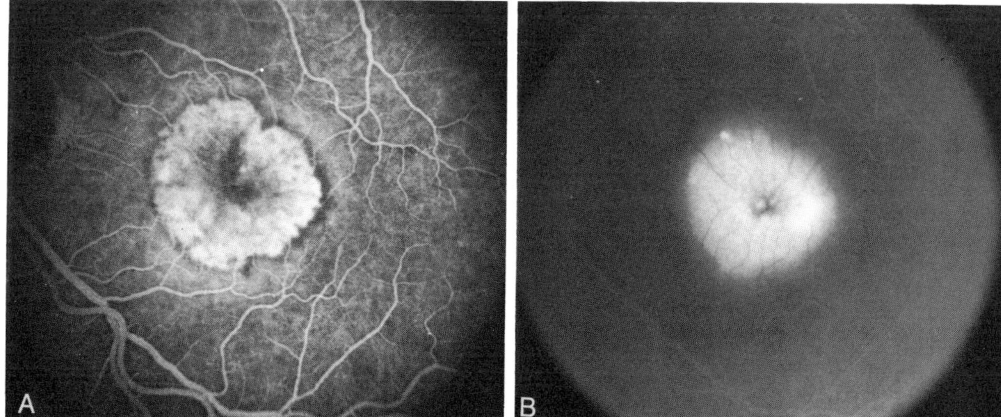

FIGURE 3–92 **Age-related macular degeneration: classic CNV.** *A,* Early phase of fluorescein angiogram of classic CNV in which boundaries of the neovascular lesion are well demarcated. *B,* Late phase of angiogram showing pooling of dye in subsensory retinal space, obscuring the boundaries of CNV demarcated in an earlier phase of the angiogram. (*A* and *B,* From Macular Photocoagulation Study Group: Subfoveal neovascular lesions in age-related macular degeneration. Guidelines for evaluation and treatment in the Macular Photocoagulation Study. Arch Ophthalmol 109:1242–1257, 1991. Copyright 1991, American Medical Association.)

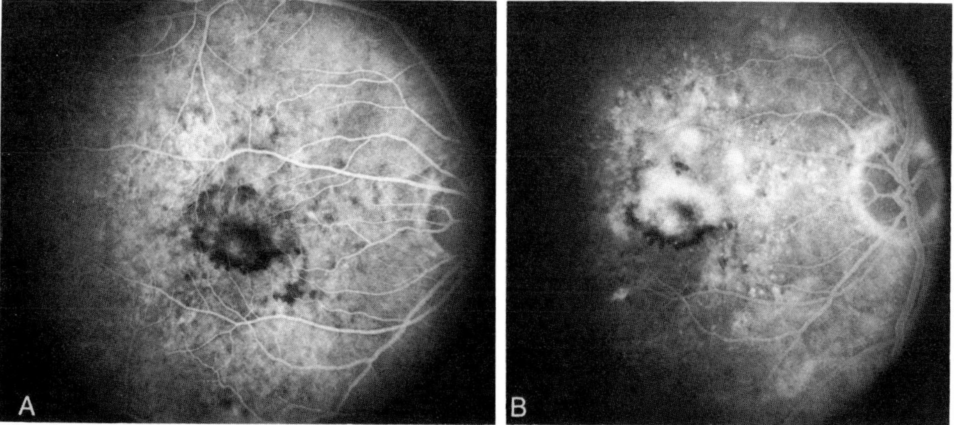

FIGURE 3–93 **Age-related macular degeneration: occult CNV with late leakage of undetermined source.** *A,* Early-phase angiogram. *B,* Middle phase of angiogram shows pinpoints of speckled hyperfluorescence and larger areas of hyperfluorescence with accumulation of fluorescein leakage in the overlying subsensory retinal space. The source of the leakage cannot be discerned from earlier phases of the angiogram. This poorly demarcated lesion does not meet Macular Photocoagulation Study eligibility criteria for laser photocoagulation. (*A* and *B,* From Macular Photocoagulation Study Group: Subfoveal neovascular lesions in age-related macular degeneration. Guidelines for evaluation and treatment in the Macular Photocoagulation Study. Arch Ophthalmol 109:1242–1257, 1991. Copyright 1991, American Medical Association.)

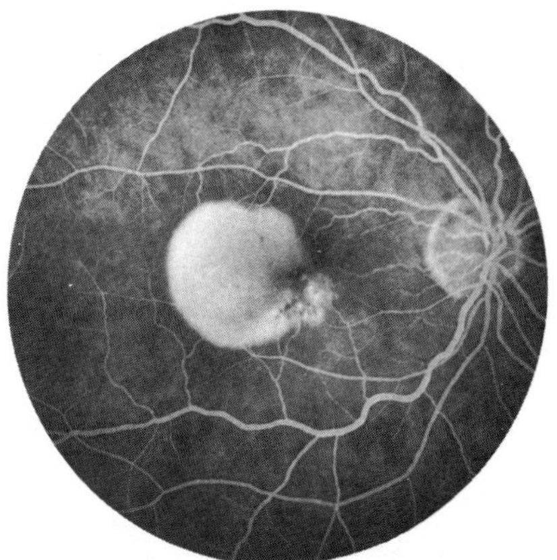

FIGURE 3–94 **Age-related macular degeneration: serous detachment of the retinal pigment epithelium owing to CNV.** Early-phase fluorescein angiogram of a serous detachment of the retinal pigment epithelium. A uniform elevation of the retinal pigment epithelium, with uniform pooling of fluorescein dye, and smooth contour to the surface of the elevated retinal pigment epithelium, with well-demarcated borders in the early phase of the angiogram, are noted. Persistent bright hyperfluorescence continued within these well-demarcated boundaries in the late phase of the angiogram (not shown).

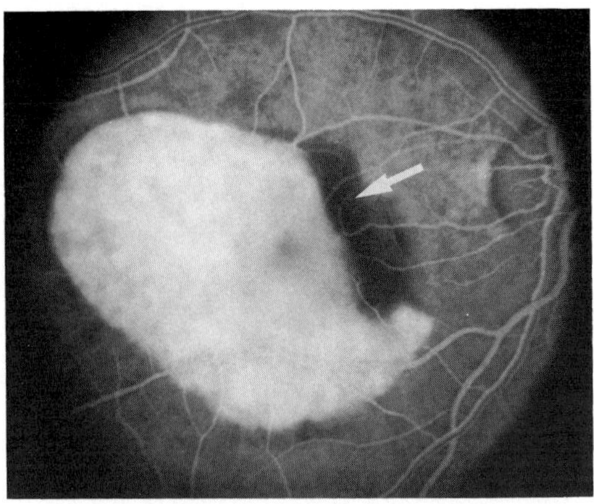

FIGURE 3–95 **Age-related macular degeneration: retinal pigment epithelial tear caused by CNV.** Retinal pigment epithelial tear seen on early-transit phase of fluorescein angiogram demonstrating extremely sharp, well-demarcated hyperfluorescence. Continued intense staining was seen in the late phase of the angiogram with no leakage. Early blocked fluorescence *(arrow)* presumably corresponds to the redundant, folded, torn pigment epithelium. (From Bressler NM, Finkelstein D, Sunness JS, et al: Retinal pigment epithelial tears through the fovea with preservation of good visual acuity. Arch Ophthalmol 108:1694–1697, 1990. Copyright 1990, American Medical Association.)

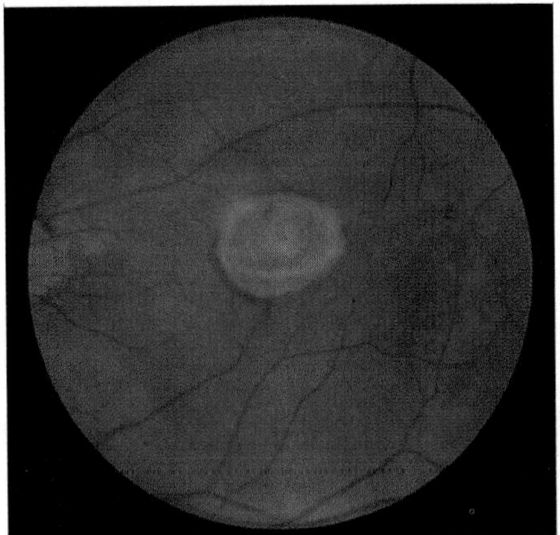

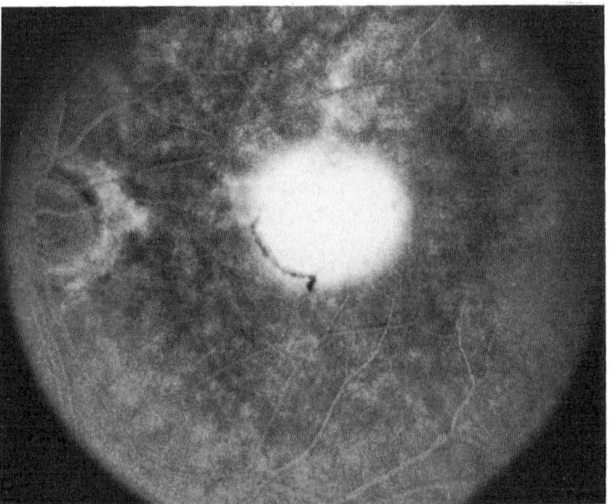

B

FIGURE 3–96 **Age-related macular degeneration: disciform scarring caused by CNV.** *A,* Subretinal and sub–retinal pigment epithelial fibrosis as well as subretinal fluid and hemorrhage is seen on color photograph. The latter presumably are indicative of persistent vascular tissue within the fibrosis. *B,* Fluorescein angiography of CNV scarring demonstrates that some blocked fluorescence corresponds to the fibrotic tissue. There is leakage toward the periphery of the lesion, presumably from CNV associated with scarring. (*A* and *B,* From Macular Photocoagulation Study Group: Subfoveal neovascular lesions in age-related macular degeneration. Guidelines for evaluation and treatment in the Macular Photocoagulation Study. Arch Ophthalmol 109:1242–1257, 1991. Copyright 1991, American Medical Association.)

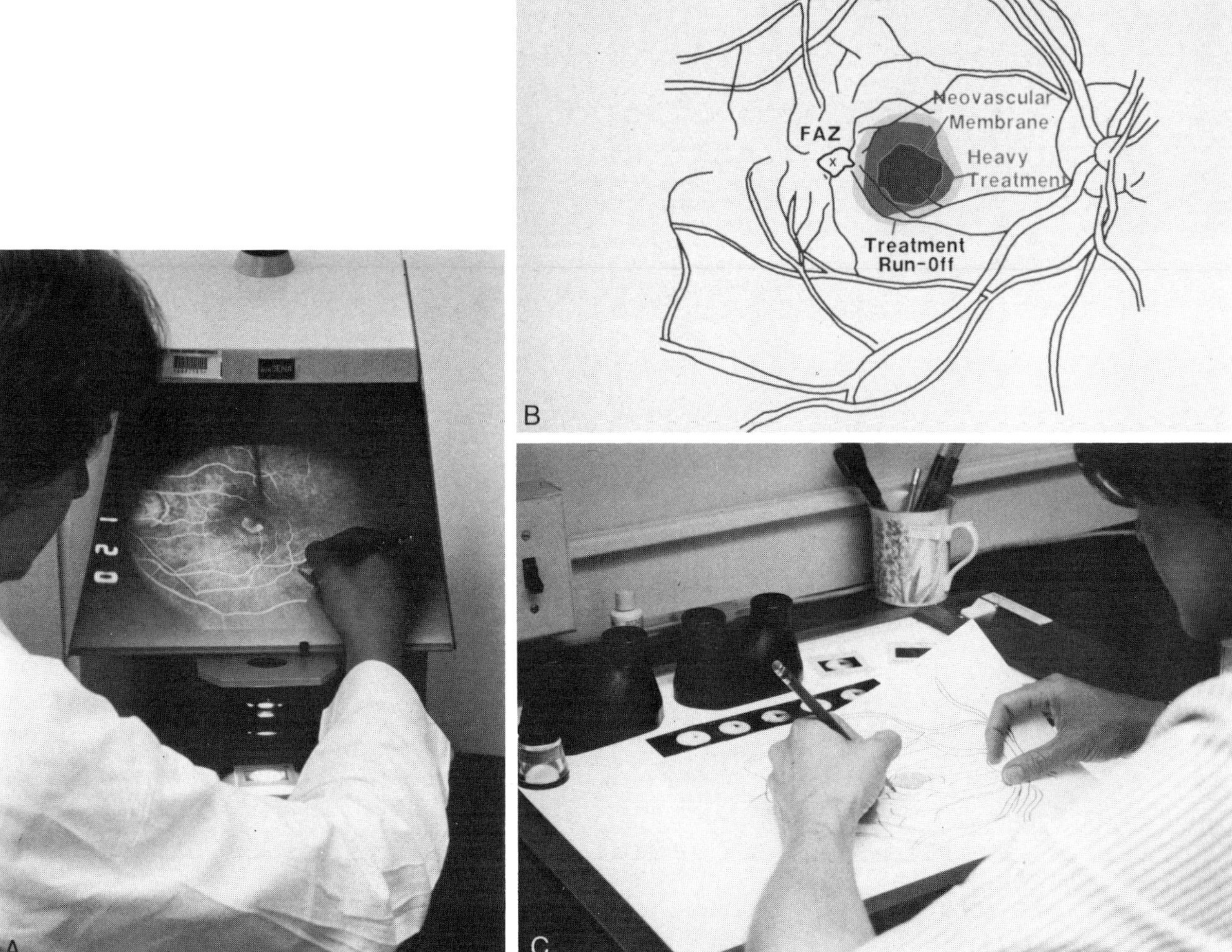

FIGURE 3–97 **Age-related macular degeneration: evaluation and treatment of CNV.** Angiogram is projected onto an apparatus (such as microfilm reader or slide viewer) such that the CNV and key landmarks around the CNV, such as subretinal blood, retinal vessels, and foveal center, can be drawn *(A)*. *FAZ* indicates foveal avascular zone and *x* indicates foveal center *(B)*. A posttreatment photograph is then projected, and the area of heavy treatment and the same landmark vessels can be outlined on a separate sheet of paper *(C)*. Evaluation of photocoagulation treatment can be determined by placing the treatment drawing *(C)* under the pretreatment drawing *(A)* on a light box. The area of heavy treatment can then be traced onto the pretreatment drawing to determine whether the treatment has covered the CNV entirely. (*A–C*, From Bressler NM, Bressler SB, Fine SL: Age-related macular degeneration. Surv Ophthalmol 32:375–413, 1988.)

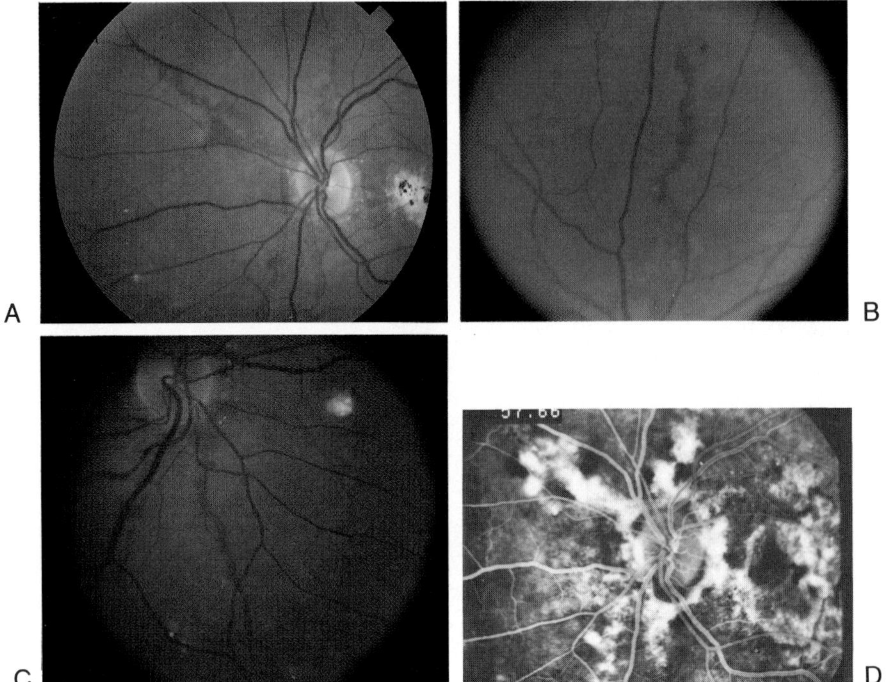

FIGURE 3–98 **Angioid streaks.** Angioid streaks are defects in the thickened, calcified elastic layer of Bruch's membrane often associated with secondary changes in the choriocapillaris, retinal pigment epithelium, and photoreceptors. *A–C,* Clinically, angioid streaks are irregular, curvilinear, reddish brown streaks that radiate out from the peripapillary area and lie beneath the retina but above the choroidal vasculature. *D,* Fluorescein angiography reveals the typical early hyperfluorescence and late staining of the streaks.

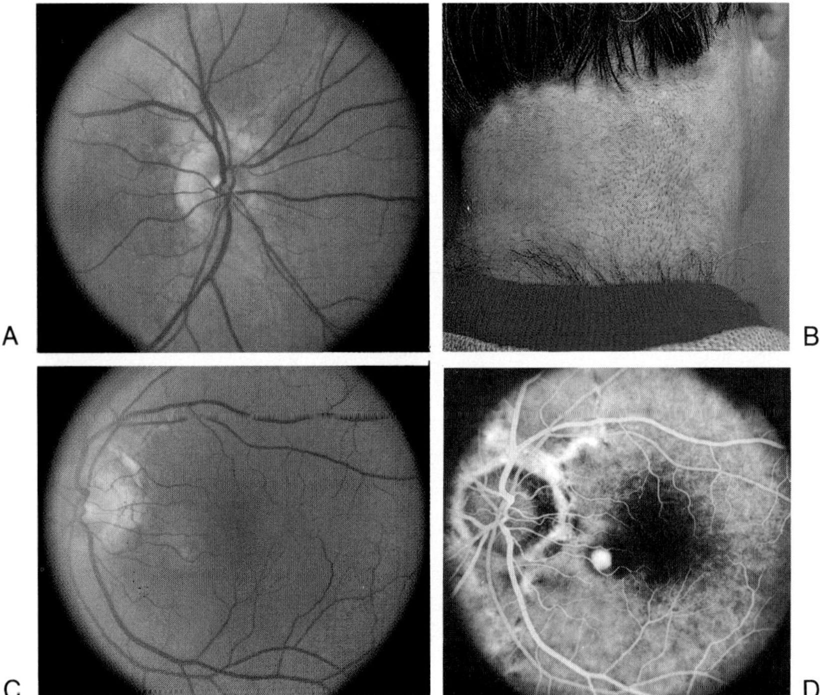

FIGURE 3–99 **Angioid streaks in pseudoxanthoma elasticum.** This patient with angioid streaks *(A)* has the characteristic "plucked-chicken" skin lesions *(B)* of pseudoxanthoma elasticum. The patient developed CNV (*C* and *D*), which is associated with a defect in the thickened, calcified elastic layer of Bruch's membrane.

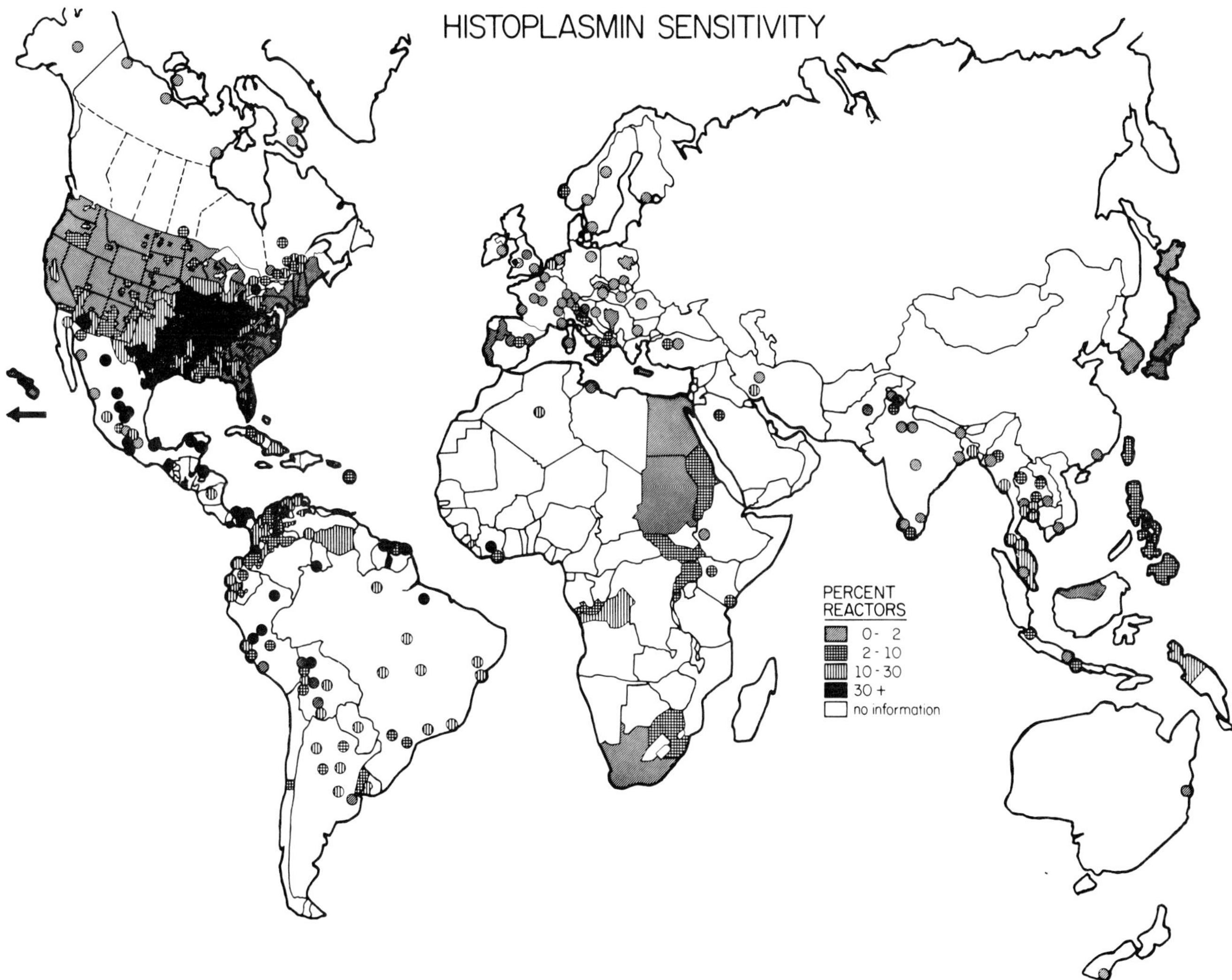

FIGURE 3–100 **Geographic localization of ocular histoplasmosis syndrome (OHS).** This world map demonstrates areas where histoplasmosis infection is endemic. (From Ellis FD, Schlaegel TF: The geographic localization of presumed histoplasmic choroiditis. Am J Ophthalmol 75:953–956, 1973. Published with permission from the American Journal of Ophthalmology. Copyright by The Ophthalmic Publishing Company.)

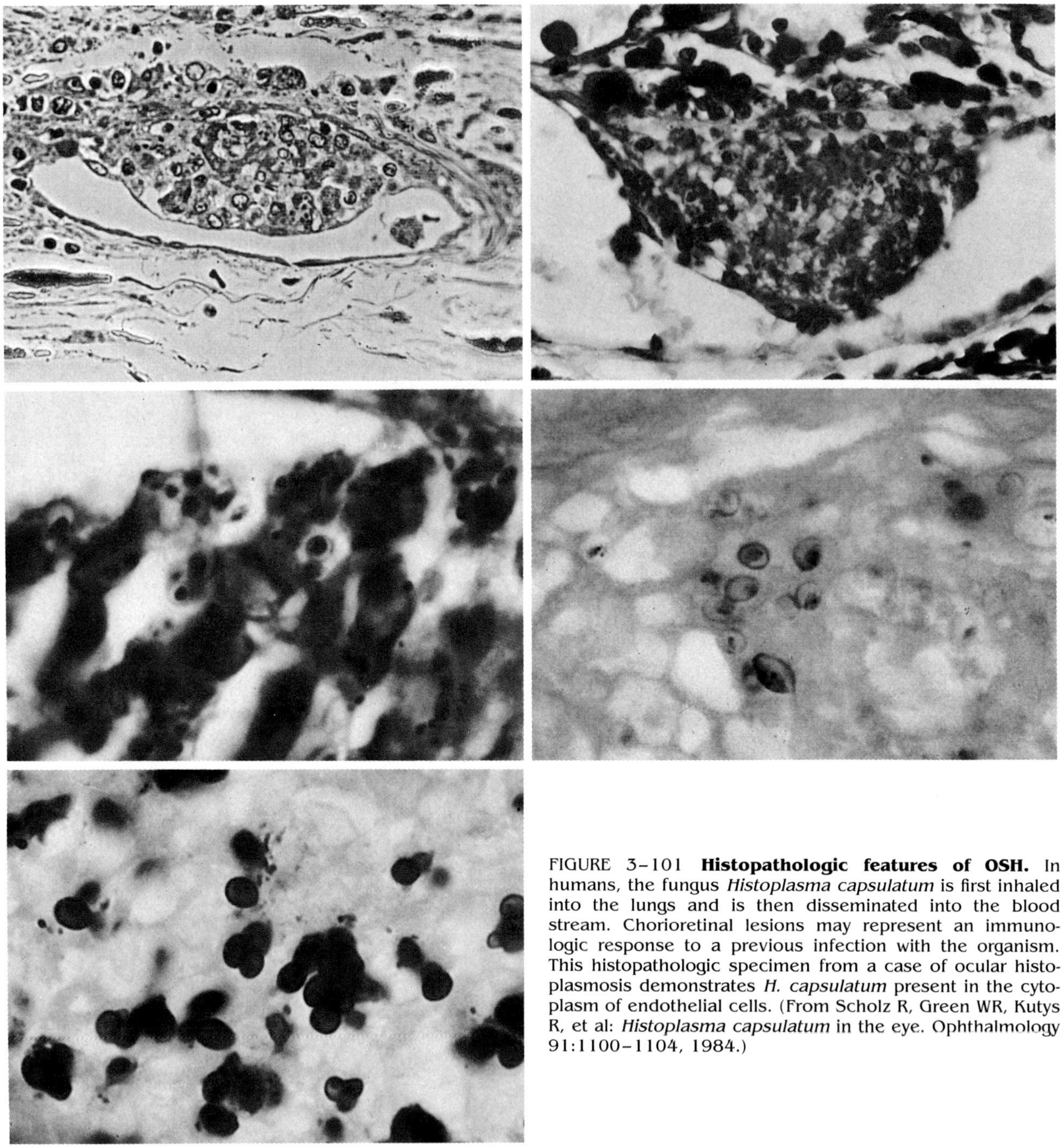

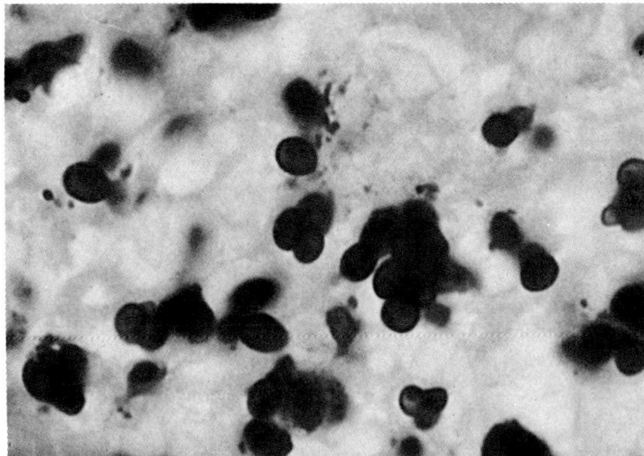

FIGURE 3–101 **Histopathologic features of OSH.** In humans, the fungus *Histoplasma capsulatum* is first inhaled into the lungs and is then disseminated into the blood stream. Chorioretinal lesions may represent an immunologic response to a previous infection with the organism. This histopathologic specimen from a case of ocular histoplasmosis demonstrates *H. capsulatum* present in the cytoplasm of endothelial cells. (From Scholz R, Green WR, Kutys R, et al: *Histoplasma capsulatum* in the eye. Ophthalmology 91:1100–1104, 1984.)

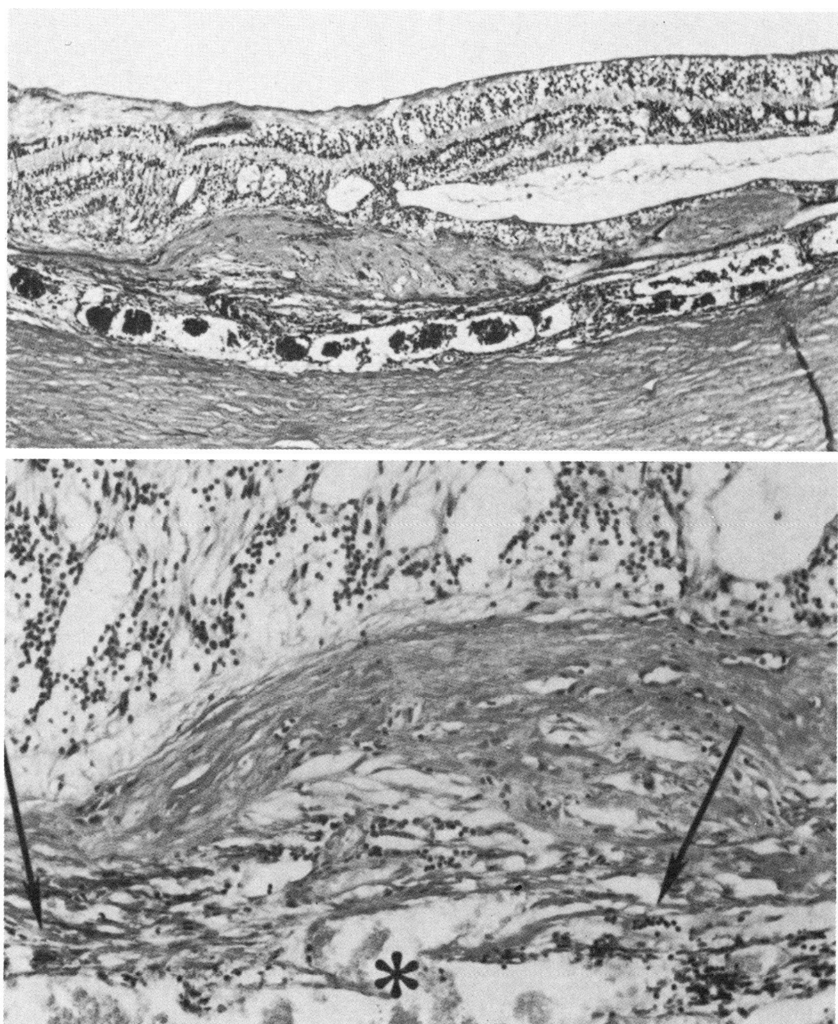

FIGURE 3–102 **Histopathologic features of OHS.** Histopathologic specimen from a case of ocular histoplasmosis. Discontinuities in Bruch's membrane *(between arrows in bottom figure)* allow choroidal blood vessels *(asterisk)* to grow into the subretinal or subretinal pigment epithelial space. (From Meredith TA, Green WR, Key SN, et al: Ocular histoplasmosis: Clinicopathologic correlation of 3 cases. Surv Ophthalmol 22:189, 1977.)

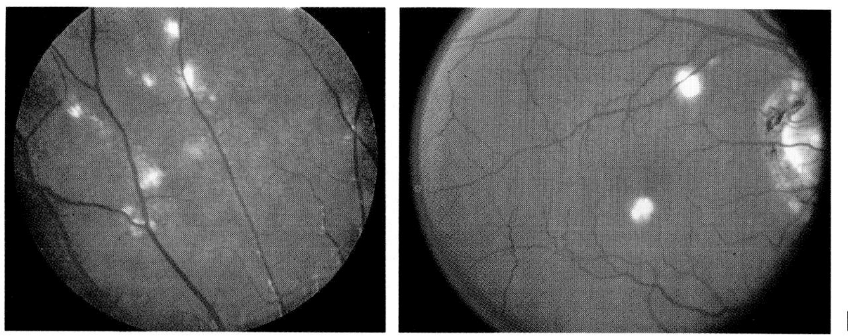

FIGURE 3–103 **Ophthalmoscopic features of OHS.** *A,* Fundus photographs of peripheral, punched-out lesions typical of the OHS. *B,* Fundus photograph of atrophic macular lesions and juxtapapillary chorioretinal atrophy.

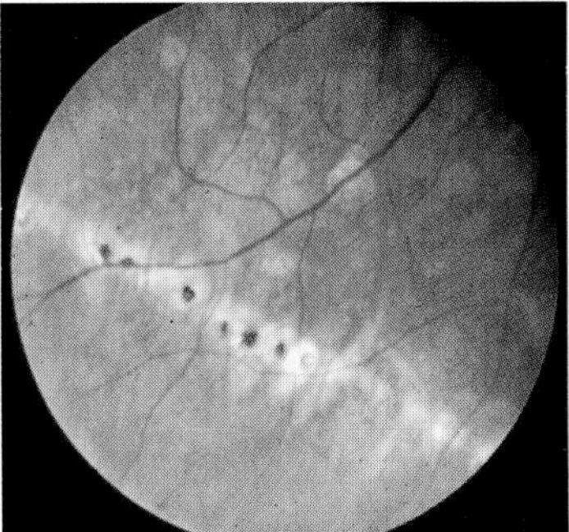

FIGURE 3–104 **Ophthalmoscopic features of OHS.** Fundus photograph shows peripheral linear streak of histoplasmosis spots. These are equatorial, parallel to the ora, and approximately 3 clock hours in length.

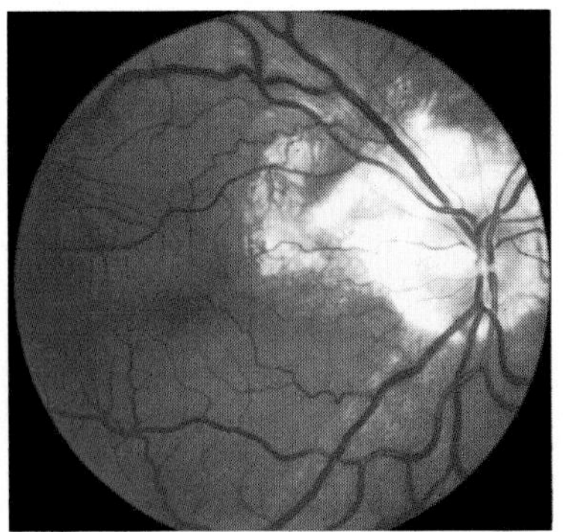

FIGURE 3–105 **Ophthalmoscopic features of OHS.** Juxtapapillary changes in OHS are probably due to asymptomatic juxtapapillary choroiditis. This figure depicts juxtapapillary retinal pigment epithelial hypertrophy and atrophy, which is present in the vast majority of patients with OHS.

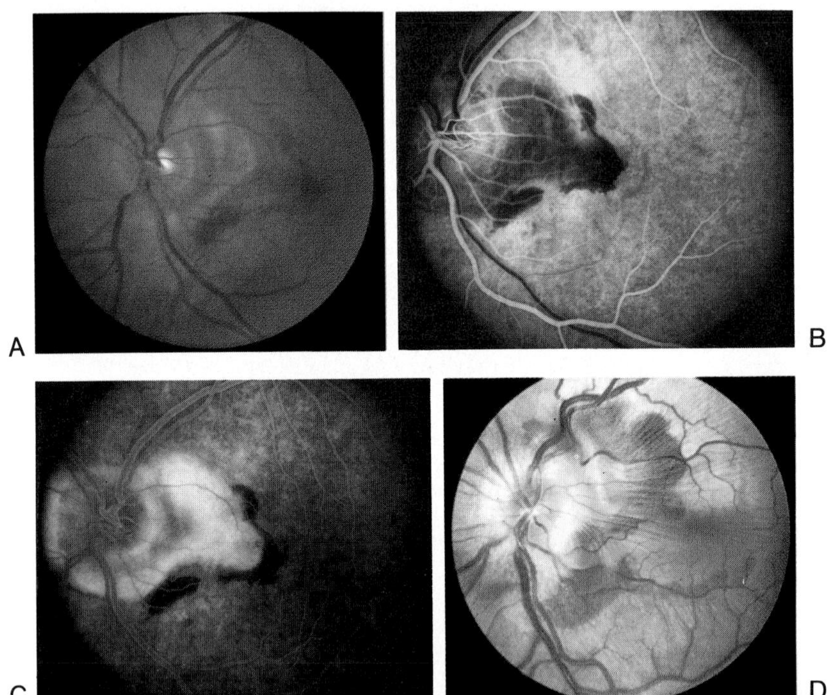

FIGURE 3–106 **CNV in OHS.** In this eye, juxtapapillary changes led to the development of CNV. *A,* The fundus photograph shows evidence of gray subretinal lesions along with subretinal blood, both of which are signs of CNV. *B,* An early frame of the fluorescein angiogram shows early hyperfluorescence. *C,* A later frame shows massive leakage from the new vessel membrane. *D,* In another patient, a juxtapapillary choroidal neovascular membrane causes extensive retinal striae.

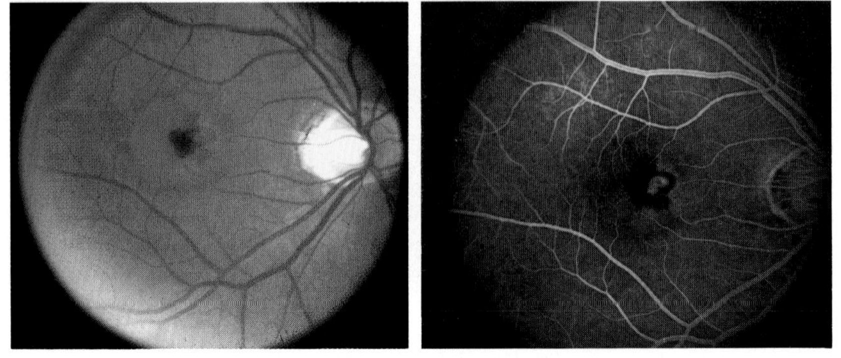

FIGURE 3–107 **CNV in OHS.** *A,* Fundus photograph of CNV, with a gray membrane, subretinal hemorrhage, subretinal fluid, and pigment ring. *B,* An early frame of a fluorescein angiogram with early hyperfluorescence demonstrates a juxtafoveal CNV.

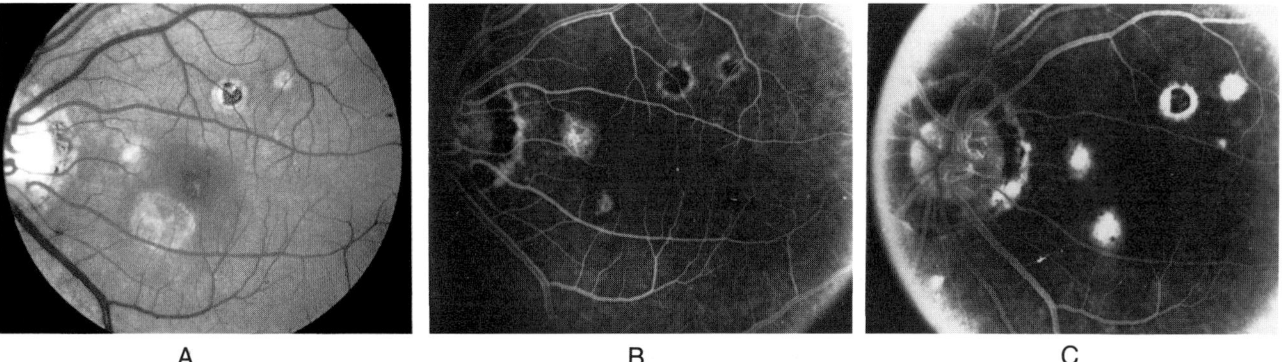

FIGURE 3-108 **CNV in OHS.** *A,* Fundus photograph of CNV (inferior to the fovea) and histoplasmosis spots (superior to the fovea). *B* and *C,* Fluorescein angiograms of histoplasmosis spots. *B* shows early hypofluorescence, and *C* shows late staining. Note how the new vessel membrane leaks fluorescein dye and develops fuzzy margins late in the study. The histoplasmosis spots show staining of the sclera but stay sharply demarcated.

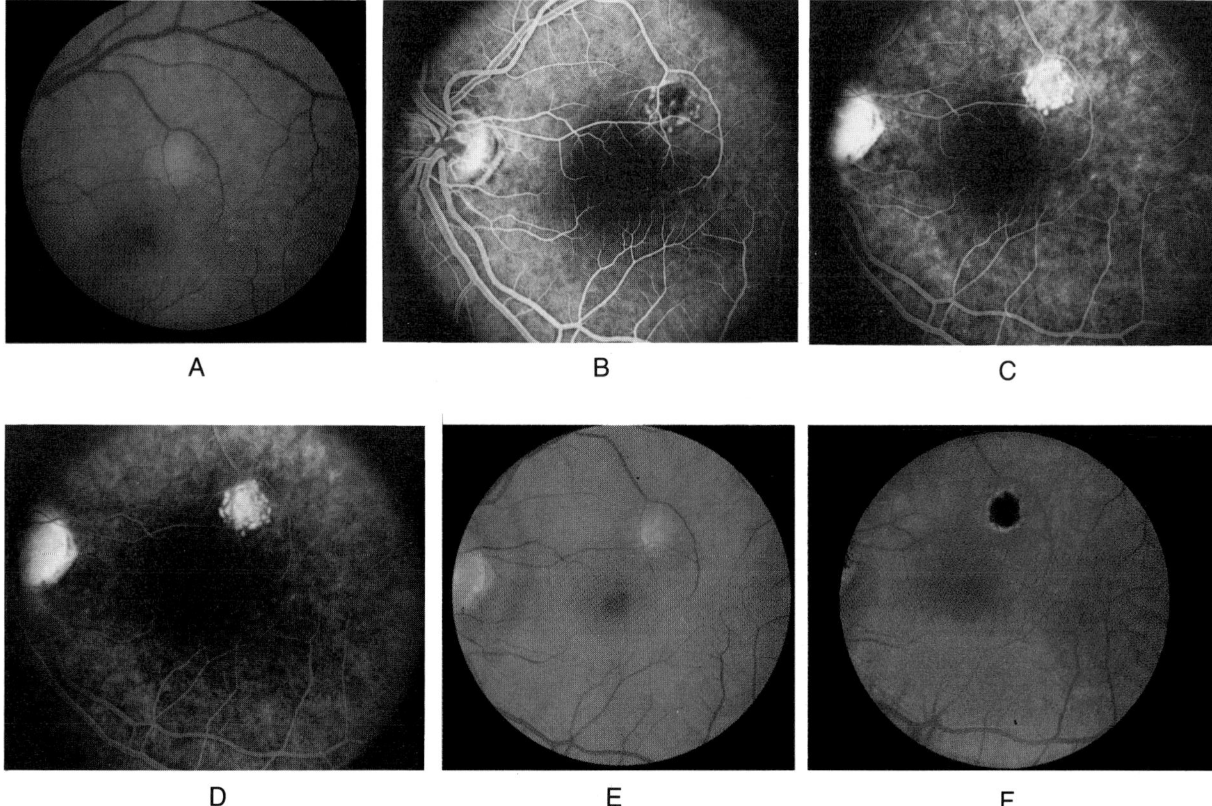

FIGURE 3-109 **Disseminated histoplasmic choroiditis.** Disseminated histoplasmic choroiditis usually occurs in immunocompromised patients. *A,* Histoplasmic choroiditis causes yellow choroidal infiltrates with a surrounding pigment ring. Fluorescein angiography demonstrates early blocked fluorescence *(B)* and intermediate *(C)* and late *(D)* staining of these lesions. The lesions can become atrophic with time *(E)* and ultimately may develop secondary reactive hyperplasia of the pigment epithelium *(F).* The foci of choroiditis may develop into CNV, with serous retinal detachment, hemorrhage, and retinal striae.

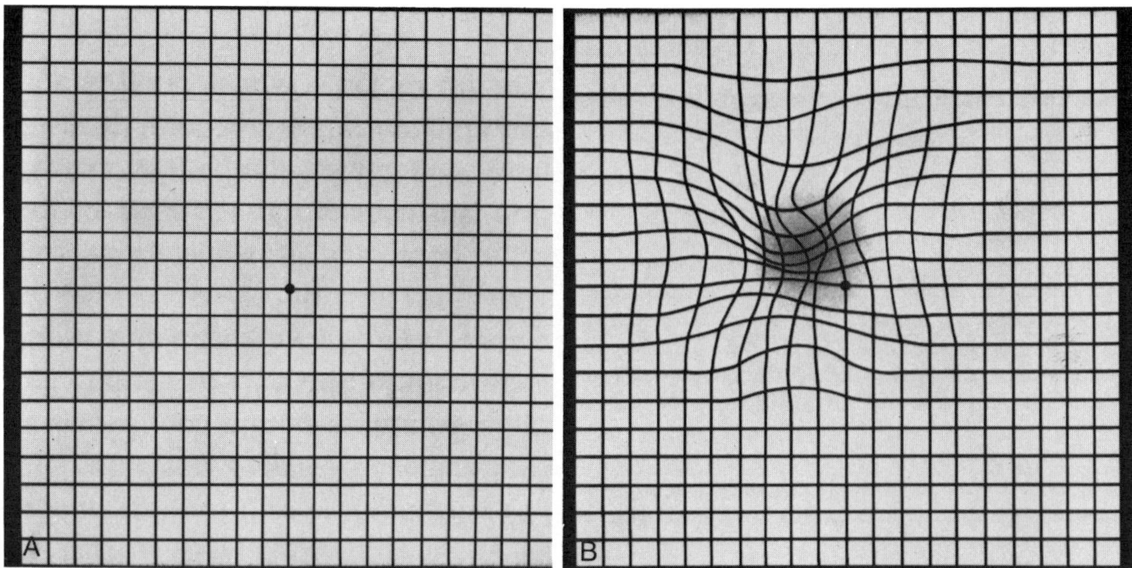

FIGURE 3–110 **Patient self-assessment in ocular histoplasmosis.** *A,* An Amsler grid is used for diagnosis of CNV. This grid can be used at home by patients at risk for developing new vessel membranes. *B,* An artist's demonstration of metamorphopsia and relative scotoma seen by a patient with new CNV. The ocular histoplasmosis section of the Macular Photocoagulation Study identified subgroups of patients with CNV who derive a clear benefit from laser photocoagulation.

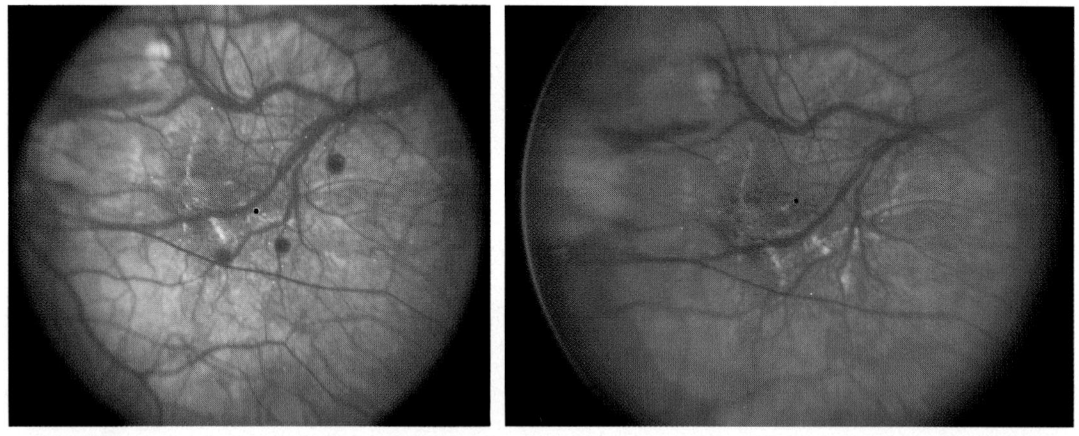

FIGURE 3–111 **Pathologic myopia.** The pathogenesis of pathologic myopia is not well understood. The disease is progressive, and vision may be compromised by retinal detachment, posterior staphyloma, retinal degeneration, or CNV. *A,* This patient demonstrates pathologic myopia with characteristic lacquer cracks reflecting breaks in Bruch's membrane and associated asymptomatic macular hemorrhages. *B,* Resolution of hemorrhages and extension of lacquer cracks in the same eye 15 months later demonstrates the progressive nature of this disease.

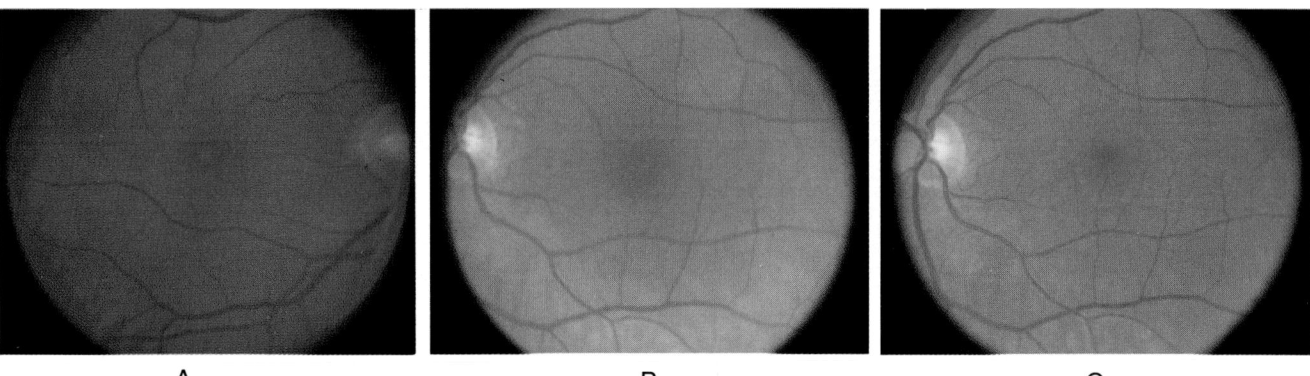

FIGURE 3-112 **Stage 1 idiopathic macular hole.** Premacular hole lesions or stage 1 lesions appear as either a yellow spot *(A)* or a yellow ring *(B)* lesion. This is thought to be due to vitreous traction causing a foveal detachment, with improved visibility of the underlying xanthophyll pigment. *B,* This patient initially presented with a visual acuity of 20/80 and a stage 1B lesion. *C,* Sixteen months later, a flat, reddish lesion was present; the yellow ring had disappeared; and the visual acuity had improved to 20/30. (*A–C,* From Guyer DR, de Bustros S, Diener-West M, Fine SL: The natural history of idiopathic macular holes and cysts. Arch Ophthalmol 110:1264–1268, 1992. Copyright 1992, American Medical Association.)

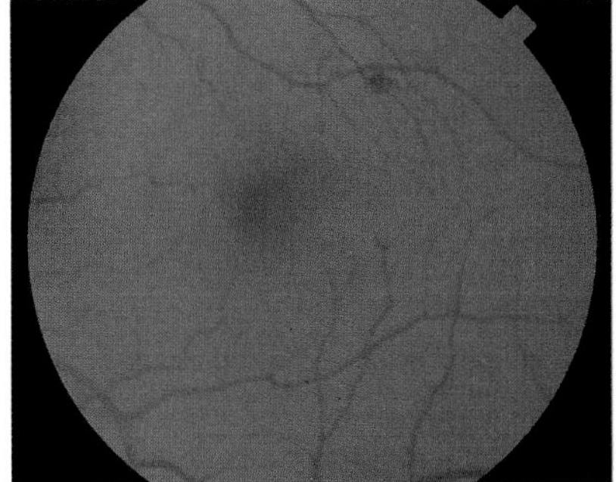

FIGURE 3-113 **Stage 2 idiopathic macular hole.** A stage 2 lesion is an eccentric full-thickness retinal break, which often has minimal accumulation of subretinal fluid. (Courtesy of Donald J. D'Amico, M.D.)

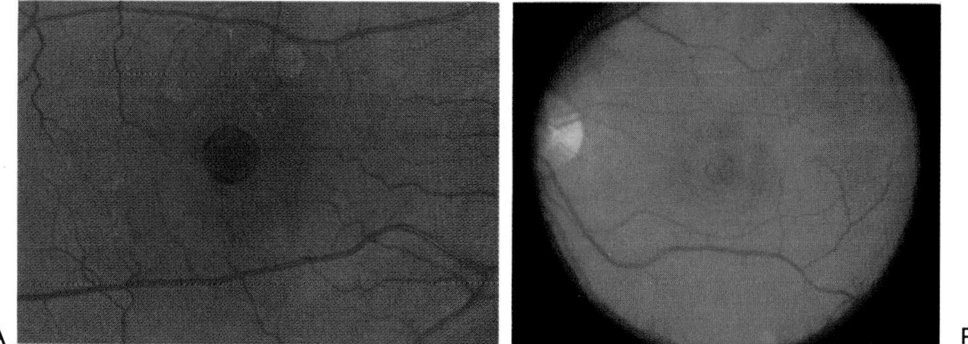

FIGURE 3-114 **Stage 3 idiopathic macular hole.** *A,* A stage 3 lesion is a full-thickness macular hole, which consists of a central area devoid of neurosensory retinal tissue with a surrounding halo of subretinal fluid and cystoid macular edema. *B,* Yellow lesions at the level of the retinal pigment epithelium are often observed in patients with full-thickness macular holes.

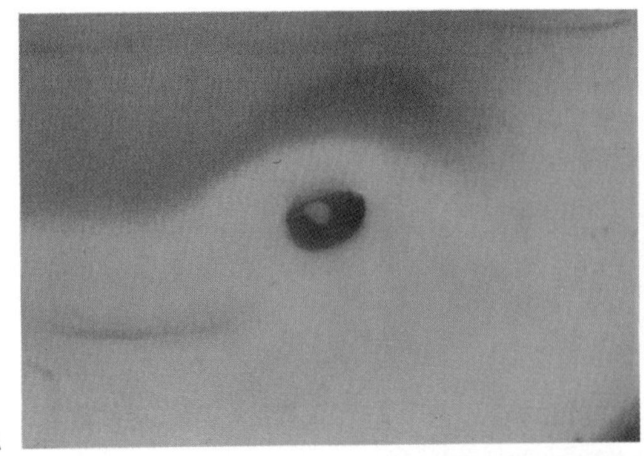

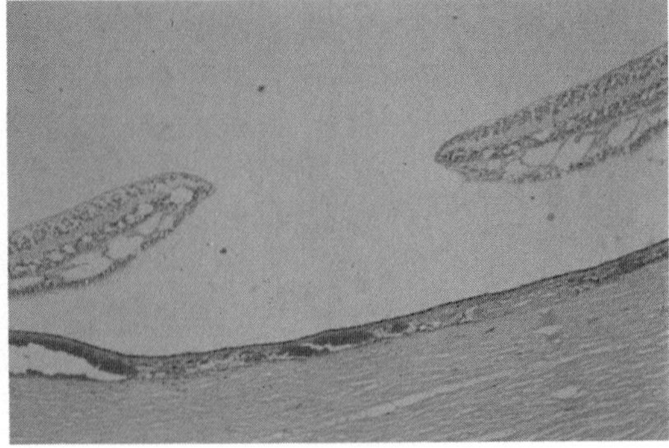

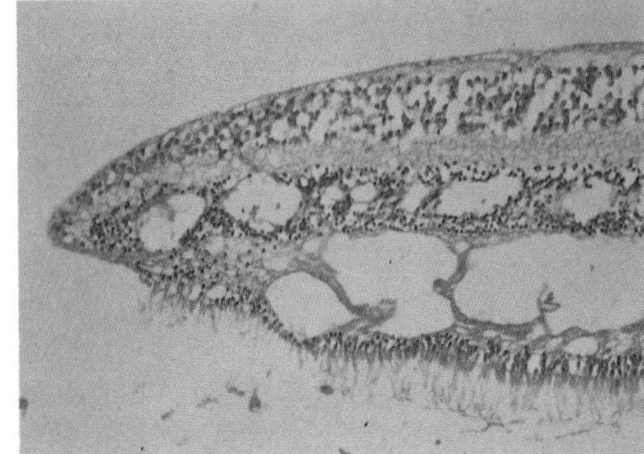

FIGURE 3–115 **Pathology of idiopathic macular hole.** *A,* Gross examination of this autopsy eye reveals a full-thickness macular hole with an overlying operculum. *B,* Histopathologic examination of this macular hole demonstrates the rounded edges of retina at the edges of the hole. Underlying subretinal fluid and cystoid macular edema are present. *C,* Higher magnification of one edge of the macular hole shows marked cystoid macular edema and photoreceptor atrophy. (*A–C,* From Guyer DR, Green WR, deBustros S, Fine SL: Histopathologic features of idiopathic macular holes and cysts. Ophthalmology 97:1045–1051, 1990.)

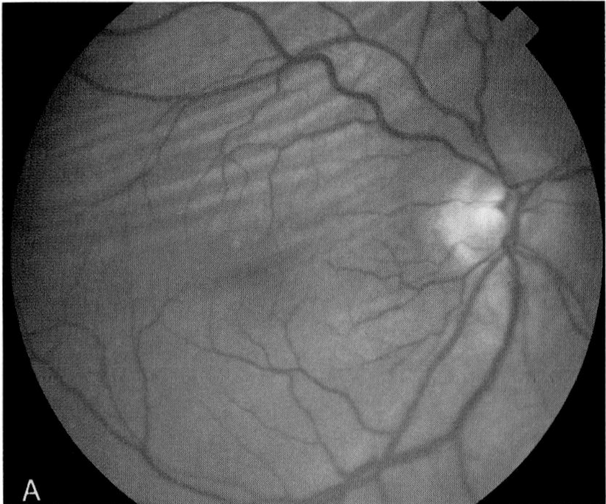

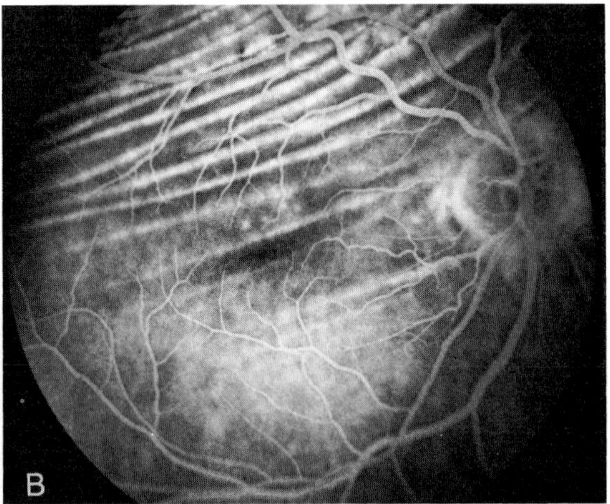

FIGURE 3–116 **Fundus findings of choroidal folds.** *A,* Fundus appearance of choroidal folds caused by an extraconal tumor located within the superior temporal quadrant of the orbit. Histopathologic specimens demonstrate undulations of the inner choroid, Bruch's membrane, and retinal pigment epithelium. *B,* On fluorescein angiography, the folds are much more dramatic, appearing as alternating light and dark streaks corresponding to the crests and troughs of the choroidal folds. The retinal pigment epithelium is thin on the crests causing greater fluorescein transmission compared with the compressed retinal pigment epithelium in the troughs. Note that the retinal vessels are not distorted by the underlying choroidal folds.

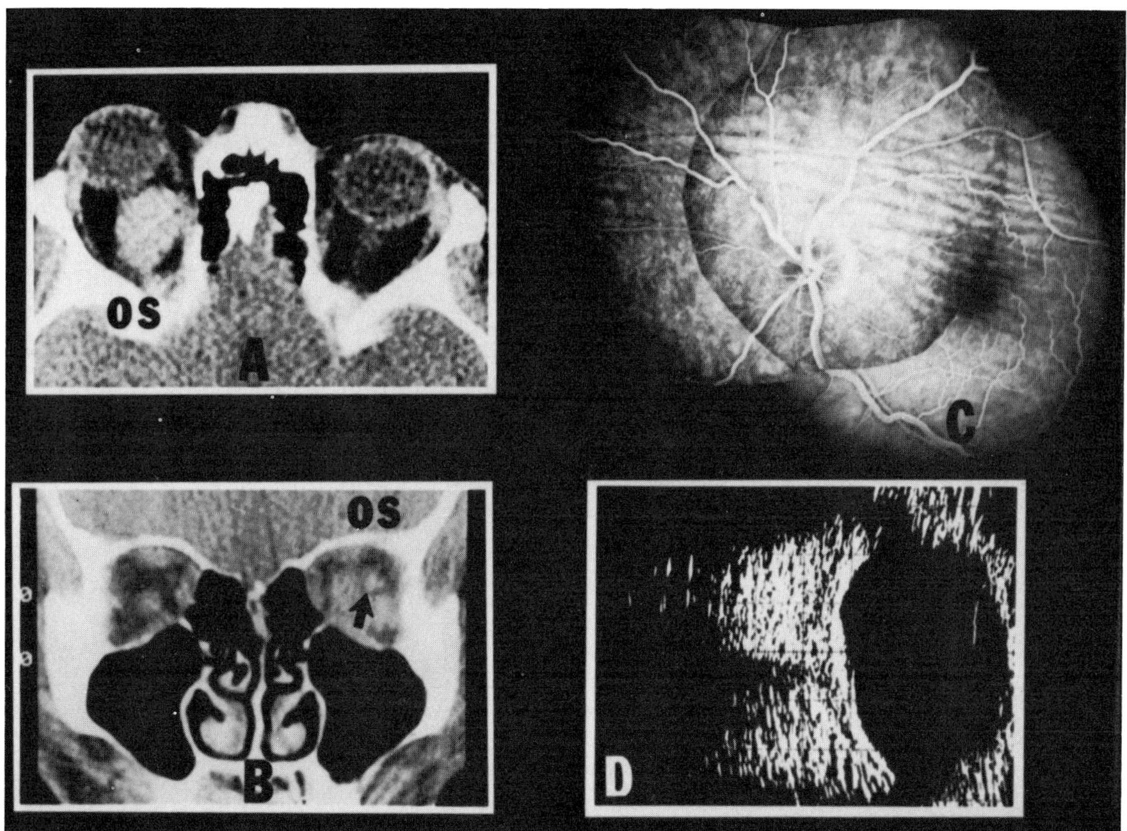

FIGURE 3-117 **Imaging studies of choroidal folds.** *A* and *B,* These computed tomograms show the superior displacement of the left globe and optic nerve owing to an intraconal tumor, in this case an orbital hemangioma. *C,* The associated choroidal folds are primarily located superior to the optic nerve, whereas some folds radiate from the disc and extend into the macula. *D,* A B-scan ultrasonogram demonstrates characteristic flattening of the posterior sclera. (From Friberg TR, Grove AS: Choroidal folds and refractive errors associated with orbital tumors. An analysis. Arch Ophthalmol 101:598–603, 1983. Copyright 1983, American Medical Association.)

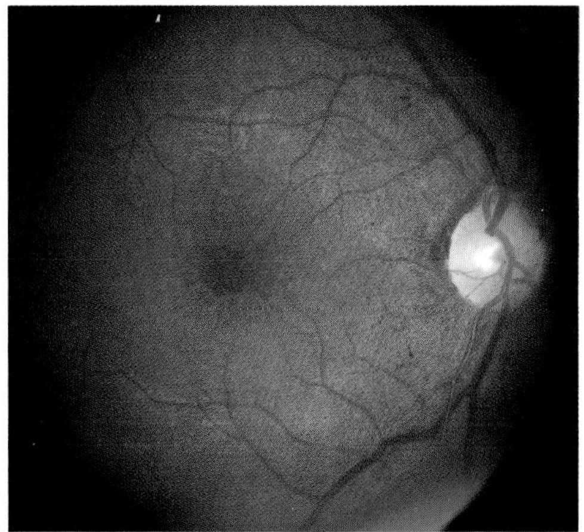

FIGURE 3-118 **Aphakic cystoid macular edema.** In this fundus photograph, note the fine lines outlining the cystoid spaces in the foveal area, including a central cystoid space. A few small intraretinal hemorrhages are seen just inferior to the first branch of the major superotemporal vein near the bifurcation.

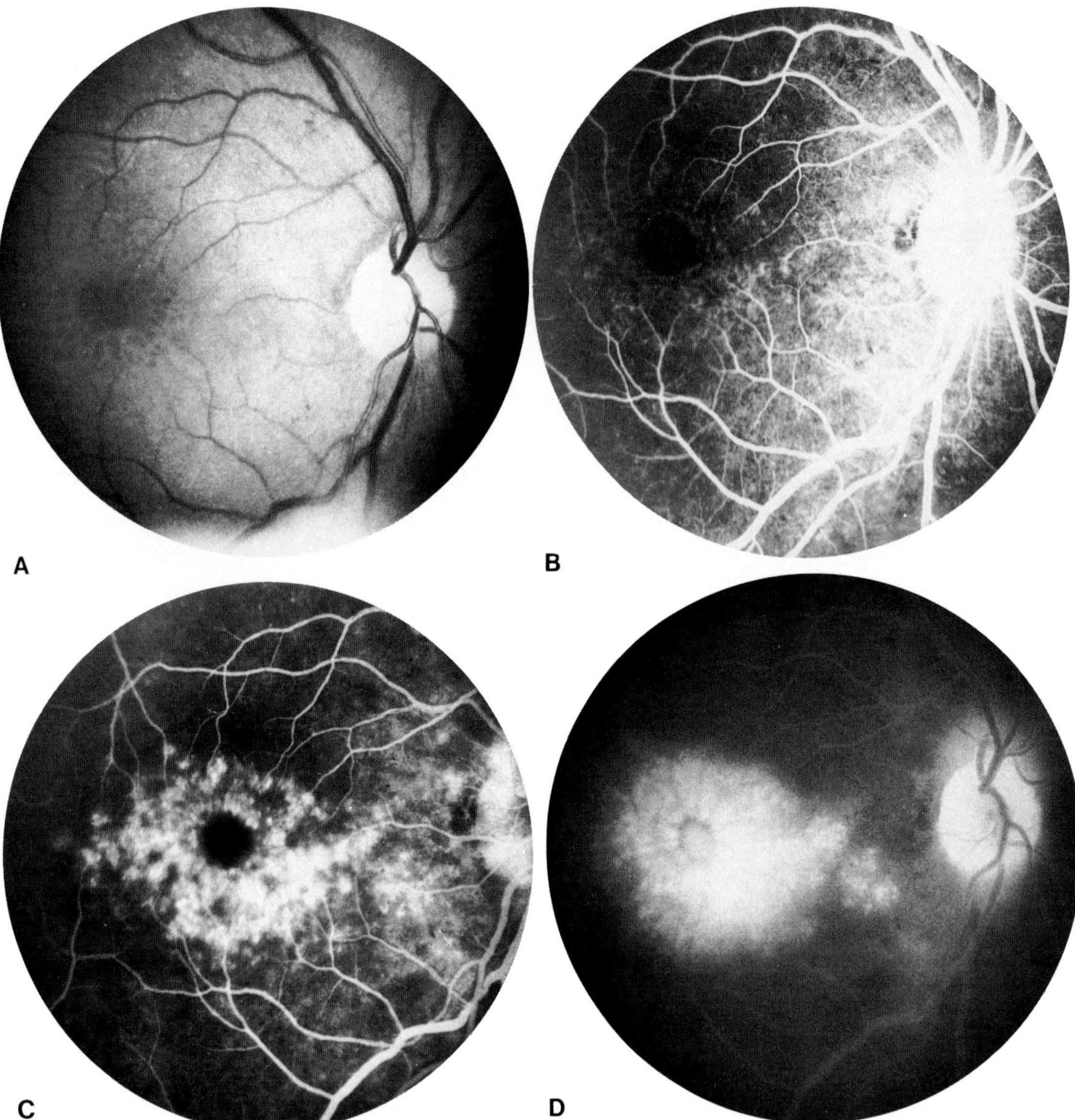

FIGURE 3–119 **Fluorescein angiography of cystoid macular edema.** The fluorescein angiogram is of the patient seen in Figure 3–118. *A,* Red-free photograph demonstrates the septae outlining the cystoid spaces. *B,* Early-phase photograph reveals some leakage from the perifoveal capillaries. *C,* Midphase photograph shows extensive, diffuse leakage from the perifoveal capillaries. Note also the leakage from the temporal aspect of the optic disc. *D,* Late-phase photograph demonstrates a well-developed petaloid pattern of cystoid macular edema. Note the central cystoid space and disc leakage.

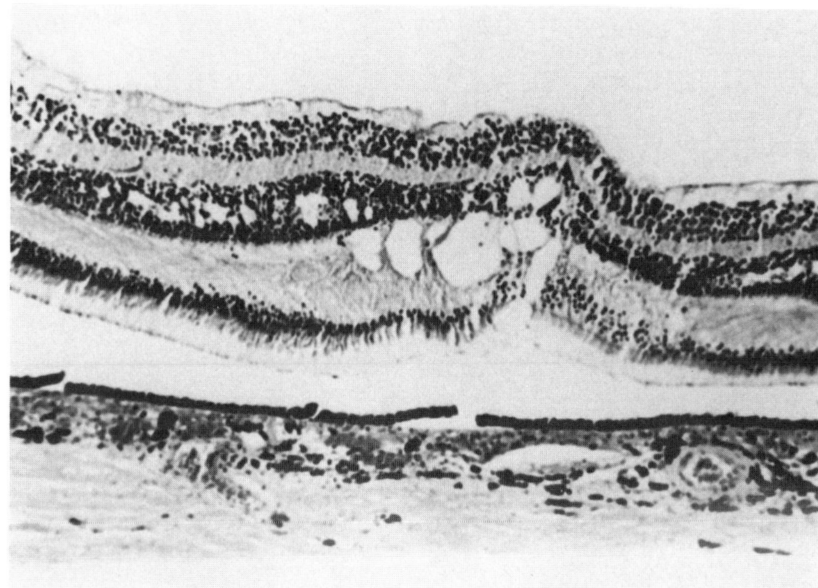

FIGURE 3–120 **Pathology of cystoid macular edema.** Photomicrograph of an eye with aphakic macular edema demonstrating large cystoid spaces in the outer plexiform layer. Smaller cystoid spaces are seen in the inner nuclear layer. Note the attenuation of the outer nuclear layer adjacent to the cystoid spaces. H&E, ×90. (From Tso MO: Pathology of cystoid macular edema. Ophthalmology 89:902–915, 1982.)

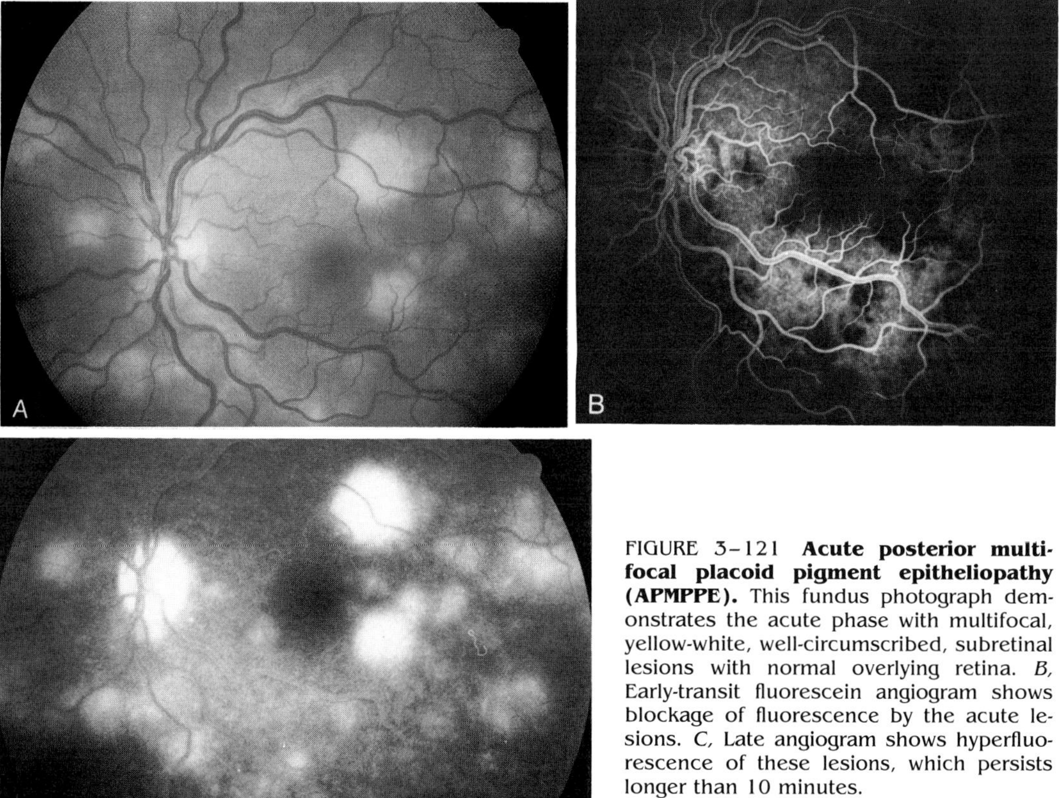

FIGURE 3–121 **Acute posterior multifocal placoid pigment epitheliopathy (APMPPE).** This fundus photograph demonstrates the acute phase with multifocal, yellow-white, well-circumscribed, subretinal lesions with normal overlying retina. *B,* Early-transit fluorescein angiogram shows blockage of fluorescence by the acute lesions. *C,* Late angiogram shows hyperfluorescence of these lesions, which persists longer than 10 minutes.

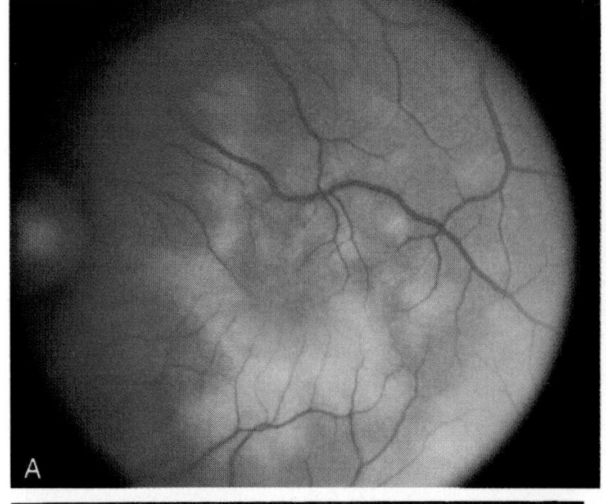

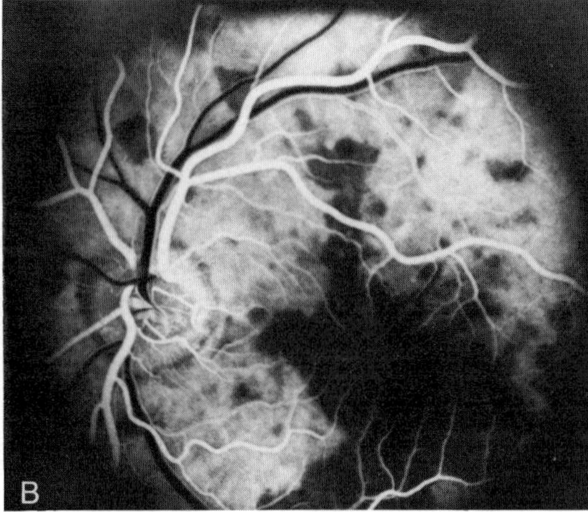

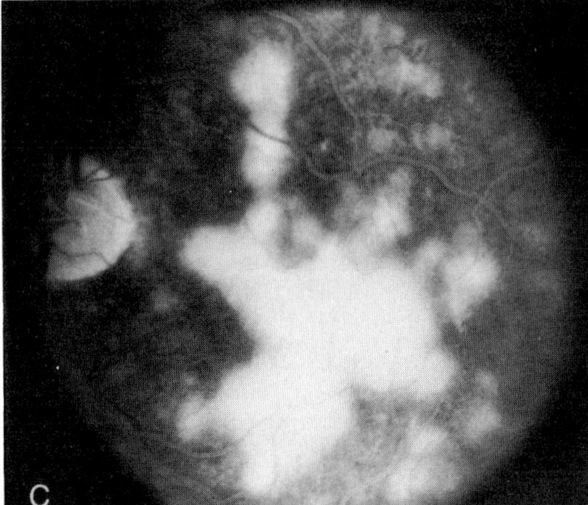

FIGURE 3-122 **APMPPE.** *A,* Fundus photograph is of a patient with a visual acuity of 20/400 and multiple, confluent lesions. *B,* Early angiogram shows blockage corresponding to the exact pattern of the acute lesions. *C,* Late staining is evident in this angiogram. (*A–C,* Courtesy of Robert J. Brockhurst, M.D.)

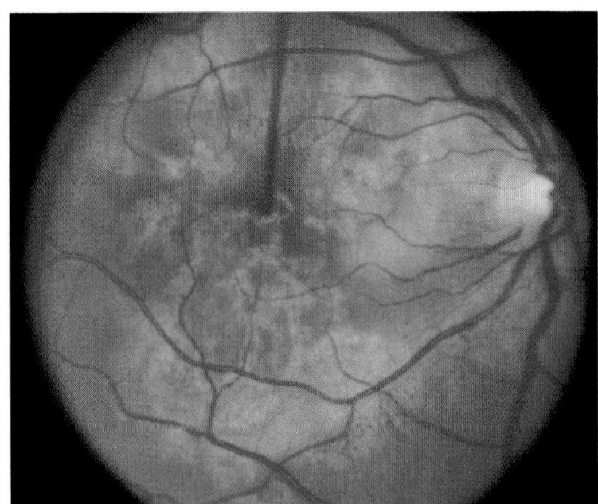

FIGURE 3-123 **Resolution of APMPPE.** The fundus photograph was taken 1 month after the acute onset of APMPPE. There are scattered areas of retinal pigment epithelial atrophy and clumping, and the visual acuity is 20/30. (Courtesy of Robert J. Brockhurst, M.D.)

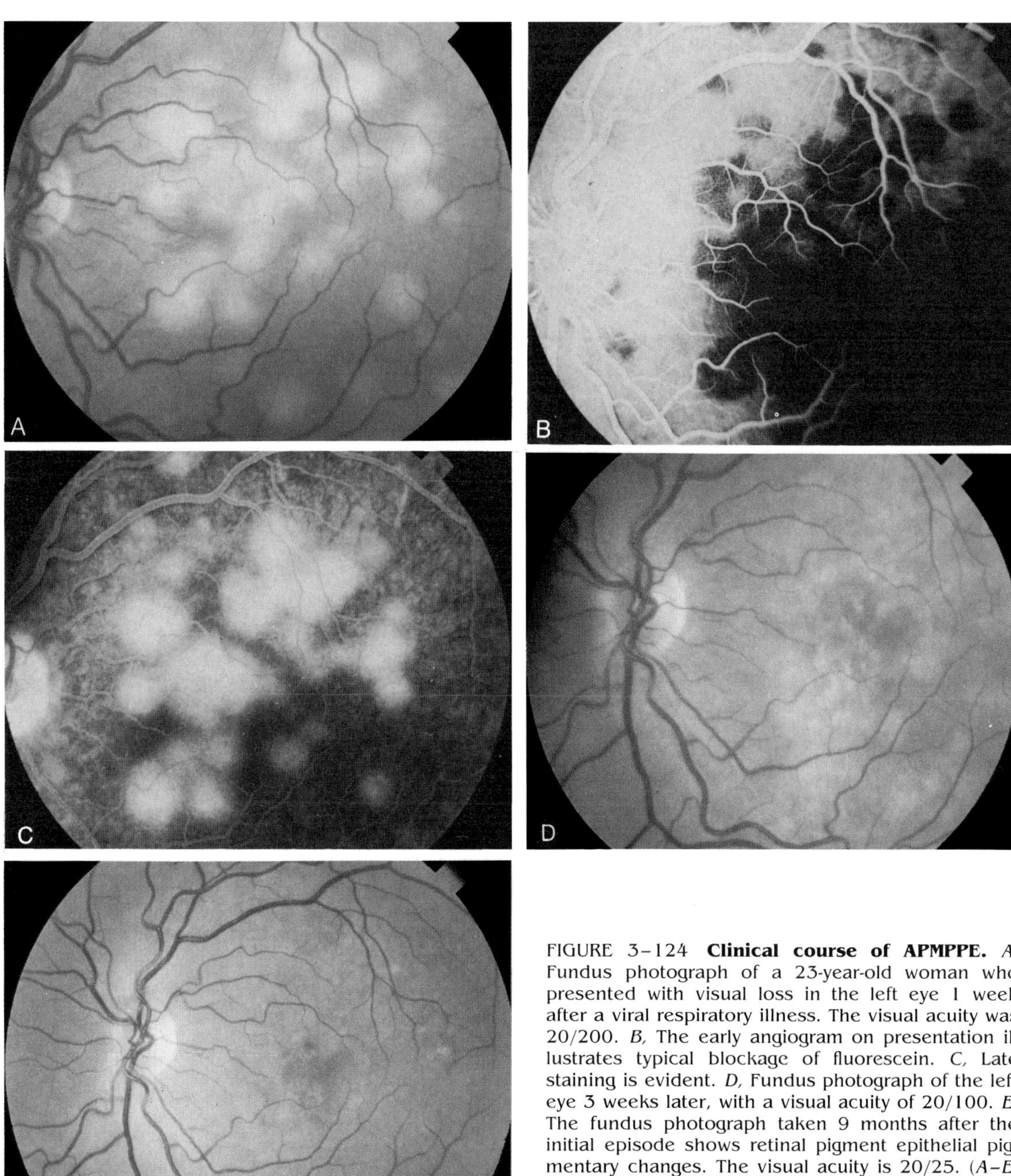

FIGURE 3–124 **Clinical course of APMPPE.** *A,* Fundus photograph of a 23-year-old woman who presented with visual loss in the left eye 1 week after a viral respiratory illness. The visual acuity was 20/200. *B,* The early angiogram on presentation illustrates typical blockage of fluorescein. *C,* Late staining is evident. *D,* Fundus photograph of the left eye 3 weeks later, with a visual acuity of 20/100. *E,* The fundus photograph taken 9 months after the initial episode shows retinal pigment epithelial pigmentary changes. The visual acuity is 20/25. (*A–E,* Courtesy of Mark W. Balles, M.D.)

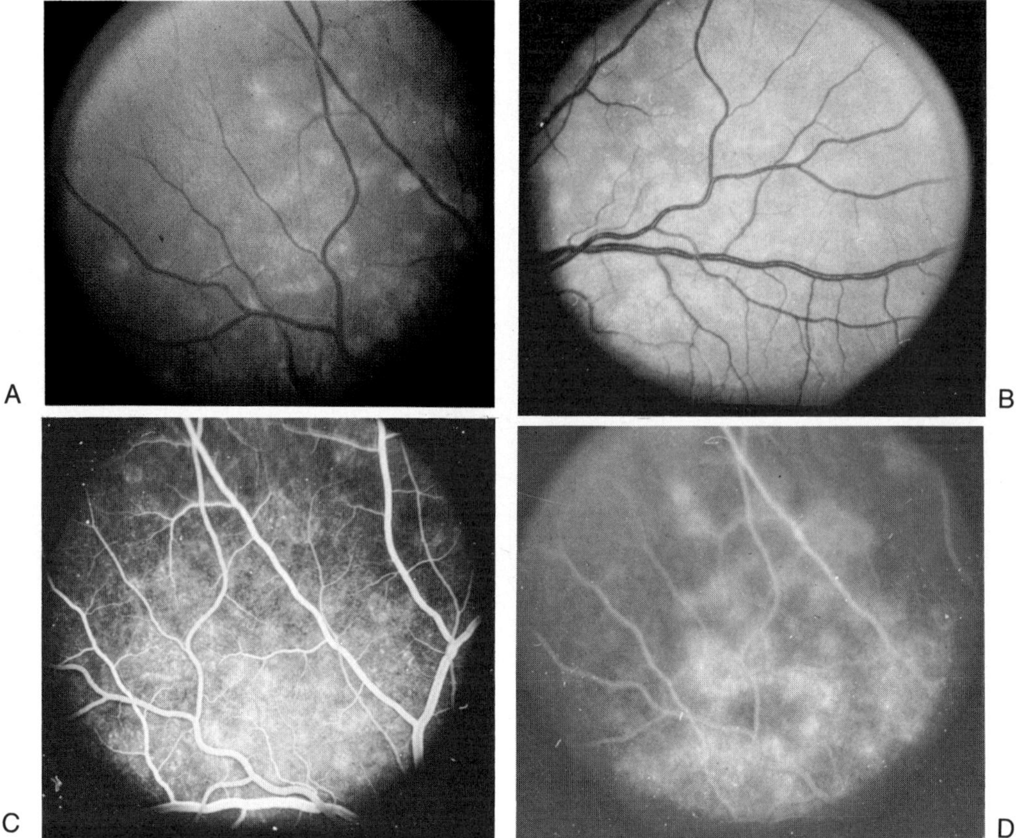

FIGURE 3-125 **Multiple evanescent white dot syndrome (MEWDS).** *A,* Note the prominent lesions at the level of the deep retinal or retinal pigment epithelium, or both. *B,* A monochromatic photograph of the same patient highlights the white spots in the fundus. *C,* An early fluorescein angiogram in this patient reveals the characteristic hyperfluorescent dots in the region of the pigment epithelium, most of which correspond to the white lesions. *D,* The late-stage fluorescein angiogram reveals staining of the retinal pigment epithelium and outer retina. In this patient, there has been alteration of the posterior blood-retinal barrier from extensive neuroretinitis involving the pigment epithelium.

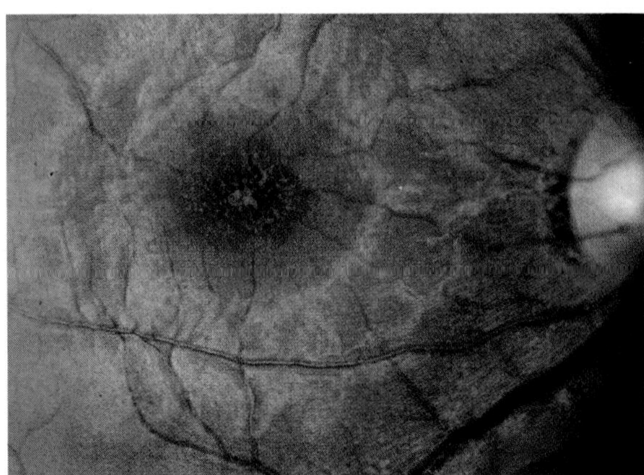

FIGURE 3-126 **Macular changes in MEWDS.** The granular appearance of the retinal pigment epithelium in the macula is demonstrated, which is characteristic of this disease and is exceedingly prominent in this patient. This is presumably due to a perifoveal neuroretinitis.

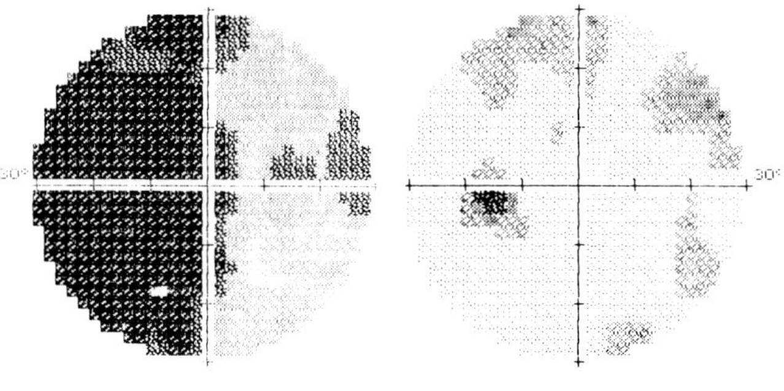

FIGURE 3–127 **Visual field in MEWDS.** *A,* A 24-year-old woman with a visual acuity of 20/40− had a Humphrey's visual field of the left eye 1 week after the onset of symptoms. The field demonstrates marked visual loss in the entire visual field, most profound temporally (giant blind spot). *B,* A visual field of the same patient 4 months later is nearly normal, although the patient still complained of dim vision. The visual acuity had returned to 20/20, and the white spots were completely gone. Eight months after the initial onset of symptoms, this patient still complained of dim vision in the left eye.

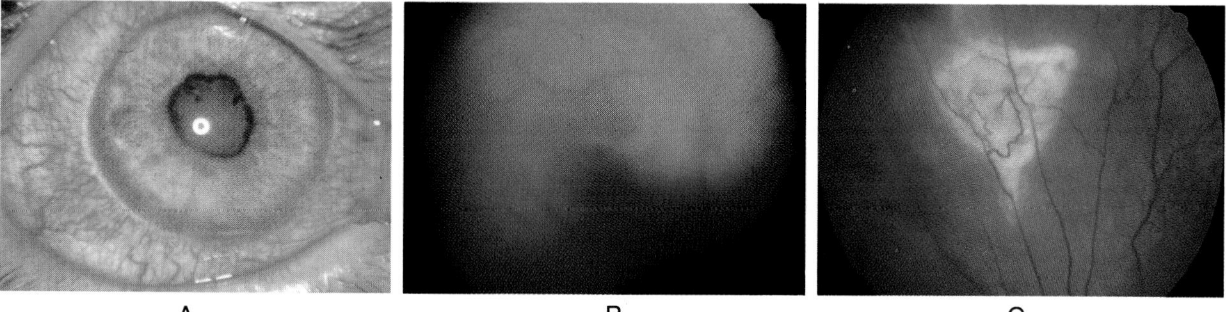

FIGURE 3–128 **Subretinal fibrosis and uveitis syndrome.** Subretinal fibrosis and uveitis syndrome is a rare form of idiopathic, bilateral, posterior uveitis, usually affecting young, healthy females. This 26-year-old woman presented with decreased vision, redness, and pain in both eyes. Note the conjunctival injection, posterior synechiae, and cataract secondary to anterior segment inflammation *(A)*. Fundus examination shows vitritis and round, discrete, yellowish white lesions at the level of the retinal pigment epithelium or choriocapillaris *(B)*. These lesions may fade or enlarge and coalesce to create multiple areas of whitish subretinal fibrosis *(C)*.

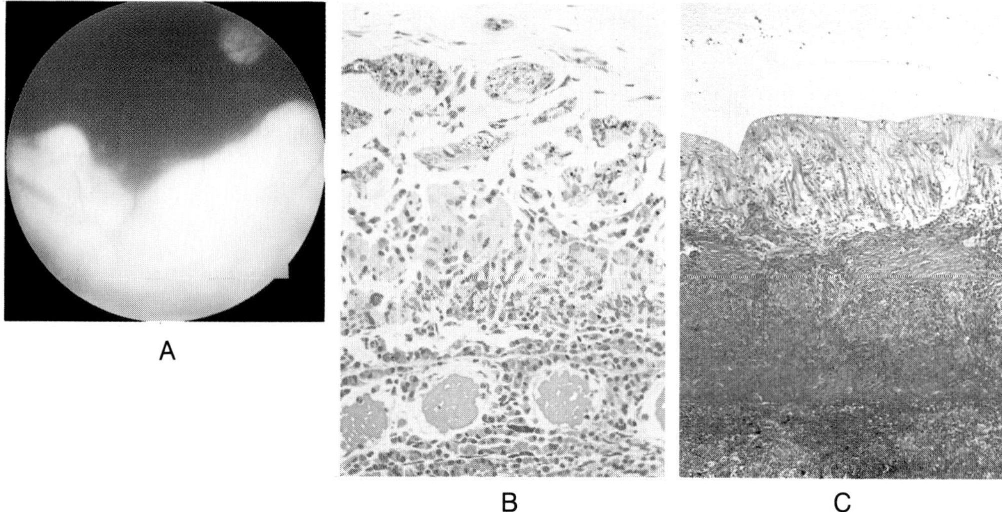

FIGURE 3–129 **Pathologic features of subretinal fibrosis and uveitis syndrome.** A chorioretinal biopsy was performed in an 18-year-old woman who presented with subretinal fibrosis and uveitis syndrome *(A)*, and histopathologic examination revealed a thickened choroid containing numerous lymphocytes and plasma cells *(B)* and gliosis of choroid and overlying retina (*B* and *C*). No virus or circulating antiretinal antibody was found. Electron microscopy suggests that the subretinal fibrotic tissue shows characteristics of both retinal pigment epithelium and Muller cells. (*A–C,* Courtesy of Chi-Chao Chan, M.D., and Robert Nussenblatt, M.D.)

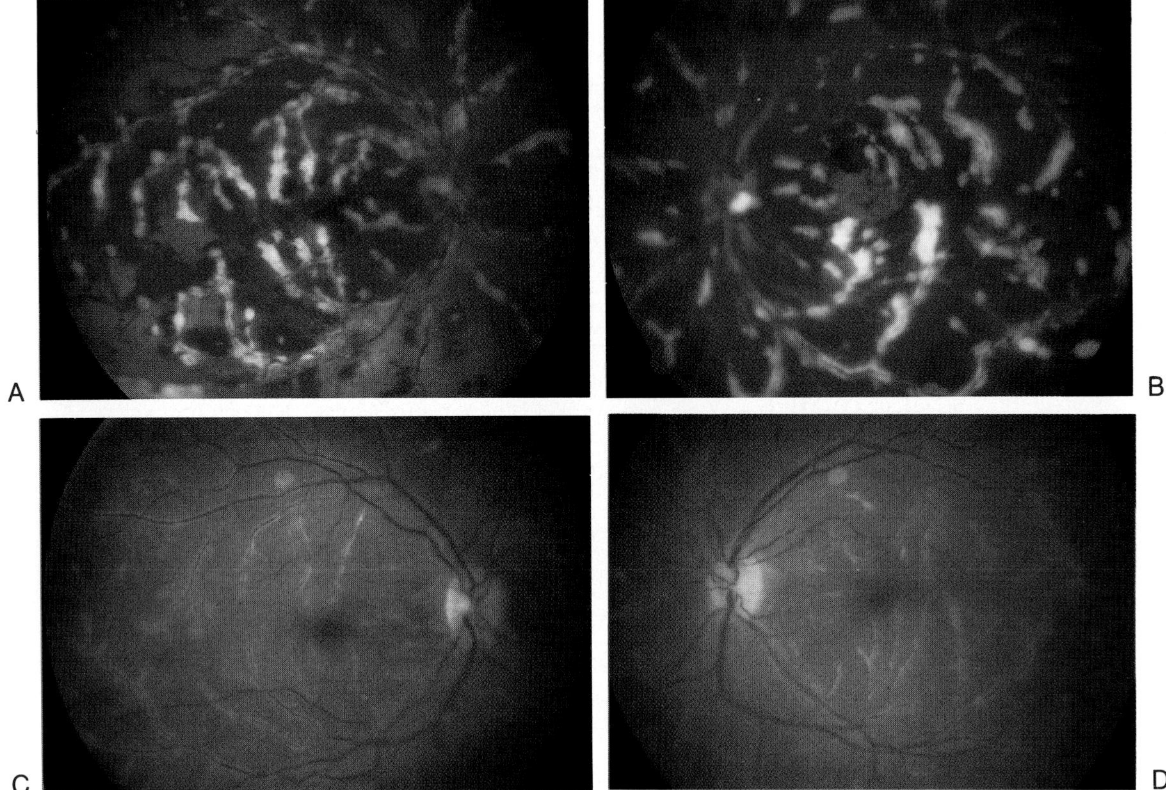

FIGURE 3–130 **Frosted branch angiitis.** *A, B,* Bilateral retinal phlebitis extends from the posterior pole to the periphery with uninterrupted severe sheathing of all the vessels, resembling the frosted branches of a tree. Extensive perivenous exudates associated with intrarenal hemorrhage are noted in this patient. *C, D,* The most frequent presentation, however, is bilateral extensive venous sheathing. There is mild pallor of the left optic disc. (*Left figures,* right eye; *right figures,* left eye.)

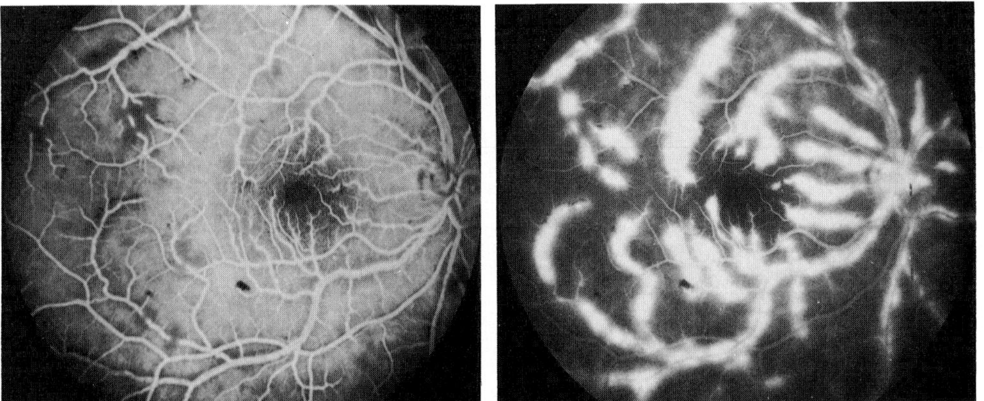

FIGURE 3–131 **Fluorescein angiographic findings in frosted branch angiitis.** The fluorescein angiogram demonstrates normal venous flow in the early phase *(left)* and diffuse staining of the vein walls in the late phase *(right).*

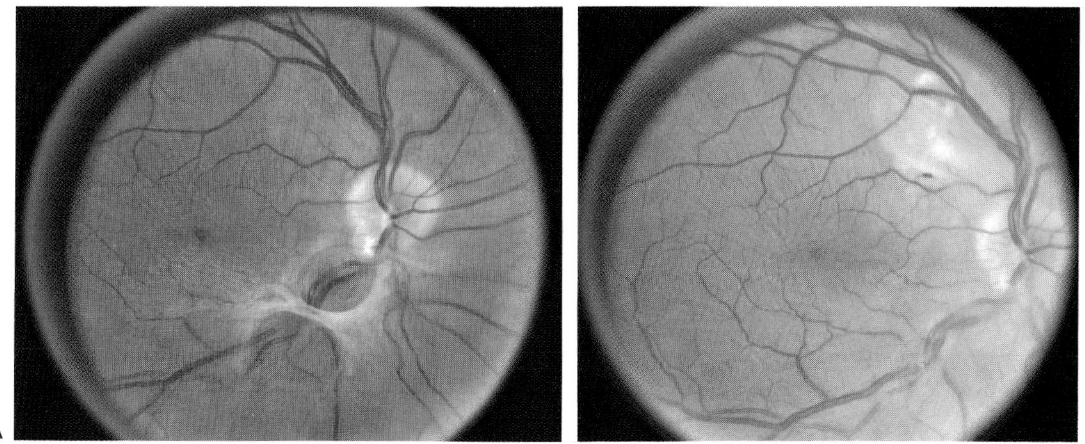

FIGURE 3–132 **Macular pseudohole with an epiretinal macular membrane.** *A,* Idiopathic epiretinal membrane with a macular pseudohole in a 35-year-old woman with a visual acuity of 20/100. Histopathologic studies suggest that the membranes are composed of retinal pigment epithelial cells and retinal glial cells. *B,* Postoperatively the macular pseudohole has disappeared, and the vision improved to 20/40.

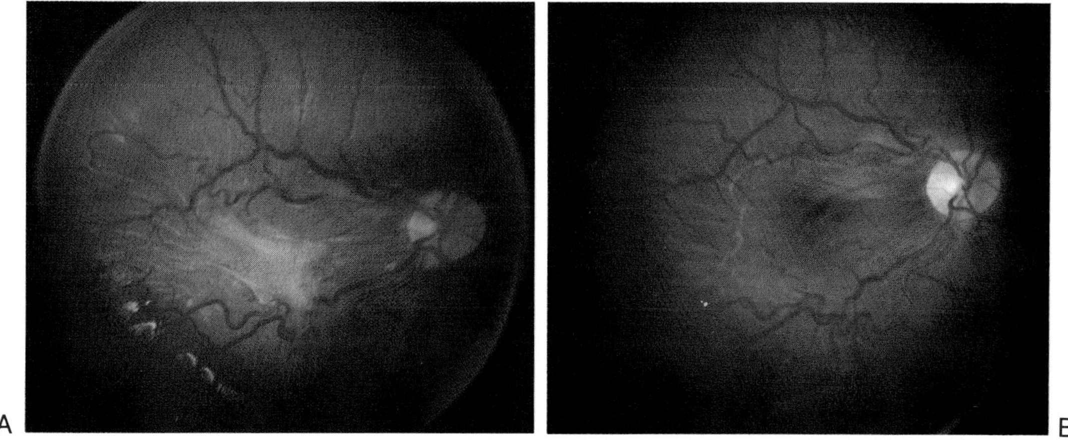

FIGURE 3–133 **Epiretinal macular membrane.** *A,* This 10-year-old boy had a thick epiretinal membrane and a vision of counting fingers following trauma. Note how the retinal details underlying the membrane are obscured. *B,* Postoperatively, after removal of the epiretinal tissue, the vision improved to 20/100. Note the improved view of the fundus.

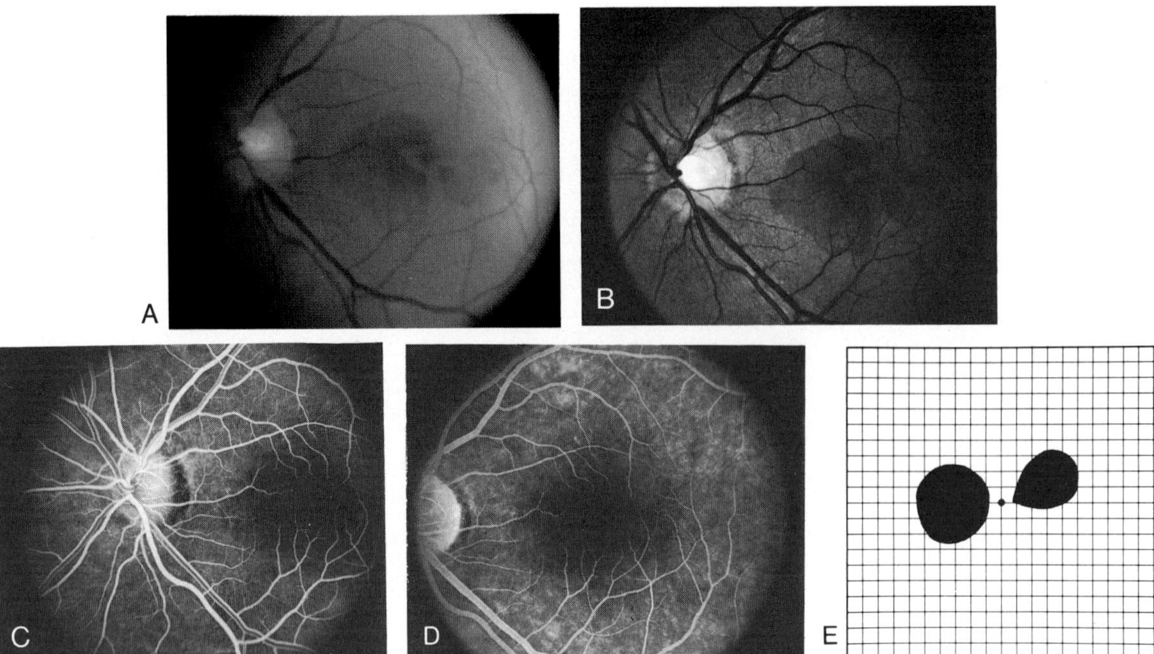

FIGURE 3–134 **Acute macular neuroretinopathy.** *A,* This 42-year-old woman presented with a 3-week history of a flulike syndrome before the onset of paracentral scotomas in the left eye and a visual acuity of 20/20. Her medical history was significant for she had undergone a hysterectomy and oophorectomy 2 years previously and had since been using an estradiol transdermal (Estroderm) patch. Note the dark, red lesions centered around the fovea, which are present in the outer retinal layers. *B,* The macular lesions are better appreciated with red-free light. The fluorescein angiogram of the early phase *(C)* and late phase *(D)* is essentially normal. *E,* Amsler grid testing demonstrates two paracentral scotomas. The scotomas may become less dense with time but usually persist. (*A–E,* Courtesy of Jack F. Bowers, M.D.)

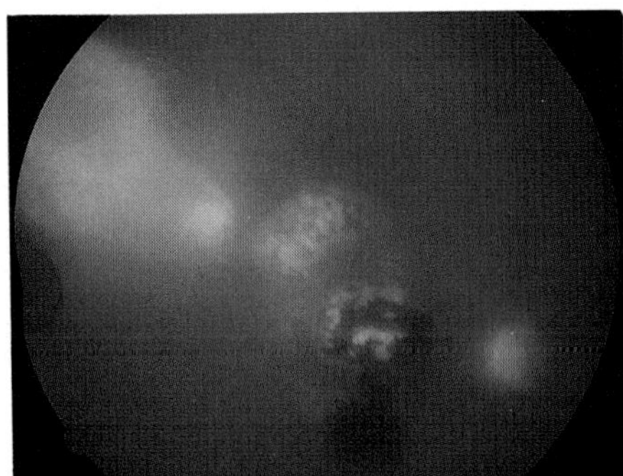

FIGURE 3–135 **Toxoplasmosis.** The multiple atrophic and hyperpigmented chorioretinal scars are signs of previous episodes of active toxoplasmosis. Note the fresh area of active chorioretinitis with overlying vitreal inflammatory cells and vitreal "haze." The areas of retinitis are due to *Toxoplasma* tissue cysts bursting and releasing bradyzoites, which transform into tachyzoites and invade adjacent cells.

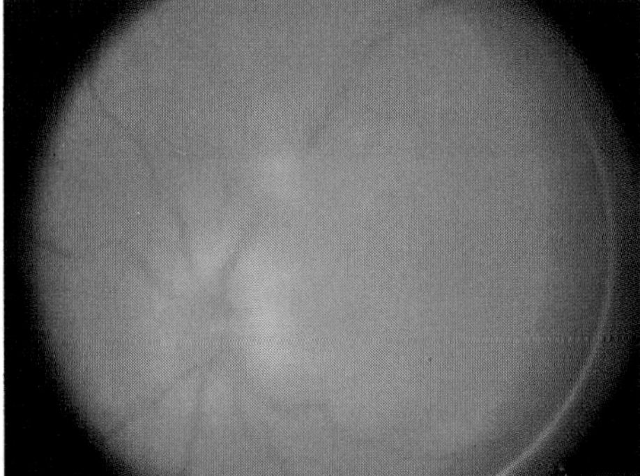

FIGURE 3–136 **Active toxoplasmosis.** Papillitis with vitreal inflammatory cells anterior to the optic nerve, making visualization of the optic nerve slightly difficult. The enzyme-linked immunosorbent assay test for *Toxoplasma* antibodies gave the following results: the IgG titer was 1 : 496, and the IgM titer was 1 : 64 at the time this photograph was taken; 2 weeks later, the IgM titer was 1 : 256.

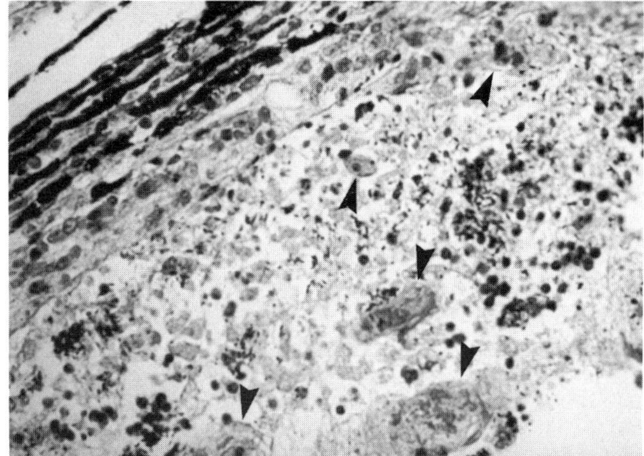

FIGURE 3–137 **Histopathology of toxoplasmosis.** This histopathologic specimen demonstrates destruction of the retinal architecture and the underlying choroid. Note the *Toxoplasma gondii* cysts *(arrows)*. The infiltrate consists predominantly of lymphocytes, macrophages, and epithelioid cells.

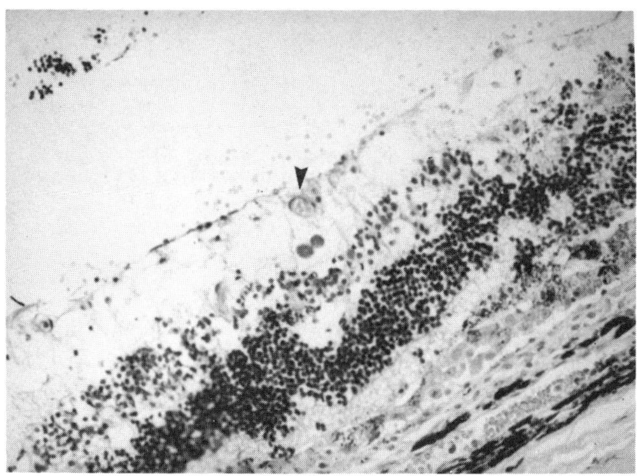

FIGURE 3–138 **Histopathology of toxoplasmosis.** The parasite has a propensity for neural tissue, and the *T. gondii* cysts are frequently found in superficial retinal layers, as seen here *(arrow)*.

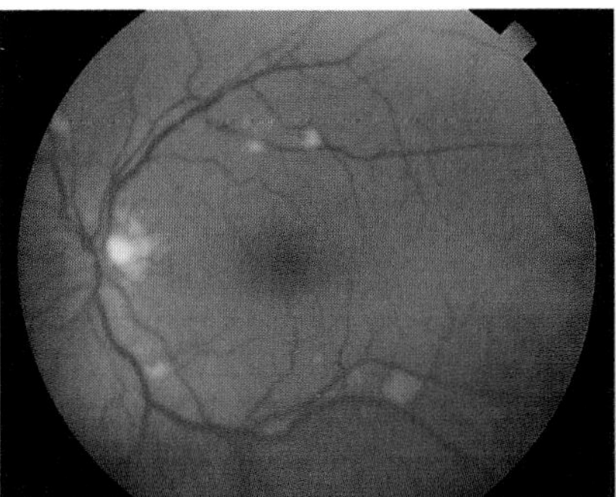

FIGURE 3–140 **Human immunodeficiency virus (HIV) associated retinopathy.** This fundus photograph shows cotton-wool spots but not scattered retinal hemorrhages, microaneurysms, or Roth spots, which can also be seen in this entity. The microangiopathy is due to focal ischemia.

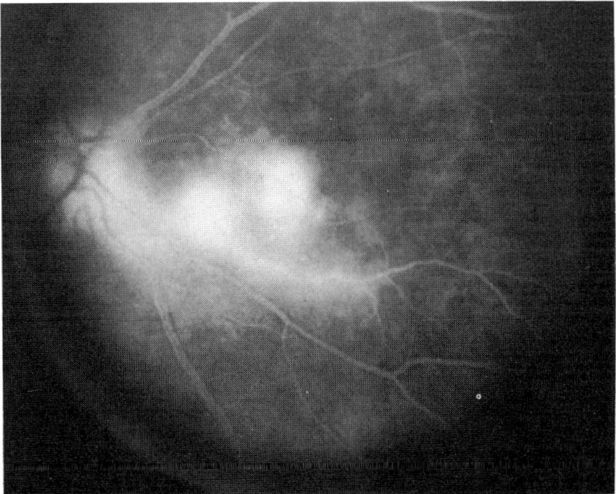

FIGURE 3–139 **Toxoplasmosis.** This fluorescein angiogram shows dye accumulation in two foci representing areas of active *Toxoplasma* retinochoroiditis, papillitis with dye staining of the nerve head, and associated retinal vasculitis with late vascular staining.

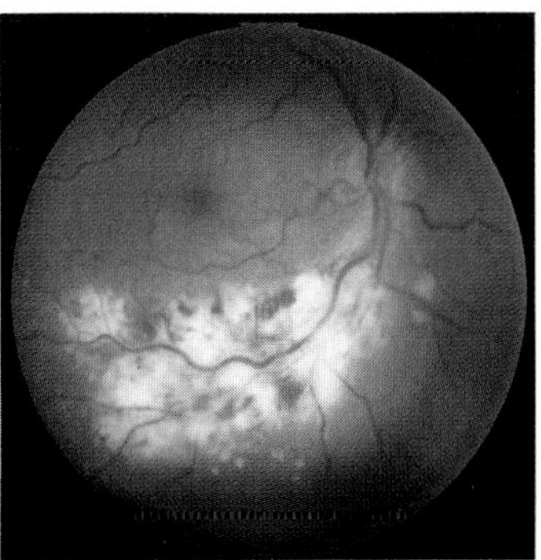

FIGURE 3–141 **Cytomegalovirus retinitis.** This fundus photograph demonstrates a posterior pole lesion that consists of whitish retinal necrosis and retinal hemorrhages that follow retinal blood vessels. This retinitis is associated with infection of the inner retina.

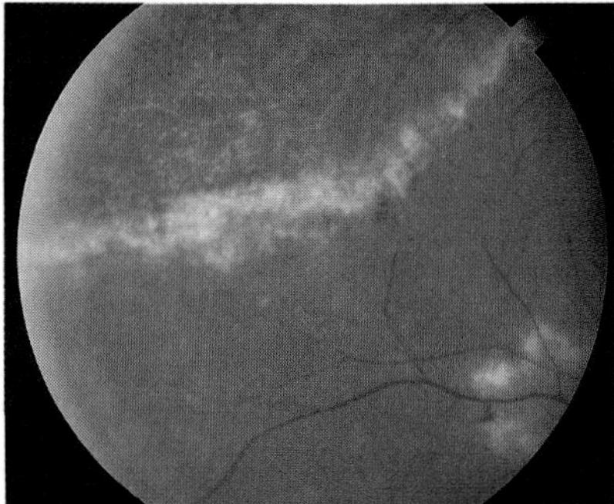

FIGURE 3–142 **Cytomegalovirus retinitis.** Peripheral infection results in atrophic retina anteriorly and a posterior advancing border that is yellow and granular with little or no hemorrhage. This is the "brush-fire" form of retinitis.

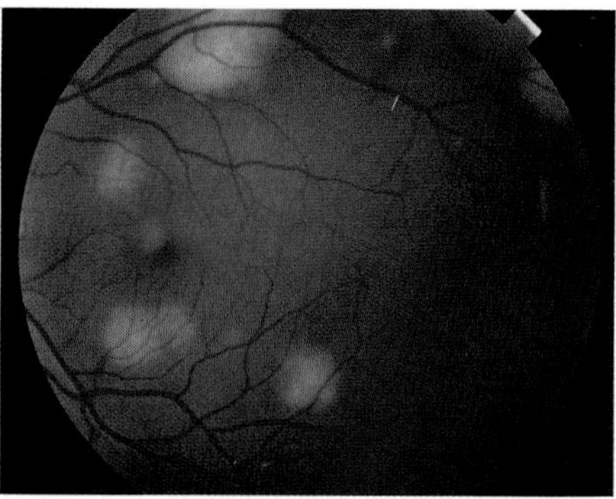

FIGURE 3–143 ***Pneumocystis carinii* choroiditis.** Note the large, plaquelike, cream-colored choroidal lesions in the posterior pole. The infiltrates grow slowly but progressively without treatment. *P. carinii* trophozoites and cysts have been demonstrated in the choroid by histopathology.

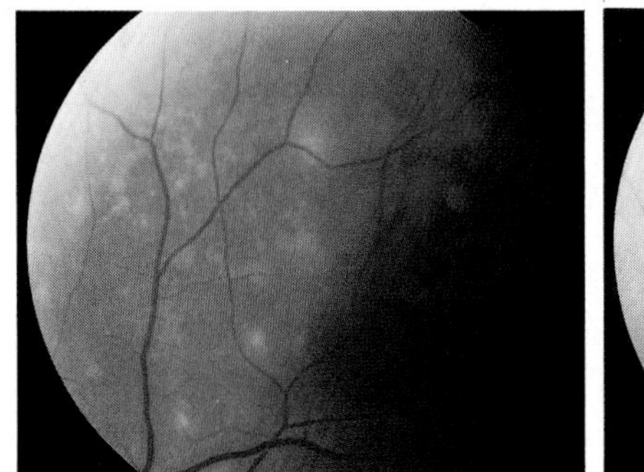

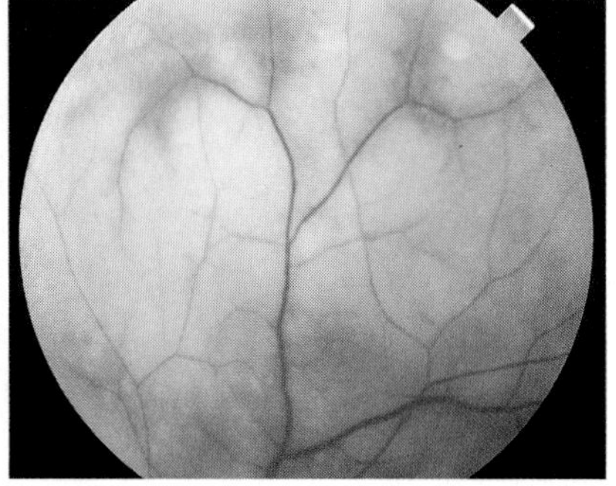

FIGURE 3–144 **Acute retinal necrosis (ARN)—presumed herpes zoster retinitis.** *A,* The initial lesions are small and yellowish and in the outer retina. The inner retina and retinal vessels are spared early in the course of this retinitis. *B,* The lesions spread within 3 weeks to form large, geographic areas of outer retinal necrosis. The appearance of retinal hemorrhage is variable.

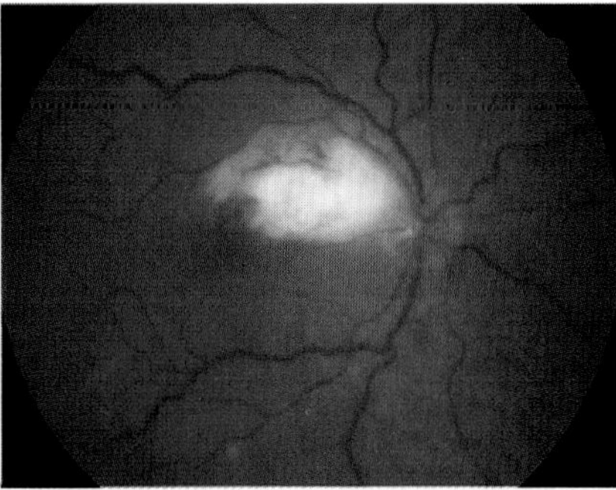

FIGURE 3–145 **Toxoplasmic retinitis.** This large, white, solitary lesion of the outer retina is seen in more severely immunocompromised patients. The retinal lesions may also be large, yellow, single or multifocal, at the level of the inner retina, and with overlying vitritis, as is seen in nonimmunocompromised hosts.

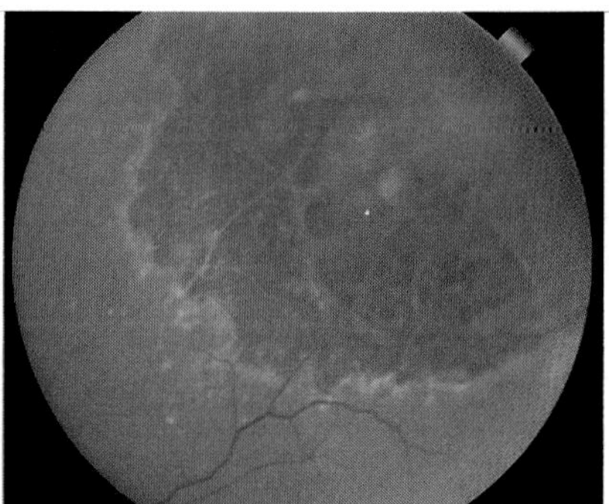

FIGURE 3–146 **Vitreoretinal surgery in AIDS patients.** This fundus photograph shows retinitis associated with multiple retinal breaks involving large areas of detached retina, as is seen in cytomegalovirus retinitis and ARN. A vitrectomy with silicone oil tamponade is often recommended as the initial procedure to keep the retina in place despite further hole formation.

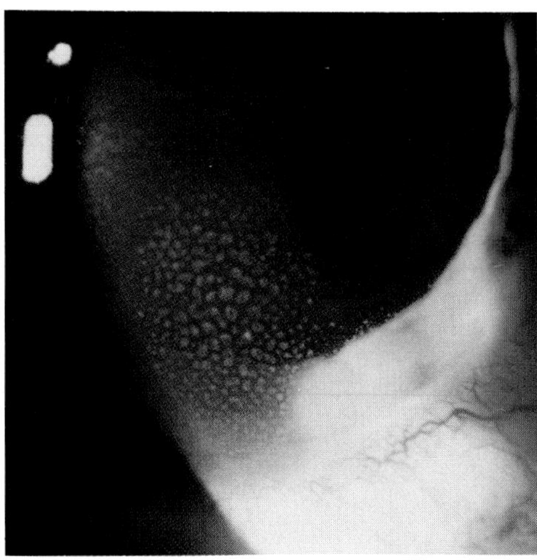

FIGURE 3–147 **Anterior segment findings in ARN.** Granulomatous keratic precipitates seen in a slit-lamp photomicrograph of a middle-aged man with the early phases of ARN. Note the limbal flush.

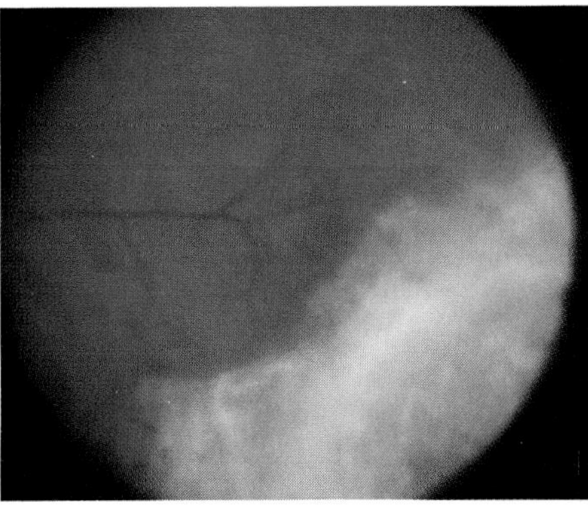

FIGURE 3–149 **Regression of ARN.** This photomicrograph demonstrates regression of necrotizing retinitis with an atrophic pigmented zone corresponding to the area of prior retinitis and fibroglial proliferative change overlying the center of the scar. Clearing of the ocular media opacities results in improved visibility of retinal vascular detail.

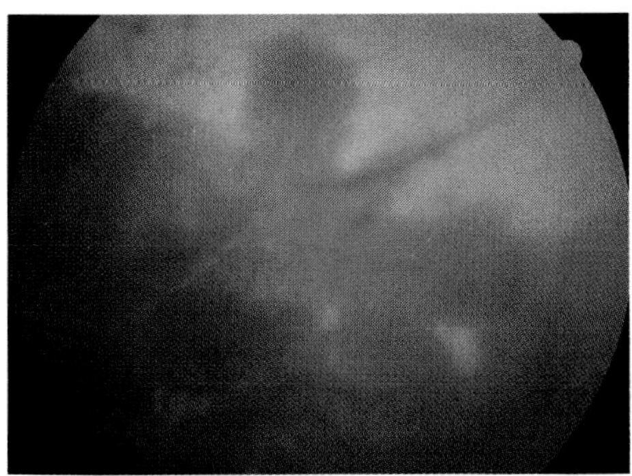

FIGURE 3–148 **ARN.** A typical peripheral lesion of ARN demonstrates a confluent white-yellow zone with an irregular scalloped posterior margin and a sharp transition between involved and noninvolved areas. The opalescent retina is due to full-thickness retinal necrosis.

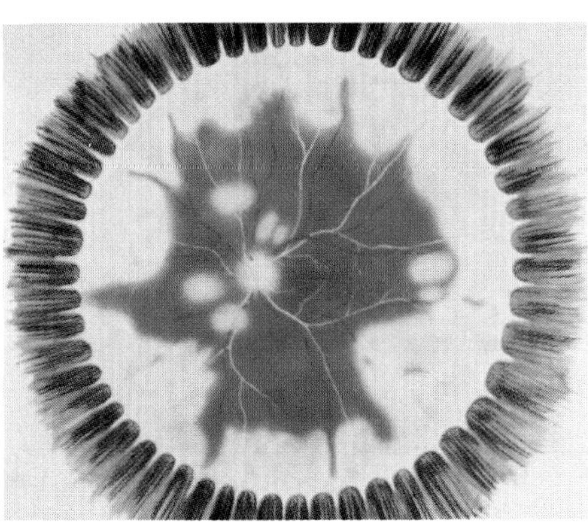

FIGURE 3–150 **ARN.** Artist's representation of a patient with the classic features of ARN, including confluent necrotizing retinitis, posterior nummular infiltrates, and retinal arteritis (with involved vessels seen in yellow).

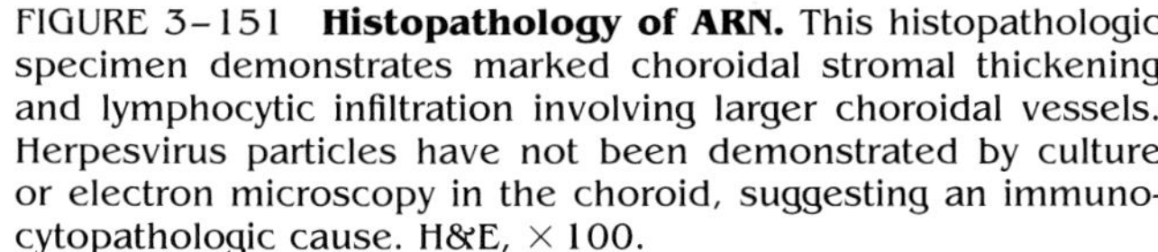

FIGURE 3–151 **Histopathology of ARN.** This histopathologic specimen demonstrates marked choroidal stromal thickening and lymphocytic infiltration involving larger choroidal vessels. Herpesvirus particles have not been demonstrated by culture or electron microscopy in the choroid, suggesting an immunocytopathologic cause. H&E, × 100.

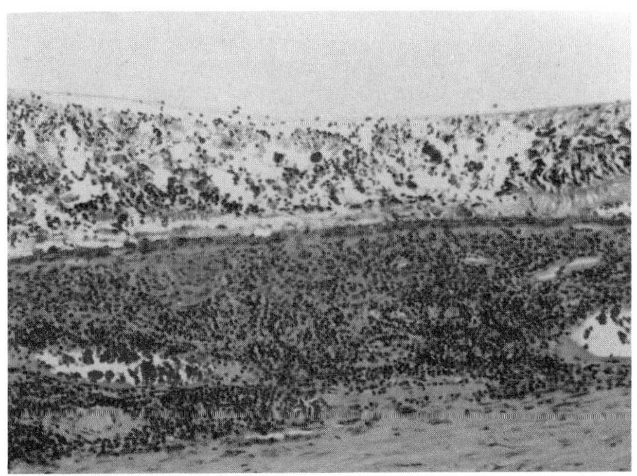

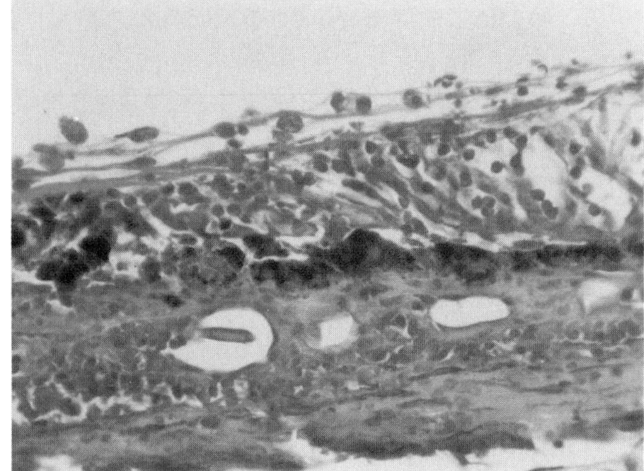

FIGURE 3–152 **Histopathology of ARN.** The cicatricial stage of ARN is demonstrated on histology by the zone of retinal pigment epithelial proliferation and migration underlying thinned necrotic peripheral retina. Note the presence of a non-pigmented epiretinal membrane on the surface of the necrotic retina. H&E, ×250.

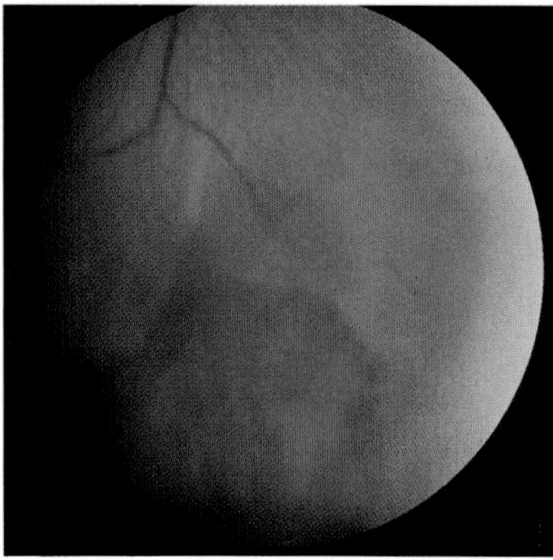

FIGURE 3–153 **Proliferative vitreoretinopathy in ARN.** Secondary cicatricial changes have led to the development of a large tear in the inferior posterior retina in this patient with ARN. The concurrence of peripheral retinal thinning, epiretinal membrane formation, and vitreous contraction contributes to the development of proliferative vitreoretinopathy.

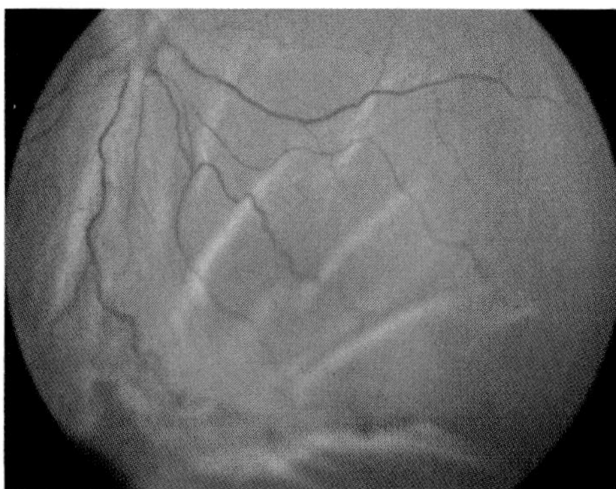

FIGURE 3–154 **Proliferative vitreoretinopathy with ARN.** Retinal folds in stage C2 proliferative vitreoretinopathy associated with ARN. Note the pigmented epiretinal membranes in the lower left corner of this photograph.

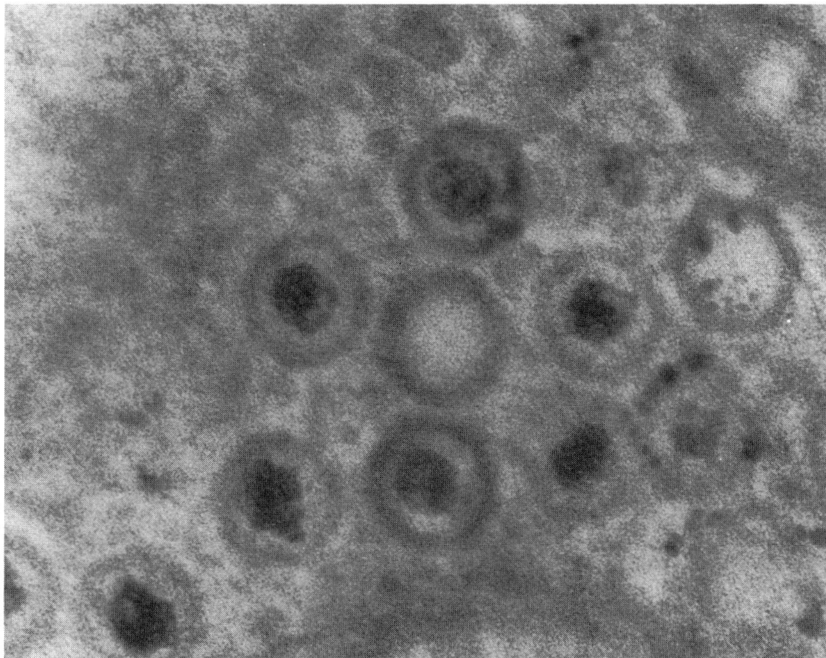

FIGURE 3–155 **Diagnostic studies in ARN.** This transmission electron micrograph shows viral particles in the necrotic retina of a middle-aged man with ARN. Note the complete and incomplete viral particles, with and without a central nucleocapsid, and with an outer lipid envelope. ×87,000.

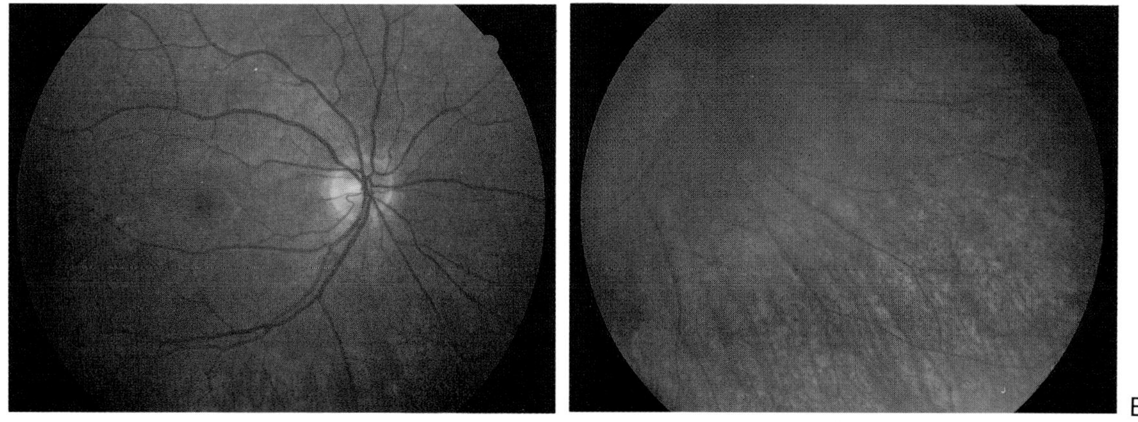

FIGURE 3–156 **Congenital rubella retinopathy.** Note the "salt-and-pepper" pigmentary mottling of the macula *(A)*, which can also affect the periphery *(B)*. The retinopathy may be progressive. Histopathology shows foci of increased and decreased pigmentation of the retinal pigment epithelium. (Courtesy of William Mieler, M.D.)

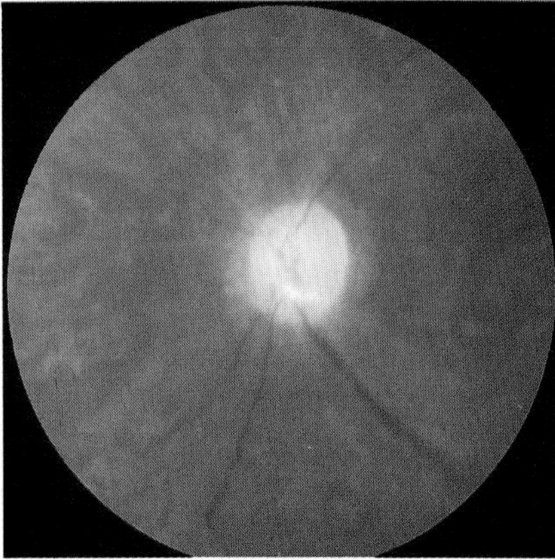

FIGURE 3–157 **Neonatal herpes simplex retinitis.** This fundus photograph demonstrates optic atrophy, which occurs in severe cases. An associated chorioretinitis may be fulminant, but evidence of healed, atrophic chorioretinal lesions suggests that a milder form occurs. Most neonatal infections are acquired at the time of delivery, by exposure in the birth canal. (Courtesy of Robert Petersen, M.D.)

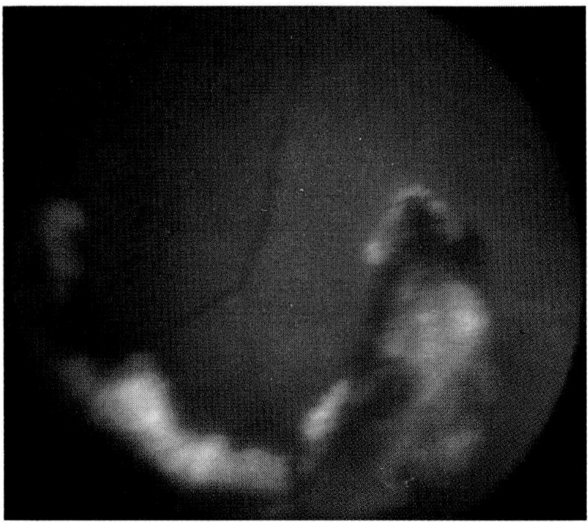

FIGURE 3–158 **Congenital varicella syndrome.** Note the large, peripheral chorioretinal scars with intense pigmentation along the edge of the lesions and central hypopigmentation. This results from maternal infection during the first or early second trimester of pregnancy.

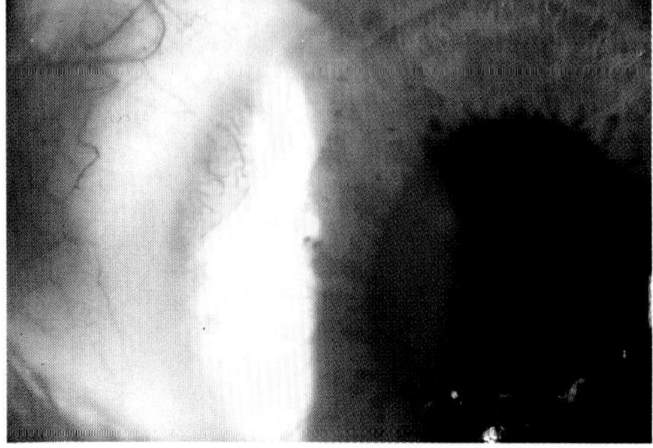

FIGURE 3–159 **Syphilitic uveitis nodosa.** This anterior segment photograph shows a mass in the substance of the peripheral iris at the 8 to 9 o'clock positions. This iris lesion may be relatively restricted to cases associated with secondary syphilis with extraocular manifestations.

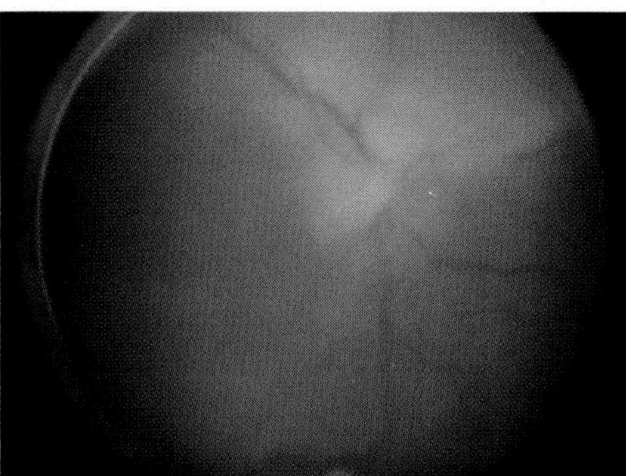

FIGURE 3–160 **Syphilitic sector retinitis.** Note the sector of retina, beginning at the disc and extending superiorly, with infiltrative retinitis and associated retinal vasculitis.

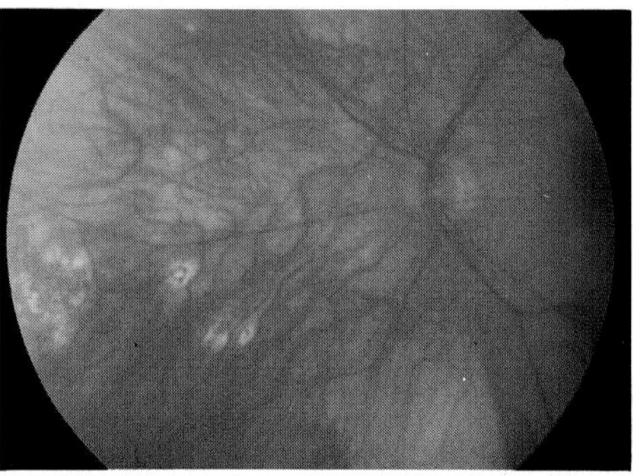

FIGURE 3–161 **Syphilitic multifocal choroiditis.** Multifocal chorioretinal lesions, now healed, in a patient with previously active syphilis and multifocal choroiditis.

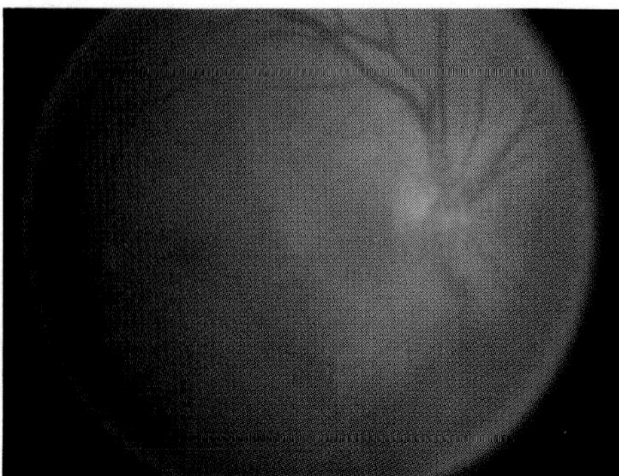

FIGURE 3–162 **Syphilitic vitritis and papillitis.** Note the swelling of the optic nerve and the hazy view of the nerve secondary to the associated inflammatory cells in the vitreous anterior to the disc.

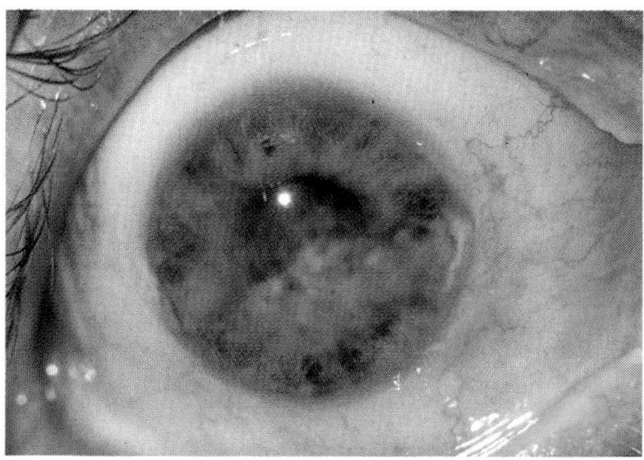

FIGURE 3-163 **Syphilitic sector interstitial keratitis.** Note the inactive sector interstitial keratitis with stromal scarring in the inferonasal quadrant in a patient with previously treated syphilis. Syphilitic interstitial keratitis may be diffuse or, as seen here, localized. Histopathology shows a nonulcerative, nonsuppurative inflammation of the corneal stroma.

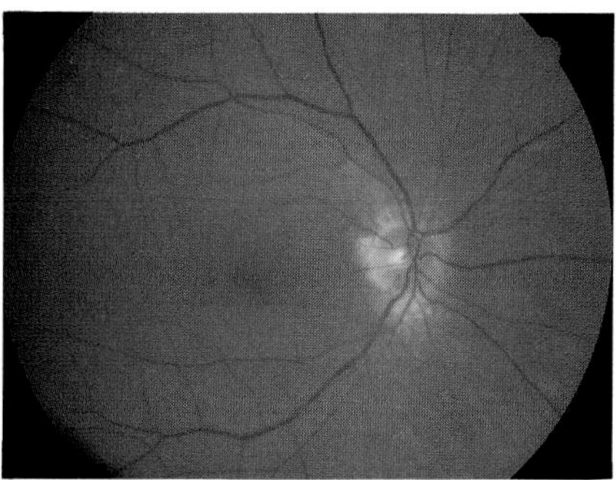

FIGURE 3-165 **Early stage of diffuse unilateral subacute neuroretinopathy (DUSN).** DUSN is characterized by widespread, unilateral inflammatory destruction of the neuroretina presumed secondary to one or more nematodes. Note the mild optic disc swelling and peripapillary pigment thinning in the active phase of diffuse unilateral subacute neuroretinitis. During this stage, the visual loss is out of proportion to visible changes in the retina or the optic nerve. Although multiple transient yellow-white lesions may be seen in the deep retina, the fundus often appears unremarkable except for a few viteous cells and mild optic disc swelling.

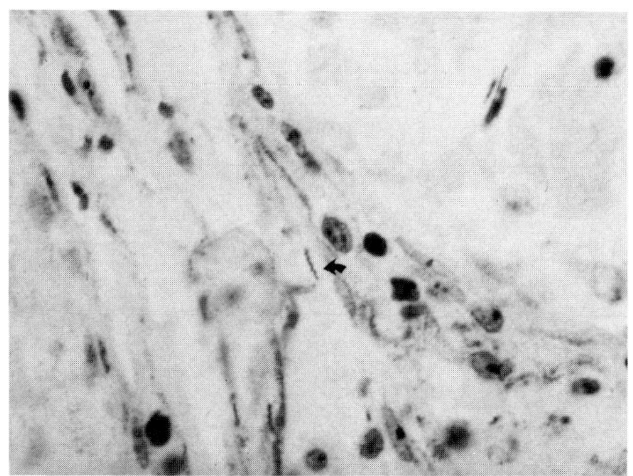

FIGURE 3-164 **Histopathology of ocular syphilis.** This specimen is from a patient with secondary syphilis and active interstitial keratitis who had a penetrating keratoplasty. The spirochetes in the cornea are demonstrated by silver stain.

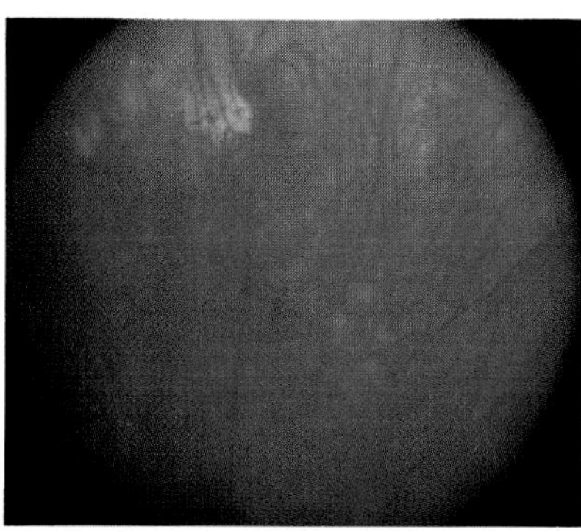

FIGURE 3-166 **Late stage of DUSN.** The late or inactive stage of the disease is characterized by patches of retinal pigment epithelial atrophy. Vision declines to 20/200 or less, and dense central and patchy peripheral scotomas develop. The optic disc becomes pale, and the retinal blood vessels become narrow.

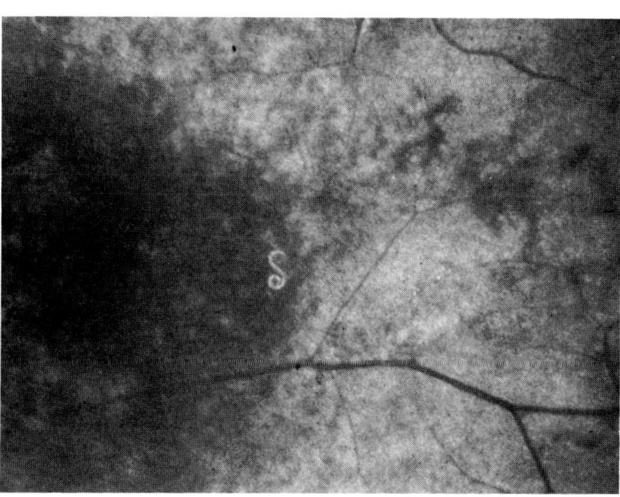

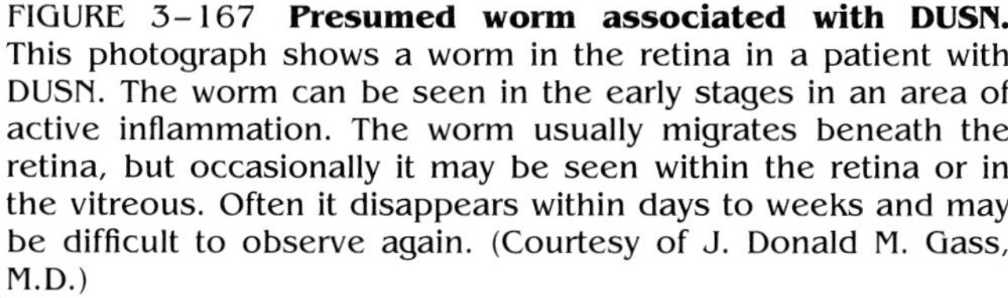

FIGURE 3-167 **Presumed worm associated with DUSN.** This photograph shows a worm in the retina in a patient with DUSN. The worm can be seen in the early stages in an area of active inflammation. The worm usually migrates beneath the retina, but occasionally it may be seen within the retina or in the vitreous. Often it disappears within days to weeks and may be difficult to observe again. (Courtesy of J. Donald M. Gass, M.D.)

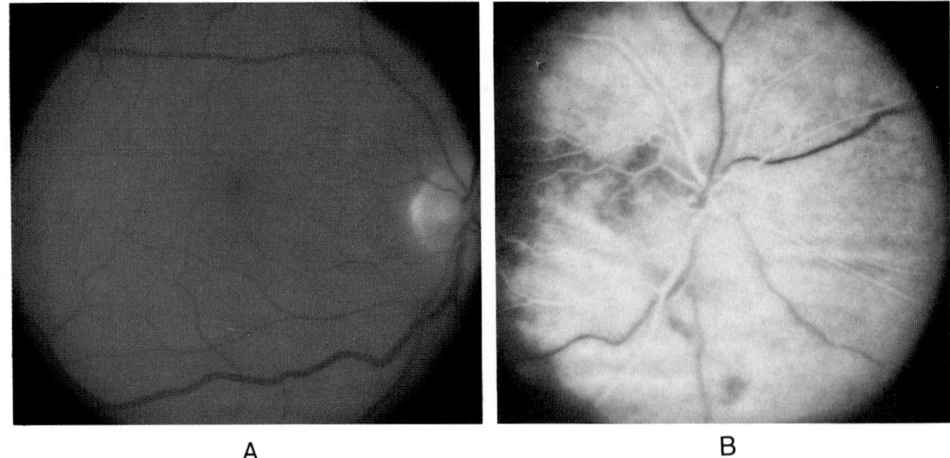

FIGURE 3–168 **Retinal manifestation of rheumatoid arthritis.** Separate connective tissues and structures within the eye can become inflamed in the various rheumatic diseases. *A,* In this fundus photograph of a patient with posterior scleritis secondary to rheumatoid arthritis, there is thickening of the choroid in the posterior pole and peripapillary area with chorioretinal striae in the macula. *B,* Fluorescein angiogram shows alternating hypofluorescent and hyperfluorescent linear streaks corresponding to the chorioretinal striae.

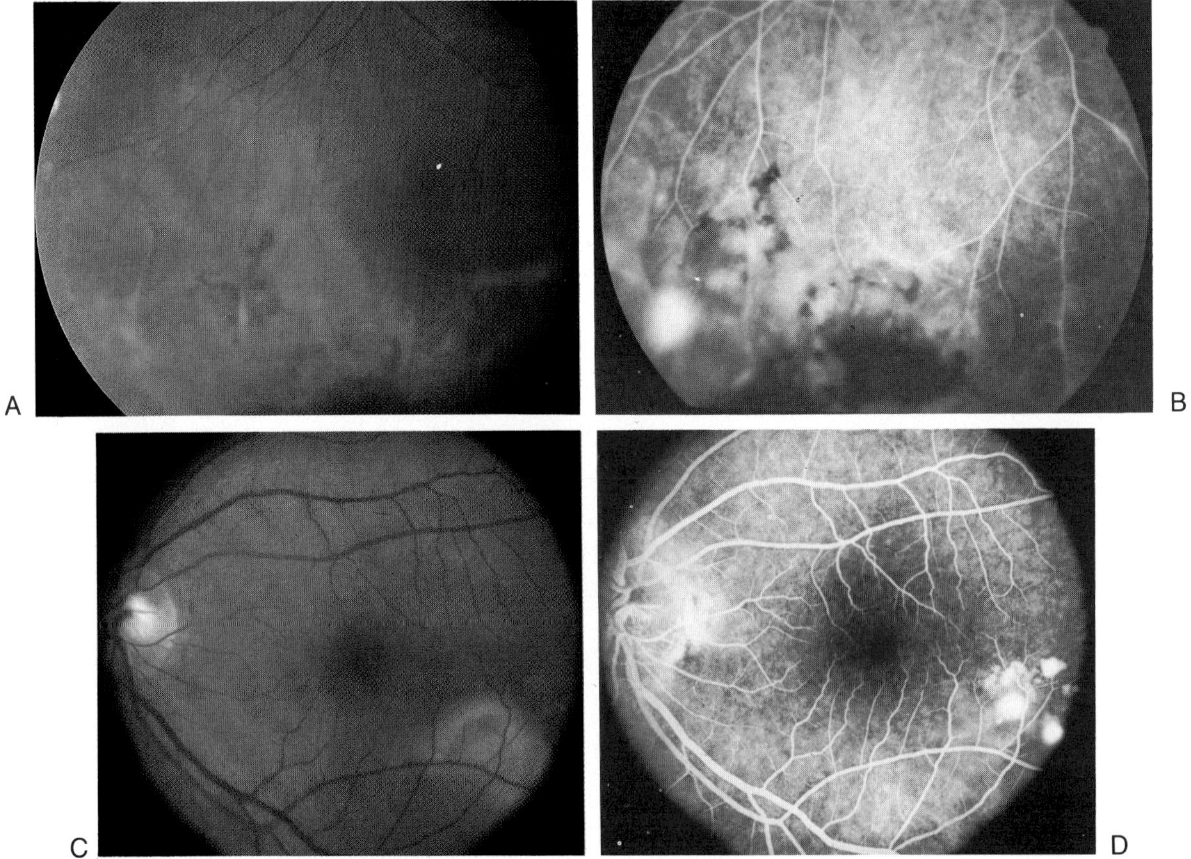

FIGURE 3–169 **Retinal manifestation of systemic lupus erythematosus.** *A* and *B,* There is peripheral retinal vasculitis with areas of intraretinal hemorrhage, retinal nonperfusion, and retinal neovascularization in this patient with systemic lupus erythematosus. *C* and *D,* Note focal area of serous elevation of the retinal pigment epithelium and sensory retina in a patient with lupus-related choroidopathy.

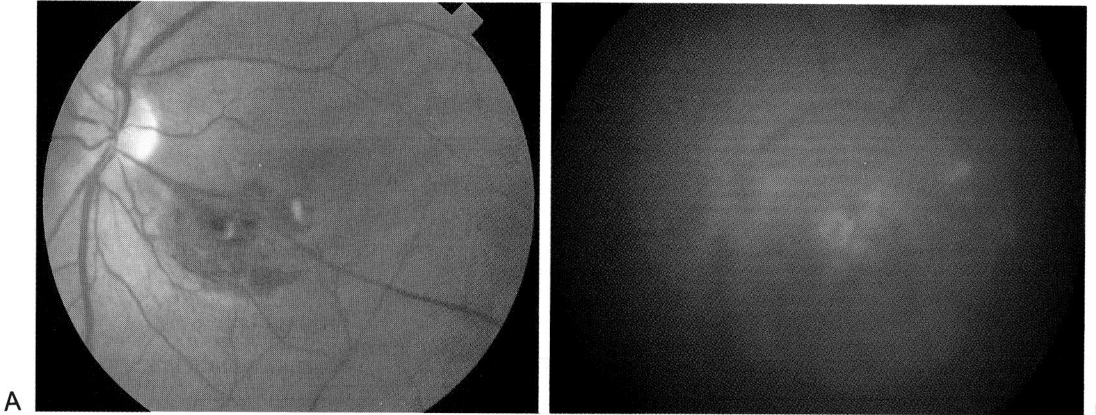

FIGURE 3–170 **Retinal manifestation of polyarteritis nodosa.** *A,* Note the localized area of necrotizing retinal vasculitis associated with intraretinal hemorrhages, cotton-wool spots, and retinal edema in this patient with polyarteritis nodosa. *B,* The media is hazy owing to vitritis associated with progressive ischemic retinal vasculitis.

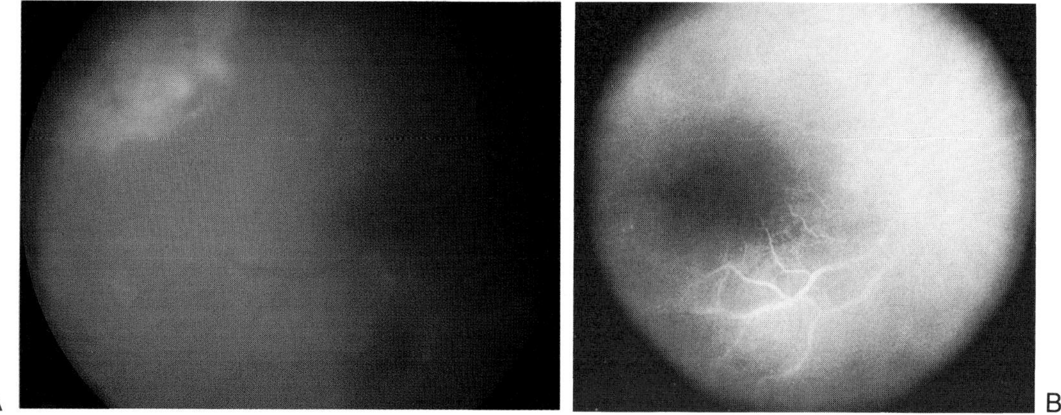

FIGURE 3–171 **Retinal manifestation of Wegener's granulomatosis.** *A,* Note an area of retinitis and retinal vasculitis characterized by retinal whitening and hemorrhage in a patient with biopsy-proven Wegener's granulomatosis. *B,* The fluorescein angiogram illustrates an area of segmental vascular staining and leakage of dye.

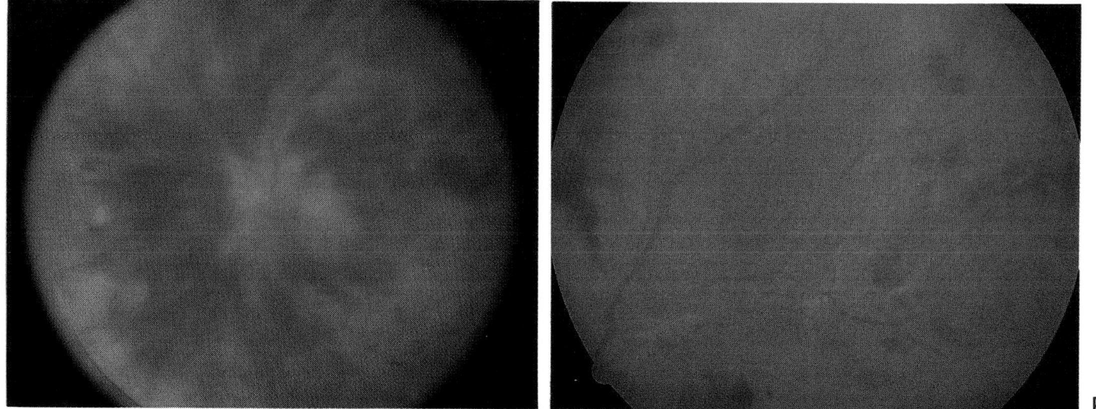

FIGURE 3–172 **Retinal manifestation of Behçet's disease.** *A,* Occlusive retinal vasculitis associated with Behçet's disease results in intraretinal edema, hemorrhages, and retinal nonperfusion. *B,* Note the marked attenuation of the retinal arterioles resulting from progressive damage to the sensory retina.

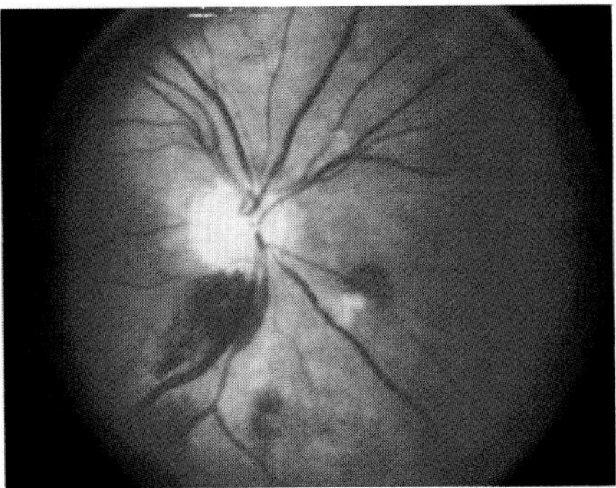

FIGURE 3–173 **Retinopathy associated with anemia.** Fundus findings in anemia may include hemorrhages, cotton-wool spots, and retinal edema. The retinal vessels are usually normal. Note the superficial intraretinal hemorrhages and cotton-wool spots in a patient with severe anemia.

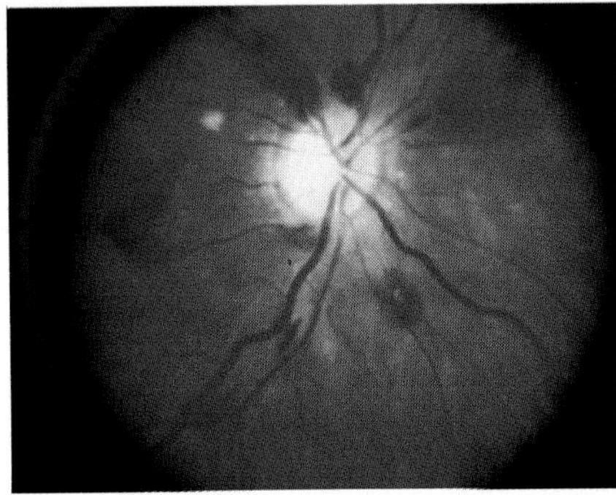

FIGURE 3–174 **Retinopathy associated with anemia.** Note the intraretinal hemorrhages, white-centered hemorrhages (Roth's spots), and cotton-wool spots in a patient with aplastic anemia. The incidence of retinal hemorrhage increases with the severity of the anemia. White-centered hemorrhages may be seen more often in patients with aplastic or pernicious anemia.

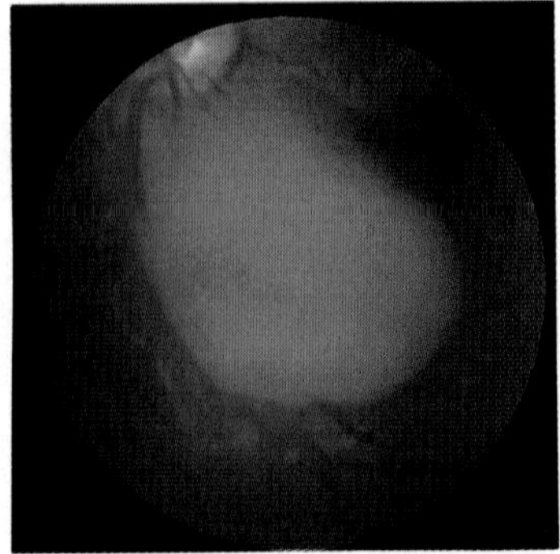

FIGURE 3–175 **Retinopathy associated with leukemia.** The fundus in patients with leukemia may show venous dilatation and tortuosity, preretinal and vitreous hemorrhages, cotton-wool spots, retinal hemorrhages, and leukemic infiltrates. Note the large intraretinal infiltrate in a patient with leukemia. (From Schachat AP, Markowitz JA, Guyer DR, et al: Ophthalmic manifestations of leukemia. Arch Ophthalmol 107:698, 1989. Copyright 1989, American Medical Association.)

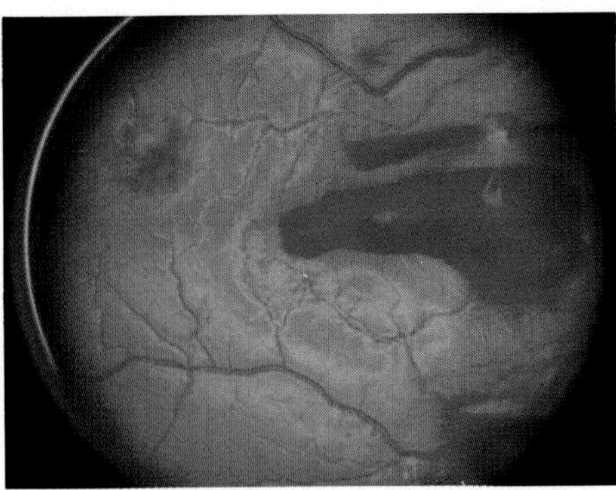

FIGURE 3–176 **Retinopathy associated with leukemia.** Note the intraretinal and preretinal hemorrhages in a patient with acute lymphocytic leukemia. The hemorrhages are likely to result from associated anemia and thrombocytopenia.

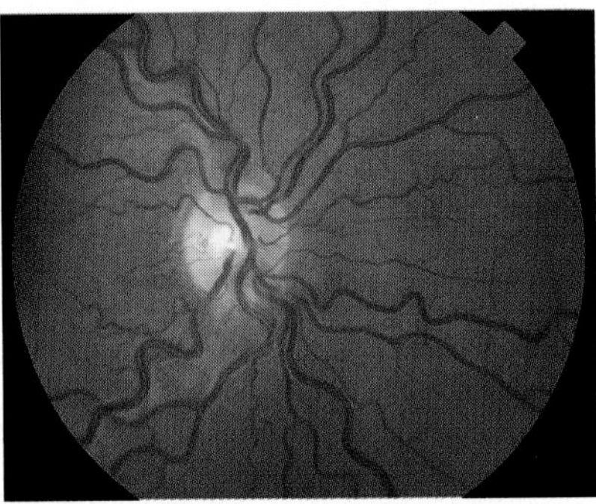

FIGURE 3–177 **Retinopathy associated with polycythemia.** This fundus photograph of a patient with secondary polycythemia shows retinal vascular dilatation and tortuosity. The disc is usually hyperemic and swollen. Central or branch retinal vein occlusion may occur and result in loss of vision. A similar fundus picture is seen in patients with other conditions that result in blood hyperviscosity.

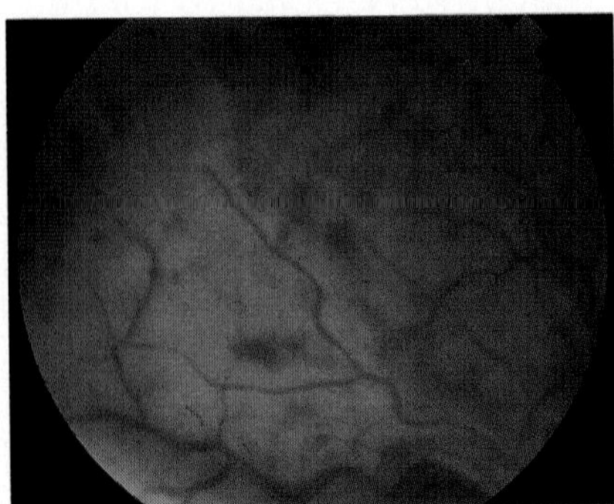

FIGURE 3–178 **Retinopathy associated with dysproteinemia.** Retinal vascular dilatation and tortuosity, with intraretinal hemorrhage, is noted in a patient with hyperviscosity owing to dysproteinemia. Conditions associated with blood hyperviscosity include multiple myeloma, cryomacroglobulinemia, hypergammaglobulinemia, and Waldenström's macroglobulinemia. The incidence of retinopathy correlates with the degree of anemia but not with the level of total serum protein.

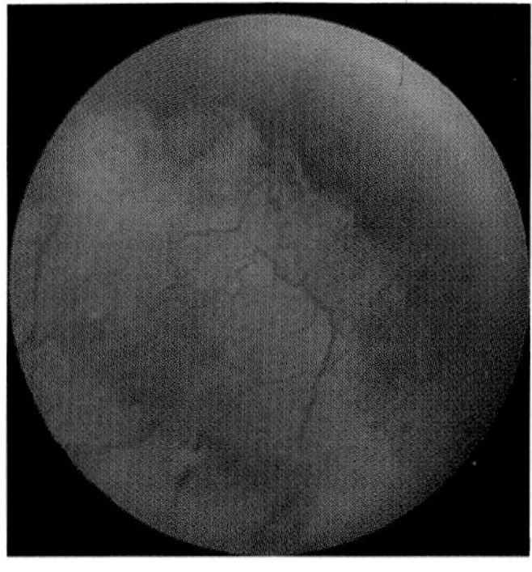

FIGURE 3–195 **Nonproliferative sickle cell retinopathy.** Areas of whitening of peripheral retina similar to the white-without-pressure sign seen in the general population have been described in patients with sickle cell disease.

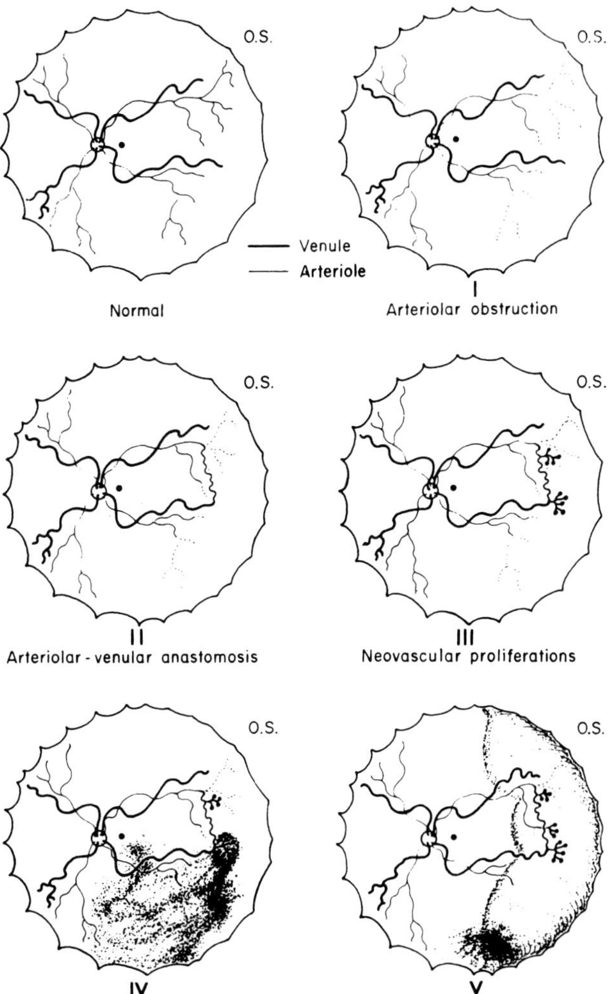

FIGURE 3–196 **Stages of proliferative sickle cell retinopathy.** Proliferative sickle retinopathy can be classified into five stages. Stage I is characterized by peripheral retinal arteriolar occlusion. Stage II is characterized by peripheral arteriolar-venular anastomoses. Stage III is characterized by neovascular proliferation at the interface of vascular and avascular retina. Stage IV is characterized by vitreous hemorrhage caused by bleeding from the peripheral neovascular tufts. Stage V is characterized by retinal detachment resulting from vitreous traction bands. (From Goldberg MF: Classification and pathogenesis of proliferative sickle retinopathy. Am J Ophthalmol 71:654, 1971. Published with permission from The American Journal of Ophthalmology. Copyright by The Ophthalmic Publishing Company.)

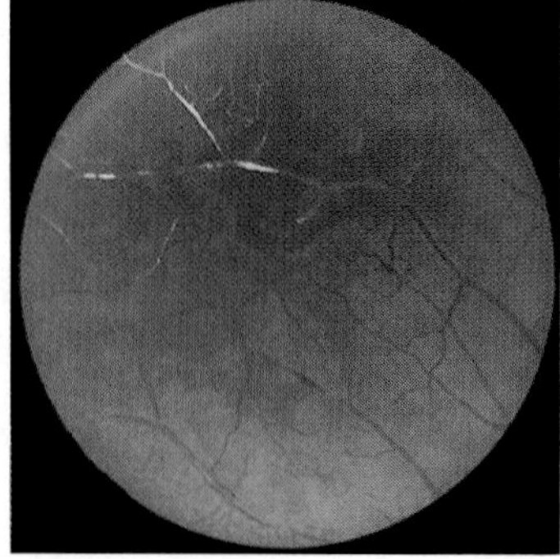

FIGURE 3-197 **Proliferative sickle cell retinopathy.** Stage I of proliferative sickle retinopathy is characterized by peripheral arteriolar occlusions seen as "silverwire" vessels.

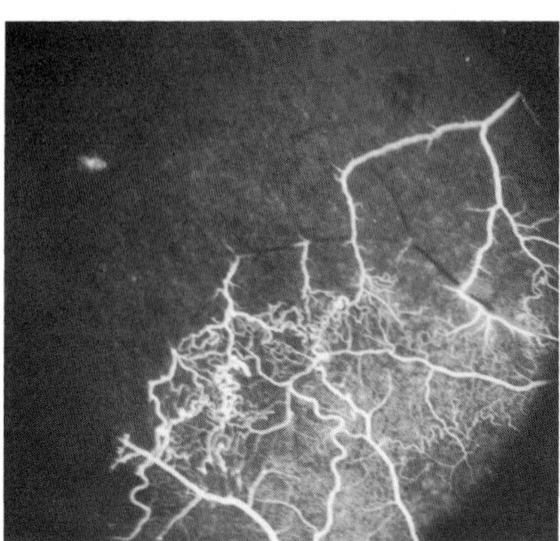

FIGURE 3-198 **Fluorescein angiographic findings in proliferative sickle cell retinopathy.** Fluorescein angiography of stage I of proliferative sickle retinopathy shows occluded peripheral retinal vessels with adjacent areas of avascular retina.

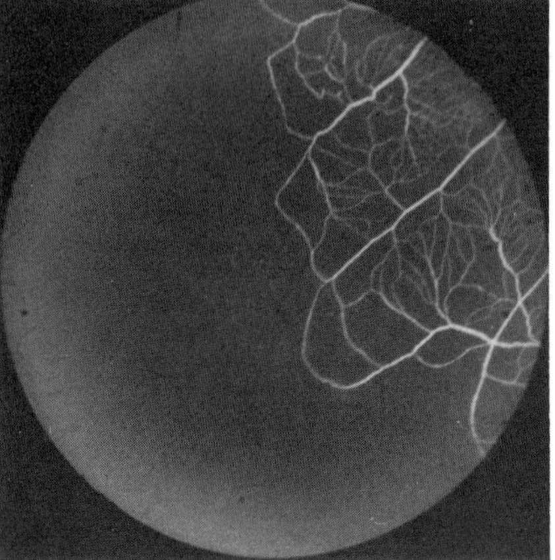

FIGURE 3-199 **Fluorescein angiographic findings in proliferative sickle cell retinopathy.** Fluorescein angiography of stage II of proliferative sickle retinopathy shows characteristic arteriolar-venular anastomoses adjacent to areas of avascular retina.

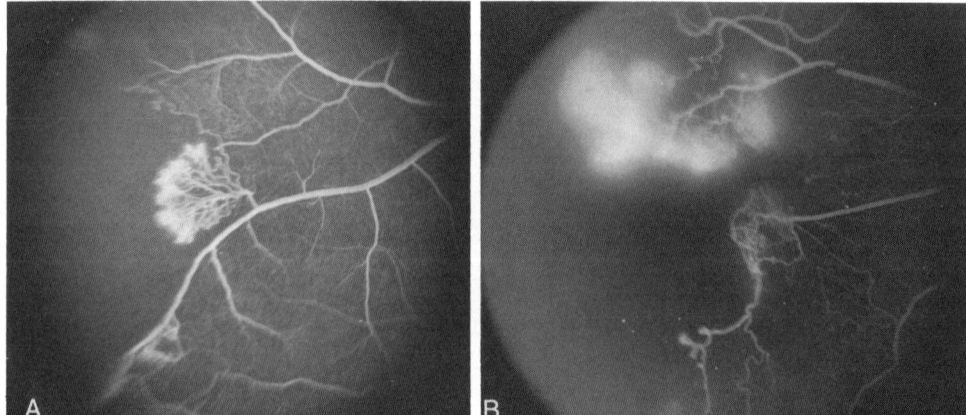

FIGURE 3-200 **Proliferative sickle cell retinopathy.** Stage III of proliferative sickle retinopathy is characterized by neovascular proliferation at the peripheral interface between vascular and avascular retina. *A,* Fluorescein angiography shows characteristic sea fan neovascularization in the peripheral retina. *B,* In late-phase angiogram, leakage of dye is seen in areas of neovascularization. Inferior to the sea fan, arteriolar-venular anastomosis is seen also with early neovascularization.

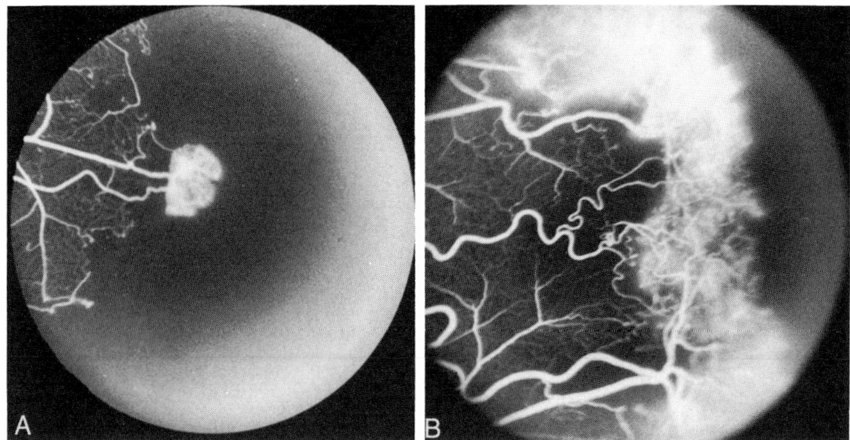

FIGURE 3-201 **Fluoroangiographic findings in proliferative sickle cell retinopathy.** *A,* Fluorescein angiogram of sea fan neovascularization shows a single feeder vessel and two draining venules. *B,* Sea fan neovascularization may have multiple feeder arterioles and draining venules.

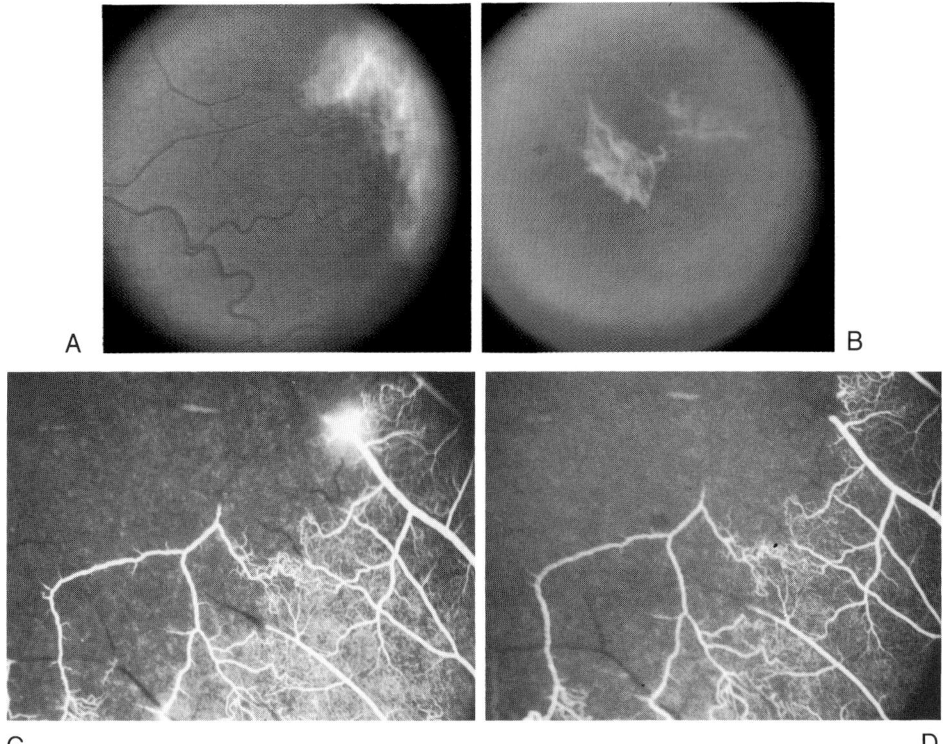

FIGURE 3-202 **Proliferative sickle cell retinopathy.** *A* and *B,* Color fundus photographs show white peripheral patches of gliotic tissue that represent autoinfarcted areas of sea fan neovascularization. *C,* Fluorescein angiogram of peripheral avascular retina shows a patch of neovascularization that is leaking fluorescein. *D,* Fluorescein angiogram of the same area several days later shows no leakage of fluorescein owing to autoinfarction of the neovascular tissue. (*C* and *D,* From Nagpal KC, Patrianakos D, Asdourian GK, et al: Spontaneous regression (autoinfarction) of proliferative sickle retinopathy. Am J Ophthalmol 80:886, 1975. Published with permission from The American Journal of Ophthalmology. Copyright by The Ophthalmic Publishing Company.)

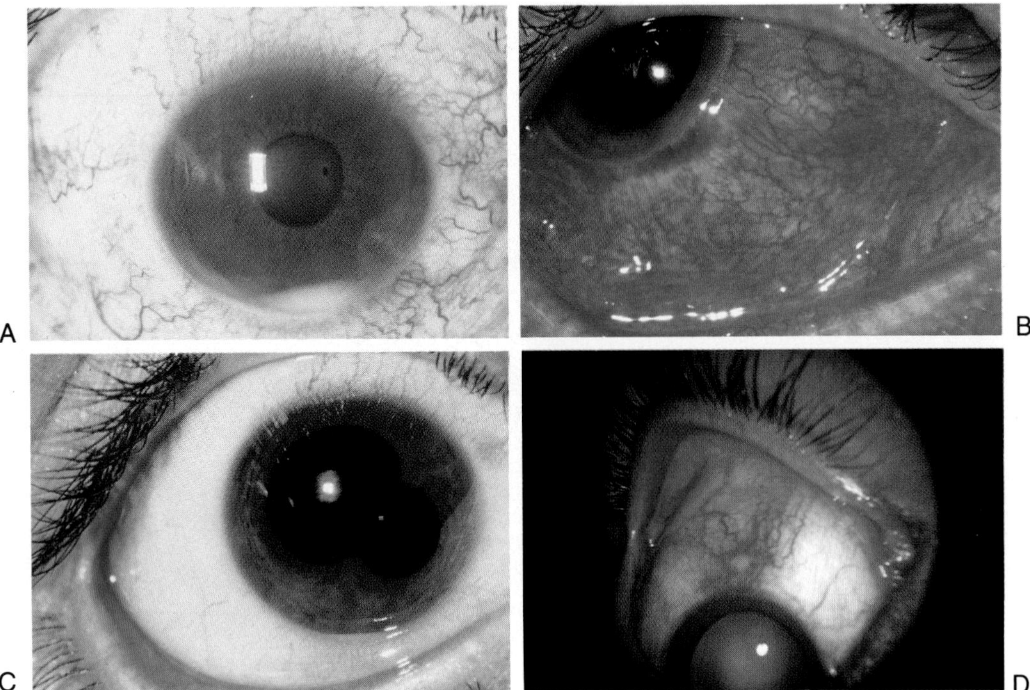

FIGURE 3-203 **Anterior segment findings of Behçet's disease.** Behçet's disease is characterized by nongranulomatous inflammation with necrotizing vasculitis, which can involve the anterior or posterior segments of the eye. *A,* The classic anterior segment finding in ocular Behçet's disease is iridocyclitis with hypopyon, which is present in 19 to 31 percent of cases. *B,* A more common anterior segment finding is iridocyclitis without hypopyon because the hypopyon may disappear rapidly or change with position. Note the subconjunctival hemorrhage, which also can be seen in these patients. *C,* Iris atrophy and posterior synechiae can result from chronic or recurrent iridocyclitis. *D,* Episcleritis is a less frequent finding. Note the sectoral dilation and injection of episcleral tissue.

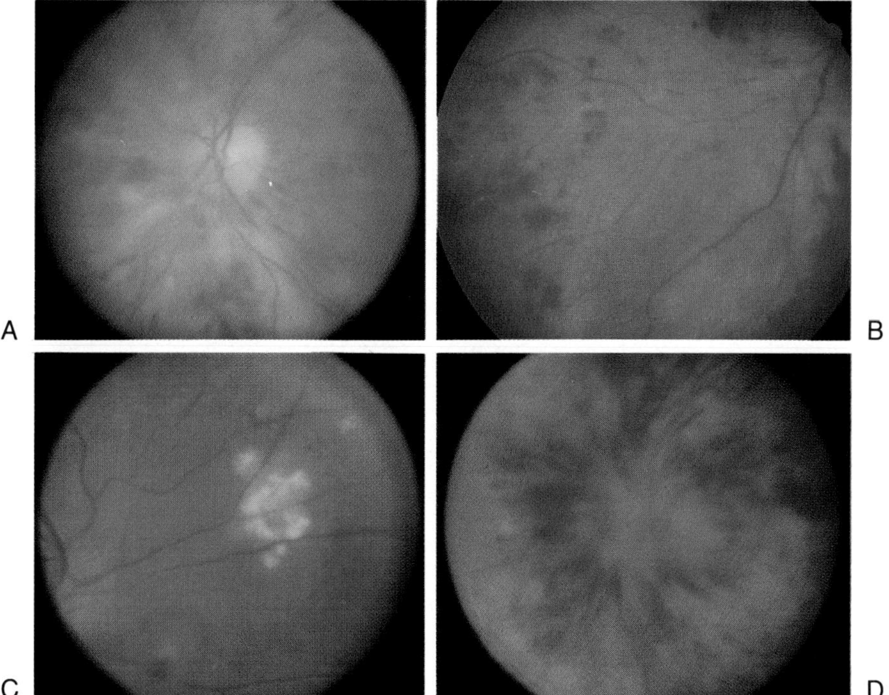

FIGURE 3–204 **Posterior segment findings of Behçet's disease.** The posterior segment findings during the acute phase include vitritis and retinal vasculitis affecting both the arteries and veins. *A,* Note the vitreous haze, retinal vessel engorgement, and retinal hemorrhages. *B,* Note the patchy, perivascular sheathing with surrounding retinal hemorrhages involving the inferotemporal vessels. *C,* Yellow and white inflammatory exudates are seen in the deeper layers of the retina. *D,* Severe retinal vasculitis can lead to thrombosis of the vessels, resulting in a retinal artery or vein occlusion.

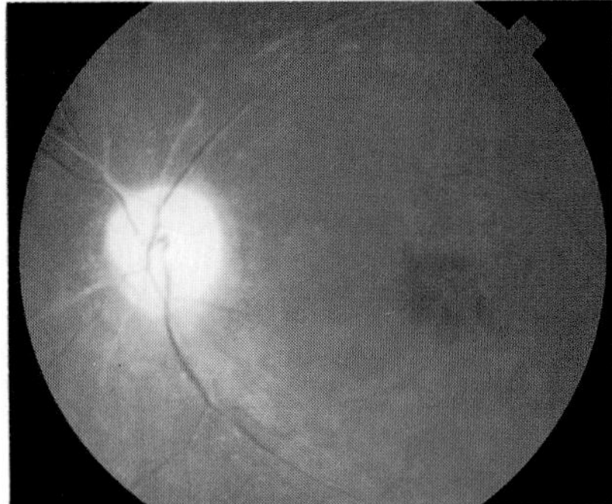

FIGURE 3–205 **Chronic phase of Behçet's disease.** During the chronic phase of the disease, optic atrophy, macular pigmentary degeneration, and attenuation of the retinal vessels are seen in the fundus. Slit-lamp biomicroscopy may show a few cells in the anterior chamber, patchy iris atrophy, and posterior synechiae.

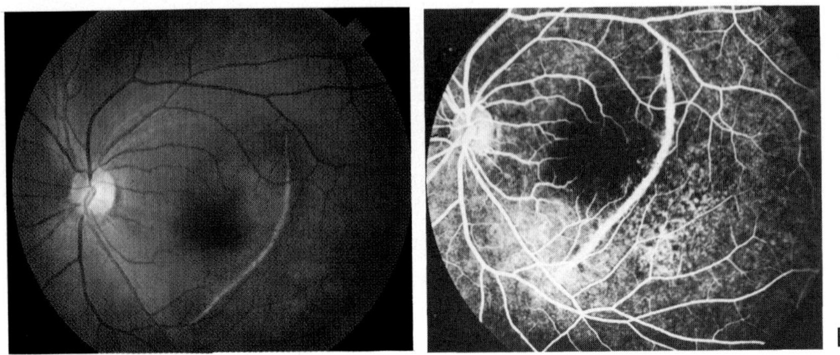

FIGURE 3–206 **Choroidal rupture: fundus and angiographic findings.** *A,* An oblique linear choroidal defect is seen temporal to the fovea in this patient who sustained blunt ocular trauma. *B,* The choroidal defect is hyperfluorescent on fluorescein angiography. Anterior choroidal ruptures are usually oriented parallel to the ora serrata. Posterior choroidal ruptures are often crescentically oriented around the optic nerve.

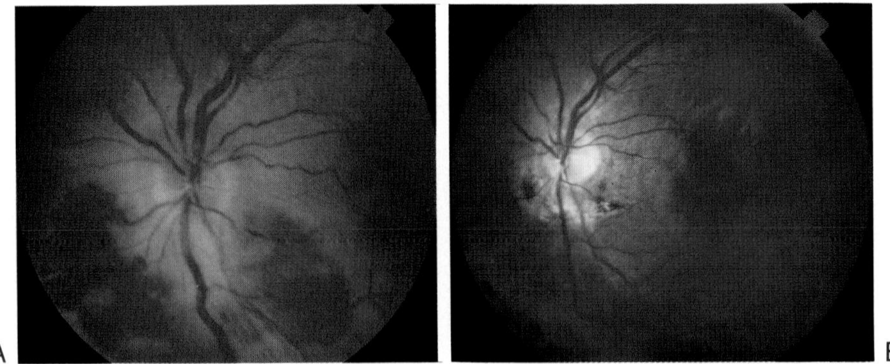

FIGURE 3–207 **Choroidal rupture: acute and chronic appearance.** *A,* Acutely, there is commotio retinae with retinal and subretinal hemorrhage. *B,* Two months later, after clearing of the hemorrhage, a choroidal rupture is seen. Patients with choroidal rupture are at risk for the development of choroidal neovascularization months or years following the initial injury.

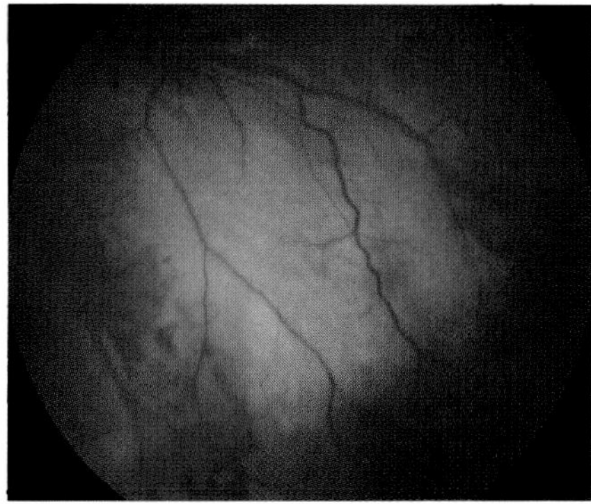

FIGURE 3–208 **Commotio retinae.** There is retinal whitening in the extramacular retina, which by histopathology represents disruption of photoreceptor cells and outer segments. One month later, the retinal whitening had resolved, but there is residual pigment migration into the retina.

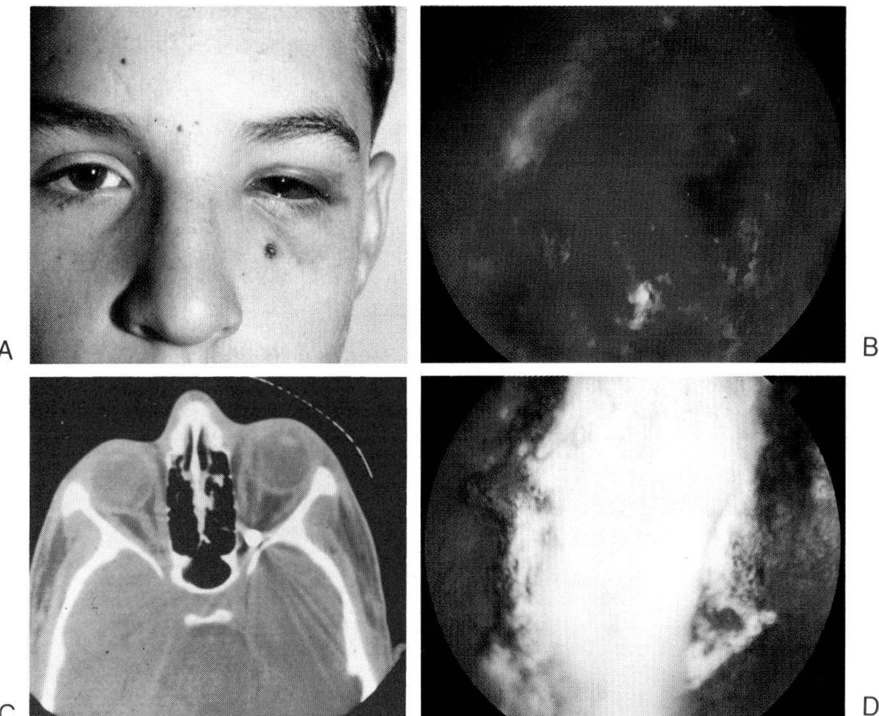

FIGURE 3–209 **Chorioretinitis sclopetaria.** *A,* This 16-year-old boy was shot through the eyelid with a BB gun. Visual acuity was 8/200, and there is eyelid edema and subconjunctival hemorrhage. *B,* Fundus photograph of the inferonasal quadrant shows the acute appearance of retinal and choroidal rupture in the absence of a scleral laceration. *C,* A computed tomogram showed the BB to be located at the orbital apex with no evidence of globe perforation. *D,* Seven months later, the vision had improved to 20/70. A white scar with pigment proliferation and intraretinal pigment migration is seen in the same area as *B.* Trauma to the choroid and retina in chorioretinitis sclopetaria is caused by transmitted shock waves from a high-velocity projectile penetrating the orbit but not the globe.

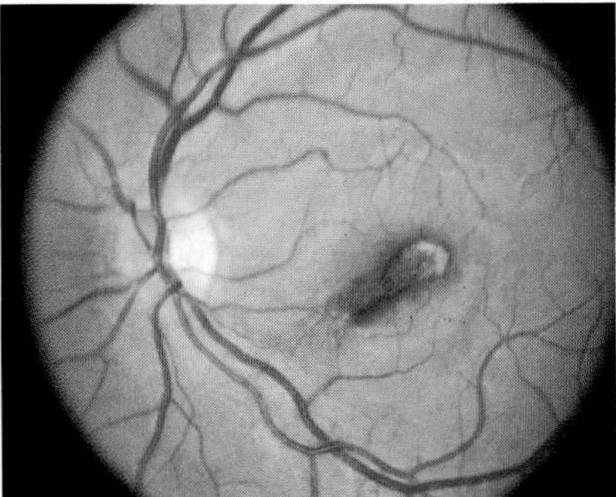

FIGURE 3–210 **Valsalva maculopathy.** This 22-year-old man noted decreased vision and a central scotoma after a coughing episode 3 weeks before presentation. The vision is 20/50, and there is preretinal hemorrhage in the macula, which is partially hemolysed. One month later, the hemorrhage was nearly resolved, and the visual acuity had improved to 20/25. Valsalva retinopathy may be associated with heavy lifting, coughing, vomiting, or straining at stool. The rupture of superficial retinal capillaries is presumed secondary to increases in retinal venous pressure caused by a rapid rise in intrathoracic or intra-abdominal pressure.

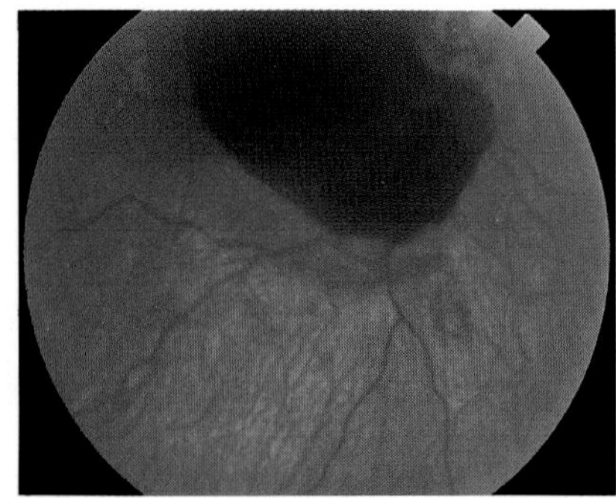

FIGURE 3–211 **Shaken baby syndrome.** This 1-month-old infant was hospitalized with subarachnoid and subdural hemorrhages after child abuse. A fundus photograph shows a large macular subinternal limiting membrane hemorrhage. There is associated intraretinal hemorrhage temporally. Retinal hemorrhages and cotton-wool spots may be seen after sustained violent shaking or after direct eye, head, or chest trauma. Vitreous hemorrhage and papilledema may occur in isolation or may be associated with subdural or subarachnoid or cerebral contusions.

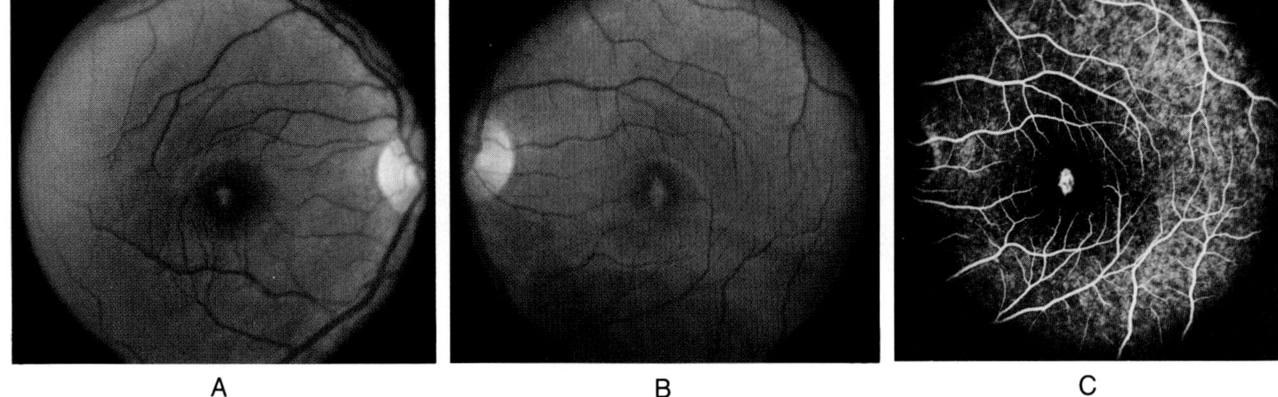

FIGURE 3–212 **Solar retinopathy: remote findings.** *A* and *B,* Fundus photographs of a 27-year-old man with a history of sun gazing 1 year before presentation. There is a reddish yellow discoloration of the foveal reflex in both eyes. *C,* Fluorescein angiography of the left eye shows increased fluorescence in the fovea, which corresponds to the foveal lesion seen on the color photographs. The mechanism of solar retinopathy is thought to be photochemical damage caused by high-energy shortwave-visible blue light and ultraviolet radiation or near ultraviolet (320 – to 400 nm) radiation. (*A* and *B,* Courtesy of Mark W. Balles, M.D.)

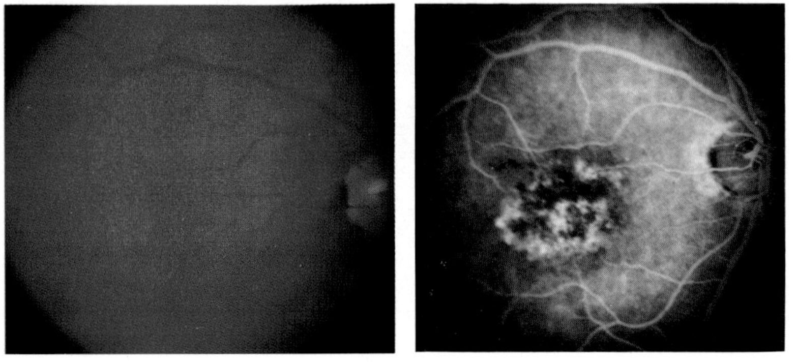

FIGURE 3–213 **Photic retinopathy from operating room microscope: remote findings.** *A,* This 67-year-old man underwent cataract extraction 2 years earlier. The visual acuity is 20/50, and there is a subtle rounded area of depigmentation in the macula. *B,* On fluorescein angiography, there is mottled hyperfluorescence corresponding to the lesion seen on the color photographs. Prolonged operating times and high-intensity light sources are risk factors for the development of photic retinopathy.

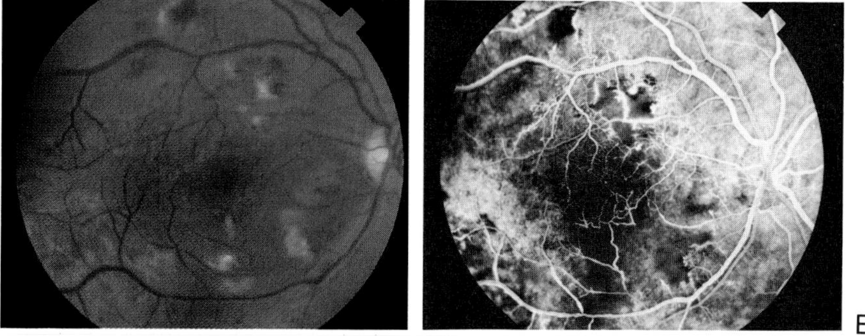

FIGURE 3-214 **Radiation retinopathy after proton beam irradiation of choroidal melanoma.** *A,* Fundus photograph shows cotton-wool spots, retinal hemorrhages, microaneurysms, and telangiectatic vessels. *B,* Fluorescein angiography of the same eye highlights the microvascular changes, including capillary nonperfusion, microaneurysms, and telangiectasia. The histopathologic features of radiation retinopathy are occlusion of retinal vessels and thickening of vessel walls by fibrillar and hyaline material.

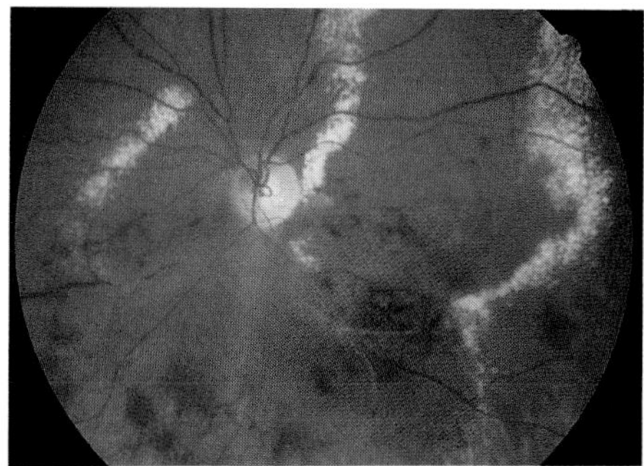

FIGURE 3-215 **Radiation retinopathy after proton beam irradiation of choroidal melanoma.** Fundus photograph shows extensive macular edema, vascular occlusions, intraretinal hemorrhages, and retinal exudation. Macular edema may precede other findings early in the course of radiation retinopathy.

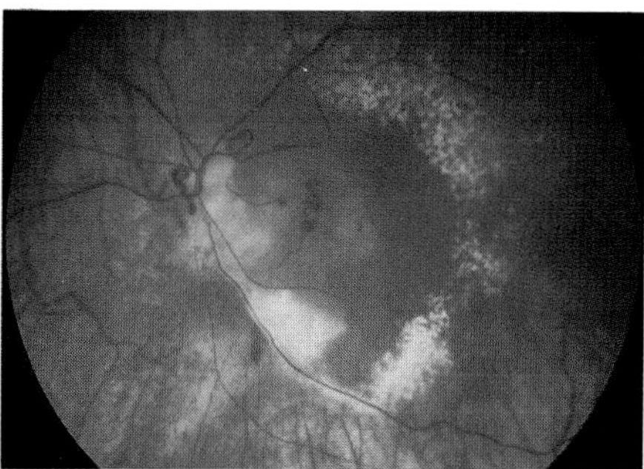

FIGURE 3-216 **Radiation retinopathy with severe macular edema.** There is extensive retinal exudation at the interface between edematous and nonedematous retina. Vascular sheathing is visible along the inferotemporal arcade. Vascular changes in radiation retinopathy usually become apparent months to years after treatment.

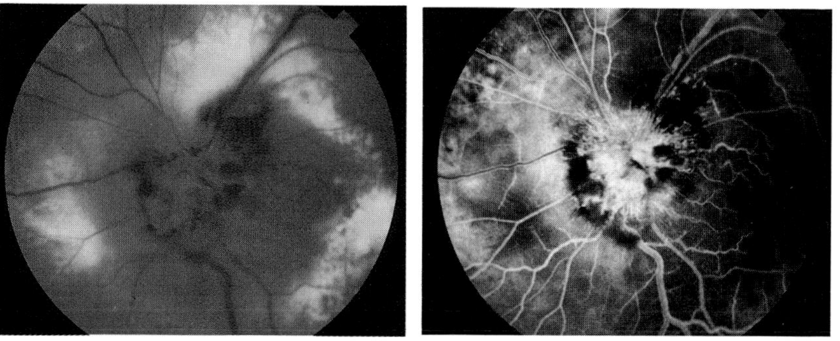

FIGURE 3-217 **Radiation papillopathy.** *A,* There is extensive disc edema with hemorrhages and peripapillary retinal exudation. *B,* Fluorescein angiography of the same optic disc shows dilatation and tortuosity of disc capillaries as well as areas of capillary nonperfusion. Other findings that may occur after radiation therapy include optic disc pallor and, less commonly, optic disc neovascularization.

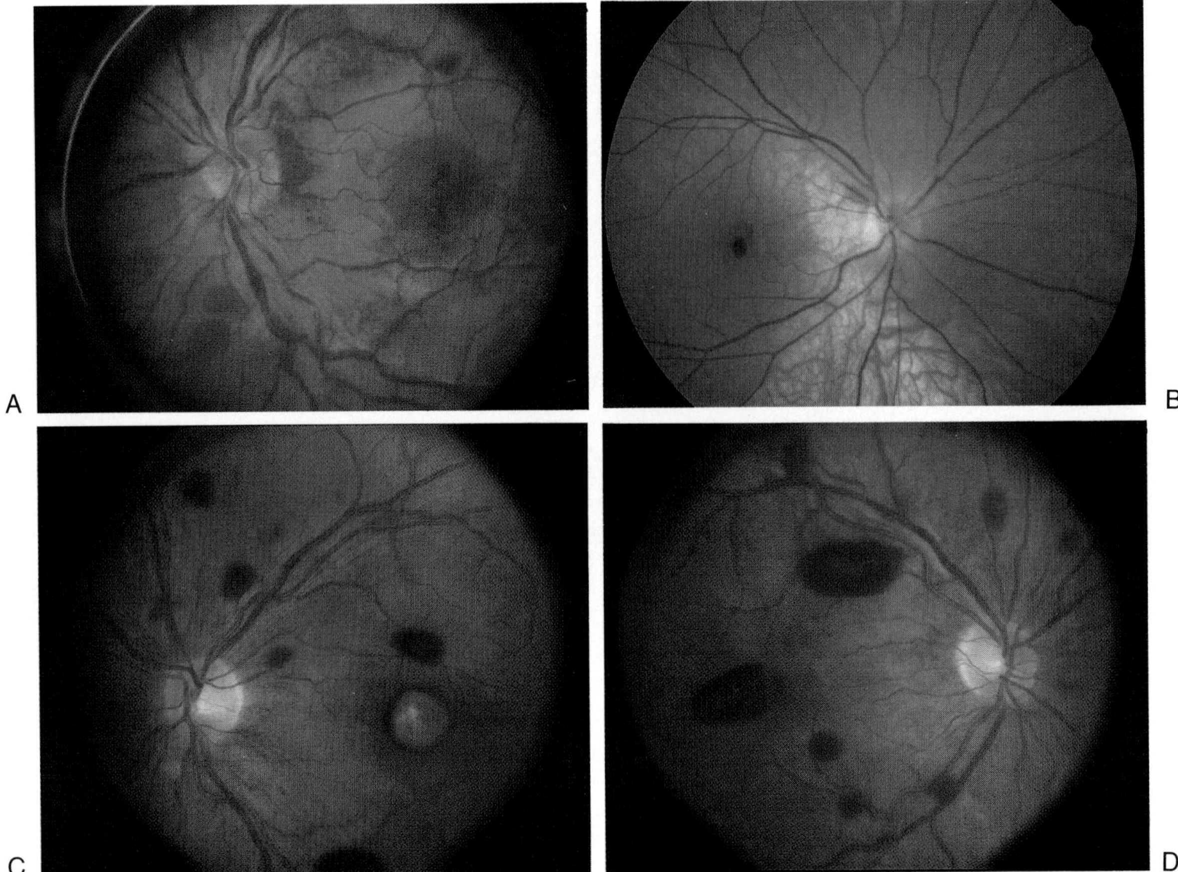

FIGURE 3–218 **High altitude retinopathy (HAR).** *A,* A florid example in a 26-year-old male physician caused by hypoxia sustained at 25,000 feet altitude on Mount Everest. Extensive intraretinal hemorrhages and early papilledema were present in both eyes. Concurrent high altitude cerebral edema (HACE) rapidly improved on descent. Treatment regimen included oxygen, diuretics, and prednisone. HAR resolved over 6 weeks, with normal vision in both eyes. *B,* Solitary macular hemorrhage noted in 28-year-old male on summitting Mount McKinley (20,320 feet). Spontaneous onset of metamorphopsia and blurred vision of 20/400 in the right eye, without antecedent Valsalva exertion, occurred during resting. Two years later, residual superofoveal pigment dispersion and Amsler chart distortion remained, with a vision of 20/30-. *C,* At relatively moderate altitudes of 10,000 to 15,000 feet in hiking, skiing, and amateur climbing areas, altitude retinopathy can occur. A 20-year-old male sustained marked left macular and peripheral retinal hemorrhages and transudates at 14,000 feet with a vision of 10/200. *D,* In the right eye, the vision was 20/30 in the same patient as shown in *C.* HAR is always bilateral, varying only in degree. At 1 year follow-up, vision was OD 20/250 and OS 20/40. This hiker had concurrent mild HACE and high altitude pulmonary edema of the altitude illness syndrome. (Courtesy of Michael Wiedman, M.D.)

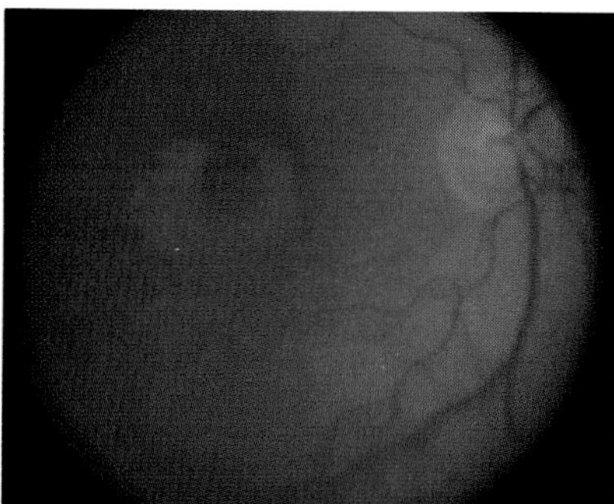

FIGURE 3–219 **Bull's eye maculopathy secondary to chloroquine and hydrochloroquine toxicity.** Fundus photograph shows circular zone of depigmentation surrounding the fovea. This zone is typically horizontally oval and may be more prominent inferiorly. Advanced cases of chloroquine or hydroxychloroquine toxicity may also show peripheral pigmentary abnormalities, vascular attenuation, and optic disc pallor.

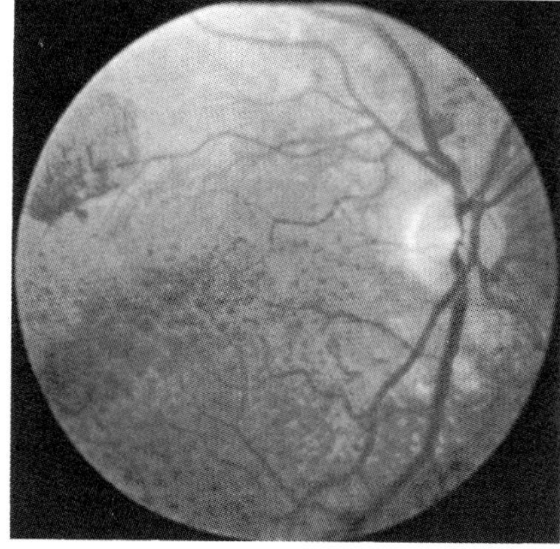

FIGURE 3–220 **Thioridazine retinal toxicity.** Fundus photograph showing coarse pigment granularity and larger pigmented plaques in a patient treated with large doses of thioridazine. Patients with acute thioridazine retinal toxicity may complain of blurred vision, nyctalopia, or a brownish discoloration in vision, which usually improves after discontinuation of the drug. (From Davidorf FH: Thioridazine pigmentary retinopathy. Arch Ophthalmol 90:251–255, 1973. Copyright 1973, American Medical Association.)

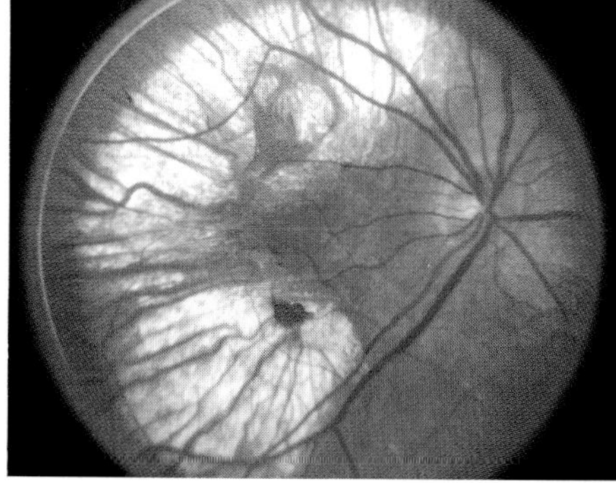

FIGURE 3–221 **Advanced thioridazine retinopathy.** Fundus photograph shows large geographic areas of atrophy of the retina, pigment epithelium, and choriocapillaris. These areas of geographic atrophy may enlarge and become more confluent over time.

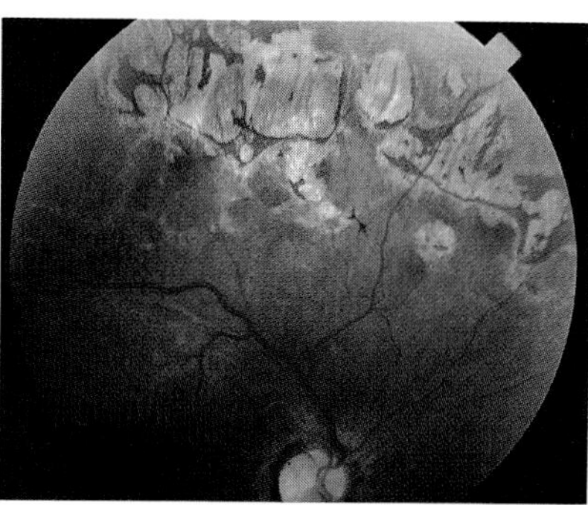

FIGURE 3–222 **Thioridazine retinopathy associated with chronic use (nummular retinopathy).** Fundus photograph shows rounded areas of retinal pigment epithelial depigmentation and hyperplasia posterior to the equator. In contrast to more acute forms of toxicity, the macula is often spared. (Courtesy of Lee M. Jampol, M.D.)

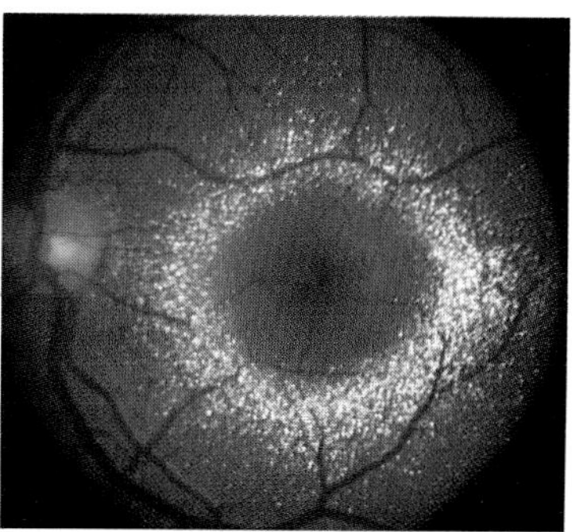

FIGURE 3–223 **Canthaxanthin retinopathy.** Fundus photograph shows innumerable iridescent crystals in the inner retina. These crystals are deposited in a ring around the fovea. Histopathologically the birefringent crystals are located in the nerve fiber layer and are most prominent paracentrally. (Courtesy of Paul Arrigg, M.D.)

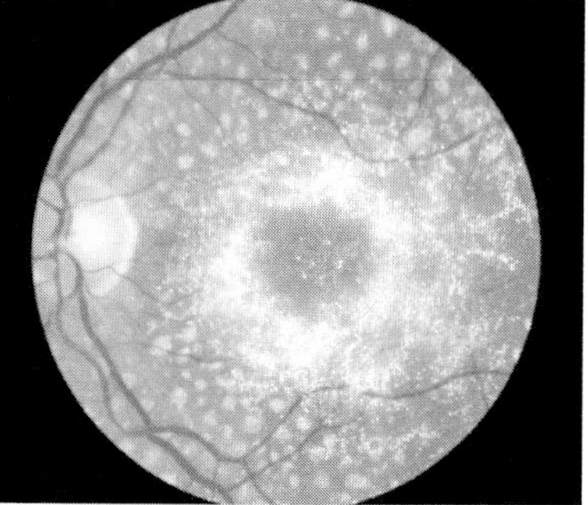

FIGURE 3–224 **Tamoxifen retinopathy.** Fundus photograph shows fine refractile intraretinal crystals and granular deposits at the level of the retinal pigment epithelium in a patient on high-dose tamoxifen chemotherapy for breast cancer. There was cystoid macular edema present on fluorescein angiography. White whorl-like subepithelial corneal deposits have also been described after tamoxifen therapy. (From McKeown CA, Swartz M, Blom J, Maggiano JM: Tamoxifen retinopathy. Br J Ophthalmol 65:177–179, 1981.)

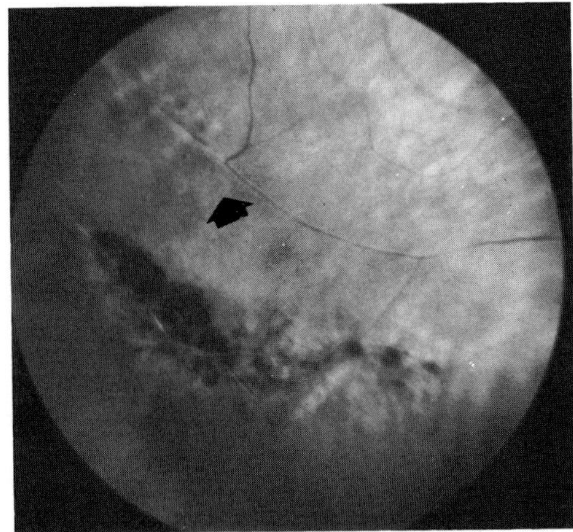

FIGURE 3–225 **Clinical appearance of lattice degeneration.** The fundus photograph shows two parallel rows. The upper *(arrow),* paravascular in orientation without pigmentation, shows surface white dots and vascular sheathing. The lower pigmented patch of lattice degeneration shows a prominent interlacing pattern of white lines, representing hyalinized blood vessels.

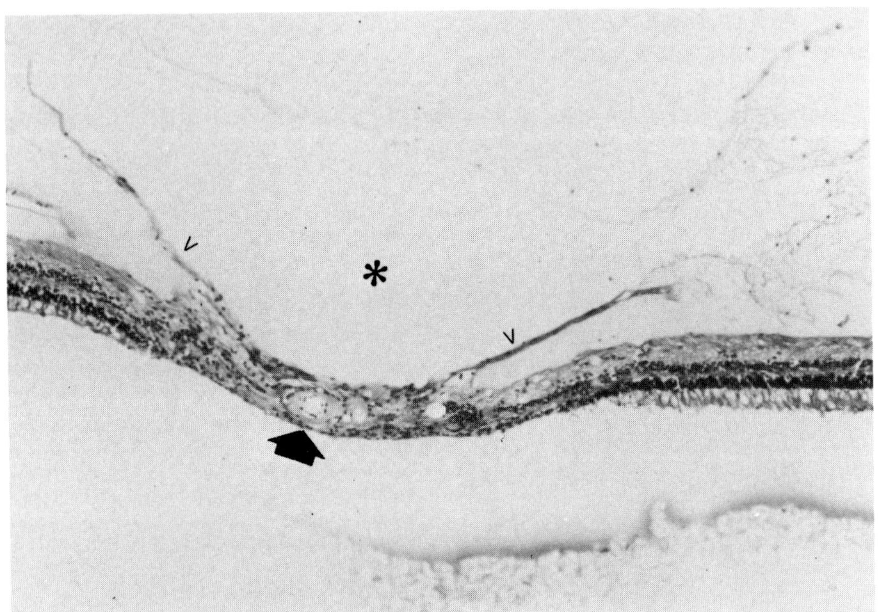

FIGURE 3–226 **Histopathology of lattice degeneration.** Cross-sectional view with anterior border to the left. Separation of the sensory retina from the retinal pigment epithelium is fixation artifact. *V* indicates condensed sheets of vitreous collagen firmly adherent to the anterior and posterior borders. The *asterisk* represents an overlying pool of liquefied vitreous. The *arrow* shows a thick-walled, hyalinized blood vessel.

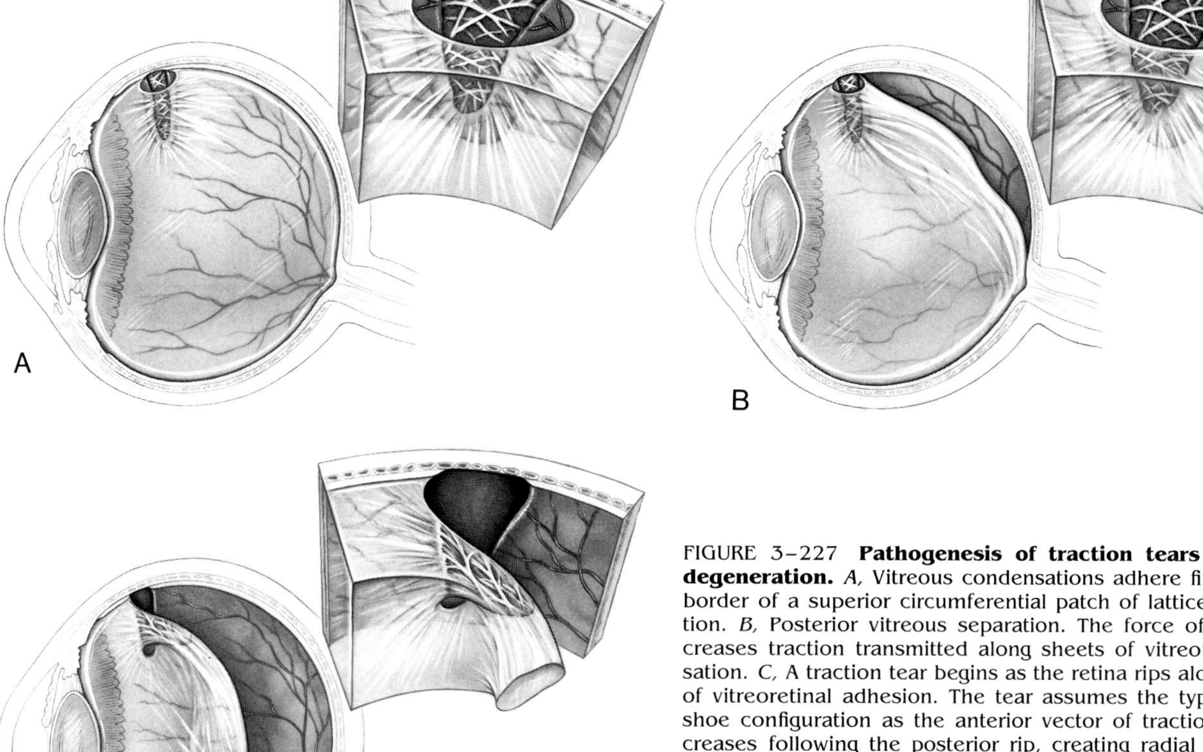

FIGURE 3–227 **Pathogenesis of traction tears in lattice degeneration.** *A,* Vitreous condensations adhere firmly to the border of a superior circumferential patch of lattice degeneration. *B,* Posterior vitreous separation. The force of gravity increases traction transmitted along sheets of vitreous condensation. *C,* A traction tear begins as the retina rips along the line of vitreoretinal adhesion. The tear assumes the typical horseshoe configuration as the anterior vector of traction force increases following the posterior rip, creating radial extensions toward the ora serrata at each end of the patch of lattice degeneration.

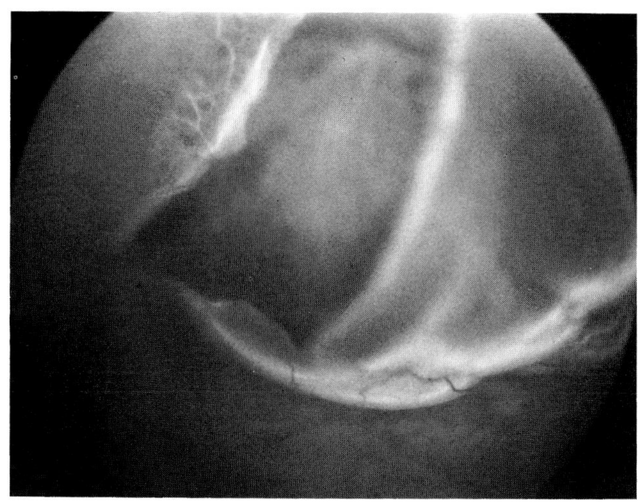

FIGURE 3–228 **Traction tears in lattice degeneration.** Fundus photograph shows a bullous retinal detachment associated with a large retinal tear occurring at the border of lattice degeneration. Strong vitreoretinal adhesions at the borders or edge of lattice degeneration may cause retinal tears after posterior vitreous detachment.

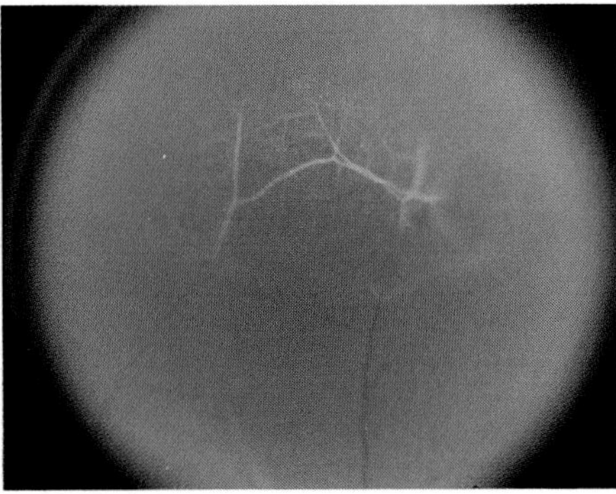

FIGURE 3–229 **Lattice retinal degeneration.** Fundus photograph of detached retina shows an oval, equatorially oriented patch of thinned retina with criss-crossing white lines (sclerotic vessels) and pigment clumps. Histopathologically the retina is thinned, the overlying vitreous is liquefied, and there is strong vitreous adhesion at its margins.

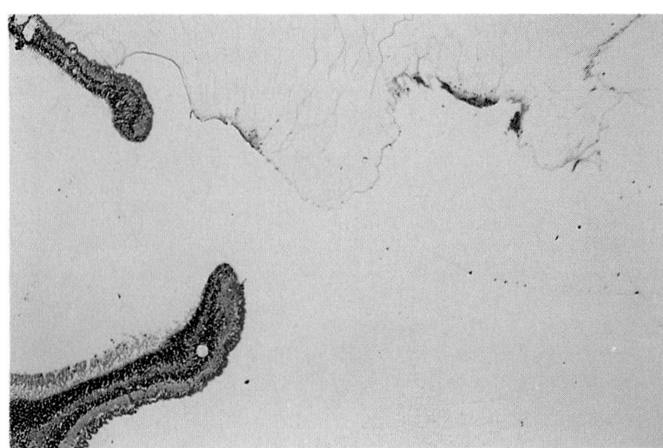

FIGURE 3–232 **Histopathology of retinal horseshoe tear.** The vitreous is adherent to the anterior flap of the tear, exerting traction on it. There is artifactual elevation of the posterior retina. PAS stain.

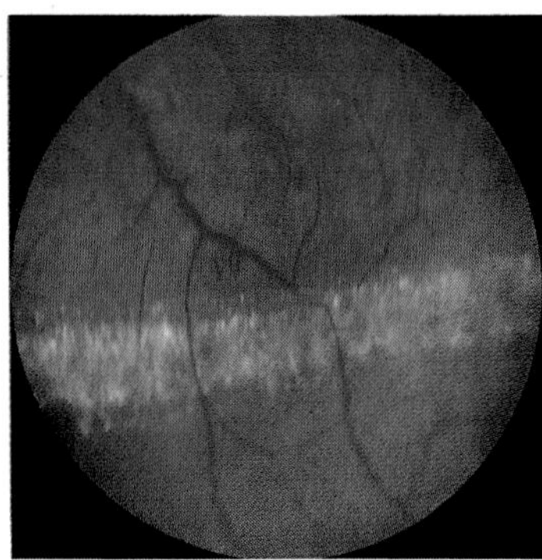

FIGURE 3–230 **Snail track degeneration.** Fundus photograph shows a linear band of yellow-white flecks at the level of the retina. Although generally acknowledged to be a form of lattice degeneration, snail track degeneration lacks the characteristic criss-crossing white lines.

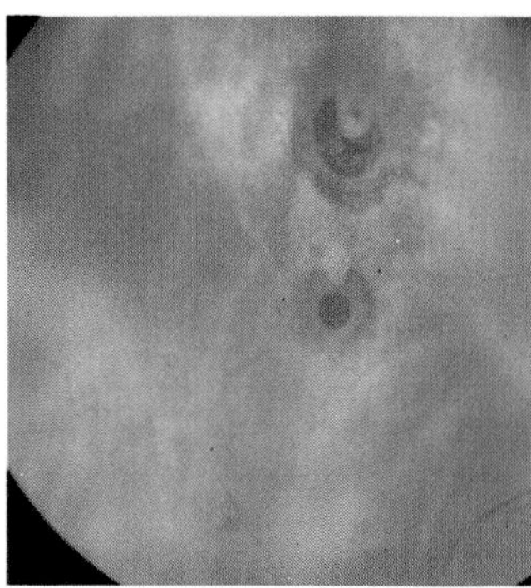

FIGURE 3–233 **Horseshoe and operculated retinal tears.** These two retinal tears were produced in an eye bank eye. The more anterior horseshoe tear was produced with less vitreoretinal traction than was required to produce the operculated retinal hole. Operculated retinal holes exert less vitreous traction than horseshoe tears and may be less likely to lead to retinal detachment.

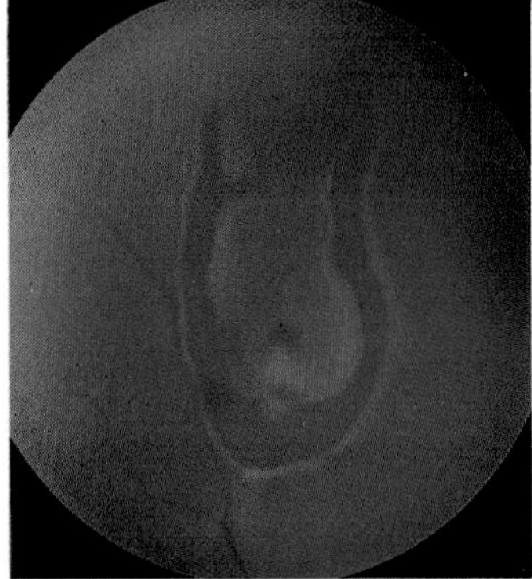

FIGURE 3–231 **Retinal horseshoe tear (flap tear).** Fundus photograph shows a horseshoe retinal tear caused by localized vitreoretinal traction. There are flecks of hemorrhage on the margins of the tear indicating disruption of small retinal vessels. Disruption of retinal vessels may also lead to vitreous hemorrhage, which sometimes obscures visualization of the retinal break.

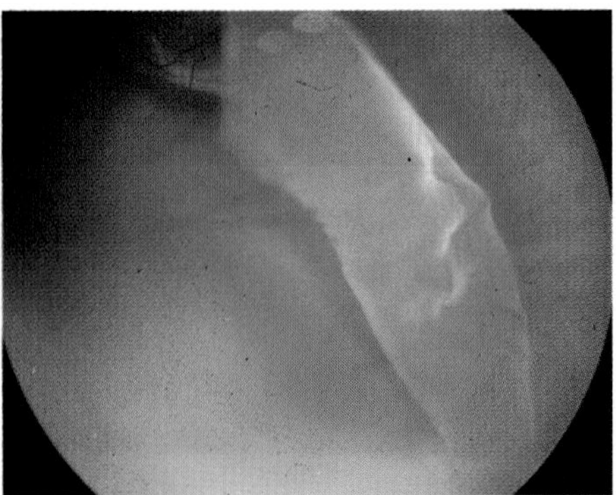

FIGURE 3–234 **Giant retinal tear.** This fundus photograph shows a giant (3 clock hours or greater) retinal tear with a rolled posterior border. These circumferential retinal tears may result from widespread vitreoretinal traction exerted at the vitreous base. The posterior border of the tear is not attached to the vitreous and may roll on itself, allowing the examiner to see the posterior surface of the retina.

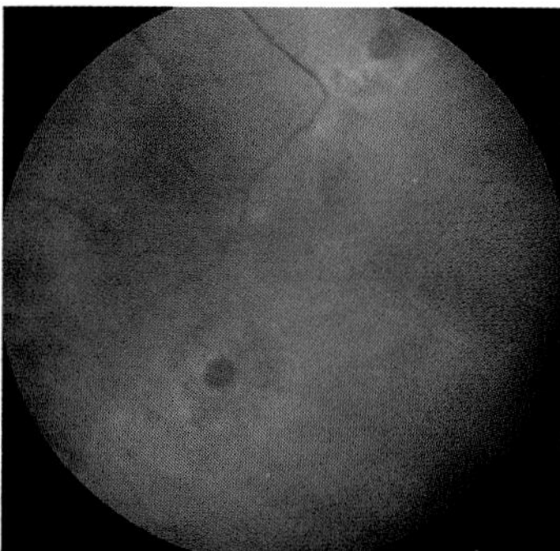

FIGURE 3–235 **Retinal holes.** This fundus photograph demonstrates two round retinal holes within lattice degeneration. Round retinal holes may also be seen in the absence of lattice degeneration. In contrast to retinal tears, retinal holes are not associated with vitreous traction and have no associated flap or operculum.

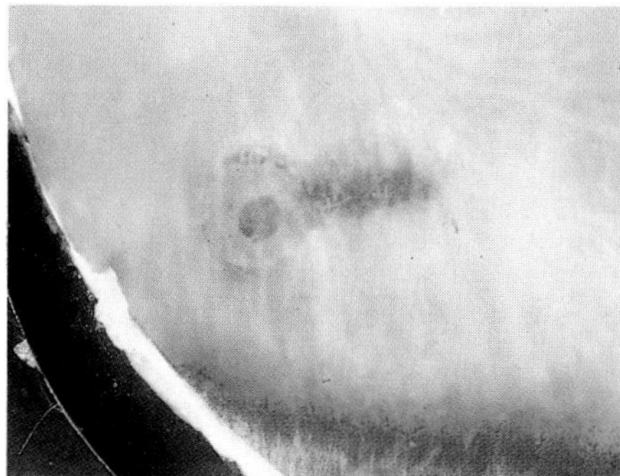

FIGURE 3–236 **Pigmented lattice degeneration with associated retinal hole and localized retinal detachment.** The localized retinal detachment surrounding the hole in this eye bank eye has a pigmented demarcation line, suggesting chronicity. Formalin has opacified the retina.

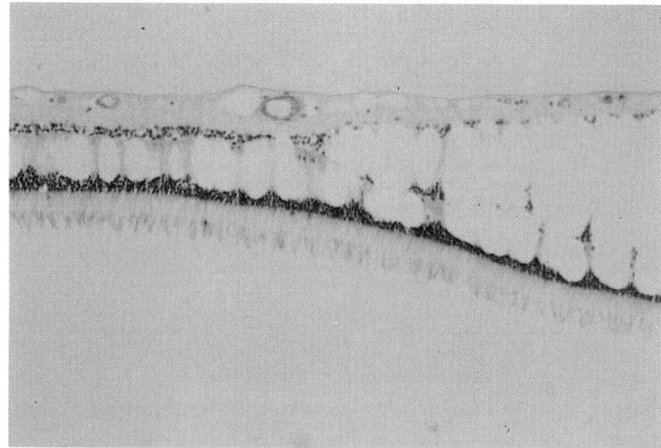

FIGURE 3–237 **Peripheral retinoschisis.** This histopathologic specimen shows the transition zone between peripheral cystoid degeneration *(left)* and degenerative retinoschisis *(right),* which is formed when the peripheral cystoid spaces coalesce to produce an internal splitting of the retina. PAS stain.

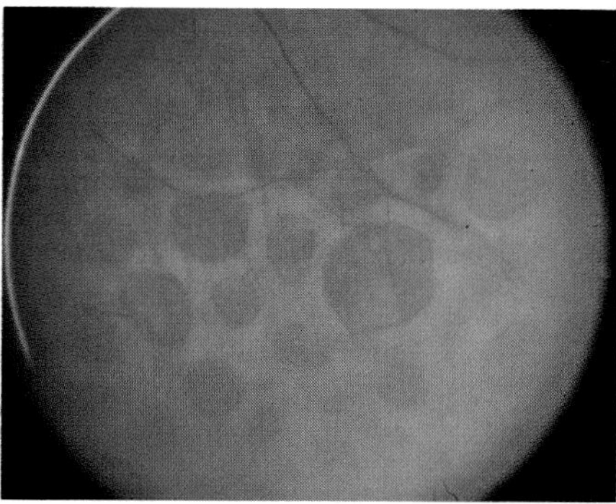

FIGURE 3–238 **Outer layer holes in peripheral retinoschisis.** This fundus photograph shows multiple round outer retinal holes in an area of degenerative retinoschisis. These holes may be single or multiple and are of variable size. They occur more frequently in the outer layer than in the inner layer of retinoschisis.

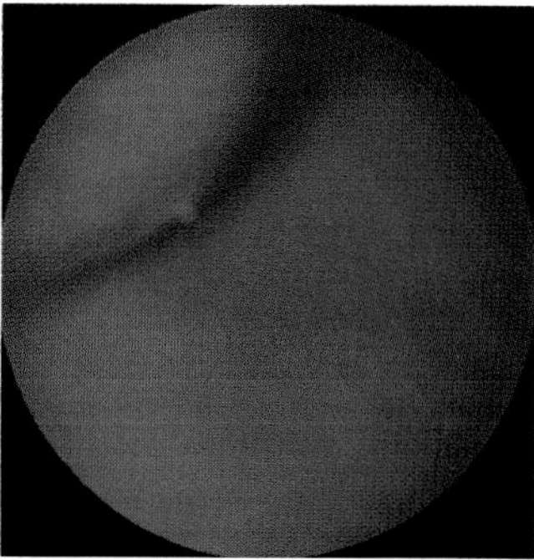

FIGURE 3–239 **Cystic retinal tuft.** This fundus photograph shows a cystic retinal tuft present in a 48-year-old woman. Cystic retinal tuft is a congenital peripheral vitreoretinal abnormality consisting primarily of glial tissue. (From Byer NE: The Peripheral Retina in Profile—A Stereoscopic Atlas. Torrance, CA, Criterion Press, 1952, p. 21.)

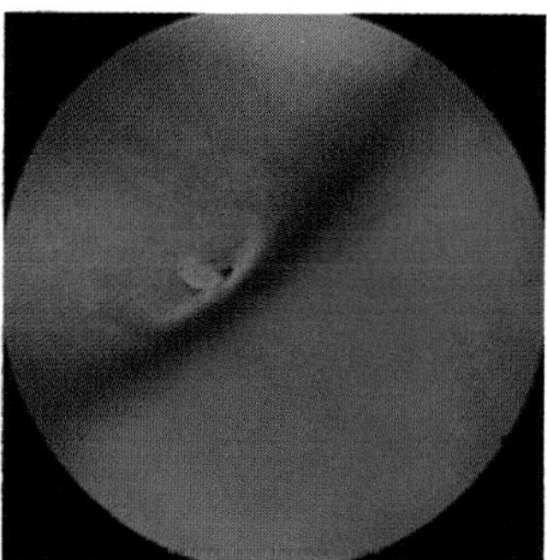

FIGURE 3–240 **Cystic retinal tuft associated with a retinal hole.** This cystic retinal tuft is associated with an atrophic retinal hole and a small localized area of subretinal fluid. (From Byer NE: The Peripheral Retina in Profile—A Stereoscopic Atlas. Torrance, CA, Criterion Press, 1952, p. 23.)

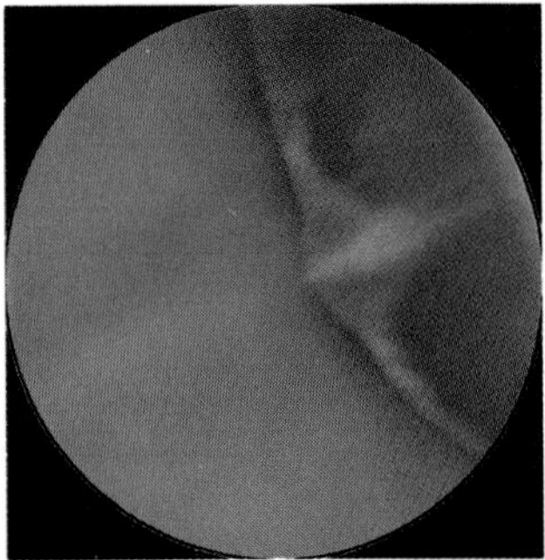

FIGURE 3-241 **Meridional folds.** Meridional folds are radially oriented, linear elevations of the peripheral retina that are aligned with a dentate process of the ora serrata (most cases) or with an ora bay. This fundus photograph shows a meridional fold at the nasal ora serrata, near the horizontal meridian. They are most commonly found superonasally. (From Byer NE: The Peripheral Retina in Profile—A Stereoscopic Atlas. Torrance, CA, Criterion Press, 1952, p. 14.)

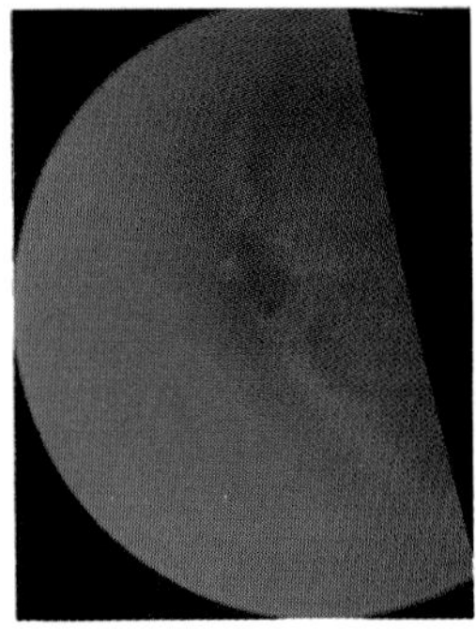

FIGURE 3-242 **Enclosed ora bay.** This is a developmental abnormality in which an island of nonpigmented pars plana epithelium becomes isolated and completely or nearly completely surrounded by peripheral retinal tissue.

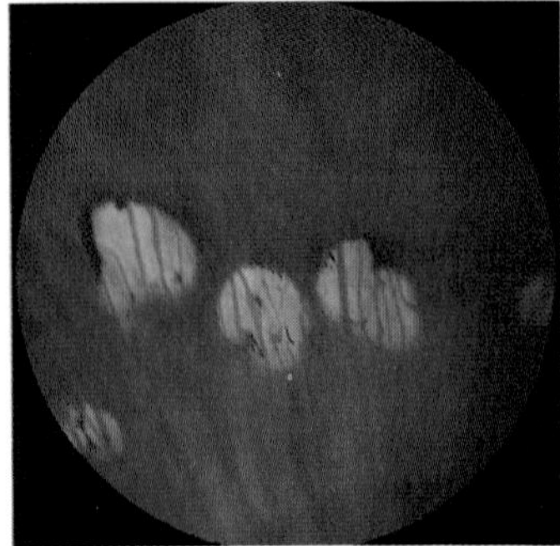

FIGURE 3-243 **Paving stone degeneration of the retina.** There are discrete, rounded, yellow-white lesions between the ora serrata and the equator with pigment borders. Histopathologically, there is circumscribed outer retinal thinning and absence of the retinal pigment epithelium and (variably) choriocapillaris.

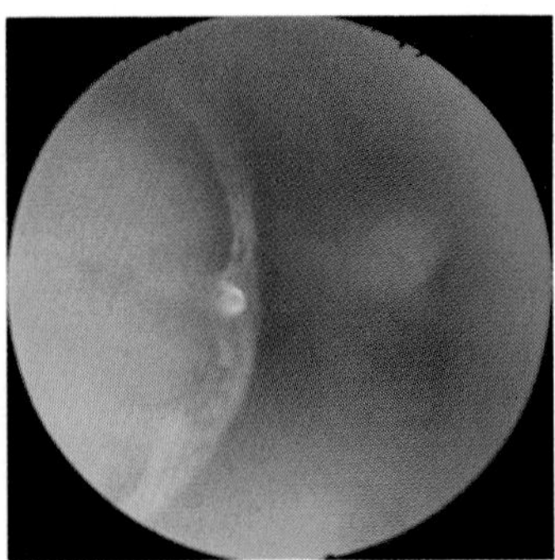

FIGURE 3-244 **Clinical appearance of a pearl of the ora serrata.** A pearl of the ora serrata is located at a dentate process of the ora serrata. Histopathologically, these lesions appear to be drusen-like structures on the inner surface of Bruch's membrane. (From Byer NE: The Peripheral Retina in Profile—A Stereoscopic Atlas. Torrance, CA, Criterion Press, 1952, p. 127.)

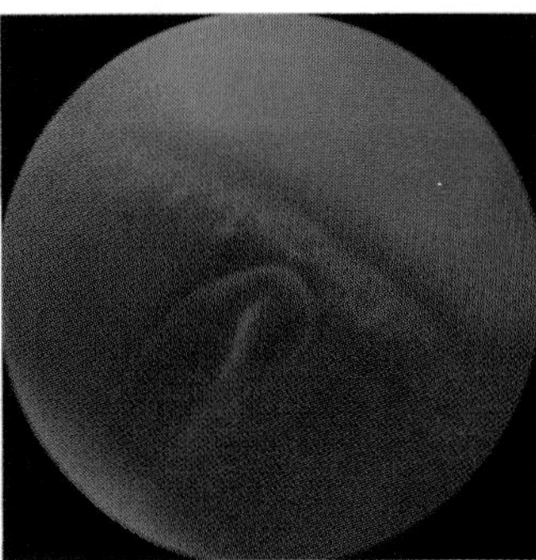

FIGURE 3-245 **Pars plana cyst.** These are smooth cystic lesions that are adjacent and just anterior to the ora serrata. Histopathologically, they may be seen to arise from vacuoles within the nonpigmented epithelial cells or, more frequently, as a separation of the nonpigmented from the pigmented cell layer of the pars plana epithelium. (From Byer NE: The Peripheral Retina in Profile—A Stereoscopic Atlas. Torrance, CA, Criterion Press, 1952, p. 148.)

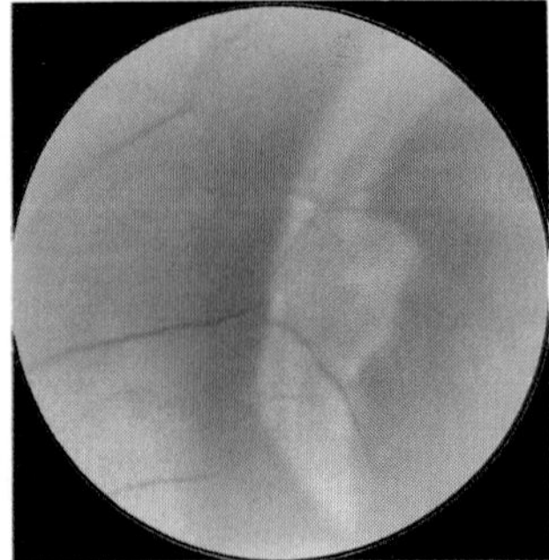

FIGURE 3-246 **White-with-pressure phenomenon.** During scleral indentation, the fundus changes from the customary orange-red color to an opaque yellow-orange or yellow-white color often with loss of visibility of the choroidal pattern. The involved areas have boundaries that are variable in configuration. (From Byer NE: The Peripheral Retina in Profile—A Stereoscopic Atlas. Torrance, CA, Criterion Press, 1952, p. 135.)

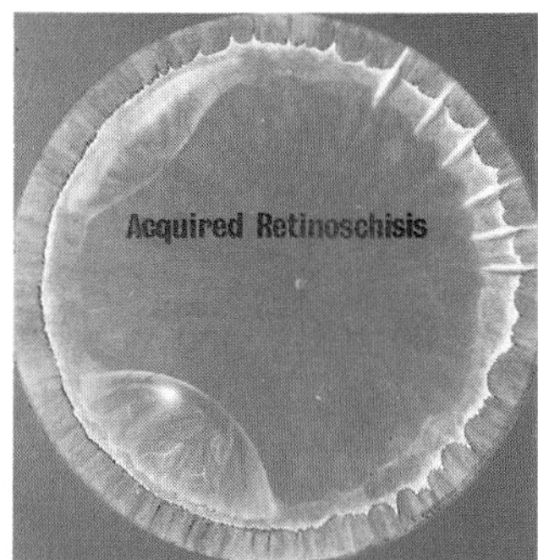

FIGURE 3–247 **Fundus drawing of acquired retinoschisis.** There is a flat dome-shaped area of retinal elevation. The elevated retina represents the inner layer of retinoschisis and contains retinal blood vessels. Retinoschisis usually begins in the extreme peripheral fundus near the ora serrata, usually in the lower temporal quadrant.

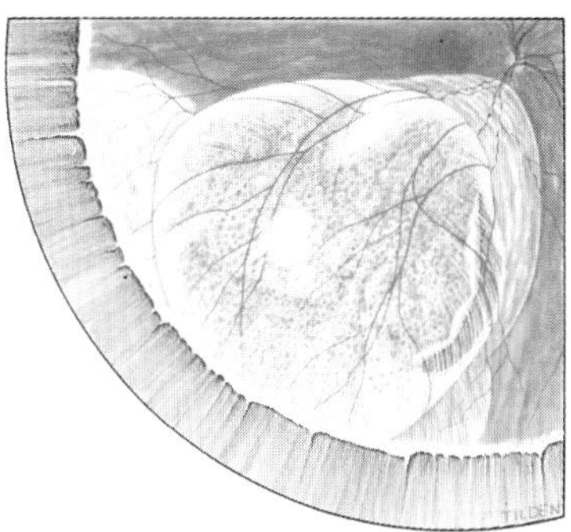

FIGURE 3–250 Fundus drawing of full-thickness retinal detachment caused by a large outer layer break in retinoschisis. The outer layer break has rolled edges and is often located at the edge of the retinoschisis.

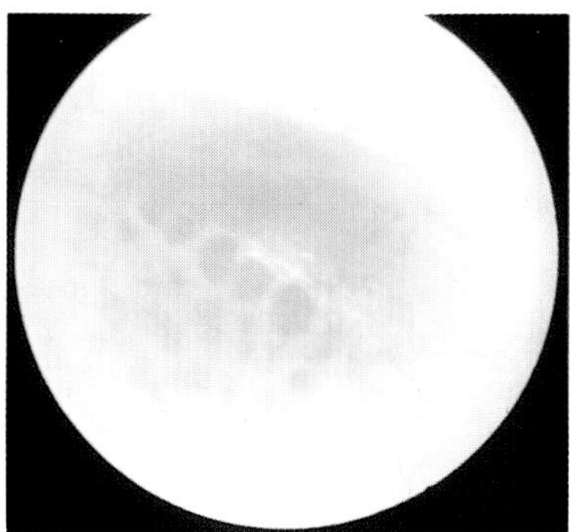

FIGURE 3–248 **Outer layer holes in acquired retinoschisis.** This fundus photograph demonstrates multiple outer layer holes giving a fish or frog egg appearance.

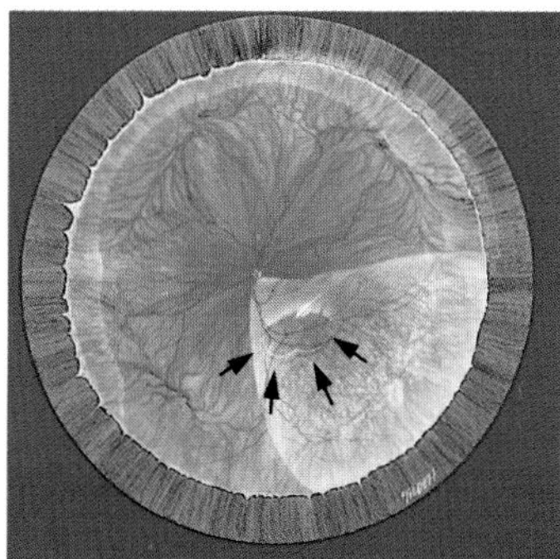

FIGURE 3–251 Fundus drawing of full-thickness retinal detachment in the posterior pole caused by a large outer layer break *(arrows)* in retinoschisis. The outer layer of retinoschisis, which is not detached from the pigment epithelium, shows a fish egg appearance. No inner layer break is found.

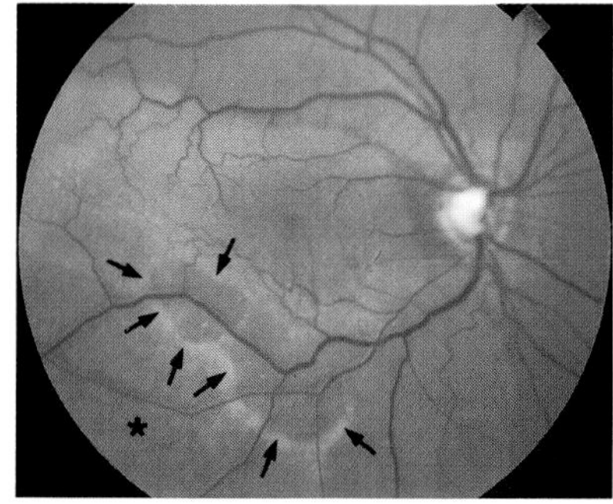

FIGURE 3–249 Full-thickness retinal detachment caused by outer layer breaks *(arrows)* in retinoschisis. The outer layer in the area anterior to the breaks is still attached to the retinal pigment epithelium and has a fish egg appearance *(asterisk)*.

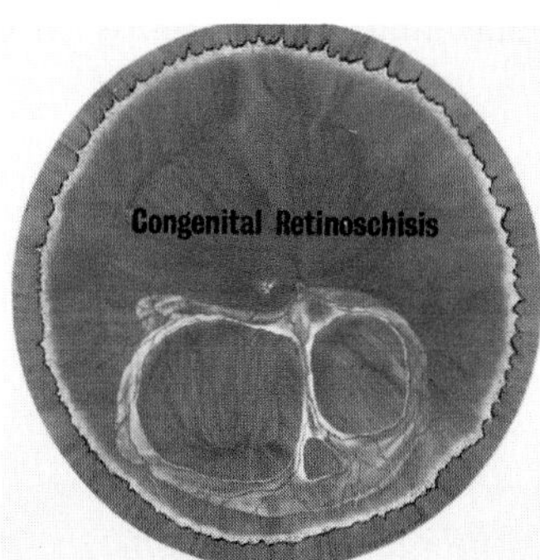

FIGURE 3–252 **Fundus drawing of congenital retinoschisis.** Large inner layer breaks are seen. In congenital retinoschisis, the inner layer breaks are larger and more frequent than in acquired retinoschisis, in which outer layer breaks are more common.

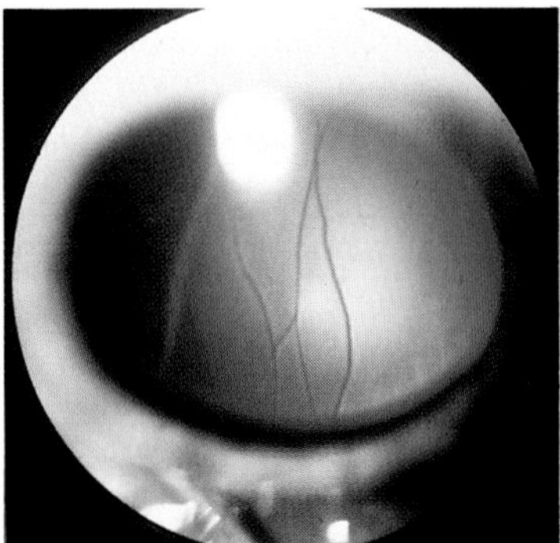

FIGURE 3-253 **Congenital retinoschisis.** The highly elevated inner layer is visible behind the lens. In some cases of congenital retinoschisis, the inner layer holes can become quite large or lead to loss of the inner layer of the retina. The resulting appearance of retinal vessels floating in the vitreous cavity has been termed *congenital vascular veil.*

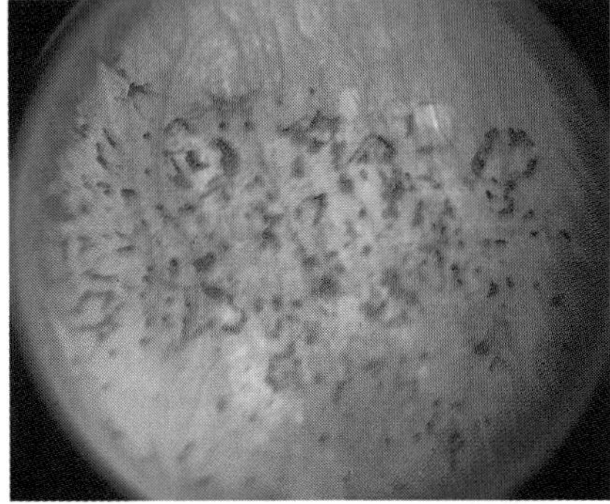

FIGURE 3-254 **Advanced congenital retinoschisis.** Late in the course of congenital retinoschisis, the retinal vessels may become invisible. Degeneration of the outer retinal layer leads to extensive pigmentation of the fundus.

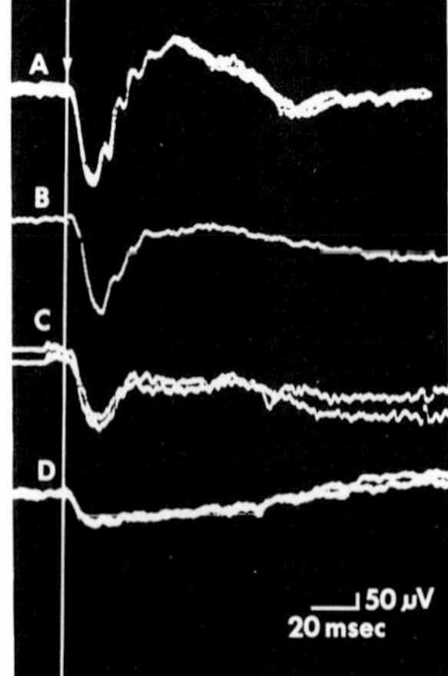

FIGURE 3-255 **Electroretinogram (ERG) findings in congenital retinoschisis.** The following recordings were made with a relatively bright single flash of light under dark adaptation. *A,* Normal ERG shows b:a wave amplitude ratio larger than 1 with good oscillatory potential. *B,* ERG in an eye with macular but no peripheral retinoschisis shows selective depression of the b-wave amplitude. Oscillatory potentials are also diminished. *C,* The a wave is depressed with more marked b-wave reduction in this patient with both macular and peripheral retinoschisis. *D,* ERG in far-advanced retinoschisis. There is a small negative wave (a wave) with complete loss of the b wave.

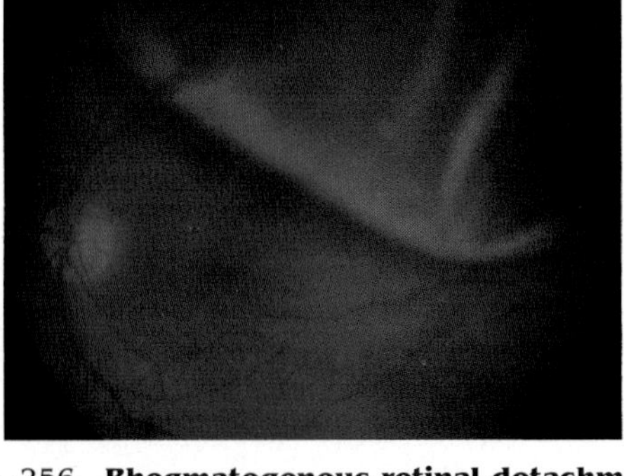

FIGURE 3-256 **Rhegmatogenous retinal detachment.** Note the superotemporal rhegmatogenous retinal detachment involving the macula. This is the most common type of retinal detachment. It occurs when fluid from the vitreous cavity enters the subretinal space through a retinal break.

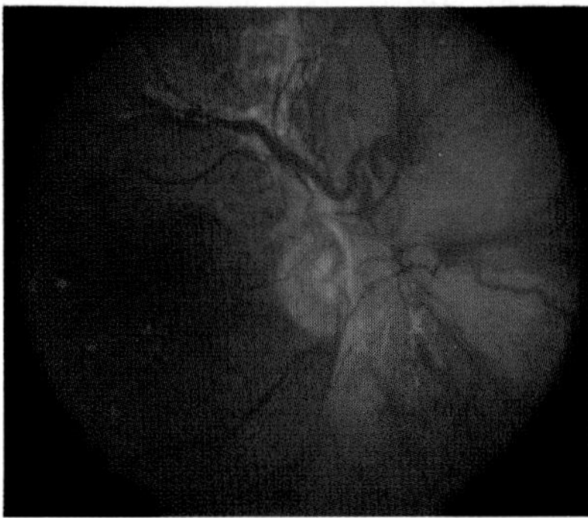

FIGURE 3-257 **Tractional retinal detachment.** Note the tractional detachment that has occurred nasal to the disc. Tractional retinal detachments are second in prevalence. They are caused by vitreoretinal fibroproliferative membranes that mechanically pull the retina away from the underlying retinal pigment epithelium.

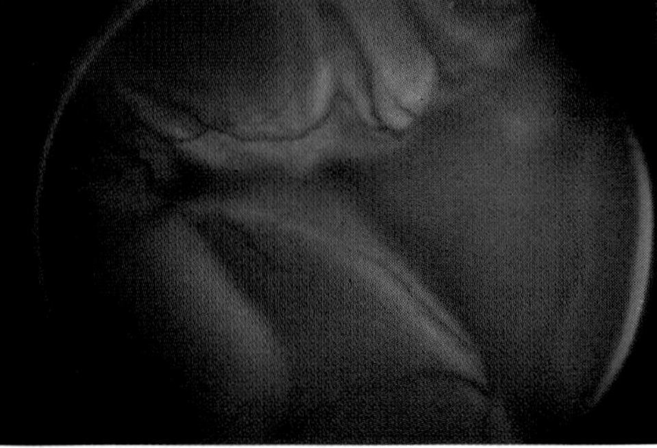

FIGURE 3-258 **Exudative retinal detachment.** Exudative retinal detachments are caused by retinal or choroidal conditions that disturb the retinal pigment epithelium or blood-retinal barrier, thus allowing fluid to accumulate in the subretinal space. These detachments generally resolve without surgery if the underlying condition can be treated. (Courtesy of Robert J. Brockhurst, M.D.)

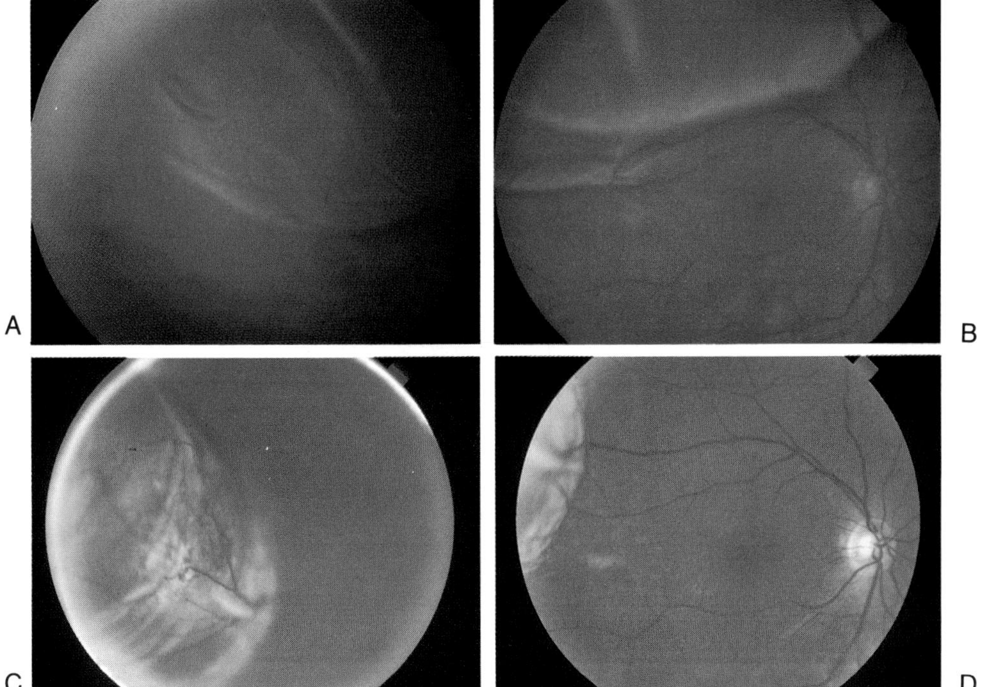

FIGURE 3–259 **Rhegmatogenous retinal detachment repaired with scleral buckle.** *A,* Right eye with superotemporal horseshoe tear resulting in a superior retinal detachment. *B,* Note the characteristic corrugated retina in the superior detachment, which involves the macula. *C,* Four months after repair with scleral buckle, the retinal break is supported on a radial element. *D,* Note the reattached posterior pole of the same eye; visual acuity improved from 20/400 to 20/25.

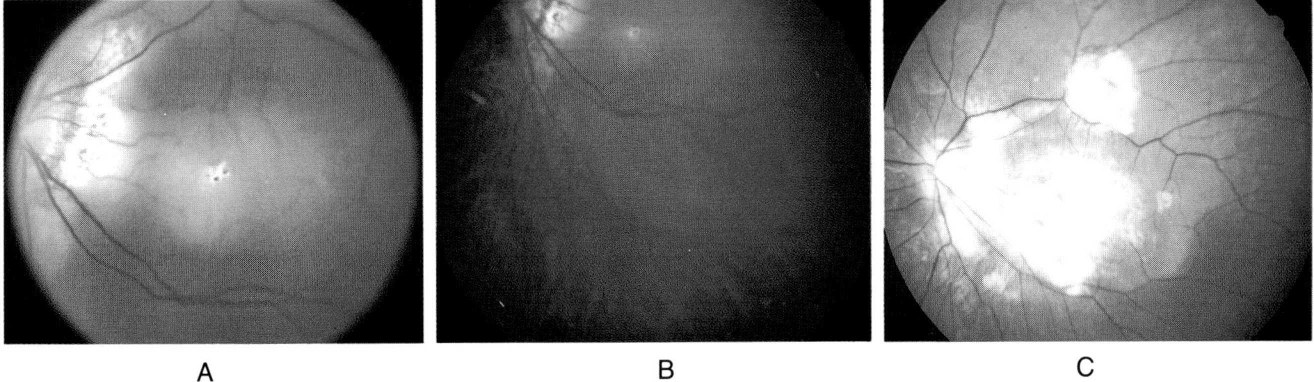

FIGURE 3–260 **Repair of rhegmatogenous retinal detachment caused by a macular hole in a patient with high myopia.** Retinal detachment can occur after a posterior pole retinal break. These detachments are uncommon and are typically seen in the following clinical situations: myopia, aphakia, and following blunt trauma. *A,* Left eye with retinal detachment due to macular break in a patient with high myopia. *B,* These detachments are typically confined to the posterior pole. *C,* Postoperative appearance of the same eye after vitrectomy with endodrainage of subretinal fluid, endolaser, and silicone oil tamponade shows resolution of the detachment. Most of these detachments can be managed in either one of two ways: vitrectomy and the intravitreal injection of long-lasting gases or the intravitreal injection of long-lasting gases alone.

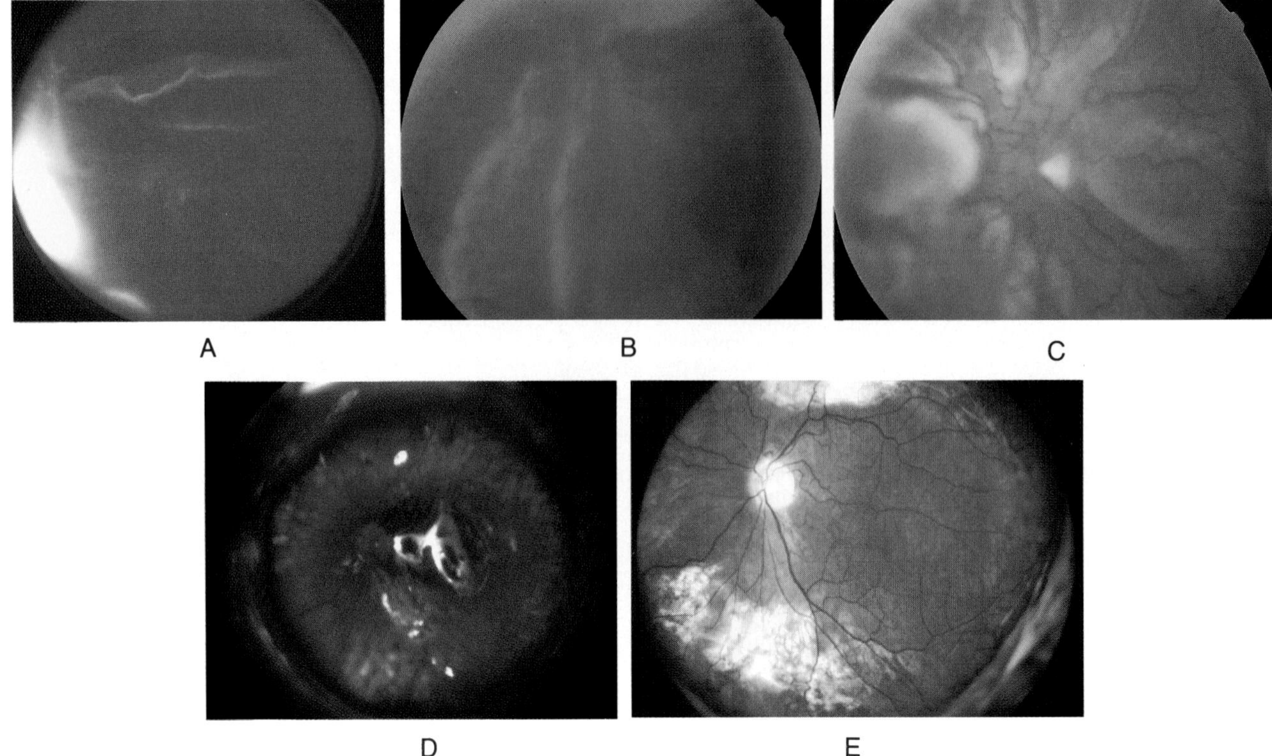

FIGURE 3–261 **Retinal detachment caused by giant retinal tear.** *A,* Wide-angle photograph displays total retinal detachment with superior giant break from the 10 to the 2 o'clock position in the left eye. *B,* Preoperative photograph from another patient with a total retinal detachment caused by a giant break from the 12 to the 6 o'clock positions in the left eye. *C,* Posterior pole of the same eye as in *B;* visual acuity is at the hand motions level. *D,* Postoperative photography 2 days after surgery from the same patient; an encircling scleral buckle, cryopexy, vitrectomy, and prone fluid-air exchange were performed, and the reattached retina is seen through perfluoropropane gas tamponade. *E,* Posterior pole in the same eye 4 months later; visual acuity is 20/200.

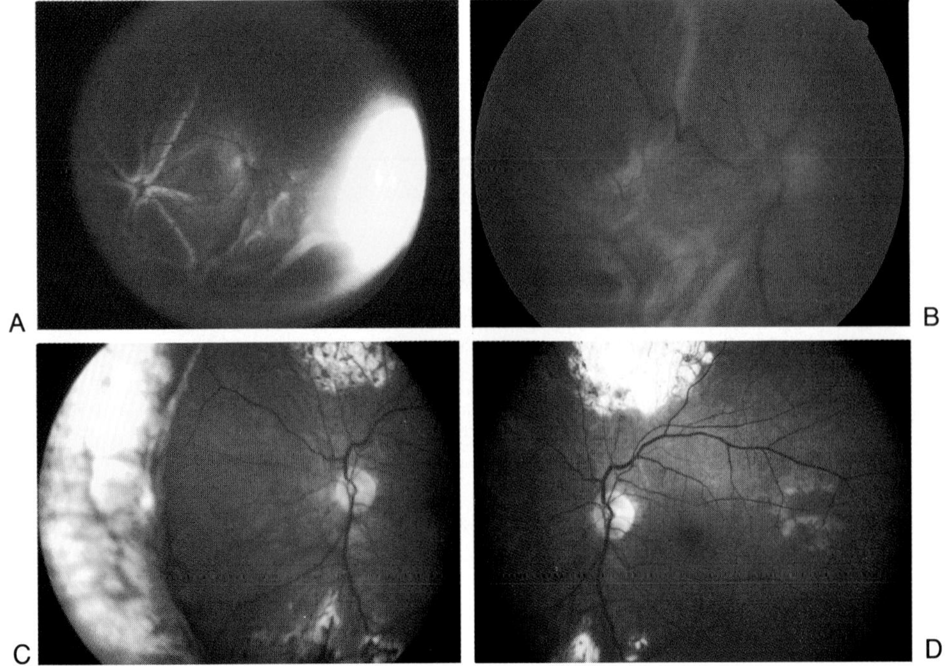

FIGURE 3–262 **Retinal detachment associated with proliferative vitreoretinopathy (PVR).** *A,* This wide-angle view demonstrates a total detachment with PVR. Note the temporal star fold and numerous inferior folds. PVR is typically managed with the use of an encircling scleral buckle combined with vitrectomy and intraocular tamponade (perfluorohydrocarbons/silicone oil) as needed. *B,* Preoperative photograph from a different patient with retinal detachment in the left eye and retinal folds caused by PVR. *C,* Postoperative photograph 3 months after a scleral buckle, vitrectomy, membrane removal, endodrainage, endolaser, and perfluoropropane gases tamponade were performed. Note the indent caused by the buckle in the nasal periphery. *D,* Reattached retina demonstrating pigment fallout in the macula and superior to the disc at the site of the drainage retinotomy. Visual acuity is 20/50.

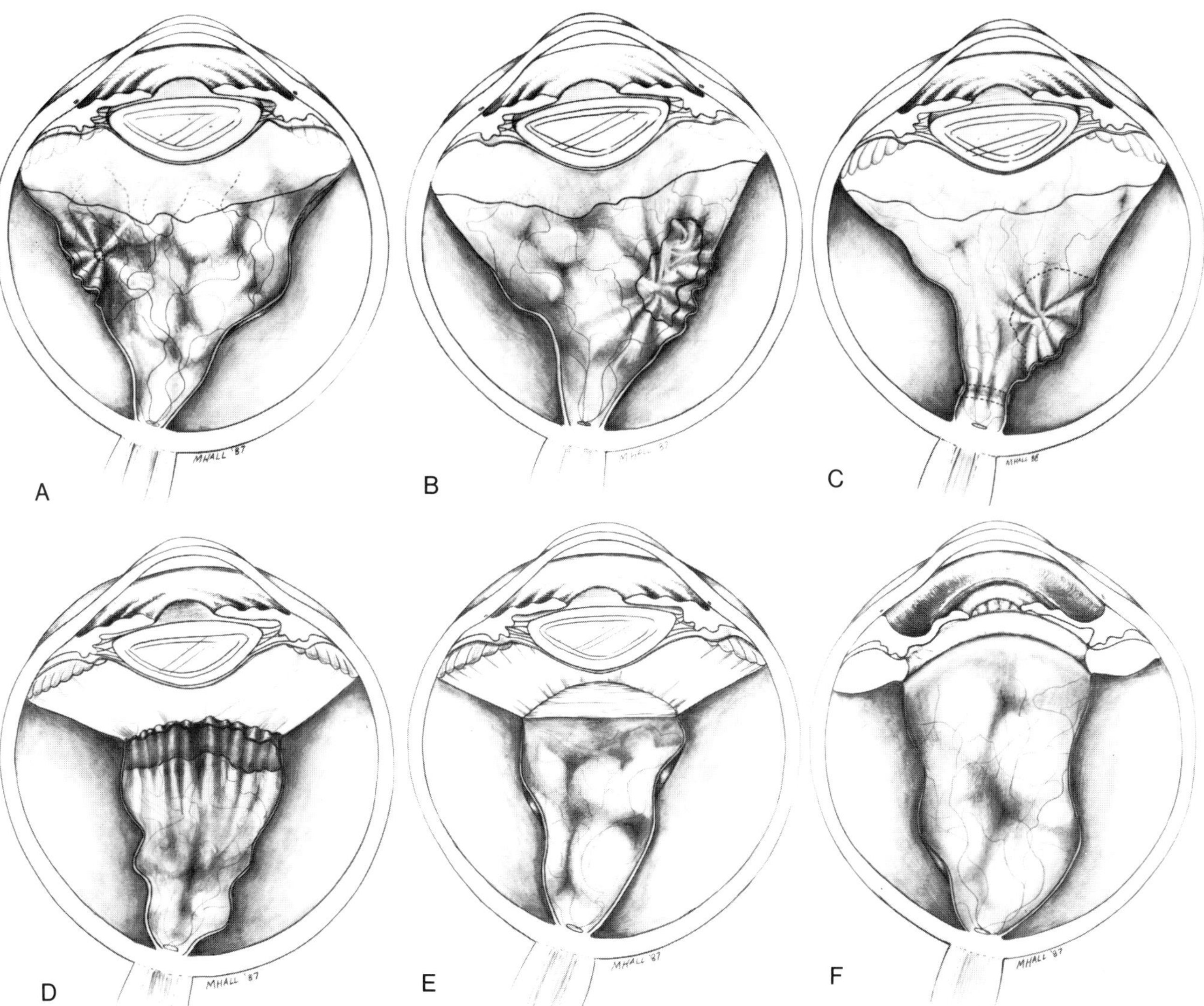

FIGURE 3-263 **PVR.** Types of grade C PVR are as follows: *A,* Type 1. Regular folds radiate ("star fold") from a focal area of PVR; traction is exerted centripetally toward the area of PVR. *B,* Type 2. Irregular folds are present in the posterior retina. The retina is contracted in an anteroposterior direction, which flattens its normally bullous convex curvature, and in circumferential direction, which creates a series of radial folds in the anterior retina. Traction is exerted on the remainder of the retina, pulling it in both a posterior direction and a circumferential direction. Traction in a perpendicular direction pulls the retina toward the center of the vitreous cavity, narrowing the funnel of retinal detachment over the optic disc. *C,* Type 3. Subretinal membrane creates an annular constriction around the disc ("napkin ring") or irregular folds more anteriorly. In the napkin ring configuration, traction in a circumferential direction gathers the posterior retina together anterior to the optic disc. With irregular folds, traction is mainly perpendicular to the retinal surface, elevating the retina toward the center of the vitreous cavity. *D,* Type 4. Irregular folds are present in the retina immediately behind the vitreous base, and the adjacent posterior hyaloid is contracted. Contraction of the retina in a circumferential direction causes radial folds posterior to the area of PVR. The anterior retina within the vitreous base is stretched inward to form a fold in the coronal plane because circumferential contraction exerted along the concavity of the retina produces a secondary traction vector perpendicular to the retinal surface, toward the center of the vitreous cavity. *E,* Type 5. The posterior hyaloid is contracted. The anterior retina is pulled in a perpendicular direction toward the center of the vitreous cavity. Radial folds are also formed as a result of contraction in a circumferential direction. *F,* Type 6. The anterior retina is pulled forward as a result of contraction in an anteroposterior direction of the posterior hyaloid, the anterior hyaloid, and the vitreous base that remain after vitrectomy. The underlying retina forms a trough within the vitreous base.

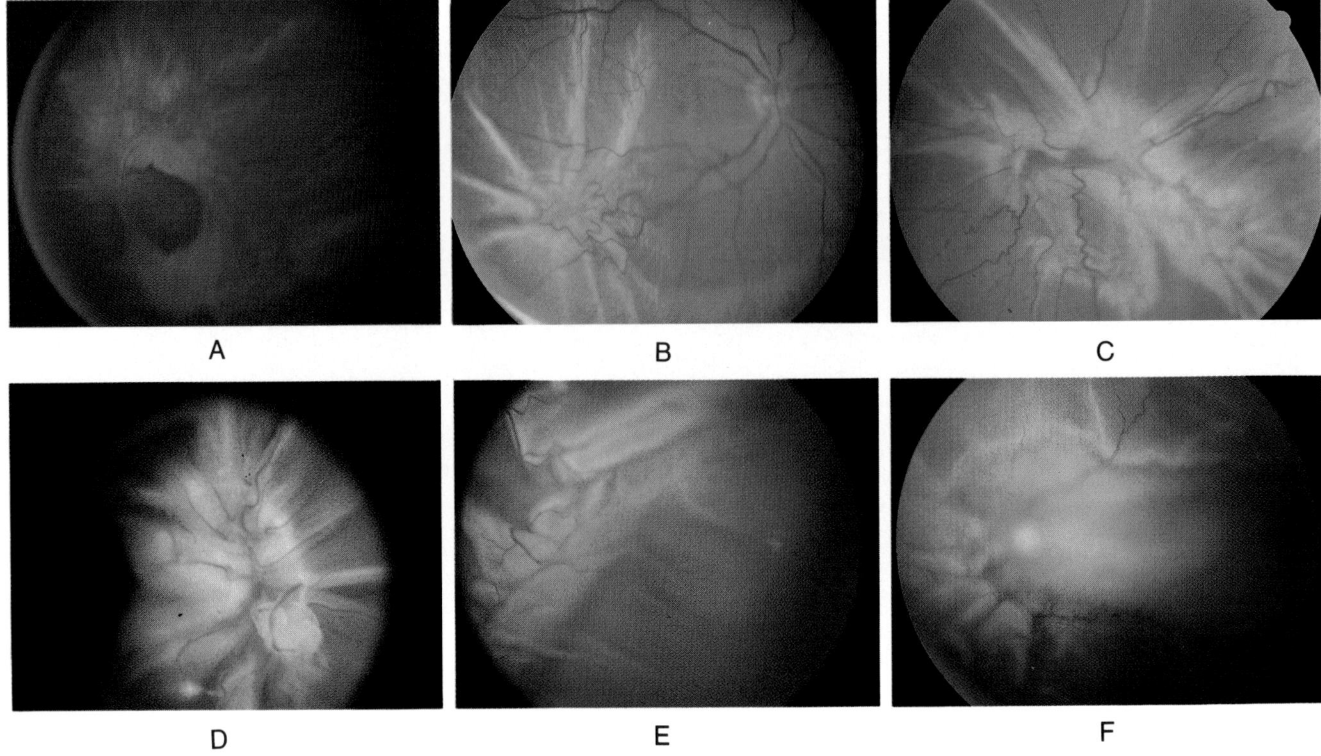

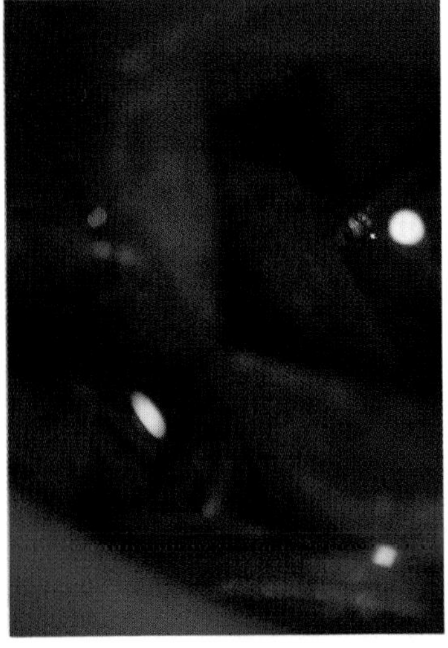

FIGURE 3-264 **Clinical photographs illustrating different types of PVR.** Membranes occurring in PVR are composed of cells originating from the retinal glia and retinal pigment epithelium, inflammatory macrophages, and collagen. Continued dispersal and proliferation of retinal pigment epithelium cells from the exposed pigment epithelium ultimately result in a contracted collagenous membrane that covers both surfaces of the retina and the exposed vitreous matrix. *A,* Grade B. The posterior lip of a large tear is rolled inward by PVR localized at its edge. *B,* Grade C, type 1. A single epicenter of PVR creates a star fold in the posterior retina. *C,* Grade C, type 2. Diffuse PVR is present in the posterior retina. *D,* Grade C, type 3. Subretinal PVR closes the funnel of retinal detachment anterior to the disc. *E,* Grade C, type 4. PVR at the retinal equator produces a circumferential fold immediately behind the insertion of the posterior hyaloid *(left side of photograph);* peripheral retina within the vitreous base is stretched inward *(right side of photograph). F,* Grade C, type 5. Contraction of the posterior hyaloid (located more posteriorly than usual in this case, as indicated by the line of pigment immediately behind its insertion inferiorly) creates a circumferential fold in the coronal plane. *G,* Grade C, type 6. An operative photograph showing a trough of retina anteriorly (immediately to the left of the vitrectomy probe), covered by an opaque PVR membrane.

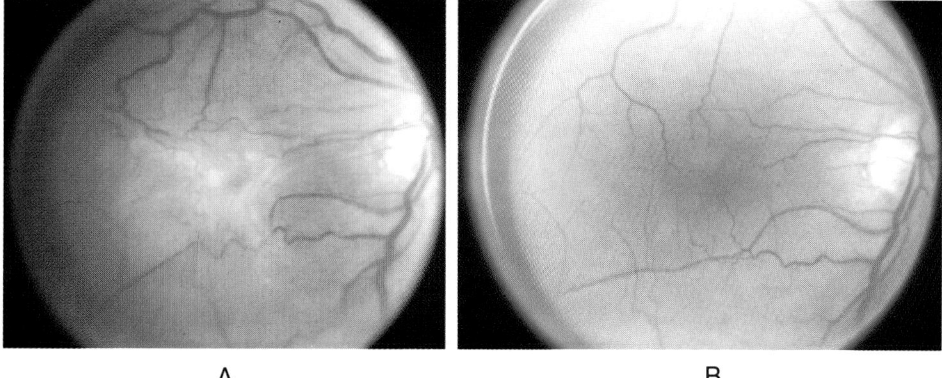

A B

FIGURE 3–265 **Epiretinal membrane secondary to the peripheral cryopexy.** Surface traction on the retina in its purest form can only be relieved by vitrectomy. This form of traction is caused by (1) membranes on either surface of the retina, (2) horizontal traction from a flat contraction of the posterior hyaloid (as may occur in macular hole formation), or (3) incarceration or intrinsic contraction of the retina. *A*, Epiretinal membrane in the right eye following peripheral retinal cryopexy; visual acuity is 20/200. *B*, Postoperative appearance of the same eye following vitrectomy with membrane peeling. Note the absence of the membrane over the central macula with release of the traction on the macular vessels; visual acuity is 20/25.

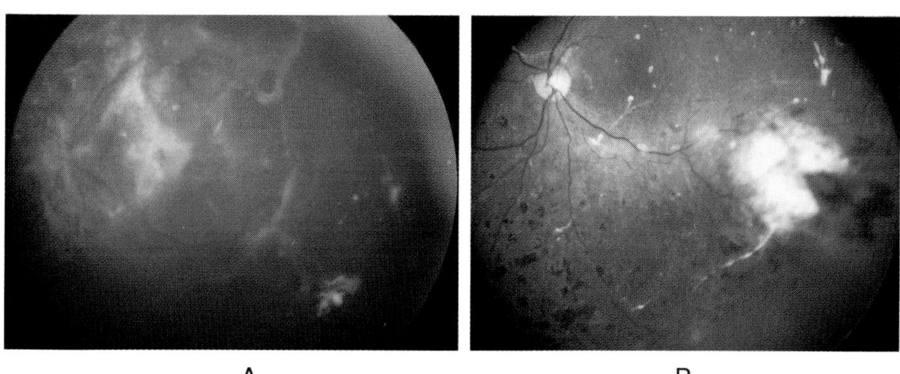

A B

FIGURE 3–266 **Management of diabetic rhegmatogenous tractional retinal detachment.** Diabetic retinal detachments can be complicated by both tractional and rhegmatogenous components. In many of these cases, the two methods of transvitreal traction relief, scleral buckling and vitrectomy, are combined to achieve the necessary relief of traction. *A*, This is the left eye of a diabetic patient with a combined tractional/rhegmatogenous retinal detachment involving the fovea caused by a retinal break along the inferotemporal arcade. *B*, Clinical photograph showing retinal reattachment and closure of the break following vitrectomy combined with a localized scleral buckle. The vision improved from counting fingers at 2 feet to 20/200.

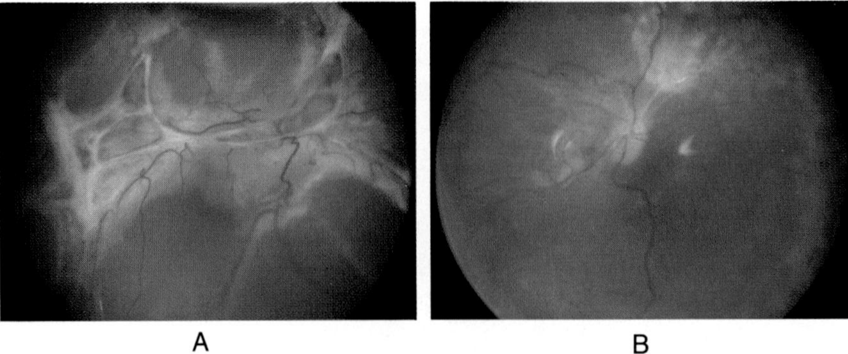

FIGURE 3-267 **PVR following traumatic retinal detachment.** Fundus photograph showing severe PVR in the right eye of a patient following a motor vehicle accident. Dispersal and proliferation of retinal pigment epithelium cells, combined with glial cell proliferation, result in contracted membranes that cover both surfaces of the retina. *A*, This photograph demonstrates the failure of previous reattachment surgery owing to PVR. *B*, A postoperative photograph 1 month after vitrectomy, membrane peeling, pneumohydraulic reattachment, endolaser, and silicone oil tamponade. The retina is attached but distorted owing to residual subretinal membranes and contracture.

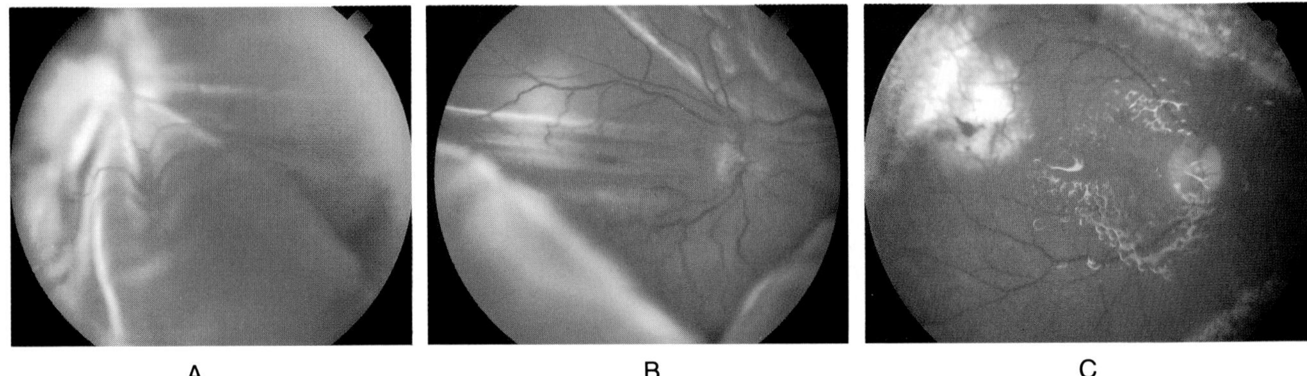

FIGURE 3-268 **Vitreoretinal surgery in the management of a retinal incarceration.** *A*, Clinical photograph demonstrating a retinal incarceration and total retinal detachment with PVR in the right eye following penetrating trauma. The incarceration site in the temporal equator is shown. *B*, The posterior pole of the same eye, demonstrating tight folds extending toward the incarceration. *C*, Clinical appearance 2 months after vitrectomy with a retinotomy, endolaser, and silicone oil tamponade. The posterior pole is reattached and demonstrates the characteristic silicone oil reflex.

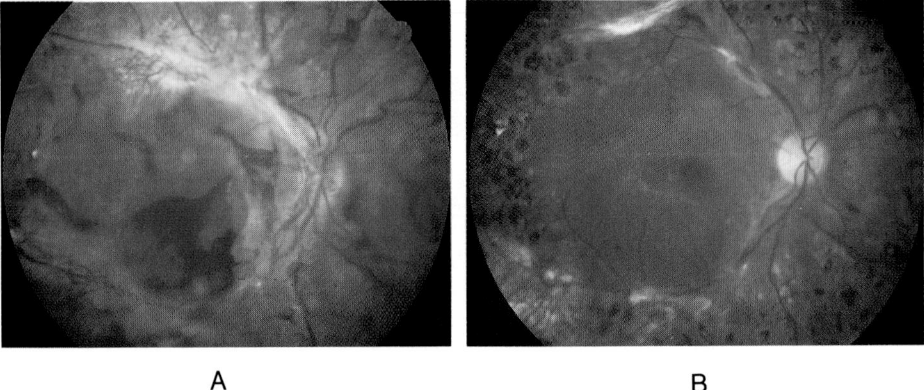

FIGURE 3-269 **Vitreoretinal surgery for diabetic tractional detachment.** *A*, Proliferative diabetic retinopathy with traction retinal detachment involving the fovea of the right eye is present. The strong attachment of the posterior hyaloid to the neovascular proliferations arising from the retinal vessels creates a complex array of transvitreal and surface traction that cause the detachment. Management of these cases requires the release of these forces. *B*, Clinical appearance 1 year after vitrectomy with segmentation of the posterior vitreous face demonstrating reattachment of the retina. The visual acuity improved from 20/125 to 20/40.

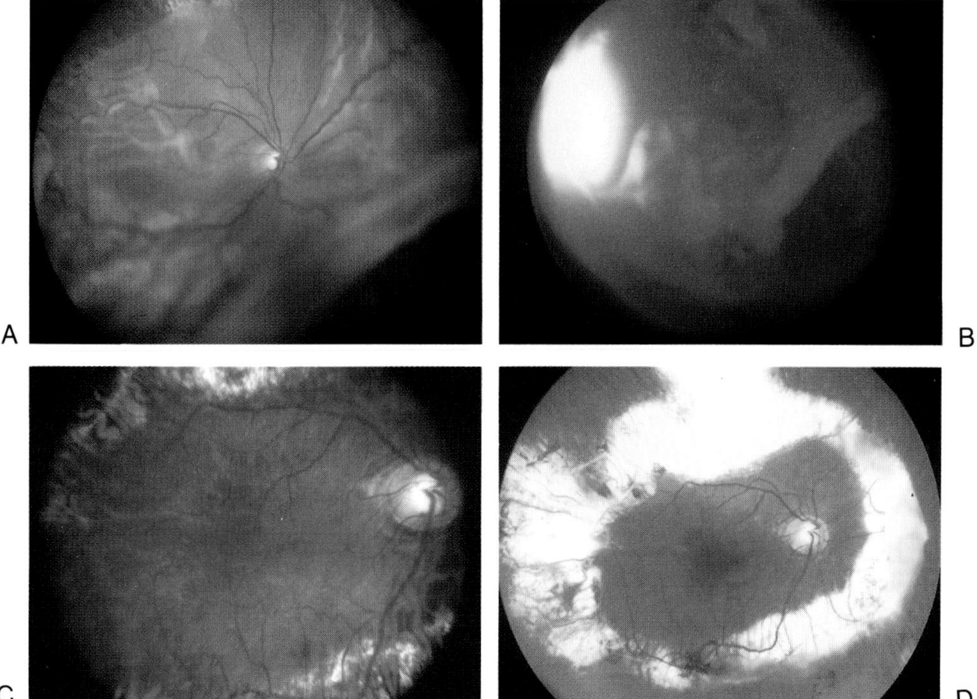

FIGURE 3-270 **Vitreoretinal surgery in the management of giant retinal tears.** *A*, Clinical photograph demonstrating a total retinal detachment in association with dual giant retinal breaks and proliferative vitreoretinopathy in the right eye. The posterior pole is bounded by giant breaks superiorly and inferiorly. These tears usually begin along the posterior margin of the vitreous base and are due to the anterior collapse of the vitreous gel resulting in traction. *B*, This wide-angle photograph of the same eye shows a giant break from the 9 to 11 o'clock positions and a second giant break with a rolled posterior edge from the 2:30 to the 5:30 clock positions. *C*, Postoperative photograph 5 months after vitrectomy with a 360-degree retinotomy, supine fluid-air exchange with direct retinal manipulation, endolaser, and perfluoropropane gas tamponade. *D*, This photograph, taken 1 year postoperatively, displays the healed 360-degree retinotomy and attached retina; visual acuity is 20/80.

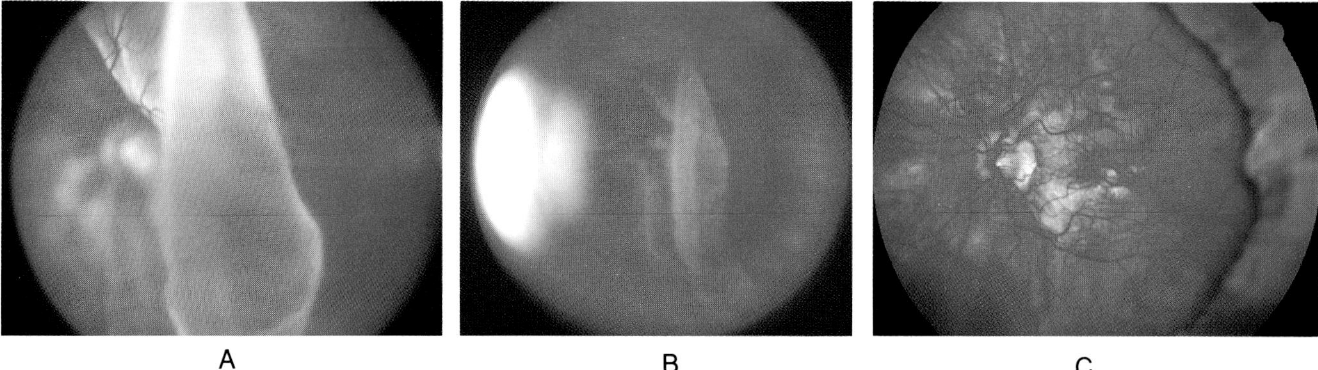

FIGURE 3-271 **Vitreoretinal surgery for giant retinal breaks.** *A*, Clinical photograph demonstrating a giant retinal break with total retinal detachment after an extracapsular extraction in the left eye. The break extends for 6 clock hours. *B*, This wide-angle photograph of the same eye demonstrates the temporal break. *C*, This postoperative photograph was taken after performing a vitrectomy, scleral buckle, cryopexy, and prone fluid-air exchange. The retina is reattached. The temporal segment of the buckle is noted.

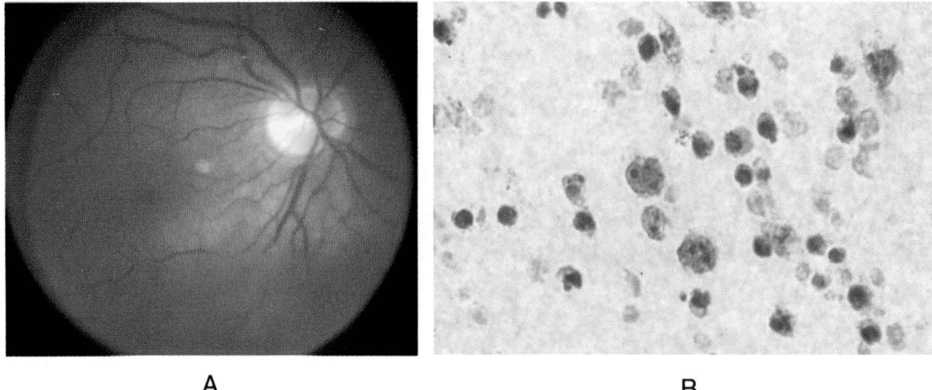

FIGURE 3–272 **Clinical and histologic features of non-Hodgkin lymphoma.** Diagnostic vitrectomy and retinal biopsy techniques can be applied to help in the diagnosis of difficult cases. *A*, Fundus photograph displaying inferior vitreous opacification in a 37-year-old woman with unexplained vitreous cellular infiltrates bilaterally. *B*, Vitreous cytology reveals undifferentiated lymphoid cells with large nuclei characteristic of non-Hodgkin lymphoma (reticulum cell sarcoma).

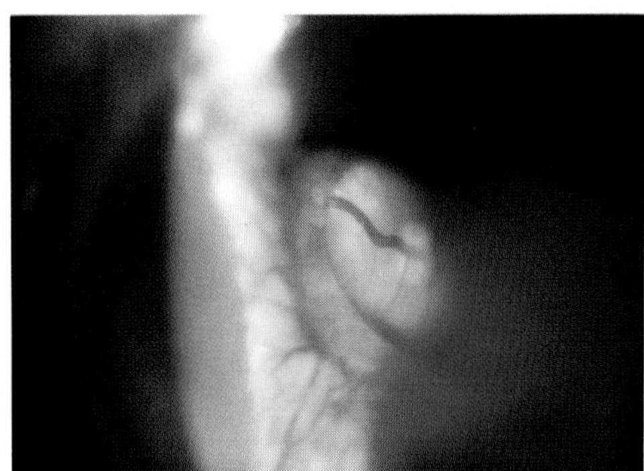

FIGURE 3–273 **Rubeosis after chronic retinal detachment.** Rubeosis and total retinal detachment with retina organized to the iris after failed vitrectomy for traumatic retinal detachment. Neovascularization of the iris is often seen in association with chronic retinal detachments, especially in patients with compromised retinal blood flow such as diabetics.

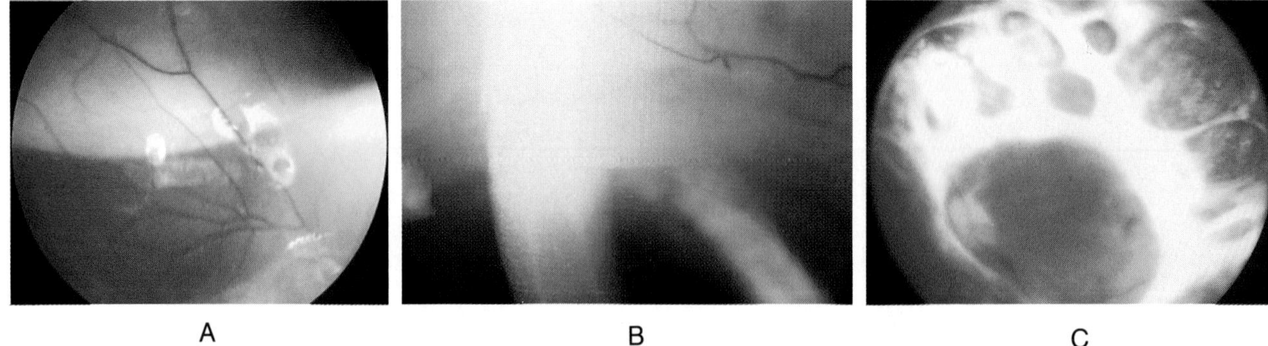

FIGURE 3–274 **Complications of silicone oil.** Use of this type of tamponade may result in pupillary block, reduction in the corneal endothelial cell density, emulsification of the oil, anterior segment inflammation, glaucoma, hypotony, cataracts in phakic patients, epiretinal membrane formation, and entrapment in the subretinal space. *A*, Note the emulsified silicone oil visible under the detached superior retina. *B*, This anterior chamber photograph demonstrates the superior meniscus of emulsified silicone oil. This patient has acute elevation of intraocular pressure. *C*, Recurrent membranes under silicone oil tamponade after vitreoretinal surgery for retinal detachment that resulted after acute necrosis syndrome.

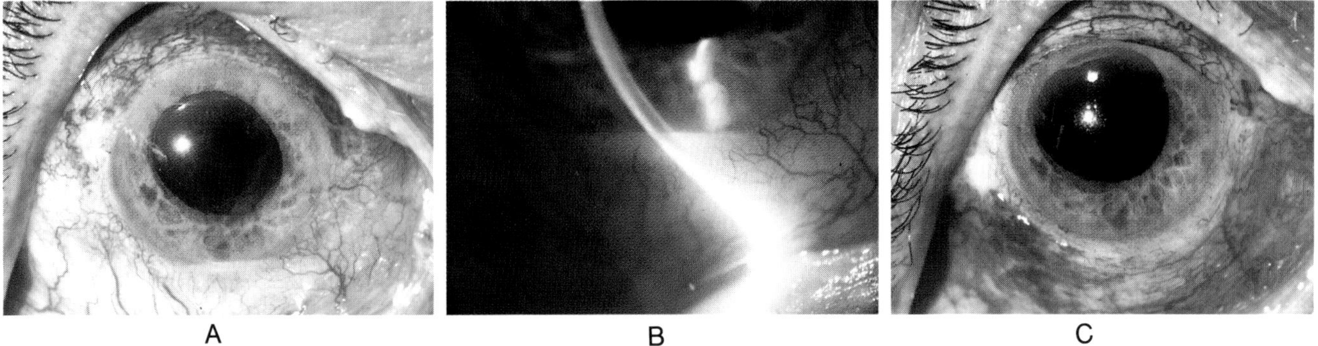

FIGURE 3–275 **Postoperative endophthalmitis.** *A*, Postoperative endophthalmitis due to *Staphylococcus epidermidis* presenting 6 days after extracapsular cataract extraction with posterior chamber lens implantation. Note the conjunctival hyperemia, hypopyon, and inflammatory membrane on the intraocular lens. *B*, Slit-lamp photograph of the hypopyon in this patient. *C*, This photograph, 2 weeks following a vitrectomy with intravitreal administration of vancomycin (1 mg), amikacin (400 μg), and dexamethasone (200 μg), illustrates resolution of the hypopyon. Approximately 64 percent of eyes with a clinical diagnosis of infectious endophthalmitis have a positive culture result. Fifty-six to 90 percent of isolates in these patients are gram-positive; 7 to 9 percent are gram-negative; and 3 to 13 percent are fungal.

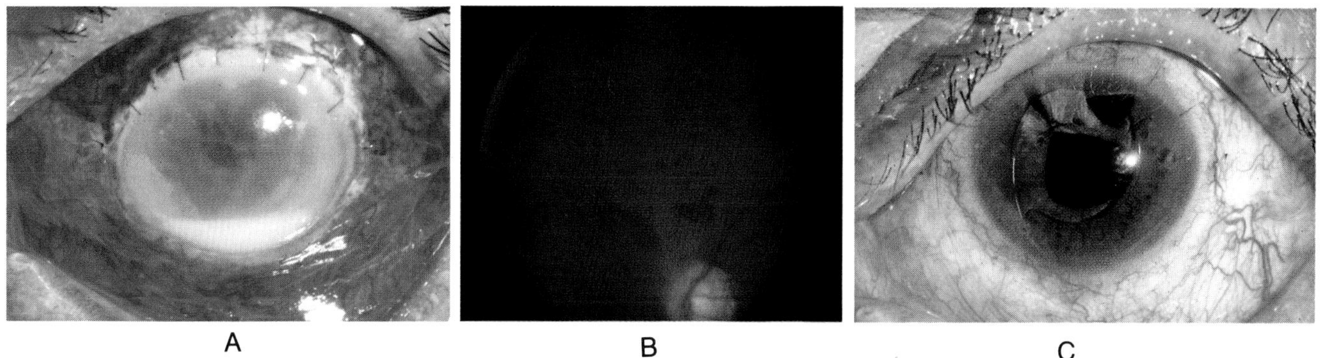

FIGURE 3–276 **Postoperative endophthalmitis after extracapsular cataract extraction.** *A*, Postoperative endophthalmitis due to *Staphylococcus epidermidis* presenting 4 days after extracapsular cataract extraction, complicated by vitreous loss, with anterior lens implantation. Conjunctival hyperemia, mild corneal edema, hypopyon, and inflammatory membranes on the iris and both surfaces of the intraocular lens are evident. *B*, Fundus photograph after vitrectomy documents the petechial hemorrhages frequently observed in association with active endophthalmitis. *C*, Clinical photograph, 2 months after vitrectomy with intravitreal administration of amikacin (400 μg), cefazolin (2.25 mg), and dexamethasone (200 μg), demonstrates resolution of hypopyon and corneal edema. The intraocular lens is preserved following intraoperative removal of the inflammatory membranes noted preoperatively.

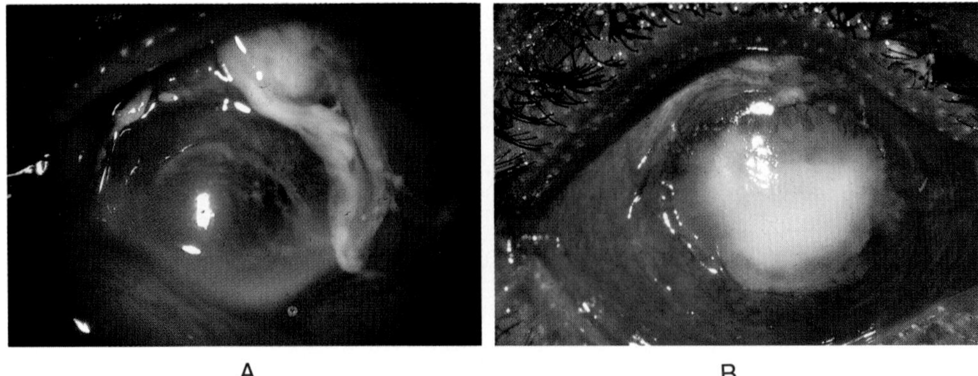

FIGURE 3–277 **Postoperative endophthalmitis due to *Streptococcus*.** Eyes with endophthalmitis associated with filtering blebs have a dismal prognosis. The cause of this condition is believed to be related to the creation of a markedly reduced tissue barrier by the filtration fistula. The two organisms most commonly encountered in this entity include *Streptococcus* and *Haemophilus influenzae*. *A,* Endophthalmitis due to *Streptococcus* in an eye with a long-standing filtering bleb. This photograph displays a purulent discharge, opacification of the bleb, anterior chamber cells and hypopyon, and loss of the red reflex. *B,* A rapid clinical deterioration over the subsequent 2 weeks occurred despite immediate and repeated therapy, including intravitreal antibiotics and vitrectomies; the eye lost all light perception.

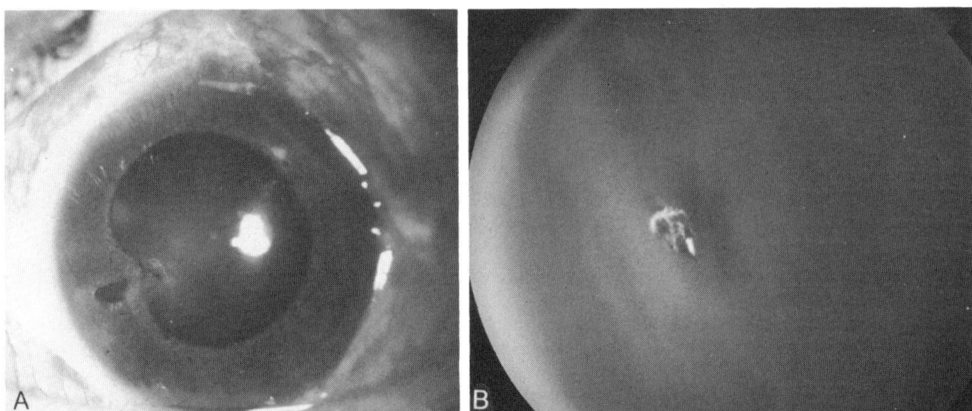

FIGURE 3–278 **Intraocular foreign body.** *A,* The track of a foreign body through the cornea, iris, and lens. *B,* The foreign body is seen in the vitreous with an associated dense hemorrhage. It is important to determine the composition of intraocular foreign bodies because certain metals, such as copper and iron, are toxic to ocular structures and require emergent removal.

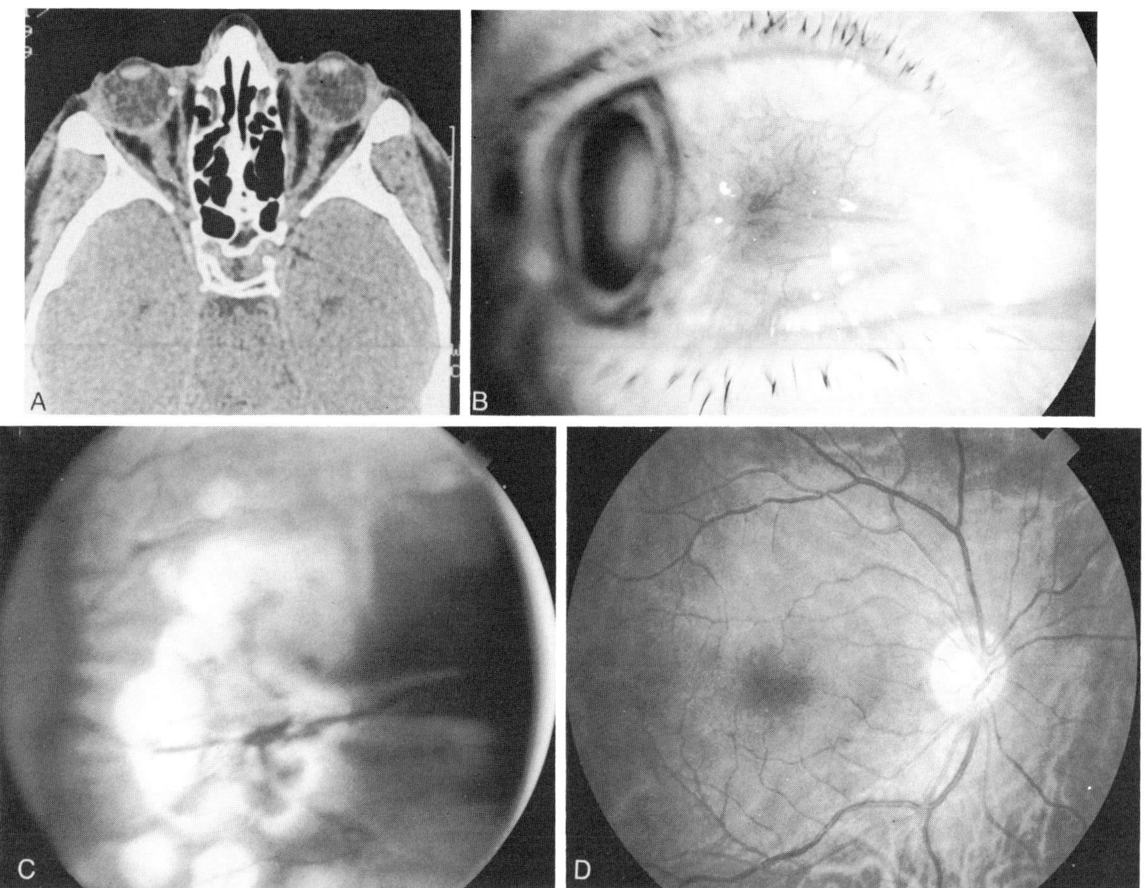

FIGURE 3-279 **Radiologic and clinical findings of an intraocular foreign body.** *A*, Computed tomography (CT) scan of a foreign body in the retina at the nasal equator. In contrast to the routine plain film, the CT scan is useful in the three-dimensional localization of intraocular radiopaque foreign bodies. *B*, Note the subconjunctival hemorrhage at the entry site. *C*, A scleral buckle has been placed at the site of the transscleral posterior extraction. *D*, Normal posterior pole; visual acuity is 20/20.

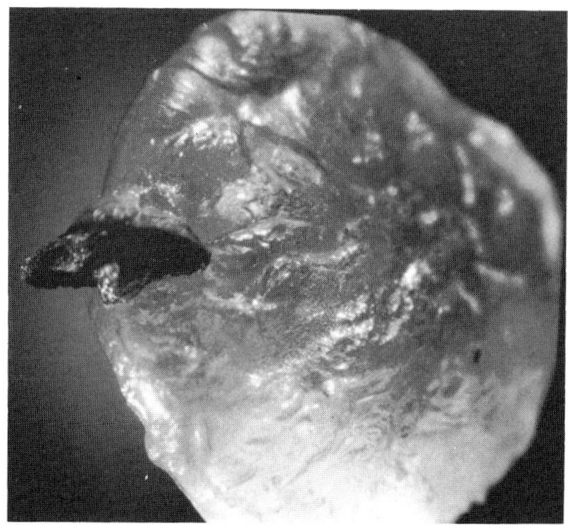

FIGURE 3-280 **Intraocular foreign body in a cataractous lens.** An intracapsular cataract extraction was performed to remove an intraocular foreign body deeply embedded in a cataractous lens.

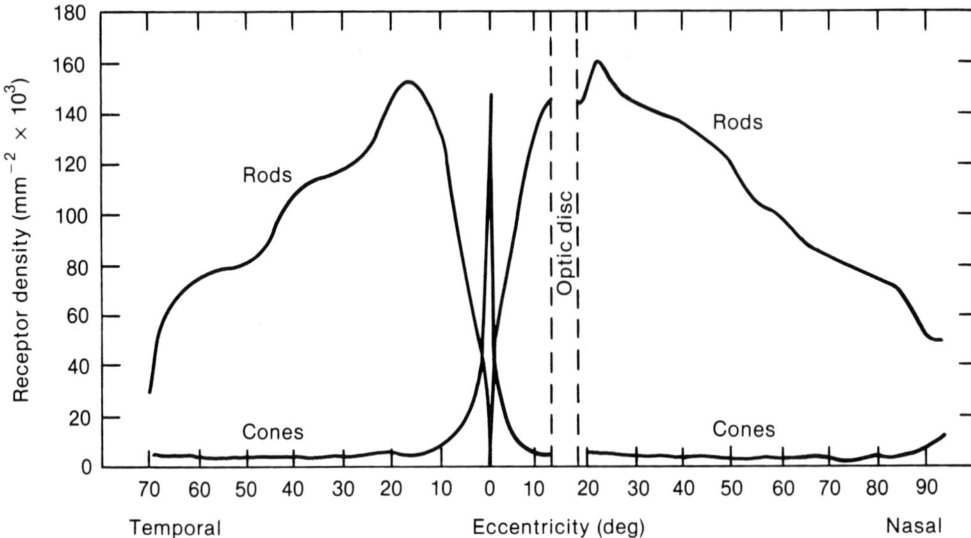

FIGURE 3-281 **Graph of photoreceptor distribution in the normal retina.** Distribution of rods and cones in the normal retina corresponding to perimetric angles from the fovea at zero degrees as given. Note the large number of rods at the retinal periphery and the high concentration of cones in the macular region. (After Østerberg. From Pirenne MH: Vision and the Eye. London, Chapman & Hall, 1967.)

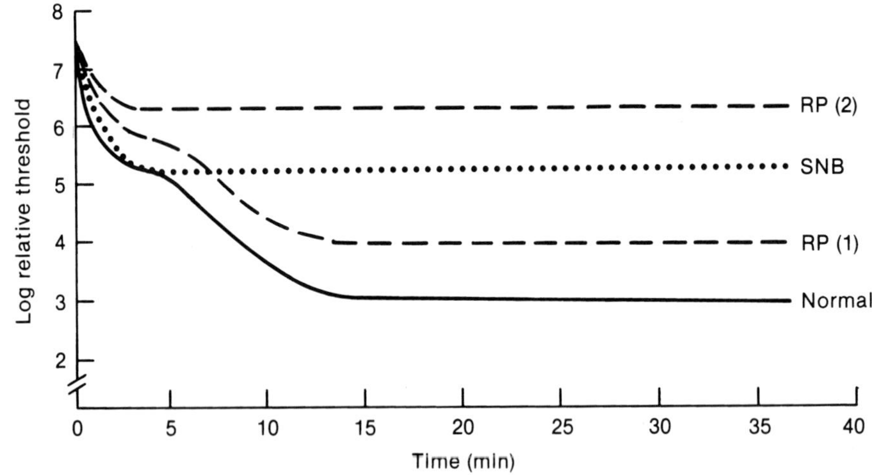

FIGURE 3-282 **Dark adaptation curves for normal subjects and patients with hereditary retinal diseases.** Representative dark-adaptation curves for a normal subject; a patient with congenital stationary night blindness (SNB); and two patients with moderately advanced retinitis pigmentosa, RP(1) and RP(2). In the patient with SNB, note the normal cone limb and the absent cone-rod break owing to the abnormal rod response. The patients with retinitis pigmentosa both have impairment of the initial cone limb of dark adaptation in contrast to the patient with SNB. (From Berson EL: Night blindness: Some aspects of management. *In* Faye E (ed): Clinical Low Vision. Boston, Little, Brown & Company, 1976.)

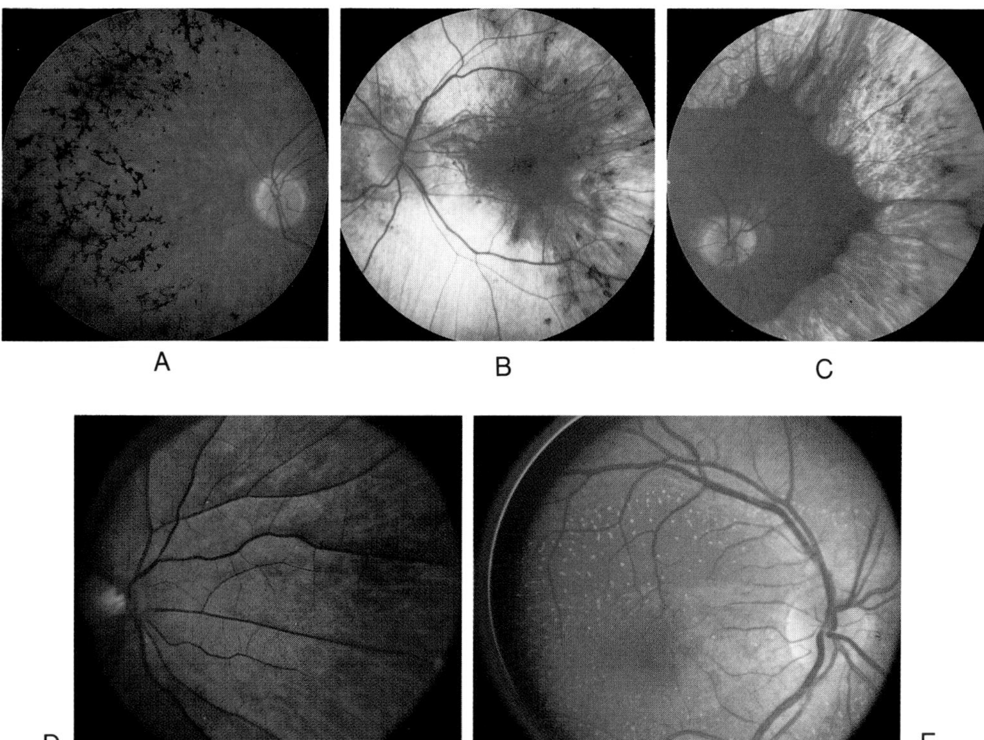

FIGURE 3–283 **Clinical photographs of retinitis pigmentosa, choroideremia, gyrate atrophy, Oguchi's disease, and fundus albipunctatus.** *A,* Moderately advanced retinitis pigmentosa demonstrating characteristic midperiphery pigmentary hypertrophy. Retinitis pigmentosa is a group of diseases caused by abnormal genes at various loci within the human genome, some of which include the X, 3, 6, and 8 chromosomes. These patients characteristically experience night blindness and difficulty with their midperipheral visual field in adolescence. *B,* This man demonstrates the characteristic findings of moderately advanced choroideremia, which include large patches of retinal pigment epithelium and choroidal atrophy with areas of pigment migration. The female carrier of this X-linked disorder demonstrates normal visual acuity, visual fields, dark adaptation studies, and electroretinographic findings. With few exceptions, the carriers show characteristic retinal pigment epithelium mottling and depigmentation that is most marked in the midperiphery. *C,* Fundus photograph of a patient with gyrate atrophy of the choroid and retina demonstrating garland-shaped, sharply defined zones of chorioretinal atrophy involving the midperiphery of the fundus. Elevated levels of ornithine in the plasma, urine, cerebrospinal fluid, and aqueous humor have been demonstrated in these patients. The enzyme ornithine ketoacid transaminase is deficient in these patients. *D,* Photograph demonstrating the clinical appearance of the fundus in a patient with Oguchi's disease without dark adaptation. Note the greenish yellow color to the fundus. This form of stationary night blindness achieves a normal fundus color after dark adaptation. Histopathologic studies demonstrate abnormally large cones in an area extending 20 degrees temporal from the optic nerve and an additional layer of granular pigment between the photoreceptors and the retinal pigment epithelium. *E,* Fundus appearance of a patient with fundus albipunctatus. Note the characteristic large number of discrete, small, punctate, white spots at the level of the retinal pigment epithelium. This autosomal recessively inherited disorder is typically nonprogressive.

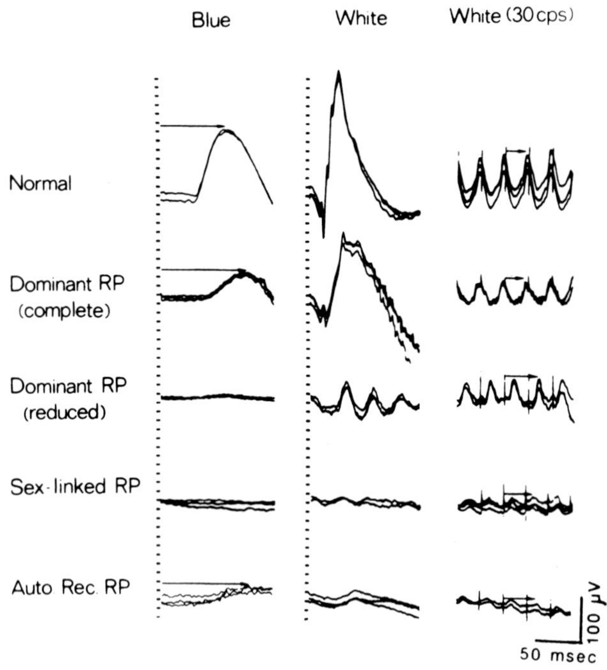

FIGURE 3–284 ERG responses for a normal subject and four patients with retinitis pigmentosa (age 13, 14, 14, and 9 years). Responses were obtained after 45 minutes of dark adaptation to single flashes of blue light *(left column)* and white light *(middle column)*. Responses *(right column)* were obtained to 30 c.p.s. (or 30 Hz) white flickering light. Calibration symbol *(lower right corner)* signifies 50 msec horizontally and 100 μV vertically. Rod b-wave implicit times in column 1 and cone implicit times in column 3 are designated with *arrows*. Rod responses to dim blue light under dark adapted conditions are reduced in all genetic types and when detectable, the b-wave implicit time is delayed as designated by horizontal *arrows* in the figure. Cone responses to 30 Hz white flickering light are normal or reduced in amplitude, and the cone implicit times may be normal or delayed. (From Berson EL: Retinitis pigmentosa and allied diseases: Electrophysiologic findings. Trans Am Acad Ophthalmol Otolaryngol 81: OP659–666, 1976.)

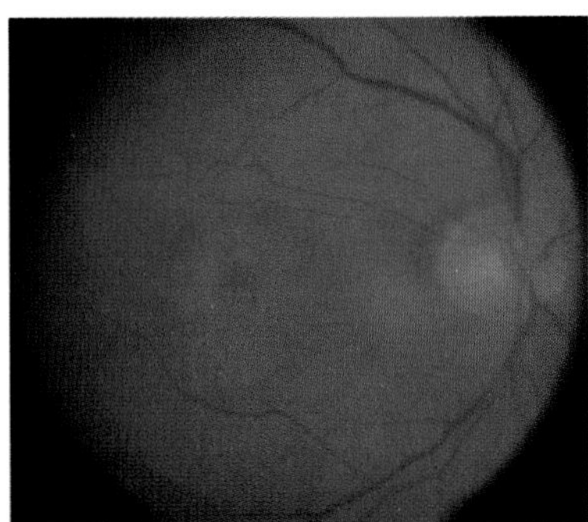

FIGURE 3–285 **Autosomal dominant cone degeneration.** Right eye of a 79-year-old man with autosomal dominant cone degeneration demonstrates the characteristic bull's eye maculopathy; visual acuity is 20/400. Patients with this condition typically present in the first two decades of life with complaints of declining central vision and photophobia. Abnormalities in the ERG are cone mediated, and color vision defects can be identified.

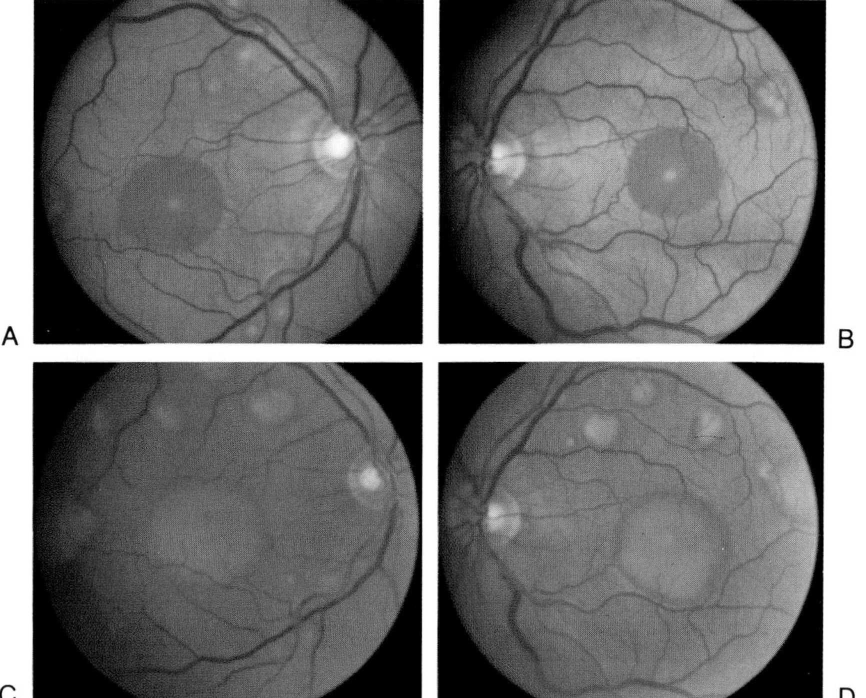

FIGURE 3–286 **Best's disease.** *A* and *B*, Fundus photographs of a 62-year-old man with a variant of Best's disease that show multifocal lesions in the posterior pole. Electro-oculogram showed a light-peak: dark-trough of 1.0 in both eyes. Visual acuity was 20/20 at the time of this photograph. *C* and *D*, Examination 8 months later revealed a typical vitelliform lesion in both eyes. Fluorescein angiography in these patients reveals blockage of choroidal fluorescence by the vitelliform lesion. Histopathologic studies of eyes from patients with Best's disease demonstrate retinal pigment epithelium cells with excessive amounts of lipofuscin-like material accumulation.

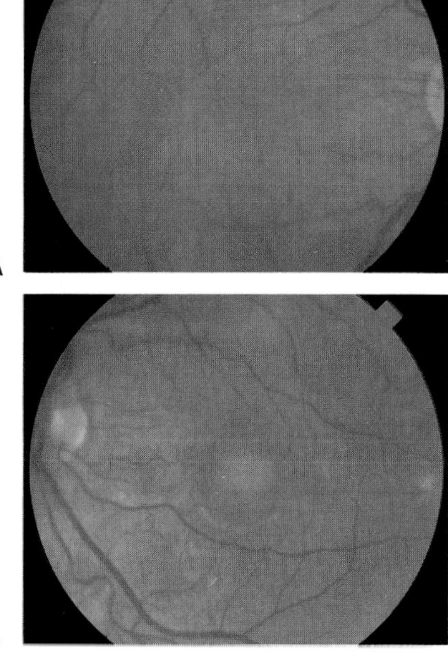

FIGURE 3–287 **Adult-onset foveomacular dystrophy.** *A* and *B*, Fundus photographs of a 30-year-old man with adult-onset foveomacular dystrophy. Note the pseudovitelliform macular lesion O.S. These patients can be distinguished from those with Best's disease by their older age at presentation and their normal electro-oculograms. Histopathologic evaluation of one eye in a patient with adult-onset vitelliform showed focal loss of photoreceptors and atrophy and partial loss of the retinal pigment epithelium in the fovea.

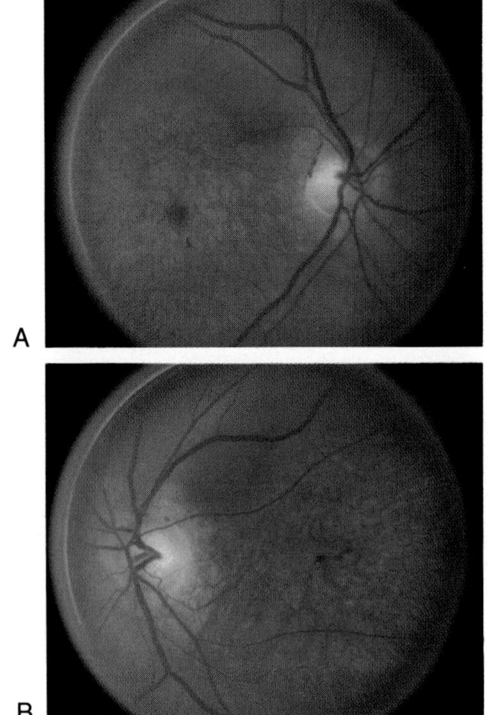

FIGURE 3–288 **Central areolar choroidal dystrophy.** Right fundus (*A*), and left fundus (*B*) of a 59-year-old woman with central areolar choroidal dystrophy O.U. Full-field cone and rod ERGs were reduced 60 percent below normal in both eyes. Dark adaptation was normal. The patient was hypermetropic and had no signs of drusen or other stigmata of age-related macular degeneration.

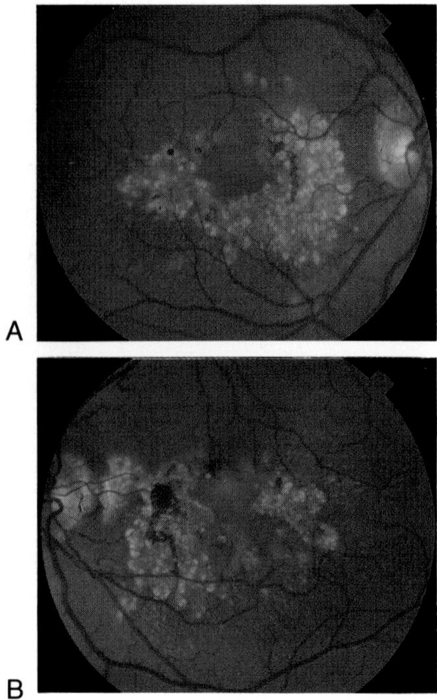

FIGURE 3–289 **Doyne's honeycomb macular dystrophy.** Fundus photographs of a 37-year-old man diagnosed with Doyne's honeycomb macular dystrophy. Visual acuity was 20/20 O.D. and 20/100 O.S. *A*, Right eye. *B*, Left eye. Note the typical honeycomb appearance of multiple confluent drusen with associated pigmentary changes. Full-field and focal ERG testing was normal.

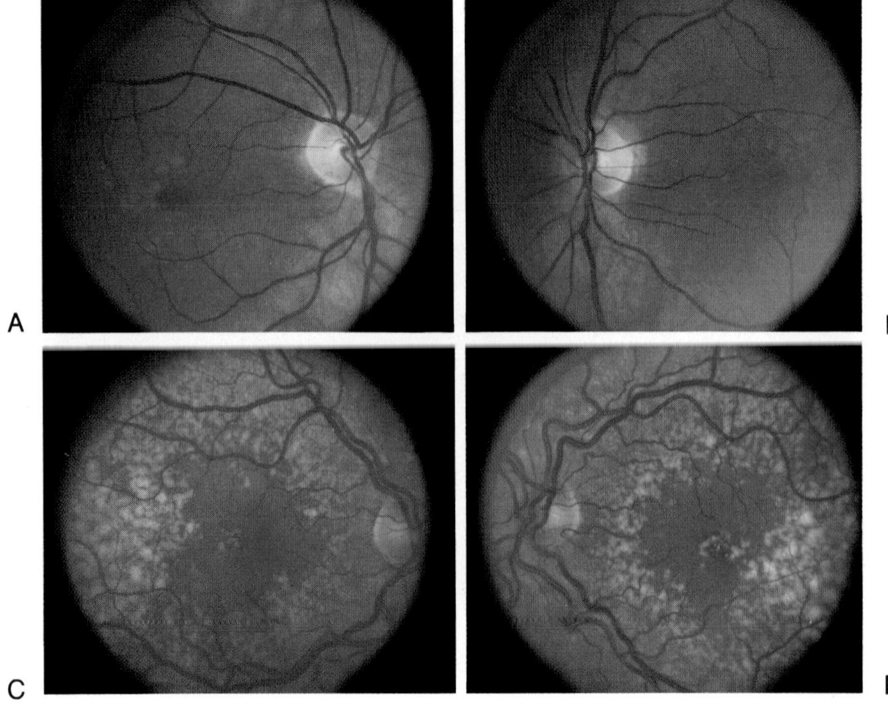

FIGURE 3–290 **Dominant drusen.** *A* and *B*, Fundus photographs of a 21-year-old woman with dominant drusen of both eyes. The visual acuity was 20/50 O.D. and 20/40 O.S. Her 57-year-old mother had 20/20 vision O.U. There were drusen in the posterior poles of both eyes (*C* and *D*). Patients with dominant drusen typically present at an early age (second to third decade of life) and usually have a family history of the disease in several generations. The drusen was distributed mainly in the macula and around the optic nerve head, often with a nasal predominance.

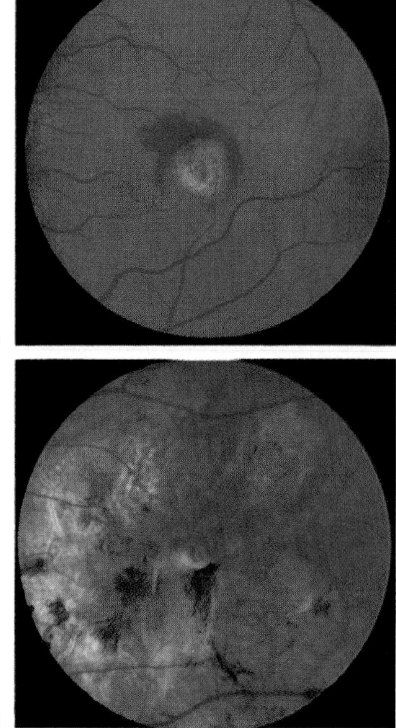

FIGURE 3–291 **Sorsby's pseudoinflammatory dystrophy.** Fundus photograph of a 40-year-old man with autosomal dominant hemorrhagic dystrophy (Sorsby's pseudoinflammatory dystrophy). *A,* A choroidal neovascular membrane is seen in the left eye. Twelve months later, a choroidal neovascular membrane developed in the right eye. *B,* His 63-year-old mother currently shows extensive retinal scarring and loss of retinal pigment epithelium and choriocapillaries. (Courtesy of Steven A. Boskovich, M.D., and Paul A. Sieving, M.D.)

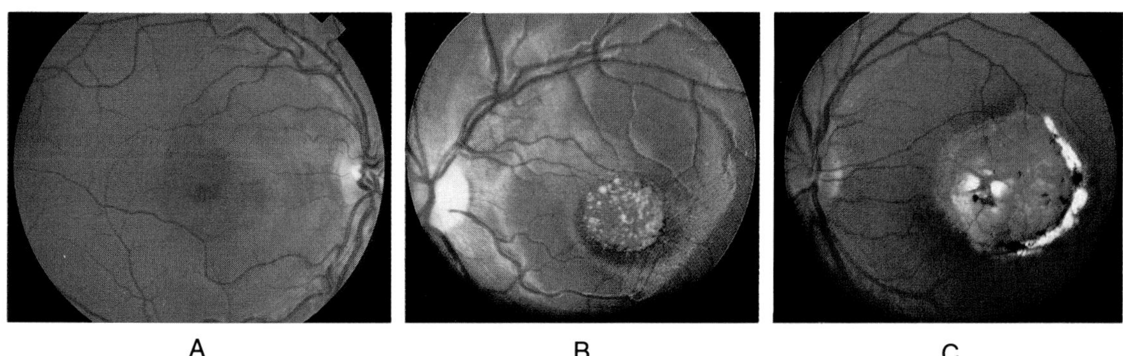

FIGURE 3–292 **North Carolina macular dystrophy.** Fundus photographs of three individuals from one family with North Carolina macular dystrophy. *A,* Left eye of a 22-year-old woman with 20/20 vision (grade 1 fundus). *B,* Right eye of a 7-year-old girl with 20/30 visual acuity (grade 2 fundus). *C,* Right eye of a 29-year-old man with 20/40 visual acuity and grade 3 fundus. In general, this condition is slowly progressive. Staphylomas with outpouching of the area of atrophy have been observed. Choroidal neovascular membranes can occur in these patients. (From Small KW, Killian J, McLean WC: North Carolina's dominant progressive foveal dystrophy: How progressive is it? Br J Ophthalmol 75:401, 1991.)

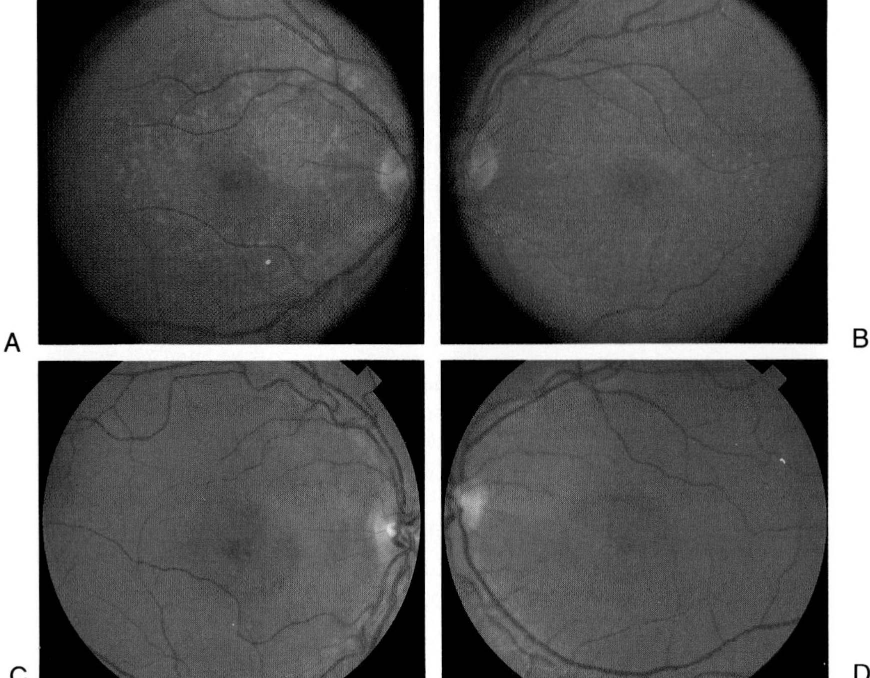

FIGURE 3–293 **Stargardt's disease.** Fundus photographs of two sisters with Stargardt's disease. The older sister (*A* and *B*), aged 17 years, had 20/200 visual acuity O.U. and showed white flecks at the level of the retinal pigment epithelium. Note the granular retinal pigment epithelial changes in the fovea. Her 10-year-old sister (*C* and *D*) had a 20/200 visual acuity O.U. with granular retinal pigment epithelial changes in the fovea and no retinal flecks. In contrast to drusen, these flecks do not fluoresce or show only an irregular pattern of fluorescence on fluorescein angiography. A heavily pigmented retinal pigment epithelium (vermillion fundus) that shows a silent choroid on fluorescein angiography has been described in a subset of these patients.

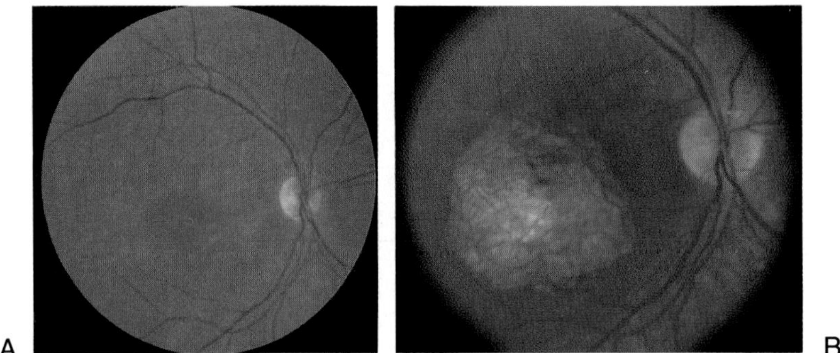

FIGURE 3–294 **Stargardt's disease.** Progression of macular changes in a patient with Stargardt's disease. *A*, Note the flecks throughout the posterior pole along with retinal pigment epithelium changes in the fovea and parafovea. Visual acuity was 20/200 at this time. *B*, Eleven years later, the visual acuity is unchanged; however, there is a large area of retinal pigment epithelium and choriocapillaris drop-out in the posterior pole. Patients can have normal full-field ERGs, whereas foveal ERGs are often abnormal even in those with near-normal visual acuity.

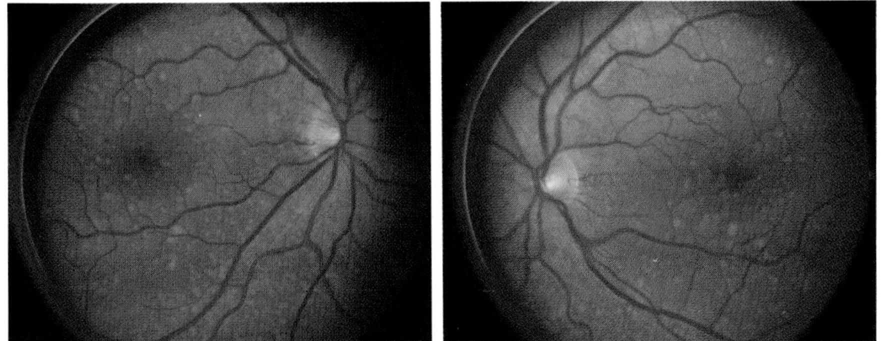

FIGURE 3–295 **Fundus flavimaculatus.** *A* and *B*, Fundus photographs of a 29-year-old woman with fundus flavimaculatus. Note the pisiform flecks at the level of the retinal pigment epithelium throughout the posterior pole. Histopathologic studies in this condition have indicated that there is an accumulation in the apex of retinal pigment epithelium cells of an acid mucopolysaccharide substance. The defects in the photoreceptors observed are believed to be secondary to the retinal pigment epithelium abnormality.

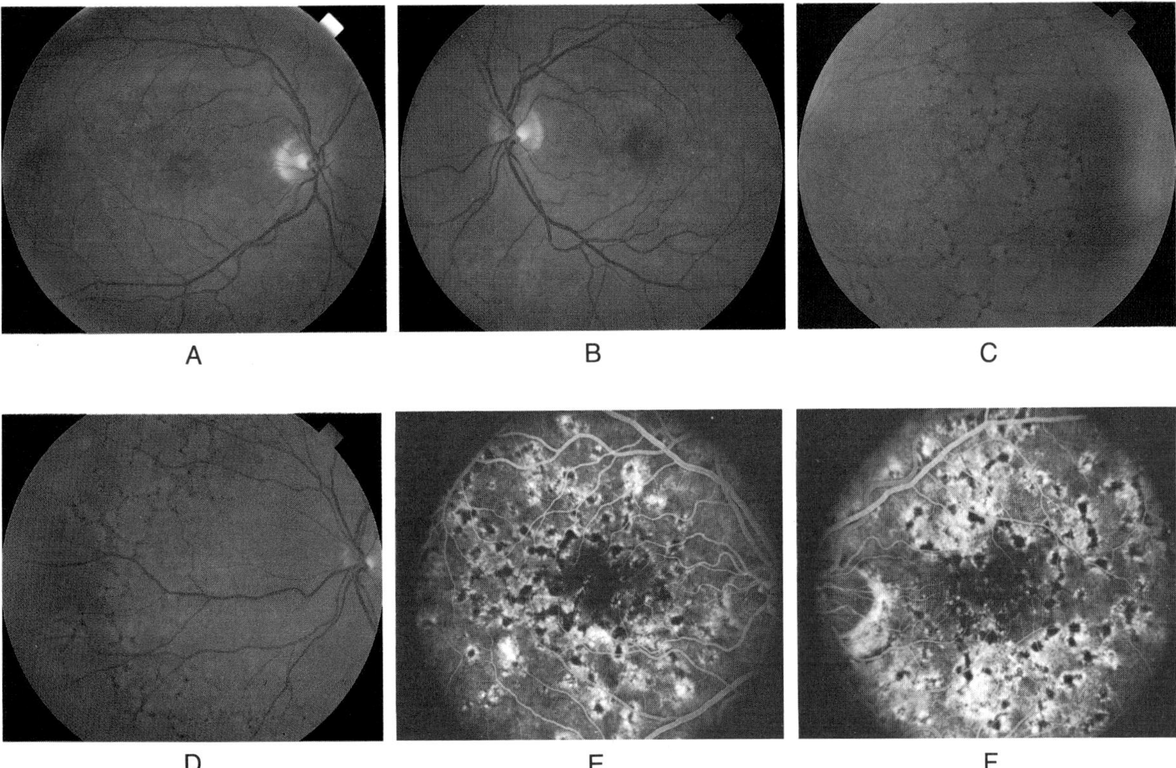

FIGURE 3–296 **Sjögren's reticular dystrophy.** Fundus photographs and fluorescein angiograms of a 32-year-old man with Sjögren's reticular dystrophy of the retinal pigment epithelium are shown. A netlike pattern of pigmentation is seen in the posterior pole and midperiphery (*A–D*). Fluorescein angiography demonstrates blockage of dye in the areas of hyperpigmentation and hyperfluorescence along with reticulated pattern corresponding to retinal pigment epithelium loss (*E* and *F*). Tests of retinal function are normal in this rare, usually autosomal recessive, condition.

SECTION 4

Glaucoma

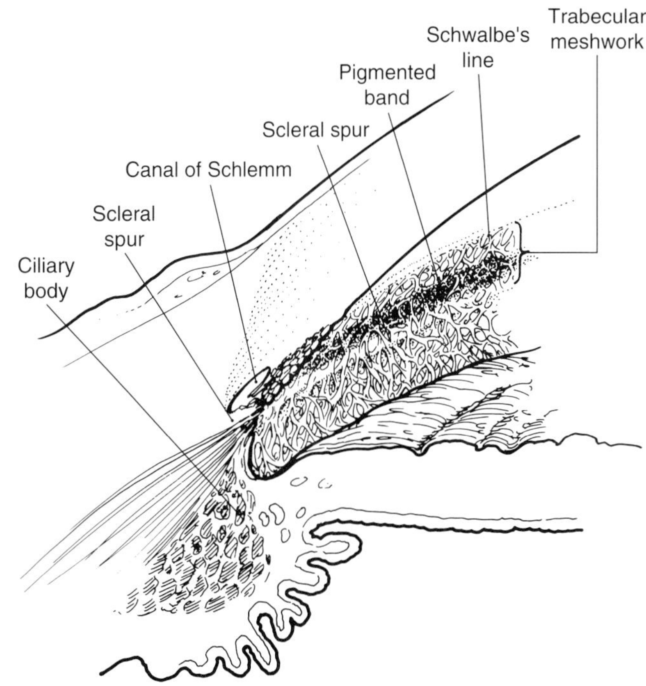

FIGURE 4–1 **Cross section of normal angle.** Posterior to the iris is the ciliary body, which produces aqueous and contributes to regulation of outflow of aqueous. The anterior extension of the ciliary body terminates at the scleral spur, which appears as a white line between the ciliary body band and the trabecular meshwork. Aqueous filters through the trabecular meshwork and exits through Schlemm's canal. A pigment band may occur in the trabecular meshwork overlying Schlemm's canal. Schwalbe's line indicates the most anterior border of the trabecular meshwork and the termination of Descemet's membrane of the cornea. If the location of this landmark is uncertain, Schwalbe's line can be identified using a slit beam and indirect gonioscopy because the slit beam is wide in the translucent cornea and converges to a single line at the more opaque tissue posterior to the end of Descemet's membrane. (Courtesy of Peter Netland, M.D.)

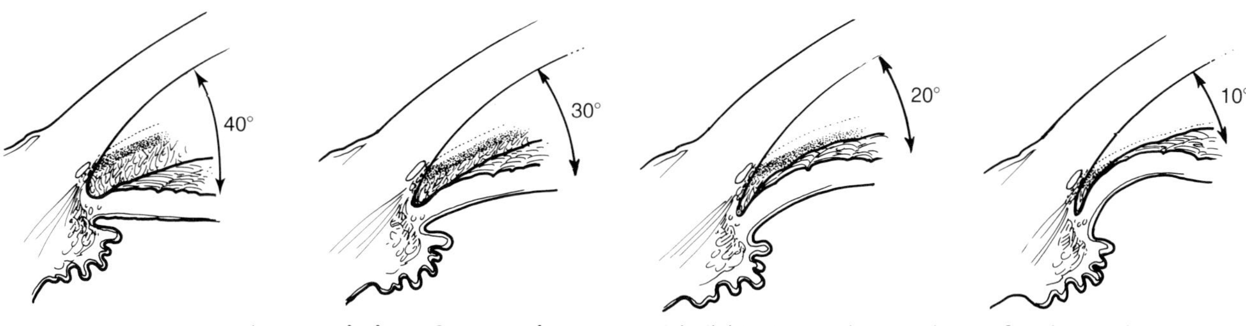

FIGURE 4–2 **Variation of angle width.** Normal individuals vary in the widths of their anterior chamber angles. The angle may be wide open, moderately narrowed, or extremely narrowed. Several classification systems have been described. The Schaffer grading system describes the wide open angle as grade 4 (>40°) or grade 3 (approximately 30°), the moderately narrow angle as grade 2 (about 20°), and the extremely narrow angle as grade 1 (about 10°). The angle may be narrowed to a slit width (grade S, <10°) or may be closed (grade 0). The likelihood of angle-closure glaucoma increases markedly when the angular width is less than 10 to 20 degrees. (Courtesy of Peter Netland, M.D.)

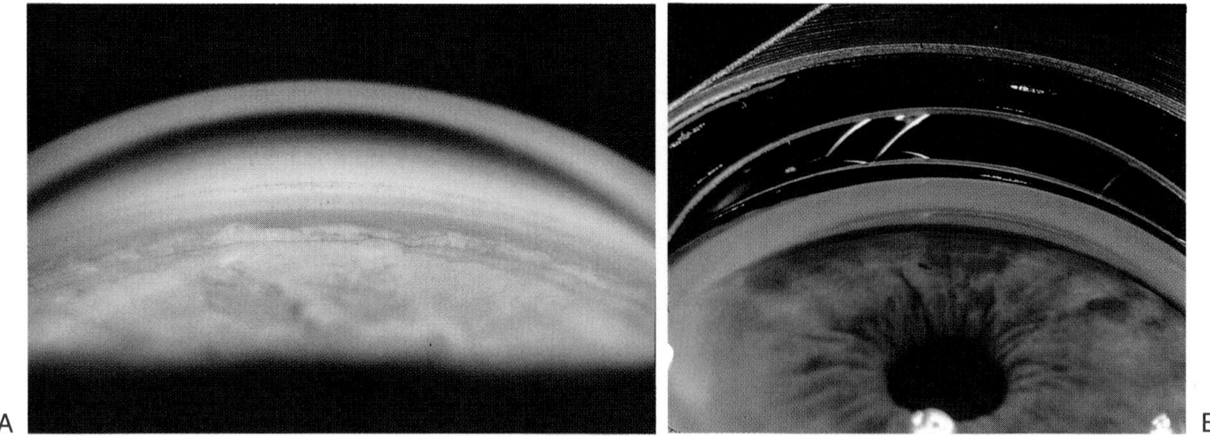

FIGURE 4–3 **Variation of angle width.** *A*, Wide open angle with a relatively flat iris contour and a broad ciliary body band. In myopic individuals, the angle is often, but not always, wide open. *B*, Convex iris and a more narrow angle with a less prominent ciliary body band. (Courtesy of Peter Netland, M.D.)

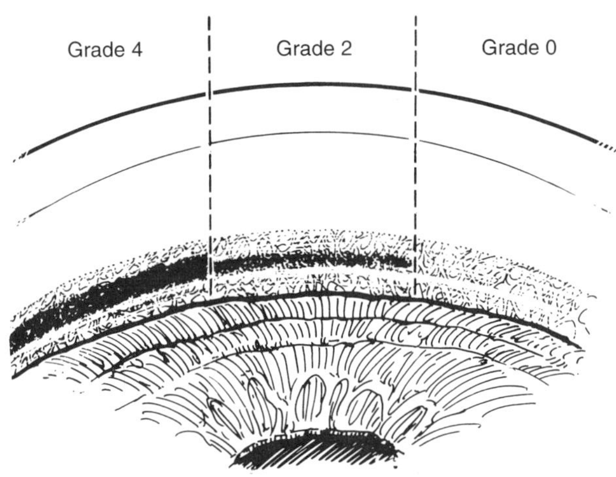

FIGURE 4–4 **Variation of angle pigmentation.** In adults, the normal angle varies in its degree of pigmentation. Pigment, which is usually more prominent in the posterior trabecular meshwork in the area overlying Schlemm's canal, may be dense, moderate, or light *(left to right in figure)*. There is a gradual accumulation of pigment in the trabecular meshwork throughout life. In younger individuals, the trabecular meshwork contains little or no pigment. (Courtesy of Peter Netland, M.D.)

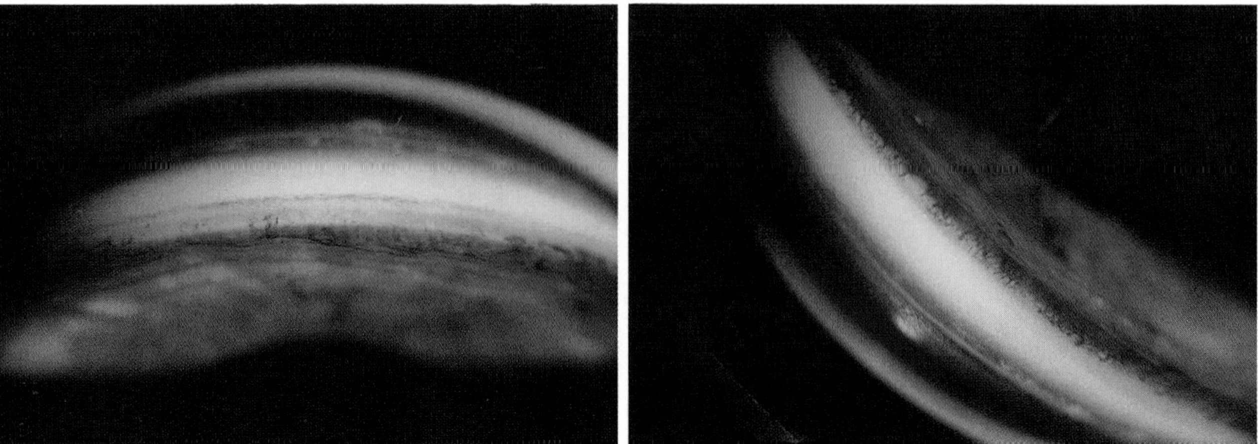

FIGURE 4–5 **Variation of angle width and pigment in the same eye.** The angle may be wider in one quadrant than another in the same eye. Often the angle is wider inferiorly than superiorly. Also, more pigment may be deposited on the inferior nasal angle. In this example, the angle is more open and is more pigmented inferiorly *(A)* compared with superonasally *(B)*. (Courtesy of Peter Netland, M.D.)

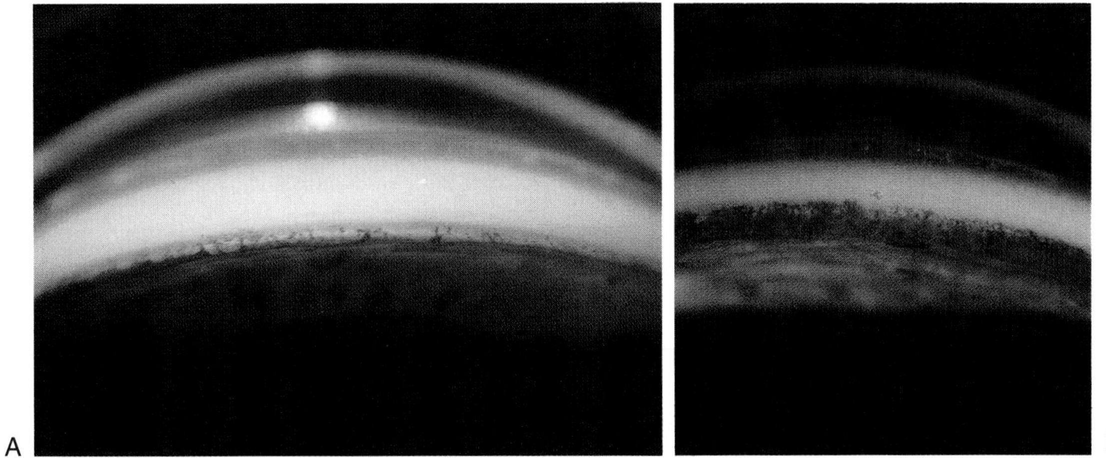

FIGURE 4–6 **Iris processes.** These delicate, irregular fibers arise from the anterior iris stroma and bridge the angle recess. Usually, iris processes terminate at the scleral spur, but they may extend more anteriorly. Normal angles vary in the distribution and appearance of these processes. Shown are sparse iris processes with blood in Schlemm's canal *(A)* and dense iris processes with lightly pigmented trabecular meshwork *(B)*. (Courtesy of Peter Netland, M.D.)

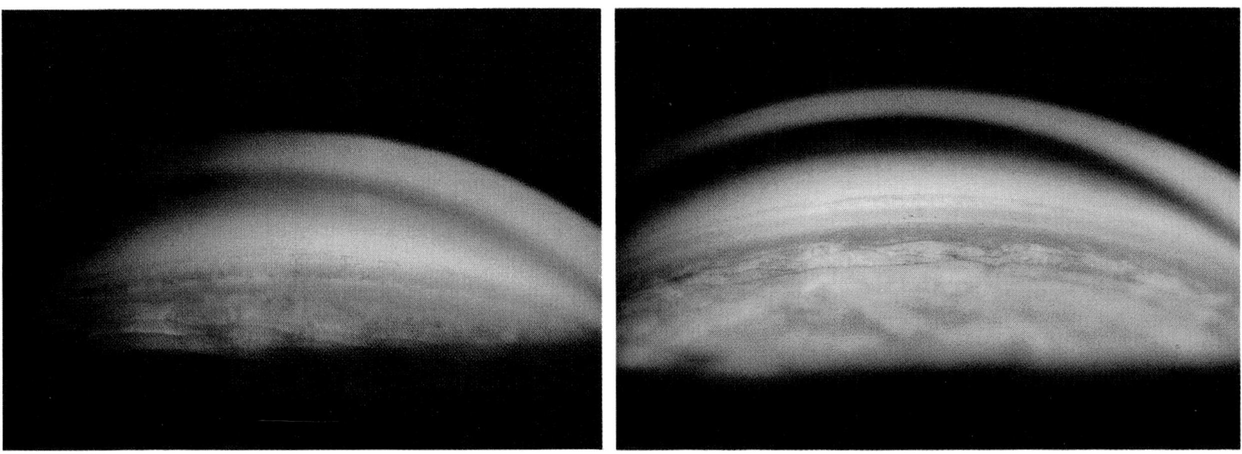

FIGURE 4–7 **Normal blood vessels.** Circumferential vessels in the peripheral iris stroma may have a sinuous, sea-serpent appearance *(A,B)*. Also seen are radial vessels in the superficial iris stroma or straight vessels in the ciliary body that disappear below the scleral spur. Vessels that extend from the iris and attach in the scleral spur or trabecular meshwork are usually abnormal. (Courtesy of Peter Netland, M.D.)

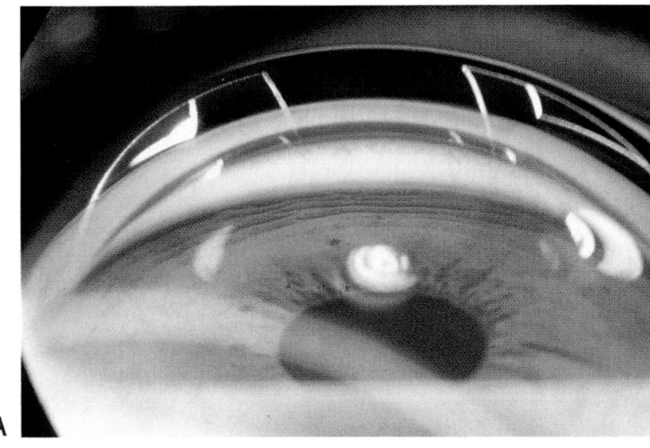

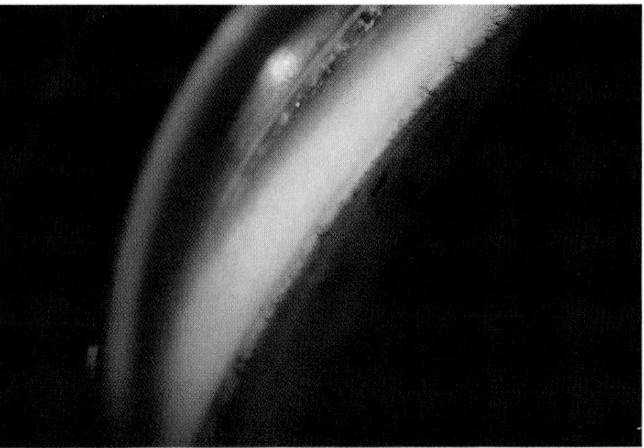

FIGURE 4–8 **Blood in Schlemm's canal.** Aqueous humor normally flows to Schlemm's canal through the trabecular meshwork. With decreased intraocular pressure or increased venous pressure (e.g., due to compression of limbal vessels with gonioscopy), blood may reflux to Schlemm's canal and into the trabecular meshwork. Blood in Schlemm's canal can be visualized by gonioscopy as a red line or band just anterior to the scleral spur, in the region of the posterior trabecular meshwork, in all or part of the circumference of the angle *(A,B)*. (Courtesy of Peter Netland, M.D.)

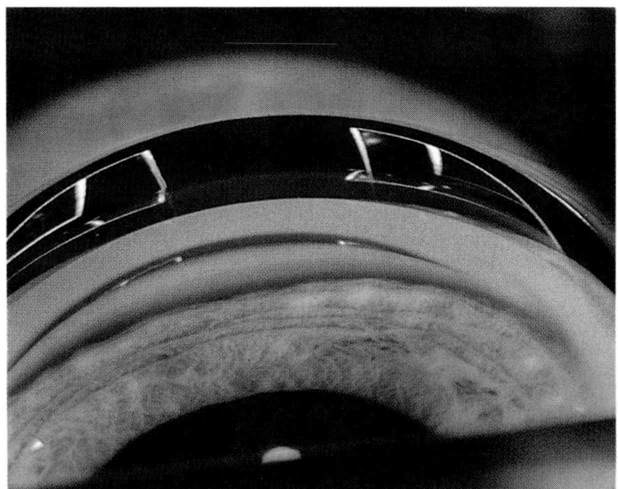

FIGURE 4–9 **Gonioscopy of primary open-angle glaucoma.** There are no known unique gonioscopic features of the anterior chamber angle in primary open-angle glaucoma. Patients with primary open-angle glaucoma cannot be distinguished from normal individuals based on the appearance of their angle. Some yet to be fully elucidated defect in aqueous outflow leads to a rise in intraocular pressure (normal in epidemiologic studies is under 21 mmHg). Damage to the retinal ganglion cells and their axons is highly unpredictable with elevations in intraocular pressure but becomes more severe with progressively rising pressure. (Courtesy of Peter Netland, M.D.)

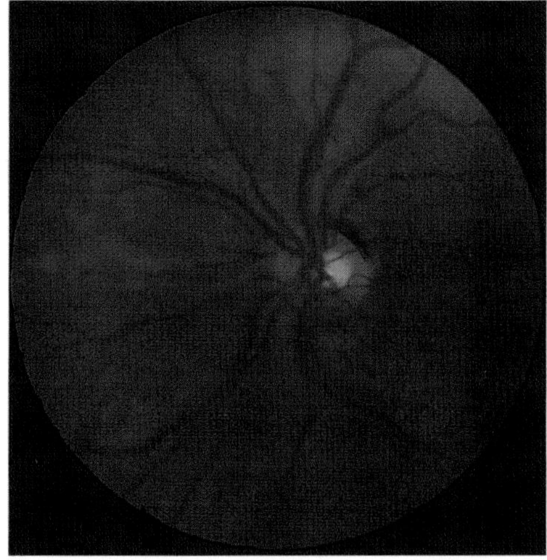

FIGURE 4–10 **Normal optic nerve head.** The optic nerve head, also referred to as the disc or the papilla, represents the exit point for all retinal ganglion cell axons from the eye. Roughly 3.5 mm nasal to the fovea, it is a 1.5 × 2 mm gap in the sclera, choroid, and retinal pigment epithelium. The normal disc contains roughly 1 million axons in the adult human eye. The disc is to date—the most sensitive index of glaucomatous pathology. It is generally believed that disc pathology can be observed before either visual field or acuity loss occurs in glaucoma. Unfortunately, however, up to half of the retinal ganglion cell axons can be lost before optic nerve pathology is detectable. Indicators of glaucoma that can be detected by examination of the disc include (1) asymmetry of the cup size between eyes; (2) notching, especially along the vertical meridian; (3) undermined sharp edges of the cup especially along the superior and inferior aspects; and (4) a cup-to-disc ratio (along the vertical meridian) of greater than 0.6. In this photograph of a healthy nerve head, the relatively greater extension of the horizontal cup when compared with the vertical extension is a normal variant. An incidental finding in this illustration is the presence of pigment along the superotemporal trim. (Courtesy of Dr. Evan B. Dreyer and Audrey C. Melanson.)

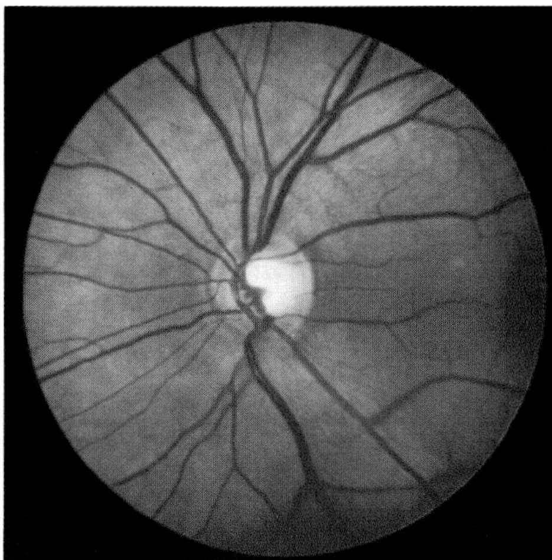

FIGURE 4–11 **Normal optic nerve head.** Although this cup is larger than that seen in (1), there is no evidence of notching, vessel displacement, or saucerization. No undermining can be seen in any quadrant. The horizontal and vertical extensions are equivalent. (Courtesy of Dr. Evan B. Dreyer and Audrey C. Melanson.)

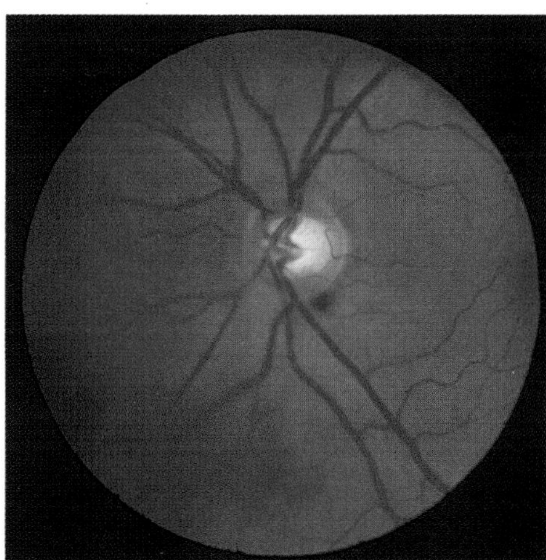

FIGURE 4–12 **Moderate glaucomatous optic nerve.** Although the cup-to-disc ratio in this nerve is similar to that depicted in (2), there is evidence of significant undermining both superiorly and inferiorly. This pathologic change is reflective of glaucoma. Furthermore, the lamina cribrosa can be clearly seen in this optic nerve head. (Courtesy of Dr. Evan B. Dreyer and Audrey C. Melanson.)

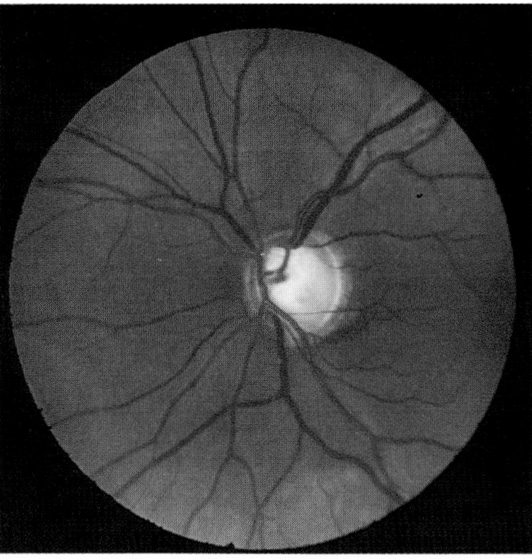

FIGURE 4–13 **Moderate glaucomatous optic nerve.** There is distinct evidence of undermining superiorly, and the cup slopes to the rim inferiorly. One can also appreciate nasal displacement of the vessels, especially inferiorly. In the normal optic nerve head, vessels should course outward in a radial fashion in all directions except temporally. In advanced glaucoma, vessels are displaced nasally. Those vessels that would in the unaffected eye have exited between 2 and 4 o'clock have been displaced by the disease process to 12 and 6 o'clock. (Courtesy of Dr. Evan B. Dreyer and Audrey C. Melanson.)

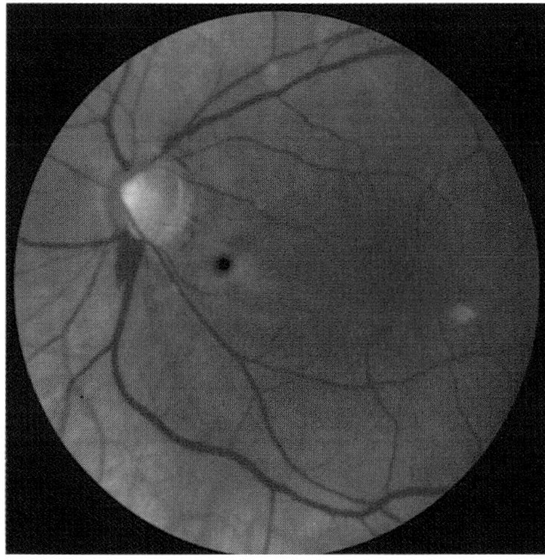

FIGURE 4–14 **Optic nerve head hemorrhage.** Most commonly found inferotemporally, optic nerve head hemorrhages are more likely to be found in patients with normal or low tension glaucoma. It can, however, represent a pathologic sign in all forms of glaucoma. Note also the pronounced nasalization of the vessels. (Courtesy of Dr. Evan B. Dreyer and Audrey C. Melanson.)

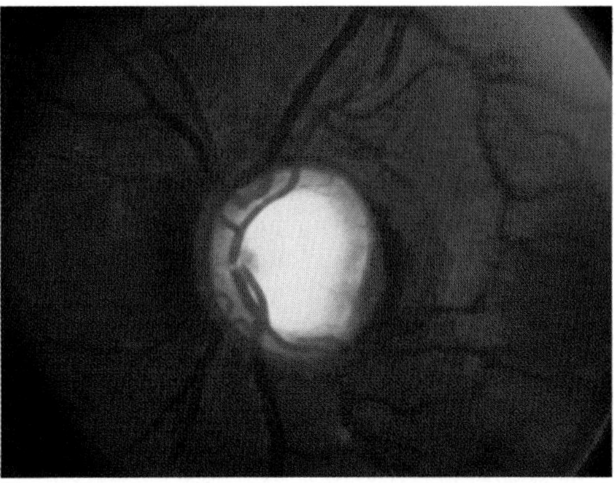

FIGURE 4–15 **Advanced glaucomatous optic nerve.** Little or no intact neural rim is seen in this photograph. The cup is enlarged in all sectors but most prominently in the vertical axis. One can also appreciate loss of the normal nerve fiber layer striations, indicative of the disease process. (Courtesy of Dr. Evan B. Dreyer and Audrey C. Melanson.)

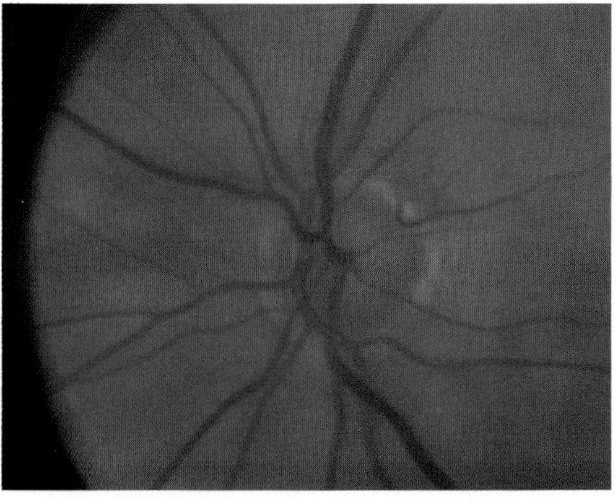

FIGURE 4–16 **Advanced glaucomatous optic nerve.** Although the optic nerve head in this photograph has no evidence of pallor, a careful evaluation of the course of the vessels reveals extension on the cup almost to the rim. This is an example of how evaluating the disc through a nuclear sclerotic cataract can be deceiving. This condition would be significantly easier to evaluate with stereophotography. (Courtesy of Dr. Evan B. Dreyer and Audrey C. Melanson.)

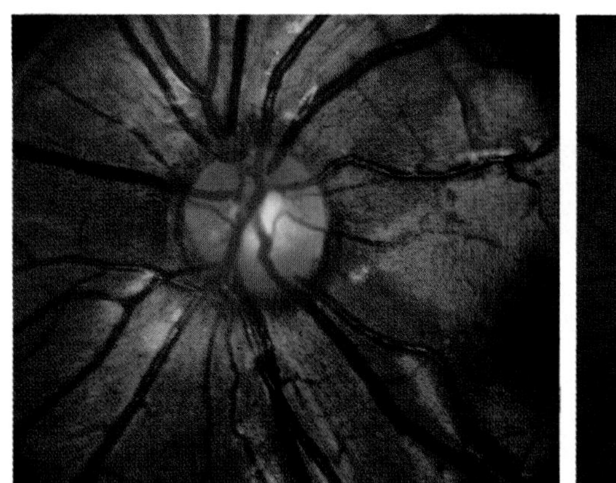

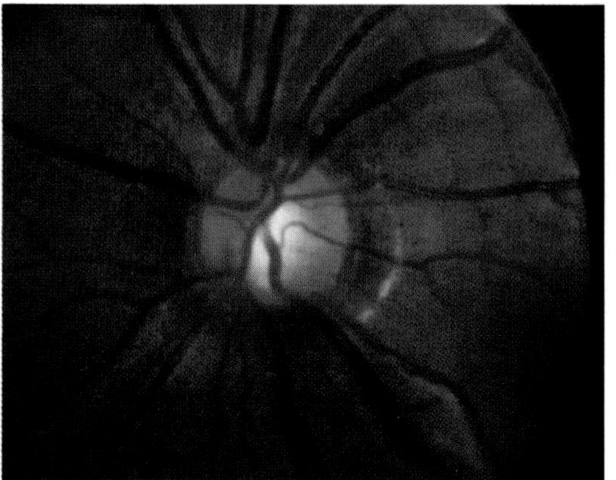

FIGURE 4–17 **Glaucomatous progression.** This illustrates the most important fact of evaluation of the optic nerve head in glaucoma—progression over time. *A* shows a healthy optic nerve head. In *B*, taken 3 years later, one can see extension of the cup inferiorly, almost to the rim. (Courtesy of Dr. Evan B. Dreyer and Audrey C. Melanson.)

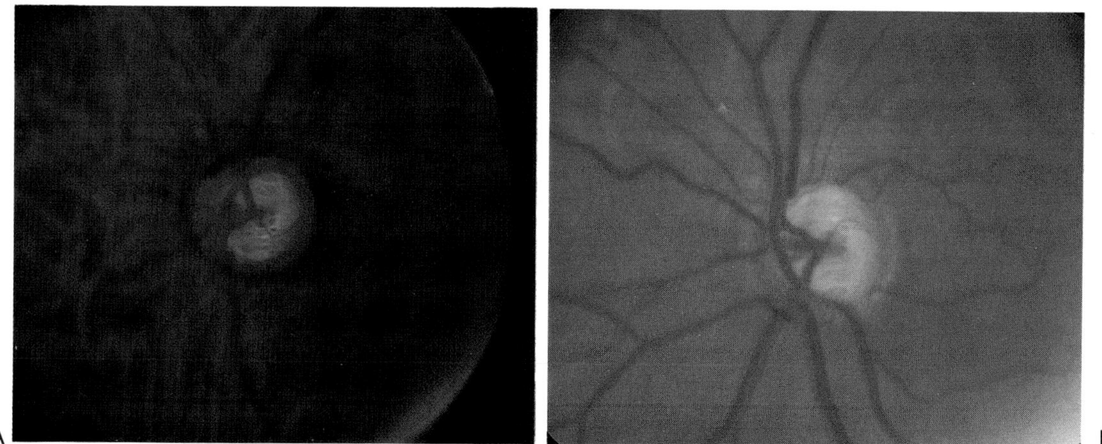

FIGURE 4–18 **Glaucomatous progression.** *A* and *B*, The inferotemporal vessels in this optic nerve head have gradually become more nasalized in these photographs, separated by 8 years. (Courtesy of Dr. Evan B. Dreyer and Audrey C. Melanson.)

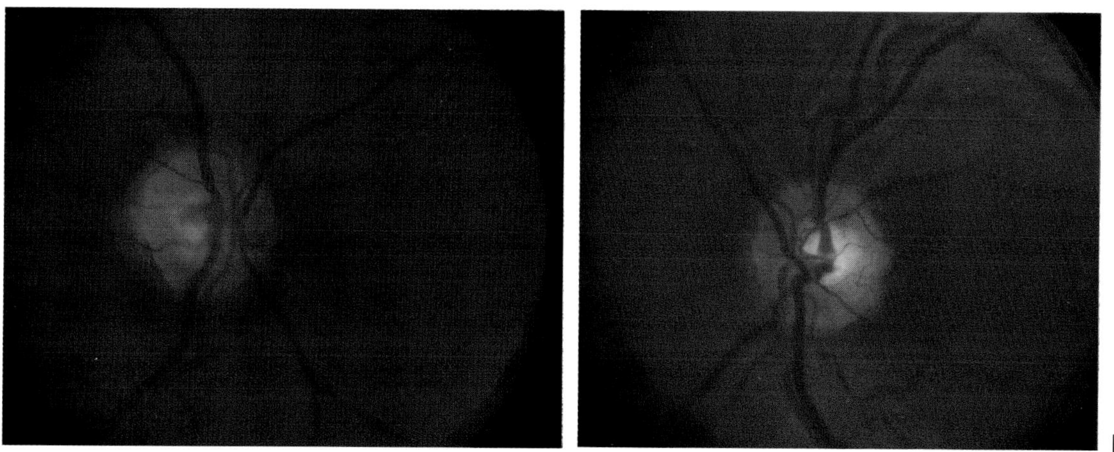

FIGURE 4–19 **Optic nerve head asymmetry.** *A* and *B*, Comparison of these photographs reveals a significantly larger cup on the right. Optic nerve head asymmetry is considered a relatively reliable indicator of the presence of glaucoma. (Courtesy of Dr. Evan B. Dreyer and Audrey C. Melanson.)

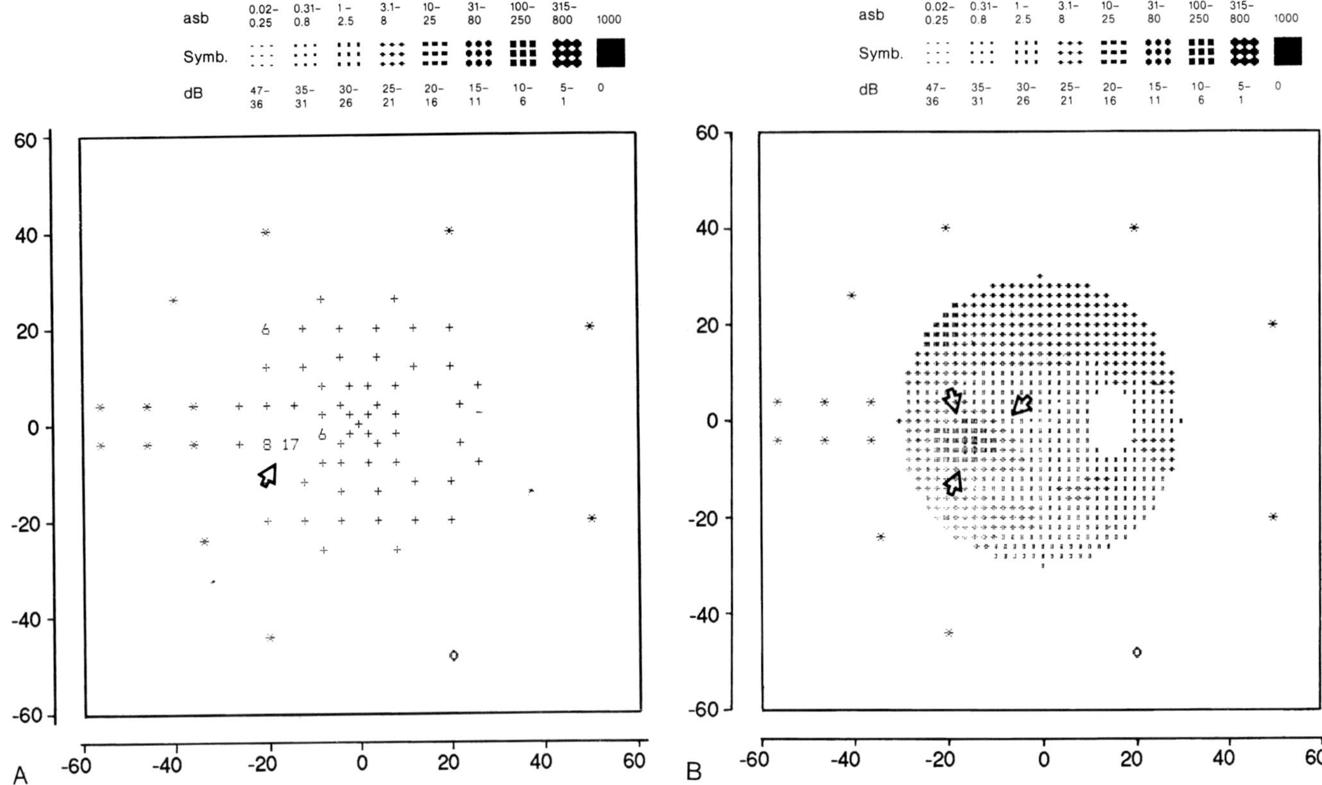

FIGURE 4–20 **Paracentral scotoma.** *A* and *B*, Octopus fields from the right eye of a 59-year-old man with open-angle glaucoma. Note the localized depression *(arrows)* just nasal to fixation, representative of an early paracentral scotoma. These paracentral scotomas develop in the nerve-fiber bundle (or arcuate area) of the visual field. The typical progression for these paracentral scotomas is to become larger and denser, eventually forming a central absolute defect, surrounded by a relative scotoma.

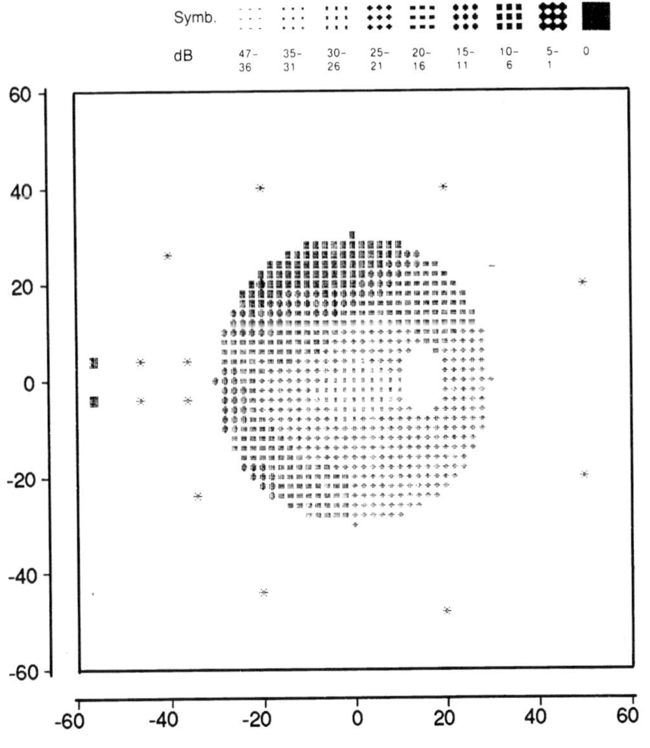

FIGURE 4–21 **Peripheral visual field depression.** A 76-year-old man with mild-to-moderate diffuse depression superiorly and mild midperipheral depression nasally. The diffuse reduction in visual threshold appears to be one of the earliest detectable alterations in the visual field of a patient with glaucoma. The diagnostic value of this phenomenon, however, is limited by its nonspecific nature, making careful correlation between the actual defect observed and the optic nerve head important. In this case, the patient has elevated intraocular pressure and an increased cup-to-disc ratio, but it is difficult to state that his field loss is entirely glaucomatous.

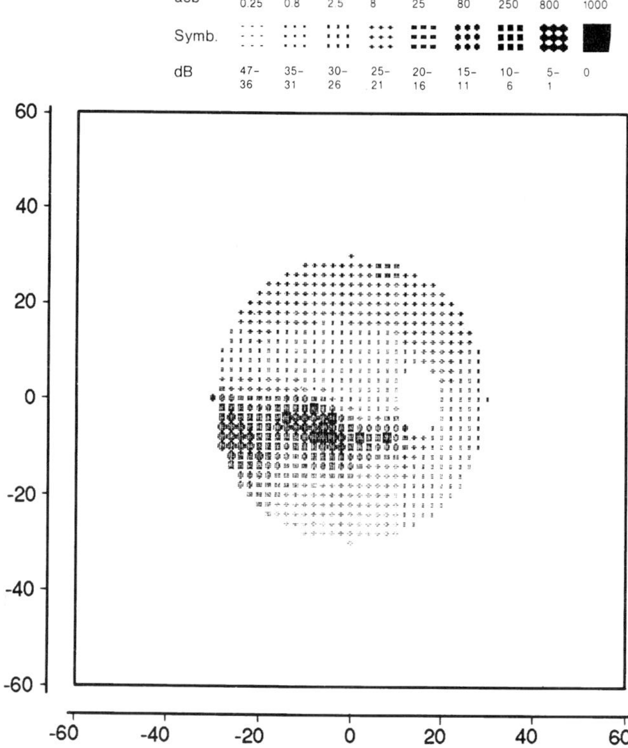

FIGURE 4–22 **Dense localized visual field defect.** The automated printout shows a dense localized defect largely surrounded by a normal area. This pattern of a dense localized defect surrounded by normal or near-normal visual field regions is characteristic of the localized visual defect pattern.

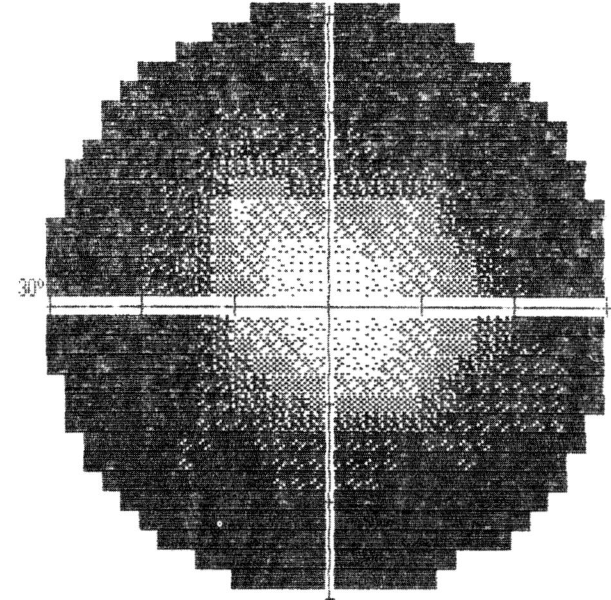

FIGURE 4–23 **Severe generalized visual field depression.** A Humphrey visual field showing severe generalized depression. In contrast to localized defects, generalized defects have a diffuse or uniform loss of field with many or most test points depressed. Areas of normal function tend to be clustered, as are areas of depressed function.

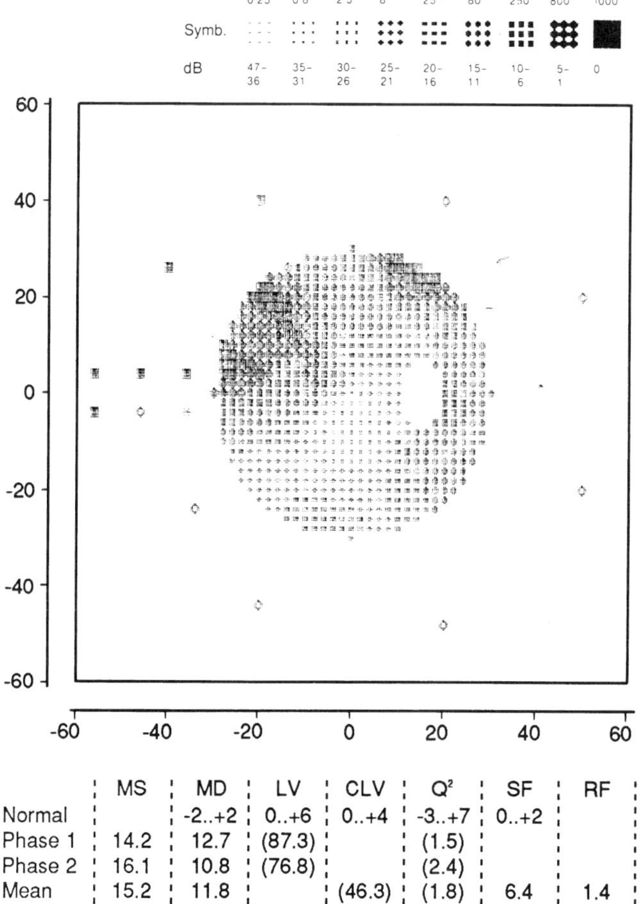

	MS	MD	LV	CLV	Q²	SF	RF
Normal		-2..+2	0..+6	0..+4	-3..+7	0..+2	
Phase 1	14.2	12.7	(87.3)		(1.5)		
Phase 2	16.1	10.8	(76.8)		(2.4)		
Mean	15.2	11.8		(46.3)	(1.8)	6.4	1.4

FIGURE 4–24 **Visual field indices from the Octopus machine.** The loss variance (LV) was high in phases 1 (first test) and 2 (second test, performed during the same examination session). In this case, the short-term fluctuation (SF), similar to measurement error, was also high. When the LV is mathematically corrected for the slightly abnormal SF, the resultant corrected loss variance (CLV) is much lower than the LV. In other words, the LV in this case was elevated substantially by measurement error; the corrected value gives a more accurate indication of the level of pathology.

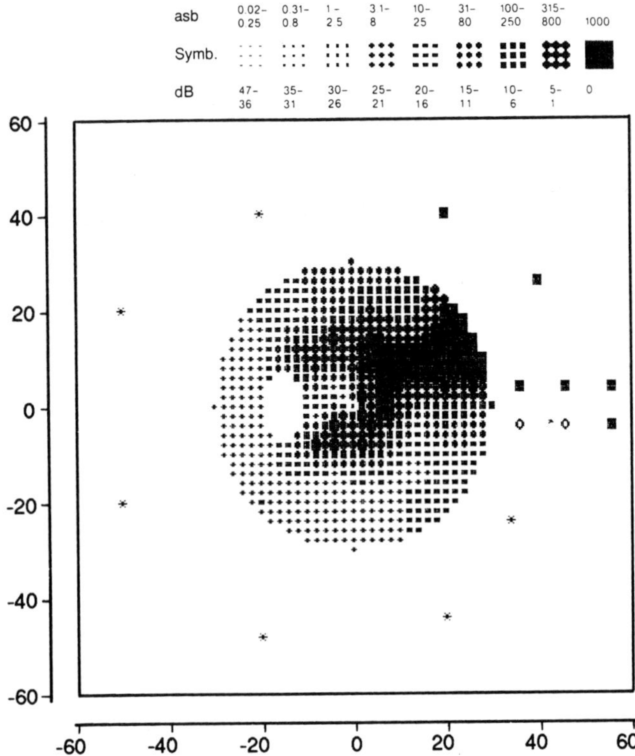

FIGURE 4-25 **Progressive glaucomatous visual field damage.** Glaucomatous visual field showing inferior and superior arcuate scotomas, superior nasal step, and superior nasal peripheral breakthrough. Central fixation and the temporal and inferior periphery are spared. The arcuate (Bjerrum) area within the visual field arches above and below fixation from the blind spot to the median raphe, and these correspond to the arcuate retinal nerve fiber orientation. Loss of corresponding bundles of peripheral nerve fibers produces unequal contraction of the peripheral isopters resulting in peripheral nasal steps.

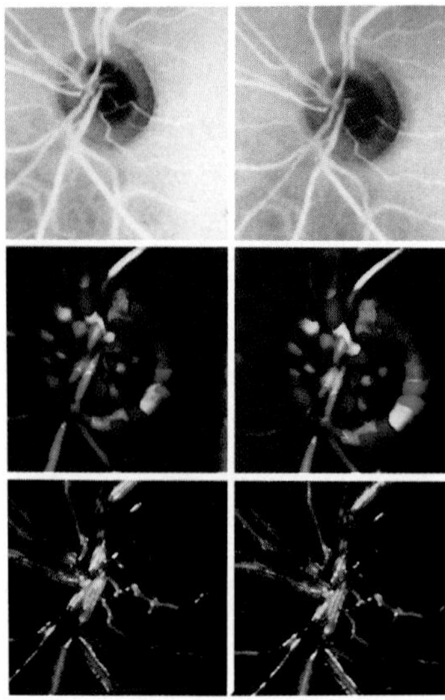

FIGURE 4-27 **Digitized stereo images of optic nerve head.** The top two images are gray scale representations of intensity values in an original pair of digitized stereo images. The middle and bottom pairs of stereo images represent digitally filtered versions of the original stereo images, with each column corresponding to the same perspective. For each location in the original stereo image pair, a series of directional filters at a given level of spatial resolution was used to evaluate the magnitude and direction of local intensity gradients at the level of spatial resolution. In these images, false colors represent these local intensity gradient direction values, and intensities represent these local gradient magnitude values. The middle pair of images was obtained at low spatial resolution, and the bottom pair of images was obtained at high spatial resolution. Note that some features of the original image are enhanced in the low-resolution images (e.g., the rim of the optic disc and larger vessels), whereas other features of the original image are enhanced in the high-resolution images (e.g., the smaller vessels). This type of multiresolution description of local image structure has been used to construct an artificial visual system. (From Coggins JM: A multiscale description of image structure for segmentation of biomedical images. Proceedings of the Conference on Visualization in Biomedical Computing. Atlanta, May 22, 1990, pp. 123–130.)

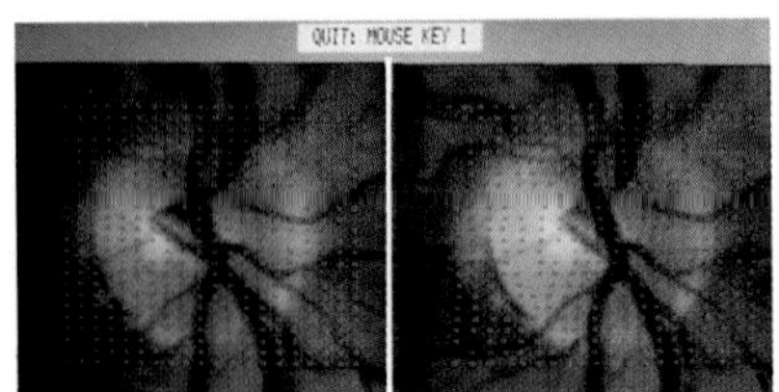

FIGURE 4-26 **Stereoscopic matching technique for optic nerve imaging.** In this example from the Humphrey retinal analyzer, a grid of points selected in the left stereo image was matched to the corresponding points in the right stereo image, using a cross-correlation operation that identifies pairs of corresponding points by the similarity of a window of intensity values around each point. After matching 400 to 650 pairs of corresponding points that have a grid correlation of their intensity windows *(shown with red crosses)*, a smooth surface is interpolated. (From Dandona DL, Quigley HA, Jampal DH: Variability of depth measurements of the optic nerve head and peripapillary retina with computerized image analysis. Arch Ophthalmol 107:1786, 1989. Copyright 1989, American Medical Association.)

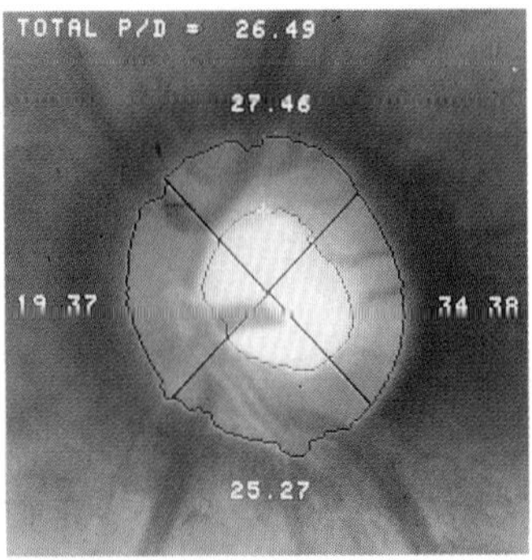

FIGURE 4-28 **A boundary-tracking algorithm for examining nerve contour.** A boundary-tracking algorithm followed the edge of the cup and disc, while ignoring edges due to crossing vessel, which are excluded by a set of local curvature constraints. The optic disc margin was determined with the red-filtered image, and the pallor margin was determined with the green-filtered image. Pallor area-to-disc area ratios were computed for each of the four illustrated quadrants and for the entire disc. (From Nagin P, Schwartz B, Nanba K: The reproducibility of computerized boundary analysis for measuring optic disc pallor in the normal optic. Ophthalmology 92:243, 1985.)

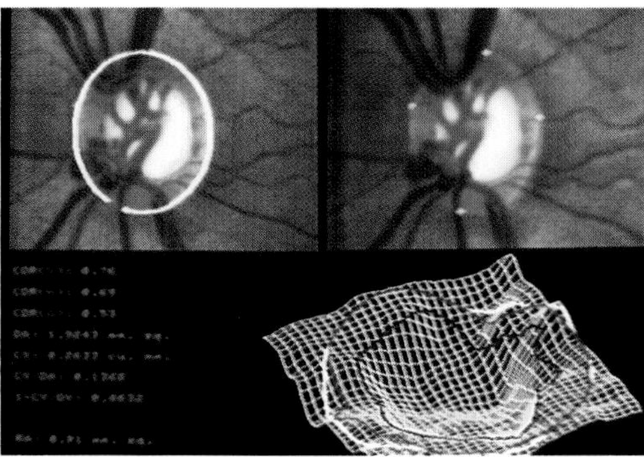

FIGURE 4–29 **Digital image analysis of the optic nerve.** In this example from the Topcon Imagenet, a pair of stereo images are shown at the top with four operator-provided control points on the right image, and the calculated cup margin and elliptical disc margin are superimposed on the left image. The three-dimensional wire basket plot was interpolated from calculated depth values and is shown with the superimposed blue cup margin determined by the cup-drop method. Using the cup-and-rim model, the optic nerve head is described in terms of several calculated statistics. (From Varma R, Spaeth GL: The PAR IS 2000: A new system for retinal digital image analysis. Ophthalmic Surg 19:183, 1988.)

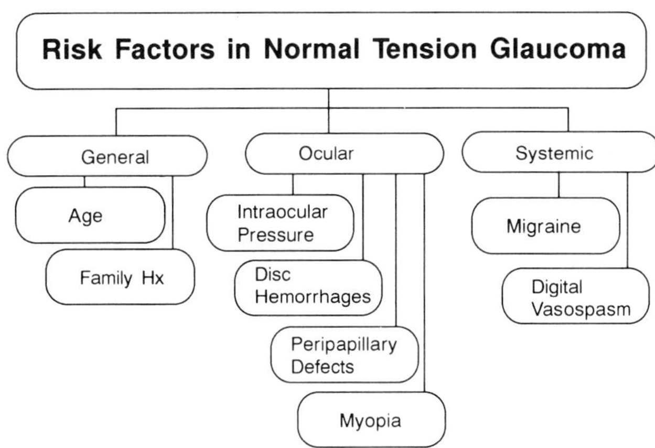

FIGURE 4–31 Flow chart illustrating risk factors to consider in normal tension glaucoma. (Hx, history.)

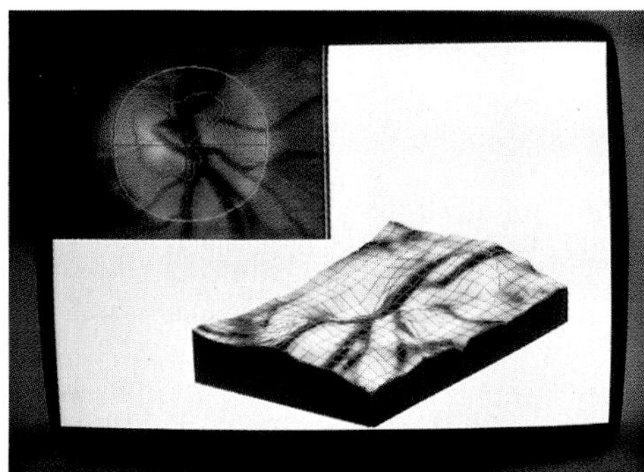

FIGURE 4–30 **Computerized image analysis of optic nerve head.** In this example from the Humphrey Retinal Analyzer, the three-dimensional wire basket plot was interpolated from calculated depth values and is shown with image intensity superimposed on a shaded surface. The green optic disc margin has an oval shape, and the red cup margin is determined by the cup-drop method. (From Dandona DL, Quigley HA, Jampal DH: Variability of depth measurements of the optic nerve head and peripapillary retina with computerized image analysis. Acta Ophthalmol 107:1786, 1989.)

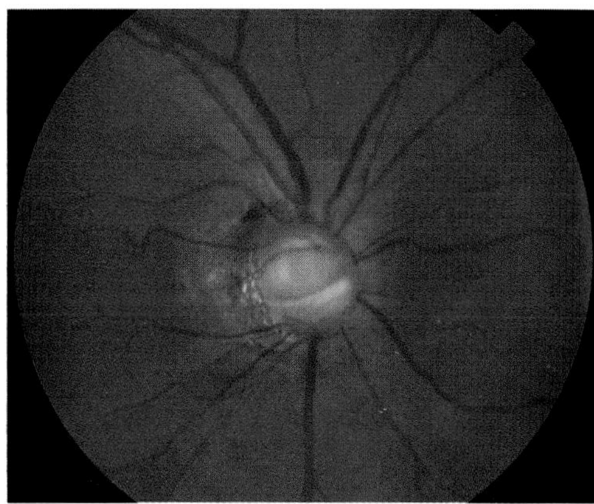

FIGURE 4–32 Right disc photograph of normal tension glaucoma in a 45-year-old woman. The excavated disc shows pit-like focal loss of lamina cribrosa centrally. Risk factors exhibited by this patient include (1) positive family history: mother with primary open-angle glaucoma, sister with normal-tension glaucoma; (2) myopia; (3) peripapillary crescent; (4) migraine; (5) digital vasospasm; and (6) disc hemorrhage noted during the initial examination.

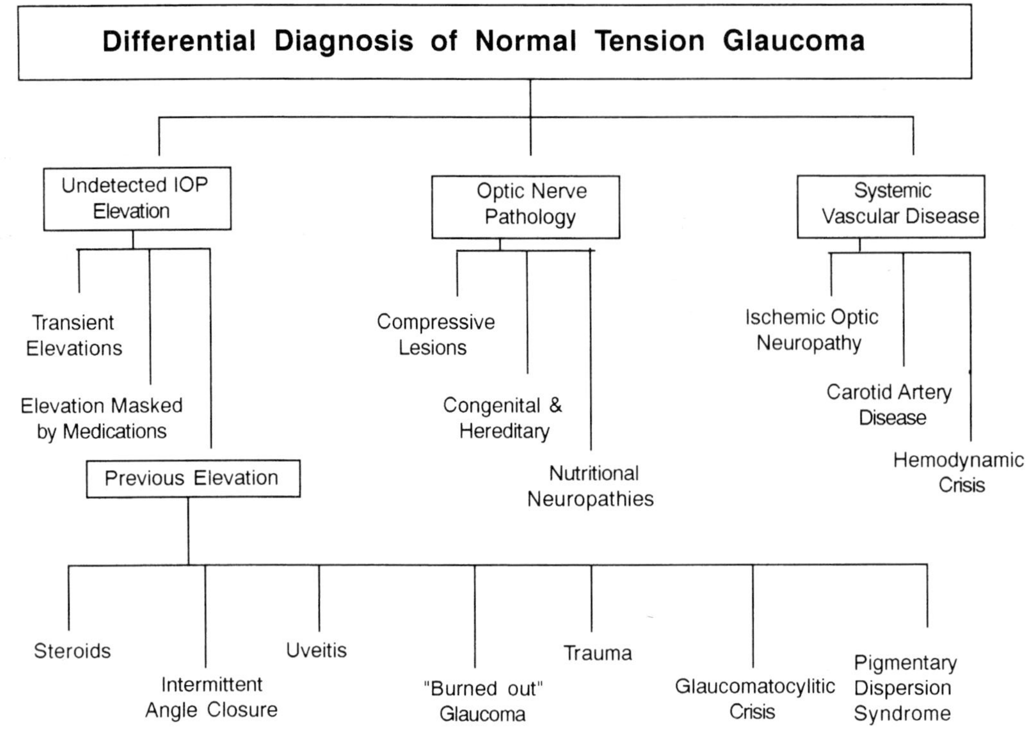

FIGURE 4–33 Flow chart providing an overview of the differential diagnosis of normal tension glaucoma.

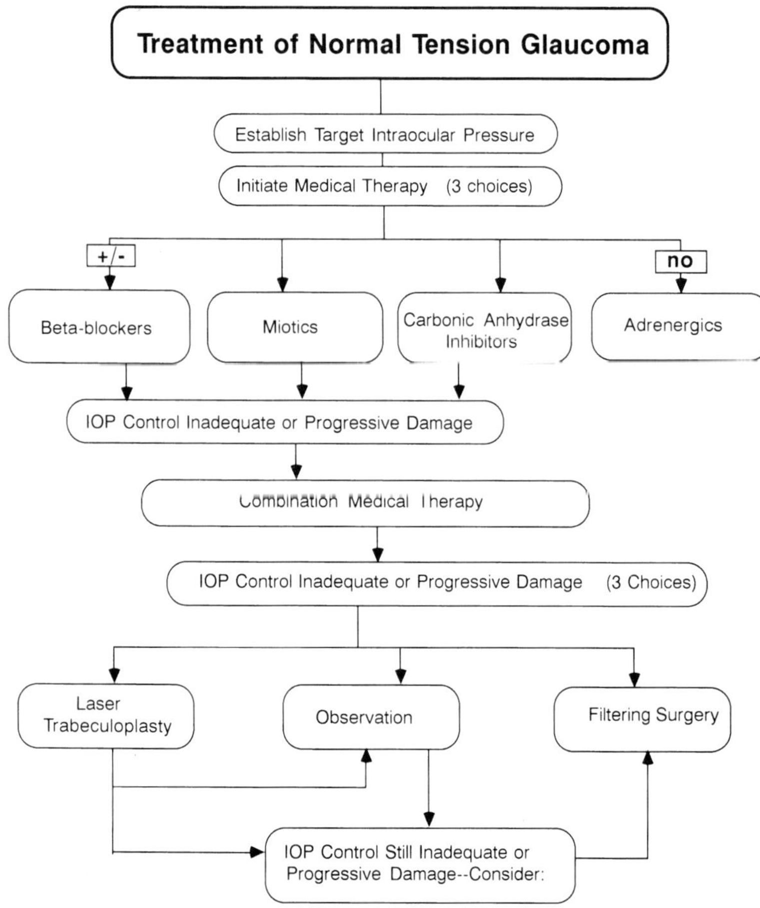

FIGURE 4–34 A flow chart illustrating one therapeutic approach for the management of normal tension glaucoma. (IOP, intraocular pressure.)

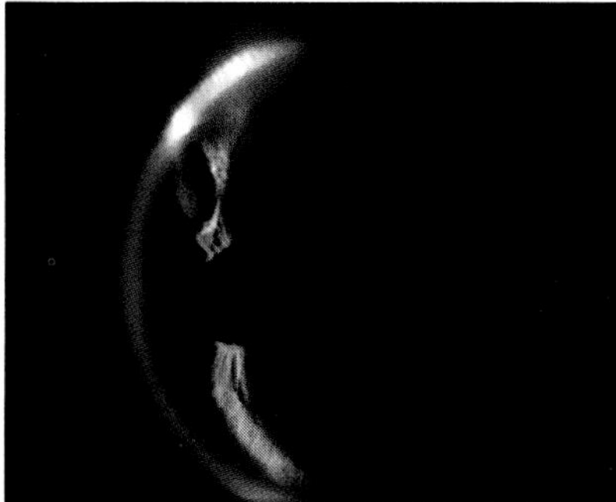

FIGURE 4–35 Slit-lamp photograph illustrating an incomplete surgical peripheral iridectomy with an intact posterior pigment layer. The layer can be seen to bulge forward into the anterior chamber owing to relative pupillary block and higher pressure in the posterior chamber. (From Campbell DG: A comparison of diagnostic techniques in angle-closure glaucoma. Am J Ophthalmol 88:199, 1979. Published with permission from the American Journal of Ophthalmology. Copyright by the Ophthalmic Publishing Company.)

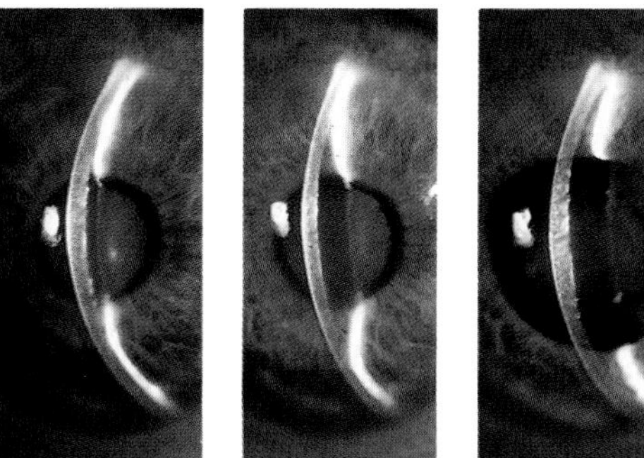

FIGURE 4–38 A patient with mobile or forward lens angle-closure glaucoma, with the lens one corneal thickness behind the iris *(left picture). The middle and right photos* show increasing deepening of the anterior chamber with mydriatic-cycloplegic therapy. (From Campbell DG: A comparison of diagnostic techniques in angle-closure glaucoma. Am J Ophthalmol 88:203, 1979. Published with permission from the American Journal of Ophthalmology. Copyright by the Ophthalmic Publishing Company.)

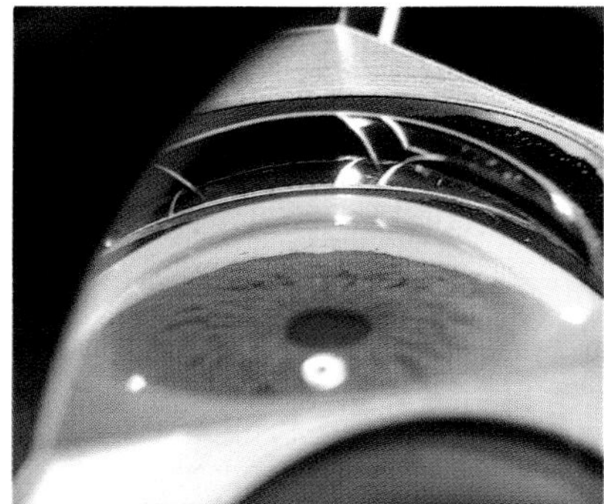

FIGURE 4–36 Gonioscopic photograph of a patient with relative pupillary block, angle-closure glaucoma. The fully distributed convexity of the iris characteristic of this type of closure is seen.

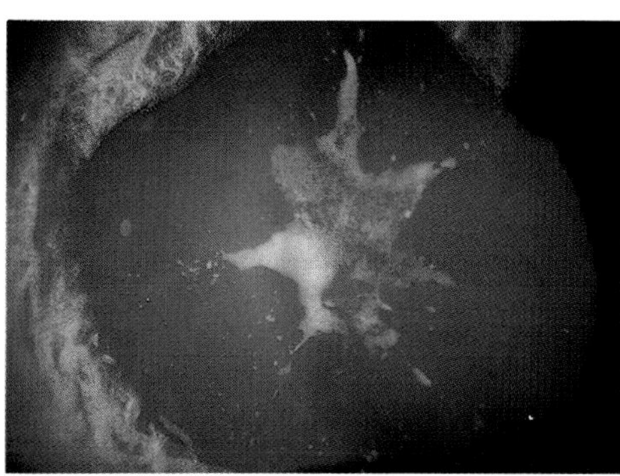

FIGURE 4–39 Glaukomflecken of the lens and an irregularly fixed and middilated pupil following an attack of acute angle-closure glaucoma. These opacities represent intraocular pressure–induced damage to the central lenticular epithelial cells and the subepithelial cortex. The opacities develop only in the exposed pupillary region.

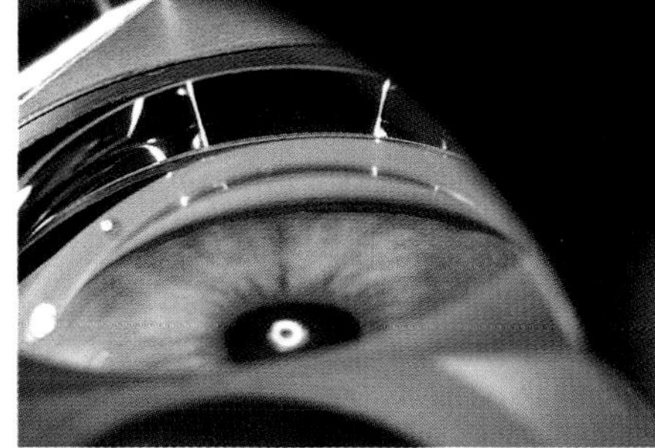

FIGURE 4–37 Gonioscopic photograph of a patient with plateau iris configuration, angle-closure glaucoma. The centrally flat iris falls off abruptly at the periphery. (From Campbell DG: A comparison of diagnostic techniques in angle-closure glaucoma. Am J Ophthalmol 88:201, 1979. Published with permission from the American Journal of Ophthalmology. Copyright by the Ophthalmic Publishing Company.)

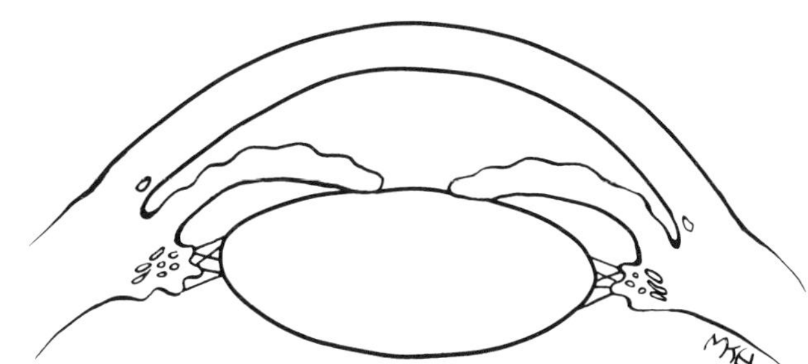

FIGURE 4–40 **Pupillary block leading to angle-closure.** The pressure in the posterior chamber is greater than the pressure in the anterior chamber, and therefore the iris is bowed forward to come into apposition to the trabecular meshwork.

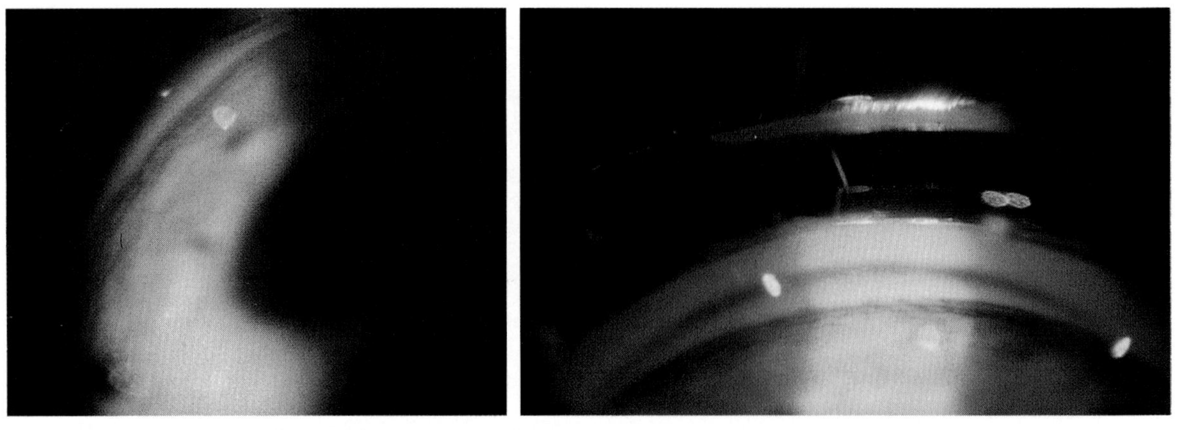

FIGURE 4–41 **Zeiss' gonioscopy.** *A*, No angle structures are identified with Zeiss' gonioscopy. *B*, With Zeiss' compression, angle structures are readily visible; no peripheral anterior synechiae are seen, and appositional closure exists.

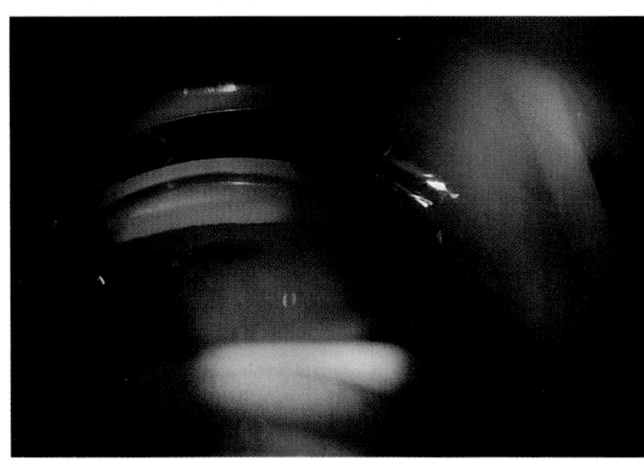

FIGURE 4–42 Appositional closure; no angle structures are identified.

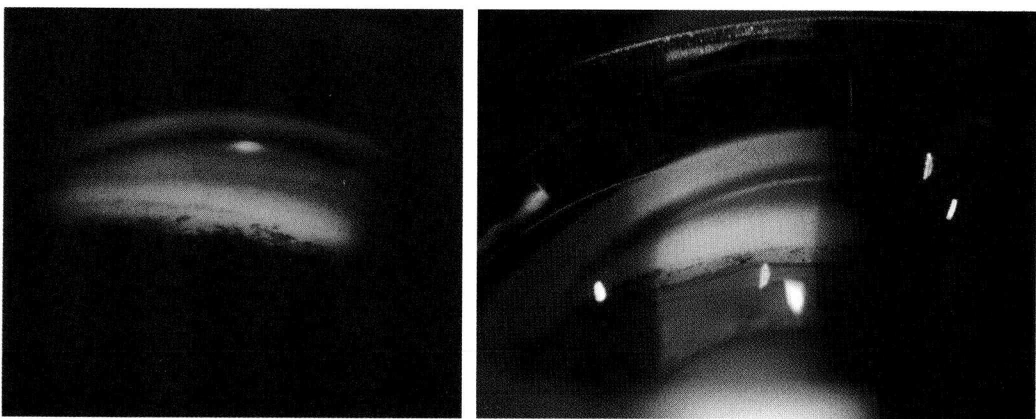

FIGURE 4–43 **Peripheral anterior synechiae.** *A*, Prominent uveal meshwork; fine branching twiglike endings with lacy, open character may be confused with peripheral anterior synechiae. *B*, Peripheral anterior synechiae, which are solid and uniform. This solidity of tissue appears to be the most consistent feature in distinguishing normal tissue from peripheral anterior synechiae.

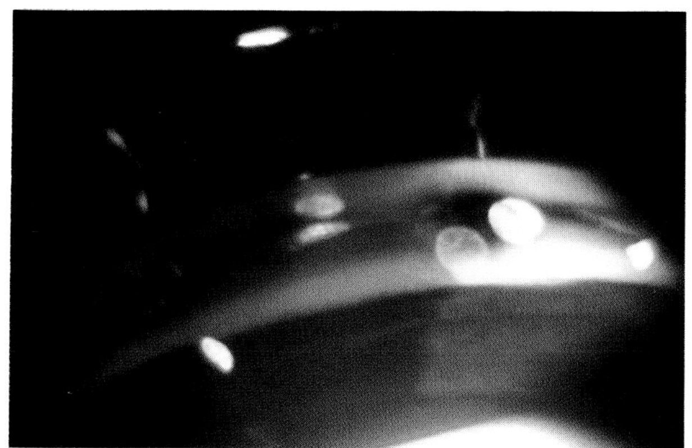

FIGURE 4–44 Low, diffuse synechial closure, typical of primary chronic angle-closure glaucoma.

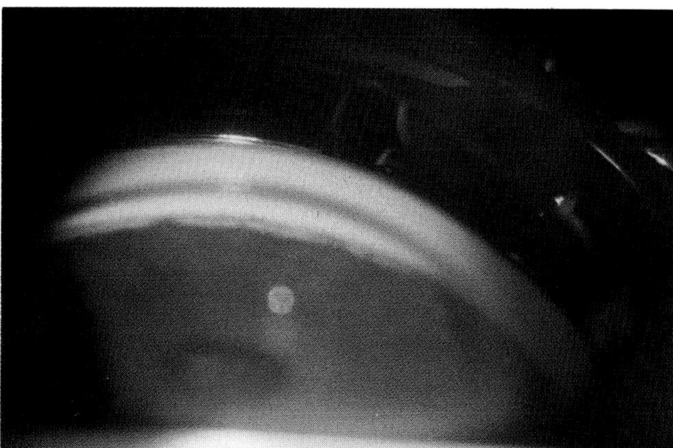

FIGURE 4–45 Small, irregular synechiae seen after argon laser trabeculoplasty. These synechiae are typically small and irregular and may occasionally extend to the posterior trabecular meshwork.

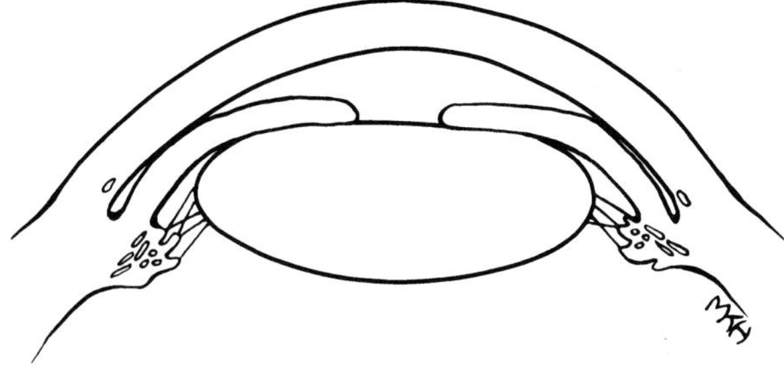

FIGURE 4–46 Pupillary block caused by the forward shift of the lens-iris diaphragm secondary to laxity of the zonules. An anterior position of the lens with respect to the ciliary body, increased lens thickness, and increased anterior lens curvature have been identified in patients with angle-closure glaucoma.

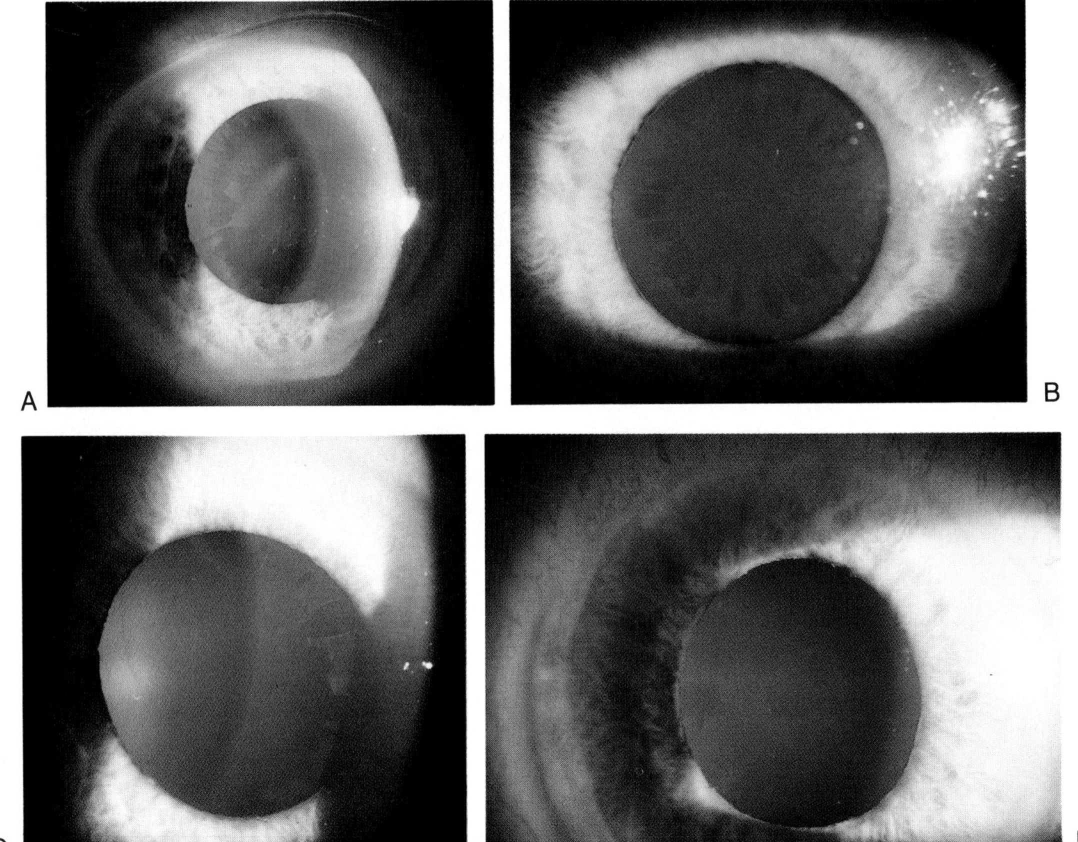

FIGURE 4–47 **Lens capsule findings in exfoliation syndrome.** *A*, Slit-lamp photograph of anterior lens capsule findings in exfoliation syndrome. Note the central disc of exfoliative material, the intermediate clear zone where most of the material has been rubbed off by the iris, and the peripheral granular zone. The pupil has been dilated. *B*, Exfoliation syndrome. The intermediate zone is not as well defined because of bridging strands of exfoliative material. *C*, Exfoliation syndrome, with no central disc of exfoliative material. The peripheral granular zone is readily seen, but only after pupil dilation. *D*, Exfoliation syndrome, subtle. The central disc and strands bridging the intermediate zone are visible through careful observation.

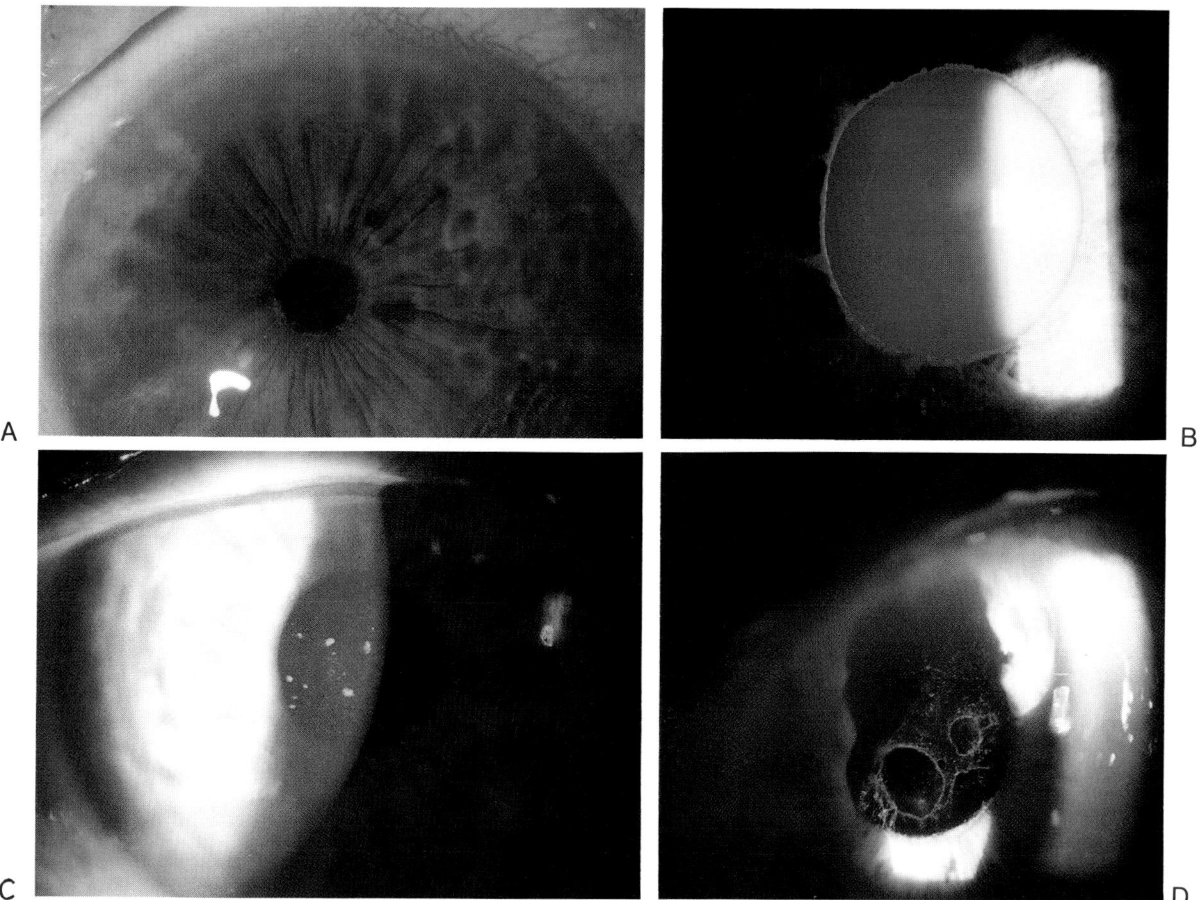

FIGURE 4-48 **Exfoliation syndrome.** Deposition of material on other anterior segment structures. *A,* Flakes of exfoliative material on the pupillary border of the iris, appearing as gray-white accumulations and small clumps of material. *B,* Peripupillary iris transillumination in exfoliation syndrome. The pupillary ruff of the pigment is missing, and scattered patchy transillumination defects with a moth-eaten appearance occur in the nearby iris. The edge of the central disc of exfoliated material appears as a whitish ring in this photograph. *C,* Flakes of exfoliative material adherent to central corneal endothelium. *D,* Whitish exfoliative material coating strands of vitreous on the anterior hyaloid face years after intracapsular cataract extraction.

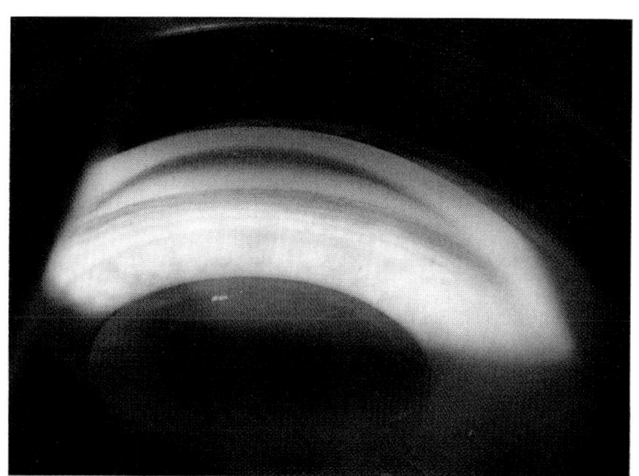

FIGURE 4-49 **Gonioscopic view of the angle in exfoliation syndrome.** Moderate-to-heavy pigmentation is evident in the trabecular meshwork. The peripheral granular zone of exfoliative material is evident on the anterior lens surface.

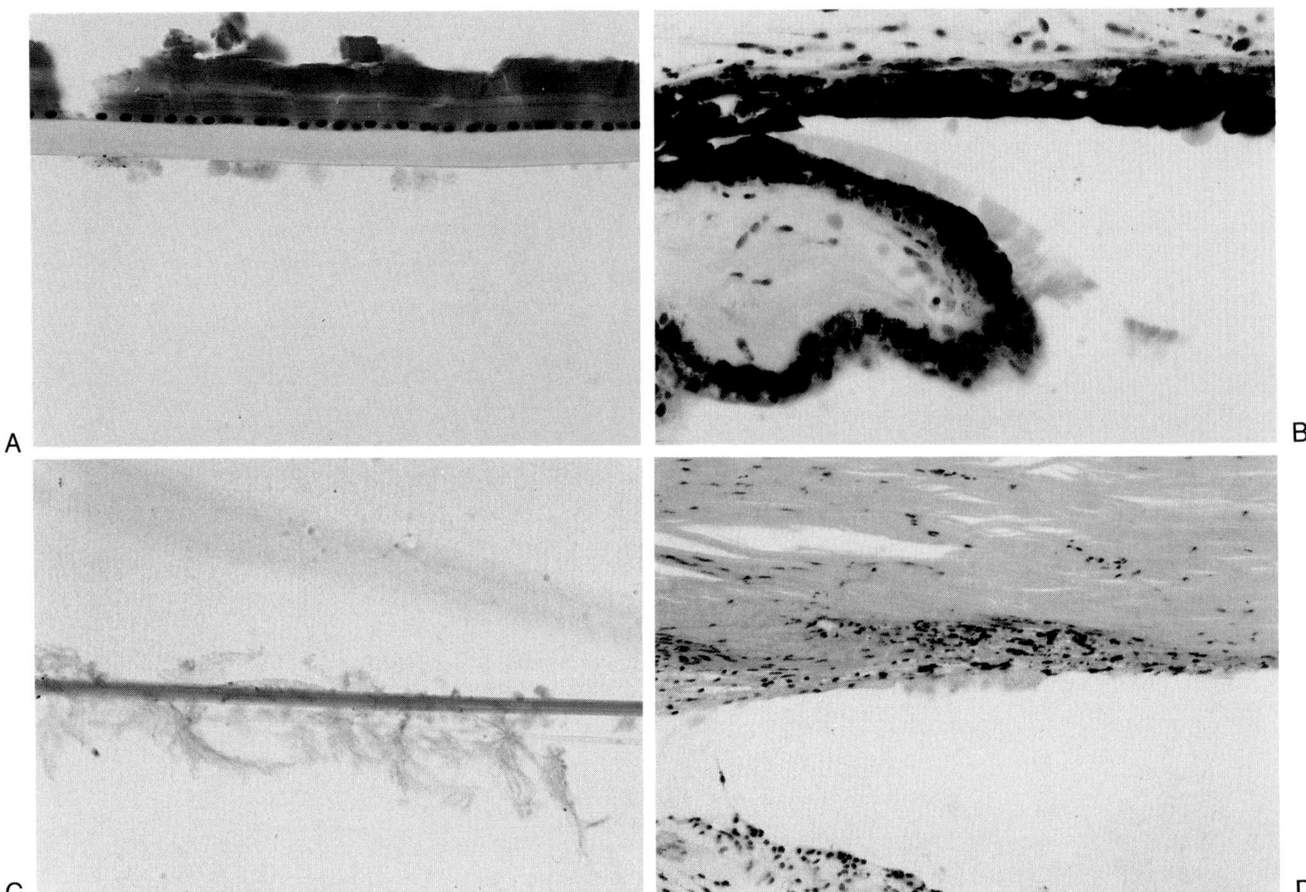

FIGURE 4–50 **Histopathology of exfoliation syndrome.** *A,* Light microscopic view of anterior lens capsule in exfoliation syndrome. Eosinophilic bushlike clumps of exfoliative material are lined up on anterior lens capsule. H&E, ×400. *B,* Ciliary process in exfoliation syndrome. The pale pink homogeneous coating of exfoliative material has been artifactually separated from ciliary process in some portions. H&E, ×400. *C,* Zonular fibers coated with exfoliative material. H&E, ×400. *D,* Trabecular meshwork in exfoliation syndrome. Clumps of material coat the uveal meshwork. H&E, ×200.

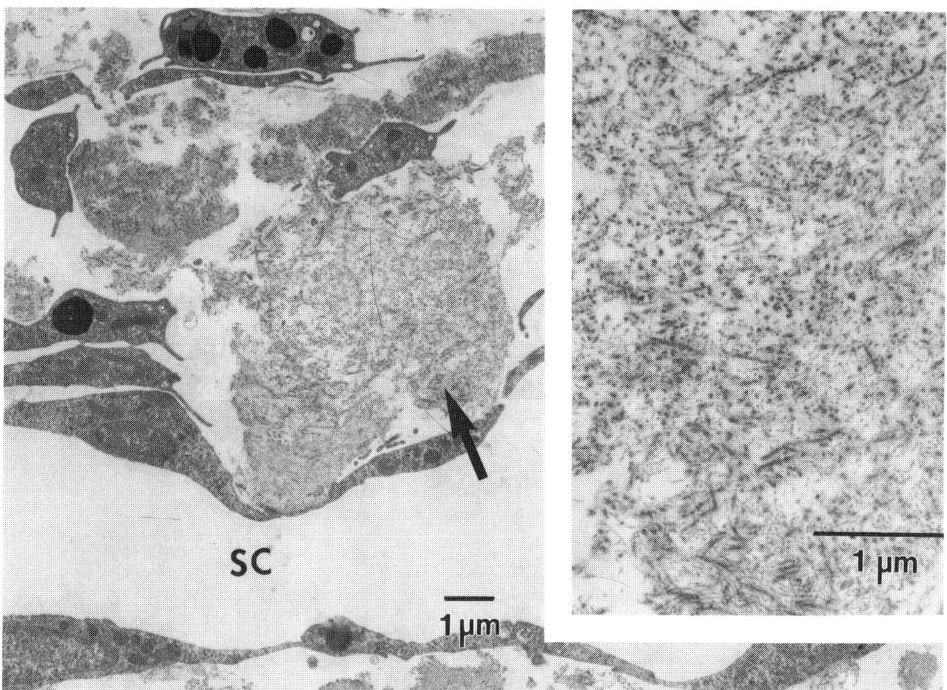

FIGURE 4–51 **Electron microscopy of exfoliation syndrome.** Exfoliative material, accumulation near Schlemm's canal (SC). The material is a randomly arranged tangle of filaments and fibrils embedded in an amorphous ground substance. Filaments are small, threadlike rods with a 10-nm diameter. Fibrils are larger rods with a 50-nm diameter. Transmission electron micrograph, ×7500. *Inset:* Magnified view of exfoliative material, ×25,000.

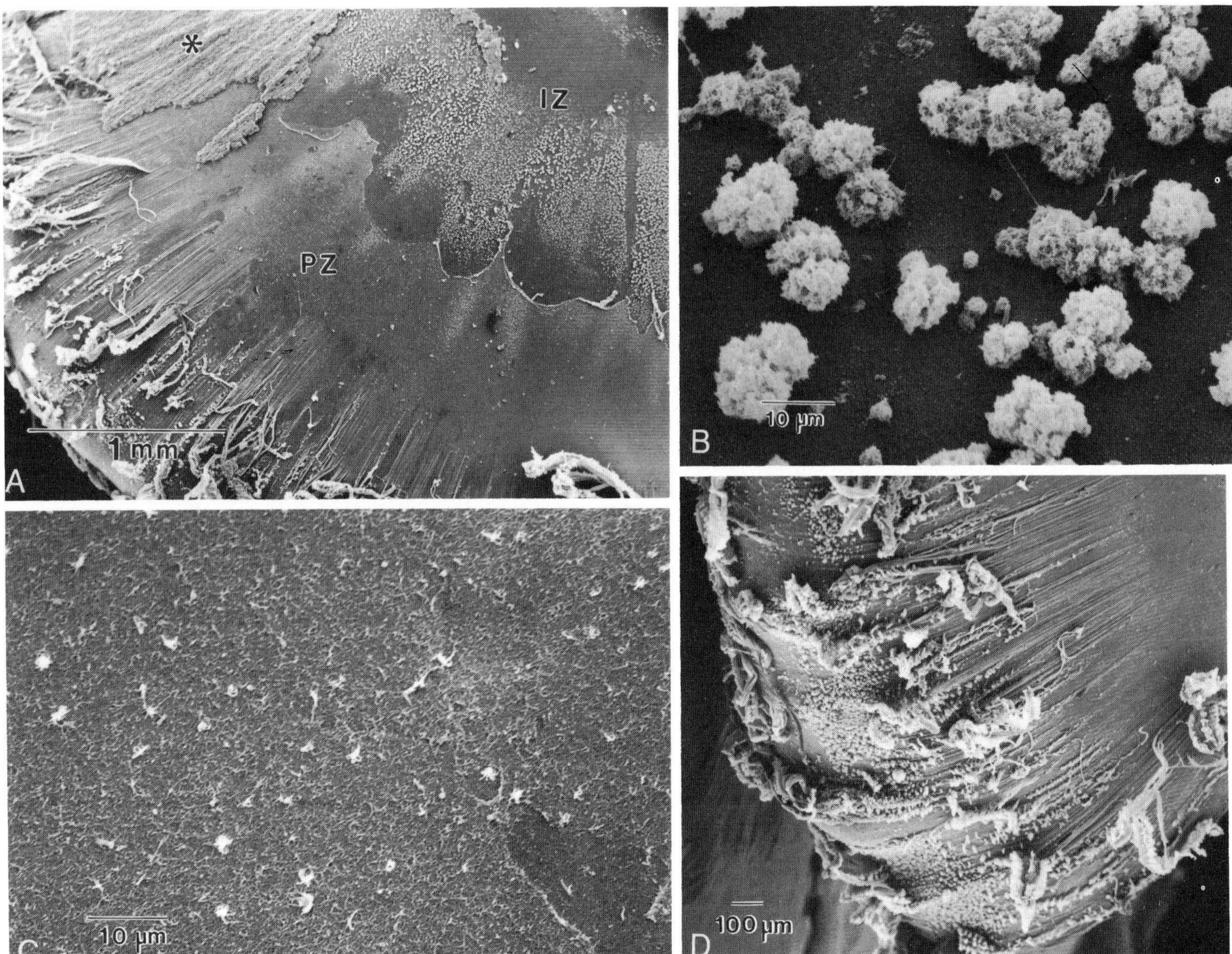

FIGURE 4-52 **Electron microscopy of exfoliation syndrome.** *A*, The anterior lens surface in exfoliation syndrome. Portions of the intermediate zone (IZ) contain granular accumulations of exfoliative material. A sharp demarcation line is evident between the intermediate zone and the peripheral zone (PZ). Zonular fibers appear as broken strands, some encrusted with exfoliative material. The iris pigment epithelium is artifactually adherent to lens surface in the upper portion of photograph *(asterisk)*. Scanning electron micrograph, ×27. *B*, Intermediate zone with rounded, bushlike accumulations of exfoliative material. Underlying lens capsule is relatively smooth and free of material. Scanning electron micrograph, ×1000. *C*, Peripheral zone. Dense feltlike mat of exfoliative material lies directly on the lens capsule. Note the lack of bushlike accumulations in contrast to the intermediate zone as shown in *B*. Scanning electron micrograph, ×1000. *D*, The equatorial zone of the lens surface in exfoliation syndrome. Granular accumulations of exfoliative material are prominent on the anterior edge of the equator, near insertion of zonular fibers. Under higher magnification, these granules of material consist of numerous fine threads (see *E*). Scanning electron micrograph, ×40.

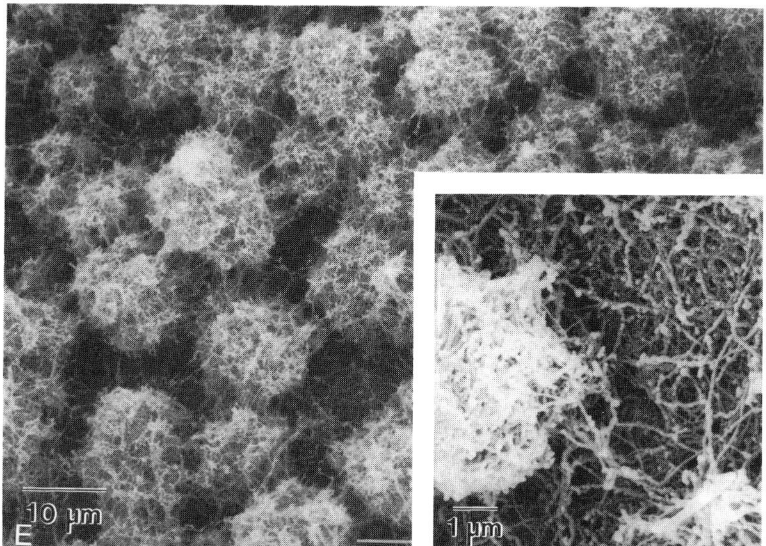

FIGURE 4–52 *Continued E,* Higher-power views of granular accumulations of exfoliative materials seen in *D.* Note that each "granule" consists of a tangle of threadlike fibrils and filaments, ×1000. *Inset:* ×9000. *F,* The anterior equatorial zone of lens surface, exfoliation syndrome. Broken zonular fibers, some encrusted with barnacle-like exfoliative material, are evident, along with granular accumulations as seen in *D.* This higher-power view also shows cobweb-like bundles of exfoliative fiber *(arrowheads).* Scanning electron micrograph, ×100. *G,* Higher-power view of cobwebs of exfoliative material covering zonular fiber insertions, as shown in *F,* ×800.

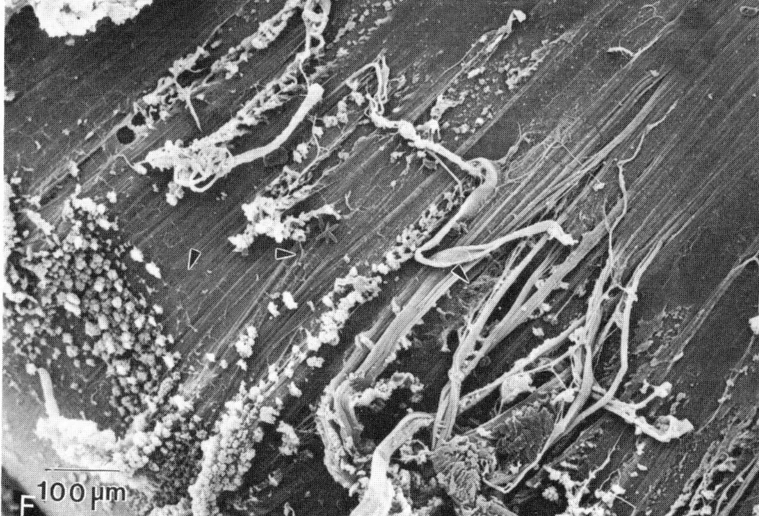

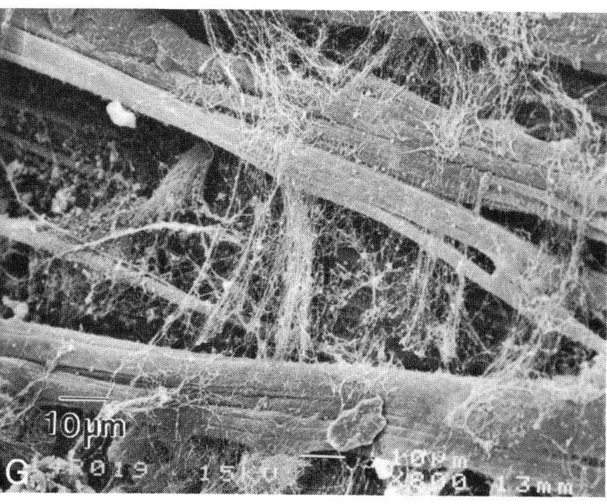

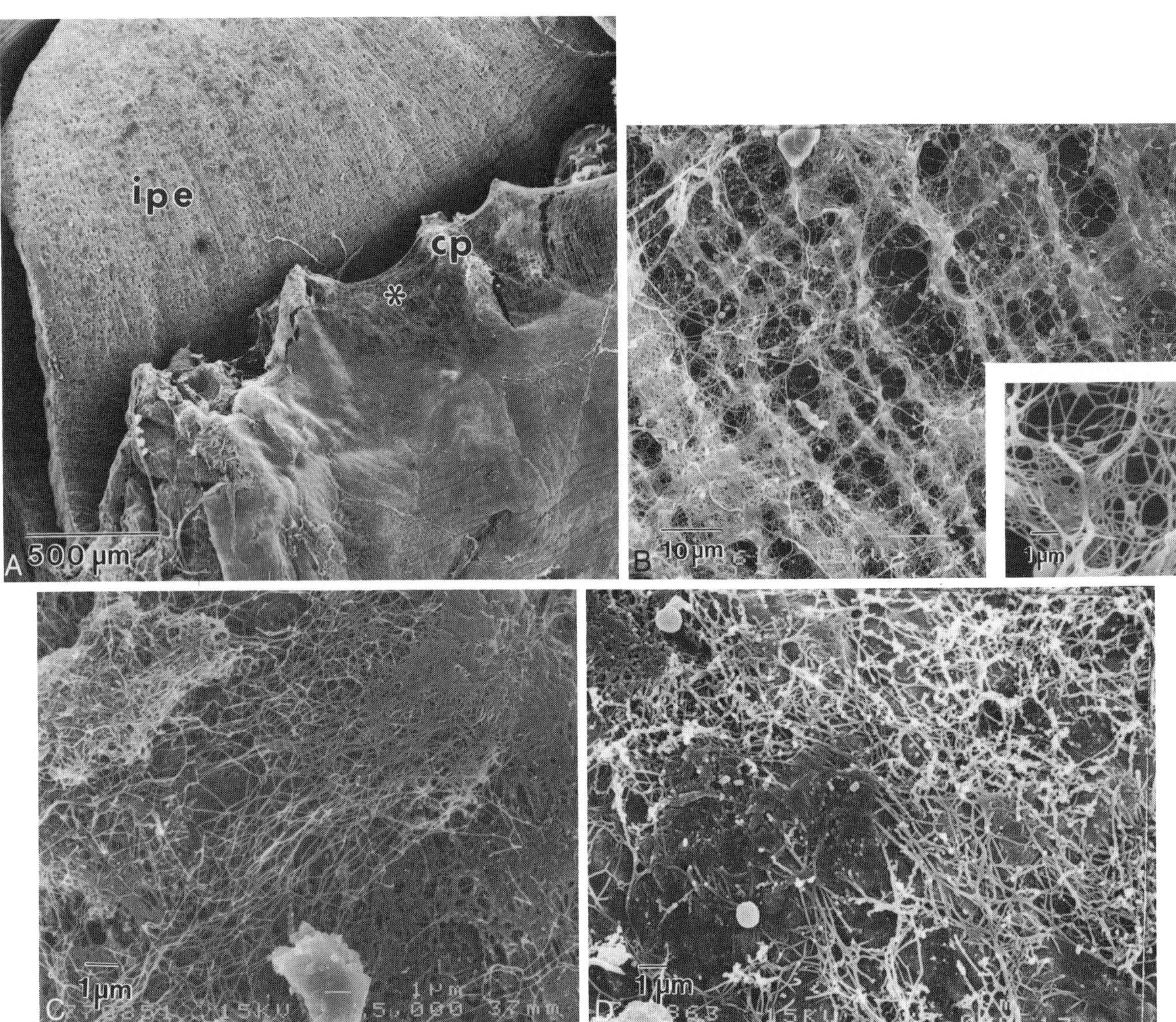

FIGURE 4–53 **Electron microscopy in exfoliation syndrome.** *A*, Posterior iris surface and ciliary processes in exfoliation syndrome. Note the dense mat of exfoliative material stretching between ciliary processes *(asterisk)*. (ipe, iris pigment epithelium; cp, ciliary processes.) Scanning electron micrograph, ×35. *B*, Higher-power views of mat of exfoliative material shown in *A*. Note tangle of fibrils forming the mat, with entrapped pigment granules scattered throughout, ×1000. *Inset:* ×5000. *C*, Exfoliative material covering ciliary process in denser tangles than in *B*, ×5000. *D*, Exfoliative material covering the posterior iris surface. Note the similarity to the material on the posterior iris surface as shown in *C*, ×5000.

FIGURE 4–54 Iris transillumination in a patient with pigmentary glaucoma; spokelike, midperipheral, radial defects result from loss of pigment from the pigment epithelium.

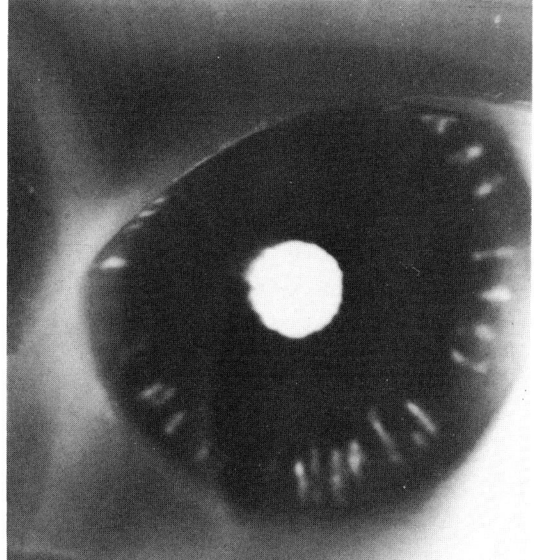

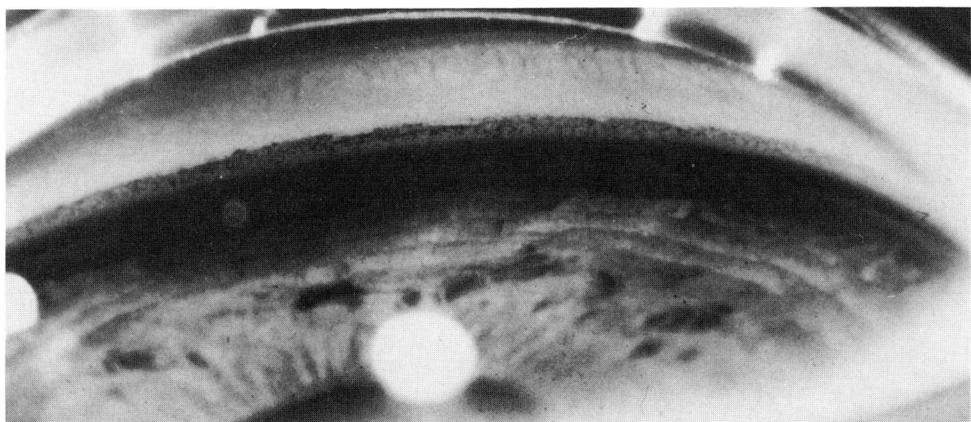

FIGURE 4–55 Goniophotograph of the anterior chamber angle from a patient with pigmentary glaucoma shows a dense band of pigment in the trabecular meshwork.

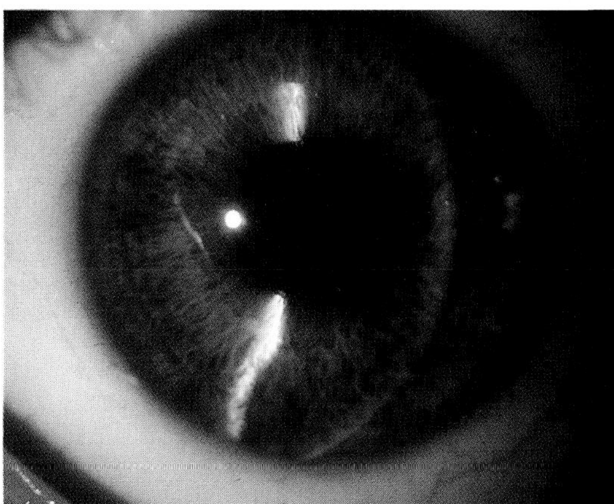

FIGURE 4–56 **Iris configuration in pigmentary dispersion syndrome.** Slit-lamp photograph of the anterior segment shows a deep anterior chamber with peripheral sagging of the iris. This iris concavity is most marked in the midperiphery.

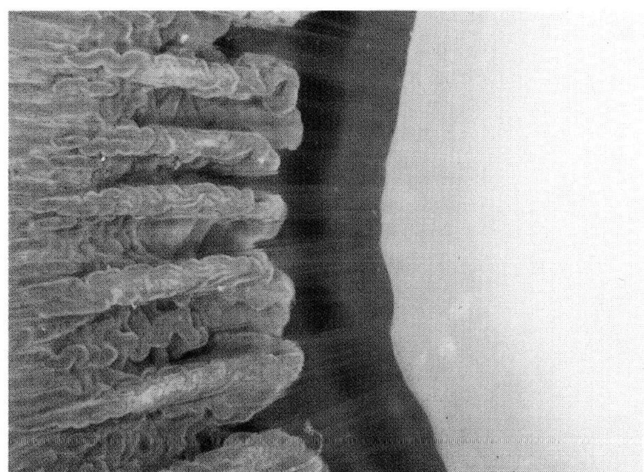

FIGURE 4–57 **Zonular fibers.** Photograph of the posterior view of the anterior segment. Zonular fibers that arise from the pars plicata and insert into the lens periphery are seen contrasted against the surface of the iris pigment epithelium.

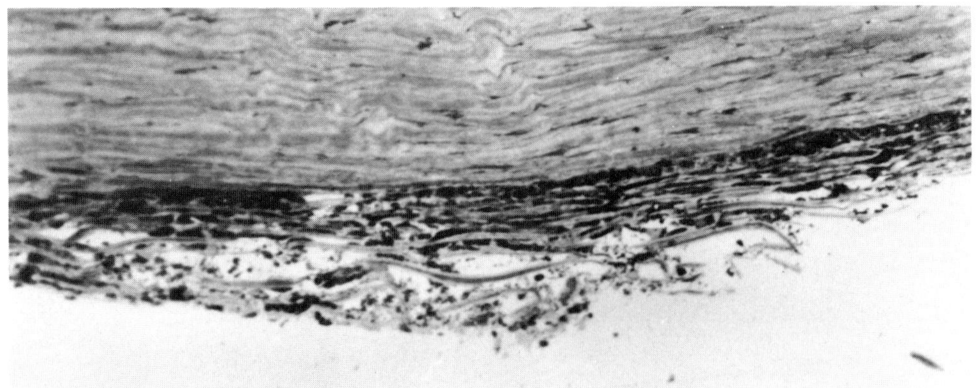

FIGURE 4–58 **Trabecular meshwork in pigmentary glaucoma.** Light microscopic view of a section through the trabecular meshwork in a case of pigmentary glaucoma. Note the heavy melanin deposits extending throughout the entire depth of the meshwork.

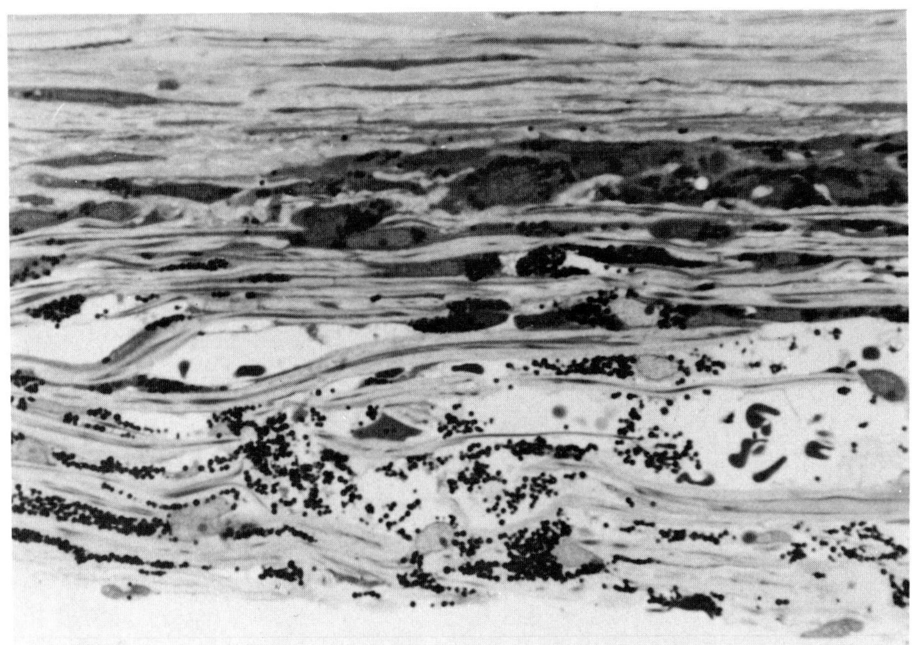

FIGURE 4–59 **Trabecular meshwork in pigmentary glaucoma.** Higher magnification of trabecular meshwork in pigmentary glaucoma. This section shows melanin pigment within and outside the trabecular meshwork cells.

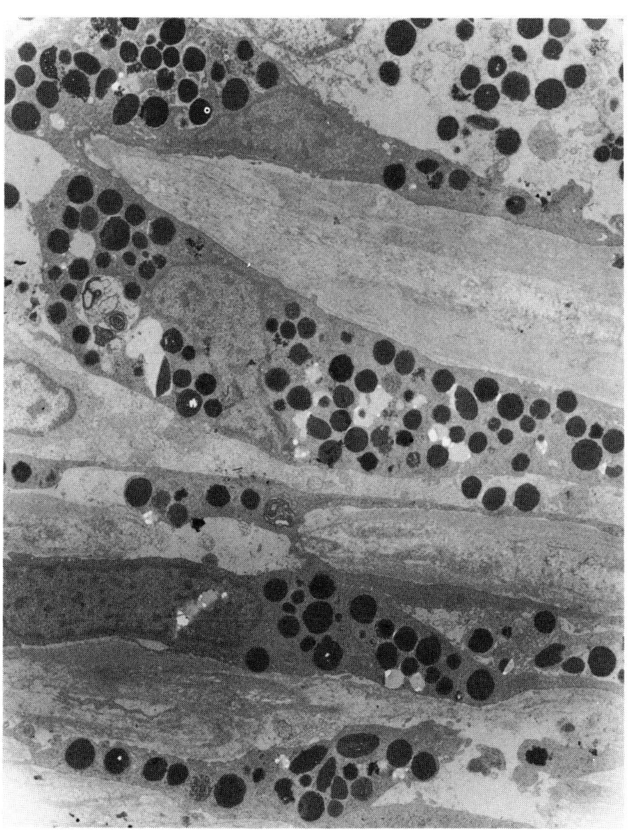

FIGURE 4–60 **Electron microscopy of trabecular meshwork in pigmentary glaucoma.** The trabecular meshwork has phagocytized pigment. Minimal intertrabecular space is available.

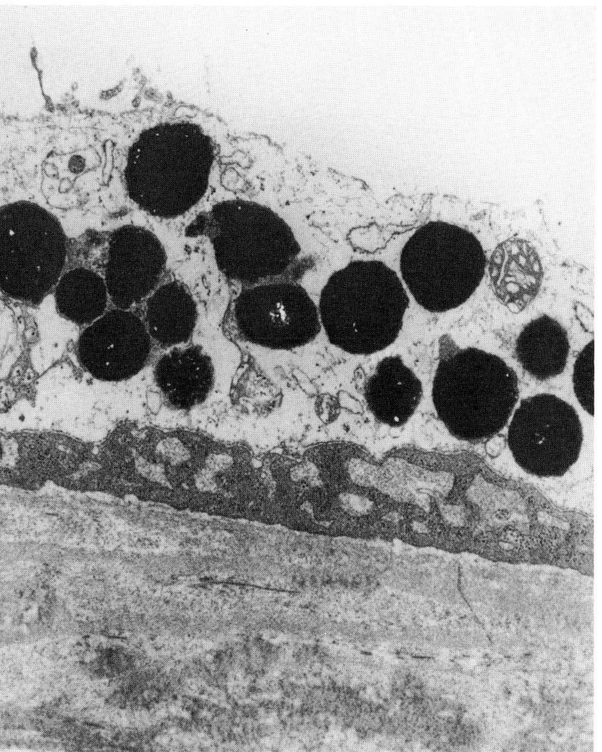

FIGURE 4–61 **Electron microscopy of trabecular meshwork in pigmentary glaucoma.** A healthy trabecular meshwork cell interposed between a degenerating cell superiorly and the trabecular beam inferiorly.

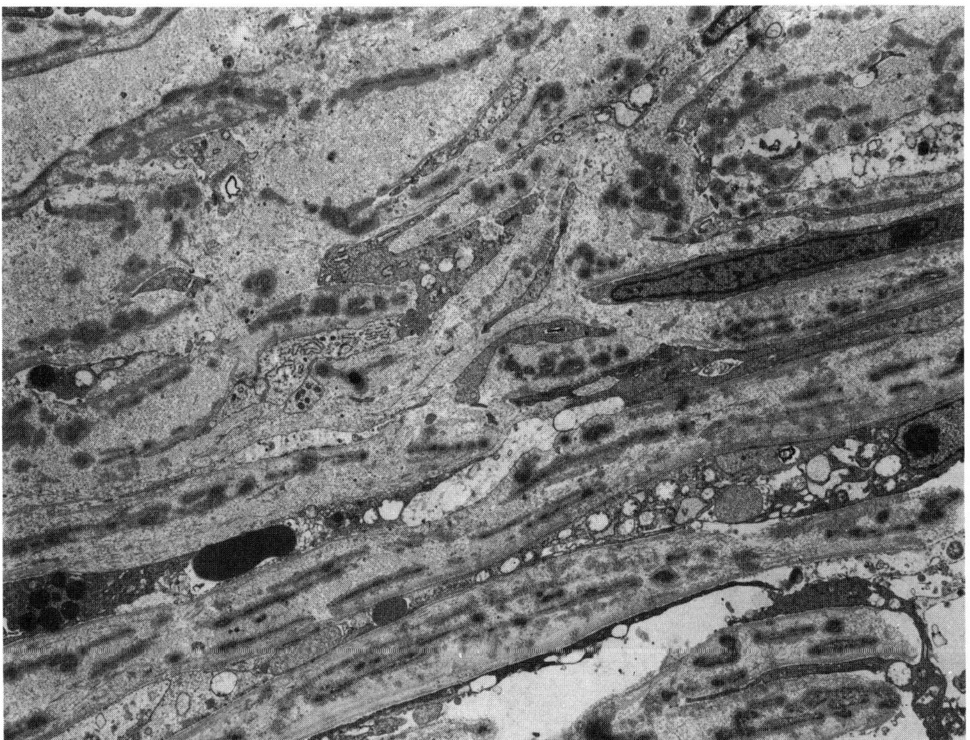

FIGURE 4–62 **Electron microscopy of trabecular meshwork in pigmentary glaucoma.** Collapse and fusion of the trabecular meshwork in a patient with advanced pigmentary glaucoma.

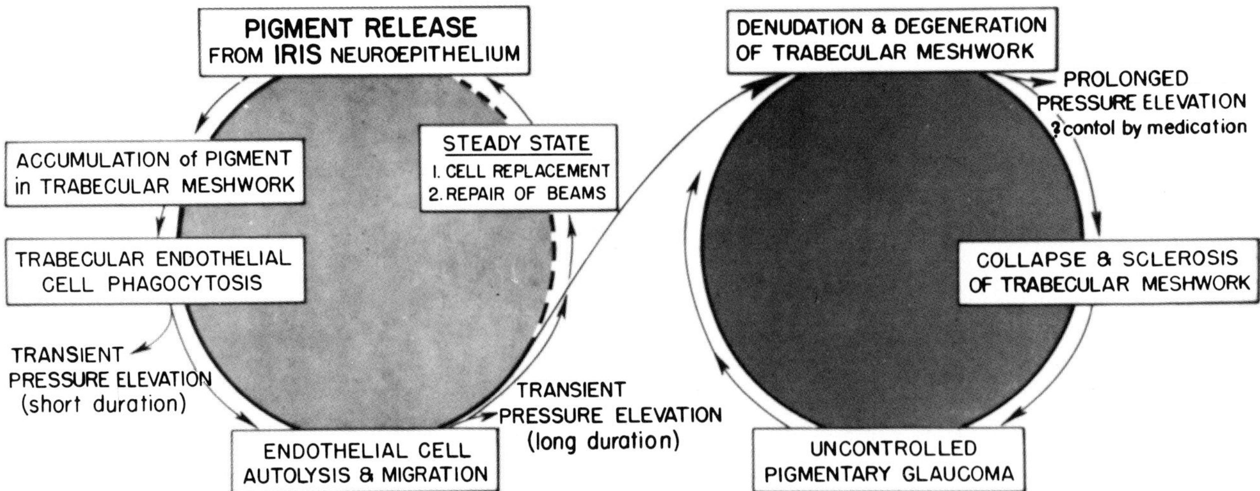

FIGURE 4–63 **Pathophysiology of pigmentary glaucoma.** This hypothetical scheme might explain the pathophysiology of pigmentary glaucoma. The first stage is clinically reversible and is characterized by transient rises in intraocular pressure. The second stage, marked by irreparable damage to trabecular tissues, is irreversible and is usually accompanied by uncontrolled glaucoma.

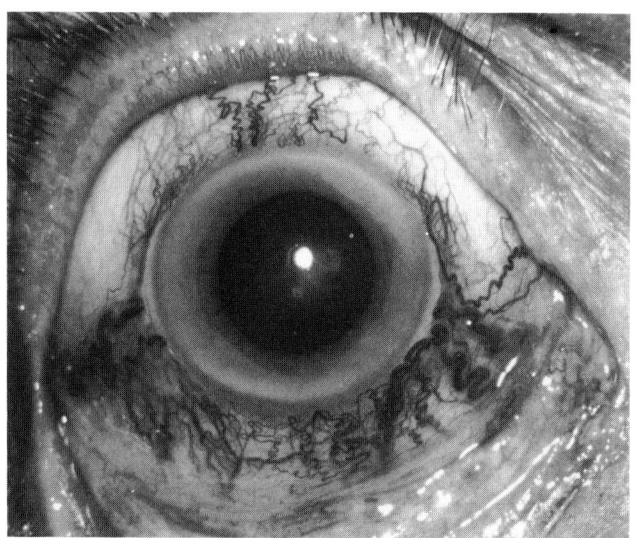

FIGURE 4–64 **Carotid cavernous fistula.** Dilated episcleral venous vessels and proptosis in a patient with a cavernous fistula. (Courtesy of Dr. W. T. Cornblath and Dr. J. D. Trobe.)

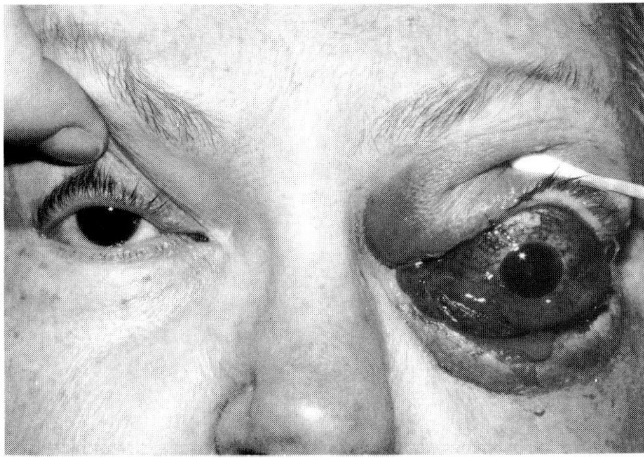

FIGURE 4–65 **Carotid cavernous fistula.** Proptosis, chemosis, and arterialization of episcleral venous vessels in a patient with a carotid cavernous fistula. (Courtesy of Dr. W. T. Cornblath and Dr. J. D. Trobe.)

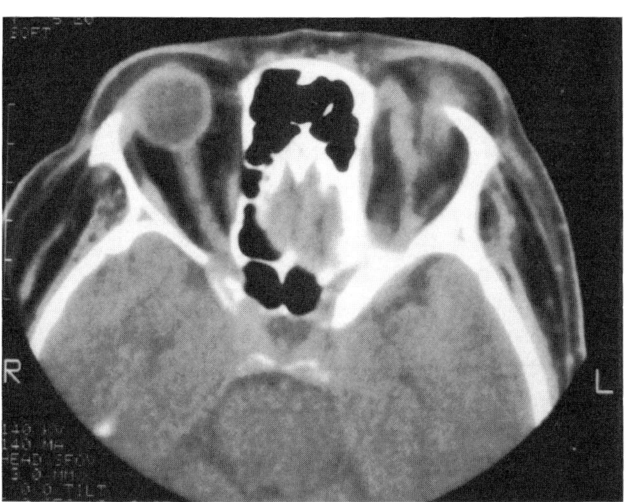

FIGURE 4-66 **Computed tomography (CT) findings in carotid cavernous fistula.** This axial CT scan shows a dilated superior ophthalmic vein on the left side in the patient depicted in Figure 4-65. (Courtesy of Dr. W. T. Cornblath and Dr. J. D. Trobe.)

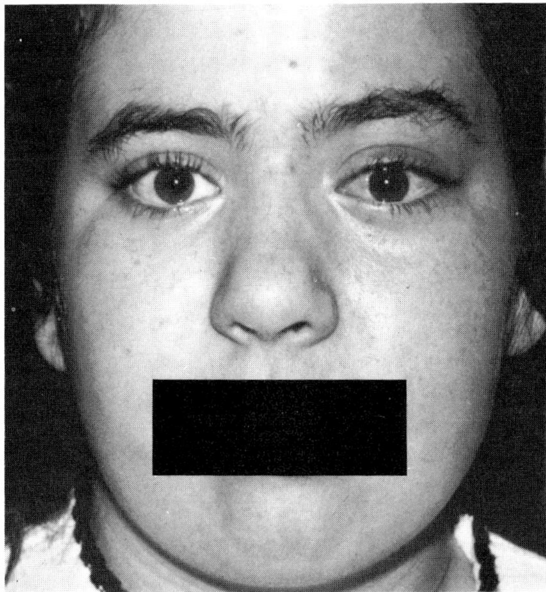

FIGURE 4-67 **Cutaneous hemifacial angioma.** This young patient has a unilateral facial angioma involving the V-1 distribution on the left side including the left upper eyelid. Glaucoma has been reported to occur in 30% of such cases. (Photograph by Frances McIver.)

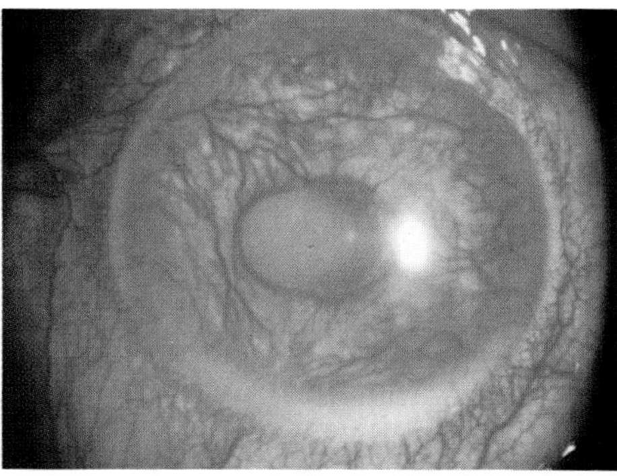

FIGURE 4-68 **Neovascular glaucoma.** Advanced fulminant neovascular glaucoma with marked conjunctival congestion, corneal haze from elevated intraocular pressure, neovascularization of the iris, and ectropion uvea.

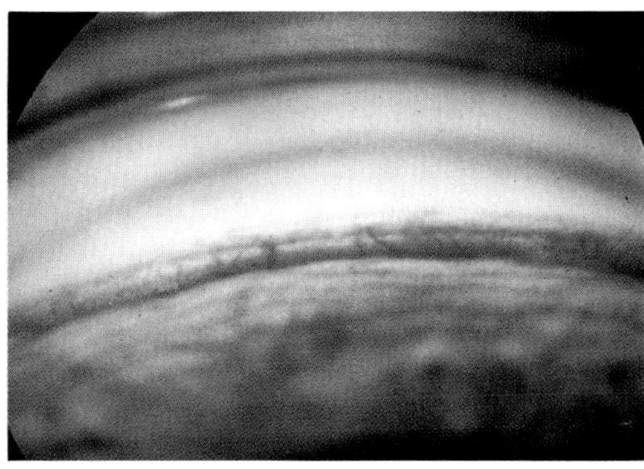

FIGURE 4-69 **Neovascularization of the angle.** Goniophotograph showing new angle vessels crossing over the ciliary body band and scleral spur and arborizing over the trabecular meshwork. (From Wand M, Hutchinson BT: The surgical management of neovascular glaucoma. Perspect Ophthalmology 4:147, 1980. Copyright ANKHO International.)

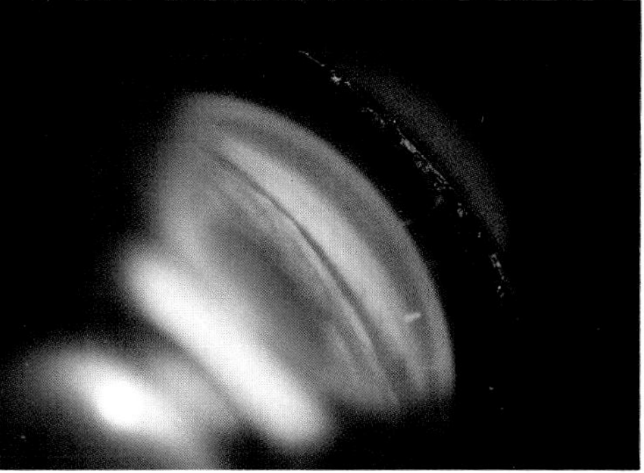

FIGURE 4-70 **Neovascularization of the angle.** Goniophotograph showing new vessels covering all of the visible trabecular meshwork with early synechial angle-closure.

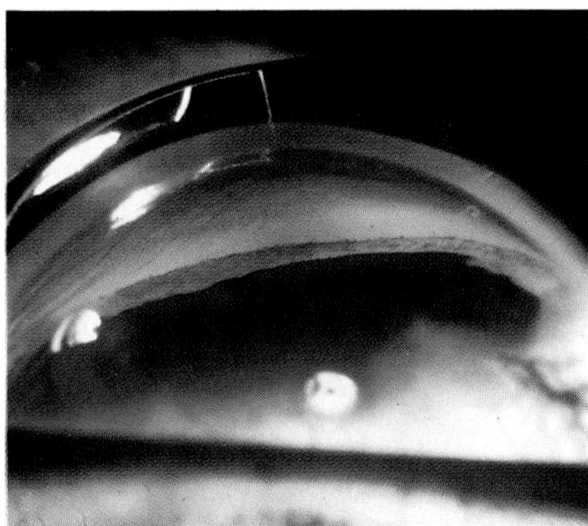

FIGURE 4–71 **Neovascular glaucoma with total synechial angle-closure.** The typical picture of a smooth line of iridocorneal adhesion is pathognomonic for total angle-closure. The irregular dark line is the edge of the ectropion uvea. (From Wand M, Hutchinson BT: The surgical management of neovascular glaucoma. Perspect Ophthalmology 4:147, 1980. Copyright ANKHO International.)

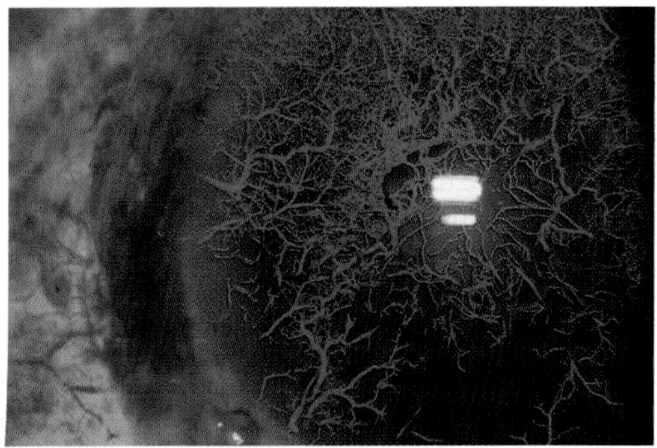

FIGURE 4–72 Liquid rubber injection mold of new vessels in an autopsy eye with neovascular glaucoma. (Courtesy of Vincente L. Jocson, M.D.)

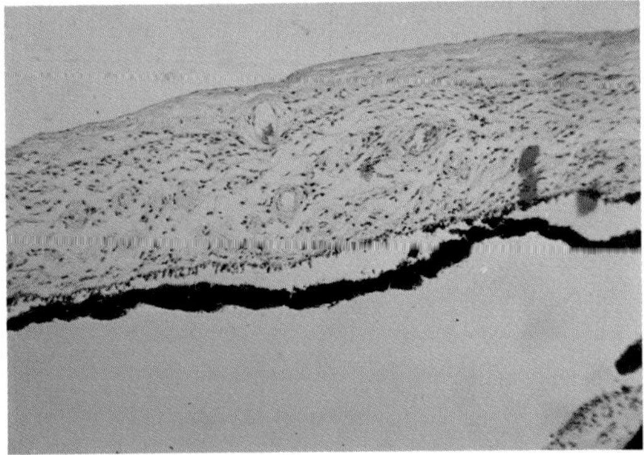

FIGURE 4–73 Histopathology of neovascularization of the iris. Note the new vessel formation on the iris surface but beneath the fibrovascular membrane. H&E, ×100.

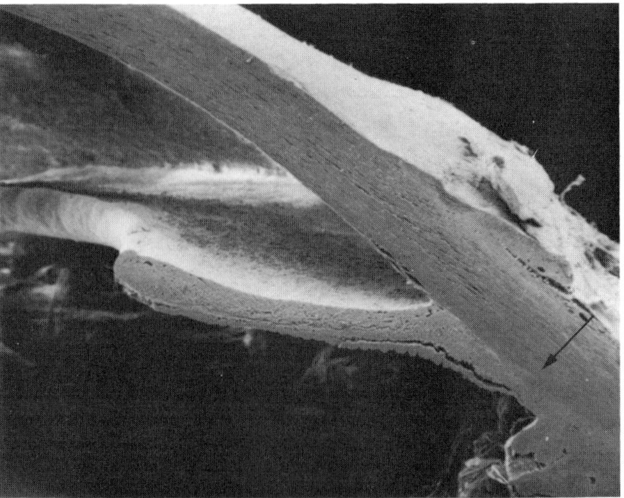

FIGURE 4–74 **Electron micrograph of neovascularization of the iris.** This scanning electron micrograph (20×) shows the fibrovascular membrane that has produced a smooth iris surface. The contraction of this membrane has completely closed the angle (*arrow* shows the compressed trabecular meshwork) and has started to pull the posterior pigment layer over the pupillary edge and onto the anterior iris surface (ectropion uvea). (From John T, Sassani JW, Eagle RC Jr: The myofibroblastic component of rubeosis iridis. Ophthalmology 90:721, 1983. Copyright American Academy of Ophthalmology.)

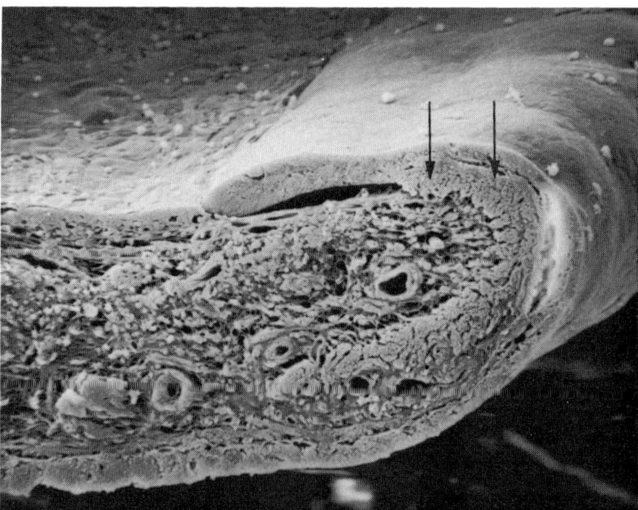

FIGURE 4–75 **Electron micrograph of ectropion uvea.** This scanning electron micrograph (160×) shows the marked ectropion uvea and ectropion of the sphincter muscle *(arrows)*. (Courtesy of Ralph C. Eagle Jr., M.D.)

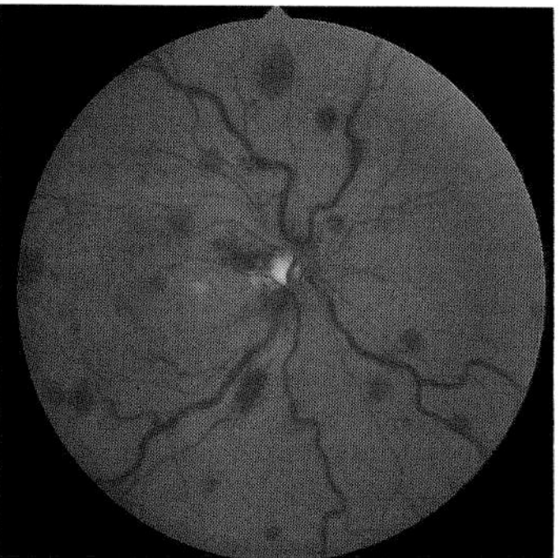

FIGURE 4–76 **Nonischemic central retinal vein occlusion.** In this scenario, the natural history of nonischemic central retinal vein occlusion is that essentially none of these eyes will progress on to neovascular glaucoma.

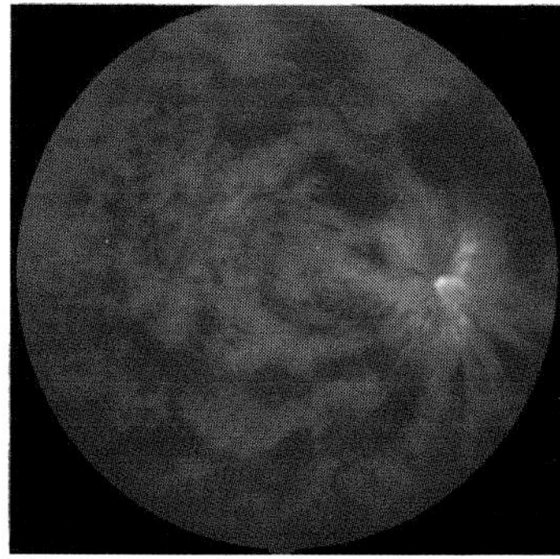

FIGURE 4–77 **Ischemic central retinal vein occlusion.** In contrast to nonischemic central retinal vein occlusion, the incidence of neovascular glaucoma in ischemic central retinal vein occlusion ranges from 18 to 60 percent. The greater the degree of capillary nonperfusion, the greater will be the chances of developing neovascularization.

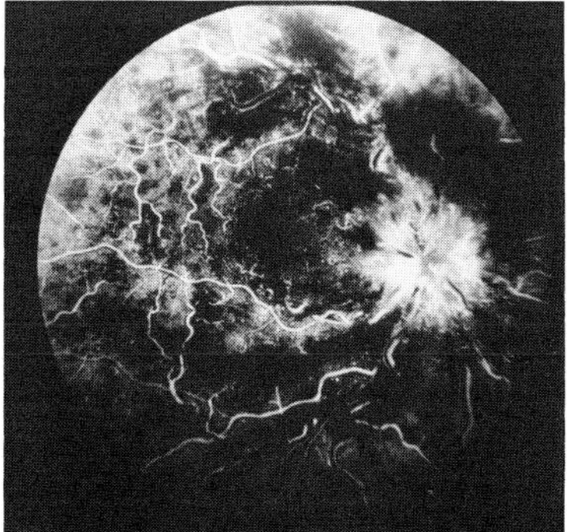

FIGURE 4–78 Fundus fluorescein angiogram of eye shown in Figure 4–77. There are extensive areas of capillary nonperfusion as well as areas of blocked fluorescence from the intraretinal hemorrhages.

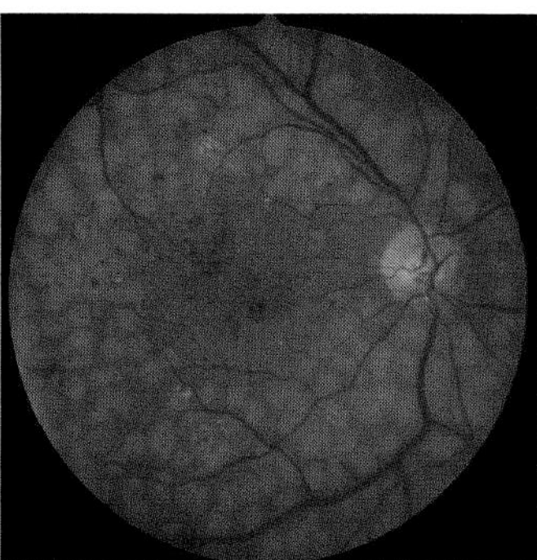

FIGURE 4–79 **Panretinal photocoagulation.** This is an example of adequate panretinal photocoagulation. Note the almost confluent areas of photocoagulation spots. A total of 1500 to 2000 spots should be applied if using the Rodenstock lens (800-μ spot size); if the Goldmann lens (500-μ spot size) is used, proportionately more spots should be applied.

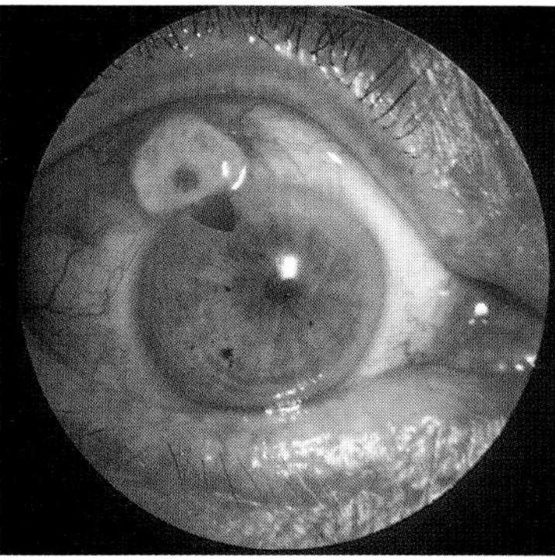

FIGURE 4–80 **Trabeculectomy in neovascular glaucoma.** Even with adequate panretinal photocoagulation, some angiogenesis factors may still be present in the eye. With successful filtration surgery, there is often a ring of injected episcleral vessels around the base of the filtration bleb. The filtration bleb also tends to be more limited in size and appears less succulent.

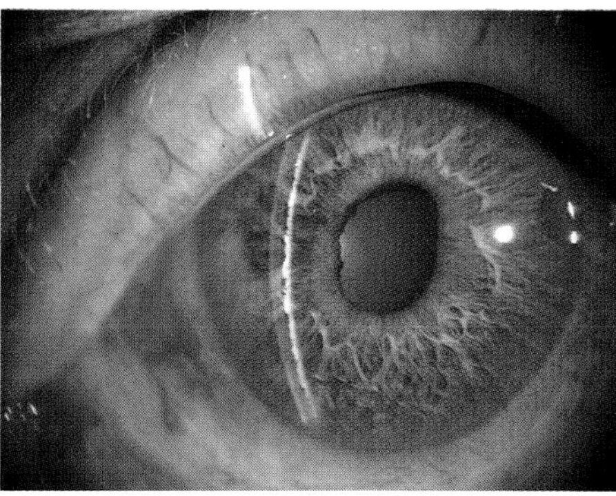

FIGURE 4–81 **Malignant glaucoma.** This photograph shows central and peripheral flat anterior chamber after a surgical peripheral iridectomy. The iridectomy site is located at the 2:30 position.

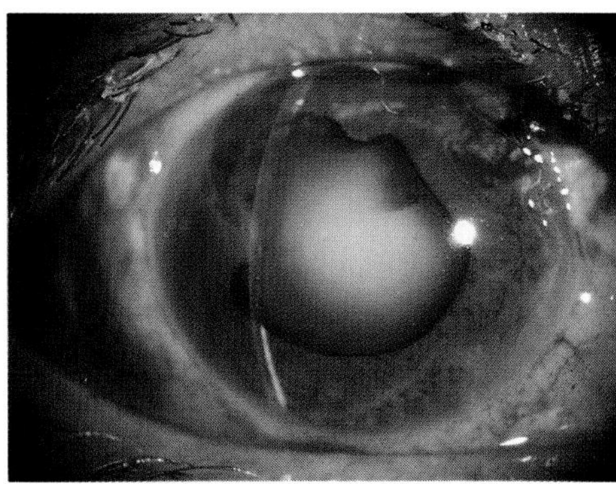

FIGURE 4–82 **Malignant glaucoma.** Central and peripheral flat anterior chambers are seen in this photograph after sector iridectomy and subsequent trabeculectomy. The onset of malignant glaucoma is attended by anterior displacement of the iris-lens diaphragm, resulting in shallowing of the central as well as peripheral anterior chamber.

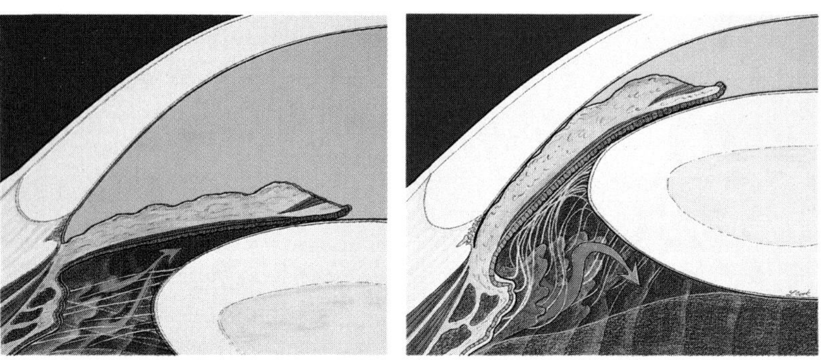

FIGURE 4–83 Diagram showing aqueous flow dynamics in malignant glaucoma. *A,* Normal pathway of aqueous flow from posterior chamber toward anterior chamber *(arrows). B,* Posterior aqueous diversion toward vitreous *(arrows)* in an eye with malignant glaucoma. The zonules are lax, the lens shifted forward, and the central and peripheral chamber shallowed. (Courtesy of Dr. B. T. Hutchinson.)

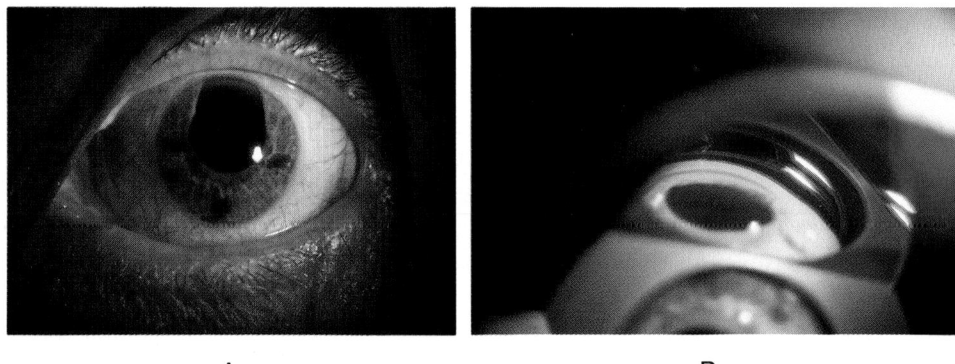

FIGURE 4–84 **Aphakic malignant glaucoma.** *A,* Aphakic malignant glaucoma, not relieved by multiple laser iridotomies, in an eye with an intact vitreous face bulging forward, totally flat anterior chamber, and intraocular pressure of 50 mmHg. *B,* Gonioscopic view of flattened ciliary processes adherent to vitreous. (Courtesy of Dr. P. A. Weber.)

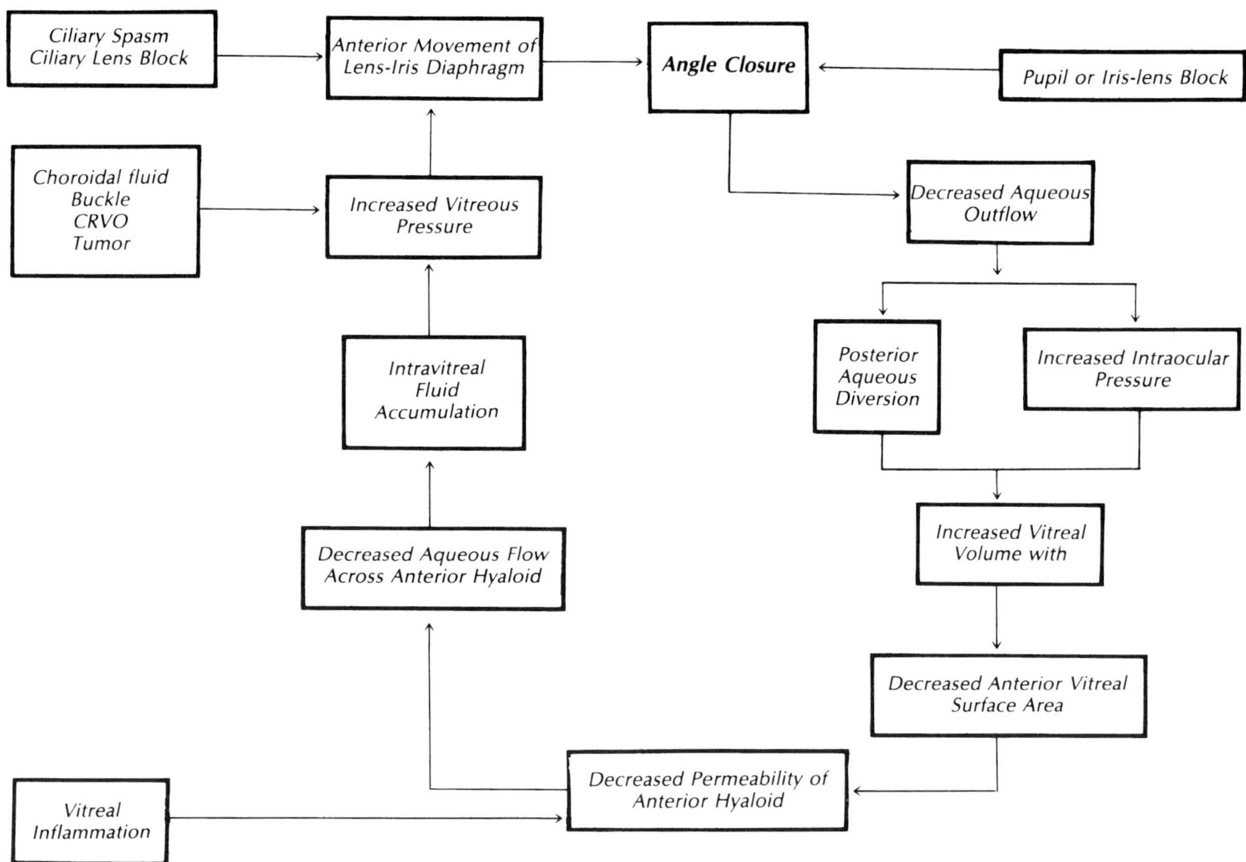

FIGURE 4–85 Possible mechanisms in malignant glaucoma emphasizing the role of the vitreous in maintaining the disease process. (From Luntz MH, Rosenblatt M: Malignant glaucoma. Surv Ophthalmol 32:73, 1987.)

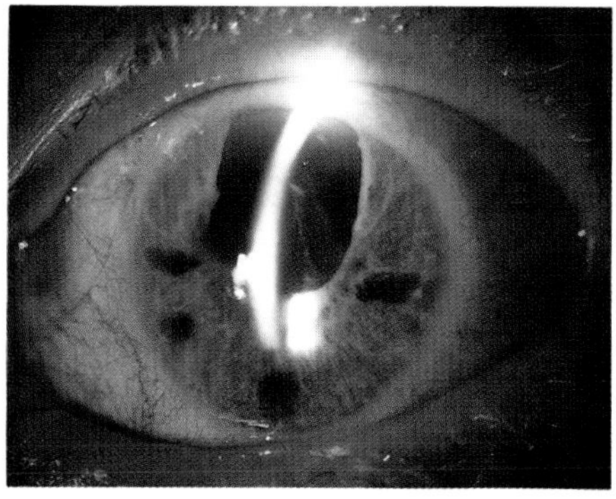

FIGURE 4–86 **Laser treatment of malignant glaucoma.** Relief of malignant glaucoma (see Fig. 4–84) with Nd.YAG laser to the superior anterior vitreous face. The anterior chamber deepened after the laser. (Courtesy of Dr. P. A. Weber.)

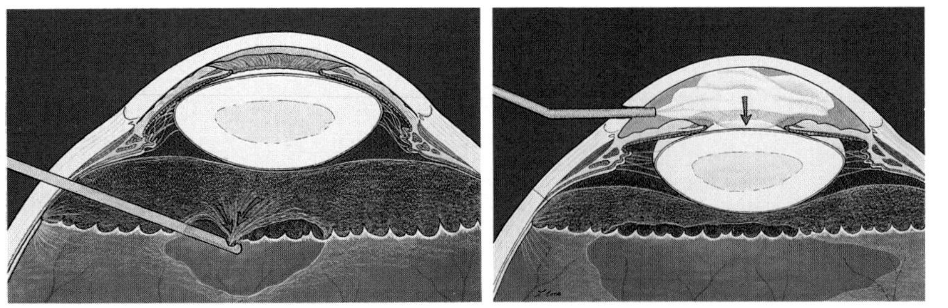

FIGURE 4–87 **Vitrectomy in malignant glaucoma.** *A,* Posterior sclerotomy with disruption of the anterior hyaloid face and automated mechanical vitrectomy for malignant glaucoma. *B,* Deepening of anterior chamber with viscoelastic agent *(arrow)* through a paracentesis after vitrectomy. (Courtesy of Dr. B. T. Hutchinson.)

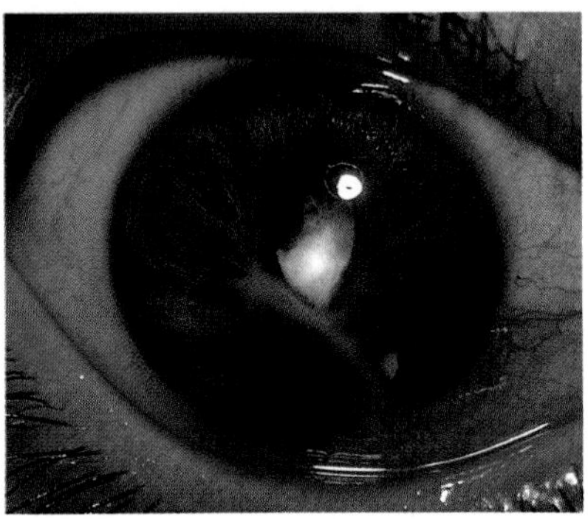

FIGURE 4–88 **Traumatic epithelial cyst.** This cyst resulted from penetrating trauma and fills the lower half of the anterior chamber. These are thought to occur when surface epithelium is implanted into the eye as a result of surgical or accidental trauma. They may demonstrate progressive growth filling the pupil and anterior chamber. (Courtesy of David Donaldson, M.D.)

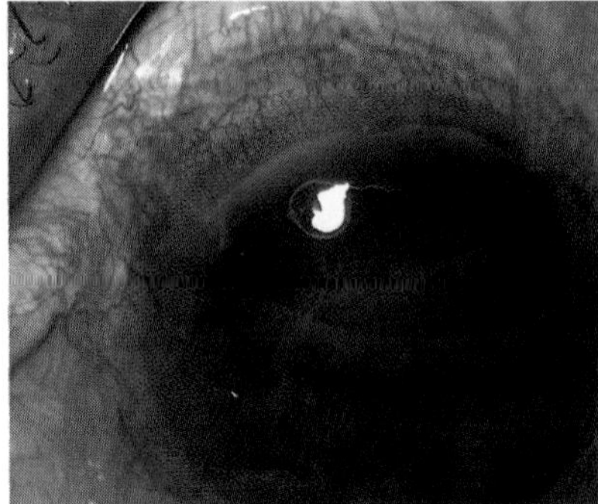

FIGURE 4–89 **Epithelial downgrowth.** Grayish retrocorneal membrane characteristic of epithelial downgrowth in an aphakic eye. A faint gray line on the posterior surface of the cornea represents the advancing edge of the epithelial sheet. This eye demonstrates ocular inflammation, which is chronic in many of these cases. (Courtesy of David Donaldson, M.D.)

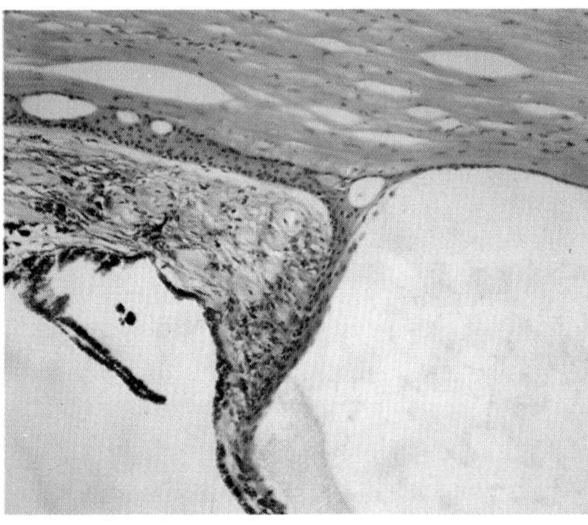

FIGURE 4–90 **Histopathology of epithelial downgrowth.** Nonkeratinized stratified squamous epithelium has formed a diffuse blanket on the iris and formed a broad surface peripheral anterior synechiae. This epithelial sheet results in destruction of underlying endothelial cells and disorganization and destruction of trabecular meshwork, leading to glaucoma. (Courtesy of David Donaldson, M.D.)

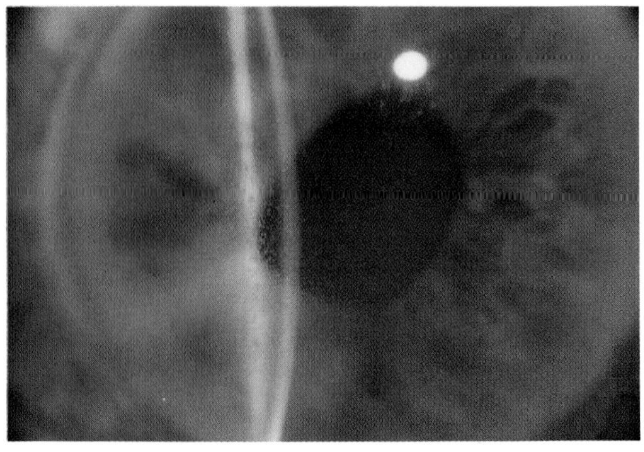

FIGURE 4–91 Inflammatory glaucoma with prominent keratic precipitates.

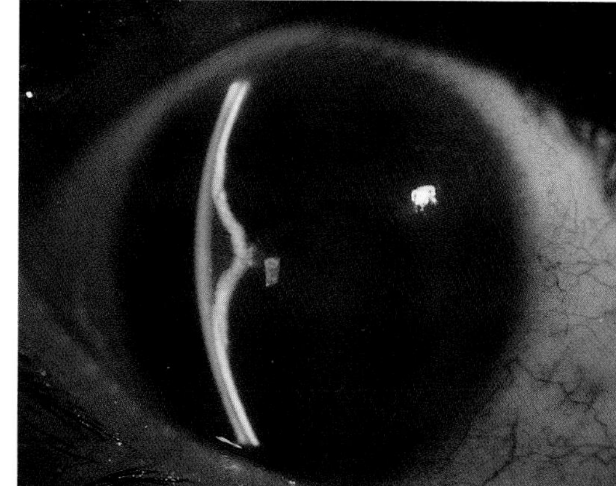

FIGURE 4–92 **Iris bombé complicating uveitis.** Note the bowing forward of the midperipheral iris toward the corneal endothelium.

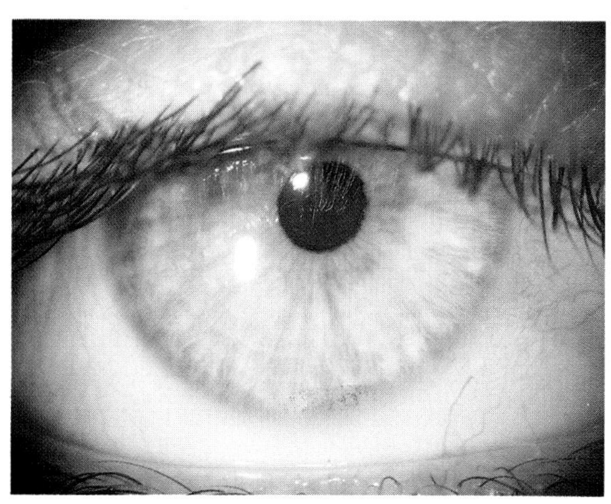

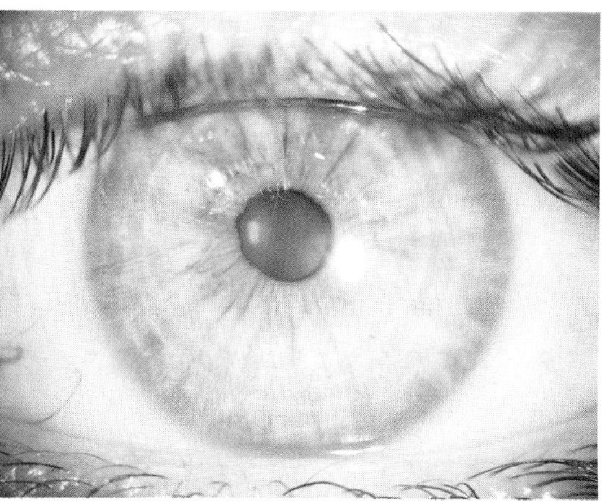

FIGURE 4–93 **Fuchs' heterochromic iridocyclitis.** *A* (right eye) and *B* (left eye), Eyes of a patient with Fuchs' heterochromic iridocyclitis in the right eye. Hypochromia is most often seen in affected eyes with dark irides caused by stromal atrophy.

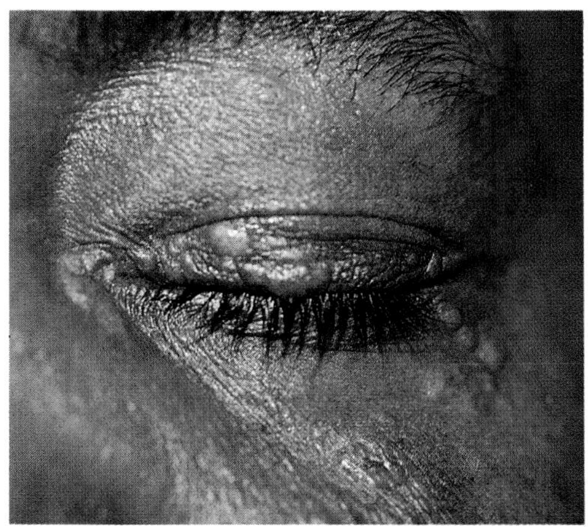

FIGURE 4–94 **Sarcoidosis.** Skin granulomas are present in a 42-year-old black man with sarcoidosis.

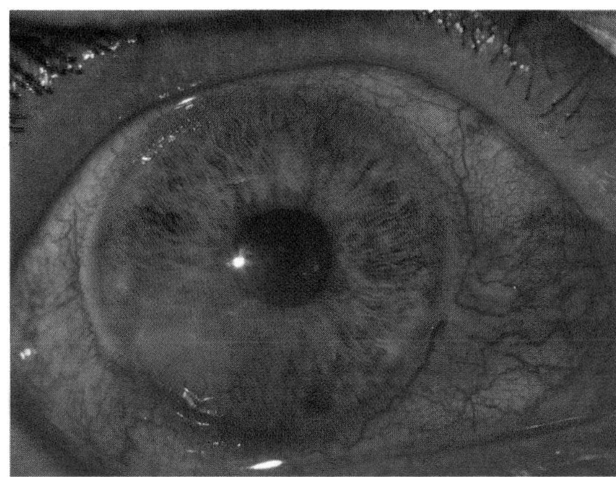

FIGURE 4–95 **Herpes simplex keratouveitis.** Glaucoma associated with herpes simplex keratouveitis is a relatively common feature, thought to be due to an associated trabeculitis.

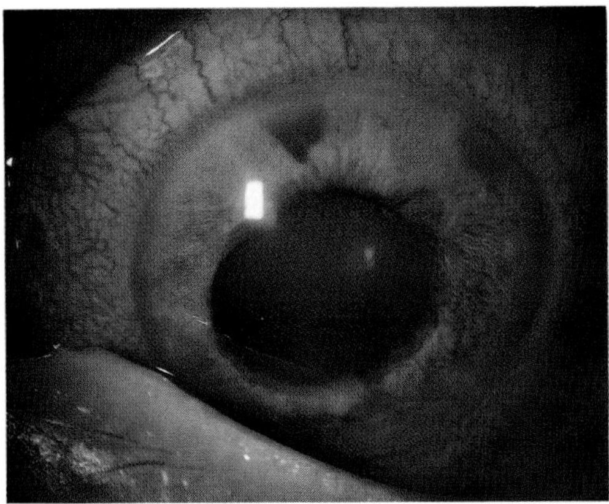

FIGURE 4–96 **Herpes zoster uveitis and glaucoma.** Note the irregular pupil and iris atrophy in this 52-year-old woman with herpes zoster uveitis and glaucoma. The patient had undergone iridectomies for angle-closure glaucoma before development of herpes zoster.

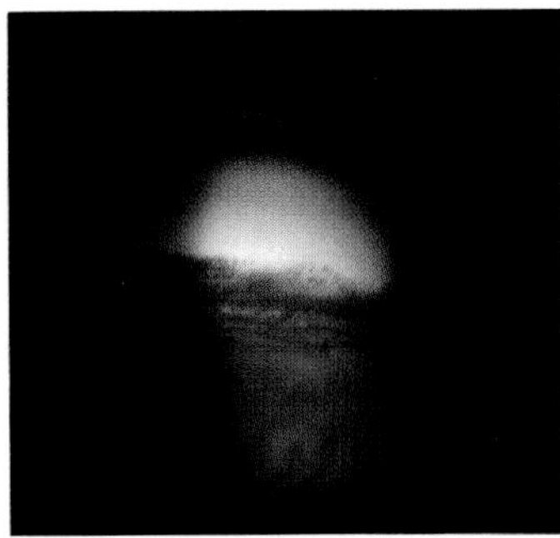

FIGURE 4–97 **Keratic precipitates in the angle.** This goniophotograph demonstrates keratic precipitates following argon laser trabeculoplasty.

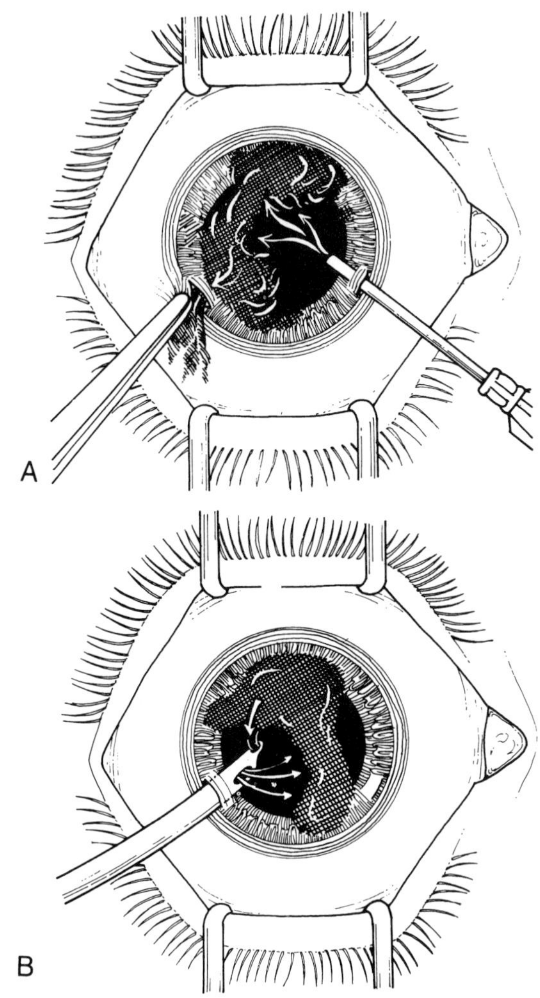

FIGURE 4–98 **Anterior chamber evacuation of hyphema.** Illustration of the technique of anterior chamber washout for hyphema with the use of direct irrigation *(A)* and the Simcoe coaxial irrigation/aspiration cannula *(B).*

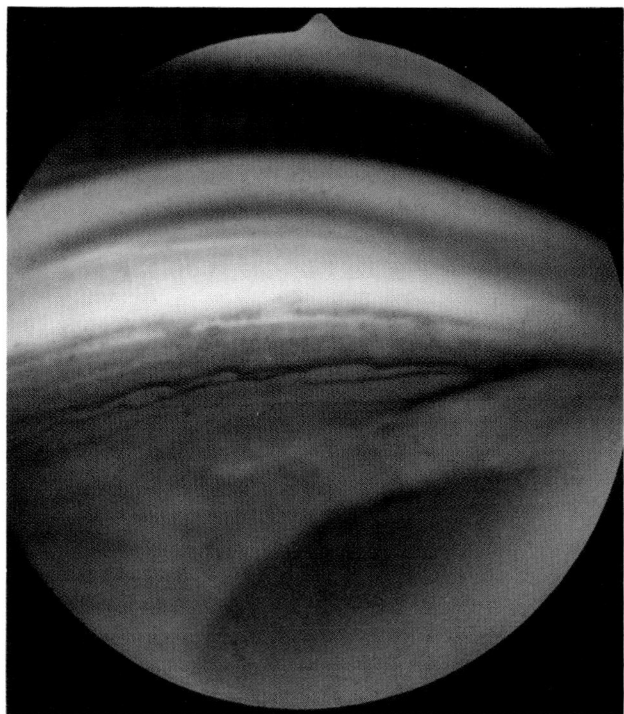

FIGURE 4–99 **Traumatic angle recession.** Gonioscopy reveals a deepening of the angle in which the exposed face of the ciliary body appears wider than is usual, and the iris root appears posteriorly displaced.

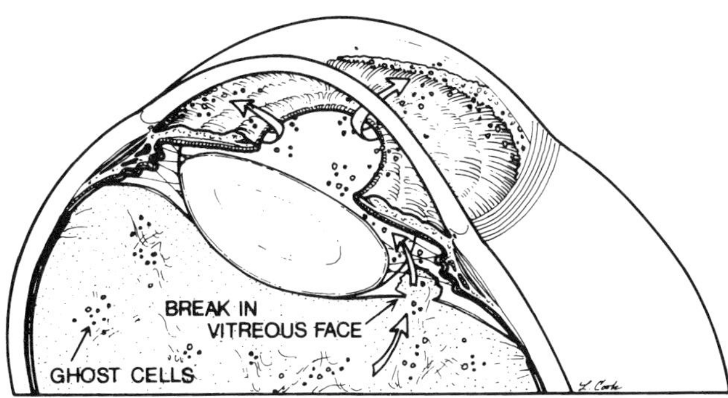

FIGURE 4–100 **Ghost cell glaucoma.** This illustration demonstrates hemorrhage within the vitreous cavity and escape of ghost cells through a break in the anterior hyaloid face into the anterior chamber.

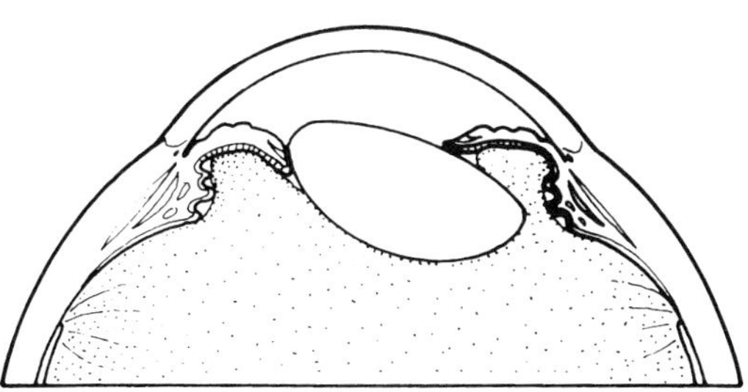

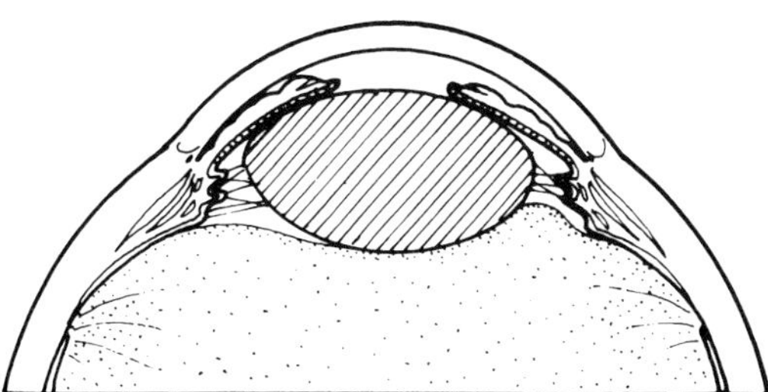

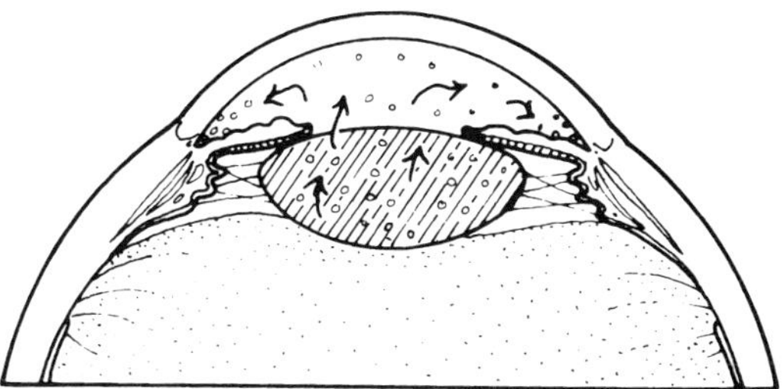

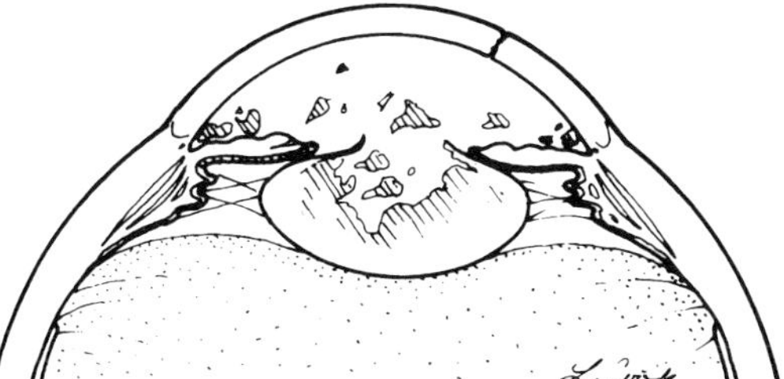

FIGURE 4–101 **Four types of lens-induced glaucoma.** *Clockwise from upper left:* lens subluxation, phacomorphic, lens particle, and phacolytic.

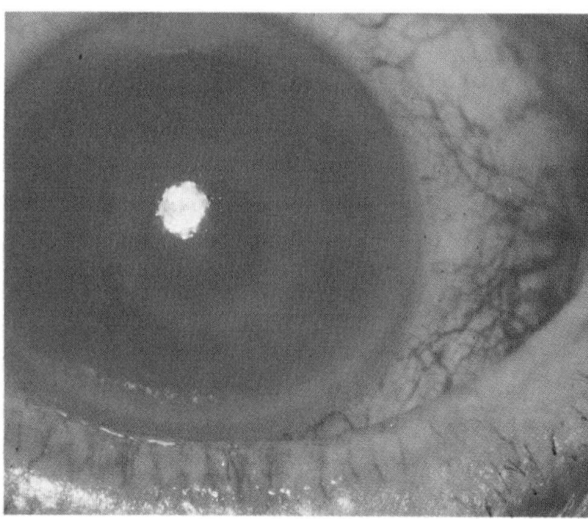

FIGURE 4-102 **Phacolytic glaucoma.** Note the perilimbal injection and the corneal edema. (Courtesy of David D. Donaldson, M.D.)

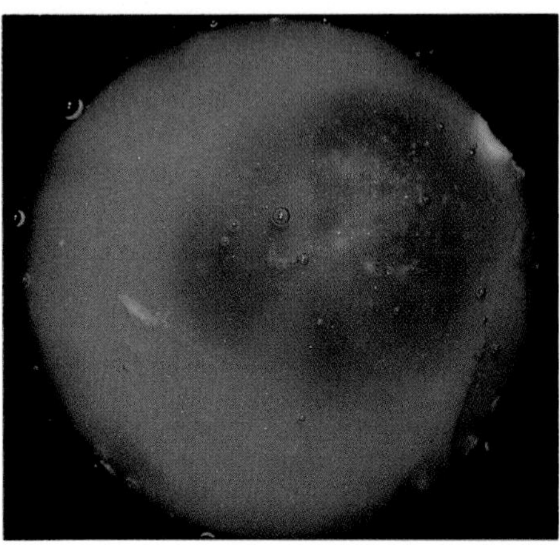

FIGURE 4-103 **Phacolytic glaucoma.** This hypermature cataract caused a secondary open-angle glaucoma. The lens protein has liquefied and leaks through an intact capsule. Lens protein induces chemotactic migration of macrophages, the principal inflammatory cell in phacolytic glaucoma. (Courtesy of David D. Donaldson, M.D.)

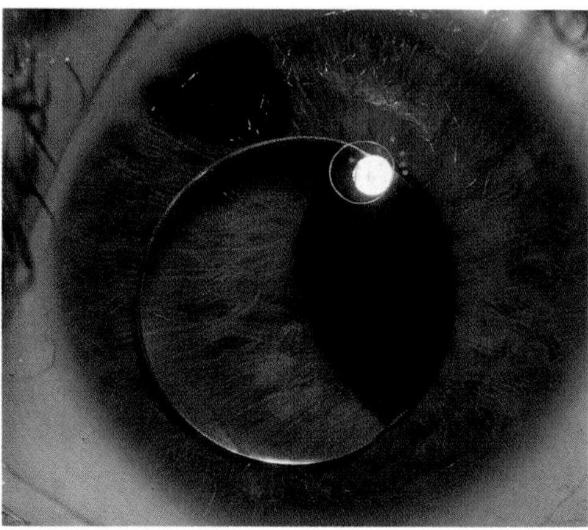

FIGURE 4-105 **Lens displacement glaucoma.** Angle-closure glaucoma caused by congenitally dislocated lens. Anterior movement of the lens or prolapse of the vitreous may result in a pupillary block glaucoma. (Courtesy of David D. Donaldson, M.D.)

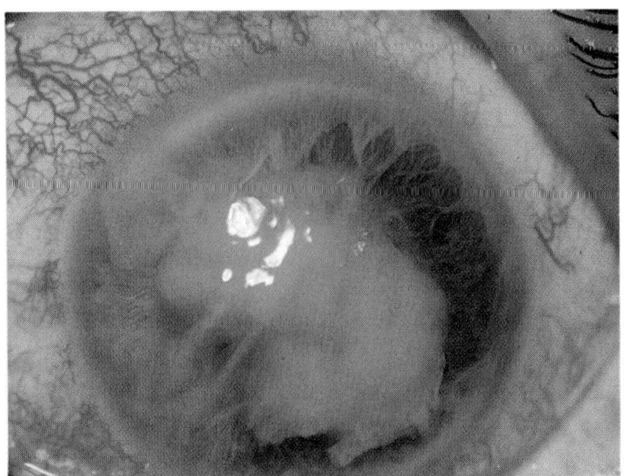

FIGURE 4-104 **Lens-particle glaucoma.** Lens-particle glaucoma requires surgical or traumatic disruption of the lens capsule with the release of cortical material into the aqueous. In this photograph, note the large amount of cortical material lying free in the anterior chamber in front of the pupillary plane. (Courtesy of David D. Donaldson, M.D.)

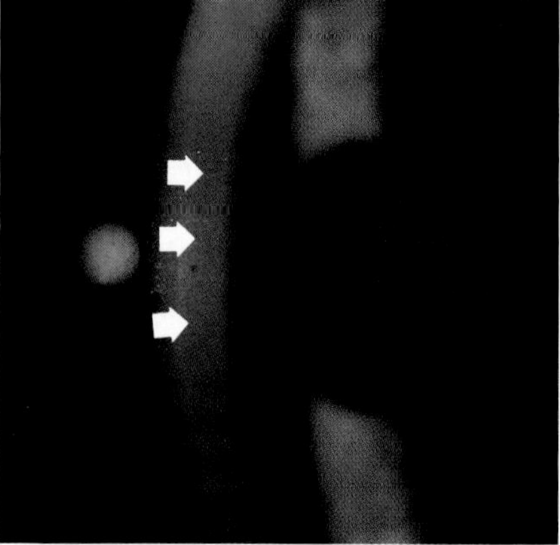

FIGURE 4-106 **Corneal endothelium in the iridocorneal endothelial (ICE) syndrome.** A slit-lamp view showing fine silver-beaten appearance of corneal endothelial abnormality *(arrow)* in the ICE syndrome. This appearance is similar to that of Fuchs' dystrophy but less coarse.

FIGURE 4–107 **Specular microscopy of endothelium in ICE syndrome.** The endothelial cells in the ICE syndrome show pleomorphism in size and shape, dark areas within the cells, and loss of clear hexagonal margins. (From Shields MB: Textbook of Glaucoma, 2nd ed, p. 222. Copyright 1987, the Williams & Wilkins Co., Baltimore.)

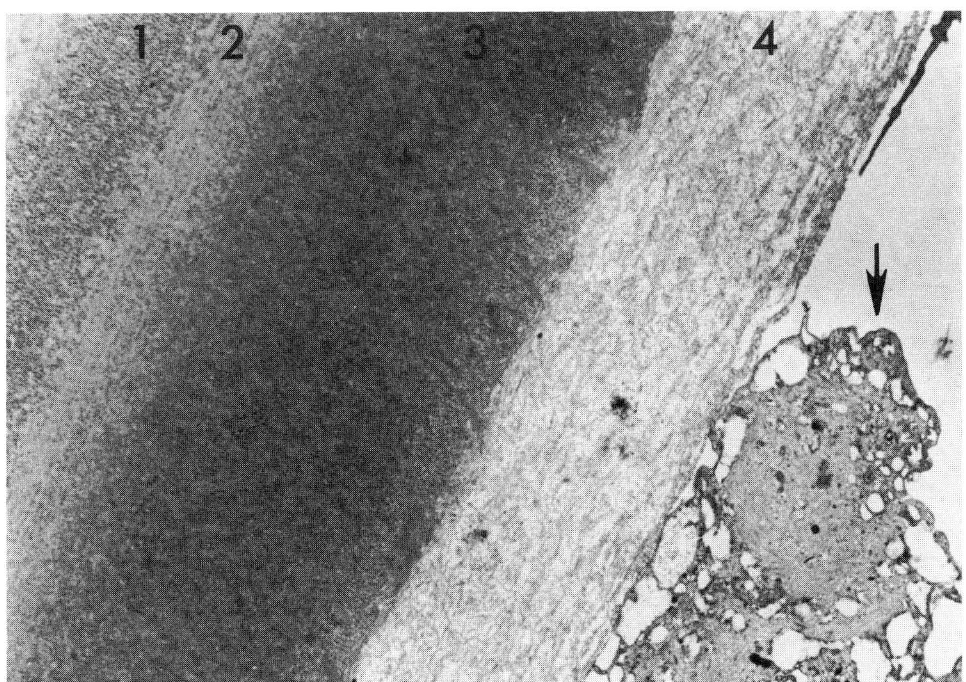

FIGURE 4–108 **Posterior cornea in ICE syndrome.** Transmission electron microscopic view of inner corneal surface in ICE syndrome, showing part of an abnormal cell *(arrow)* on a four-layered membrane composed of the anterior nonbanded (1) and posterior-banded (2) portions of Descemet's membrane with abnormal compact collagenous (3) and loose collagenous (4) layers. ×6875. (From Shields MB, McCracken JS, Klintworth KG, Campbell DG: Corneal edema in essential iris atrophy. Ophthalmology 86:1533–1550, 1979.)

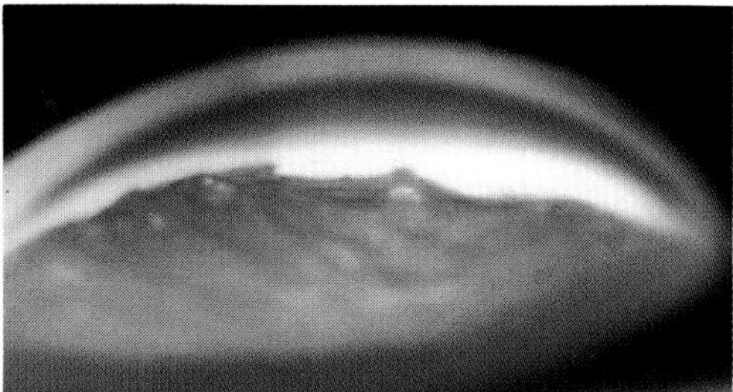

FIGURE 4-109 **Peripheral anterior synechia in ICE syndrome.** The typical gonioscopic appearance of patients with ICE syndrome is that of broad peripheral anterior synechia, often extending to or beyond Schwalbe's line.

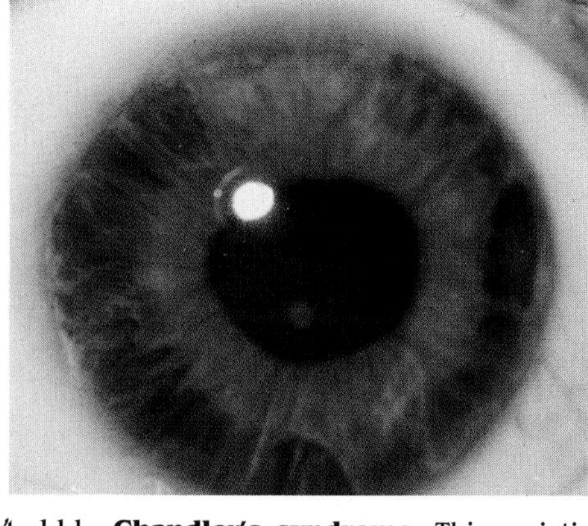

FIGURE 4-111 **Chandler's syndrome.** This variation of ICE syndrome shows an irregular pupil with stromal iris atrophy. Note that in some cases of Chandler's syndrome, the iris may appear entirely normal.

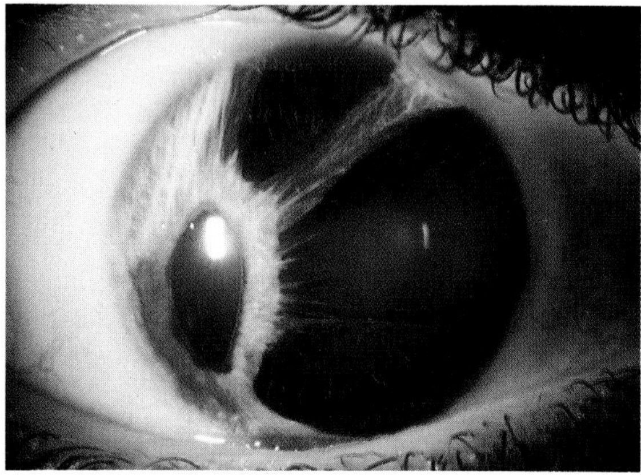

FIGURE 4-110 **Progressive iris atrophy.** This variation of ICE syndrome is characterized by marked corectopia and iris atrophy with multiple iris holes.

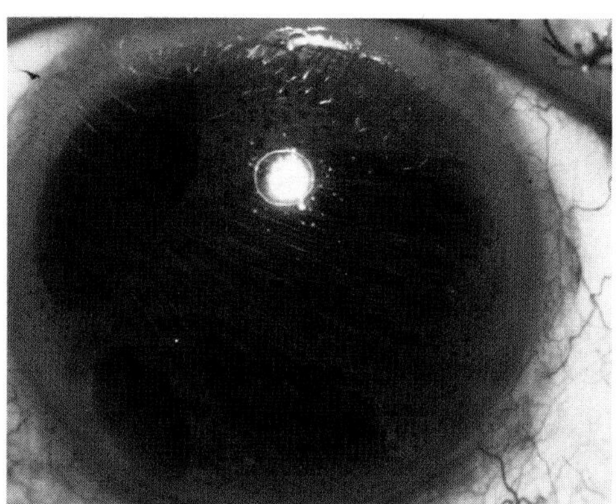

FIGURE 4-112 **Cogan-Reese syndrome.** This variation of ICE syndrome is characterized by ectropion uvea and marked corectopia with iris atrophy, hole formation, and numerous dark nodules on the iris surface. These pigmented, pedunculated nodules on the surface of the iris are the distinguishing feature in this entity. (From Shields MB, Campbell DG, Simmons RJ, Hutchinson BT: Iris nodules in essential iris atrophy. Arch Ophthalmol 94:406–410, 1976. Copyright 1976, American Medical Association.)

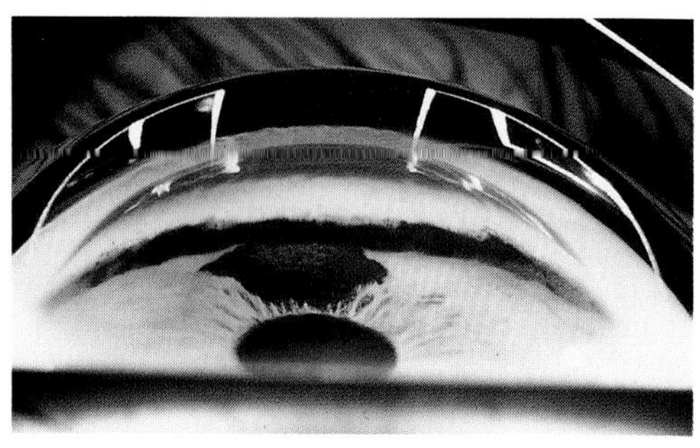

FIGURE 4-113 **Iris melanoma with extension into angle structures.** In this photograph, there is direct growth of solid tumor into the anterior chamber angle and aqueous outflow pathways causing obstruction of aqueous outflow. Diffuse iris melanomas are more likely to result in secondary glaucoma compared with smaller circumscribed tumors.

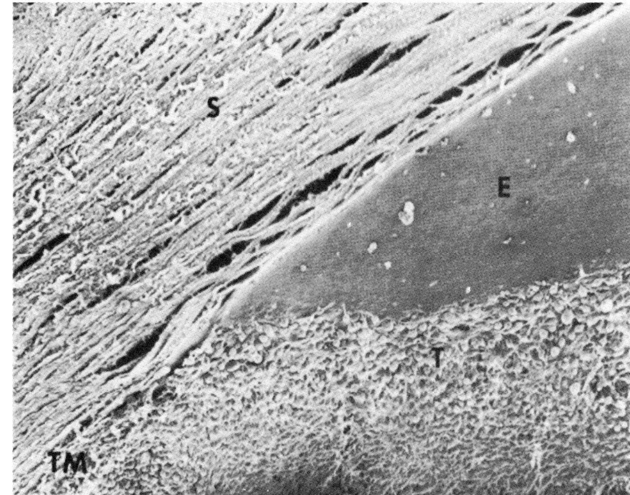

FIGURE 4–114 **Extension of melanoma from the ciliary body into trabecular meshwork.** Scanning electron microscopy of ciliary body melanoma tumor cells seeding the trabecular meshwork. E, exudate; S, sclera; TM, trabecular meshwork. (From Shields MB, Klintworth GK: Anterior uveal melanomas and intraocular pressure. Ophthalmology 87:503–517, 1980.)

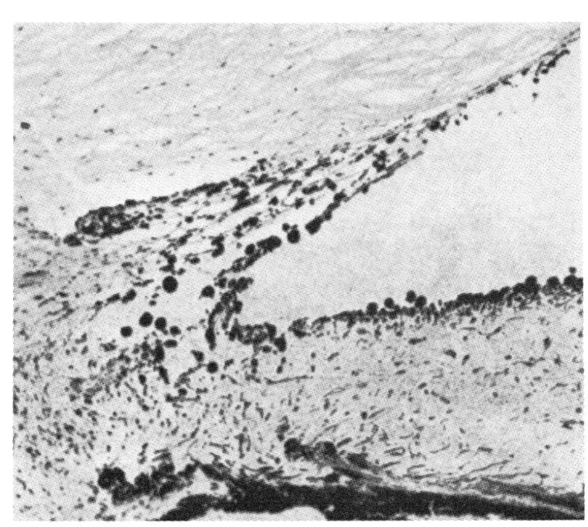

FIGURE 4–115 **Melanomalytic glaucoma.** Pigment-laden macrophages lining the anterior chamber angle with involvement of the trabecular meshwork in melanomalytic glaucoma. (From Yanoff M, Scheie H: Melanocyte glaucoma: Report of a case. Arch Ophthalmol 84:471–473, 1970. Copyright 1970, American Medical Association.)

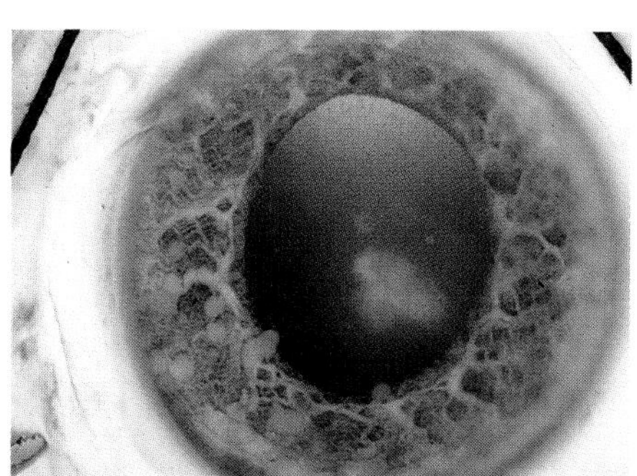

FIGURE 4–116 **Anterior segment seeding by retinoblastoma with secondary glaucoma.** Note the white globular foci of tumor lying on the iris surface. Seeding of the trabecular meshwork by these cells results in secondary glaucoma. Note that the most common mechanism of secondary glaucoma in eyes with retinoblastoma is neovascularization of the iris in angle structures with formation of peripheral anterior synechiae.

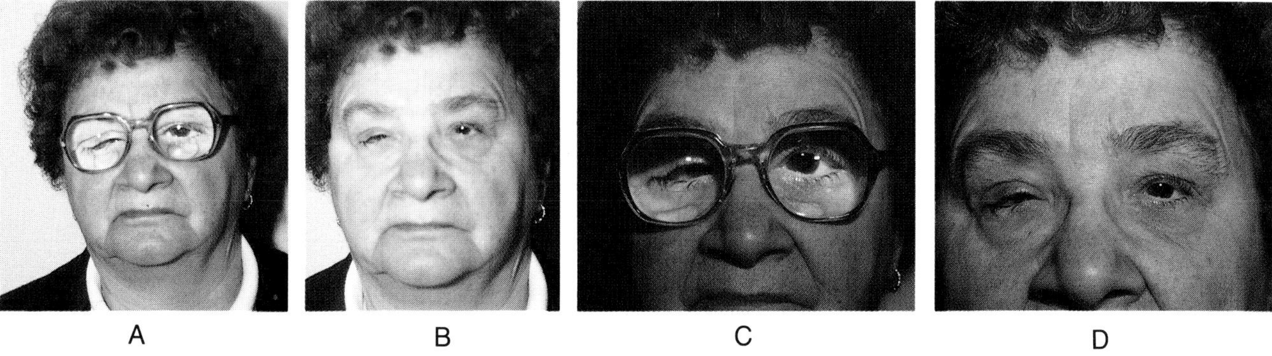

FIGURE 4–117 **Nanophthalmos.** *A–D,* A 64-year-old white woman with typical external characteristics of nanophthalmos including deeply-set eyes in small bony orbits, narrow palpebral fissures, and hyperopic refractive correction resembling aphakic spectacles.

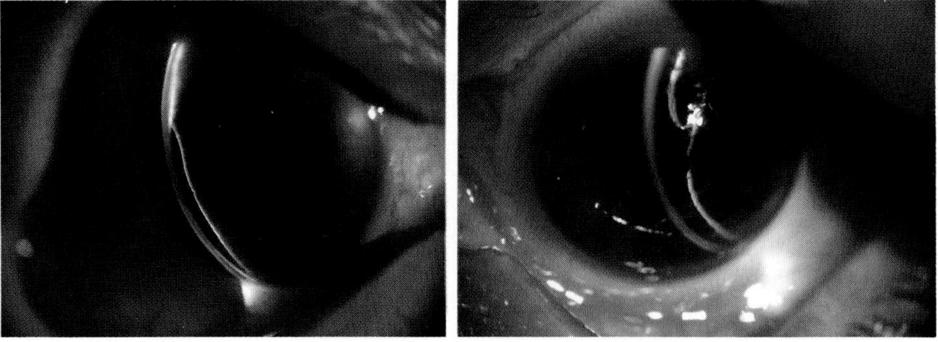

FIGURE 4–118 **Anterior chamber shallowing in nanophthalmos.** *A* and *B*, The parallelopiped of light demonstrates asymmetric stages of anterior chamber shallowing by slit-lamp examination. In the young nanophthalmic patient, the anterior chamber is open in the presence of prominent iris convexity. Progressive anterior chamber shallowing and narrowing of the angle occurs with the onset of angle closure during the fourth to sixth decades.

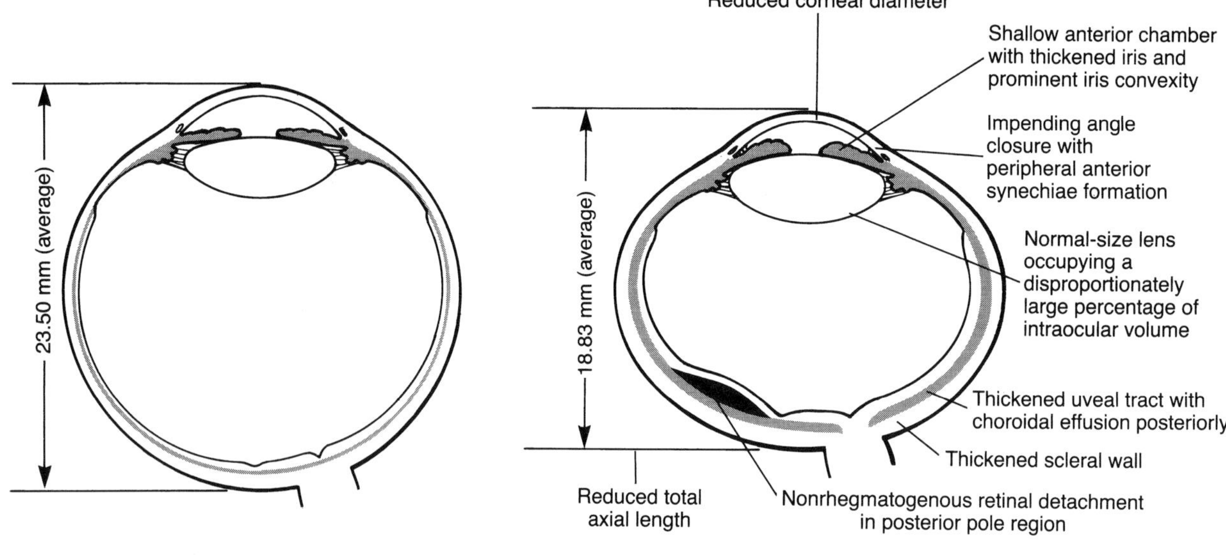

FIGURE 4–119 **Schematic diagram of the normal eye and nanophthalmic eye.** The eye in nanophthalmos has these ocular features: (1) reduced corneal diameter, (2) shallow anterior chamber with thickened iris and prominent iris convexity, (3) impending angle closure with peripheral anterior synechiae formation, (4) a crystalline lens of normal size occupying a disproportionately large percentage of intraocular volume, (5) a thickened uveal tract with choroidal effusion occurring posteriorly, (6) a thickened scleral wall, (7) nonrhegmatogenous retinal detachment affecting the posterior pole region, and (8) reduced total length of 18.83 mm (compared with the normal axial length of 23.50 mm, average).

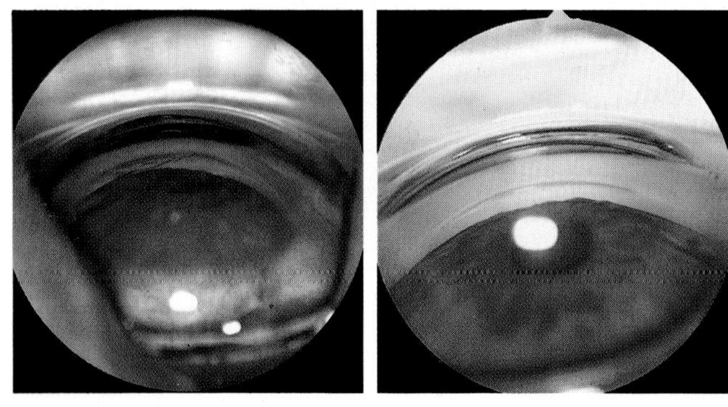

FIGURE 4–120 **Gonioscopy in nanophthalmos.** *A* and *B*, Koeppe gonioscopy demonstrates prominent iris convexity and asymmetric stages of angle closure in both eyes.

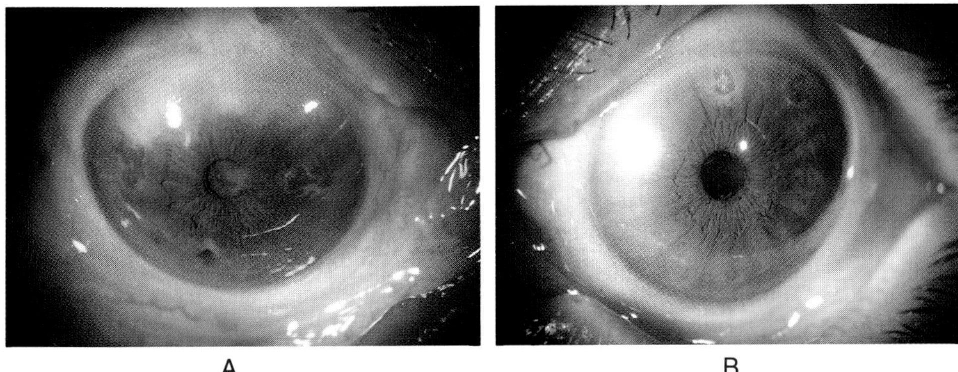

FIGURE 4–121 **Iridocorneal changes in nanophthalmos.** *A* and *B*, The anterior segment examination demonstrates superior corneal opacification corresponding to areas of iridocorneal apposition during acute angle-closure glaucoma in the right eye. Patent iridotomies present inferiorly in the right eye and superiorly in the left eye were created by argon and subsequent Nd.YAG lasers.

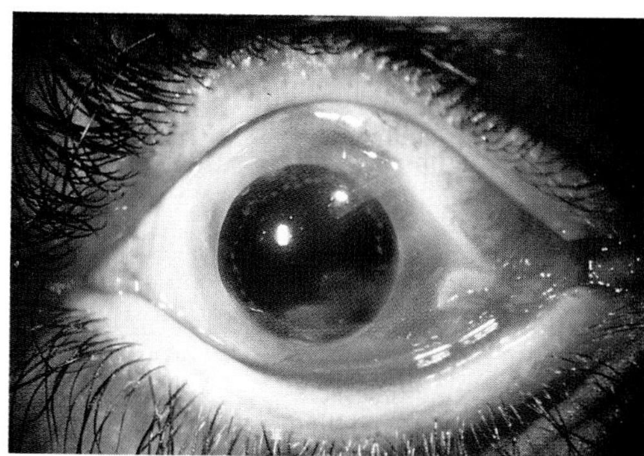

FIGURE 4–122 **Molteno's implant.** Low-power photograph of a Molteno's tube in an eye with penetrating keratoplasty. The tube is visible in the anterior chamber at approximately the 2:00 position.

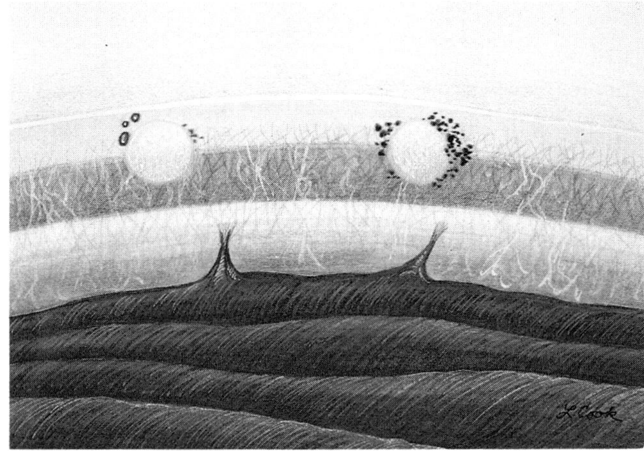

FIGURE 4–123 **Schematic diagram showing laser burn in trabeculoplasty.** The desired tissue reaction is blanching of the trabecular meshwork, with or without minimal bubble formation, demonstrated *on the left*. The laser burn *on the right* demonstrates excessive pigment scattering, and the power should be reduced.

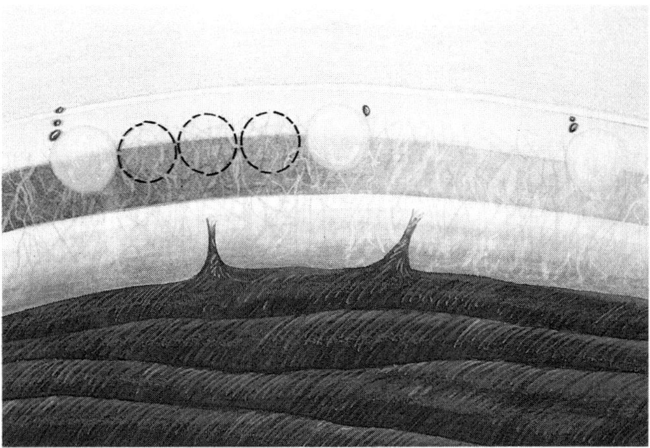

FIGURE 4–124 **Schematic diagram showing laser placement in trabeculoplasty.** The laser burns are placed at the anterior half of the trabecular meshwork, straddling the junction of the pigmented and nonpigmented meshwork. The appropriate spacing between laser burns and the effect of trabecular meshwork pigmentation on tissue reaction are also demonstrated.

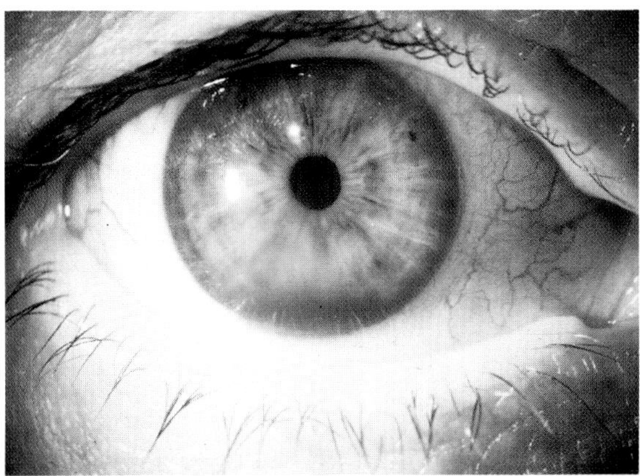

FIGURE 4–125 **Hyphema after argon laser trabeculoplasty.** Bleeding may result from reflux of blood from Schlemm's canal or inadvertent photocoagulation of an iris root vessel or a circumferential ciliary vessel. Low-power photocoagulations (200 mW, 200 μ, 0.2 sec) can be used to control bleeding from an identifiable site.

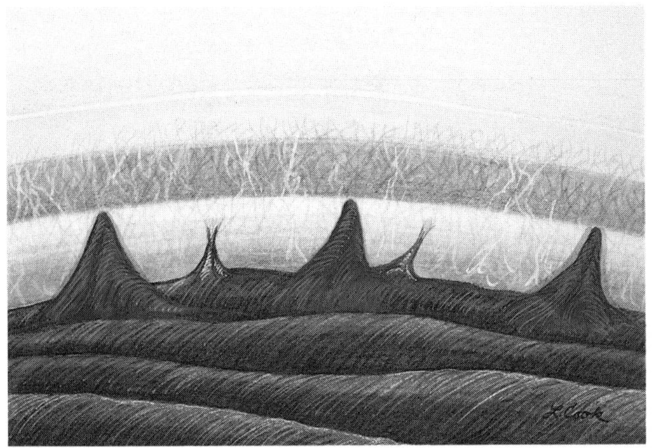

FIGURE 4-126 **Peripheral anterior synechiae posttrabeculoplasty.** Small, peaked peripheral synechiae can complicate argon laser trabeculoplasty. These synechiae can be identified in as many as 46% of eyes treated with argon laser trabeculoplasty. They may reach to the ciliary body band, scleral spur, or the trabecular meshwork.

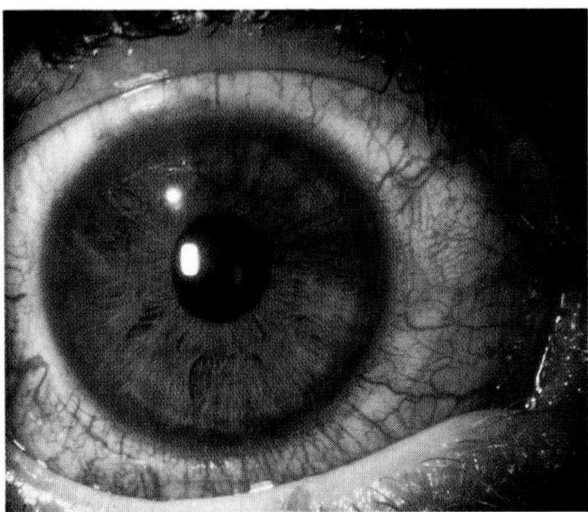

FIGURE 4-127 **Inflammation after laser trabeculoplasty.** This eye had argon laser trabeculoplasty to the inferior 180 degrees of the trabecular meshwork. Note the circumlimbal injection of vessels. The iritis is usually mild and clears rapidly with use of postoperative topical corticosteroids.

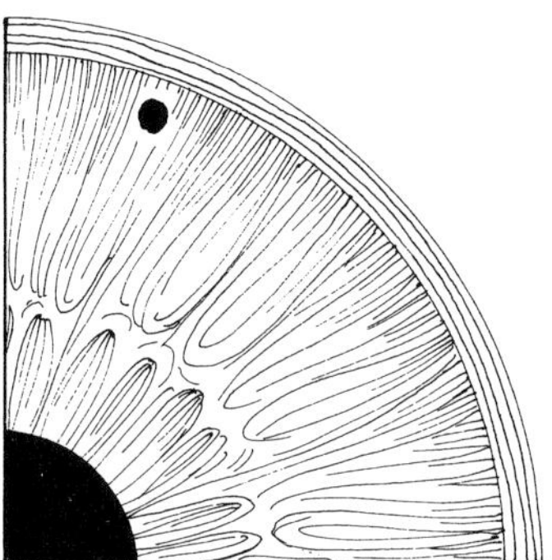

FIGURE 4-128 **Laser iridectomy location.** The ideal laser iridectomy location is in the far periphery of one of the superior quadrants of the eye.

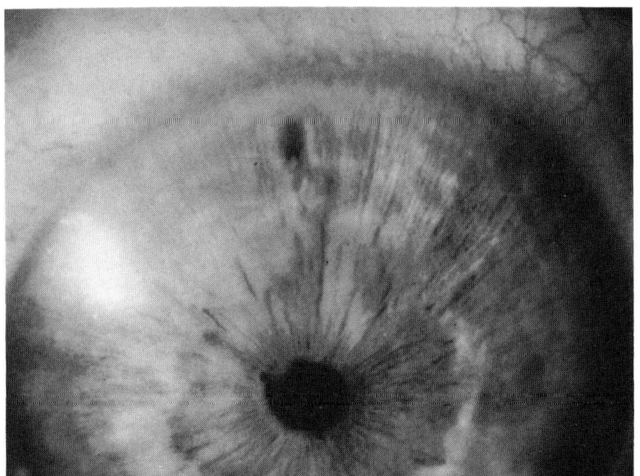

FIGURE 4-129 **Nd.YAG laser iridectomy.** When the pupil resumes its normal position, the iridectomy is located in the far periphery.

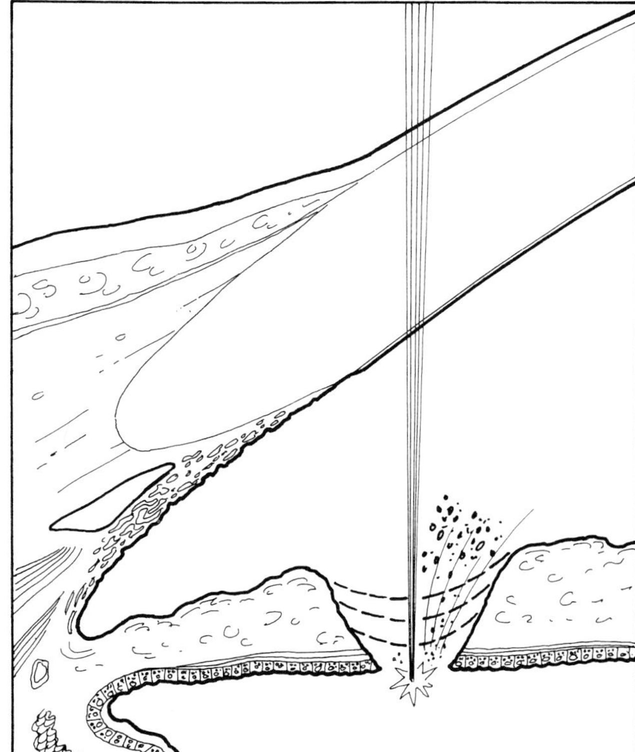

FIGURE 4–130 **Nd.YAG iridectomy.** By focusing deep into the iris stroma, optical breakdown is produced, and the shock and acoustic waves cause the iridectomy to form.

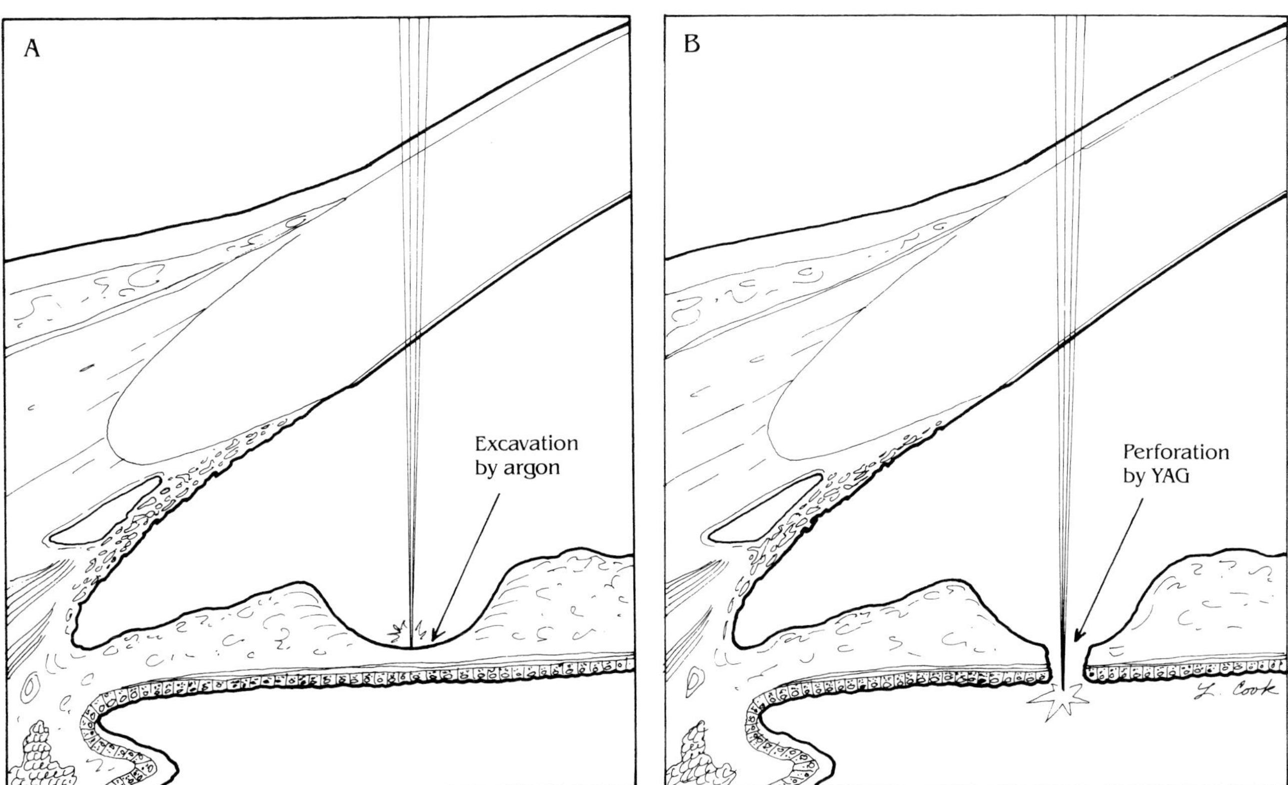

FIGURE 4–131 **Combined argon and Nd.YAG laser iridectomy.** *A,* Approximately 80% of the surface of the thick brown iris is excavated with the use of the argon laser. *B,* The Nd.YAG laser is then used to perforate the remaining iris substance.

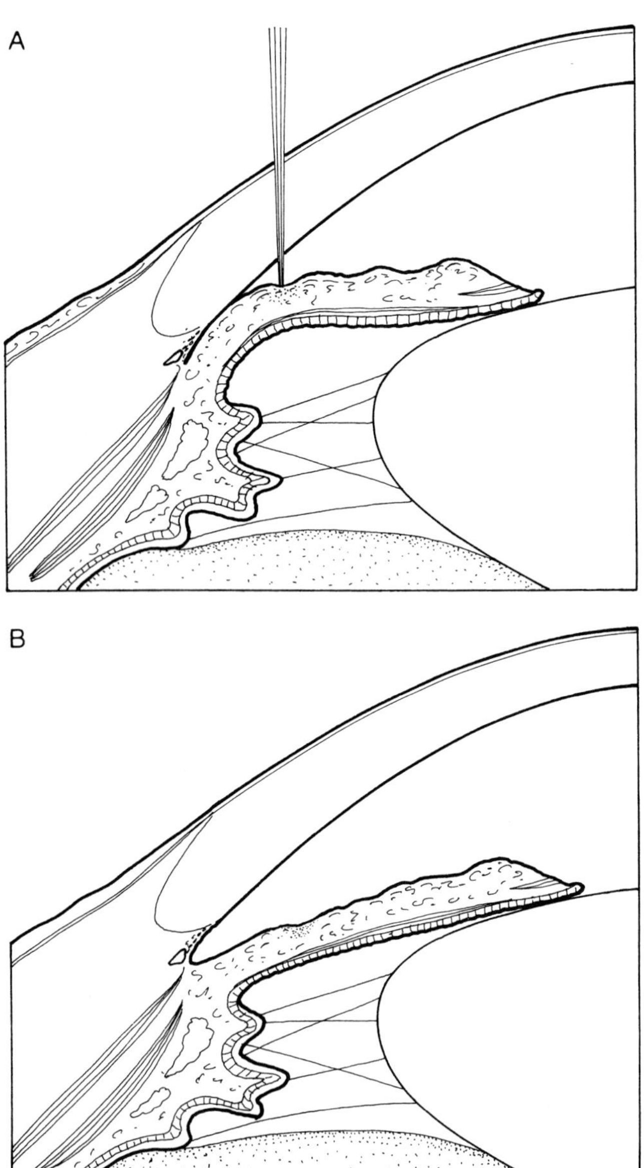

FIGURE 4–132 **Argon laser gonioplasty.** *A,* Argon laser application to the iris surface in the gonioplasty technique. The argon laser beam is directed to the peripheral iris 1.5 mm from the iris root. *B,* Widening of the angle brought about by the contracture of the iris stroma in the gonioplasty technique.

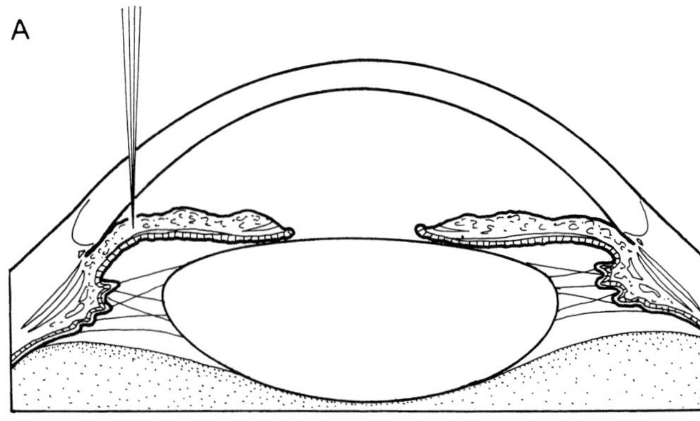

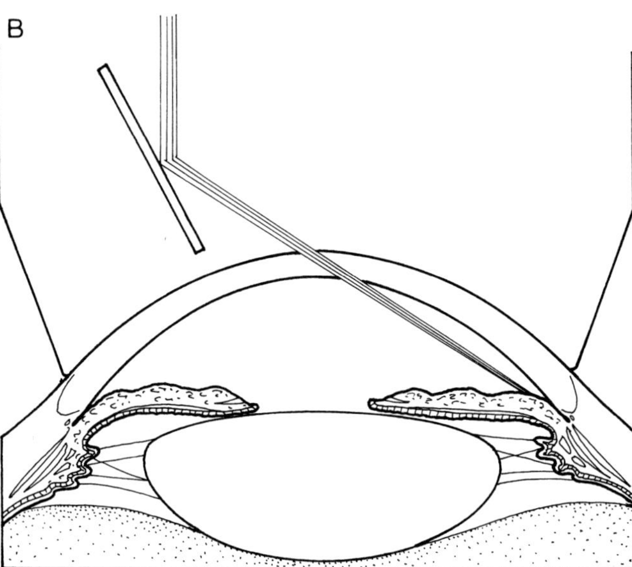

FIGURE 4–133 **Argon laser gonioplasty.** *A,* Direct applications of the argon laser in the gonioplasty technique. *B,* Indirect applications of the argon laser in the gonioplasty technique with the use of the angle mirror of the Goldmann lens.

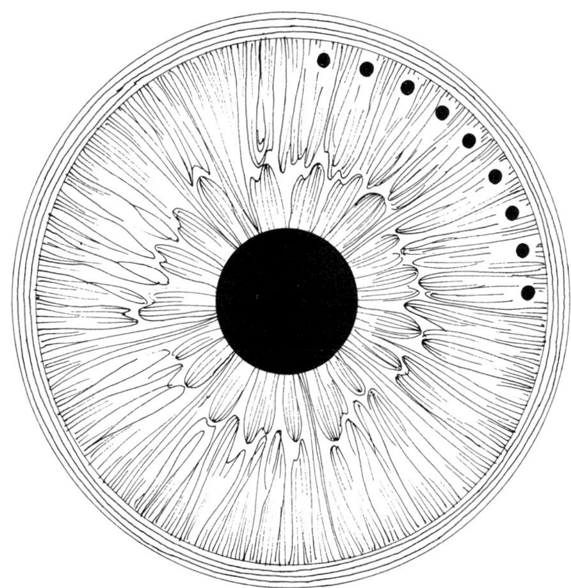

FIGURE 4–134 Location and spacing of argon laser applications in the gonioplasty technique.

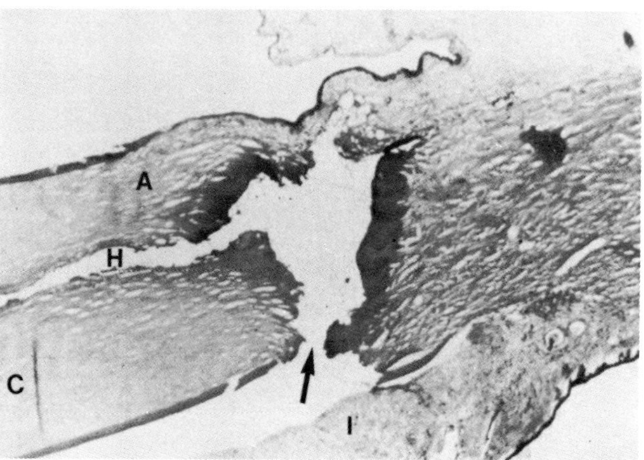

FIGURE 4–136 **Light micrograph of Nd.YAG laser sclerostomy.** Rabbit corneoscleral junction after silver-stabilized protein injection into the sclera and Nd.YAG laser sclerostomy. The *arrow* denotes a fistula. The dark color of the silver injection (A) has penetrated halfway through the rabbit sclera. C, cornea; I, iris. (From March WF: Silver oxide in YAG sclerostomy. Lasers Surg Med 7:354, 1987.)

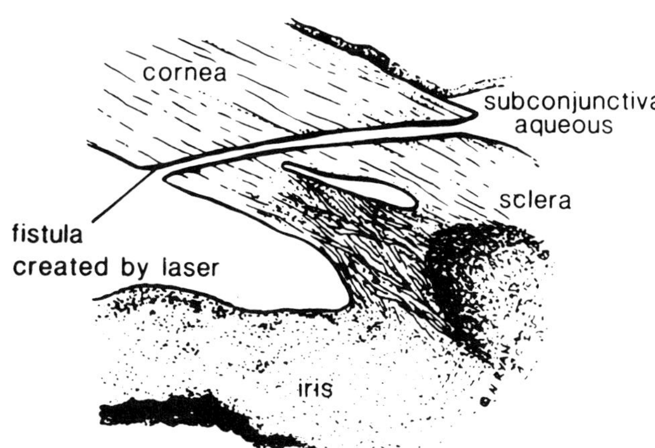

FIGURE 4–135 Diagram for sclerostomy performed using the laser. (Courtesy of W. March, M.D.)

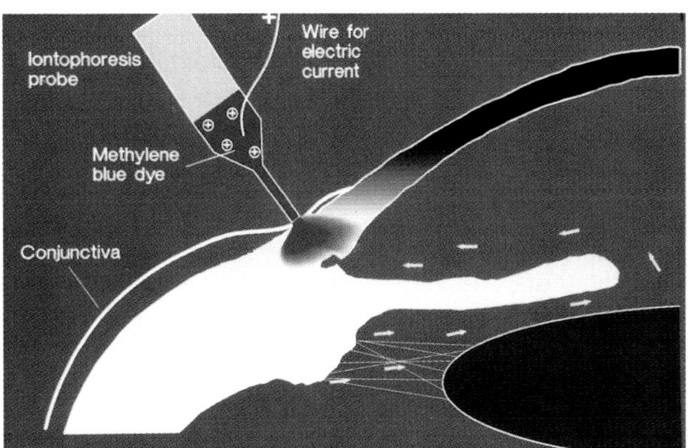

FIGURE 4–137 Schematic representation of iontophoresis of methylene blue dye into the sclera at the limbus. (From Latina MA, et al: Experimental ab-interno sclerostomies using a pulsed-dye laser and goniolens. Arch Ophthalmol 108:1747, 1990. Copyright 1990, American Medical Association.)

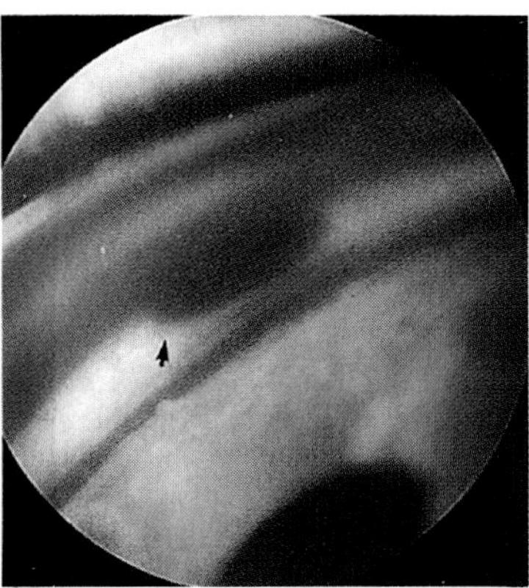

FIGURE 4–138 Gonioscopy view of methylene blue–dyed sclera *(arrow)*. Kawa Camera, ×2. (From Latina MA, et al: Experimental ab-interno sclerostomies using a pulsed-dye laser and goniolens. Arch Ophthalmol 108:1747, 1990. Copyright 1990, American Medical Association.)

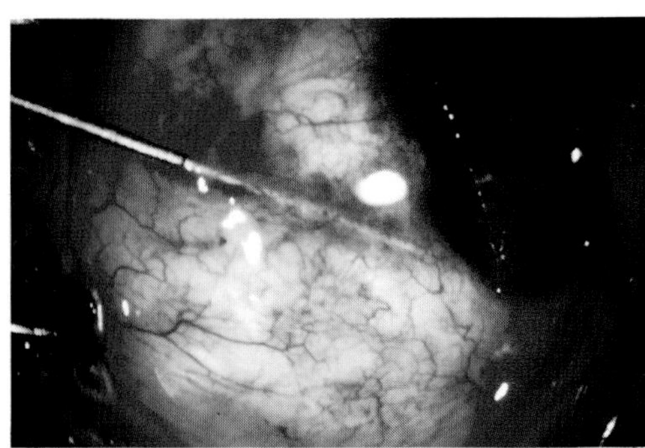

FIGURE 4–140 **Holmium laser sclerostomy.** Fiberoptic probe is introduced into subconjunctival space and advanced to the limbus. Holmium laser energy is emitted perpendicular to the axis of the probe. (Courtesy of Sunrise Technology, CA.)

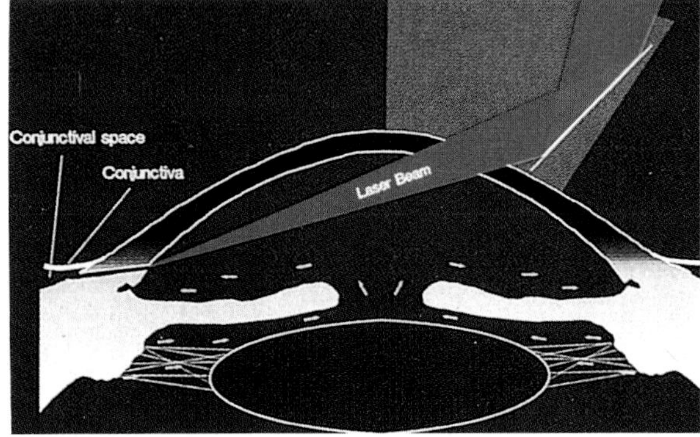

FIGURE 4–139 Schematic representation of a laser beam directed through a goniolens onto the dyed scleral region to create a full-thickness fistula. (From Latina MA, et al: Experimental ab-interno sclerostomies using a pulsed-dye laser and goniolens. Arch Ophthalmol 108:1747, 1990. Copyright 1990, American Medical Association.)

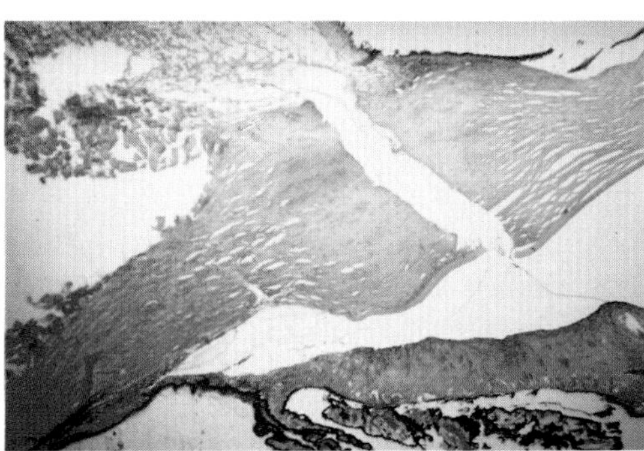

FIGURE 4–141 Histopathology of ab-externo THC:YAG laser sclerostomy without an iridectomy. (From Hoskins HD, et al: Subconjunctival THC:YAG laser limbal sclerostomy ab-externo in the rabbit. Ophthalmic Surg 21:591, 1990.)

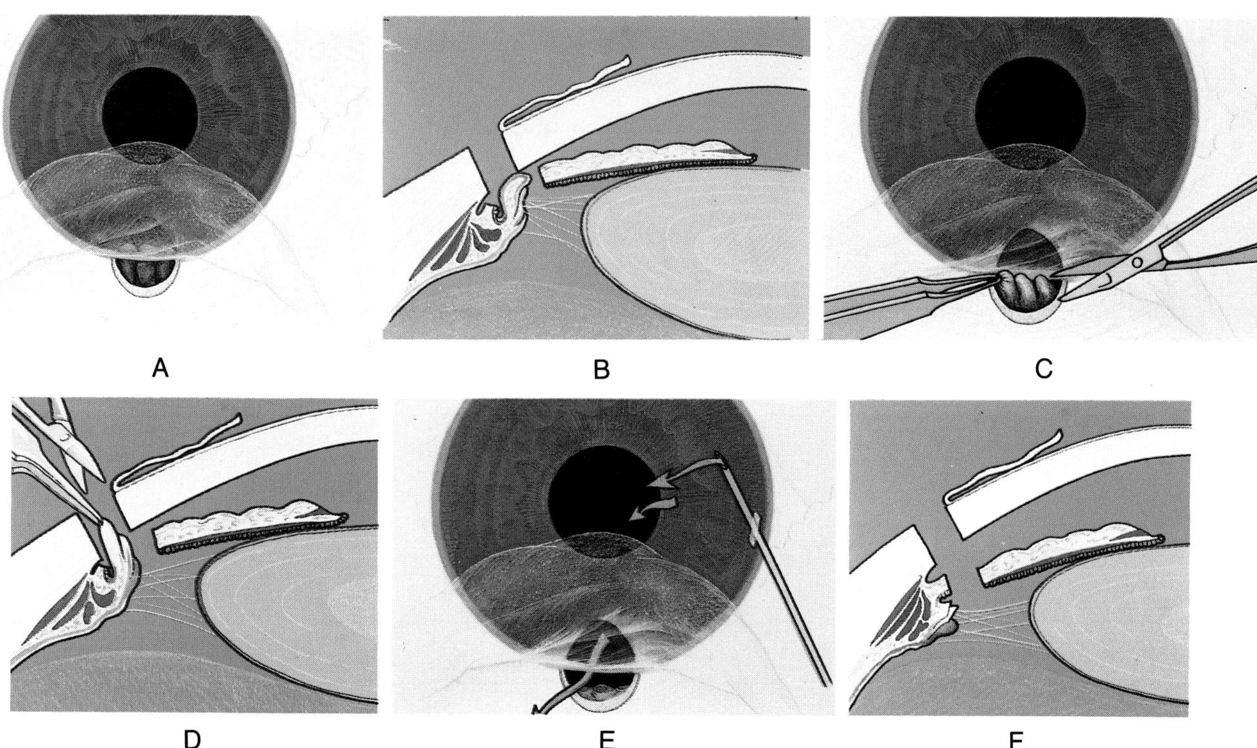

FIGURE 4–142 **Incarceration into sclerectomy site.** *A* and *B*, Front and side view. A ciliary process incarcerated into the sclerectomy, preventing flow through the sclerectomy. *C* and *D*, Excision of the obstructing ciliary processes. *E* and *F*, Amputated ciliary processes and patent sclerectomy permitting adequate aqueous flow from the anterior chamber through the sclerectomy.

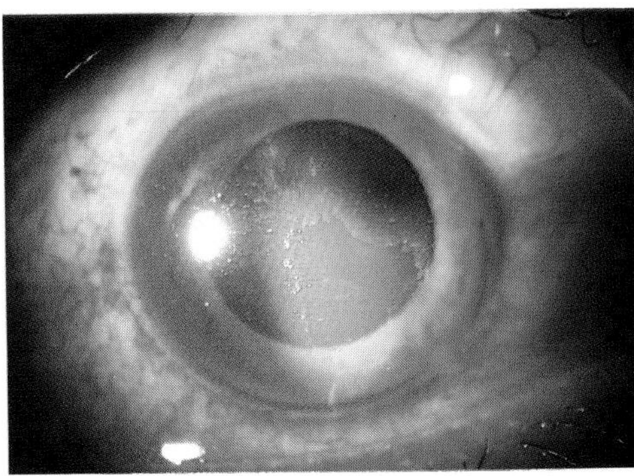

FIGURE 4–143 Corneal epithelial defect following subconjunctival injections of 5-fluorouracil. Corneal toxicity is more likely to occur in patients with previous abrasions or epithelial pathology.

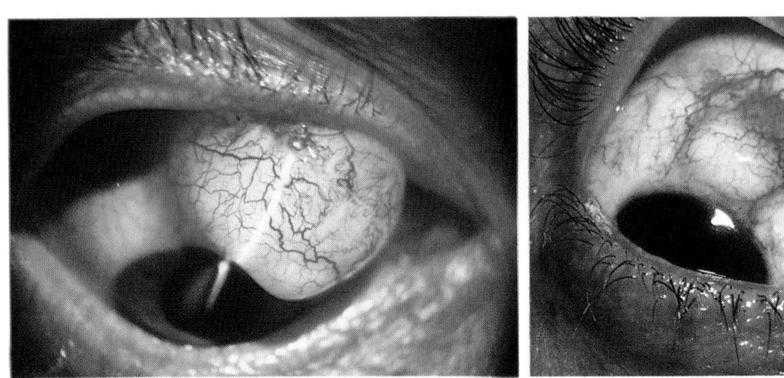

FIGURE 4–144 **Tenon's cyst.** *A,* The characteristic appearance of smooth, domed, markedly elevated, cystlike structure at the site of the filtering procedure is seen on the left. *B,* Localized encapsulated cyst with prominent vascular margin at the site of Tenon's episcleral scarring.

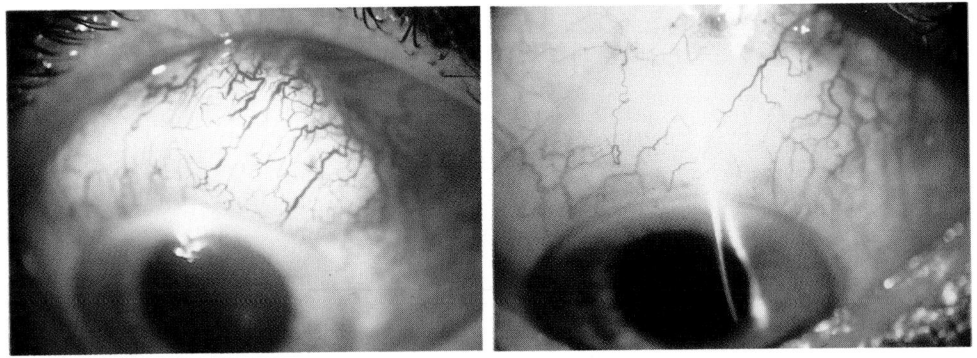

FIGURE 4–145 **Revision of Tenon's cyst.** *A,* Tenon's cyst with prominent vascularization and elevated intraocular pressure despite medical therapy. *B,* Excellent filtration following surgical revision of a Tenon's cyst with excision of a dense fibrovascular cyst wall.

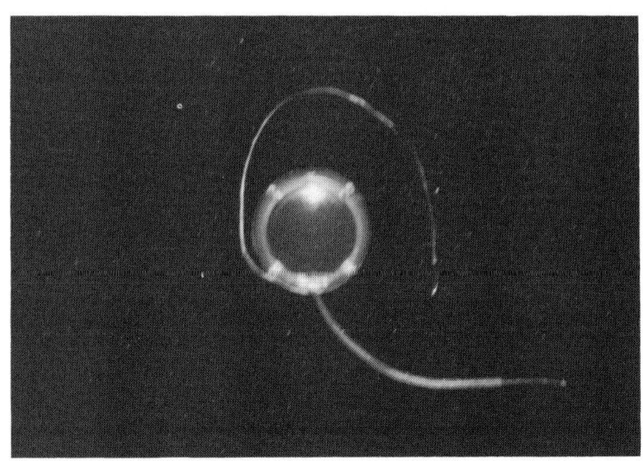

FIGURE 4–146 A single-plate Molteno implant with 4–0 collagen suture occluding the tube.

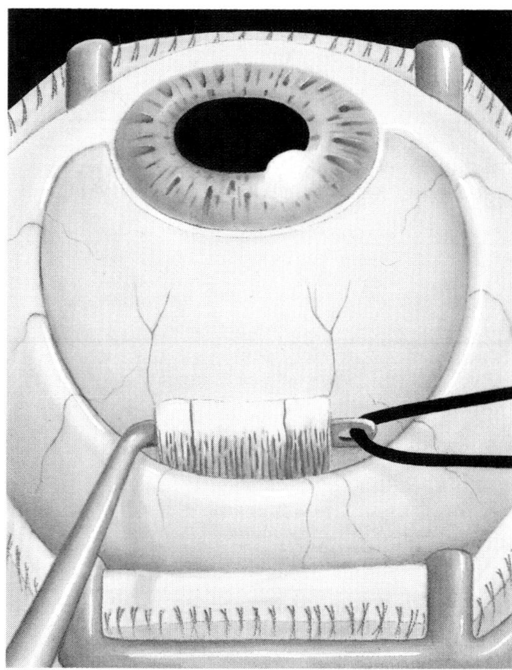

FIGURE 4–147 **Molteno implant technique.** Initial stage of the implant operation showing a large peritomy with small relaxing incisions. A 2–0 silk suture is being passed under the superior rectus muscle. The quadrants have been opened far posteriorly by blunt dissection.

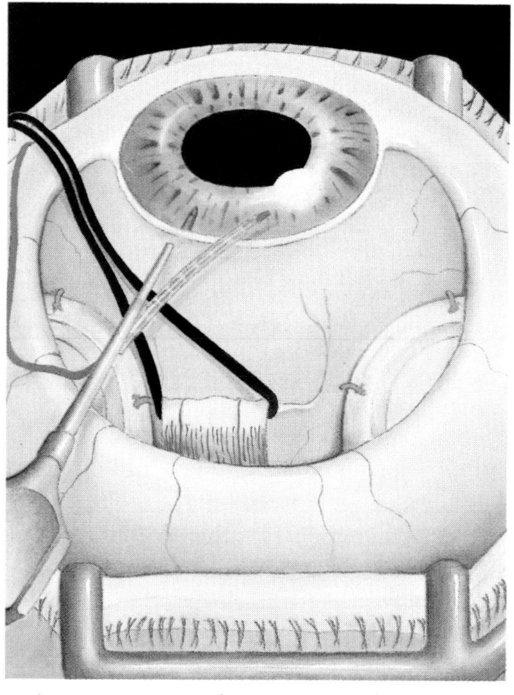

FIGURE 4–149 **Molteno implant technique.** With the implant positioned and sutured in place, the 23-gauge needle is passed into the anterior chamber parallel to the surface of the iris. The needle should pierce the sclera about 1 mm posterior to the limbus and enter the anterior chamber just posterior to Schwalbe's line.

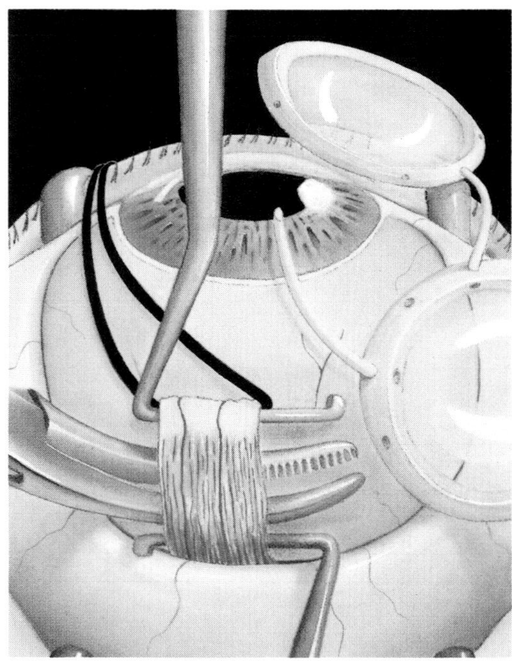

FIGURE 4–148 **Molteno implant technique.** Passing the Molteno implant beneath the superior rectus muscle.

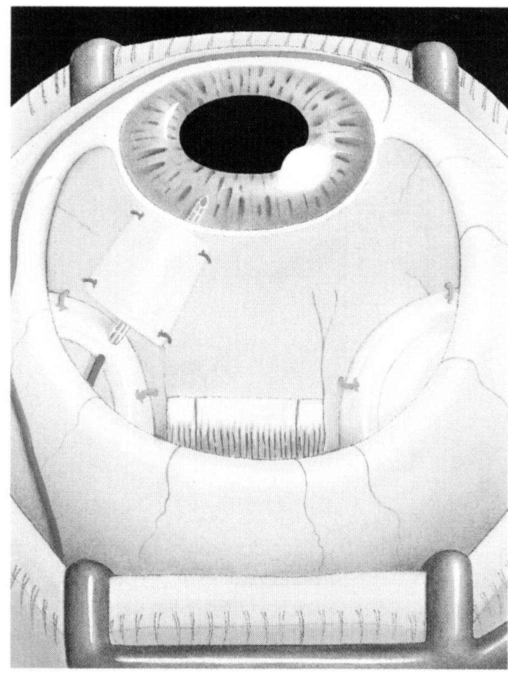

FIGURE 4–150 **Molteno implant technique.** The implant is correctly positioned, and the tube is occluded by the 4–0 collagen suture. The tube is cut bevel up to extend 2 to 3 mm into the anterior chamber. The scleral patch is sewn into place overlying the tube. The collagen suture is passed high in the fornix, exiting between the plates and tied loosely to the conjunctiva in the inferior fornix.

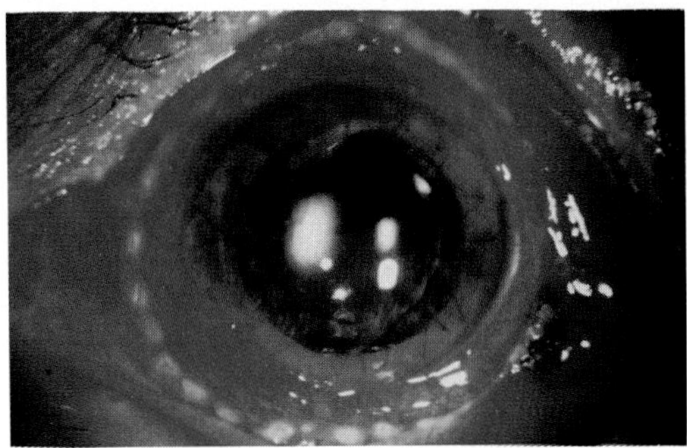

FIGURE 4-151 Postoperative noncontact cyclophotocoagulation. Note white conjunctival lesions, which fade with time.

SECTION 5

Eyelids

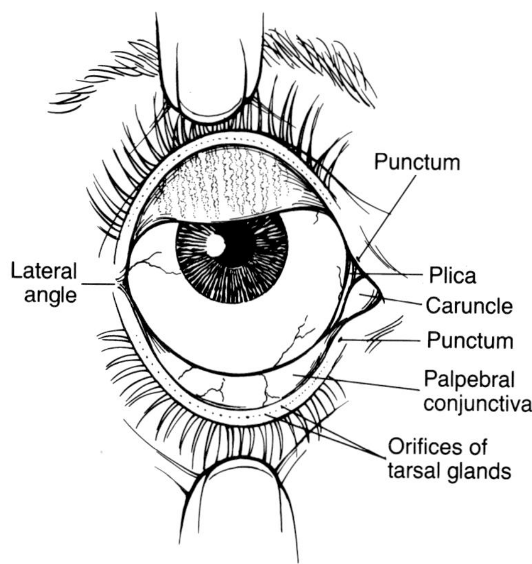

FIGURE 5–1 Right upper lid is everted and lower lid is pulled downward to demonstrate gross anatomy. The lateral angle is the point where the upper and lower eyelids fuse together. The orifices of the tarsal glands, which are meibomian oil-secreting (sebum) glands, located in the tarsus, empty at the eyelid margin next to the gray line. There are approximately 30 of these tarsal glands in the upper lid and 20 in the lower. The palpebral conjunctiva is a reflection onto the backside of both the upper and the lower eyelids of the epibulbar and forniceal conjunctiva. In both the upper and the lower medial eyelid margins, there are small orifices, referred to as the puncta, which drain the tears through the canaliculi into the lacrimal sac. The plica is a small web of tissue located medially and is regarded as a persistence of the nictitating membrane of lower species. The caruncle is a fleshy mound of tissue found medially, which contains hairs, sebaceous glands, and occasionally ectopic lacrimal tissue.

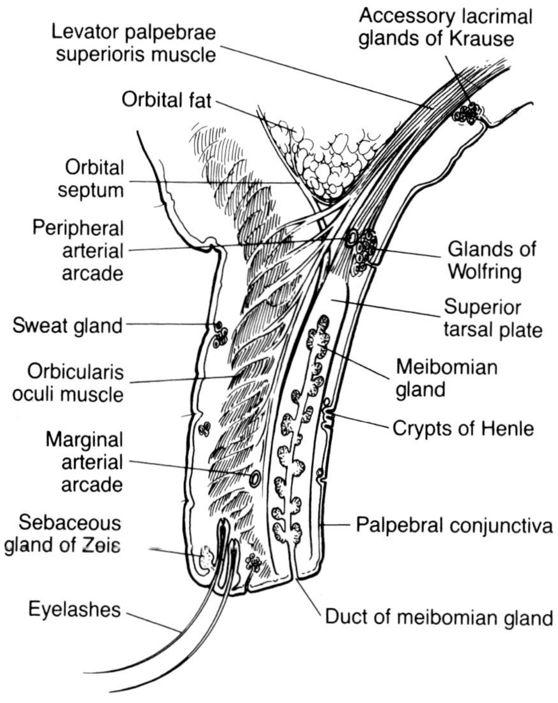

FIGURE 5–2 **Cross section of upper eyelid.** The upper eyelid is maintained in an uplifted position by the contraction of the levator palpebrae superioris muscle. A bundle of smooth muscle (Müller's) also attaches to the upper border of the tarsal plate. The orbital septum is located on the backside of the preorbital portion of the eyelid and reflects off the periorbital lining membrane at the orbital rim. Eccrine sweat glands are scattered throughout the eyelid skin, although larger apocrine glands (glands of Moll) are limited to the eyelid margin and often empty their secretion into the eyelash canals. The accessory lacrimal glands of Krause are located in the superior fornix, whereas accessory lacrimal glands of Wolfring are often embedded in the superior pole of the tarsal plate or in the immediately adjacent conjunctiva. The crypts of Henle are pseudoglandular evaginations of the palpebral conjunctiva.

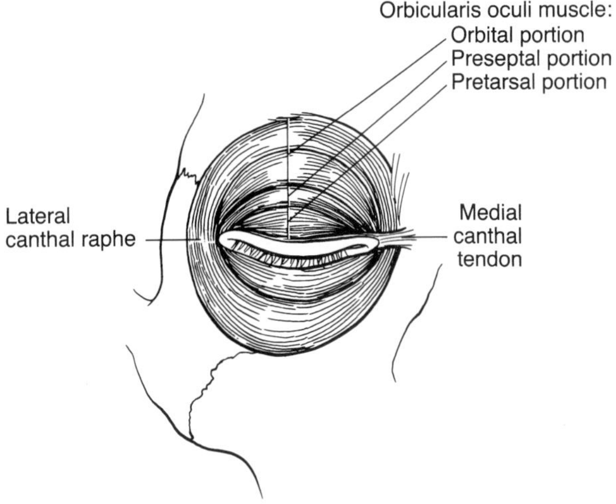

FIGURE 5–3 Frontal view of orbicularis oculi muscle, which is innervated by the facial nerve.

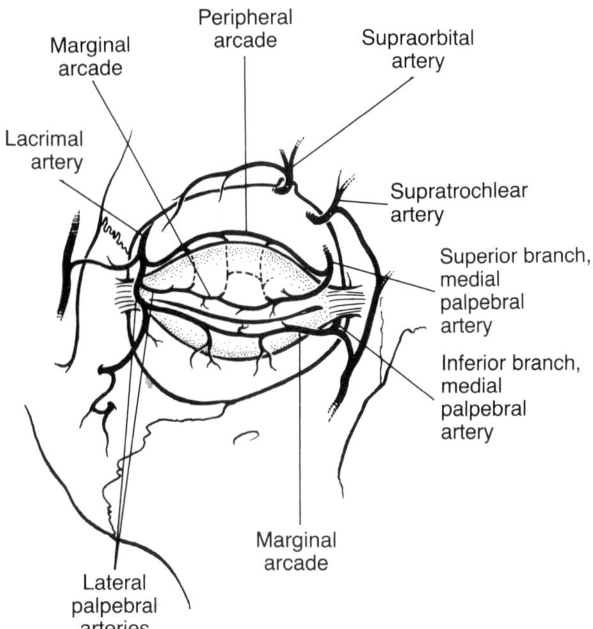

FIGURE 5–5 **Arterial supply to the eylids.** The vast majority of the arterial supply of the upper and the lower eyelids is contributed by terminal branches of the ophthalmic artery. Portions of the external carotid and facial arterial systems also anastomose with the lower eyelid network. There are two horizontal arcades in the upper eyelid, one referred to as the peripheral arcade located along the superior pole of the tarsus, and a second marginal arcade is situated at the eyelid margin. There is only one (marginal) arcade in the inferior eyelid.

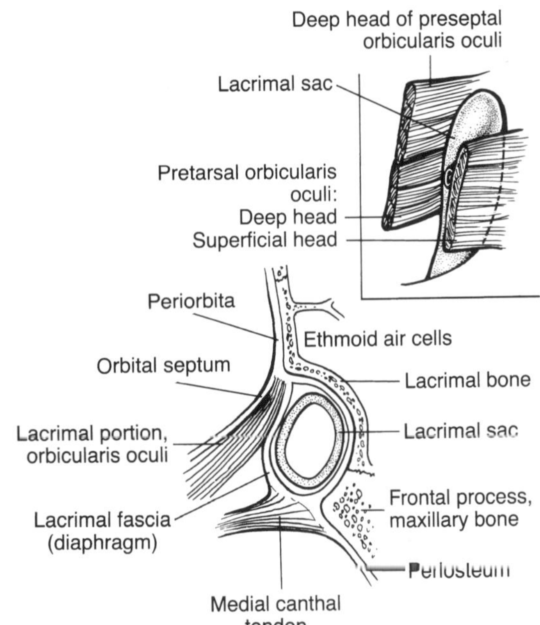

FIGURE 5–4 Cross-sectional view of medial portion of the orbicularis oculi muscle. When the eyelids are relaxed, tears enter the canaliculi via the puncta through capillary action. The canaliculi and lacrimal sac are emptied of their draining tears by virtue of contractions of the various components of the orbicularis muscle around the canaliculi and around the sac wall. The tears are thereby propeled down the nasolacrimal duct to the nose. When the orbicularis relaxes, the sac opens up and tears again collect in the canaliculi, with the sac exercising a relative negative pressure.

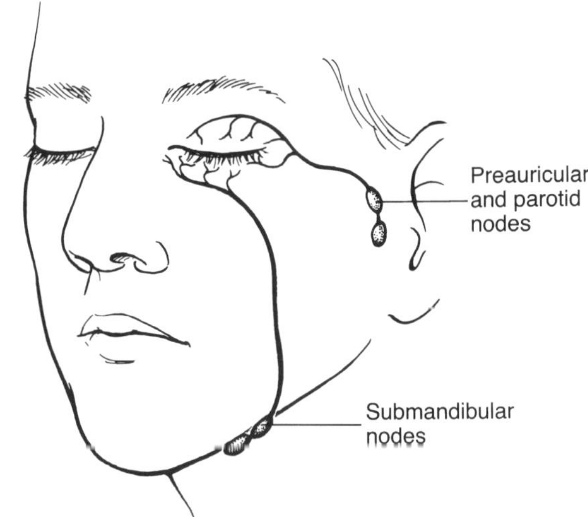

FIGURE 5–6 **Lymphatics of the eyelids.** All of the upper eyelid lymphatics and the lateralmost of the lower eyelid drain to the preauricular and parotid lymph nodes, whereas the medial two-thirds of the lower lid lymphatics drain to the submandibular nodes. It is important to palpate these regional lymph nodes in initial evaluation and follow-up evaluations of all patients with eyelid malignancies, particularly sebaceous carcinoma, squamous cell carcinoma, and malignant melanomas of both the cutaneous and the conjunctival aspects of the eyelids.

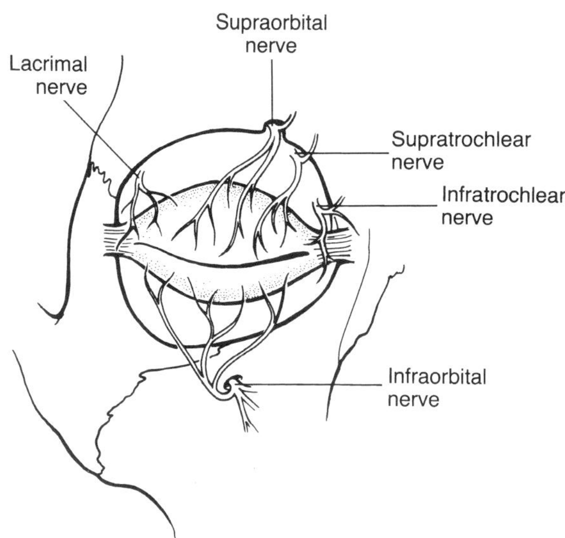

FIGURE 5-7 **Innervation of the eyelids.** The upper eyelid receives its sensory innovation from terminal branches of the ophthalmic division of the trigeminal (V-I), whereas the infraorbital nerve supplying sensation to the inferior eyelid is a branch of the second division (V-II) of the trigeminal nerve. Fractures of the floor of the orbit can lead to hypoesthesia of the lower eyelid from damage to the infraorbital nerve in its bony canal.

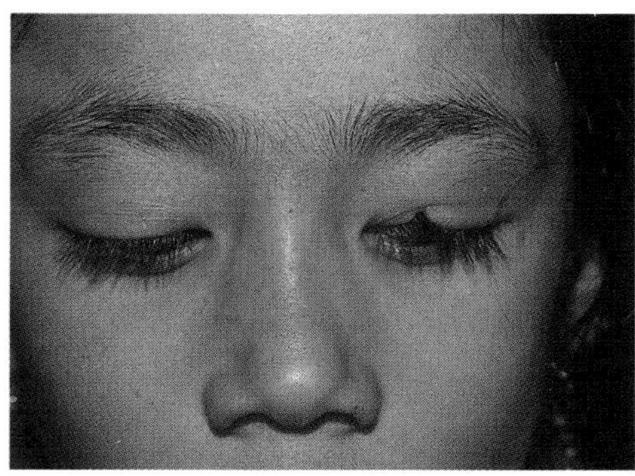

FIGURE 5-8 **Coloboma.** Typical eyelid coloboma (congenital absence of lid tissue) occurring at the junction of the medial third and lateral two-thirds of the left upper eyelid. (Courtesy of Dr. L. H. Allen.)

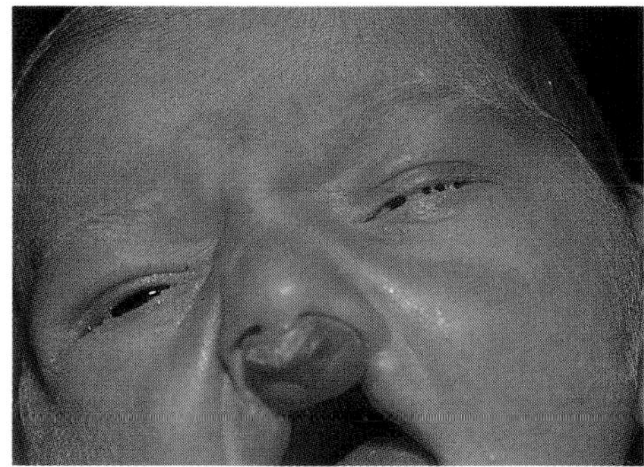

FIGURE 5-9 **Ankyloblepharon filiforme adnatum.** Strands of tissue extend between the lid margins. Note the presence of a cleft lip, an abnormality frequently associated with this condition. (Courtesy of Dr. L. H. Allen.)

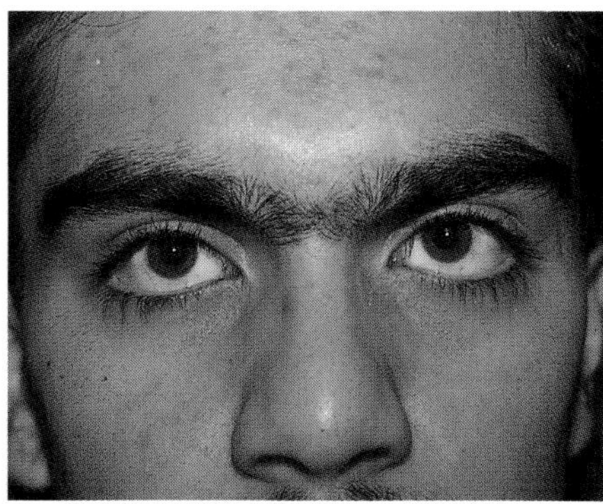

FIGURE 5-10 **Euryblepharon.** Symmetric enlargement of the palpebral apertures with anterior and downward displacement of the lateral canthal tendons. Note the loss of apposition of the lower eyelid margin to the globe. (Courtesy of Dr. L. H. Allen.)

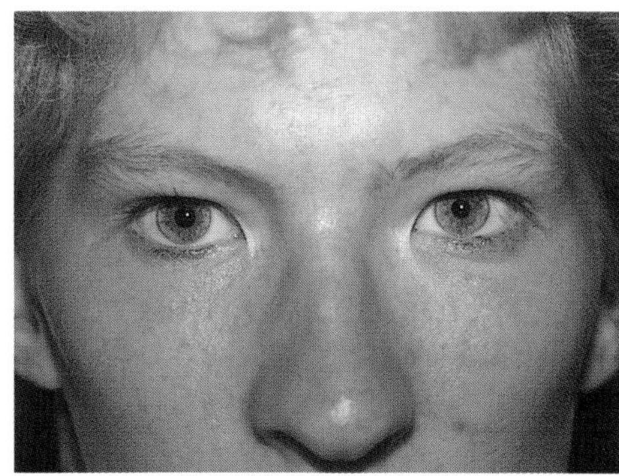

FIGURE 5-11 **Bilateral epicanthal folds.** There are vertical skin folds in the medial canthal area. (Courtesy of Dr. L. H. Allen.)

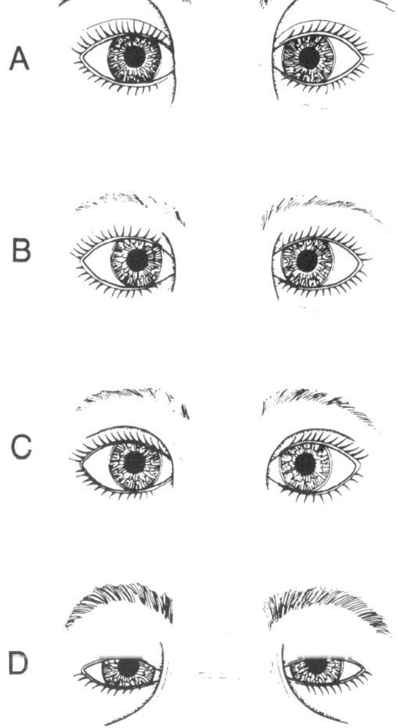

FIGURE 5-12 **Epicanthal folds.** *A*, Epicanthus superciliaris. *B*, Epicanthus palpebralis. *C*, Epicanthus tarsalis. *D*, Epicanthus inversus.

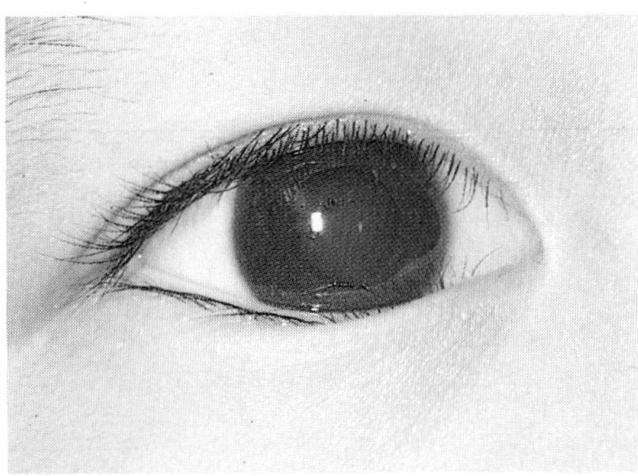

FIGURE 5-13 **Epiblepharon.** An excess of eyelid skin nasally, causing a vertical orientation of the lashes. (Courtesy of Dr. L. H. Allen.)

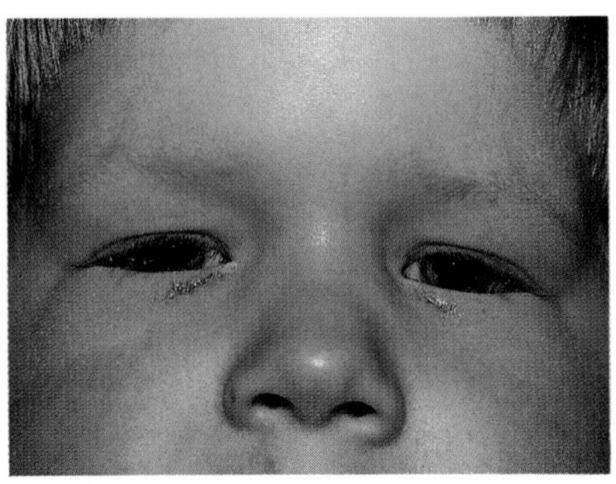

FIGURE 5-14 **Congenital entropion.** Complete inturning of the eyelid margin with secondary corneal irritation from the eyelashes. (Courtesy of Dr. L. H. Allen.)

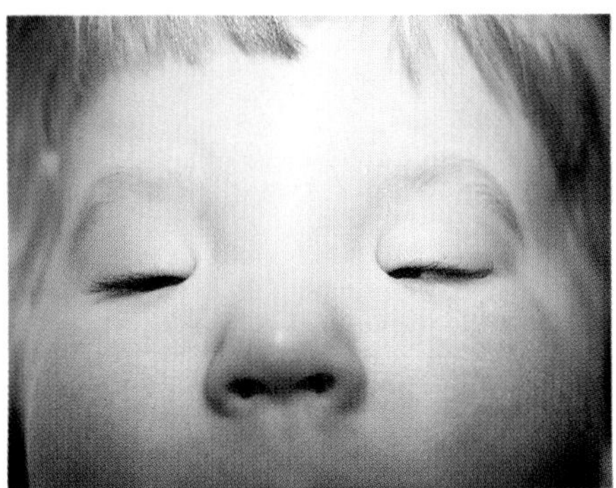

FIGURE 5-15 **Congenital tetrad syndrome.** Blepharophimosis (shortening of palpebral fissure), blepharoptosis (drooping of eyelids), epicanthus inversus, and telecanthus (widening of distance between medial canthal regions).

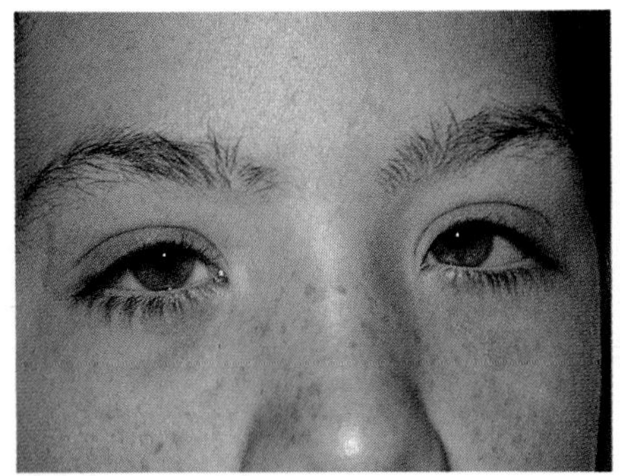

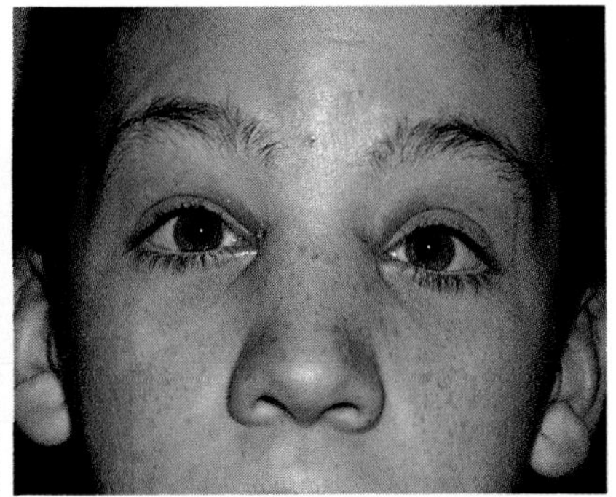

FIGURE 5-16 **Telecanthus.** *A*, Preoperative appearance of increased distance between the medial canthi. *B*, Postoperative appearance after transnasal wiring.

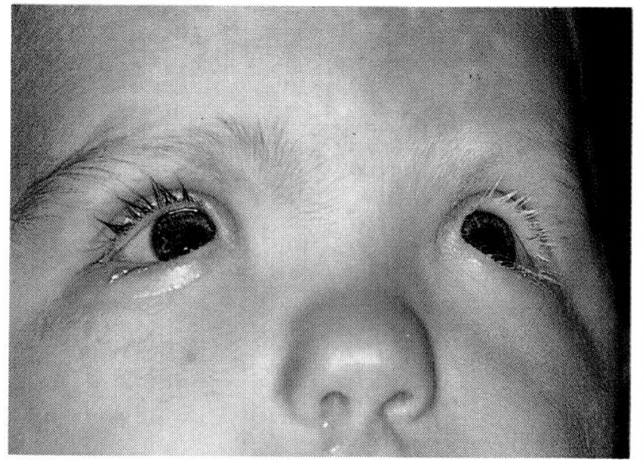

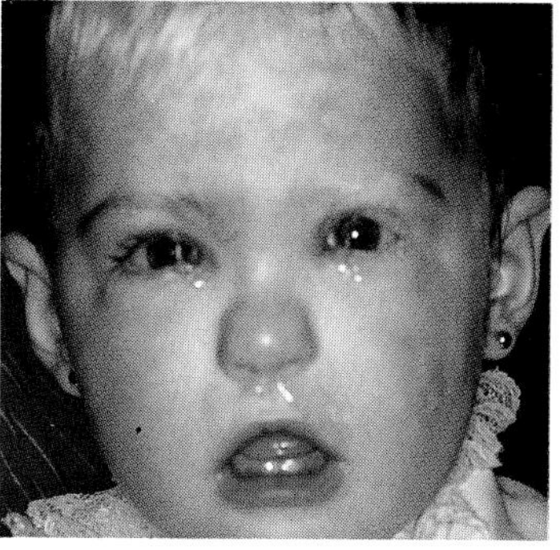

FIGURE 5-17 *A*, Medial canthal dystopia. An infant with Waardenburg's syndrome manifesting blepharophimosis, telecanthus, and medial ankyloblepharon. *B*, Postoperative appearance following reconstruction of the medial canthus and silicone intubation.

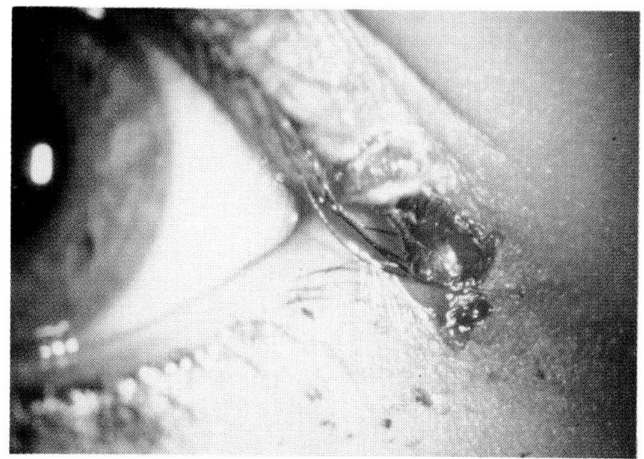

FIGURE 5-18 **Angular blepharitis.** Fissuring and exudate from the left lateral canthus, often caused by *Moraxella lacunata* or *Staphylococcus aureus.* (Courtesy of M. B. Moore, M.D.)

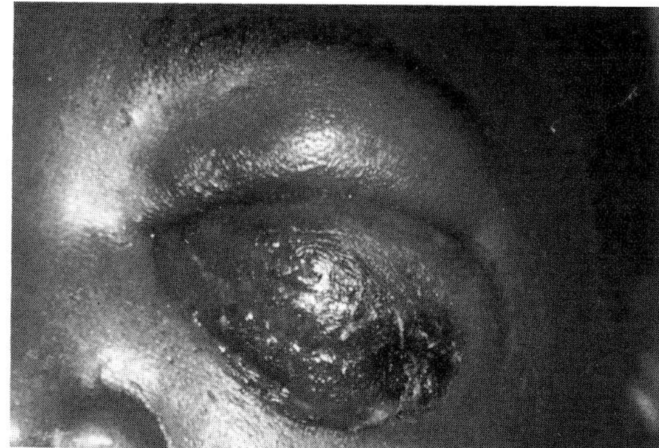

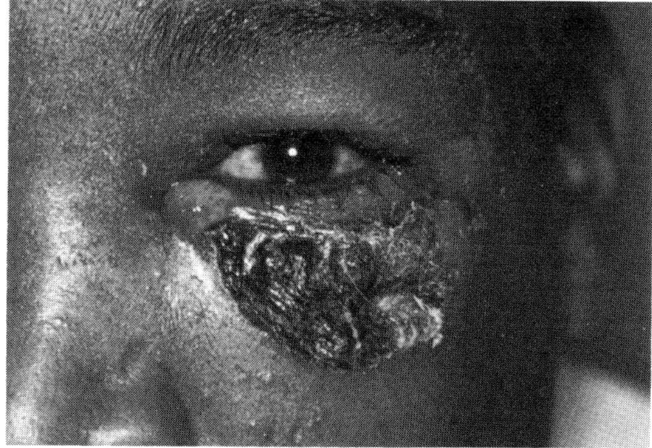

FIGURE 5-19 **Anthrax of left lower lid.** Black eschar, signifying tissue necrosis, occurs when lid edema resolves. (From Yorston D, Foster A: Cutaneous anthrax leading to corneal scarring from cicatricial ectropion. Br J Ophthalmol 73:809-811, 1989.)

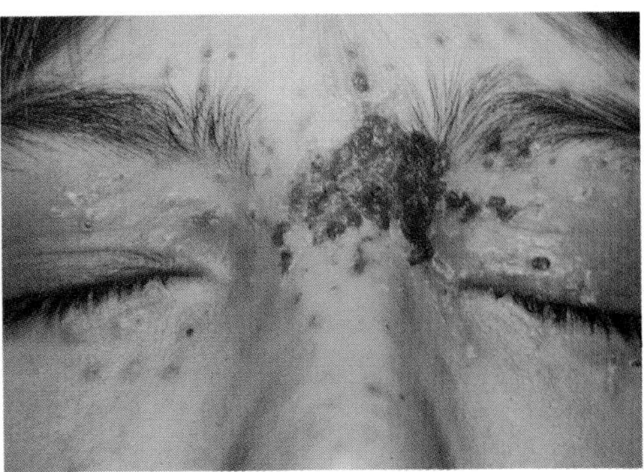

FIGURE 5–20 Herpes simplex infection, showing large number of periorbital and lid skin papules and vesicles. Note crusting of glabellar area as lesions heal. Viral infection of the epidermis causes vesicle formation (acantholysis). (Courtesy of M. J. Mannis, M.D.)

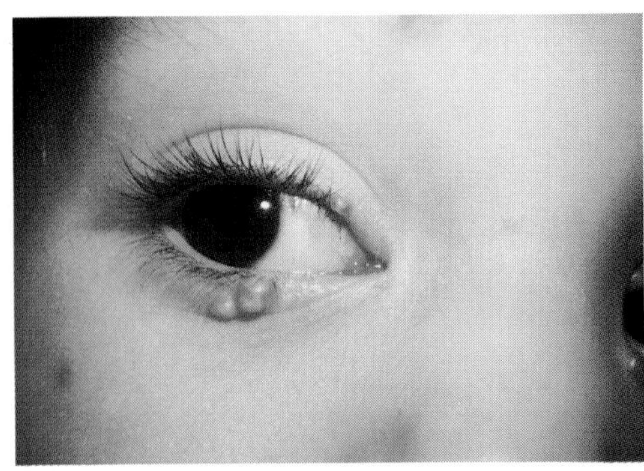

FIGURE 5–22 **Molluscum contagiosum.** Multiple, dome-shaped, umbilicated, and waxy papules are situated along the lid margin. There may be an associated follicular conjunctivitis. The poxvirus causes invasive acanthosis of the epidermis, which contains viral particles.

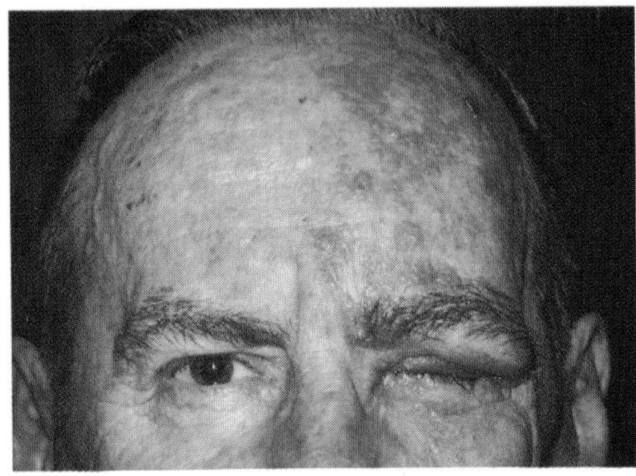

FIGURE 5–21 **Herpes zoster ophthalmicus.** Maculopapular and vesicular skin eruption in dermatomal distribution of the ophthalmic division of the trigeminal nerve. The viral particles spread to the epidermis from a latent site in the gasserian ganglion. (Courtesy of M. J. Mannis, M.D.)

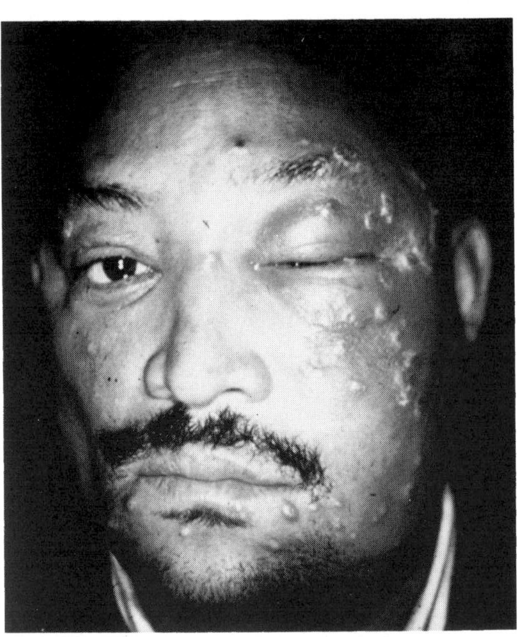

FIGURE 5–23 **Vaccinia infection of the face.** Disease is characterized by marked edema and erythema with crops of vesicles and pustules. The patient was accidentally infected by a recently vaccinated child. (Courtesy of A. P. Ferry, M.D.)

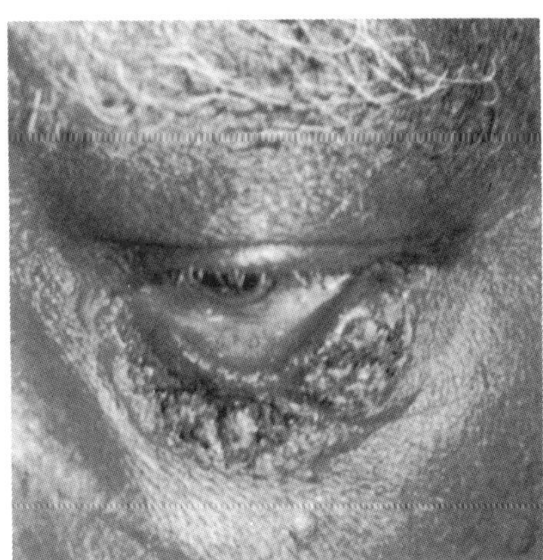

FIGURE 5–24 **Blastomycosis.** Clinical appearance of left lower lid. Note ectropion and blackish discoloration of papillomatous lesion. The causative agent is a yeastlike, dimorphic fungus. (From Barr C, Gamel JW: Blastomycosis of the eyelid. Arch Ophthalmol 104:96–97, 1986. Copyright 1986, American Medical Association.)

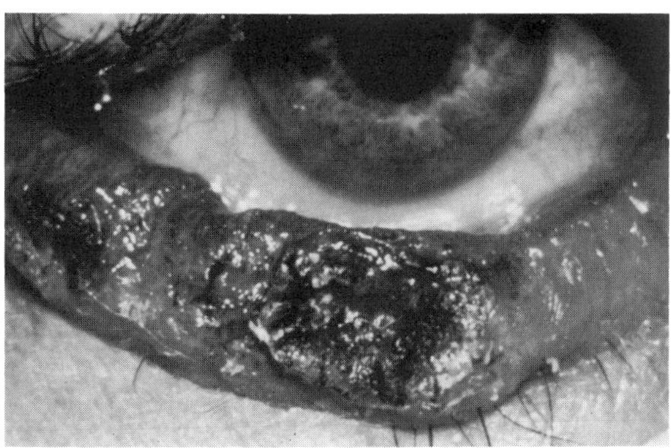

FIGURE 5–25 **Coccidioidomycosis of the eyelid.** The lateral two-thirds of the lower lid is thickened, reddened, and indurated with areas of ulceration and crusting. Pseudoepitheliomatous hyperplasia of the epidermis frequently accompanies fungal infections of the skin. Skin lesions can develop from hematogenous dissemination of fungi in pulmonary lesions. This dimorphic fungus is found in the soil of the San Joaquin Valley of southeastern California (From Font RL: Eyelids and lacrimal drainage system. *In* Spencer WA (ed): Ophthalmic Pathology, 3rd ed. Philadelphia, WB Saunders, 1986, pp. 2141–2336.)

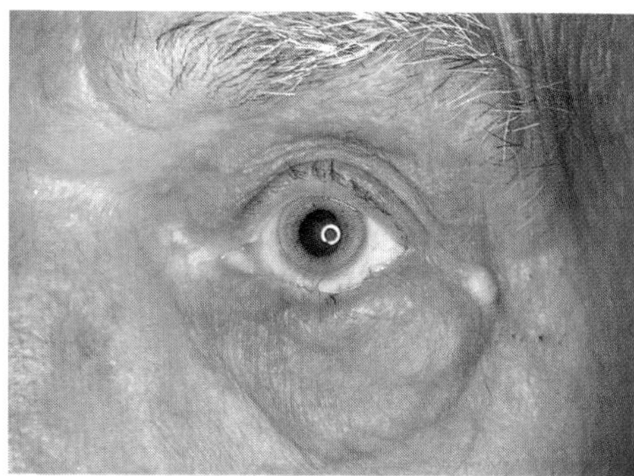

FIGURE 5–28 Epidermal inclusion cyst in the lateral canthal region. The lesion is white because it is filled with keratin shed by a lining epidermal membrane.

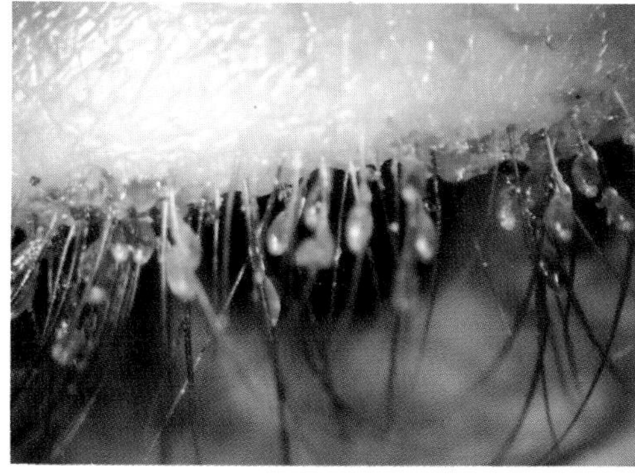

FIGURE 5–26 **Phthiriasis.** Eggs and egg cases adhering to base of eyelashes. The crab louse can be transferred by towels or sexual contact from the pubic region. (Courtesy of M. L. Mannis, M.D.)

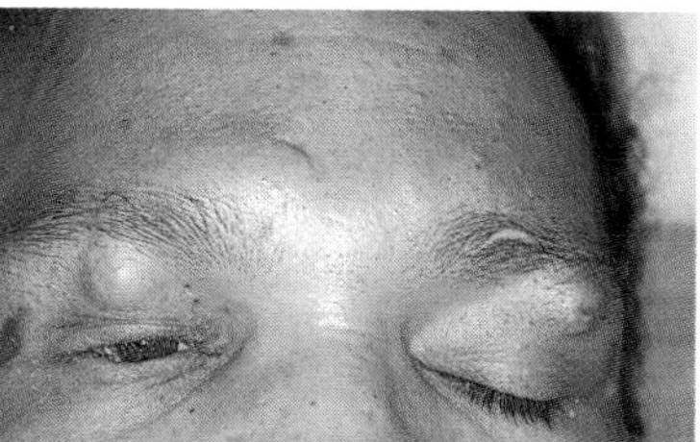

FIGURE 5–29 Epidermal inclusion cysts on both upper lids. These lesions are sometimes incorrectly referred to as "wens."

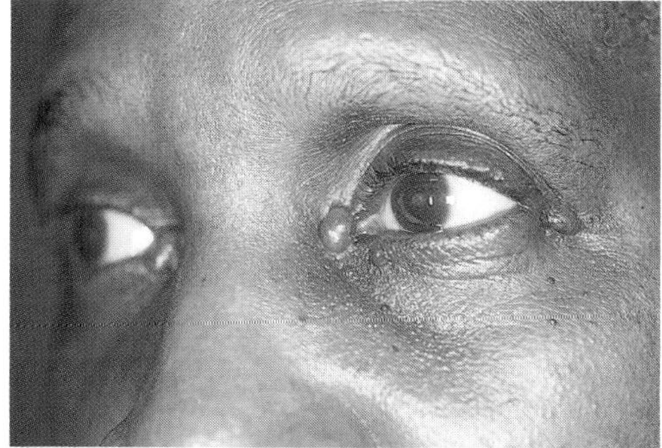

FIGURE 5–27 Multiple eccrine hidrocystomas on both eyes. These sweat gland duct cysts are filled with clear fluid. In a black individual, the pigmented epidermis obscures the cyst contents.

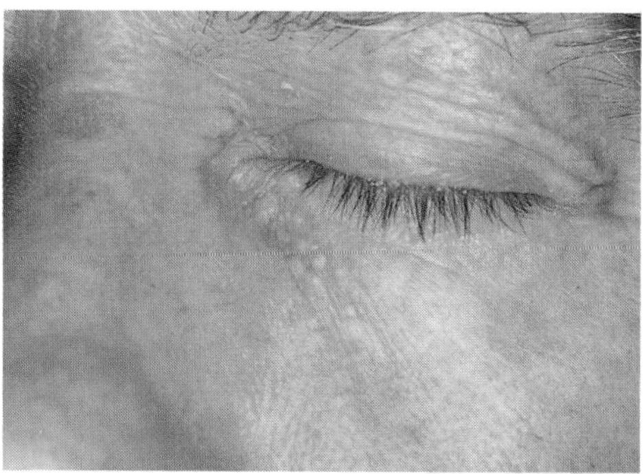

FIGURE 5–30 Multiple milia of the lower lid. These lesions are retention cysts of the pilosebaceous units.

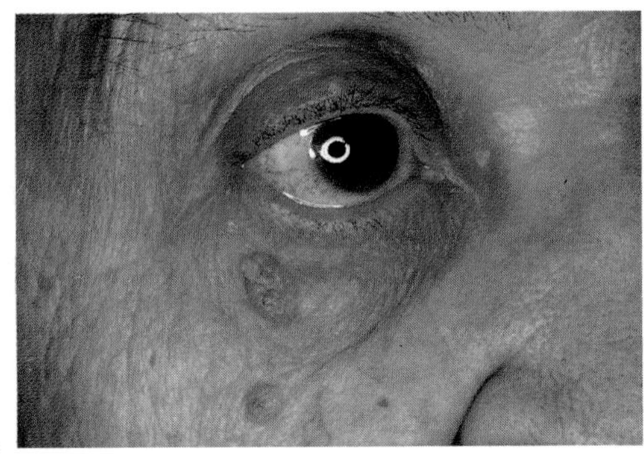

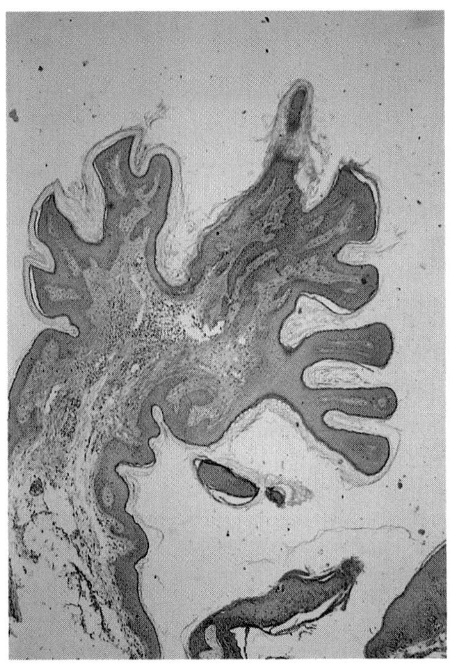

FIGURE 5–31 *A,* Sessile papilloma of the lower lid. These lesions may sometimes show features of a seborrheic keratosis. *B,* In a papilloma, there are fronds of fibrovascular connective tissue covered by slightly hyperkeratotic epidermis. *B,* H&E, ×130.

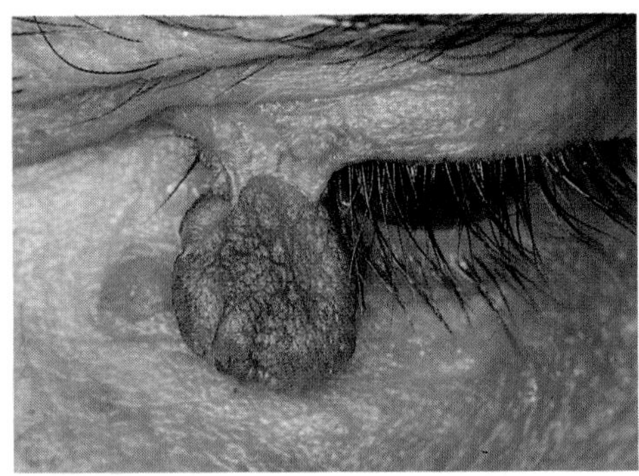

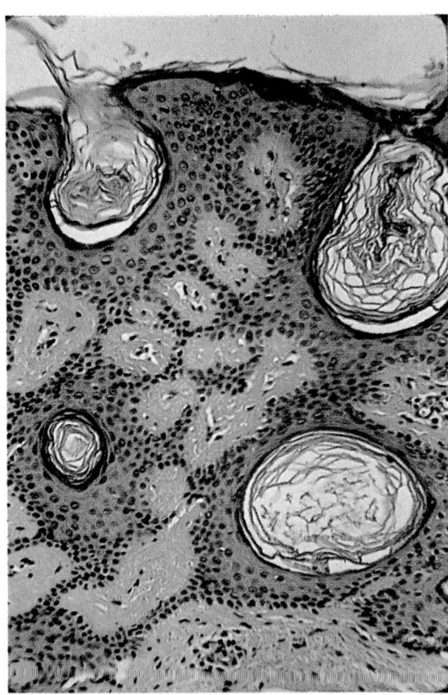

FIGURE 5–32 *A,* Pendulous seborrheic keratosis of the upper lid. Note the creased or cerebriform surface. *B,* A seborrheic keratosis is a benign proliferation of small basaloid cells. The tumor has no malignant potential. It grows above the epidermal plane and can have a stuck-on appearance. Pseudohorn cysts form at the surface or complete horn cysts in the body of the lesion. *B,* H&E, ×80.

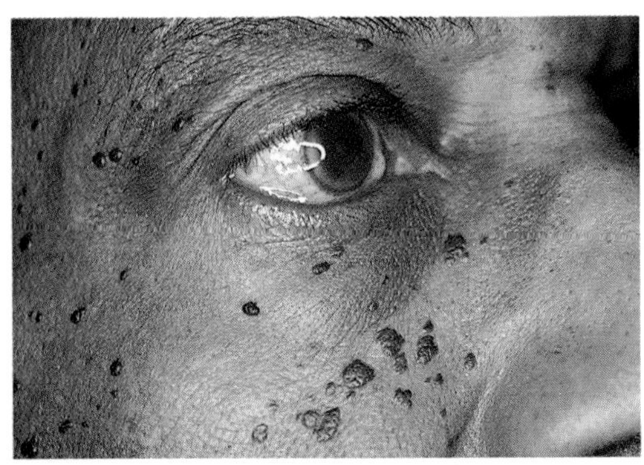

FIGURE 5–33 **Dermatosis papulosa nigra.** These are multiple pigmented seborrheic keratoses. The condition occurs predominantly in young black women and has no associated systemic implications.

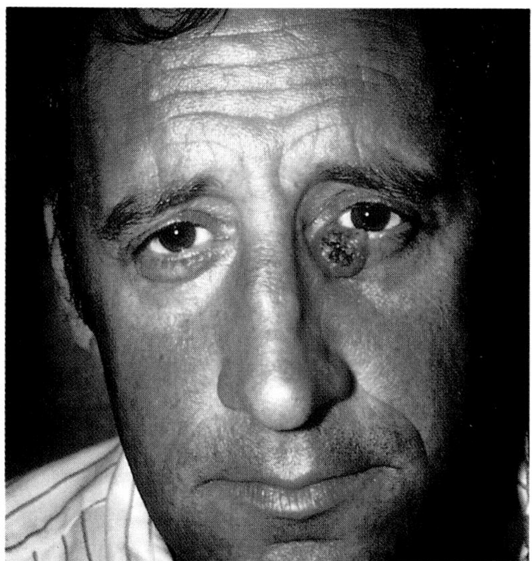

FIGURE 5–34 **Keratoacanthoma.** This is a rapidly developing (several weeks to months) pseudoepitheliomatous (pseudocancerous) hyperplasia of the epidermis in which there is a distinctive central crater of accumulated keratin. Some of these lesions have a tendency to spontaneous involution ("selfcure"). The lesion can be confused clinically and pathologically with invasive squamous cell carcinoma except that the latter tends to develop somewhat more insidiously over many months to years. When multiply eruptive, keratoacanthoma can be a cutaneous sign of the Muir-Torre syndrome with associated cancer of the colon.

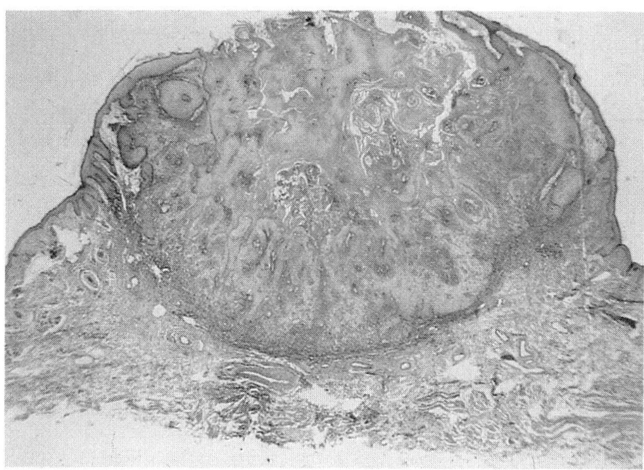

FIGURE 5–35 **Keratoacanthoma.** Histopathologically, keratoacanthoma is a highly structured variant of pseudoepitheliomatous hyperplasia in which the constituent cells are squamous and therefore stain eosinophilic. There are invasive acanthotic lobules of epidermis often with keratin pearls, and in the crateriform center of the lesion, there are masses of parakeratin (nuclei retained). The lesion blends imperceptibly on either side with the epidermis, rather than exhibiting the abrupt transition of dysplastic cells as is typical of a squamous dysplasia and squamous carcinoma. Note the narrow band of the mononuclear inflammatory cells at the base of the lesion. H&E, ×30.

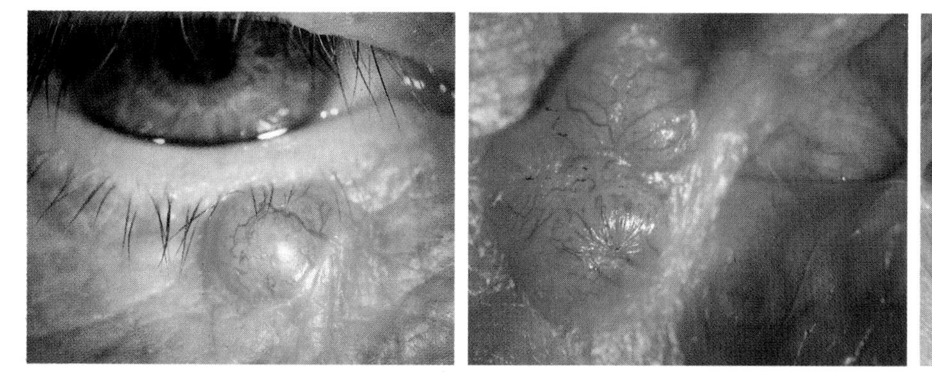

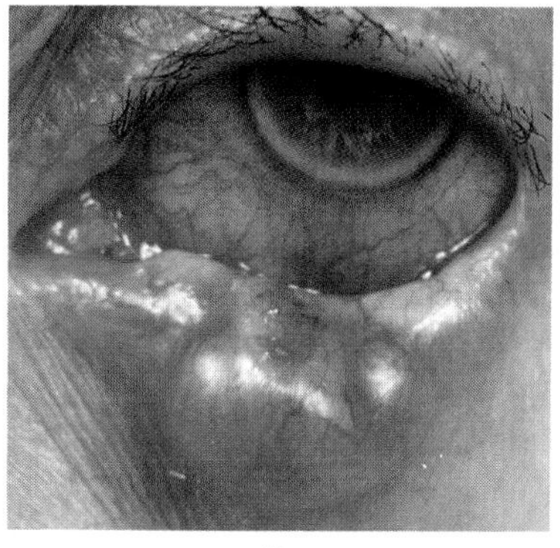

A B C

FIGURE 5–36 *A–C,* **Nodular basal cell carcinoma.** Clinical appearance, showing three different cases with firm, pearly nodules, telangiectatic vessels, and markedly thinned epidermis at the surface of the tumor. This is a nonmetastasizing tumor (except in severely immunocompromised patients) of the basal cells of the epidermis and originates most often in the lower eyelid because of its increased exposure to ultraviolet light.

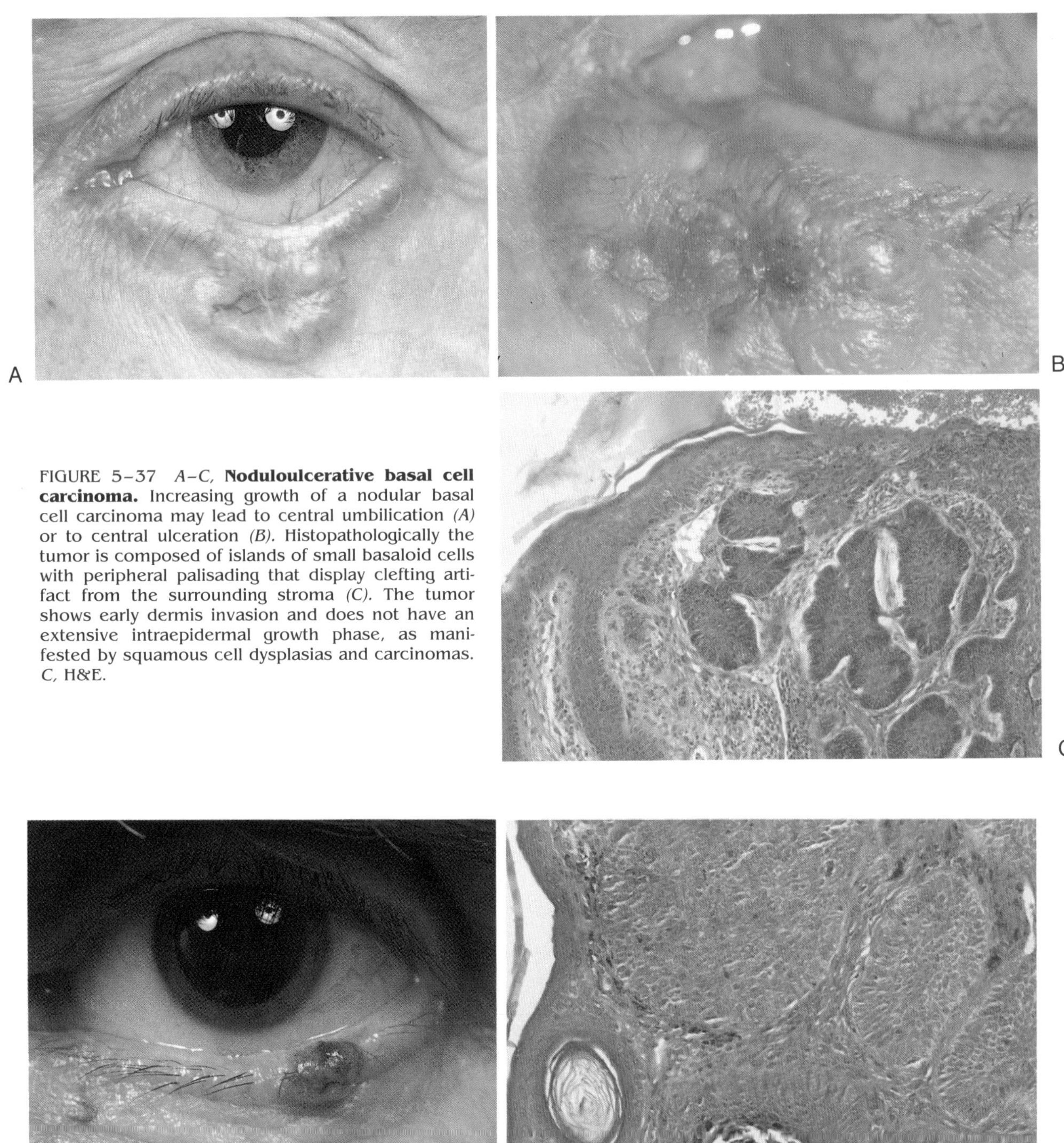

FIGURE 5–37 *A–C,* **Noduloulcerative basal cell carcinoma.** Increasing growth of a nodular basal cell carcinoma may lead to central umbilication *(A)* or to central ulceration *(B)*. Histopathologically the tumor is composed of islands of small basaloid cells with peripheral palisading that display clefting artifact from the surrounding stroma *(C)*. The tumor shows early dermis invasion and does not have an extensive intraepidermal growth phase, as manifested by squamous cell dysplasias and carcinomas. *C,* H&E.

FIGURE 5–38 *A* and *B,* **Pigmented basal cell carcinoma.** The nodular growth pattern of this tumor at the lid margin induced a loss of lid lashes at the tumor site. Histopathology reveals a marked amount of pigment from fellow-traveling nonneoplastic melanocytes. This variant tends to occur in darkly complexioned individuals. *B,* H&E.

FIGURE 5–39 **Pathology of basal cell carcinoma.** Nodular or solid basal cell carcinomas present as well-defined masses of various shapes and sizes, consisting of small hyperchromatic cells. Characteristically, they show parallel alignment of peripheral tumor cells (palisading) and separation of tumor lobules from the neighboring stroma following tissue fixation. H&E.

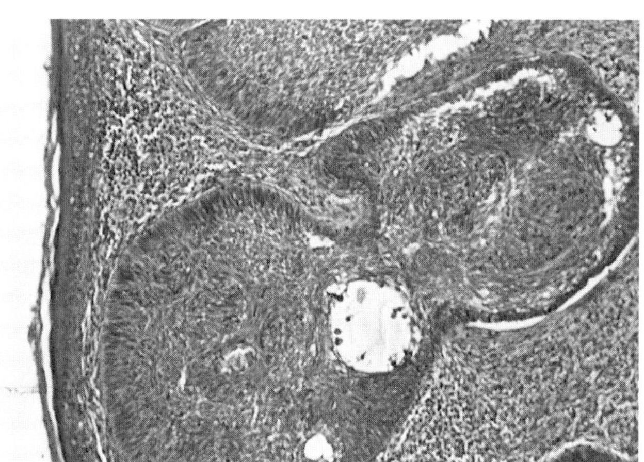

A

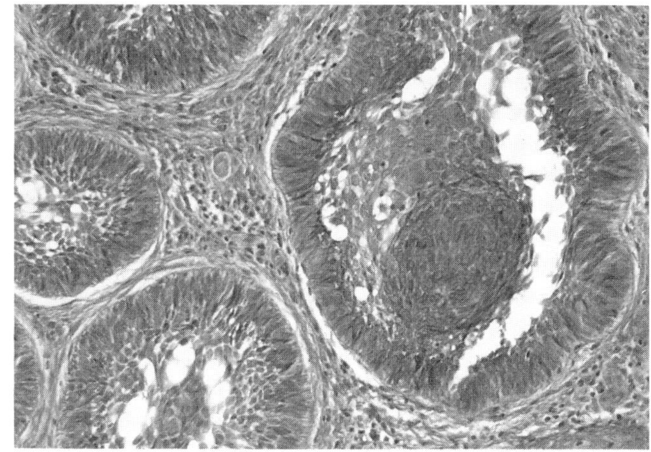

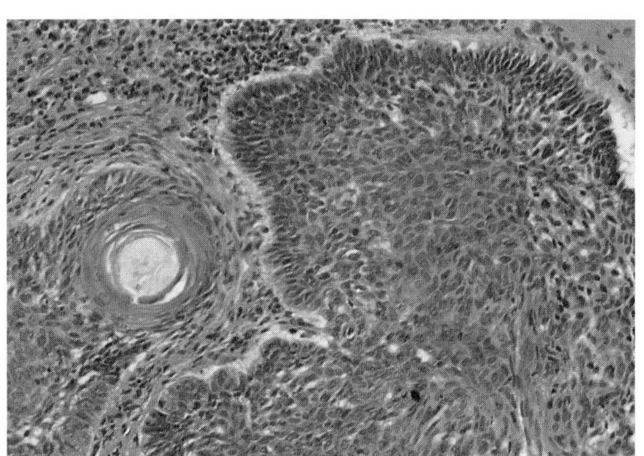

B

C

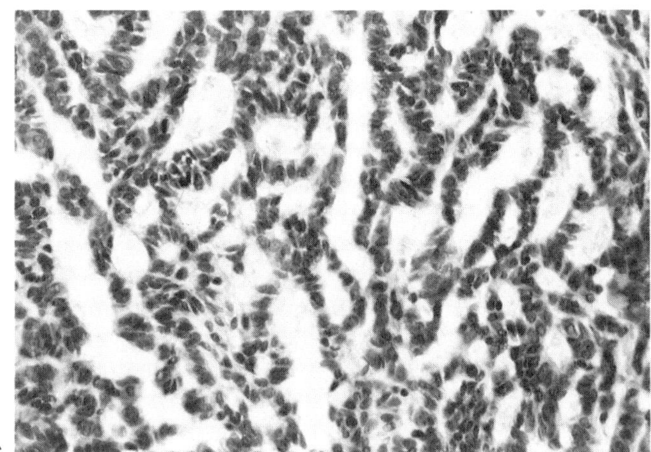

FIGURE 5–40 *A–C,* **Cystic, keratotic, and adenoid basal cell carcinoma.** Cystic degeneration of solid basal cell carcinoma is the result of central tumor cell disintegration. (*A,* ×100.) Horn cysts and parakeratotic cells are characteristic for keratotic basal cell carcinoma (*B,* ×100). Adenoid basal cell carcinoma presents with small, lacelike strands of tumor cells. H&E.

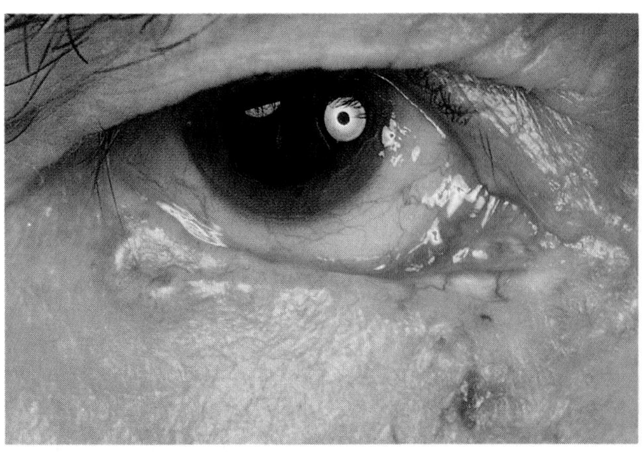
A

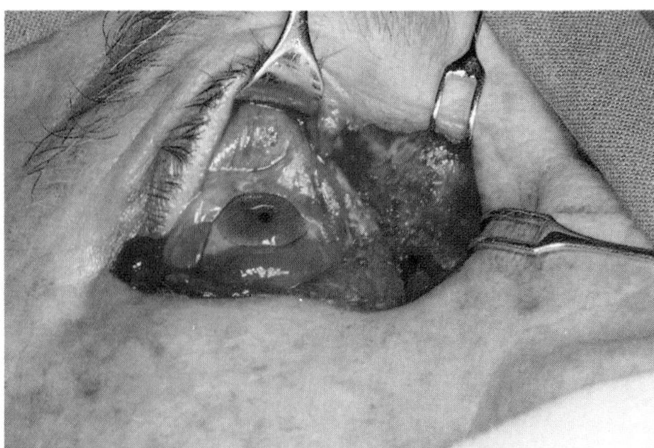
B

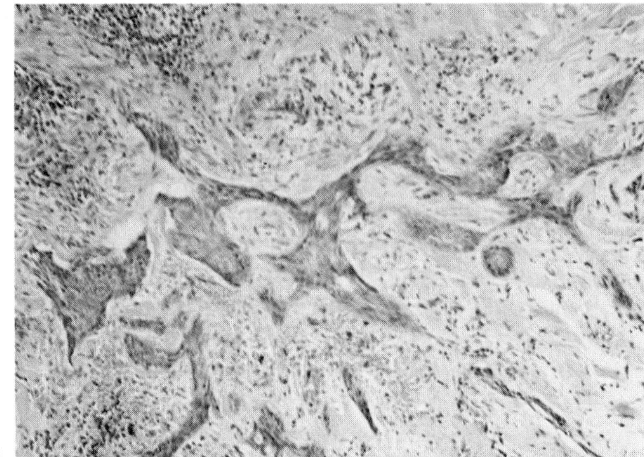
C

FIGURE 5–41 *A–C,* **Morpheaform basal cell carcinoma.** Clinically, this growth pattern leads to flat, pale, and indurated plaques. In the patient shown, tumor reaches from the inner canthal region along the entire lower lid to the lateral lid angle, leading to a total loss of lower eyelid lashes *(A).* The defect following microscopic-controlled tumor removal discloses the full extent of this lesion *(B).* Numerous groups of tumor cells, arranged in small nests or strands, are embedded in a dense fibrous stroma. *C,* H&E.

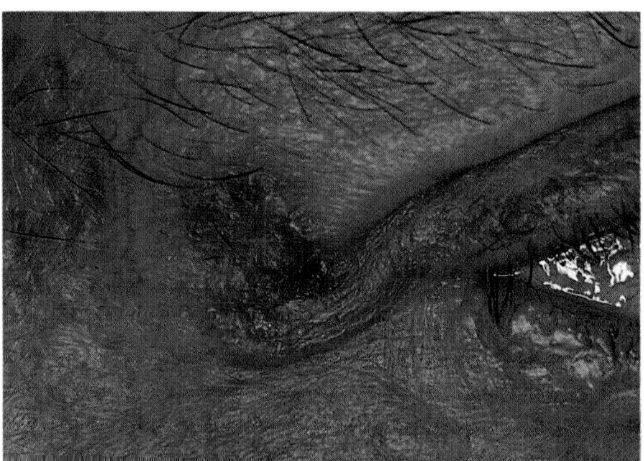

FIGURE 5–42 Actinic keratosis (i.e., due to sun or ultraviolet exposure) of the lateral canthal region showing a rounded erythematous lesion with a central keratotic plaque. This is a premalignant population of cells replacing the epidermis. The replacement occurs in a radial or horizontal fashion and may spread for several years before invading the dermis. This growth pattern differs from that of basal cell carcinoma, which early in its evolution invades the dermis.

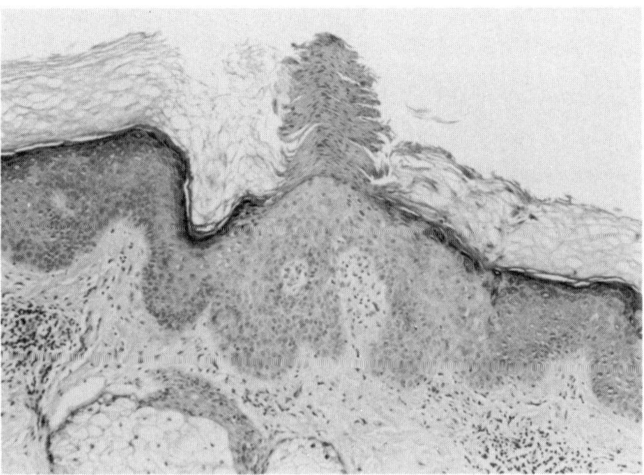

FIGURE 5–43 Typical actinic keratosis showing a central tier of parakeratosis surmounting a focus of abnormal keratinocytic (epidermal squamous cell) maturation. H&E.

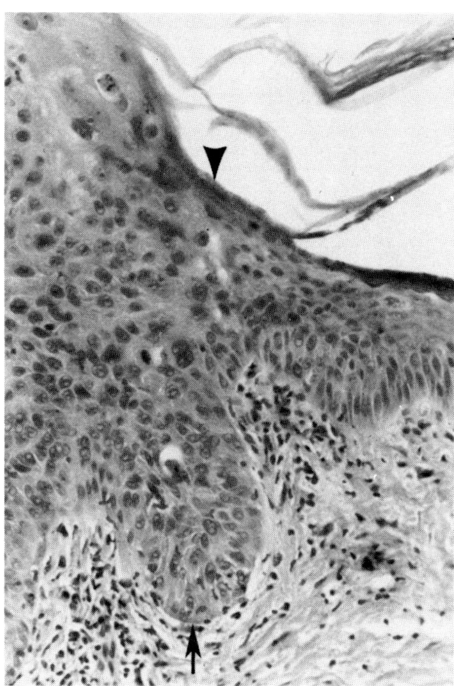

FIGURE 5–44 **Premalignant squamous dysplasia not due to sun exposure.** Note the abrupt transition *(arrowhead)* from normal epidermis on the right to the markedly acanthotic epidermis on the left. There is full-thickness cellular atypia with loss of maturation, yet the dermoepidermal basement membrane *(arrow)* remains intact (carcinoma in situ). H&E.

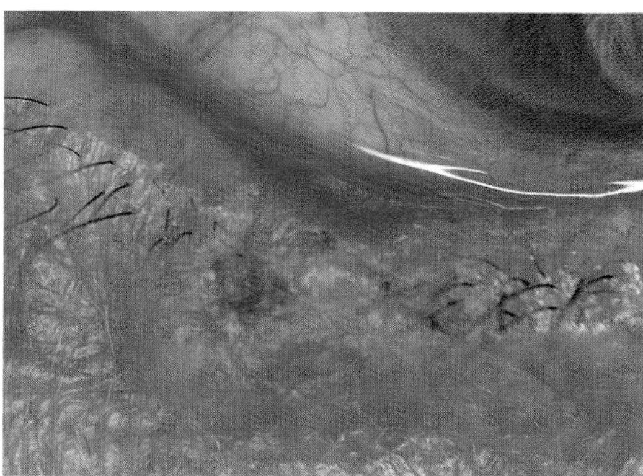

FIGURE 5–46 Clinical appearance of an early nodular squamous cell carcinoma of the lower lid with central ulceration, anterior displacement of mucoepidermal junction, and madarosis (loss of lashes). Squamous cell carcinoma indicates invasion of the dermis, when metastatic potential is acquired.

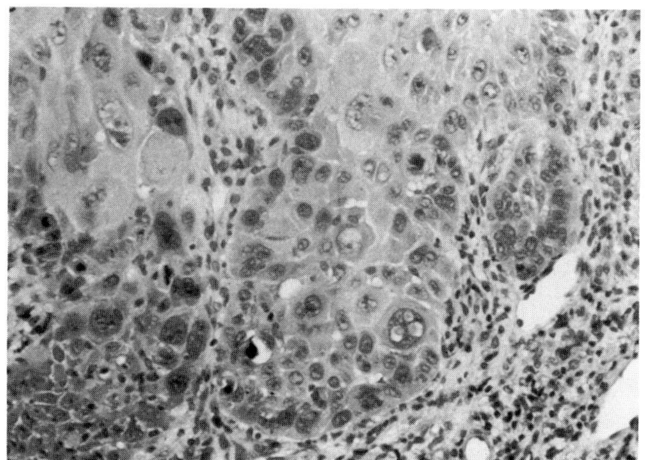

FIGURE 5–45 Same case as in Figure 5–44 demonstrating extreme cellular atypia with hyperchromatic nuclei, multinucleated giant cells, vacuolated cells, and dyskeratosis (premature individual cell keratinization). H&E, ×240.

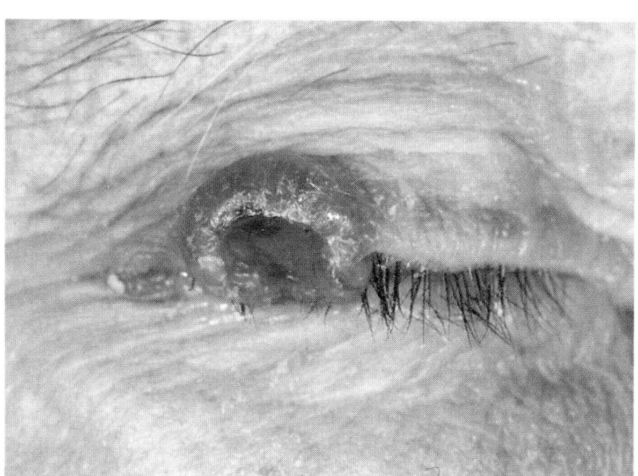

FIGURE 5–47 An erythematous nodular squamous cell carcinoma with rolled edges and central ulceration involving the upper lid margin. Invasive squamous cell carcinoma, if neglected, is capable of regional and distant metastases. It is $^1/_{20}$ to $^1/_{40}$ as common as basal cell carcinoma of the eyelids.

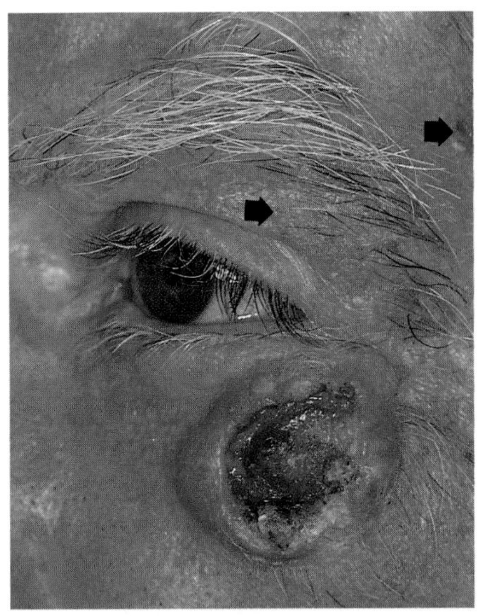

FIGURE 5–48 A large squamous cell carcinoma of the lower lid and cheek. In addition, note the actinic changes on the lateral aspect of the upper lid and forehead *(arrows)*.

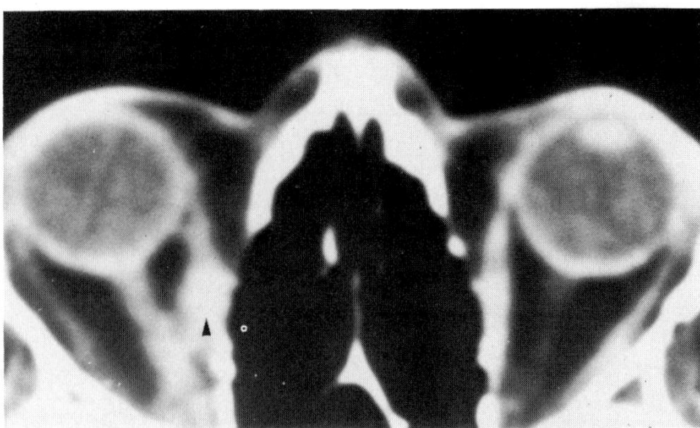

FIGURE 5–49 **Deeply invasive squamous cell carcinoma.** Computed tomographic scan demonstrates a mass adjacent to the medial wall of the right orbit *(arrow)* in a patient who had a squamous cell carcinoma previously resected from the right lower lid. The orbital lesion was biopsied and found to represent a squamous cell carcinoma with perineural infiltration of the orbit.

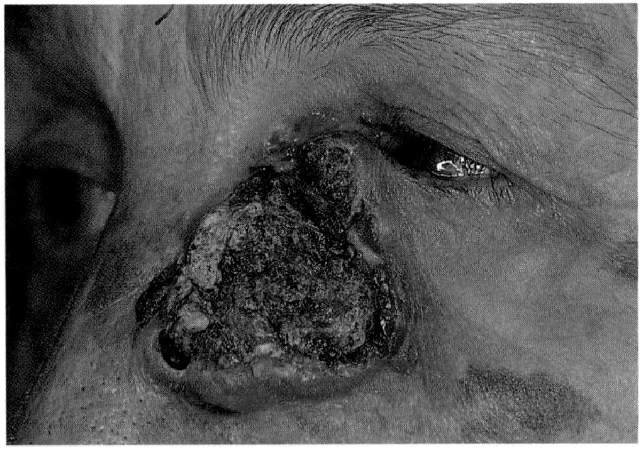

A

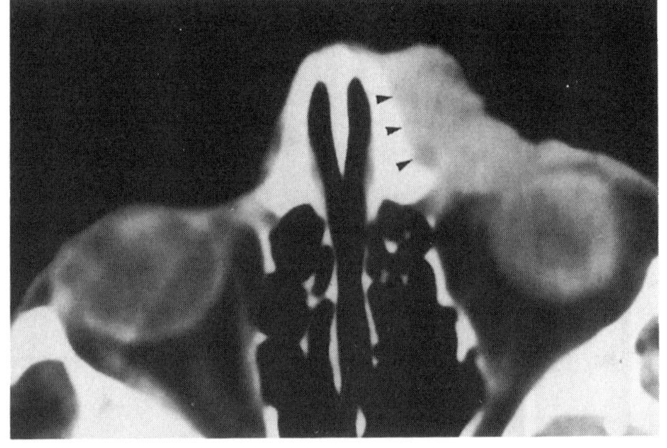

B

FIGURE 5–50 A, Clinical appearance of a large squamous cell carcinoma involving the lower lid, medial canthus, and nasal bridge. *B,* Computed tomographic scan of the same patient demonstrates the nasal bone involvement *(arrowheads)* with early orbital extension. This lesion was removed by exenteration with en bloc excision of the involved bone.

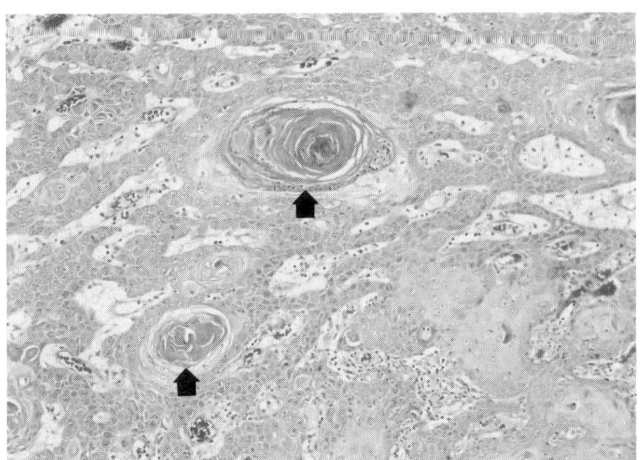

FIGURE 5–51 A moderately well-differentiated squamous cell carcinoma exhibiting mild pleomorphism and extensive interconnecting cords of tumor cells with keratin pearl formation *(arrows)*. The brightly eosinophilic cytoplasm results from abnormal intracellular keratin production. H&E.

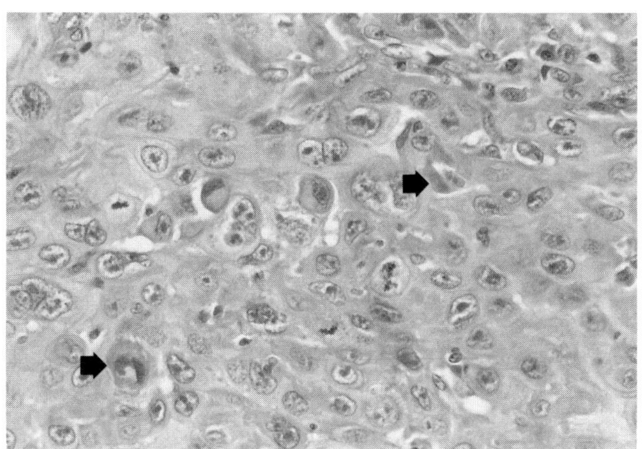

FIGURE 5–52 Squamous cell carcinoma showing dyskeratosis, moderate pleomorphism, and numerous mitotic figures *(arrows)*. H&E.

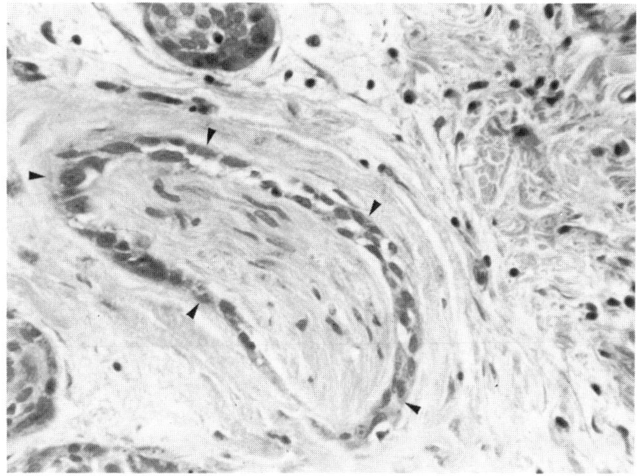

FIGURE 5–53 A branch of the trigeminal nerve containing perineural tumor infiltration by squamous cell carcinoma *(arrowheads)*. H&E.

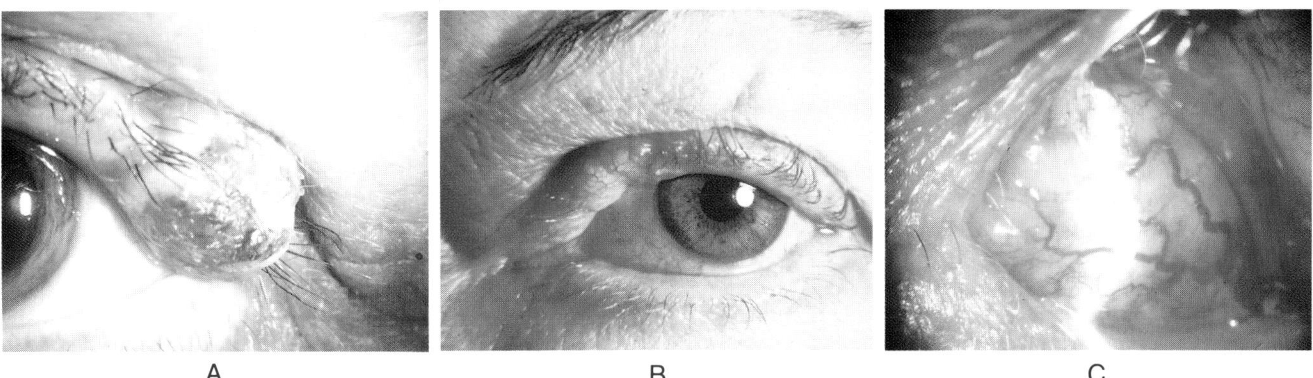

FIGURE 5–54 *A*, A sebaceous carcinoma at the eyelid margin arising from a gland of Zeis. This tumor synthesizes lipid (sebum). There is a yellow hue in addition to the superficial ulceration at the surface of the lesion. (Courtesy of Jerry Shields, M.D.) *B*, Another sebaceous carcinoma of the eyelid margin, probably arising from the Zeis gland, which has caused loss of eyelashes. (Courtesy of Lorenz E. Zimmerman, M.D.) *C*, A yellow-appearing sebaceous carcinoma arising in the sebaceous glands of the caruncle. (Courtesy of Robert Folberg, M.D., and Pathology of the Eye: An Interactive Videodisc Program, copyright Department of Ophthalmology, University of Iowa, 1991, 1992.)

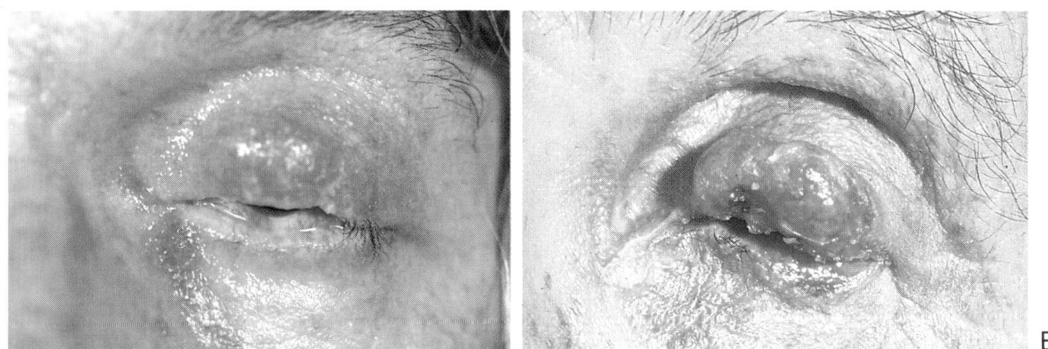

FIGURE 5–55 *A*, A sebaceous carcinoma of the upper eyelid meibomian glands (most common site of origin) has diffusely infiltrated the lid. Note the loss of eyelashes in both the upper and lower eyelids. *B*, This tumor has eroded through to the epidermis and has a yellow coloration. (*B*, Courtesy of Lorenz E. Zimmerman, M.D.)

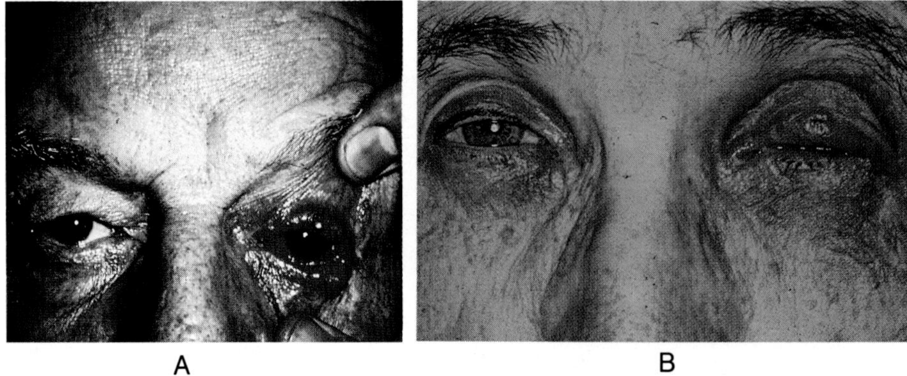

FIGURE 5-56 **Sebaceous carcinoma.** *A,* A strictly uniocular reddened left eye (blepharoconjunctivitis or masquerade syndrome) is accompanied by nodules of both the upper and the lower eyelids. This appearance is due to spread of sebaceous cells within the conjunctival epithelium. *B,* Diffuse sebaceous cell carcinoma with some thickening of the upper eyelid as well as total loss of eyelashes of the upper eyelid and of some of the lower eyelid. In this case, there is unilateral eyelid weeping or eczematous appearance without the dramatic erythema displayed in *A.* (*A* and *B,* Courtesy of Lorenz E. Zimmerman, M.D.)

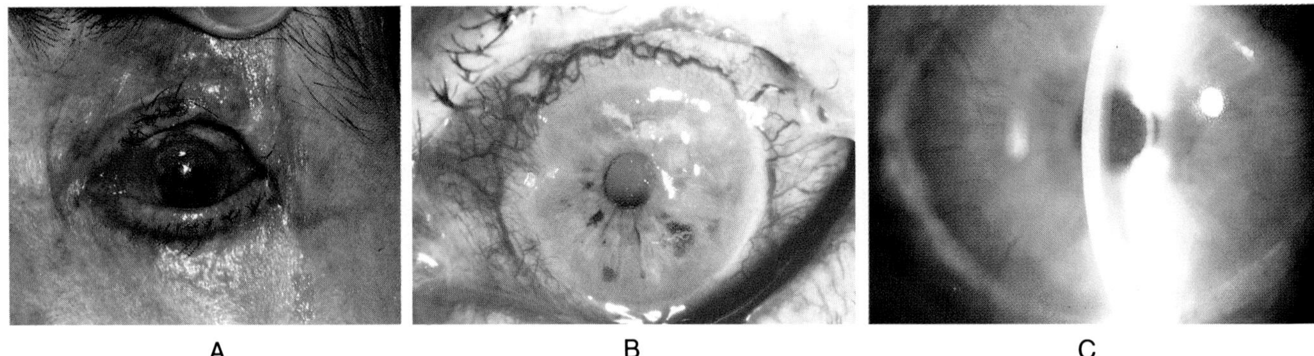

FIGURE 5-57 *A,* A uniocular, chronically reddened eye with a nodule in the upper eyelid and corneal epithelial irregularity. *B,* There is an opalescence of the corneal epithelium from the spread of sebaceous carcinoma cells within this layer. *C,* Corneal epithelial involvement with sebaceous carcinoma, causing an underlying neoplastic pannus. (*A–C,* Courtesy of John W. Shore, M.D.)

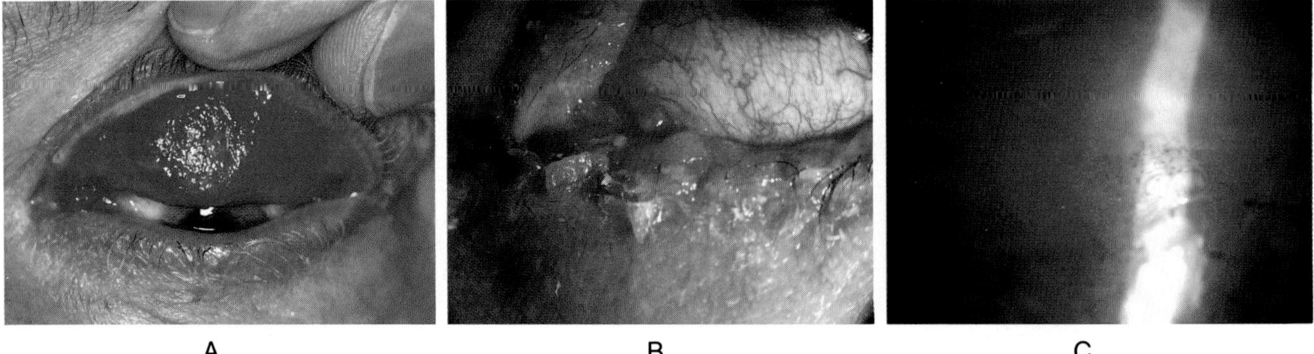

FIGURE 5-58 **Sebaceous carcinoma.** *A,* A diffusely reddened and irregular palpebral surface from spread of sebaceous carcinoma within the tarsal conjunctival epithelium. (Courtesy of John W. Shore, M.D.) *B,* An irregular lower eyelid margin with partial loss of eyelashes due to sebaceous carcinoma spread within the epithelium and glands of the eyelid margin. *C,* On everting the lower eyelid, the tarsal epithelium is thickened and beset with numerous tumor-associated curlicue or hairpin vessels, as indicated within the slit beam as well as on either side of it.

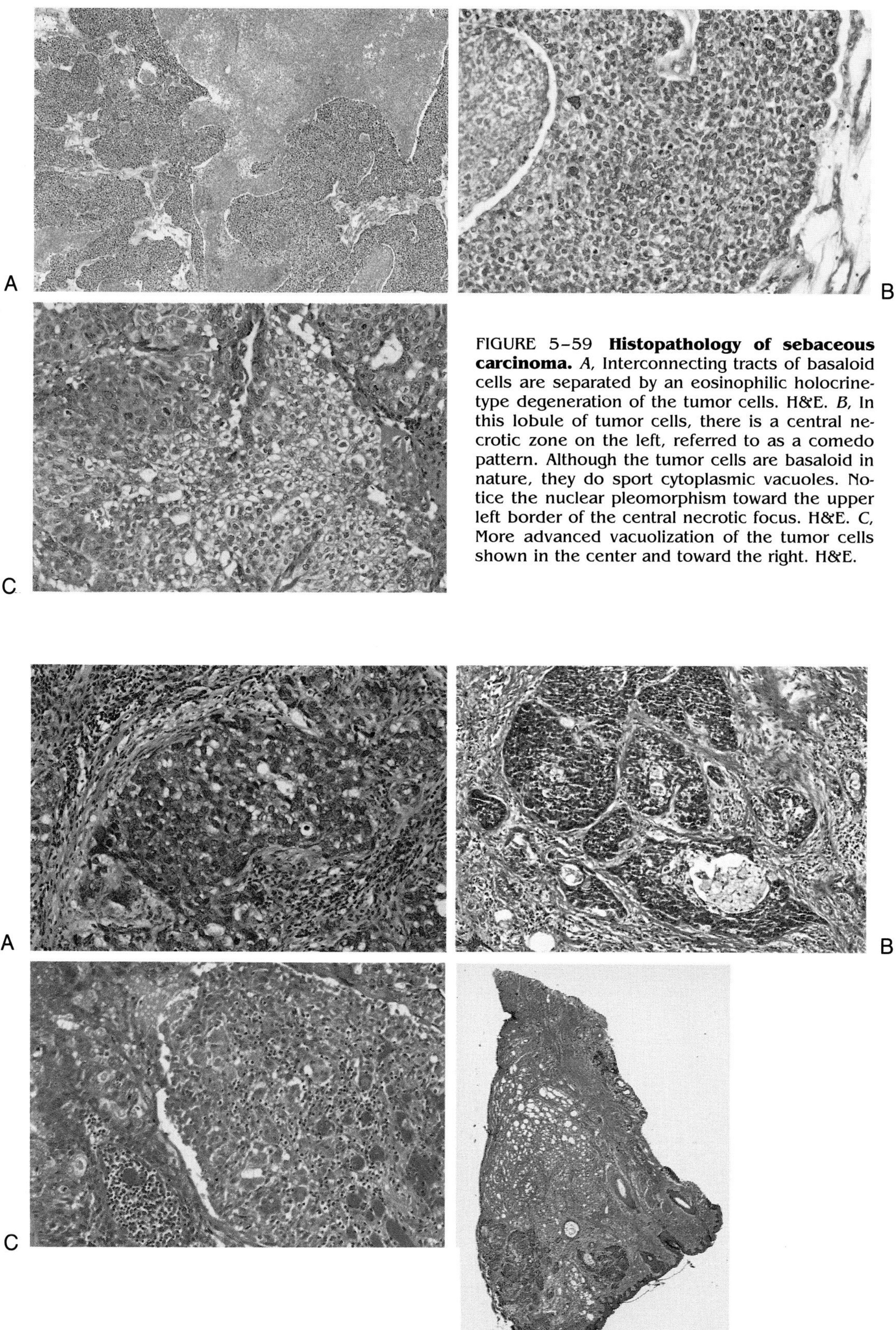

FIGURE 5–59 **Histopathology of sebaceous carcinoma.** *A,* Interconnecting tracts of basaloid cells are separated by an eosinophilic holocrine-type degeneration of the tumor cells. H&E. *B,* In this lobule of tumor cells, there is a central necrotic zone on the left, referred to as a comedo pattern. Although the tumor cells are basaloid in nature, they do sport cytoplasmic vacuoles. Notice the nuclear pleomorphism toward the upper left border of the central necrotic focus. H&E. *C,* More advanced vacuolization of the tumor cells shown in the center and toward the right. H&E.

FIGURE 5–60 **Sebaceous carcinoma.** *A,* Zone of anaplastic cells with randomly dispersed cells with vacuolization. *B,* Several small tumor cell islands possess highly vacuolated and frothy cells in their centers, shown particularly well toward the bottom right of the figure. *C,* An interstitial giant cell granulomatous response to the release of sebum-type material synthesized by tumor cells on the left. Note the eosinophilic, frothy, extracellular material toward the upper left of the figure. *D,* Full-thickness section of an upper eyelid with a sebaceous carcinoma below, presumably arising in a gland of Zeis, which has caused a lipogranulomatous chalazion reaction in the middle and upper portions of the lid. *A–D,* All H&E. (*B* and *D,* Courtesy of Lorenz E. Zimmerman, M.D.)

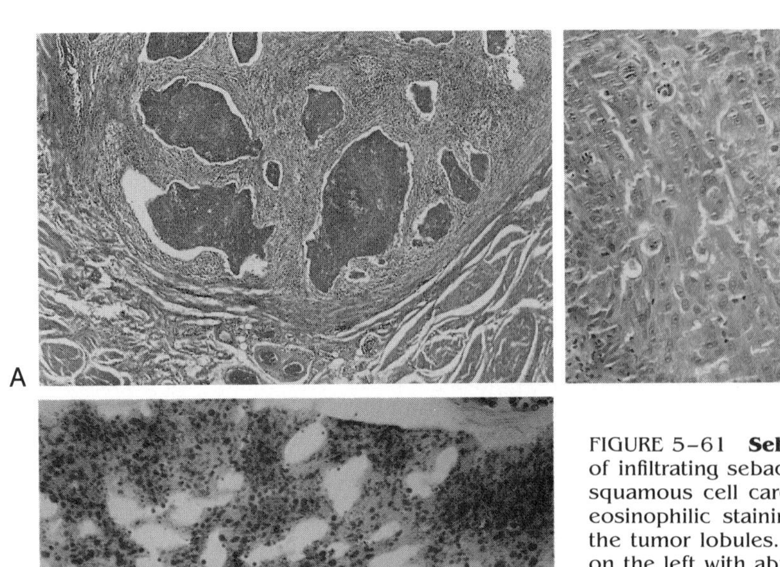

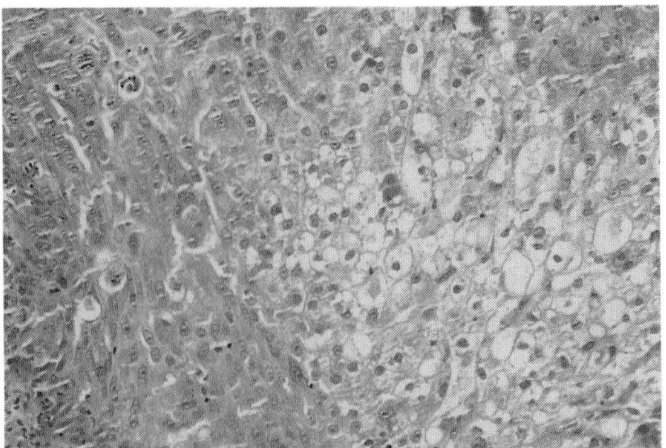

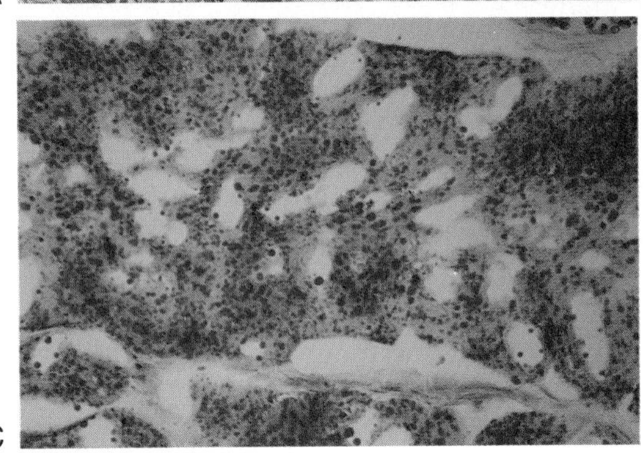

FIGURE 5-61 **Sebaceous carcinoma.** *A,* Focus of infiltrating sebaceous carcinoma suggestive of squamous cell carcinoma by virtue of the more eosinophilic staining properties of cytoplasm in the tumor lobules. H&E. *B,* Squamous-type cells on the left with abundant eosinophilic cytoplasm quickly transform into the vacuolated sebaceous cells on the right. H&E. *C,* Either fresh or frozen tissue or recently retrieved wet formalin-fixed tissue can be frozen-sectioned and stained with oil-red-O to determine if cytoplasmic lipid is present. Formalin-fixed wet tissue, oil-red-O.

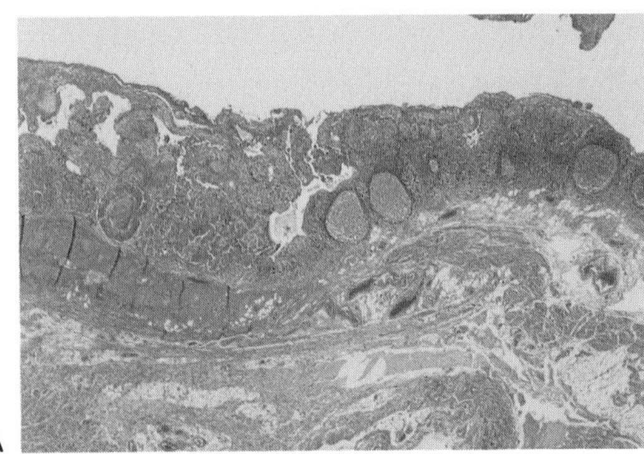

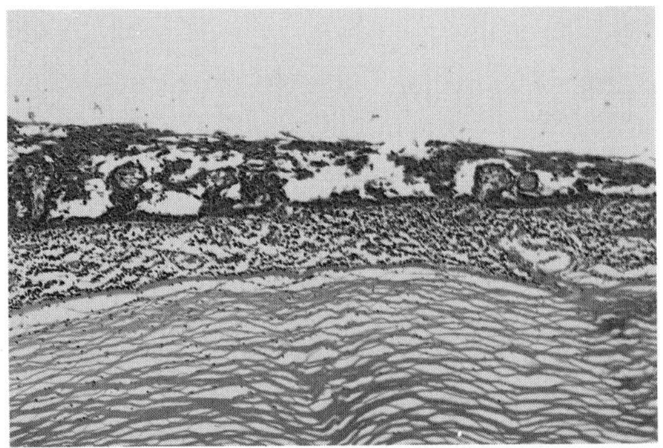

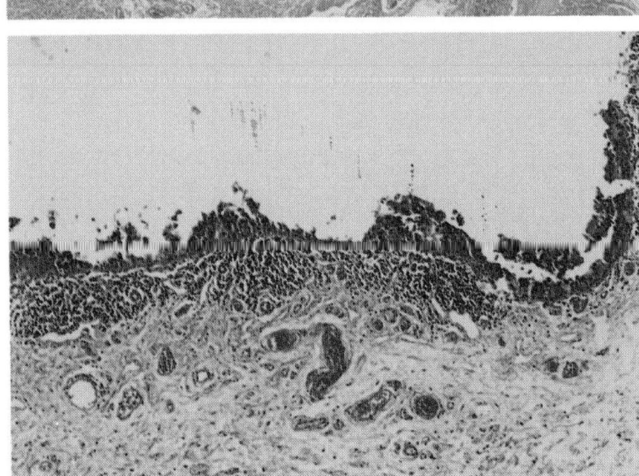

FIGURE 5-62 **Sebaceous carcinoma.** *A,* Conjunctival intraepithelial sebaceous spread with an underlying lymphocytic response that is organized into follicles. This intense type of inflammatory response is unusual in squamous lesions. *B,* Dyscohesive intraepithelial sebaceous carcinoma cells are supplied by stubby papillary units growing across the cornea. Neoplastic epithelium is friable and breaking apart. Notice there is an inflamed and vascularized pannus beneath the tumor cells, with an intact Bowman's membrane. Uninvolved corneal stroma is shown below. *C,* A desquamative and exfoliative tendency of intraepithelial sebaceous carcinoma cells with "tombstoning" of the remaining cells. *A–C,* All H&E.

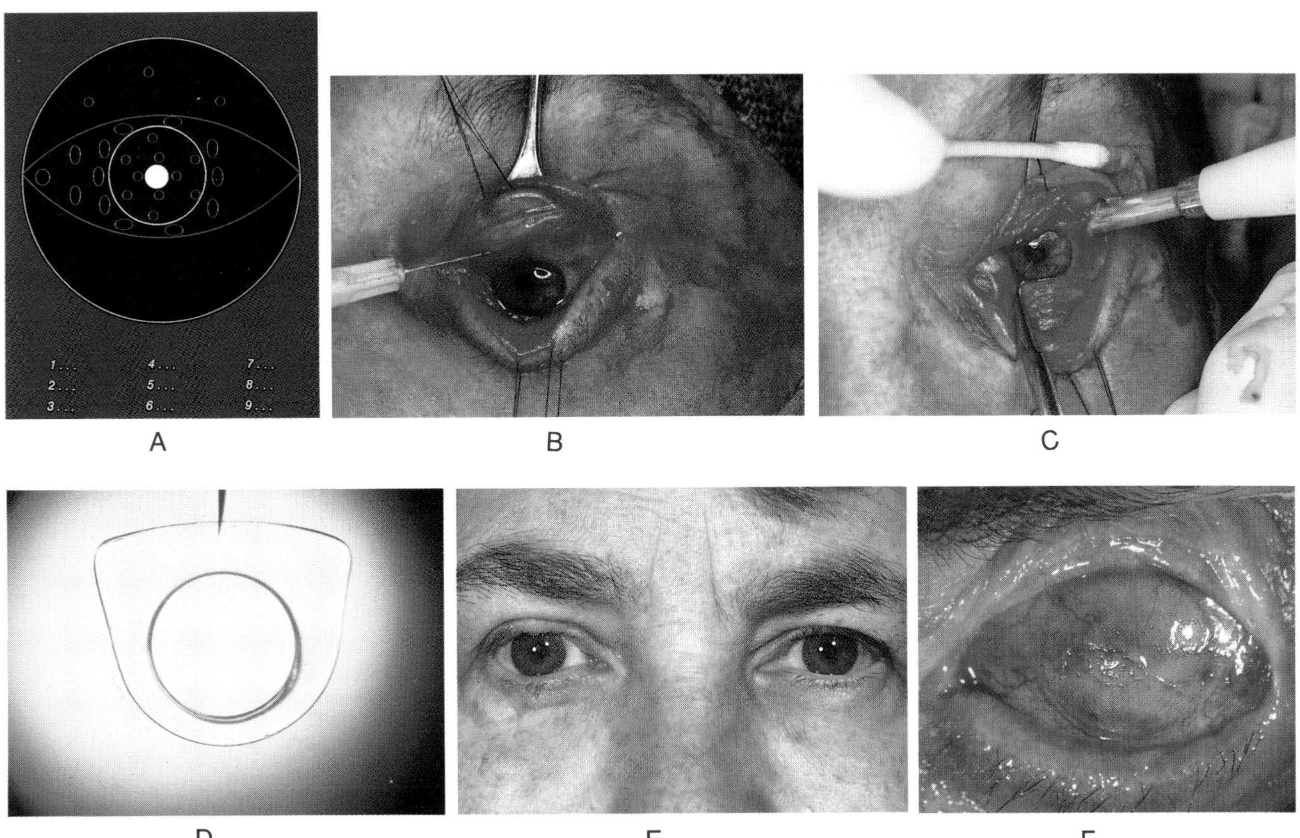

FIGURE 5-63 *A,* Before proceeding with any definitive form of surgery for an ocular adnexal sebaceous carcinoma, it is now routine to obtain permanent microscopic evaluations of multiple map biopsy specimens of the conjunctival sac. Each biopsy specimen should be placed in its own bottle with a clear label. This permits the pathologist to report normal and abnormal areas precisely. Any opalescence of the corneal epithelium should lead to cytologic scraping, with independent reports of the different corneal epithelial zones. (*A,* Courtesy of John W. Shore, M.D.) *B,* Cryotherapy has been used to treat residual intraepithelial sebaceous carcinoma of the conjunctival sac. After a Cutler-Beard first-stage procedure has been performed, the superior forniceal and epibulbar conjunctiva is ballooned up with lidocaine (Xylocaine). *C,* A double freeze-thaw application of cryotherapy is administered to the involved zones. Once the cryoprobe cannot be moved from side to side, it is an indication that the iceball has fused to the sclera and the treatment should be stopped. *D,* After the completion of the cryotherapy session, a conformer is placed in the conjunctival sac. Note the widened superior flange shape of the conformer, which is designed to deepen and broaden the superior fornix and prevent contraction from scarification. *E,* An acceptable postsurgical and adjunctive cryotherapy result in the right eye. *F,* An unsuccessful postsurgical and adjunctive cryotherapy result caused by persistent dry eye with delayed corneal healing and vascularization. Most of the epibulbar surface was treated. (*B–D,* From Lisman RD, Jakobiec FA, Small P: Sebaceous carcinoma of the eyelids: The role of adjunctive cryotherapy in the management of conjunctival pagetoid spread. Ophthalmology 96:1021–1026, 1989.)

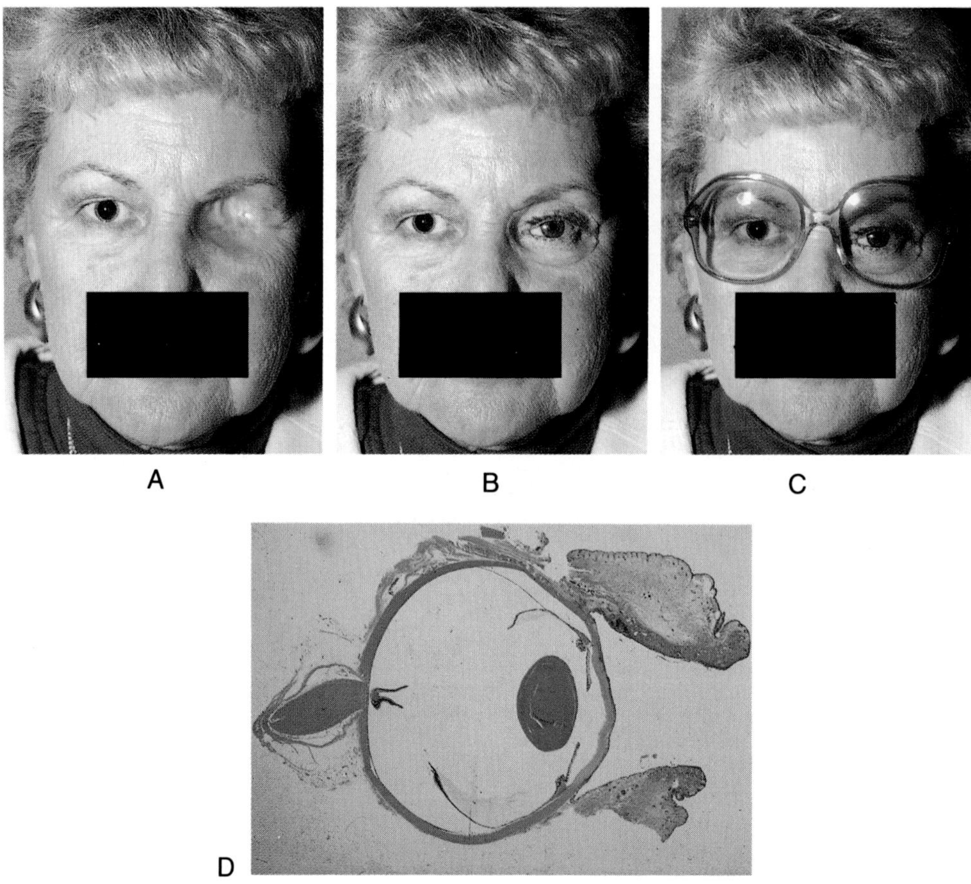

FIGURE 5–64 **Sebaceous carcinoma.** *A,* Appearance of the socket after it has healed by spontaneous granulation in a patient who had diffuse sebaceous carcinoma with an upper eyelid nodule and lower eyelid intraepithelial sebaceous spread. All of the epibulbar surface was involved. The deep orbital fat and periorbital membrane were spared. There are no lymphatic connections between the eyelid skin, the conjunctival lymphatics, and the deep orbital soft tissues (which are devoid of lymphatic channels). *B,* Appearance of the patient after placement of a prosthesis. *C,* An excellent cosmetic appearance is obtained when the patient further camouflages the prosthesis with slightly tinted glasses. *D,* An orbital exenteration specimen with sparing of the deep orbital connective tissues. Note that the eyelid skin has been taken because of the possibility of intraepidermal spread of sebaceous carcinoma. H&E. (*D,* Courtesy of Miguel Bernier, M.D.)

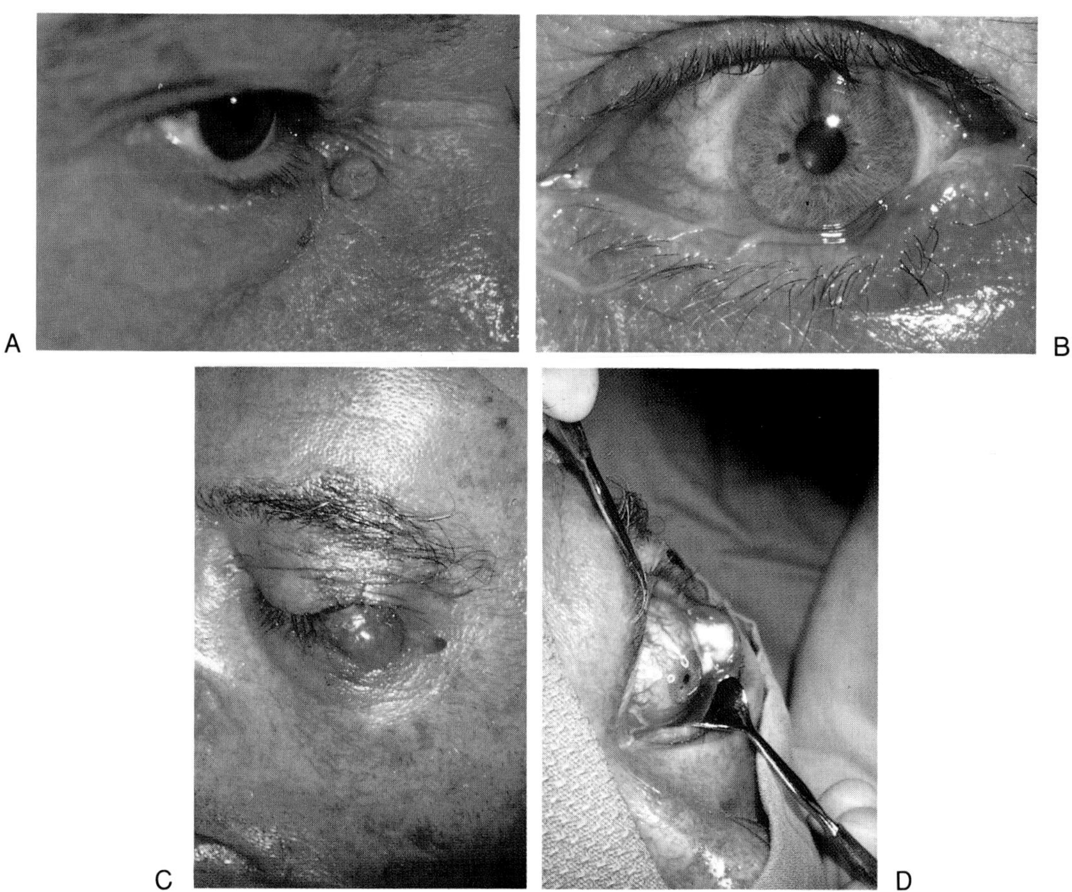

FIGURE 5–65 **Sebaceous adenoma.** *A,* Yellow-appearing sebaceous adenoma of the medial canthal skin in a patient who had multiple colonic carcinomas (Muir-Torre syndrome). *B,* The lid skin has been stretched over a benign sebaceous tumor that originated in the conjunctival epithelium. *C,* After an incomplete excision of the lesion shown in *B,* a massive and explosive growth occurred over a 1-week period. *D,* At the time of definitive surgery, a whitened inferior palpebral surface indicates an origin from the tarsal epithelium. Incompletely removed sebaceous adenomas can recur rapidly with a pseudoepitheliomatous hyperplasia featuring mostly squamous cells. (*D,* From Jakobiec FA, Zimmerman LE, La Piana F, et al: Unusual eyelid tumors with sebaceous differentiation in the Muir-Torre syndrome: Rapid clinical regrowth and frank squamous transformation after biopsy. Ophthalmology 95:1543–1548, 1988.)

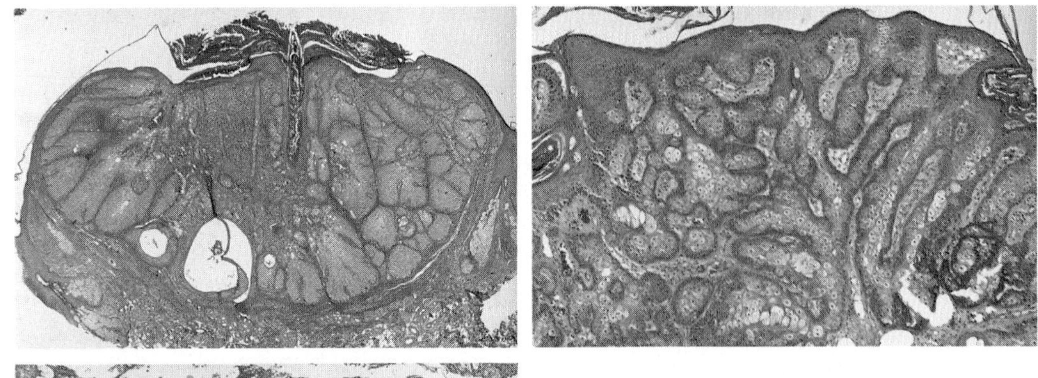

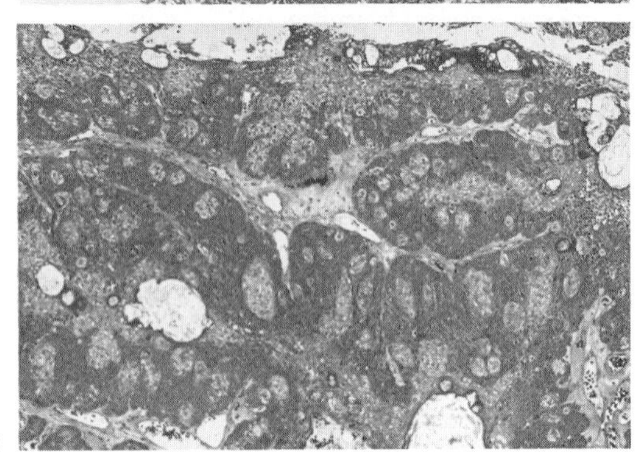

FIGURE 5–66 *A,* Classic sebaceous adenoma of the cheek in a patient who had an eyelid lesion and a colonic carcinoma in the Muir-Torre syndrome. Note the encapsulated but highly circumscribed nature of the dermal proliferation. Each lobule has an outer basal germinal cell layer, which quickly becomes lipidized centrally. Note the surface hyperkeratosis and parakeratosis. *B,* A nonlobular sebaceous adenoma taking origin in cords from the surface epidermis in the patient shown in Figure 5–65*A*. *C,* The palpebral epithelial lesion shown in Figure 5–65*B* features interconnecting units of basaloid cells with scattered nests of highly differentiated, pale-staining sebaceous cells. *A–C,* All H&E. (*B,* From Jakobiec FA, Zimmerman LE, La Piana F, et al: Unusual eyelid tumors with sebaceous differentiation in the Muir-Torre syndrome: Rapid clinical regrowth and frank squamous transformation after biopsy. Ophthalmology 95:1543–1548, 1988.)

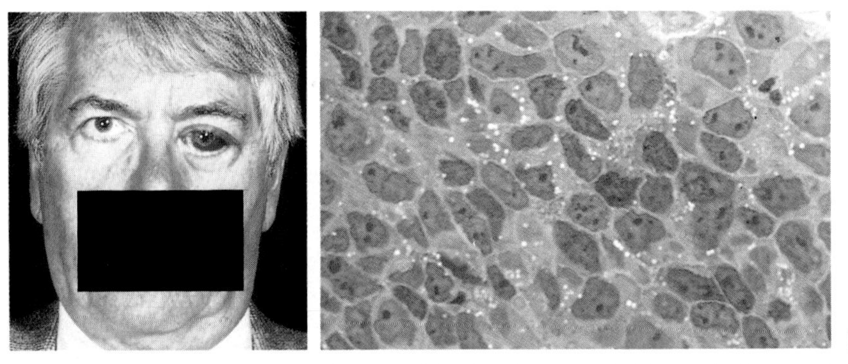

FIGURE 5–67 **Primary sebaceous carcinoma of lacrimal gland.** *A,* This patient presented with multiple left recurrent subconjunctival hemorrhages before it became apparent that there was a mass in the lacrimal fossa region that had caused proptosis as well as downward and inward displacement of the eyeball. This has been a uniformly fatal tumor to date. *B,* The tumor was composed of islands and lobules of highly undifferentiated cells, which failed to form clear-cut lumina or to secrete mucinous materials. However, 1-μ plastic sections obtained preparatory to electron microscopy revealed that most of the tumor cells possessed myriad cytoplasmic vacuoles. Methylene blue. (From Rodgers IR, Jakobiec FA, Gingold MP, et al: Anaplastic carcinoma of the lacrimal gland presenting with recurrent subconjunctival hemorrhages and displaying incipient sebaceous differentiation. Ophthalmic Plast Reconstr Surg 7:229–237, 1991.)

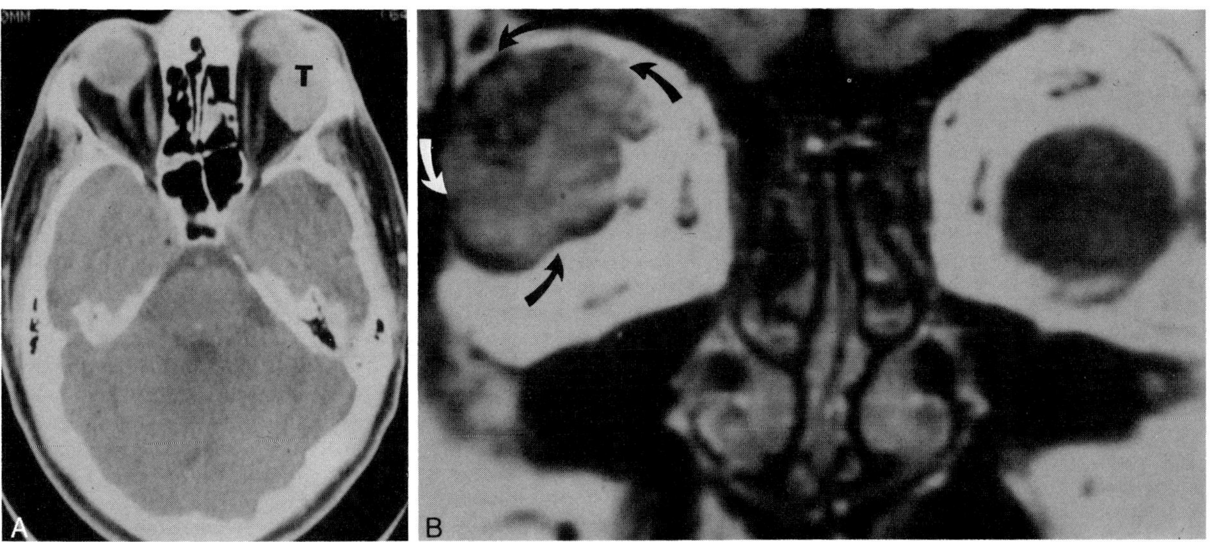

FIGURE 5–68 **Sebaceous carcinoma of lacrimal gland.** *A,* An axial computed tomographic scan of the primary lacrimal gland sebaceous carcinoma depicted in Figure 5–67. Note the overall rounded or globular outline of the tumor (*T*) in the lacrimal fossa region. *B,* A T_1-weighted coronal image from a magnetic resonance scan shows the tumor outline (*arrows*), which has more signal intensity than do most primary orbital tumors in T_1-phase images. Lipid, mucus, melanin, and blood breakdown products may all display increased signal intensity in T_1-weighted images. (From Rodgers IR, Jakobiec FA, Gingold MP, et al: Anaplastic carcinoma of the lacrimal gland presenting with recurrent subconjunctival hemorrhages and displaying incipient sebaceous differentiation. Ophthalmic Plast Reconstr Surg 7:229–237, 1991.)

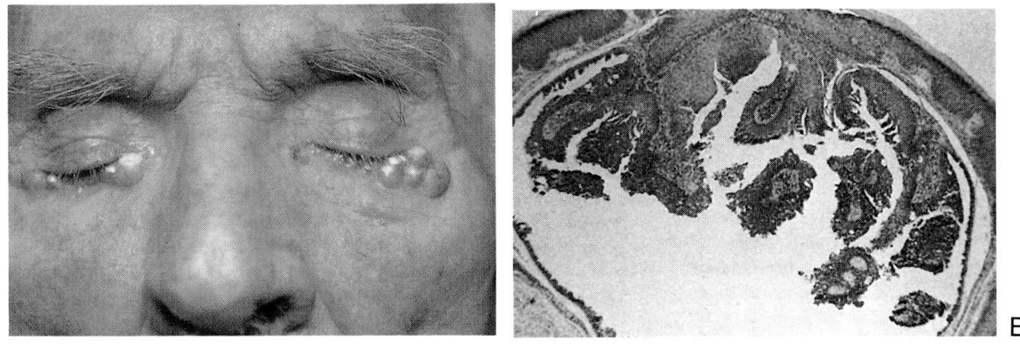

FIGURE 5–69 **Apocrine cystadenoma.** *A,* The superior border of these cystic lesions arises from the lash line and contains yellowish white lipoidal material. The lesions have confluent margins and may affect multiple eyelids. They arise from the glands of Moll, which are restricted to the eyelid margins. *B,* The excised specimen is well circumscribed and contains numerous papillary fronds projecting into a central cavity. *B,* H&E. (*A,* From Sacks E, Jakobiec FA, McMillan R: Multiple bilateral apocrine cystadenomas of the eyelid: Light and electron microscopic studies. Ophthalmology 94:65–71, 1987.)

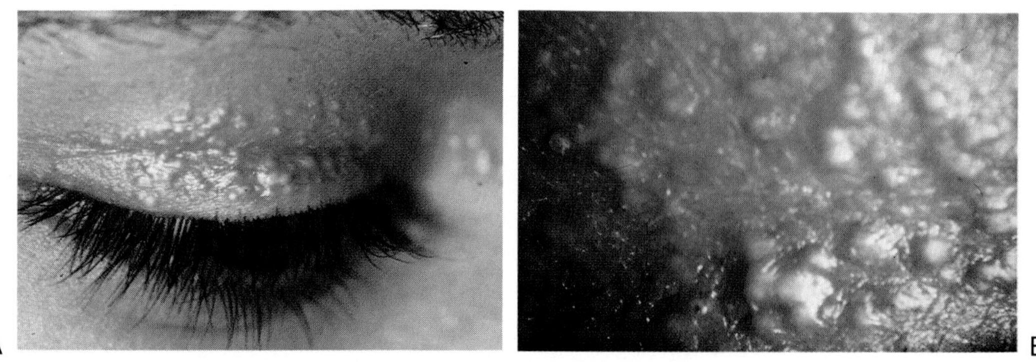

FIGURE 5–70 **Milia.** *A*, These retention cysts of pilosebaceous origin may be confused with apocrine cystadenomas. Milia, although multiple and lightly colored, arise from the eyelid and facial skin. *B*, Milia also have umbilicated centers. (*A* and *B*, Courtesy of C. Matta, M.D.)

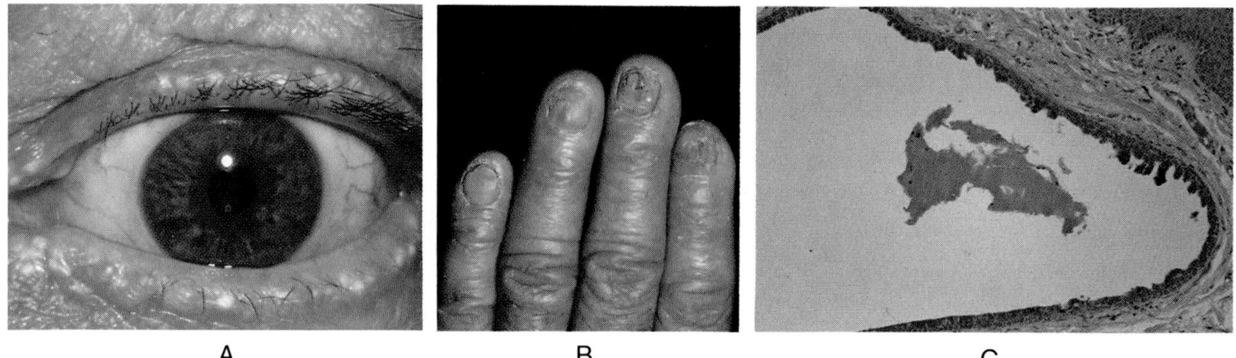

FIGURE 5–71 **Apocrine cystadenoma and ectodermal dysplasia.** *A*, Multiple 1- to 2-mm cystic lesions are found along the eyelid margin. *B*, Affected patients have dystrophic fingernails with thickened nail plates, onycholysis, and gray discoloration. *C*, Decapitation secretion occurs from a double cuboidal epithelial lined cyst. H&E. (*A–C*, From Font RL, Stone MS, Schanzer C: Apocrine hidrocystomas of the lids, hypodontia, palmar-plantar hyperkeratosis, and onychodystrophy: A new variant of ectodermal dysplasia. Arch Ophthalmol 104:1811–1813, 1986. Copyright 1986, American Medical Association.)

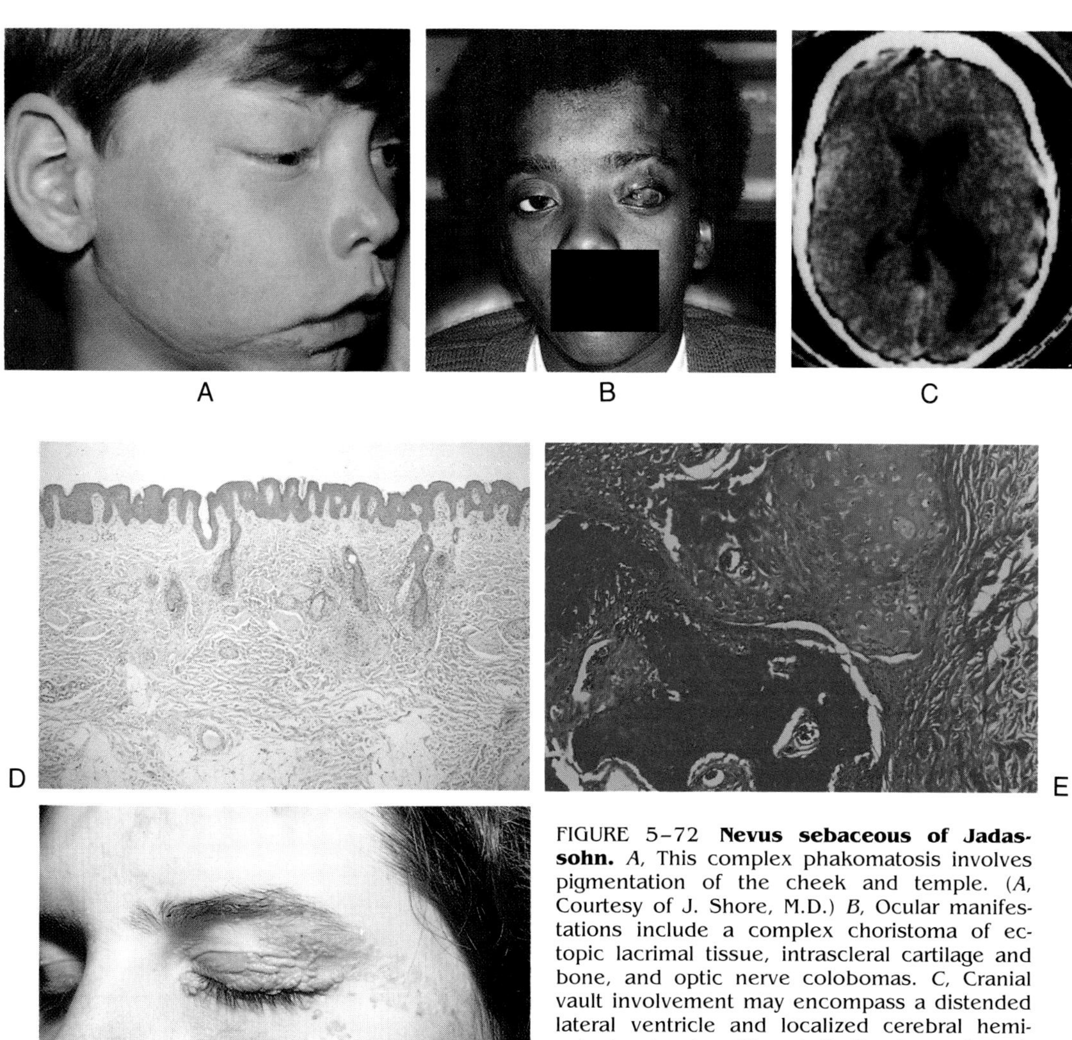

FIGURE 5–72 **Nevus sebaceous of Jadassohn.** *A*, This complex phakomatosis involves pigmentation of the cheek and temple. (*A*, Courtesy of J. Shore, M.D.) *B*, Ocular manifestations include a complex choristoma of ectopic lacrimal tissue, intrascleral cartilage and bone, and optic nerve colobomas. *C*, Cranial vault involvement may encompass a distended lateral ventricle and localized cerebral hemispheric atrophy. (*B* and *C*, Courtesy of R. J. Campbell.) *D*, A thin layer of keratin overlies surface papillations. Dermal hair follicles may be scant in number; the sebaceous glands may be hypertrophied and their cell membranes disrupted; apocrine glands may be found. H&E. (*D*, Courtesy of J. B. Crawford, M.D.) *E*, Sclera containing cartilage and bone. H&E. *F*, The clinical differential diagnosis includes linear epidermal nevus: a verrucous-appearing lesion devoid of apocrine glands.

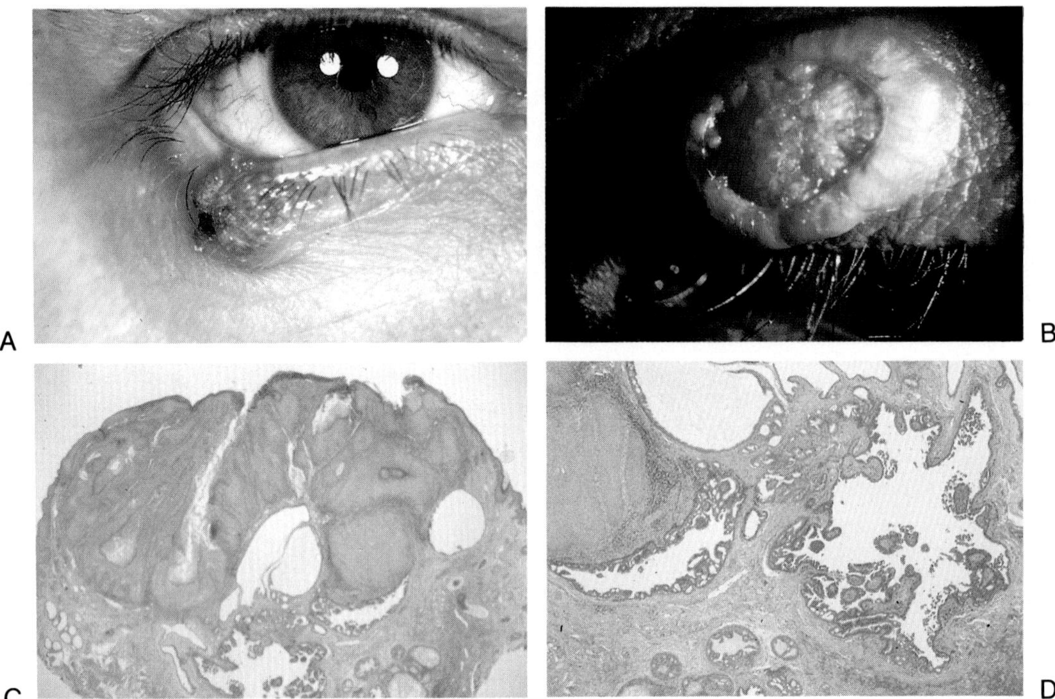

FIGURE 5–73 **Syringocystadenoma papilliferum.** *A,* The eyelid margin and skin have been replaced by a benign multilobulated, hyperkeratotic lesion. (*A,* From Jakobiec FA, Streeten BW, Iwamoto T: Syringocystadenoma papilliferum of the eyelid. Ophthalmology 88:1175–1181, 1981.) *B,* A discrete nodule with a central corrugated surface and multiple poral openings. (*B,* Courtesy of M. Tso, M.D., and R. Urban, M.D.) *C,* This low-power photomicrograph reveals a cup-shaped lesion containing a central acanthotic core and deeper dilated apocrine cysts. The epidermis displays acanthosis. *D,* On higher power, papillae project into a luminal space. Plasma cells are apparent within the papillary cores. *C* and *D,* H&E. (*C* and *D,* Courtesy of R. Eagle, M.D.)

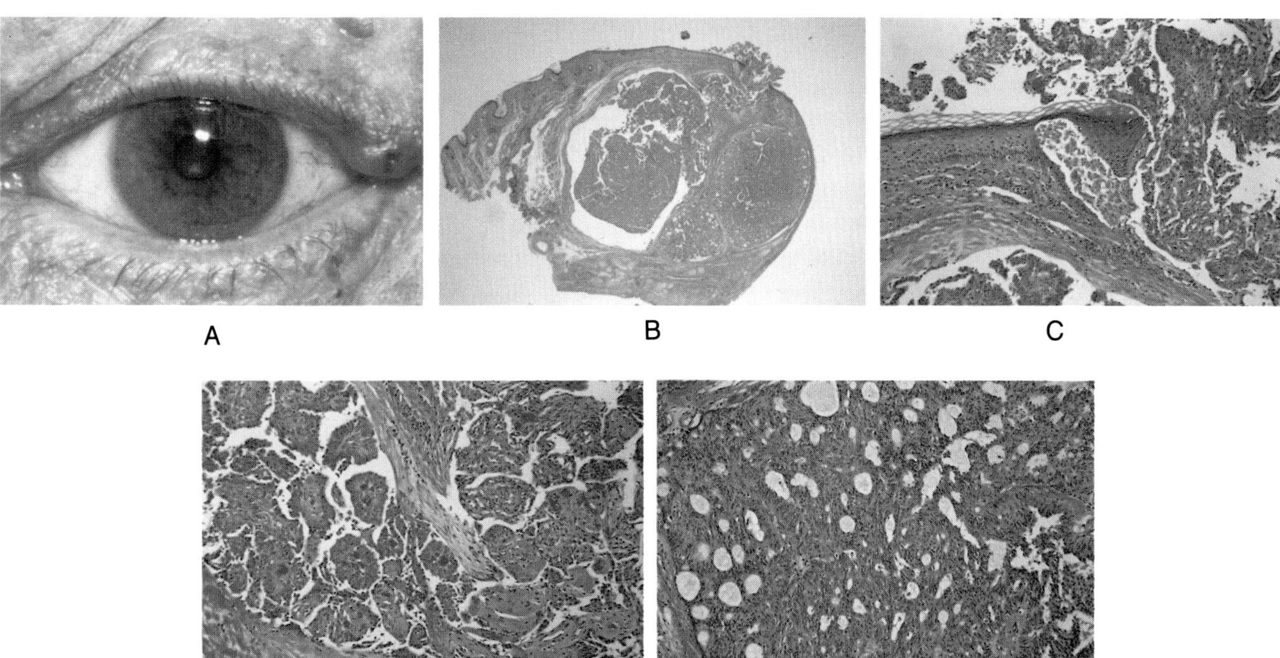

FIGURE 5–74 **Hidradenoma papilliferum.** *A*, Hidradenoma papilliferum typically presents as a benign dermal nodule with a poral opening. This umbilication may represent an ectasia of the apocrine secretion-rich pilar canal or may be the result of burrowing of tumor cells. *B*, Histologically, this well-circumscribed lesion consisting of tumor lobules has a poral connection to the epidermis. *C*, High-power photomicrograph of the poral opening through which tumor cells are extruding. *D*, The characteristic papillary configuration of the tumor cells covering fibrovascular cores. *E*, These lesions consist of solid areas of spindle-like tumor cells and tubular or glandular structures, the lumen of which contains faintly eosinophilic secretory material. *B–E*, H&E. (From Netland PA, Townsend DJ, Albert DM, Jakobiec FA: Hidradenoma papilliferum of the upper eyelid arising from the apocrine gland of Moll. Ophthalmology 97:1593–1598, 1990.)

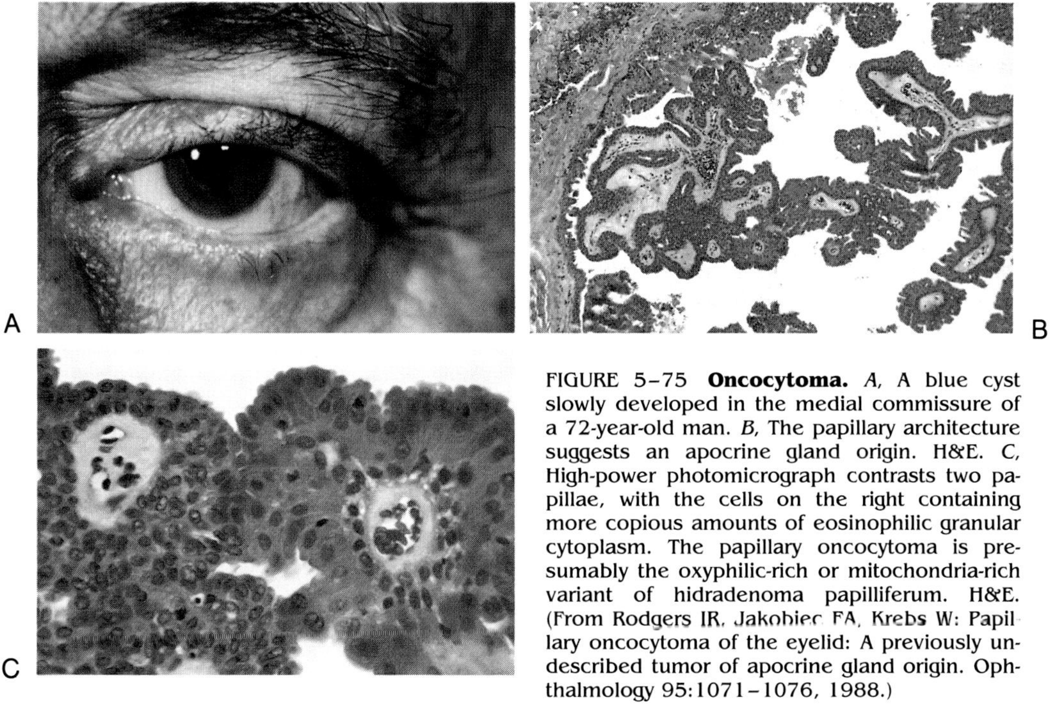

FIGURE 5–75 **Oncocytoma.** *A*, A blue cyst slowly developed in the medial commissure of a 72-year-old man. *B*, The papillary architecture suggests an apocrine gland origin. H&E. *C*, High-power photomicrograph contrasts two papillae, with the cells on the right containing more copious amounts of eosinophilic granular cytoplasm. The papillary oncocytoma is presumably the oxyphilic-rich or mitochondria-rich variant of hidradenoma papilliferum. H&E. (From Rodgers IR, Jakobiec FA, Krebs W: Papillary oncocytoma of the eyelid: A previously undescribed tumor of apocrine gland origin. Ophthalmology 95:1071–1076, 1988.)

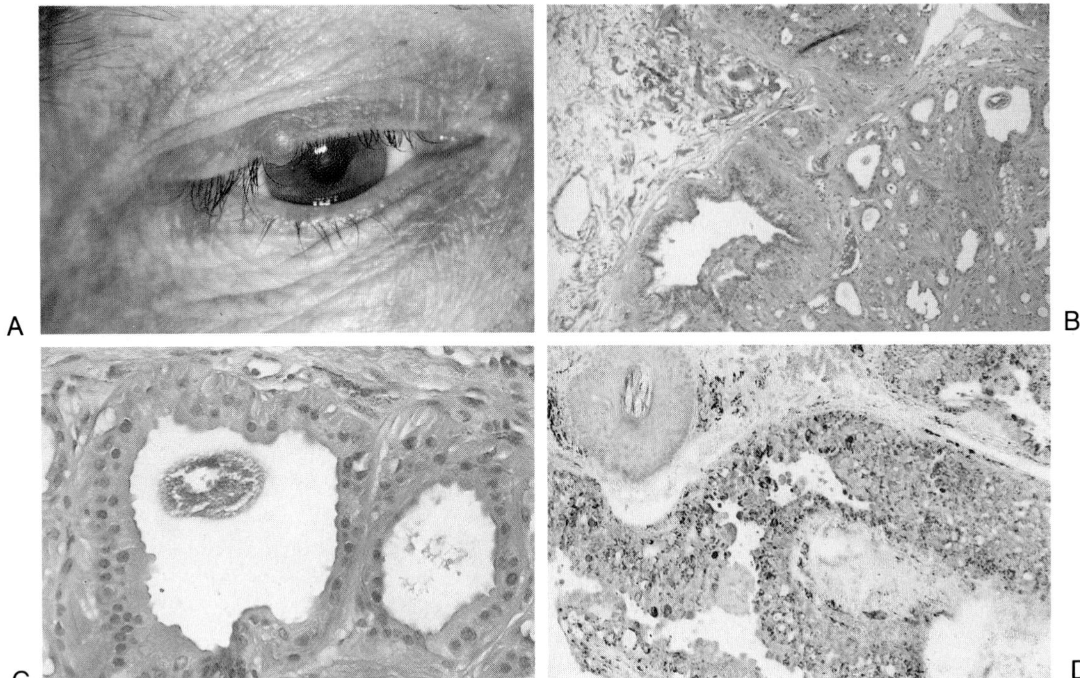

FIGURE 5–76 **Apocrine adenoma.** *A*, Flesh-colored nodule arising along the lid margin from a gland of Moll. *B*, The tumor consists of irregular glandular structures lined by a double layer of eosinophilic staining cuboidal cells. H&E. *C*, Areas of decapitation secretion are readily visible. The individual cells have a normal size and shape. H&E. *D*, Approximately one-third of these tumors contain iron-positive intracellular granules. Perls' stain. (*A*, Courtesy of D. Townsend, M.D.)

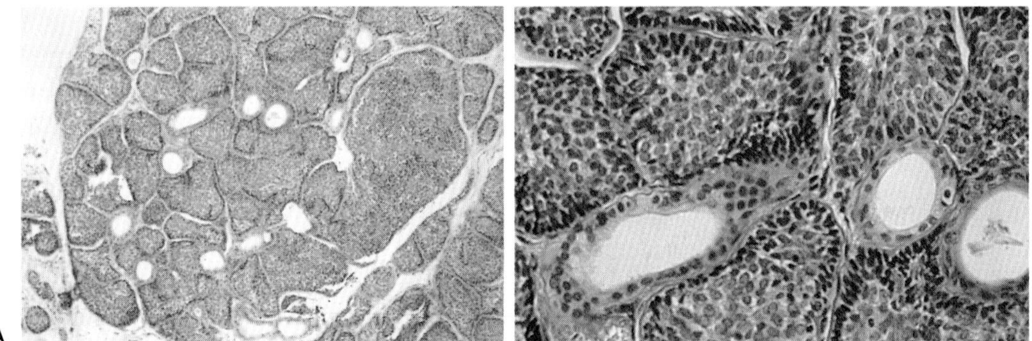

FIGURE 5–77 **Cylindroma.** *A*, This tumor is located in the dermis, is not connected to the overlying epithelium, and is not encapsulated. *B*, The tumor cell lobules are interposed in a "jig-saw" or mosaic pattern. A thickened basement membrane surrounds the lobules that contain ductal lumina. *A* and *B*, H&E.

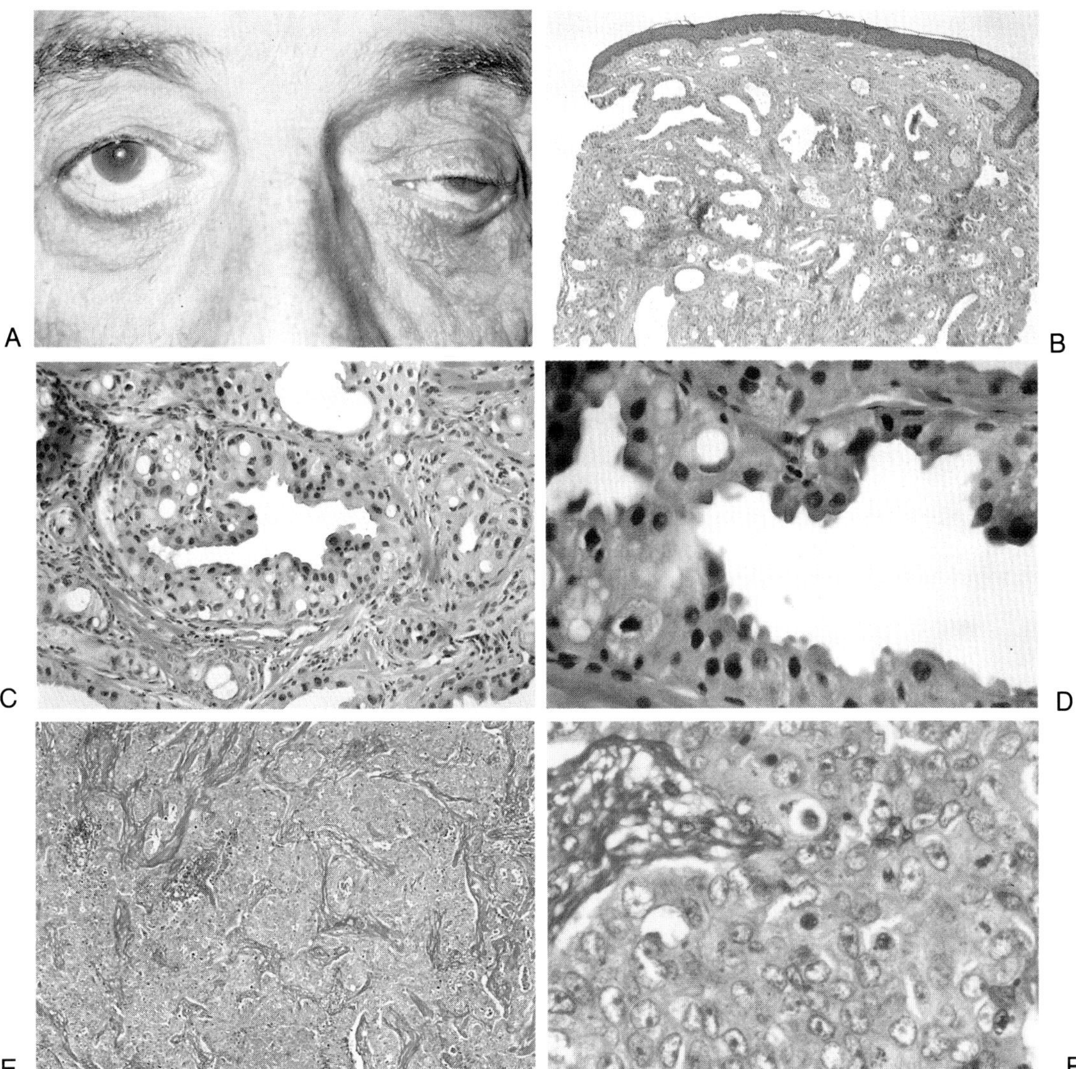

FIGURE 5-78 **Adenocarcinoma of the gland of Moll.** *A,* Chalazion-like lesion on the left lower eyelid of this man was locally excised after a biopsy proved that it was an adenocarcinoma. The lesion recurred within 1 year. *B,* The tumor consisted of adenoid tissue arranged in dilated tubules that deeply infiltrated the dermis. *C,* In contradistinction to the double layer of cuboidal cells found in benign apocrine tumors, adenocarcinoma is characterized by an irregular cellular proliferation; this "pile-up" of cells may obliterate the lumina. The tumor is capable of metastasis. *D,* The individual cells are pleomorphic. Decapitation apical secretion is present. *E,* Poorly differentiated tumors may be characterized by solid epithelial growth patterns. Papillary projections and disorganized tubular structures may not be present. *F,* This high-power photomicrograph depicts nuclear atypia, mitotic figures, and an opaque cytoplasm. *B–F,* H&E. (*A–D,* Courtesy of T. Dryja, M.D.)

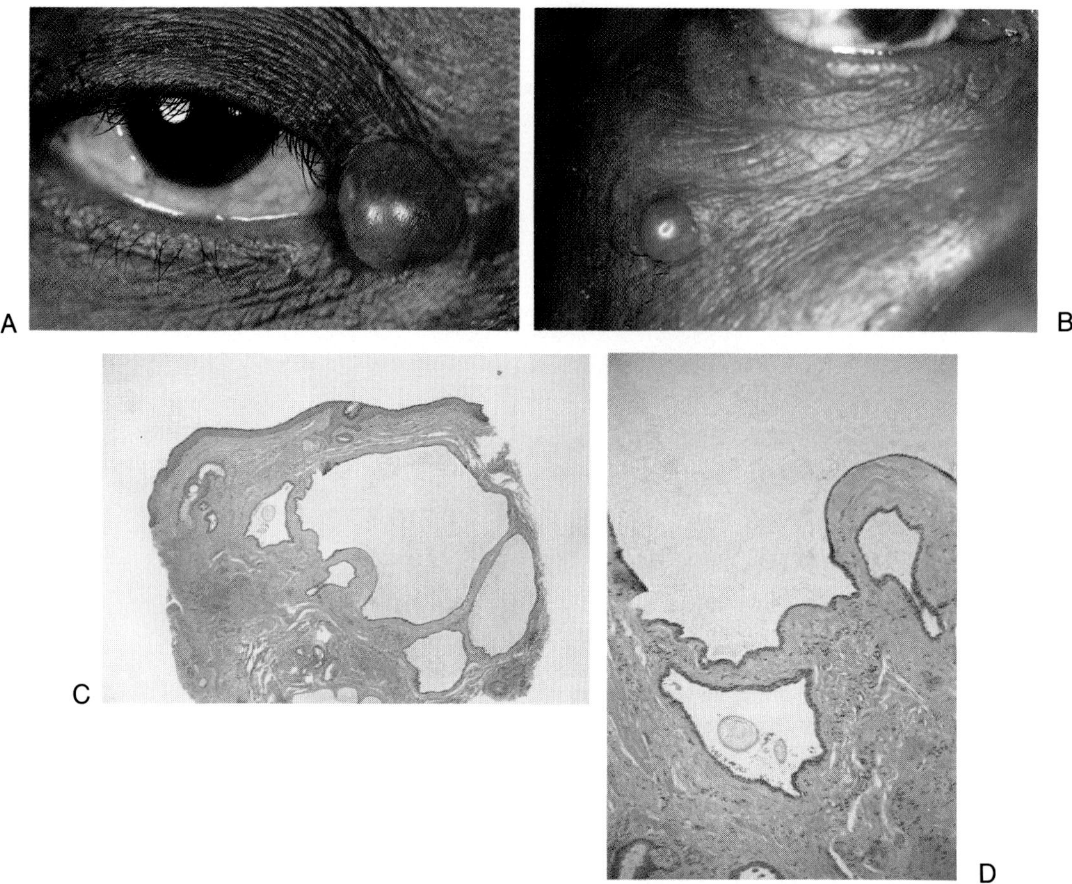

FIGURE 5–79 **Eccrine hidrocystoma.** *A,* Translucent cystic-appearing lesion arising in the medial canthus. *B,* Eccrine hidrocystomas are not limited to the eyelid margins but occur wherever eccrine glands are found throughout the eyelids. *C,* Multiple cystic spaces are lined by a double layer of low cuboidal epithelial cells. H&E. *D,* Decapitation secretion and papillations are not a feature of eccrine gland lesions. A faintly eosinophilic material may be found within the ductals. H&E. (*B,* Courtesy of S. Salasche, M.D.)

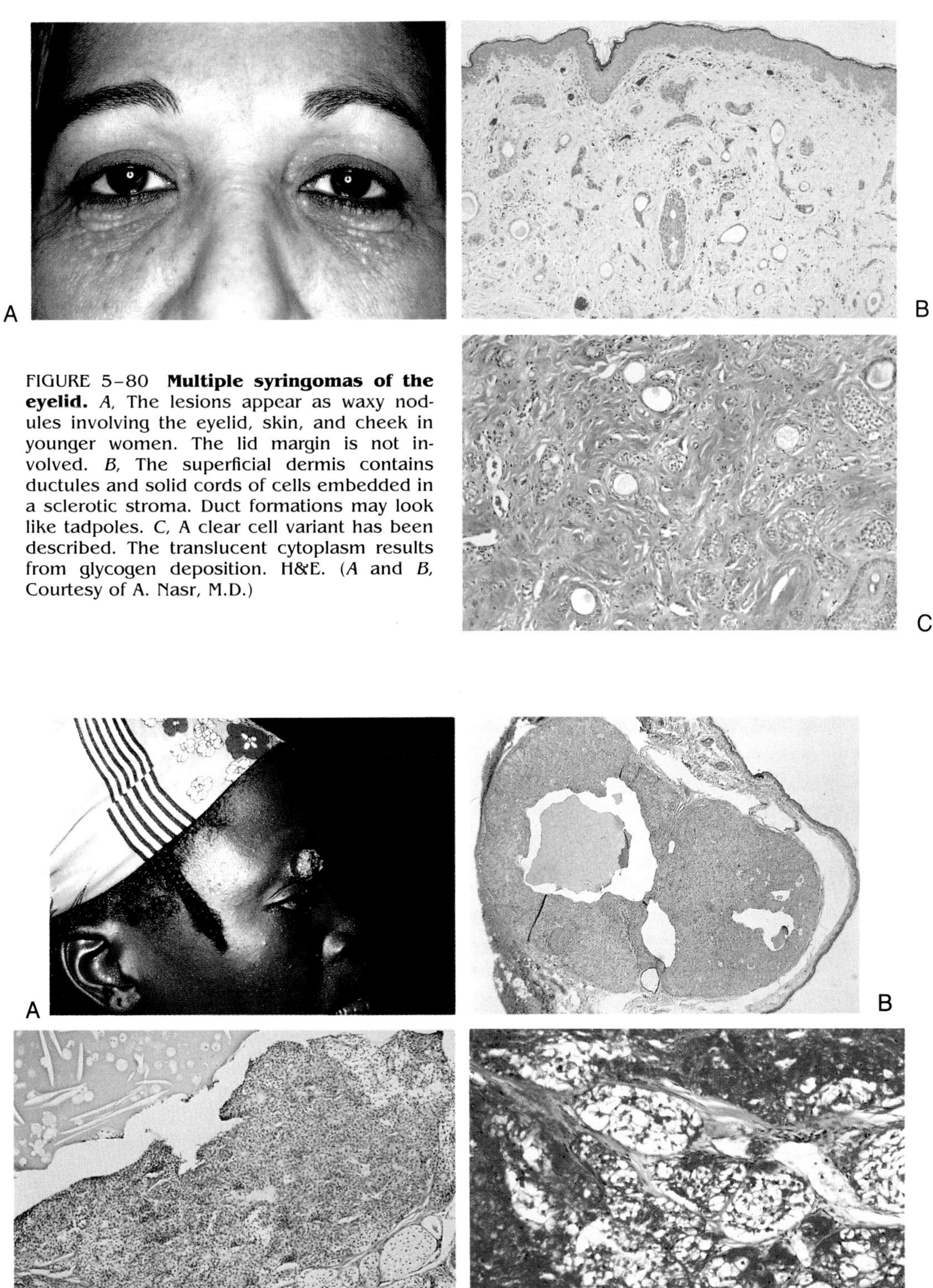

FIGURE 5–80 **Multiple syringomas of the eyelid.** *A*, The lesions appear as waxy nodules involving the eyelid, skin, and cheek in younger women. The lid margin is not involved. *B*, The superficial dermis contains ductules and solid cords of cells embedded in a sclerotic stroma. Duct formations may look like tadpoles. *C*, A clear cell variant has been described. The translucent cytoplasm results from glycogen deposition. H&E. (*A* and *B*, Courtesy of A. Nasr, M.D.)

FIGURE 5–81 **Acrospiroma.** *A*, A benign dermal tumor has caused surface hyperkeratosis. *B*, Histologically, acrospiromas are well-circumscribed dermal lesions that contain cystic spaces and solid foci of tumefaction. H&E. *C*, Small basophilic cells border an area of degenerative cystic material toward the upper left, while clear cells are present toward the bottom right. Sometimes, but not always, there may be interspersed small lumina. H&E. *D*, An abundance of periodic acid–Schiff (PAS)–positive material is found within the tumor cells, often within the clear cell regions. This material is usually glycogen and is sensitive to diastase predigestion (PAS reaction). PAS.

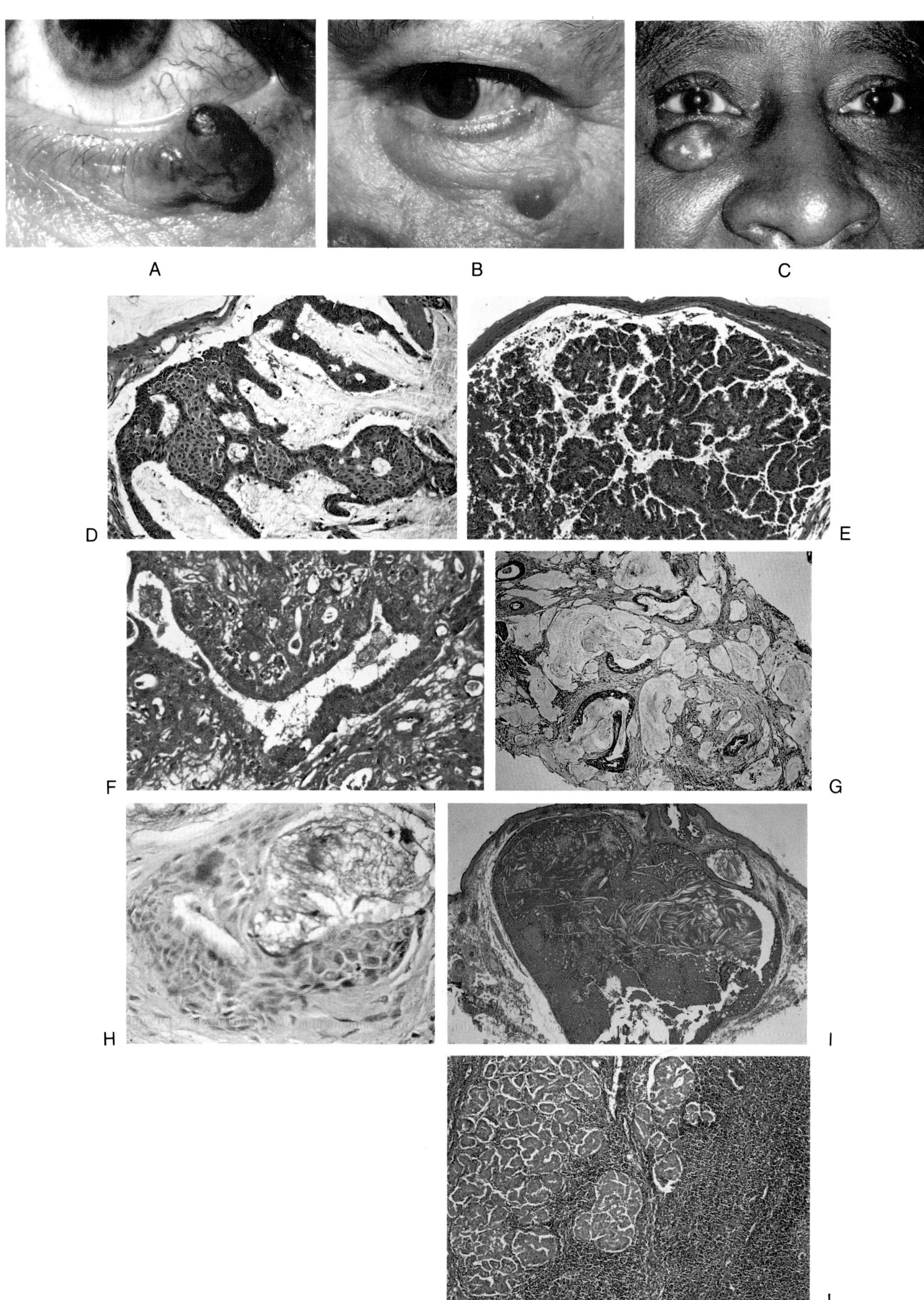

FIGURE 5–82 *See legend on opposite page*

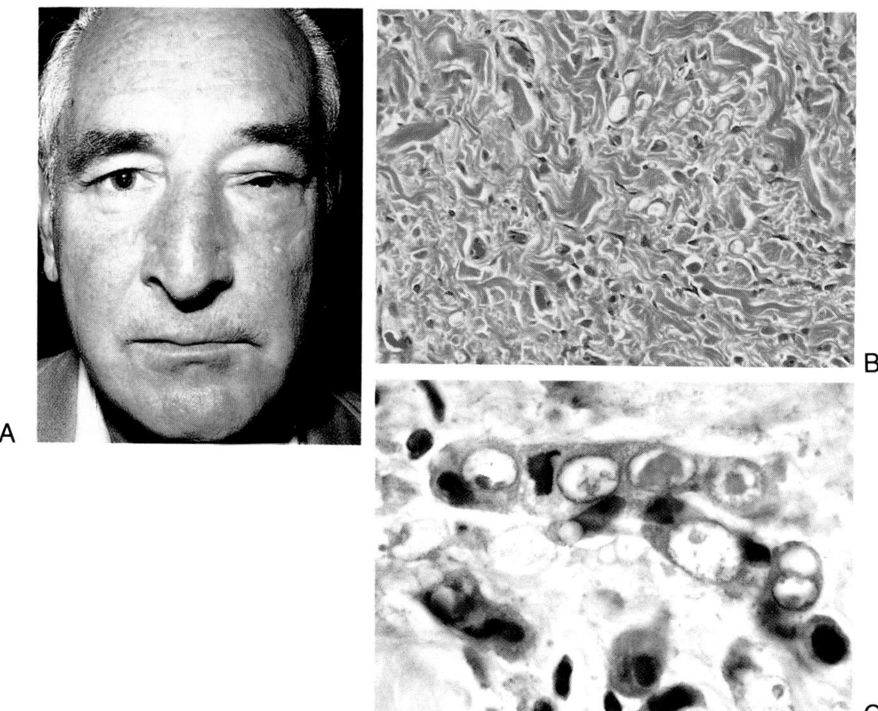

FIGURE 5–83 **Infiltrating signet ring carcinoma.** This rare tumor arises from eccrine or apocrine glands, can metastasize, and simulates a metastatic scirrhous carcinoma. *A*, The lower eyelid is involved by a diffusely infiltrating process. The vertical palpebral fissure is narrowed owing to upper eyelid involvement as well. (*A*, From Jakobiec FA, Austin P, Iwamoto T, et al: Primary infiltrating signet ring carcinoma of the eyelids. Ophthalmology 90:291–299, 1983.) *B*, Fibrotic collagenous stroma separates faintly staining epithelial cells that have invaded the deep dermis. H&E. (*B*, Courtesy of I. McLean, M.D.) *C*, The tumor cells are arranged in "Indian file," and they contain a foamy cytoplasm. A signet ring configuration is visible in cells containing a single vacuole.

◀ FIGURE 5–82 **Mucinous adenocarcinoma.** *A–C*, These illustrations demonstrate the variable clinical appearance of this potentially metastasizing eccrine gland neoplasm. The tumor can arise near the eyelid margin or from the eyelid skin in older men. Its coloration ranges from yellow to violaceous to flesh tone. *D*, This dermal nodule contains epithelial islands and cords. The clear areas contain mucin. H&E. *E*, A papillary configuration may be present. H&E. *F*, A tubular pattern may predominate. H&E. *G*, The tumor cells are separated by abundant amounts of mucin. H&E. *H*, Mucin is found both intracellularly and extracellularly. Mucicarmine. *I*, Degenerative changes including cholesterol clefts are found in tumor recurrences. H&E. *J*, This low-power photomicrograph shows a submandibular gland infiltrated by metastatic mucinous adenocarcinoma. H&E. (*A*, Courtesy of R. B. O'Grady, M.D. *B*, From Wright JD, Font RL: Mucinous adenocarcinoma of the eyelids: A clinicopathologic study of 21 cases with histochemical and electron microscopic observations. Cancer 44:1757–1768, 1979. *C*, *E–H*, Courtesy of R. L. Font, M.D.)

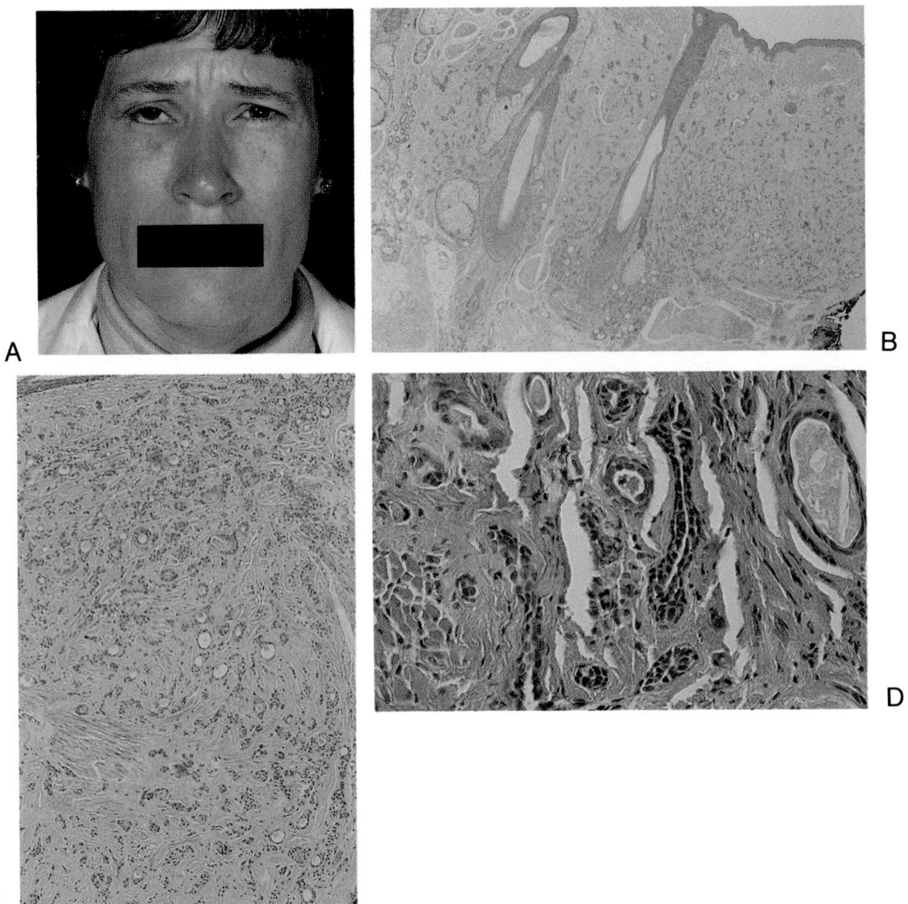

FIGURE 5–84 **Sclerosing sweat duct carcinoma.** Because of a dense collagenous stroma, lid retraction can develop, and orbital invasion can develop over a 10-year period. The tumor is generally nonmetastasizing. *A*, This woman has an indurated left lower eyelid. *B*, Low-power photomicrograph reveals a deeply infiltrative lesion composed of solid epithelial strands and microacini formed by small basaloid cells with scant cytoplasm. *C*, Small keratinous cysts with well-developed lamellar keratin alternate with the glandular lumina. *D*, Striated muscle is infiltrated by this neoplasia. *B–D*, H&E.

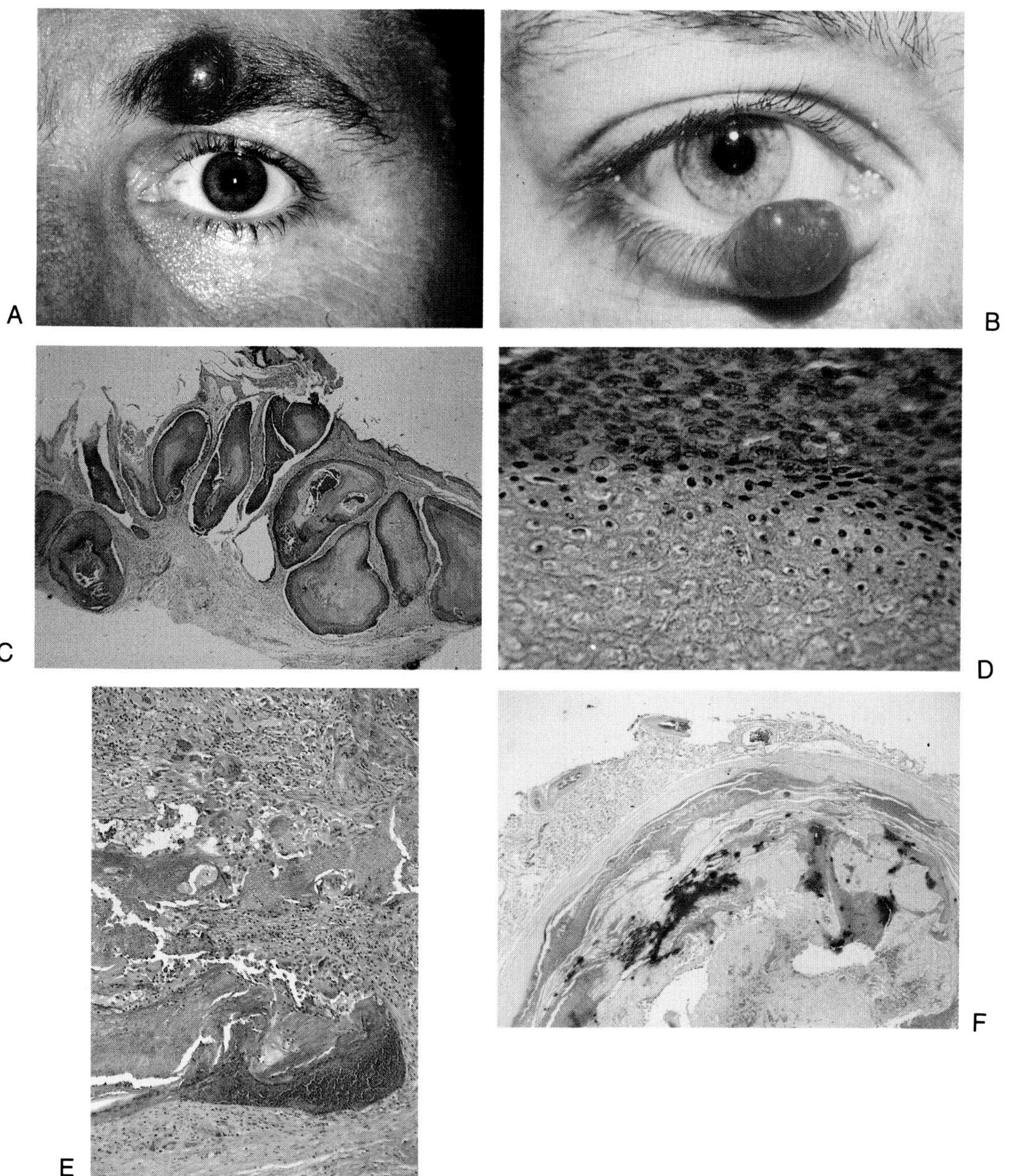

FIGURE 5-85 **Pilomatrixoma.** *A,* This young man had a freely mobile, subcutaneous mass of the left brow. Note the characteristic reddish pink color. *B,* This 24-year-old woman had a firm nodule of the lower eyelid margin. This benign tumor tends to develop in the strong hairs of the brow or eyelash regions. *C,* The excised specimen consists of several lobules limited to the dermis. Basophilic cells are found at the periphery of the lobules, and foci of calcification are present. The tumor arises deep in the dermis from the germinal cells of the hair bulb. H&E. *D,* Transition zone from basophilic cells to the more centrally located shadow cells. Intensely eosinophilic staining results from degeneration of shadow cell nuclei. H&E. *E,* The necrotic debris stimulates a granulomatous foreign body reaction. The presence of multinucleated giant cells and keratin debris can lead to confusion with dermoid cysts of the brow region. H&E. *F,* Dystrophic calcification begins as the shadow cells degenerate. Alizarin red.

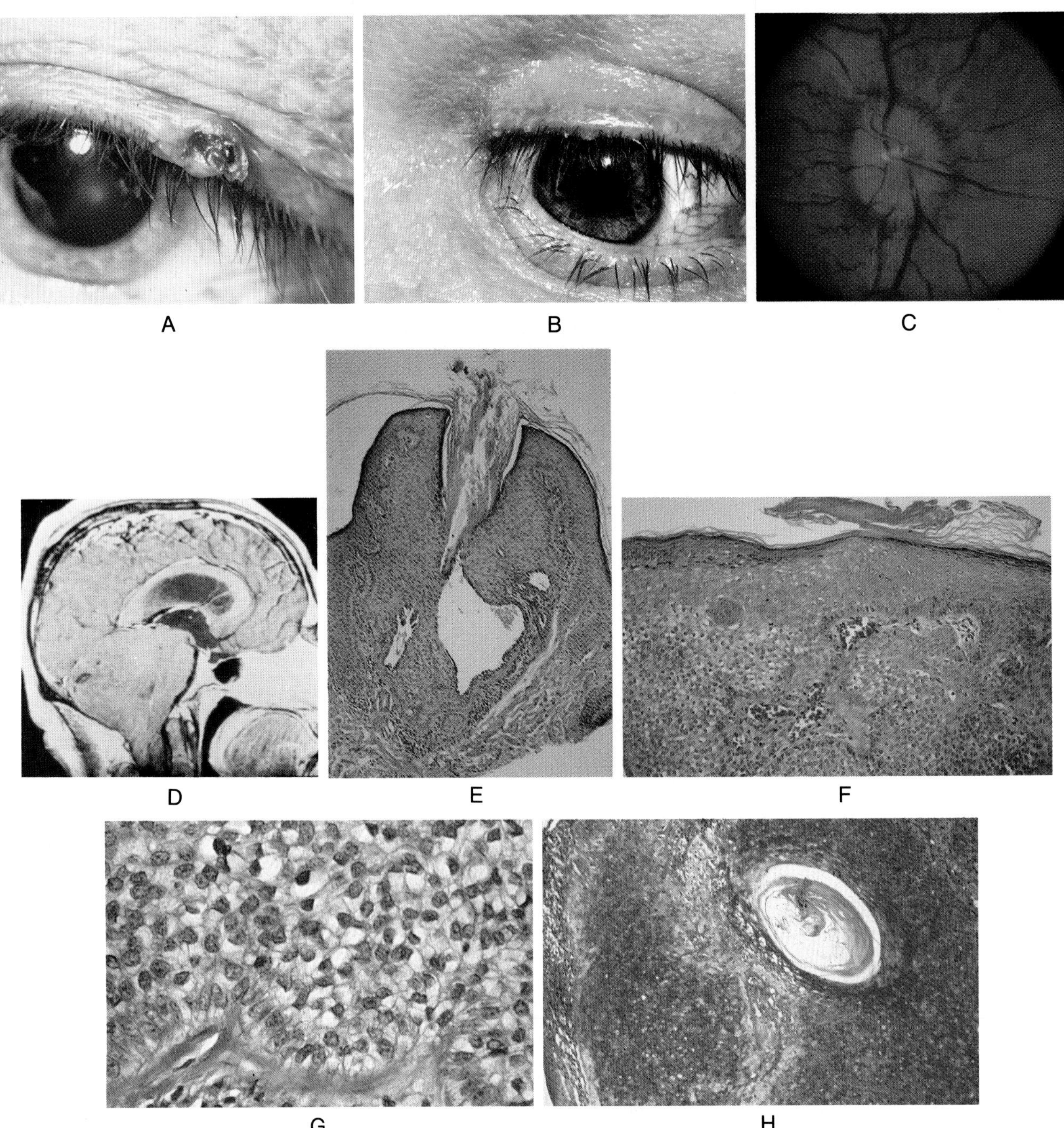

FIGURE 5–86 **Trichilemmoma.** The tumor arises from the epithelium of the hair shaft. *A,* Solitary nodule with surface ulceration and crusting. (*A,* Courtesy of R. Eagle, M.D.) *B,* Multiple flesh-colored papules resembling verrucae. *C,* Multiple trichilemmomas are associated with Cowden's syndrome. Such patients may develop breast or thyroid carcinoma. This patient suffered from papilledema. *D,* The increased intracranial pressure resulted from the cerebellar mass that characterizes the phakomatosis called Lhermitte-Duclose disease. (*C* and *D,* Courtesy of S. Lessell, M.D., and S. Hamilton, M.D.) *E,* The skin tumor displays marked acanthosis with palisading of polygonal to columnar epithelial cells at the periphery. Hyalinization is shown in the center. H&E. *F,* A thickened cuticular membrane encloses the tumor lobule. A squamous eddy and glycogen-rich clear cells are demonstrated. H&E. *G,* This high-power photomicrograph shows a relatively uniform set of small cells with round nuclei and clear cytoplasm. H&E. *H,* This periodic acid–Schiff stain demonstrates the presence of glycogen intracellularly. PAS.

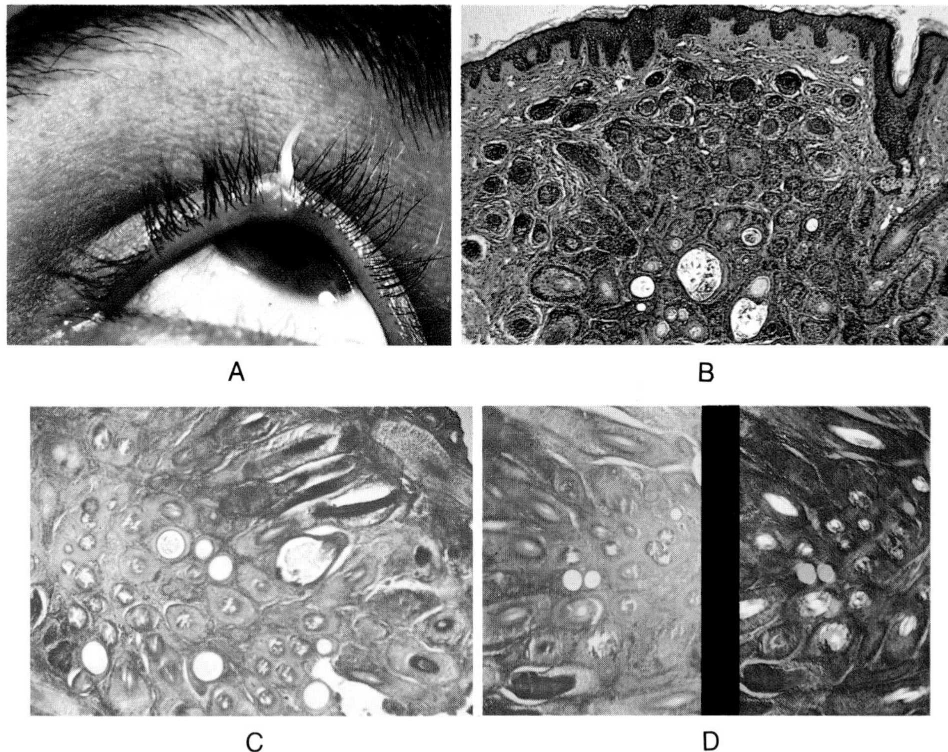

FIGURE 5–87 **Trichofolliculoma.** *A,* White wisp of lanugo hairs. This is the most highly differentiated tumor of hair origin. *B,* Several cystic spaces representing dilated hair follicles containing keratin. Attempts at hair follicle differentiation are seen radiating from these primary follicles. *C,* Differing levels of hair follicle differentiation. *D,* Polarized light depicts several small birefringent hair shafts in the lumina of the follicle. (The polarized light is on the right; the nonpolarized light is on the left.) *B–D,* H&E. (*A,* Courtesy of N. Charles, M.D.)

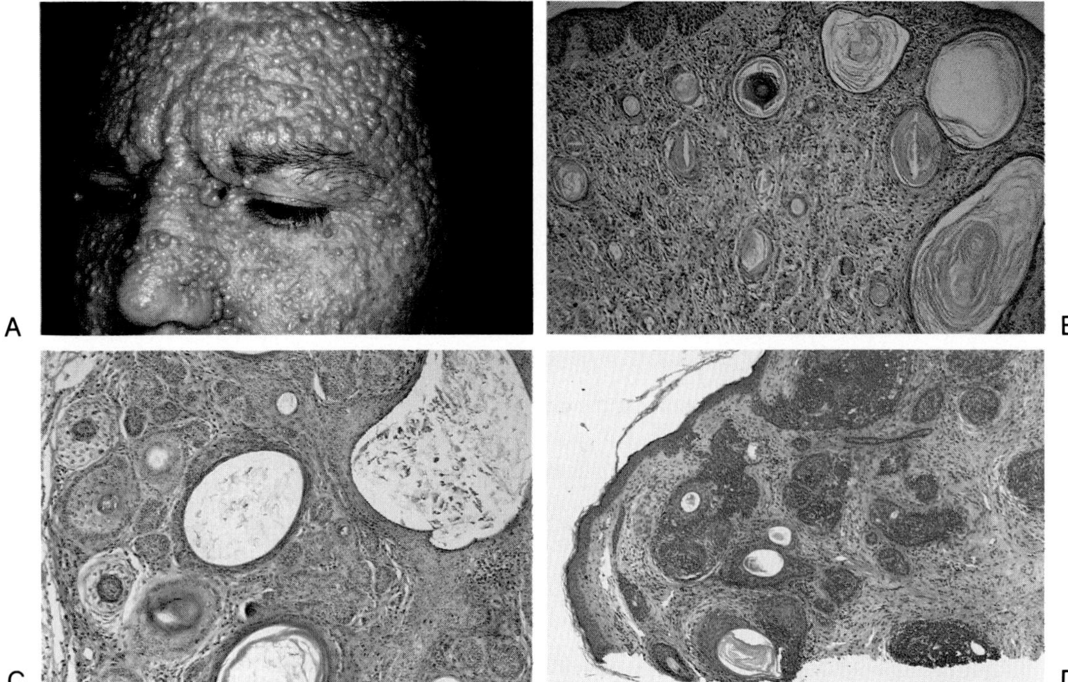

FIGURE 5–88 **Multiple trichoepitheliomas (Brooke's tumor).** This is a hair tumor with only primitive differentiation. *A*, Multiple trichoepitheliomas involving the entire face. The left medial canthal region displayed an ulceration that proved to be a basal cell carcinoma, which can rarely complicate this condition. *B*, Extensive replacement of the dermis with numerous keratin-filled cysts (abortive hair canals). H&E. *C*, Basophilic cells with peripheral palisading surround multiple horn cysts. This lesion may be histologically difficult to differentiate from keratinizing cutaneous basal cell carcinoma. H&E. *D*, A desmoplastic variant with a thickened, sclerotic stroma. This pattern is similar to sclerosing basal cell epithelioma except for the abundance of horn cysts. (*A*, Courtesy of Lewis Shapiro, M.D.)

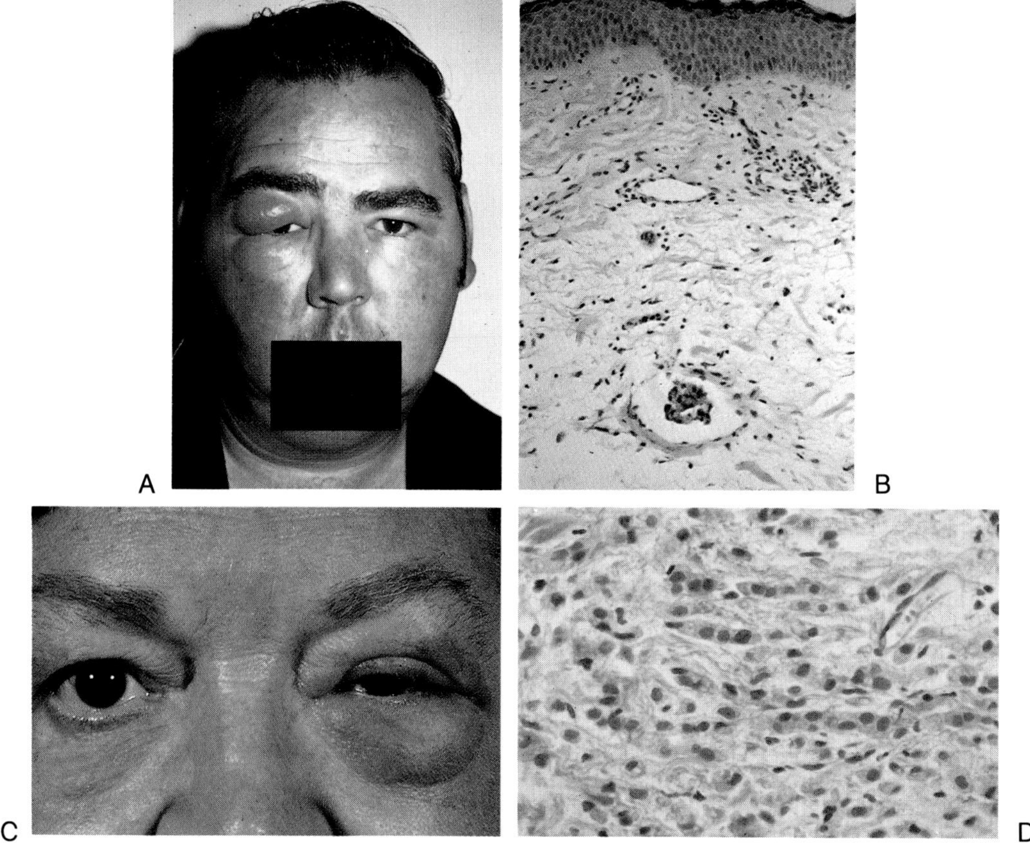

FIGURE 5–89 **Metastatic carcinoma to the eyelids.** *A,* A 54-year-old man with chemotic eyelids. The skin has a peau d'orange appearance. *B,* Carcinomatous cells within the eyelid lymphatics. The primary tumor was presumed to be of gastrointestinal origin. H&E. *C,* Painless swelling and pseudoinflammatory nodular induration of the left eyelids in a 56-year-old woman with a history of breast carcinoma. *D,* Collagen fibers separate tumor cells that contain large cytoplasmic lumina and that are arranged in an Indian file. The "histiocytoid" tumor cells contain one large intracytoplasmic vacuole (signet ring cell) rather than myriad ones of true histiocytes. H&E.

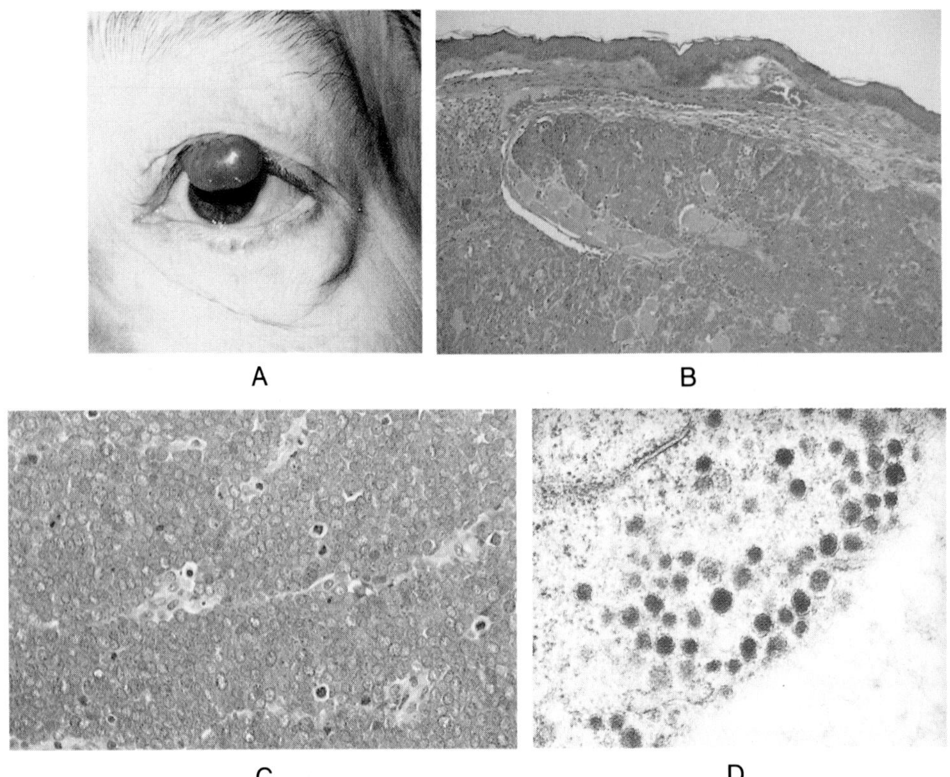

FIGURE 5–90 **Merkel cell tumor.** This tumor is capable of metastasis and arises from an intraepidermal sensory cell. *A*, Red-violaceous lid margin tumor. (*A*, Courtesy of Professor O. A. Jensen.) *B*, Trabecular pattern limited to the dermis. H&E. *C*, Sheets of tumor cells with uniform nuclei and scant cytoplasm. Numerous mitotic figures are present. The tumor can be mistakenly diagnosed as an amelanotic melanoma or a lymphoma. H&E. *D*, This electron micrograph discloses dense secretory granules that contain catecholamine products. (*D*, Courtesy of G. Klintworth, M.D.)

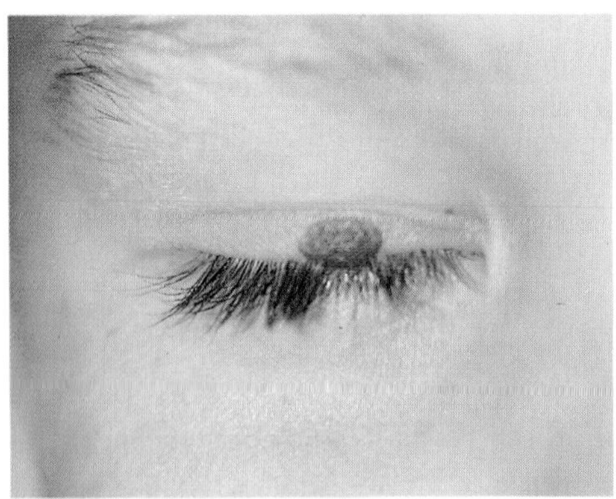

FIGURE 5–91 **Compound nevus on the upper eyelid of a young woman.** The discrete pigmented nodule encroaches on the superior lash margin. The lesion had not been growing for several years. Melanoma is rare on the eyelid skin of individuals less than 20 years of age.

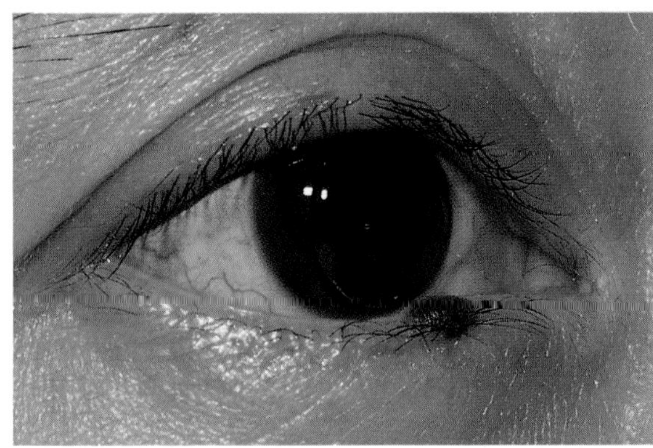

FIGURE 5–92 **Dermal nevus of the eyelid margin.** Lashes project from the surface of the pigmented nodule, which has not changed in appearance in many years.

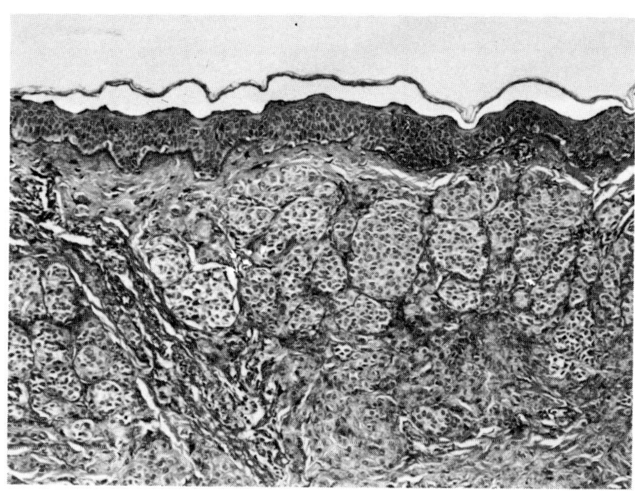

FIGURE 5–93 **Nevocellular dermal nevus.** Well-organized nests of uniform cells fill the papillary dermis. Nuclei are centrally located, and cellular cytoplasm is abundant. For a compound nevus, which occurs in younger persons, there should be intraepidermal as well as dermal nests. H&E.

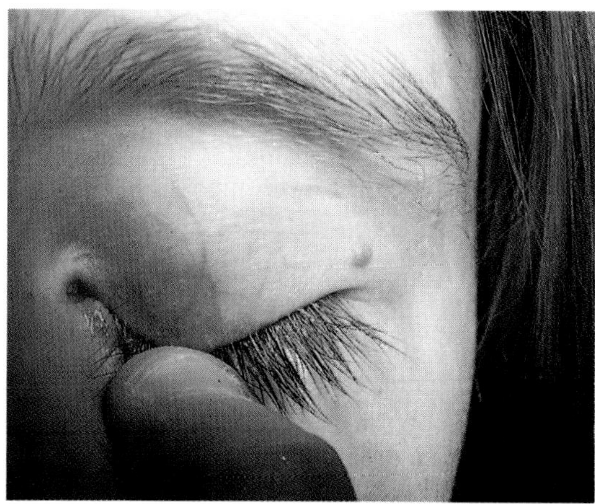

FIGURE 5–95 **Spindle and epithelioid cell nevus (Spitz nevus) of the upper eyelid.** The small flesh-colored nodule cannot be distinguished from a common nevus clinically but tends to develop more rapidly in children. The diagnosis of Spitz nevus was established by excisional biopsy. (Courtesy of Kenneth Burwell, M.D.)

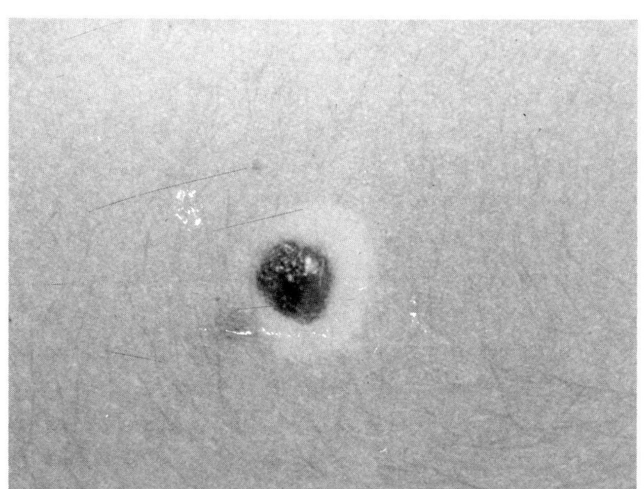

FIGURE 5–94 **Halo nevus surrounded by a rim of nonpigmented skin.** This represents an inflammatory attack (regression) on the benign tumor cells. This lesion should raise the possibility of an occult melanoma elsewhere or can be an isolated event. (Courtesy of Frank Flowers, M.D.)

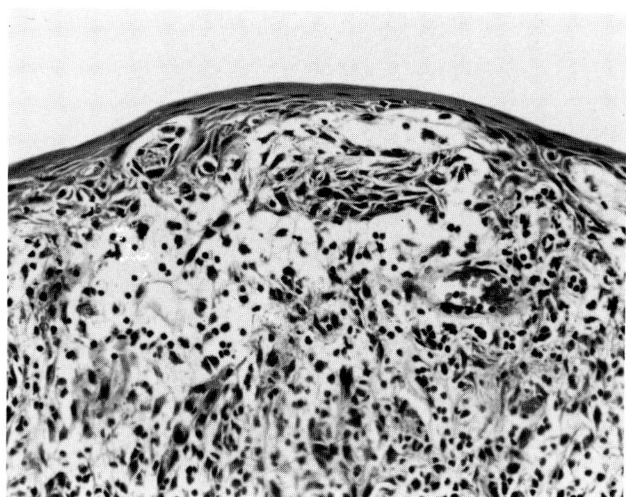

FIGURE 5–96 Histopathologic appearance of a Spitz nevus in a 9-year-old child shows loosely cohesive, round and spindle-shaped cells in the basal epithelium and upper dermis. Ill-defined nests of melanocytes are present at the dermal-epidermal junction. H&E.

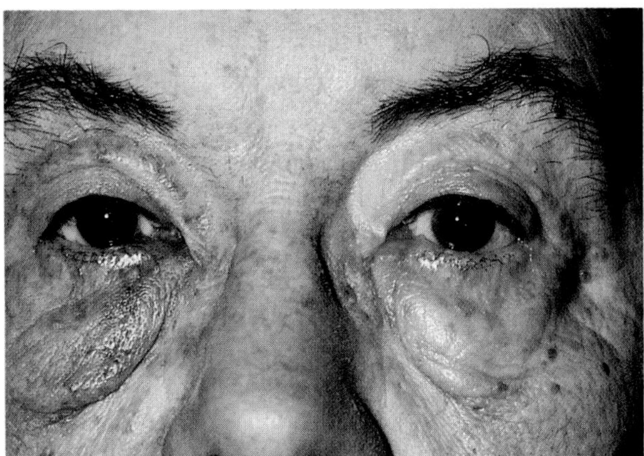

FIGURE 5–97 Nevus of Ota characterized by large gray-blue discoloration of the right lower eyelid. The lesion is congenital, impalpable, and flat and is associated with gray episcleral discoloration. The melanocytes are located in the dermis rather than the epidermis. Uveal melanocytosis with a modest chance of melanoma developing requires periodic intraocular examinations.

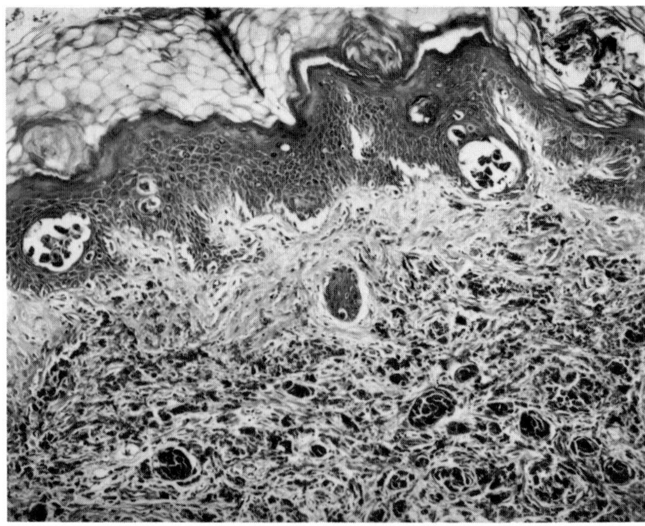

FIGURE 5–99 Histopathologic appearance of a congenital nevus that displays surface hyperkeratosis. Melanocytes are found in nests and are also found individually in the epidermis. The dermis contains heavily pigmented nevus cells. H&E.

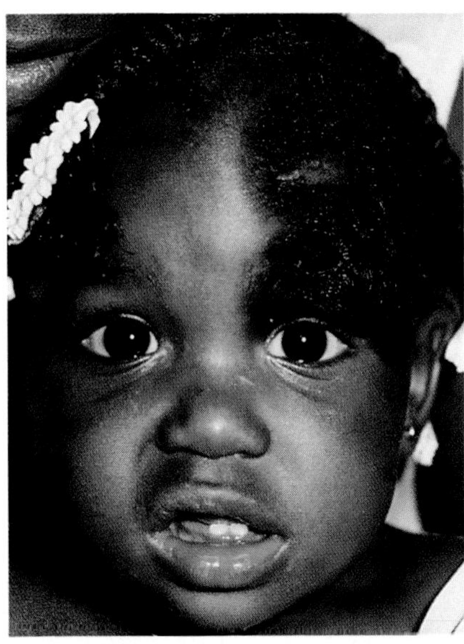

FIGURE 5–98 A large congenital nevus involving the upper eyelid and extending into the scalp. The nevus is elevated and indurated and covered with hair. It is analogous to large bathing trunk nevi of the torso. This periocular lesion has a modest potential for malignant transformation. (From Margo CE, Habal MB: Large congenital melanocytic nevus: Light and electron microscopic findings. Ophthalmology 94:960, 1987.)

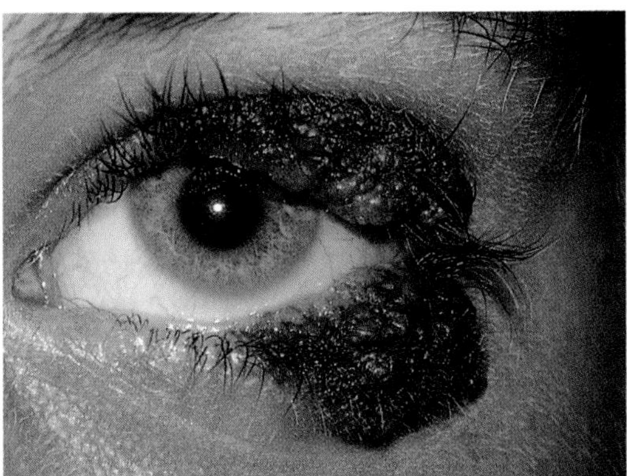

FIGURE 5–100 **Small congenital nevus of upper and lower eyelids (so-called kissing nevus).** This pigmented verrucous tumor, although large for a typical acquired eyelid nevus, is less than 2 cm at its greatest diameter and is thus considered "small" for a congenital nevus. It has a negligible potential for malignant transformation. The lesion forms when the eyelids are fused in utero and excessive numbers of neural crest melanocytes invade the lid anlagen symmetrically.

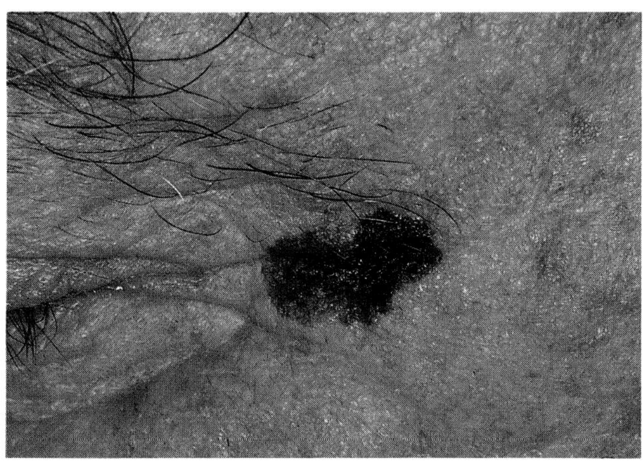

FIGURE 5–101 **Lentigo maligna of the outer canthal skin.** The dark brown lesion is flat and develops over 5 to 15 years in sun-exposed skin in older individuals. When flat, it is premalignant, and nodule formation signifies malignant transformation (lentigo maligna melanoma). (Courtesy of Frank Flowers, M.D.)

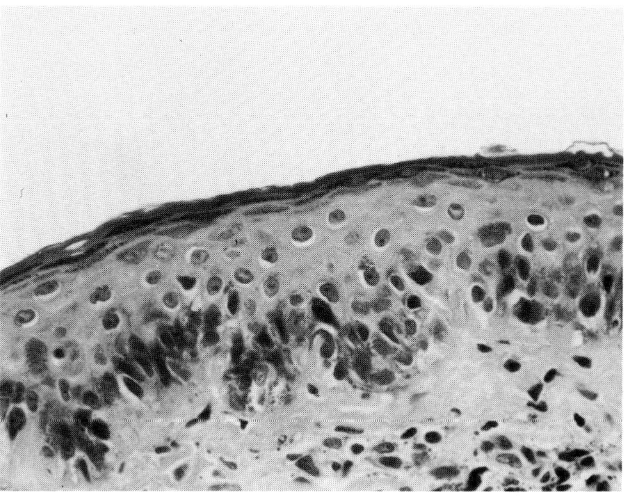

FIGURE 5–103 Histopathologic features of lentigo maligna showing a proliferation of atypical basal melanocytes entirely restricted to the basal region of epidermis. H&E.

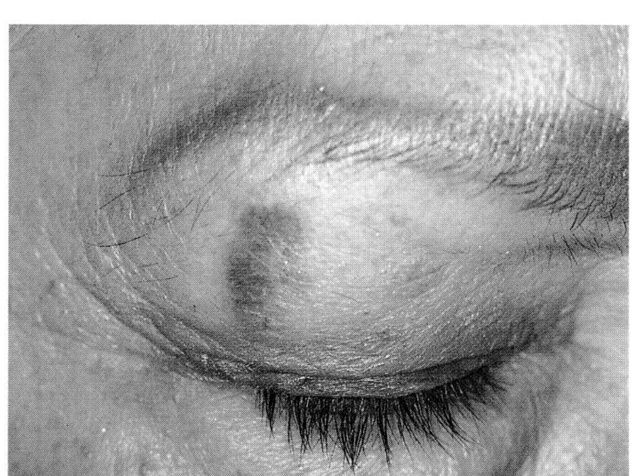

FIGURE 5–102 **Lentigo maligna of the right upper eyelid.** The macule has a patchy light tan color. It developed slowly and remained a flat, impalpable lesion.

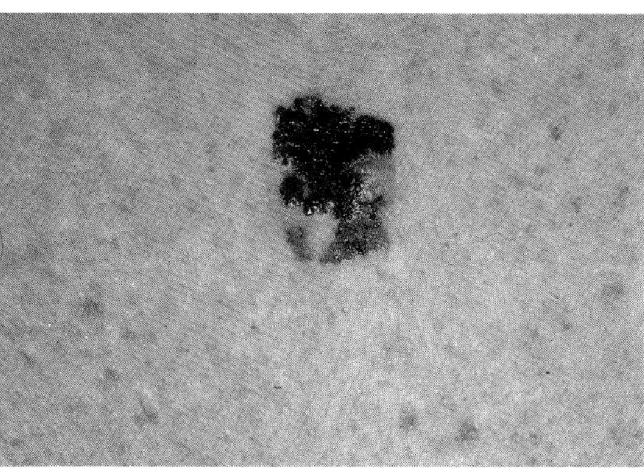

FIGURE 5–104 **Superficial spreading melanoma.** This is an aggressive lesion capable of early and late metastasis. The elevated multinodular lesion is characterized by its variegated colors and develops over 2 to 5 years, not necessarily in sun-exposed skin. Patches of pink and flesh are admixed with dark brown. The flat areas represent a radial growth phase of cells within the epidermis, and elevated areas represent vertical growth into the dermis. Lesions measuring less than 0.75 mm of thickness usually do not metastasize, whereas lesions of 3.0-mm thickness have an 80% chance of metastasizing. (Courtesy of Frank Flowers, M.D.)

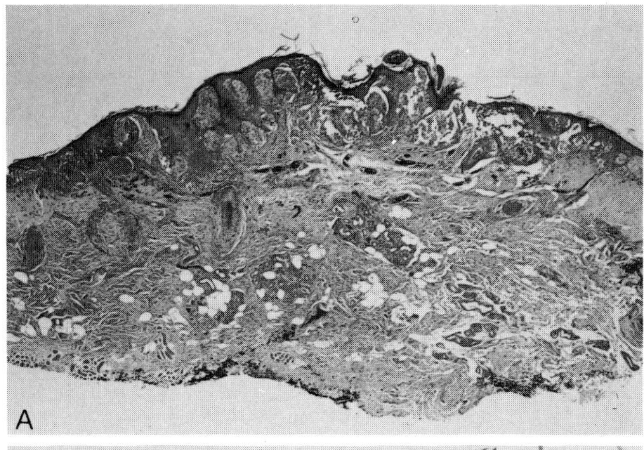

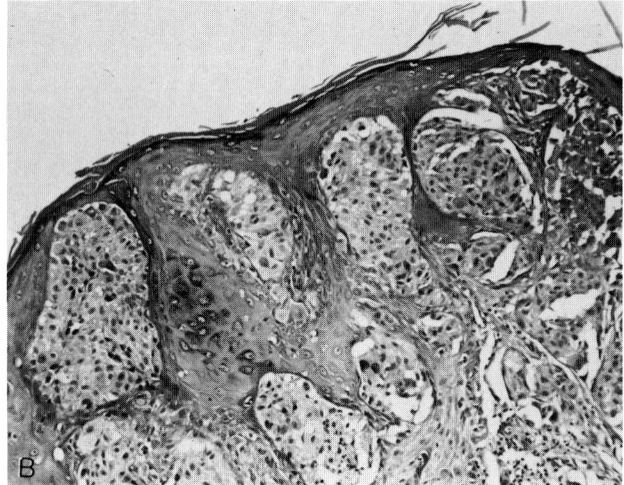

FIGURE 5-105 *A,* Histologically a superficial spreading melanoma displays clusters of atypical melanocytes in the epidermis and papillary dermis. *B,* Atypical melanocytes within the epidermis form nests. H&E.

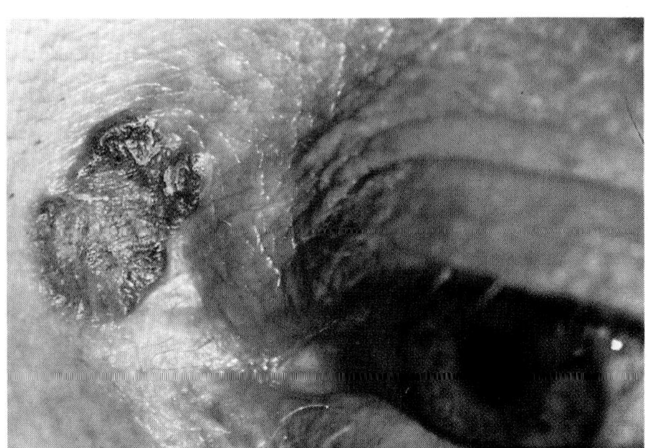

FIGURE 5-106 **Pigmented basal cell carcinoma of the medial canthal skin.** This ulcerated, infiltrated tumor cannot be clinically distinguished from a malignant melanoma except that it feels more hyperkeratotic than a melanoma. It occurs in darkly complexioned people, and the melanocytes are passively carried along by the neoplastic basal cells. (From Resnick RI, Sadun A, Albert DM: Basal cell epithelioma: An unusual case. Ophthalmology 88:1182, 1981.)

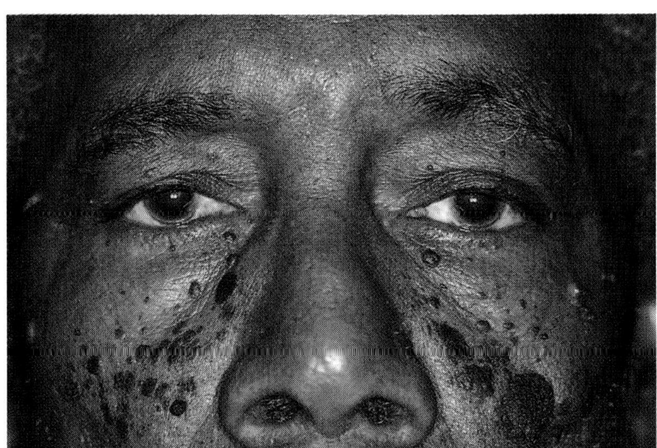

FIGURE 5-107 Multiple pigmented seborrheic keratoses in a black patient with a pulmonary plasmacytoma. The development in late adulthood of numerous seborrheic keratoses, particularly when as large as these, can be associated with visceral malignancies. Younger black women can develop clusters of smaller lesions (dermatosis papulosa nigra) without ominous systemic implications.

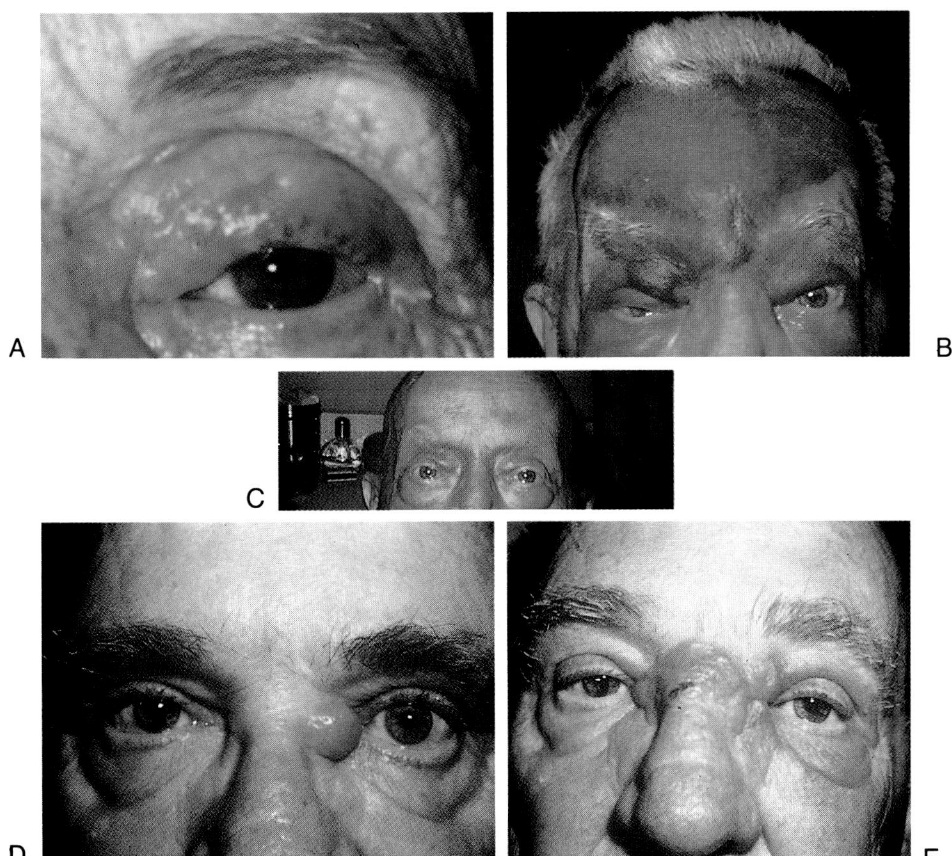

FIGURE 5–108 **Angiosarcoma.** This is an extremely rare eyelid tumor. *A,* There is a nodular thickening of the left upper eyelid extending from the medial canthus and the nose to the lateral aspect of the lid. There is also slight ptosis and periorbital edema. (*A,* courtesy of C. I. Hood, M.D.) *B,* Multicentric tumor of the forehead and eyelids with an ecchymotic appearance. *C,* The same patient shown in *B* after receiving a course of definitive external beam radiation therapy of 4600 rads. There is considerable regression of the tumor, but dermatochalasis of the eyelids persists. (*B* and *C,* Courtesy of J. Caya, M.D.) *D,* A 76-year-old man had a 1-year history of a left medial canthal lesion arising in the region of the lacrimal sac. There was patent irrigation through the nasolacrimal drainage apparatus. A wide local excision was performed. *E,* The tumor recurred and has spread across the bridge of the nose to the contralateral medial canthal region. The tumor was poorly responsive to radiotherapy, and the patient eventually succumbed from intracranial extension. (*D* and *E,* Courtesy of S. Searl, M.D., and R. Kennedy, M.D.)

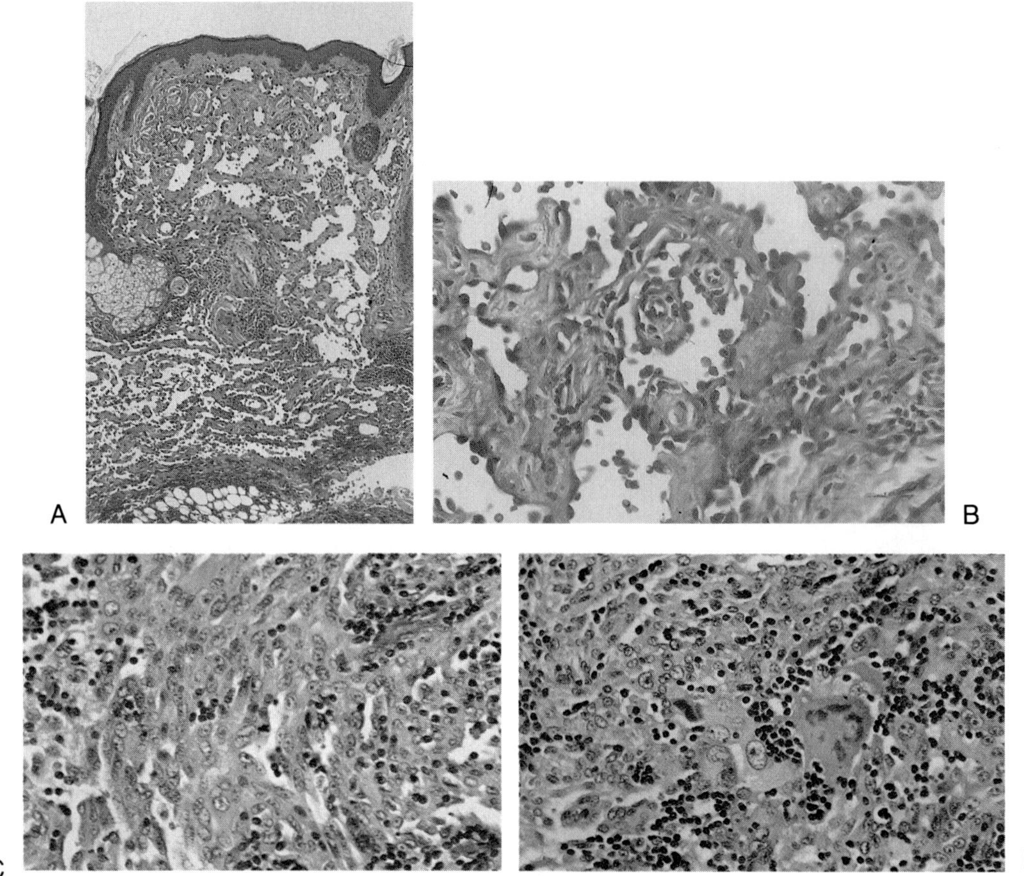

FIGURE 5–109 **Histopathologic features of angiosarcoma.** *A,* The dermis is infiltrated by a tumor composed of irregular and interanastomosing vascular channels that create a network of sinusoids. *B,* The vascular channels are lined by malignant endothelial cells with large and hyperchromatic nuclei. In some areas, the malignant cells have piled up along the lumina, creating papillations that are typical of angiosarcoma. *C,* Hyperchromatic tumor cells forming solid masses as well as slitlike vascular spaces have an eosinophilic cytoplasm, sometimes leading to the designation of epithelioid-histiocytoid malignant hemangioendothelioma. Note the background infiltration of lymphocytes. *D,* More pleomorphic region of the tumor with less obvious lumen formation and pleomorphic giant cell formation. In some instances, angiosarcomas can be high-grade tumors that are difficult to distinguish from carcinomas or pleomorphic fibrosarcomas. The demonstration of ulex or Factor VIII positivity can help to make the correct diagnosis. *A–D,* H&E. (C and *D,* Courtesy of S. Searl, M.D.)

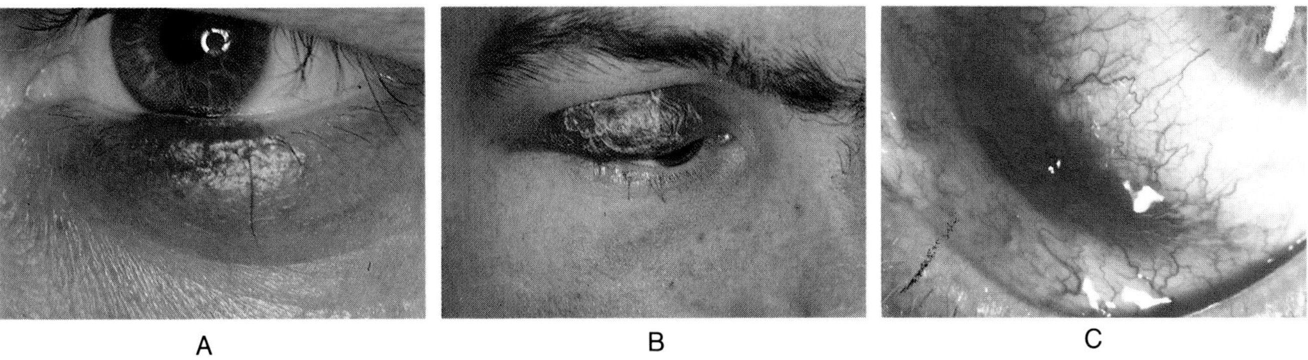

FIGURE 5–110 **Kaposi's sarcoma.** *A*, An indurated erythematous lesion of the lower eyelid in a patient with acquired immunodeficiency syndrome (AIDS). *B*, An eschar-like thickening with surface hyperkeratosis and a deep violaceous hue of the upper eyelid in Kaposi's sarcoma. *C*, In the conjunctiva, a typical location for Kaposi's sarcoma in patients with AIDS is seen in the inferior fornix, where a much brighter and beefier red lesion is presented, owing to the transparency of the overlying nonkeratinizing squamous epithelium. (*A* and *B*, Courtesy of H. Perry, M.D.)

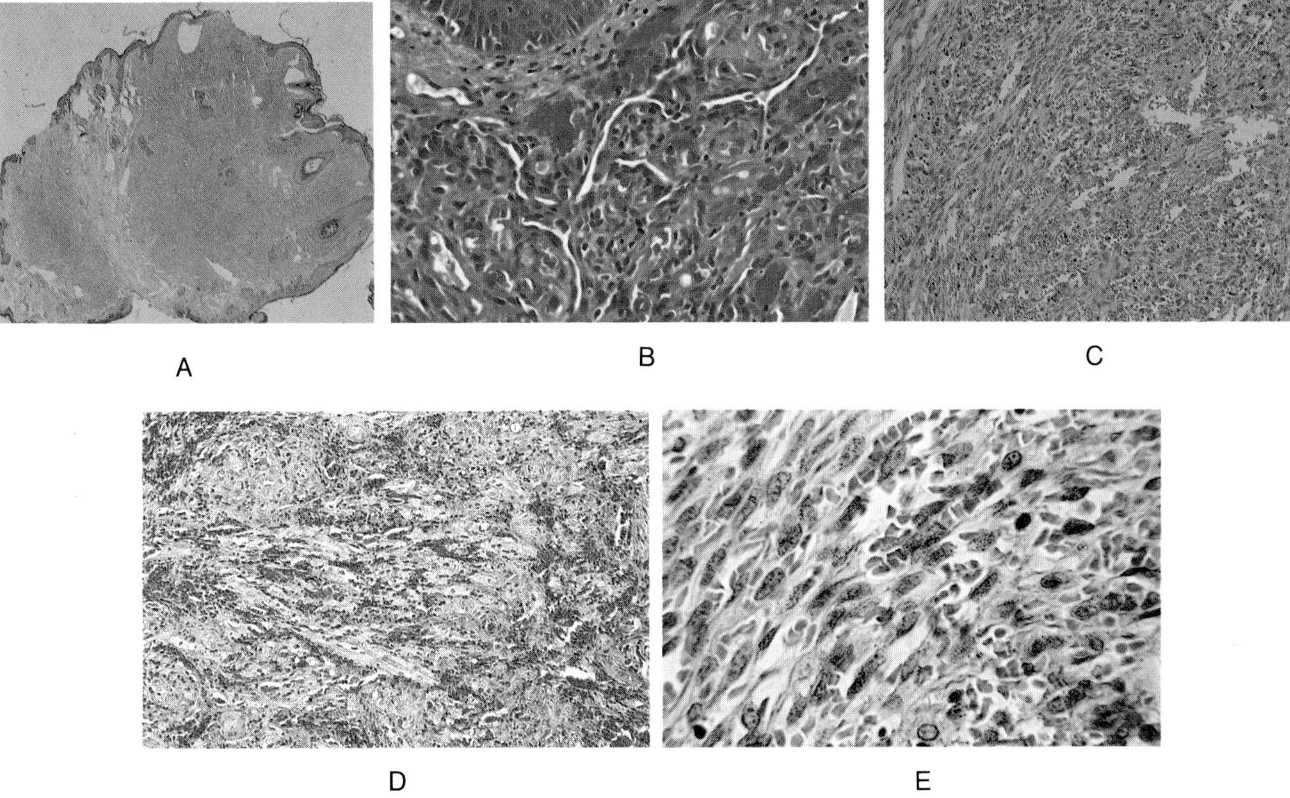

FIGURE 5–111 **Histopathologic features of Kaposi's sarcoma.** *A*, A hypercellular proliferation is situated within the dermis. *B*, The early stages of Kaposi's sarcoma may be difficult to distinguish from granulation tissue. Note above that the lesion consists of numerous proliferating capillaries with plump endothelial cells and a wispy proliferation of more immature spindle cells around the newly formed vessels. *C*, This hypercellular tumor consists of a combination of spindled areas blending with angiomatous areas. The spindled areas resemble a well-differentiated fibrosarcoma except that they manifest slitlike vascular spaces containing erythrocytes and merge with attenuated vascular lumina lined by recognizable endothelium. *D*, There is less evidence of lumen formation in this tumor, which consists predominantly of spindle cells. The extensive hemorrhagic foci and occasional clefts within the lesion are useful artifacts pointing toward the probable diagnosis of Kaposi's sarcoma. *E*, Spindle cells without clear-cut lumen formation have many percolating erythrocytes between them. Hemosiderin deposits may also form from extravasated erythrocytes. *A–E*, H&E. (*B*, Courtesy of H. Perry, M.D.)

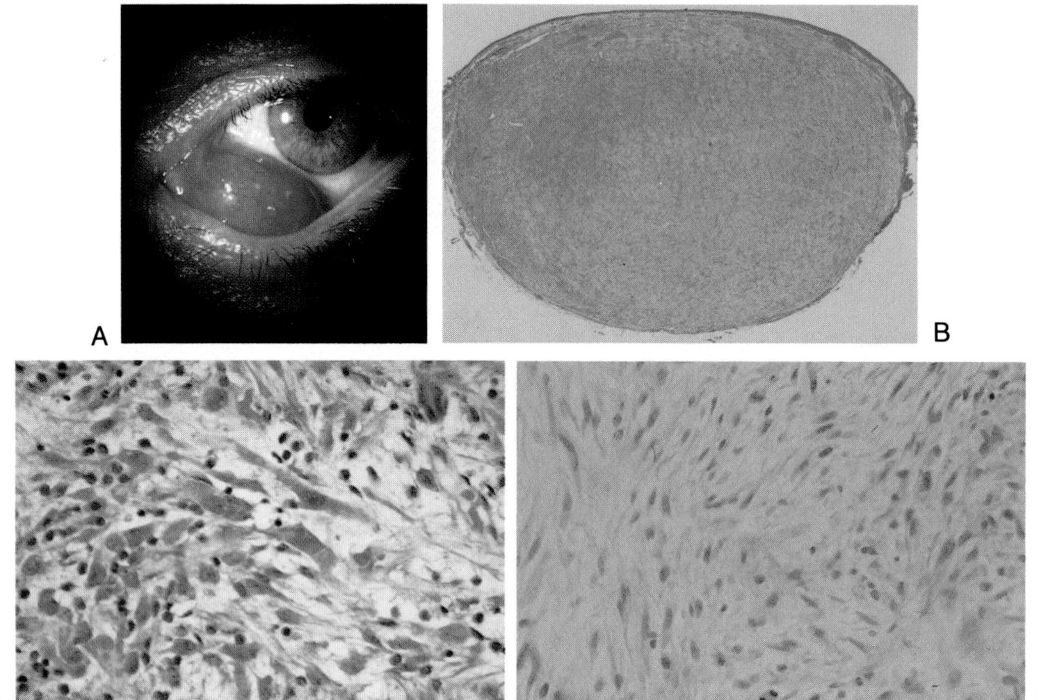

FIGURE 5–112 **Nodular fasciitis.** *A,* Rapidly developing, violaceous mass situated in the inferior fornix, anterior orbit, and inferior palpebral conjunctiva. *B,* The excised benign nodule displays cellular regions alternating with paler myxoid areas. *C,* Somewhat immature and pleomorphic-looking cells are proliferating and extending cytoplasmic processes into a loose matrix, which is often Alcian blue positive because of the presence of hyaluronic acid. Note the infiltrating lymphocytes. *D,* A looser proliferation of fibroblasts without a conspicuous inflammatory infiltrate. A mitotic figure is shown toward the bottom of the field. *B–D,* H&E. (*A–C,* Courtesy of A. Perry, M.D.)

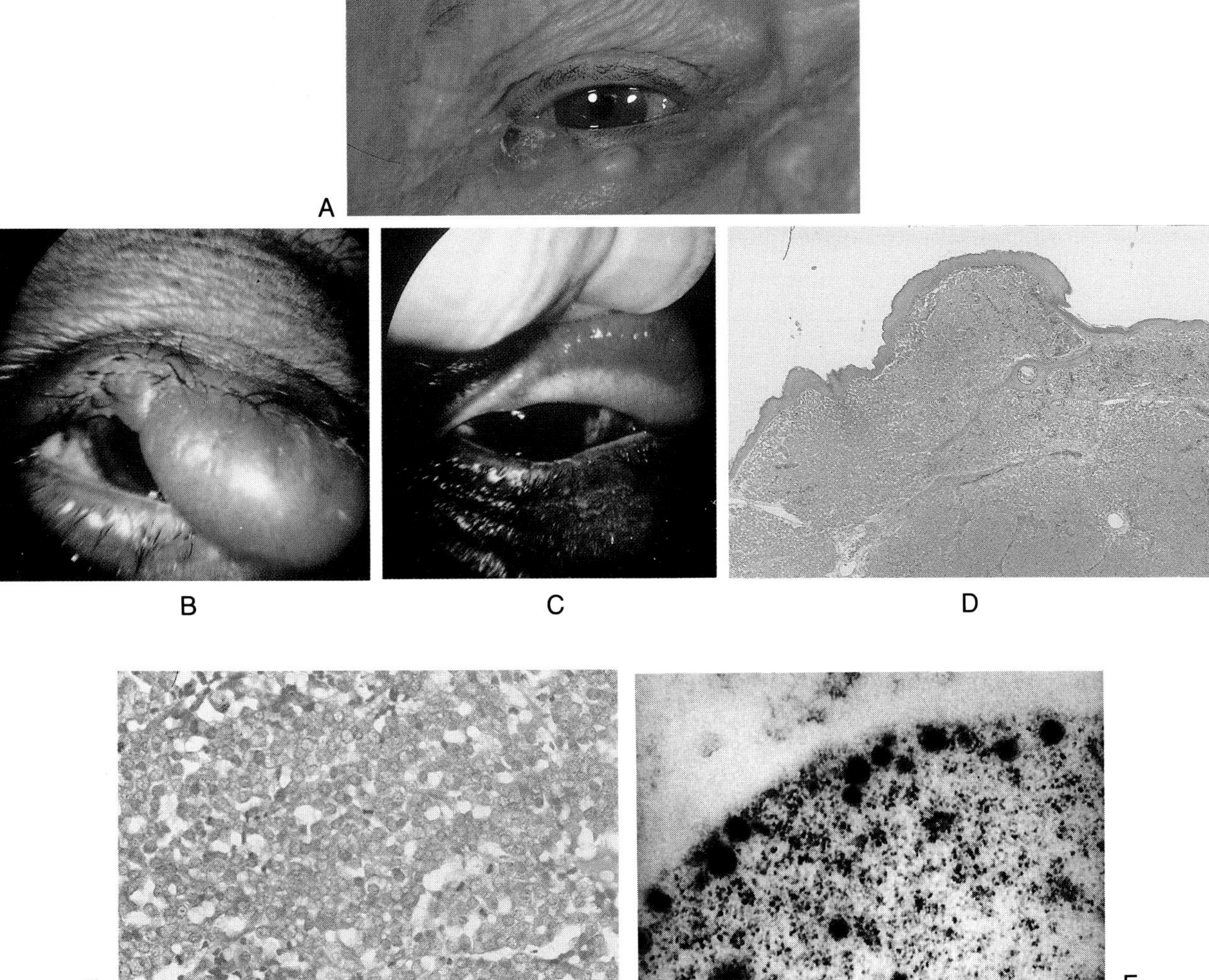

FIGURE 5–113 **Merkel cell tumors.** *A*, The red color of this tumor in an older patient is a common feature, but the partial ulceration is atypical. Adnexal carcinomas, such as mucinous adenocarcinoma, should be considered in the clinical differential diagnosis. *B*, The surface of this bulky lesion is smooth and shiny without ulceration, and there are telangiectatic vessels scattered throughout. In contrast to sebaceous carcinoma, the cilia are preserved. *C*, On eversion of the eyelid of the patient shown in *B*, a more obvious reddish discoloration of the base of the lesion is observed. *D*, The dermis is infiltrated by sheets of small round cells. *E*, The tumor consists of uniformly round cells with pale vesicular nuclei, sparse cytoplasm, and many mitotic figures. Both large round cell lymphoma and amelanotic melanoma are frequently offered as mistaken diagnoses. *F*, An electron micrograph displaying several membrane-bound neurosecretory granules along the cytoplasmic border of a tumor cell. *D* and *E*, H&E. (*A*, Courtesy of G. Klintworth, M.D.)

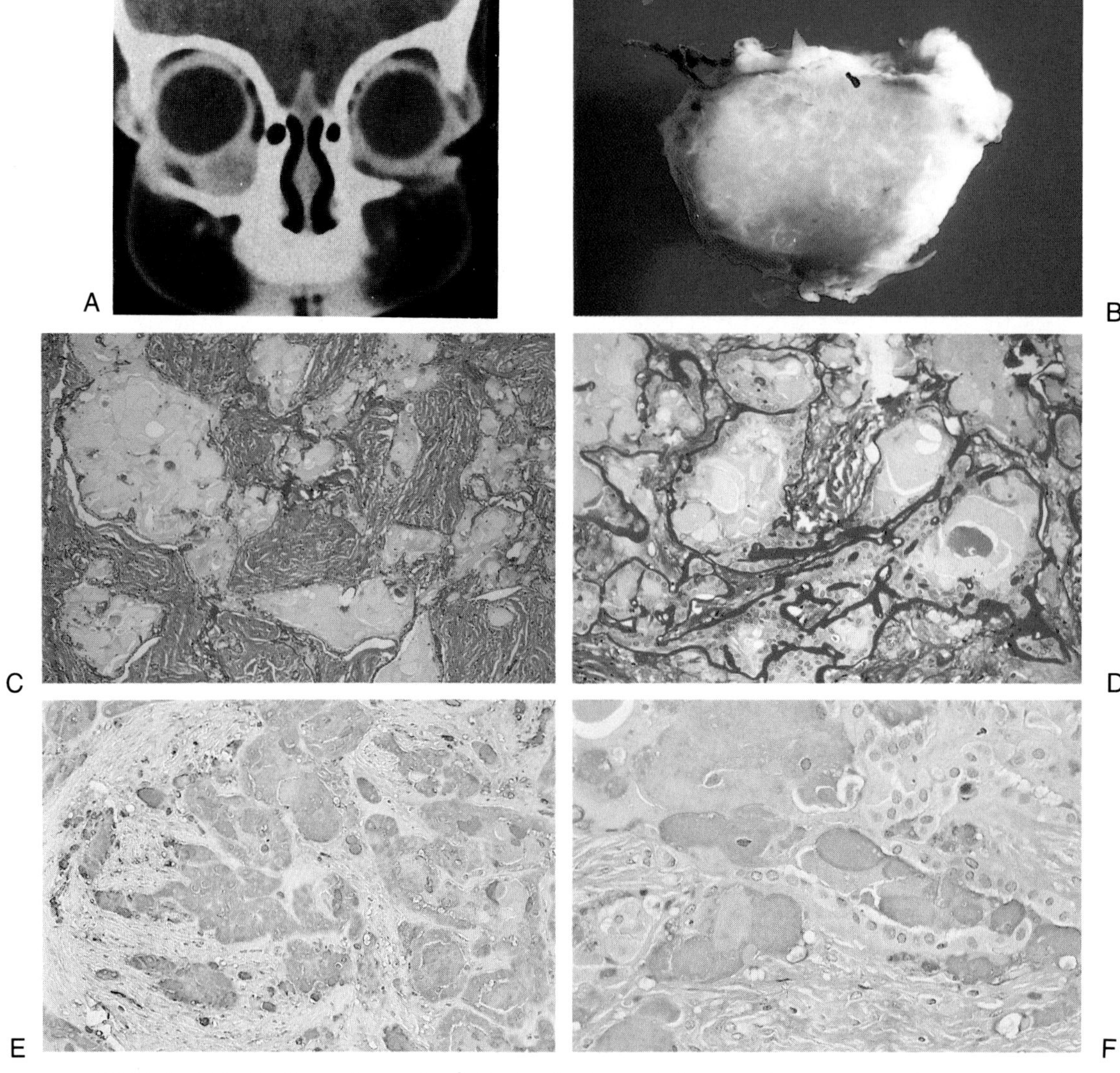

FIGURE 5–114 **Phakomatous choristoma.** *A,* Computed coronal tomogram of a congenital lesion that was palpable through the inferomedial eyelid and extends to the equator of the globe. It measured approximately 1.5 cm in greatest diameter. *B,* The excised specimen is unencapsulated but has good circumscription. Note the trabeculation throughout the cut surface, indicating the alternation of the collagen with collections of tumor cells. *C,* Large swollen bladder cells (like cataractous Wedl cells) are present in the central portions of the lobules of the tumor cells and are surrounded on their outer perimeter by a low cuboidal epithelium. Note the fibrotic stroma. *D,* The PAS stain outlines a thickened basement membrane, simulating the capsule of the lens. *E,* Positive staining of most of the lobular cellular masses with an antibody to cytoplasmic α lens protein (crystallin). *F,* Positive staining for β-protein (crystallin) tends to spare the outer cuboidal cells. C, H&E. (*A, B, E,* and *F,* Courtesy of R. Eagle, M.D., and Jerry Shields, M.D.)

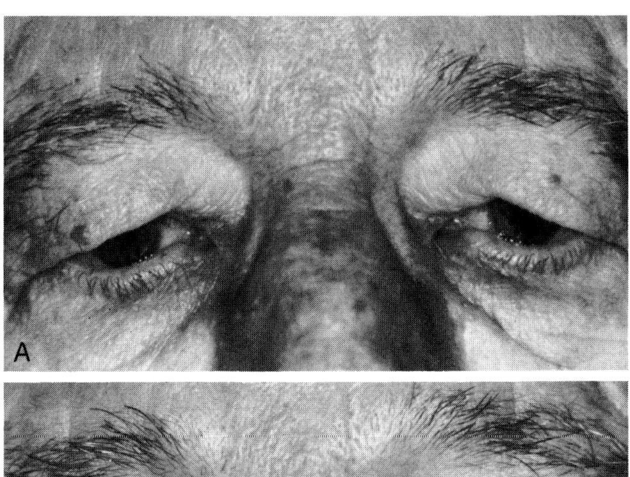

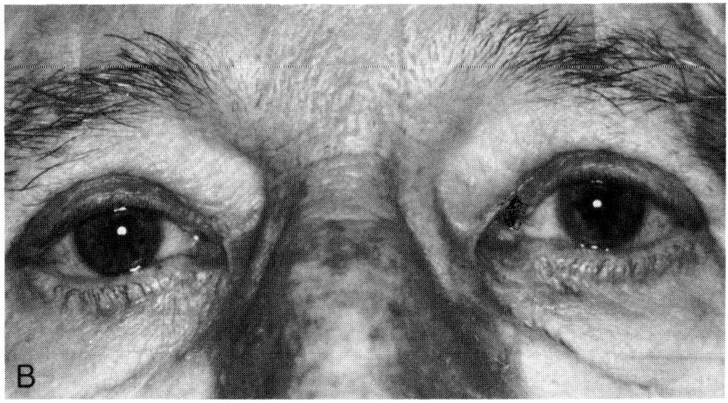

FIGURE 5–115 *A*, Pseudoptosis resulting from dermatochalasis. Excess upper eyelid skin and orbicularis muscle hang over upper lid margin of both eyes. *B*, Appearances after correction of dermatochalasis with a bilateral upper eyelid blepharoplasty.

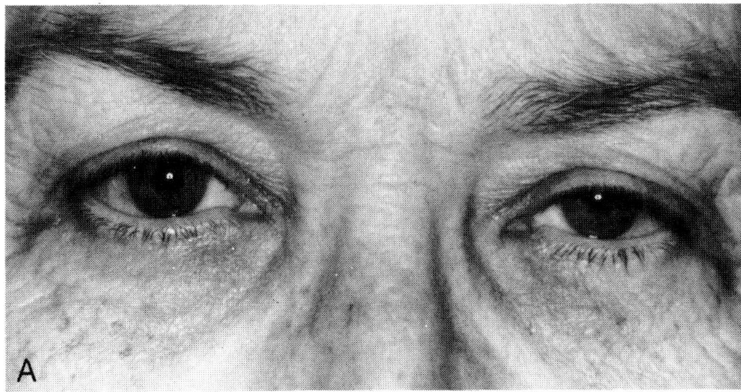

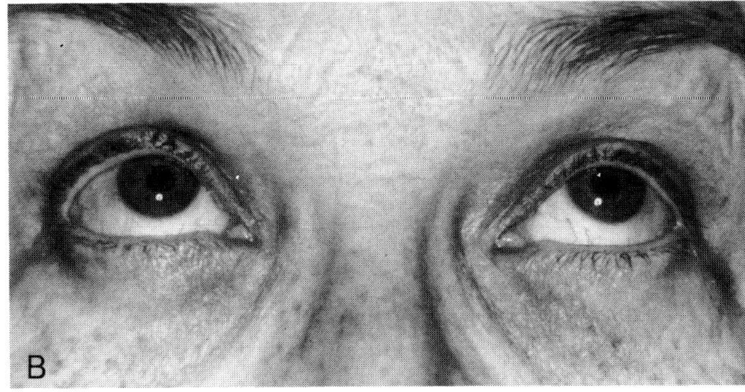

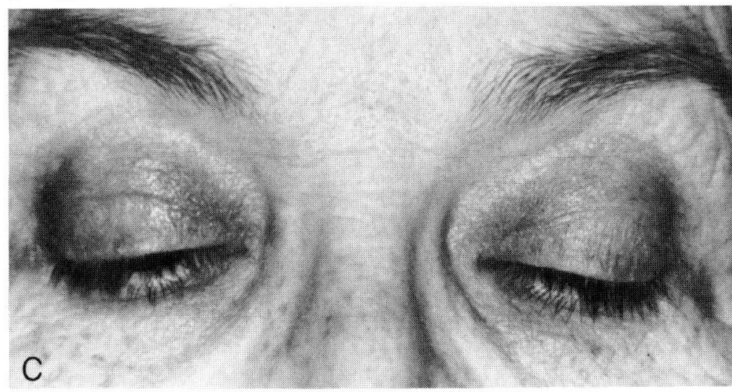

FIGURE 5–116 Asymmetric bilateral aponeurogenic ptosis. *A*, Primary gaze. *B*, Upgaze. *C*, Downgaze. Note the good upper lid excursion (levator function) and asymmetry of the upper lid creases (left upper lid crease higher than right). The condition develops from defects or dehiscences in the levator aponeurosis.

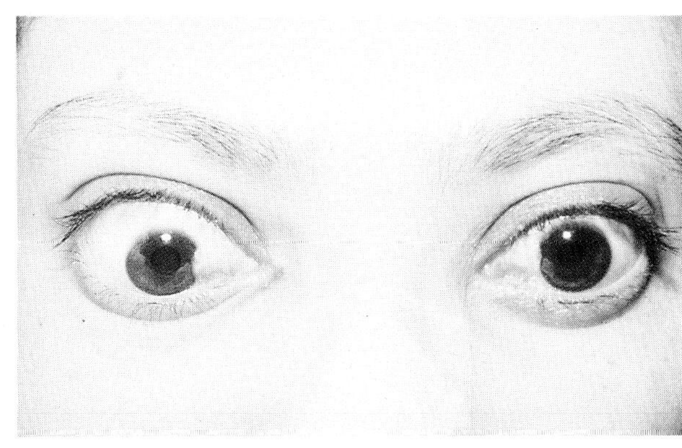

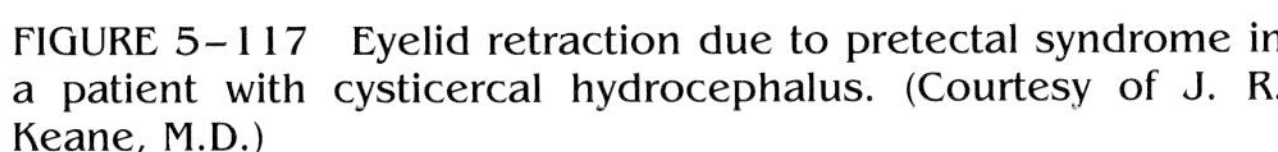
FIGURE 5–117 Eyelid retraction due to pretectal syndrome in a patient with cysticercal hydrocephalus. (Courtesy of J. R. Keane, M.D.)

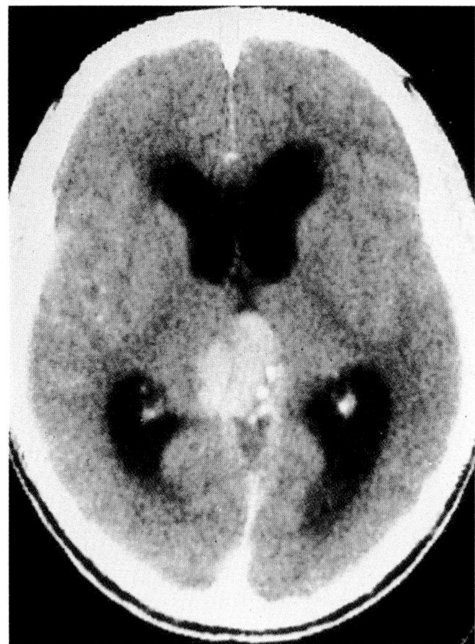

FIGURE 5–118 A pineal tumor is demonstrated in a computed tomographic scan of a patient with pretectal syndrome. (Courtesy of J. R. Keane, M.D.)

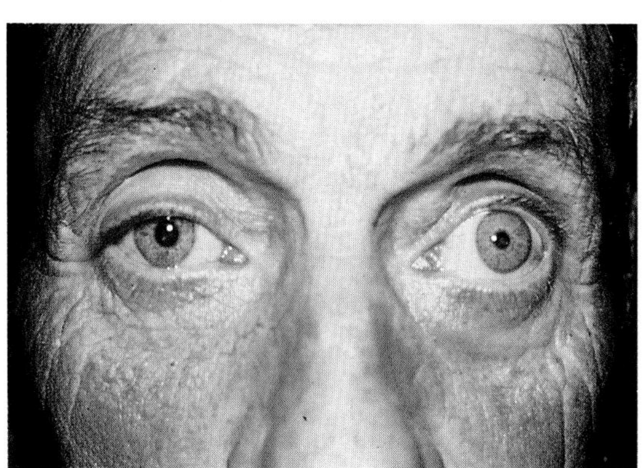

FIGURE 5–119 Pseudoretraction of the left upper eyelid in a patient with third-nerve palsy of the dominant and fixating right eye.

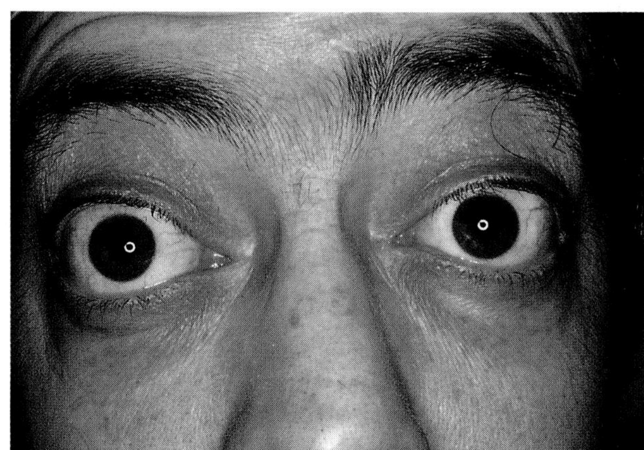

FIGURE 5–120 **Proptosis and dysthyroid eyelid retraction.** The proptosis is caused by swelling of one or more of the extraocular muscles.

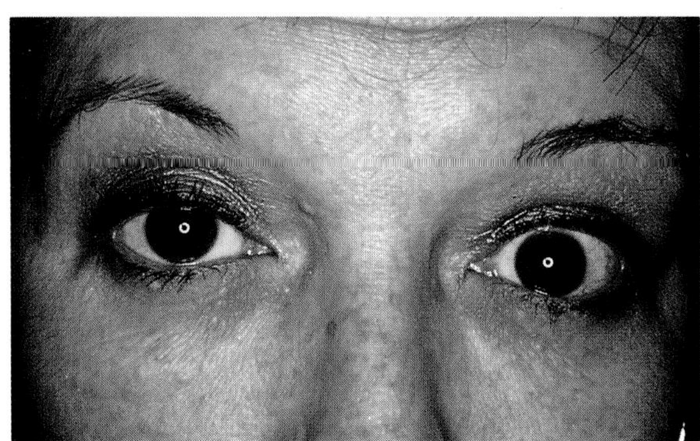

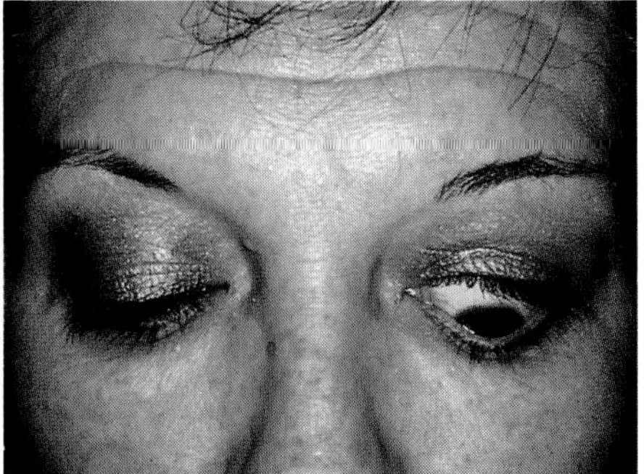

FIGURE 5–121 *A*, Left upper eyelid retraction in Graves' disease (Dalrymple's sign). *B*, On downgaze, lid lag is evident (von Graefe's sign).

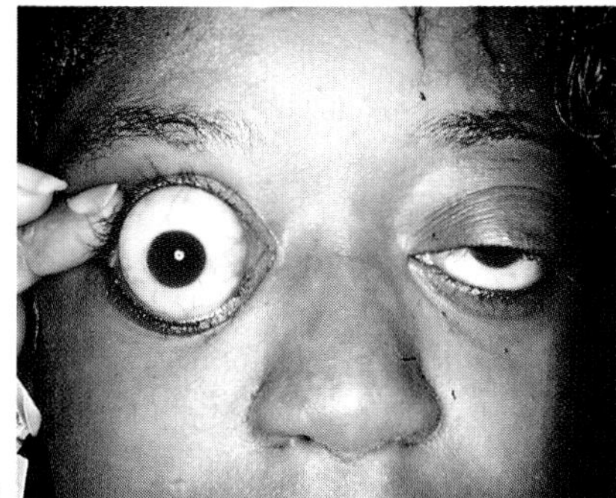

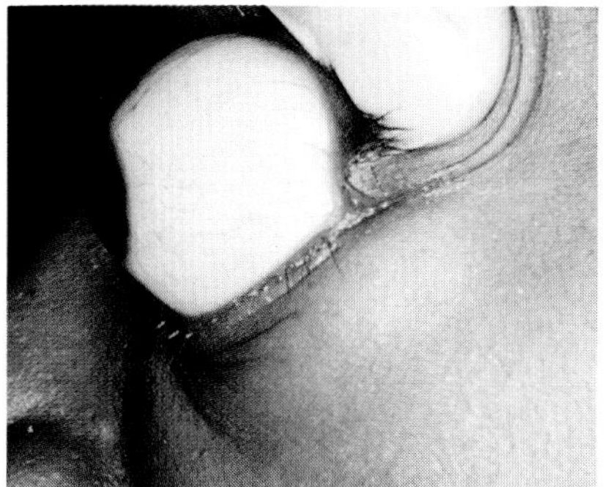

FIGURE 5–122 *A*, This patient with Graves' exophthalmos and eyelid retraction can induce luxation of the globe by increasing eyelid retraction via lateral canthal traction. *B*, Same patient, lateral view.

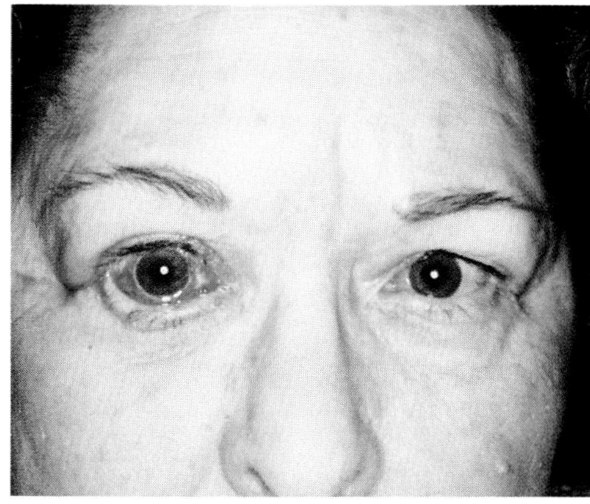

FIGURE 5–123 Right-sided exophthalmos and lid retraction due to unilateral dysthyroid orbitopathy. The conjunctiva is injected and chemotic.

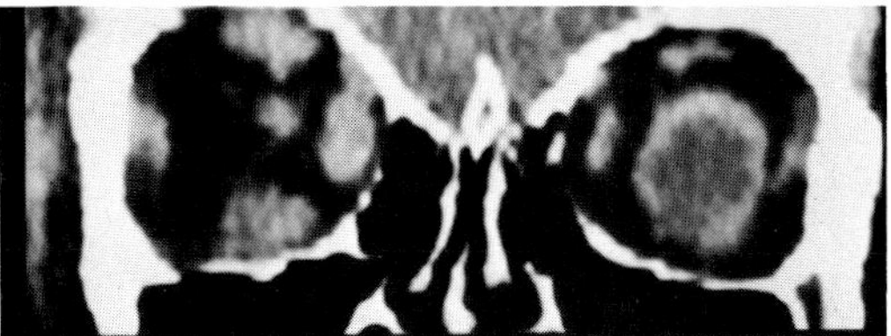

FIGURE 5–125 **Computed tomographic scan, Graves' disease.** Coronal computed tomographic scan shows enlarged extraocular muscles in the dysthyroid right orbit compared with the normal-sized muscles of the left orbit. Note that the right levator/superior rectus complex is enlarged. The posterior left globe is seen, but the right globe is displaced anteriorly owing to proptosis (same patient as in Fig. 5–124).

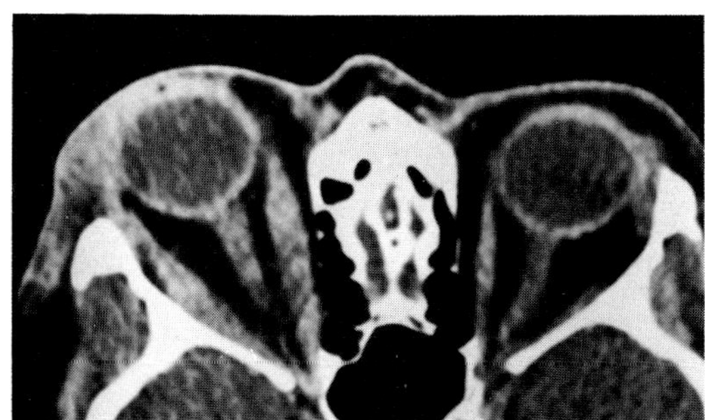

FIGURE 5–124 **Computed tomographic scan, Graves' disease.** Axial computed tomographic scan shows fusiform enlargement of horizontal rectus muscle bellies in the dysthyroid right orbit versus normal-sized muscles of the left orbit (same patient as in Fig. 5–123).

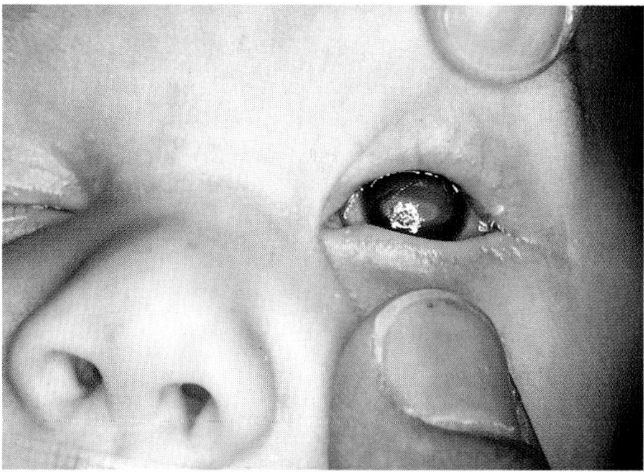

FIGURE 5–126 **Tarsal kink syndrome.** Left eyelids and opacified cornea of a 6-week-old infant who was treated since birth for unilateral left-sided conjunctivitis. The left upper eyelid margin is completely inverted owing to tarsal kink syndrome.

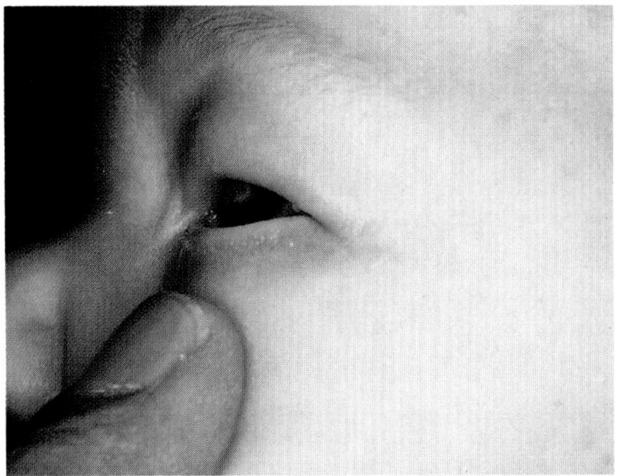

FIGURE 5-127 **Tarsal kink syndrome.** A lateral view of the patient in Figure 5-126 shows complete inversion of the distal upper eyelid.

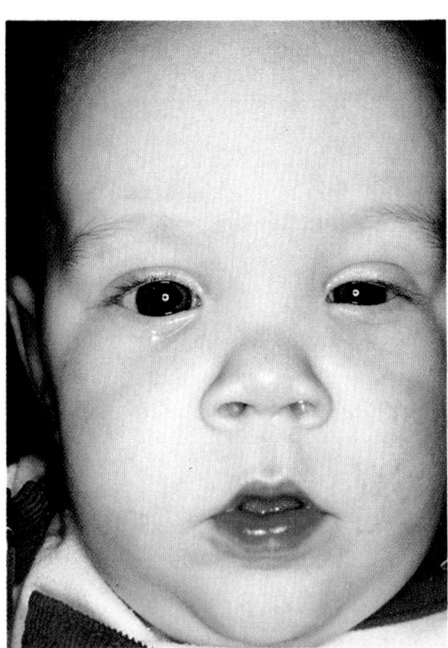

FIGURE 5-129 **Tarsal kink syndrome.** Corneal opacity and entropion correction following a posterior approach horizontal wedge resection and eyelid rotation. The residual ptosis is characteristic of tarsal kink syndrome. In anticipation of future ptosis repair, a posterior approach was used to leave the levator undisturbed.

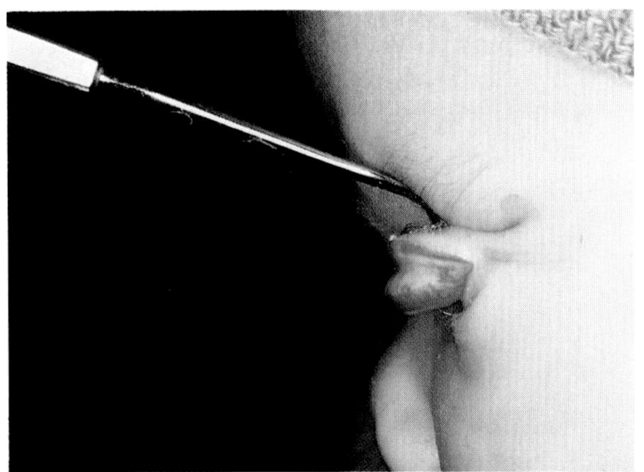

FIGURE 5-128 **Tarsal kink syndrome.** Eversion of the eyelid over a Desmarres' retractor demonstrates the horizontally oriented kink that plicates the eyelid.

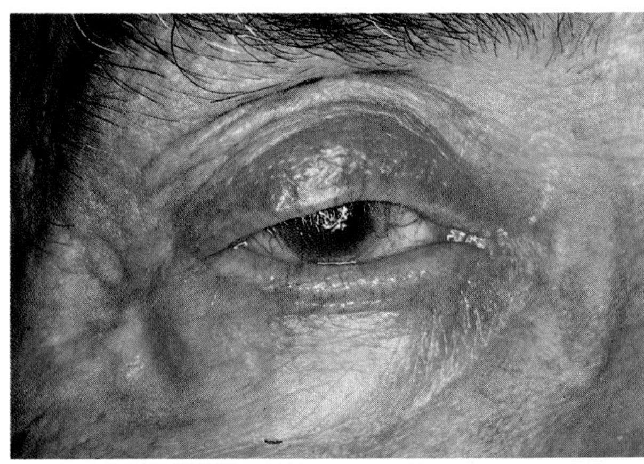

FIGURE 5-130 Moderate upper eyelid entropion secondary to scarification in trachoma. Eyelashes abrade the cornea, and there is a loss of corneal luster.

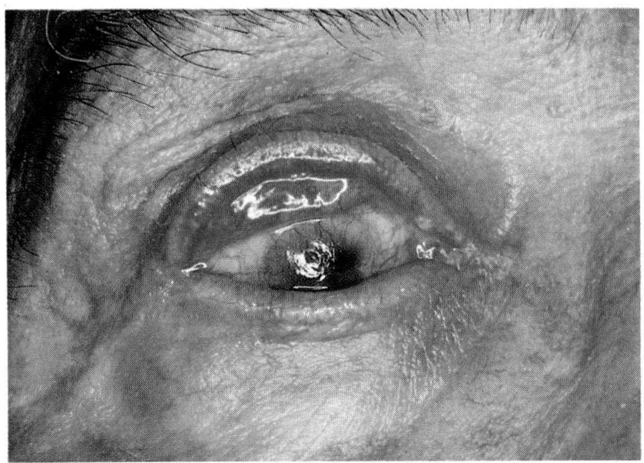

FIGURE 5-131 **Entropion in trachoma.** Eversion of the upper eyelid reveals a thickened eyelid and a curled tarsal plate.

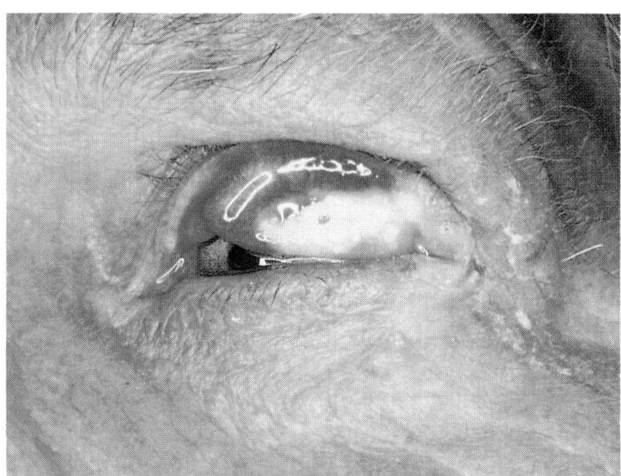

FIGURE 5–132 Frank keratinization of the tarsal conjunctiva by moist white keratin plaques called leukoplakia. This condition can be benign and associated with ectropion or may be a finding in premalignant hyperkeratotic squamous cell dysplasia.

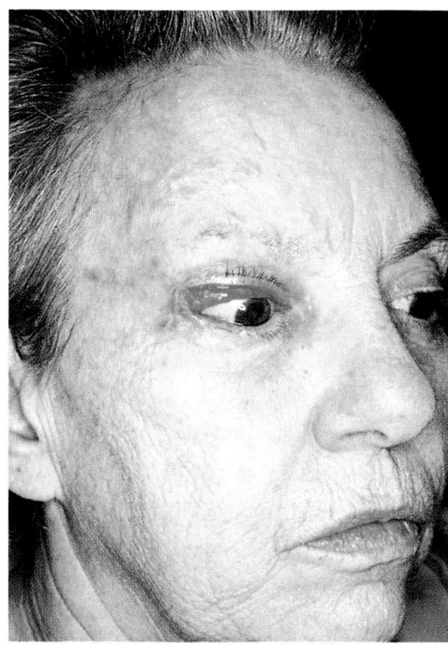

FIGURE 5–133 Upper eyelid ectropion, cutaneous scarring, and partial loss of an eyebrow in a patient with severe neuralgia following an attack of herpes zoster ophthalmicus.

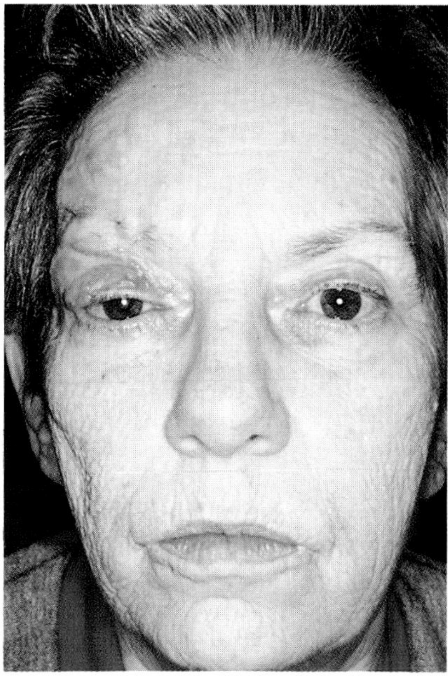

FIGURE 5–134 **Postherpetic cicatricial ectropion.** Patient after the release of cicatrix and the placement of a free skin graft. Return of eyelid to a normal position resulted in a complete cessation of neuralgia.

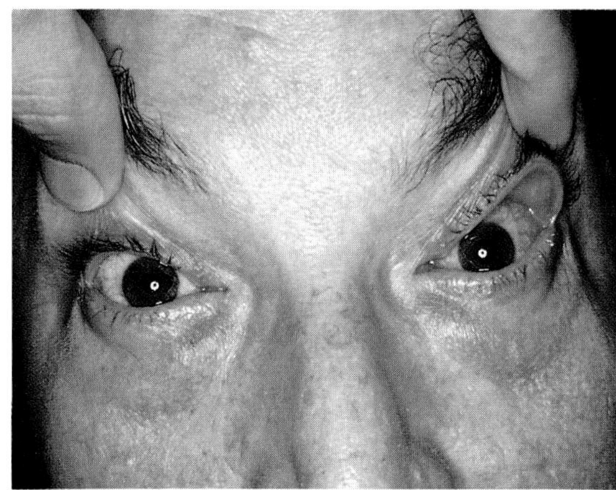

FIGURE 5–135 A patient with unilateral left chronic papillary conjunctivitis due to floppy eyelid syndrome. Superior traction on the eyelids reveals increased laxity of the eyelid that is loose, rubbery, and easily everted.

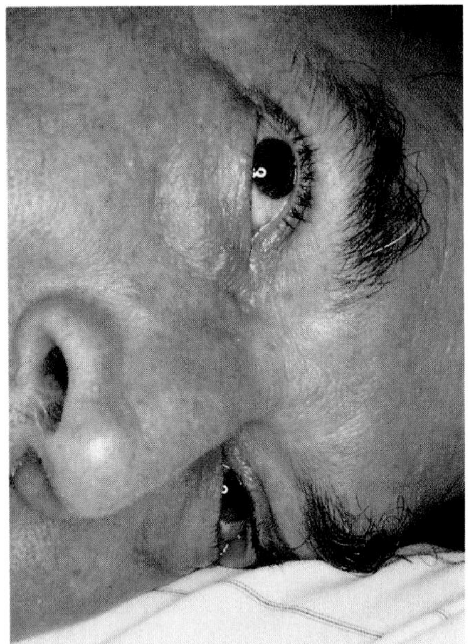

FIGURE 5–136 **Floppy eyelid syndrome.** Same patient in repose; gravity allows the loose eyelid to fall away from the globe.

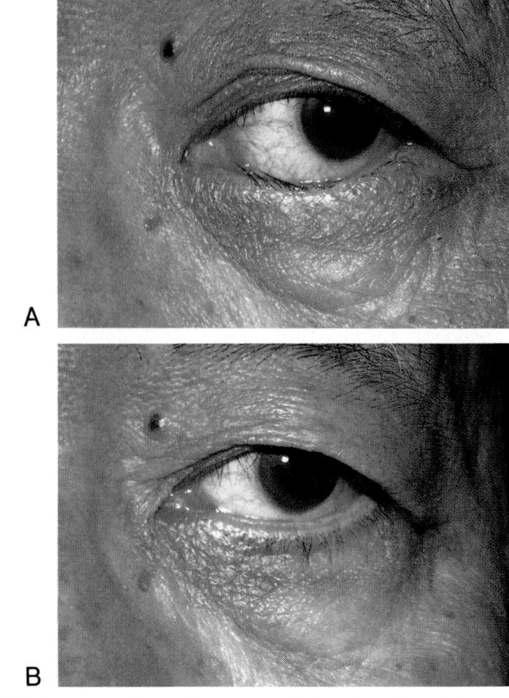

FIGURE 5–138 Right lower eyelid entropion before (*A*) and after (*B*) repair with the combined tarsal strip and Quickert sutures.

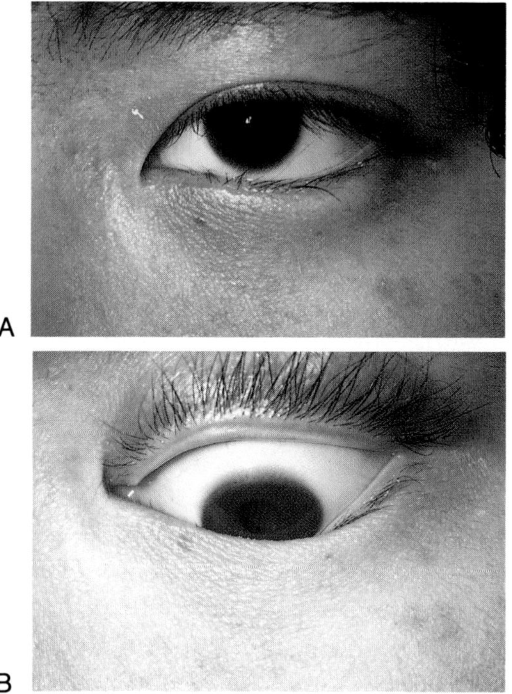

FIGURE 5–137 In this patient with epiblepharon, note the tendency toward entropion in the primary position of gaze (*A*), with frank entropion in downgaze (*B*).

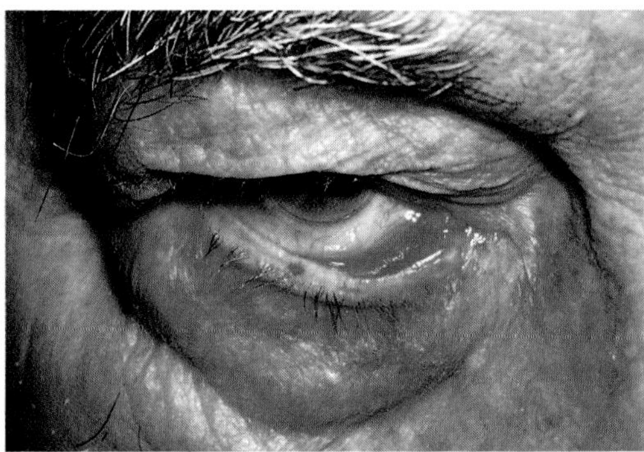

FIGURE 5–139 **Involutional ectropion.** Increased horizontal eyelid laxity with medial ectropion and punctal eversion. In this condition, the medial and canthal tendons may be lax and contribute to the outer pouting of the eyelid.

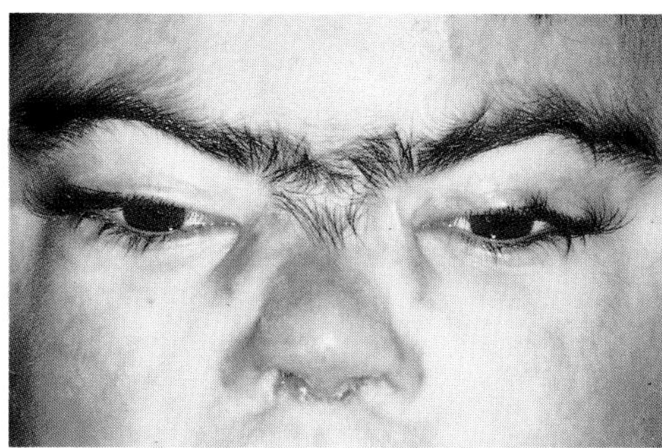

FIGURE 5-140 Synophrys, or fusion of the brows, may be an inherited familial finding or may be associated with specific congenital defects, as in this case of Cornelia de Lange's syndrome (pathologic dwarfism). (Courtesy of John Woog, M.D.)

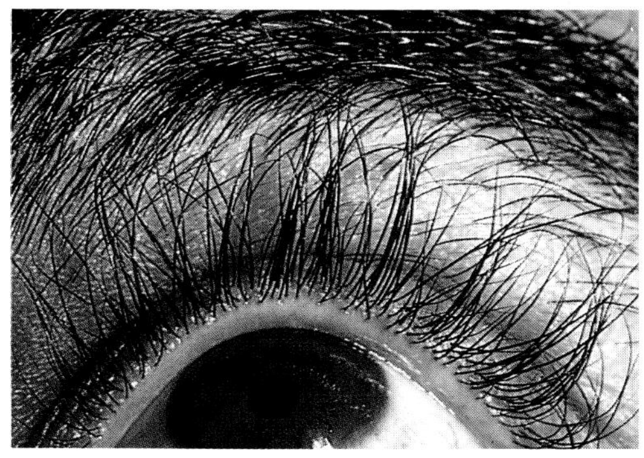

FIGURE 5-141 Trichomegaly: abnormally long and luxuriant eyelashes.

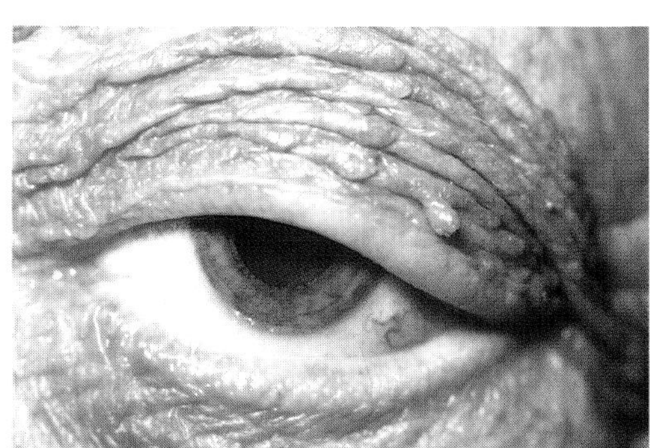

FIGURE 5-142 Alopecia areata, with complete loss of the eyelashes.

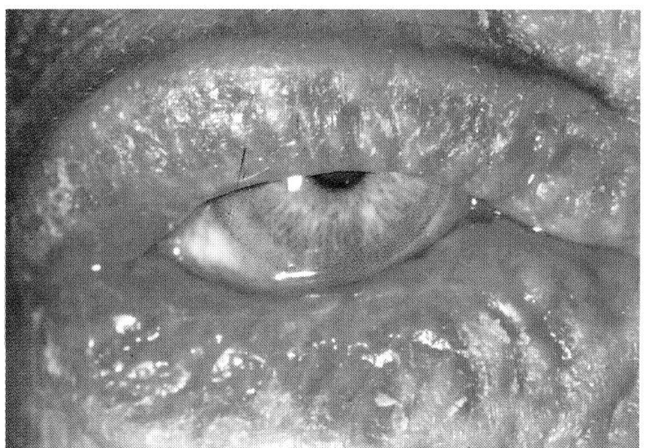

FIGURE 5-143 Chronic dermatitis with severe eczematous thickening of the eyelid margins accounts for the extensive madarosis (loss of lashes). This appearance can also be seen in diffusely spreading sebaceous carcinoma.

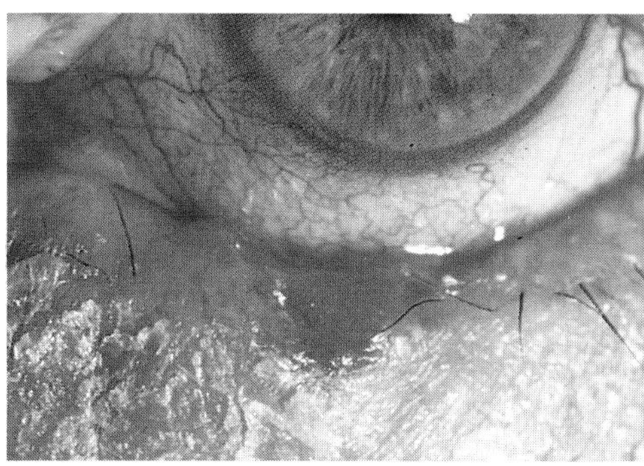

FIGURE 5-144 **Squamous cell carcinoma.** Neoplastic loss of cilia may occur from invasion and destruction of the follicles situated at the anterior face of the tarsus.

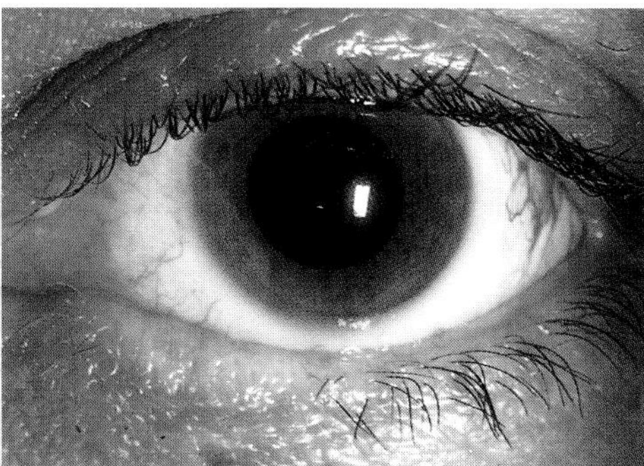

FIGURE 5-145 Radiation madarosis and focal depigmentation in the medial portion of the lower eyelid occurred after proton beam irradiation for a uveal melanoma.

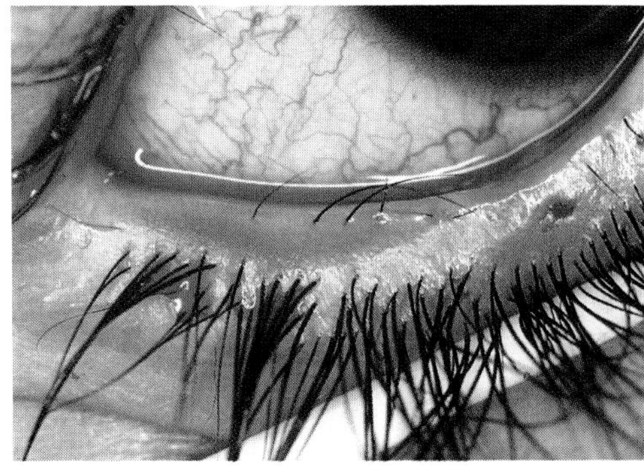

FIGURE 5-146 **Congenital distichiasis.** Normally formed cilia are emerging from meibomian gland orifices and can irritate the globe.

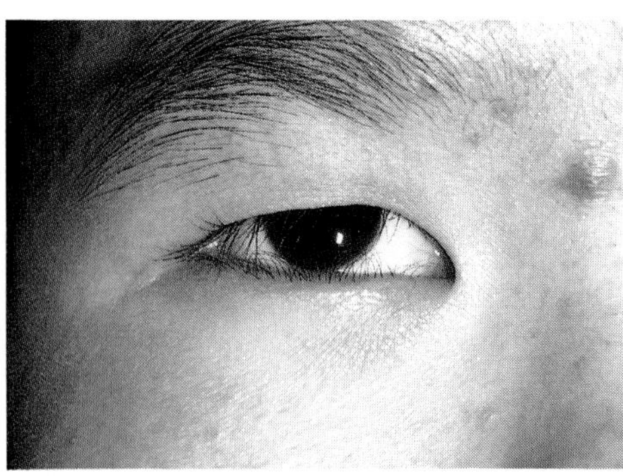

FIGURE 5-148 **Epiblepharon.** A redundant fold of pretarsal skin and underlying orbicularis muscle overrides the eyelid margin and applies the cilia of the lower eyelid against the globe. (Courtesy of J. Woog, M.D.)

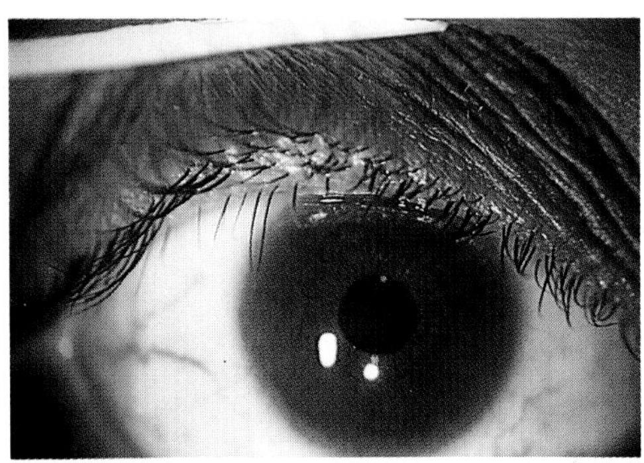

FIGURE 5-147 **Trichiasis.** Cilia emerging from a normal anterior lamellar location are misdirected toward the globe. Trichiasis in this case was due to underlying trachoma.

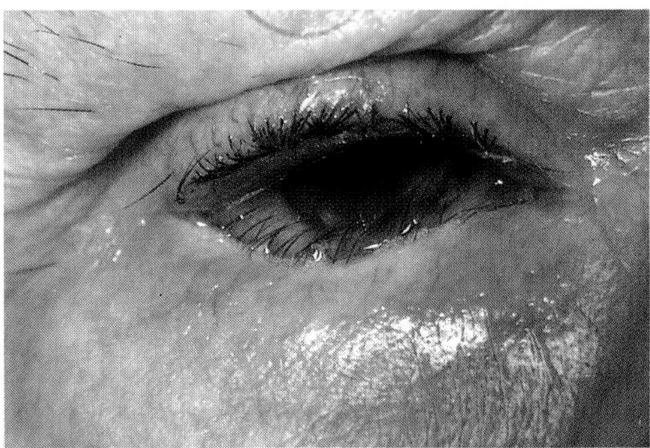

FIGURE 5-149 **Involutionary entropion.** Rotation of the entire lower eyelid margin against the globe. Thickening of the lower eyelid margin and narrowing of the horizontal palpebral aperture are reflective of an overriding preseptal orbicularis muscle and a lateral canthal dehiscence, respectively.

A 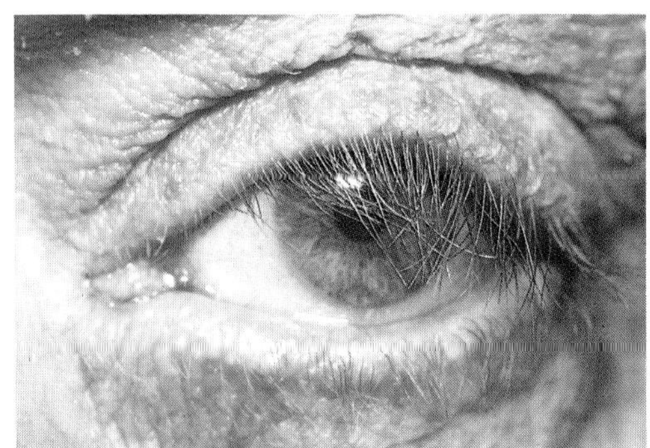

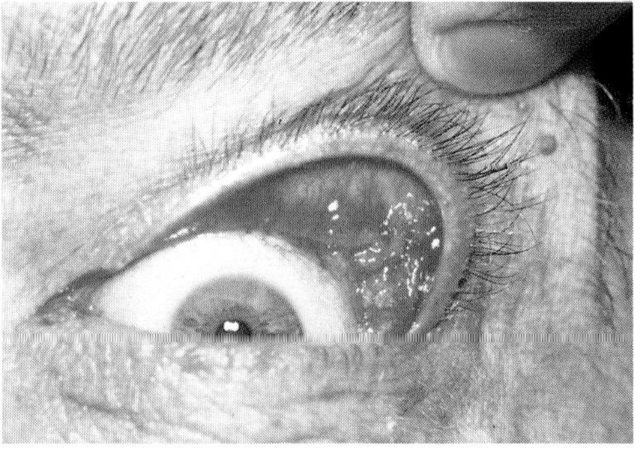 B

FIGURE 5-150 **Eyelash ptosis.** *A,* The upper eyelid cilia are in a vertical configuration yet are not contacting the ocular surface. *B,* The upper eyelid's marked laxity, contributing to the eyelash malposition, is apparent in this case of floppy eyelid syndrome.

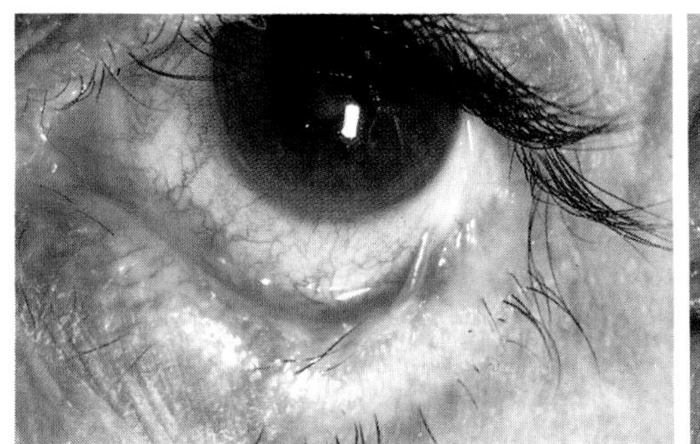
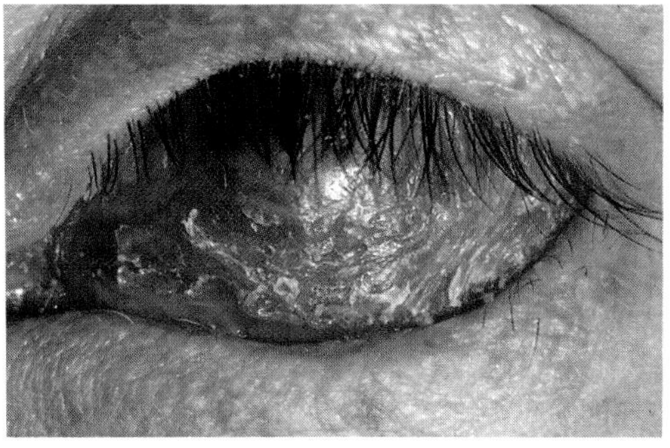

A B

FIGURE 5–151 *A*, Trichiasis and acquired distichiasis are present along with a dense inferior symblepharon in this case of ocular cicatricial pemphigoid. *B*, Severe trichiasis, cicatricial entropion, and diffuse ocular surface keratinization are found in this advanced case of Stevens-Johnson syndrome.

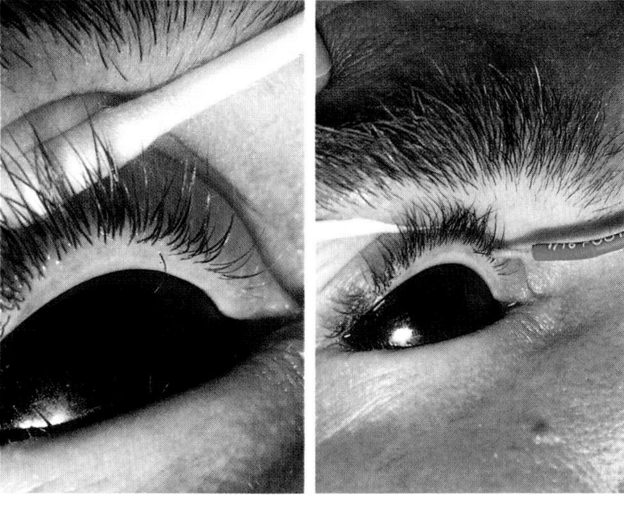

A B

FIGURE 5–152 *A*, Focal trichiasis in the upper eyelid. *B*, Electroepilation of a trichiatic cilium. A corneal/scleral shell is placed to protect the globe.

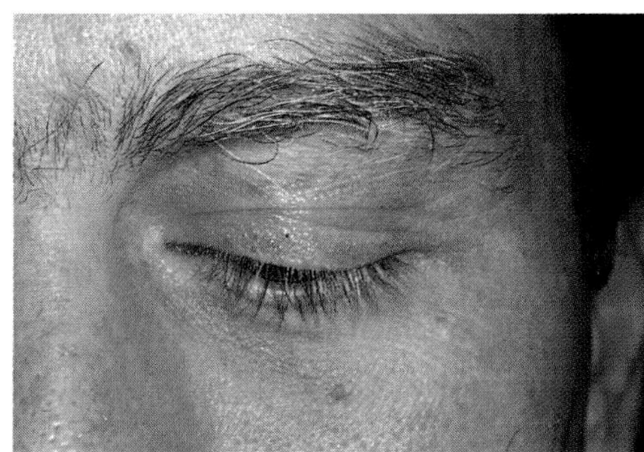

FIGURE 5–153 **Poliosis.** Segmental depigmentation of the eyelash and brow cilia. This finding can be seen in vitiligo, severe dermatitis, local irradiation, tuberous sclerosis, neurofibromatosis, and the uveitis syndrome of sympathetic ophthalmia and Vogt-Koyanagi-Harada.

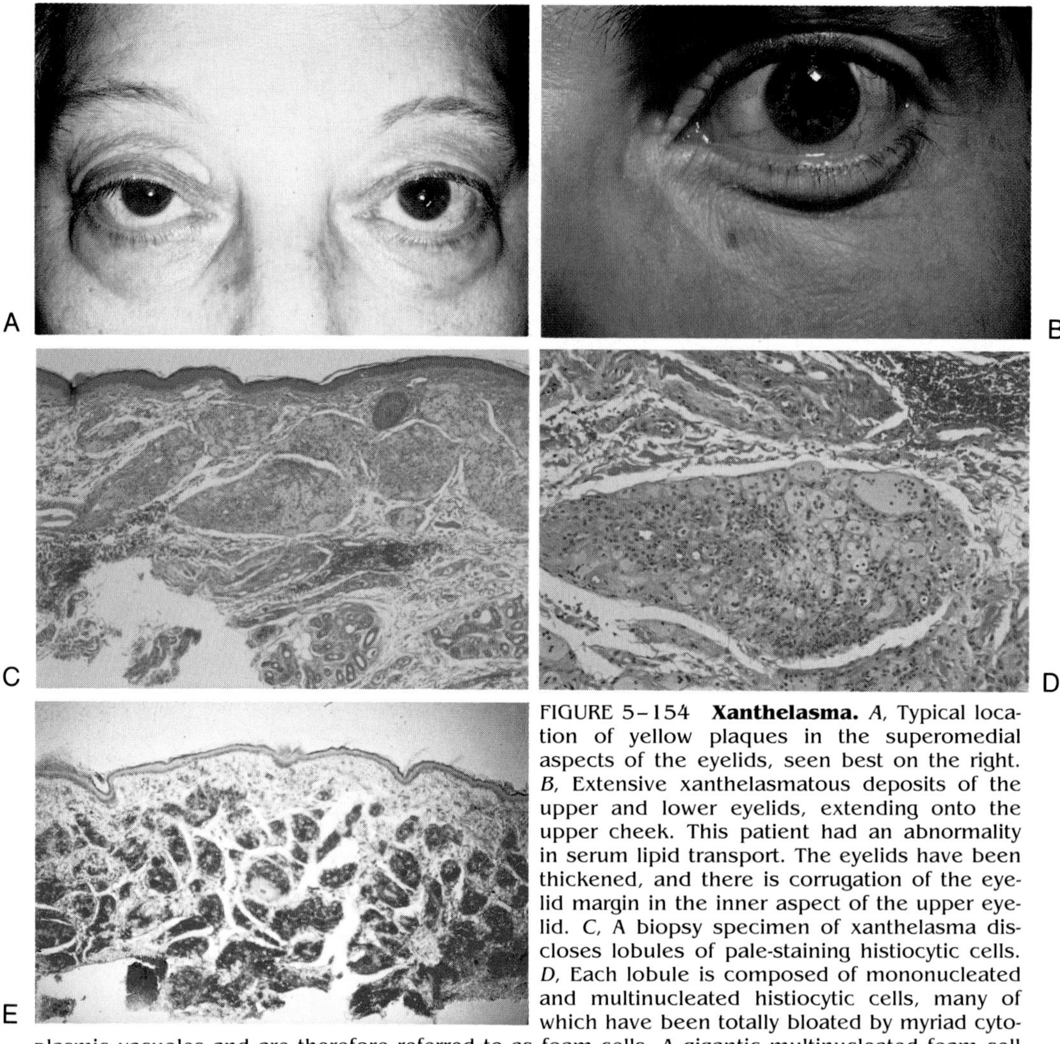

FIGURE 5-154 **Xanthelasma.** *A*, Typical location of yellow plaques in the superomedial aspects of the eyelids, seen best on the right. *B*, Extensive xanthelasmatous deposits of the upper and lower eyelids, extending onto the upper cheek. This patient had an abnormality in serum lipid transport. The eyelids have been thickened, and there is corrugation of the eyelid margin in the inner aspect of the upper eyelid. *C*, A biopsy specimen of xanthelasma discloses lobules of pale-staining histiocytic cells. *D*, Each lobule is composed of mononucleated and multinucleated histiocytic cells, many of which have been totally bloated by myriad cytoplasmic vacuoles and are therefore referred to as foam cells. A gigantic multinucleated foam cell is shown at the outer periphery on upper right. *E*, Oil-red-O stain of fresh frozen tissue demonstrates that the cytoplasmic vacuoles contain lipid. Most of the lobules are arranged around a central capillary. *C* and *D*, H&E.

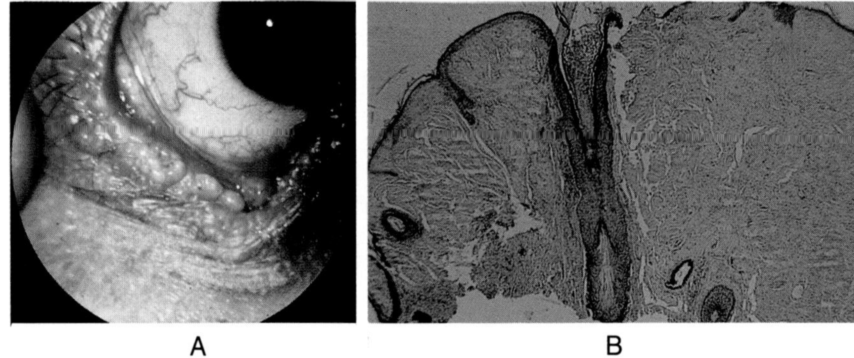

FIGURE 5-155 **Lipoid proteinosis.** *A*, All four eyelids are characteristically involved in this process. The eyelid margins are beset with confluent pearly nodules. *B*, A biopsy specimen reveals replacement of the upper and lower dermis of the eyelid by a hyaline/amorphous material that has destroyed most of the adnexal structures, with a single eyelash being preserved. This hyaline material is a PAS-positive glycoprotein that is diastase-resistant and may be the result of dermal fibroblasts synthesizing noncollagenous proteins at the expense of collagens. The material may also contain lipidic material and is weakly positive on Congo red staining. *B*, H&E.

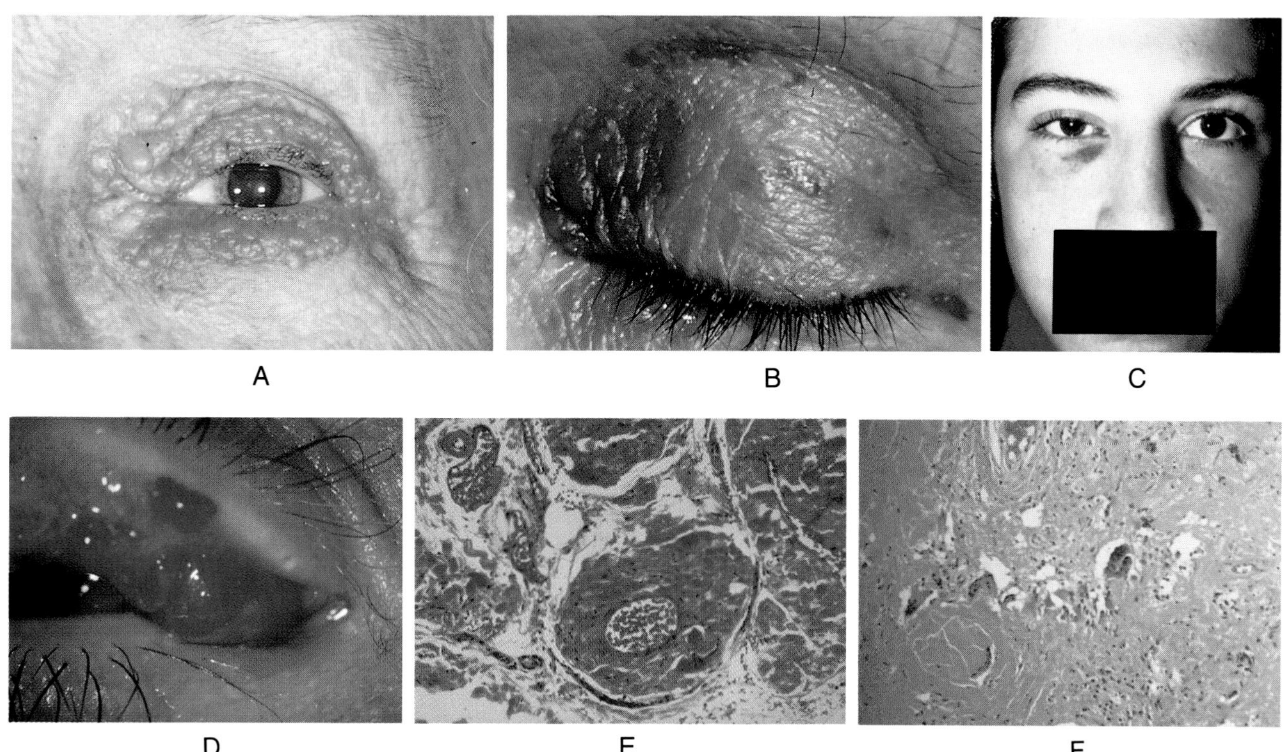

FIGURE 5-156 **Cutaneous involvement with amyloidosis.** *A,* An elderly patient presented with yellow nodules of all four eyelids and was not known to have a systemic ailment. Systemic amyloidosis was ultimately diagnosed. *B,* Hemorrhagic papules of the eyelid skin in a patient with amyloidosis. Perivascular amyloid deposits render the vessels fragile, and rubbing can cause purpura. *C,* This teenaged patient presented with a hemorrhage of the lower eyelid and a reddish mass in the caruncular region. *D,* On everting the eyelids, hemorrhagic and yellowish deposits are identified in the conjunctiva of the same patient shown in C. In contradistinction to cutaneous eyelid involvement, conjunctival amyloid deposits are generally not associated with systemic disease, which was not discovered in this patient. *E,* Characteristic Congophilic perivascular deposits of amyloid material. Congo red stain. *F,* A multinucleated foreign body giant cell response has been mounted to amorphous deposits of amyloid material. *F,* H&E. (*A,* Courtesy of Dr. Alan Proia.)

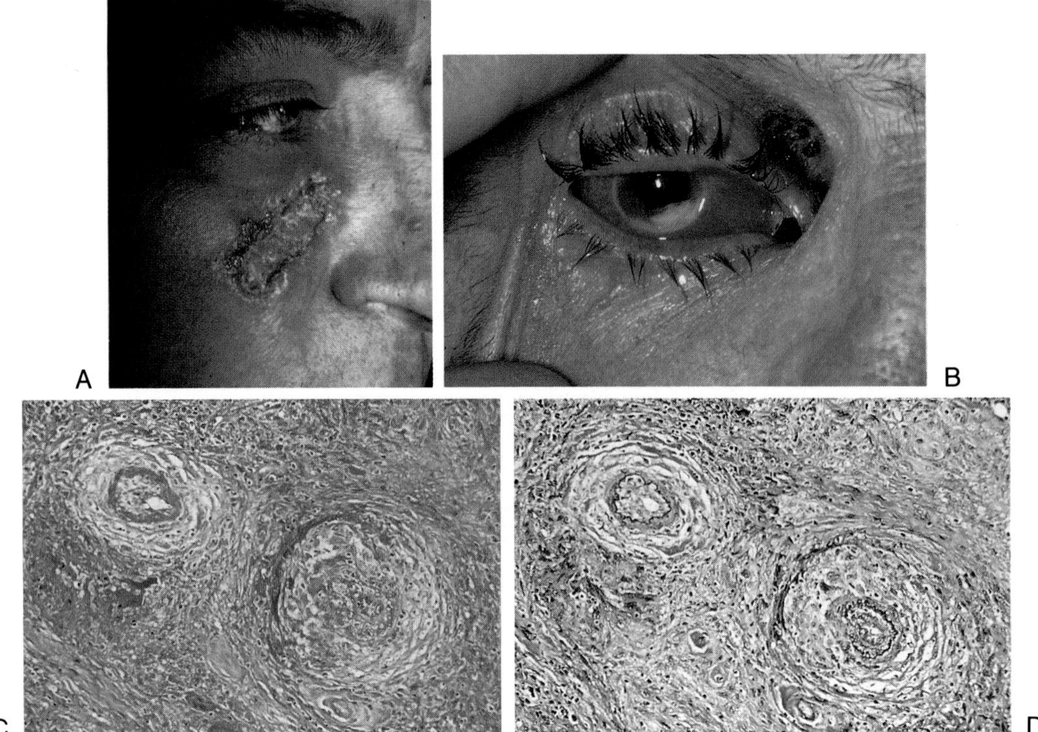

FIGURE 5–157 **Wegener's granulomatosis.** *A*, A cutaneous infarct from underlying vasculitis with ulcer formation and erythema of the eyelids. *B*, There is active scleritis with a peripheral ulcerative keratitis in this patient with retraction of the eyelids toward a fistula in the caruncular area that opens into the ethmoid sinus. This patient had extensive sinus and orbital destructive vasculitis. *C*, Two blood vessels in an orbital biopsy specimen exhibit granulomatous vasculitis as well as granulomatous elements in the adjacent interstitium. *D*, An elastic stain identifies surviving remnants of the internal elastica. *C*, H&E. (*C* and *D*, Courtesy of Dr. Ralph Eagle.)

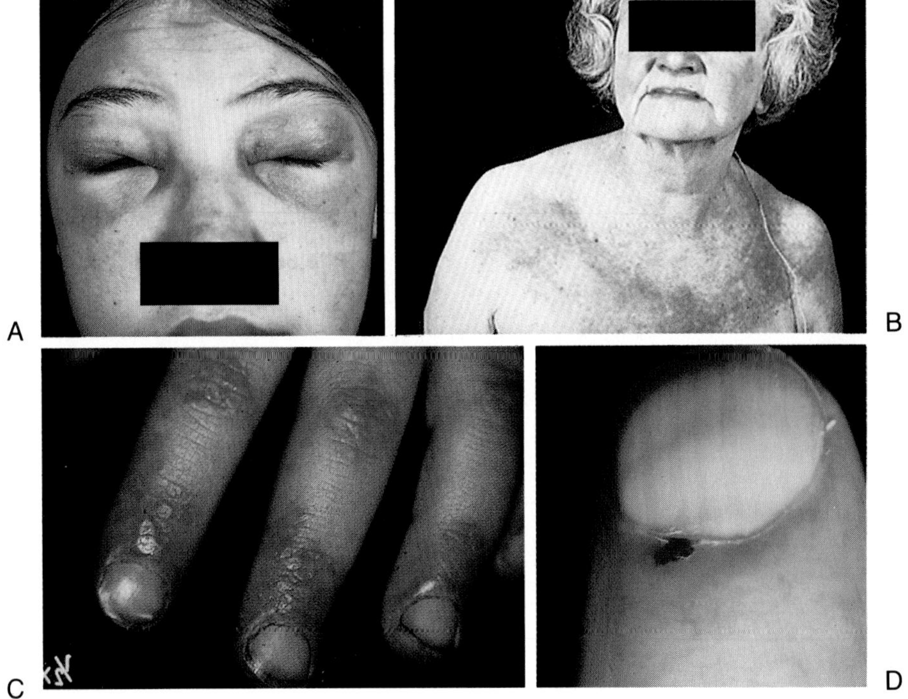

FIGURE 5–158 **Dermatomyositis.** *A*, Eyelid erythema (heliotrope sign) with a distinctive violaceous hue and profound edema. The condition may be associated with an underlying malignancy. *B*, Erythema of the chest skin associated with underlying atrophy of the muscles. *C*, Distinctive periungual erythema with erythematous nodules of the knuckles (Gottron's papules). *D*, In contradistinction to dermatomyositis, other systemic autoimmune diseases may present with focal cutaneous and periungual ulcers from an underlying vasculitis, as in this patient with systemic rheumatoid arthritis.

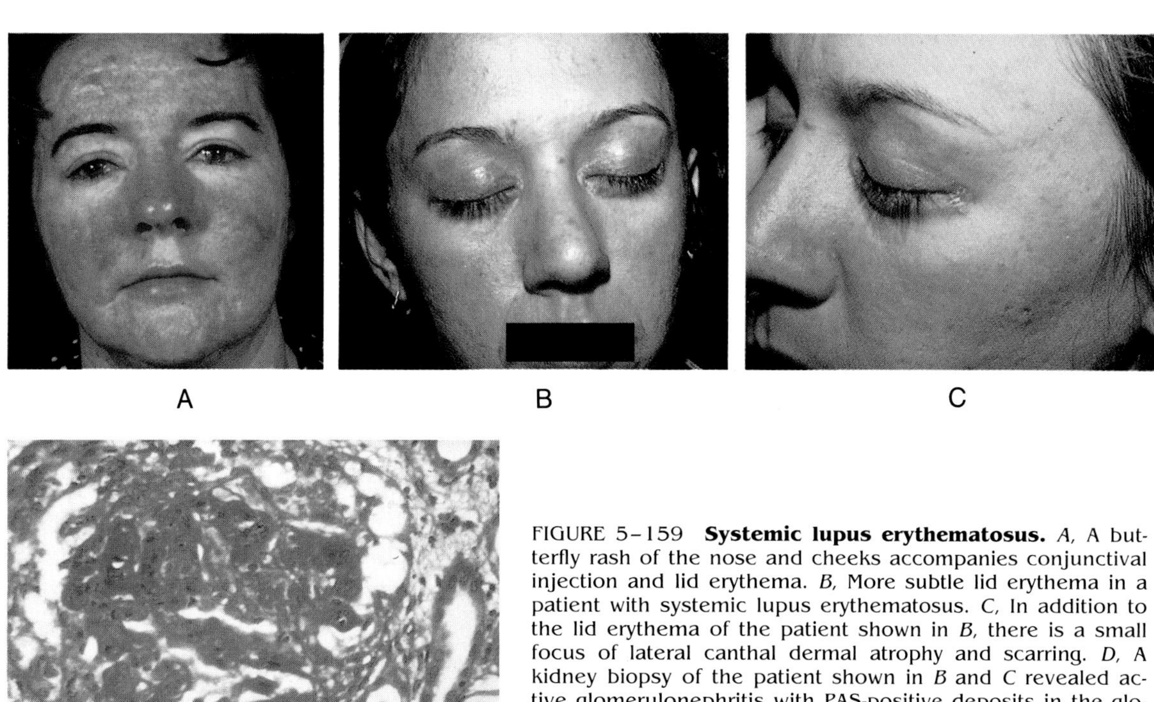

FIGURE 5-159 **Systemic lupus erythematosus.** *A,* A butterfly rash of the nose and cheeks accompanies conjunctival injection and lid erythema. *B,* More subtle lid erythema in a patient with systemic lupus erythematosus. *C,* In addition to the lid erythema of the patient shown in *B,* there is a small focus of lateral canthal dermal atrophy and scarring. *D,* A kidney biopsy of the patient shown in *B* and *C* revealed active glomerulonephritis with PAS-positive deposits in the glomeruli. (*B–D,* Courtesy of Dr. M. Bernier.)

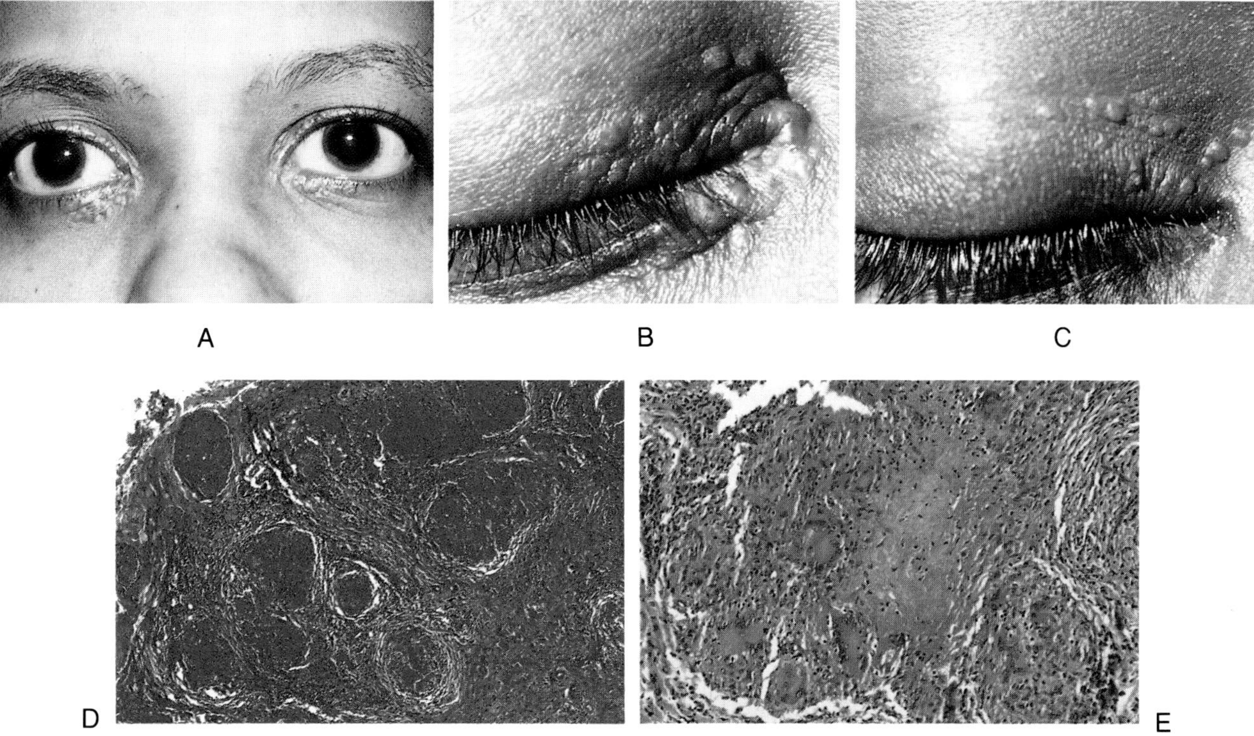

FIGURE 5-160 **Sarcoidosis.** *A,* Multiple small, confluent dermal papules of all four eyelids. *B,* The papules are nonhemorrhagic and located in the superficial lid dermis beneath the epidermis and can cause release of pigment from the epidermis (incontinentia pigmenti). (*A* and *B,* Courtesy of Dr. D. Morris.) *C,* Small nonconfluent papules of the dermis can invite the mistaken diagnosis of milia. *D,* The granulomas in sarcoidosis elicit a prominent fibroblastic response. In this modified trichrome stain, the granulomas stain intensely red, owing to the presence in the cytoplasm of filaments (vimentin) and numerous cytoplasmic organelles. *E,* Multinucleated giant cells are not infrequently associated with the sarcoid nodules. In general, there is a light lymphocytic and plasmacytic infiltrate associated with the nodules ("naked granulomas"). *E,* H&E.

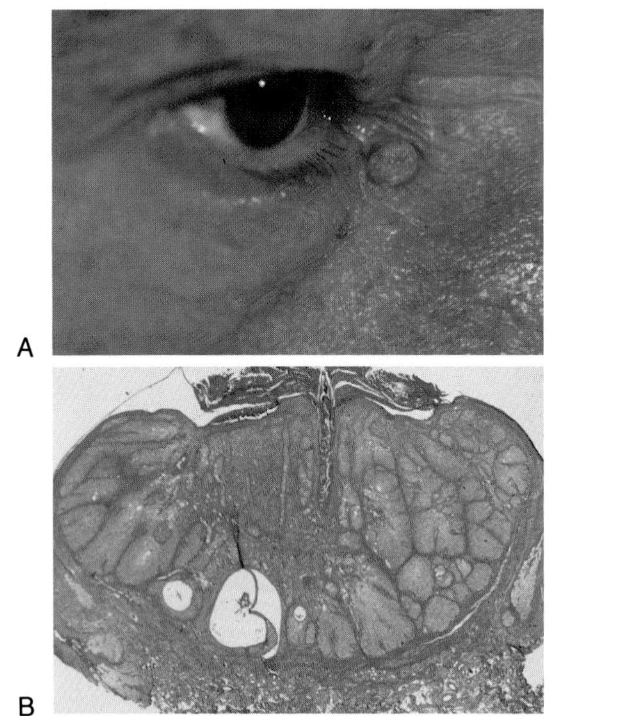

FIGURE 5–161 *A,* **Sebaceous adenoma** of the lower lid in a patient with Muir-Torre syndrome, in which there is associated colon carcinoma. *B,* Photomicrograph of a sebaceous adenoma from a patient with Muir-Torre syndrome showing central lipidization of cells and an outer single, basal germinal layer. *B,* H&E.

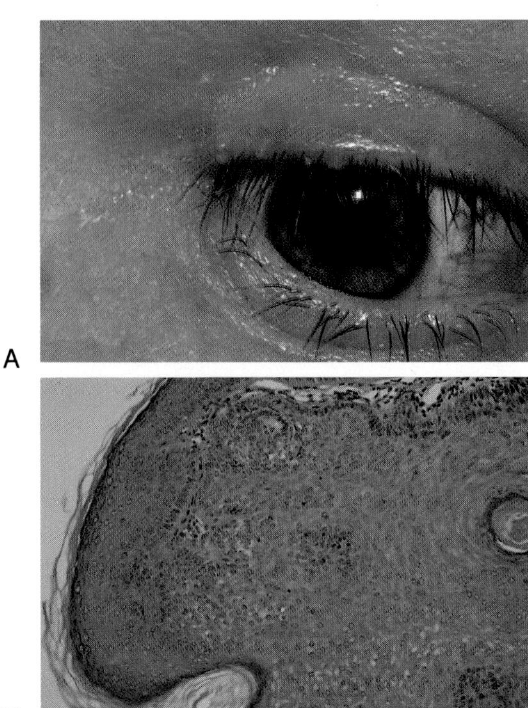

FIGURE 5–162 *A,* **Multiple trichilemmomas** of the upper lid in a patient with Cowden's disease in which breast, thyroid, and gastrointestinal neoplasms can be seen. *B,* Photomicrograph of a trichilemmoma excised from a patient with Cowden's disease. The tumor arises from the epithelium of the pilar canal. The cells toward the top exhibit peripheral palisading, the adjacent cells are small squamous, and the cells toward the bottom display early clear cell change (owing to accumulation of glycogen). *B,* H&E. (*A,* From Bardenstein D, McLean I, Nerney J, Boatwright R: Cowden's disease. Ophthalmology 95:1038, 1988.)

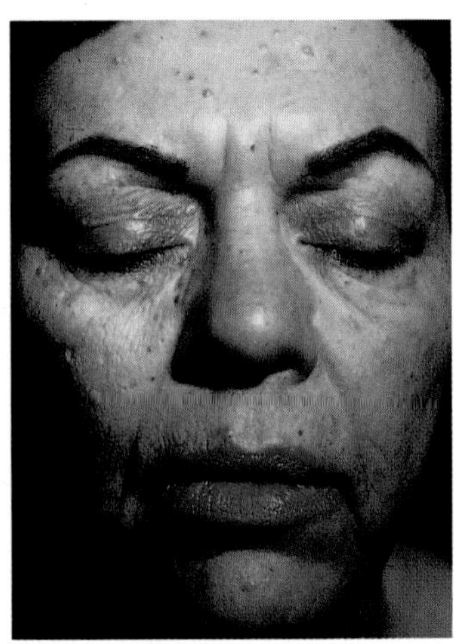

FIGURE 5–163 Multiple basal cell carcinomas in a patient with the basal cell nevus syndrome. In this condition, there can be musculoskeletal abnormalities, ovarian tumors, jaw cysts, and cerebellar medulloblastoma. (Courtesy of Dr. L. Shapiro.)

SECTION 6

Orbit

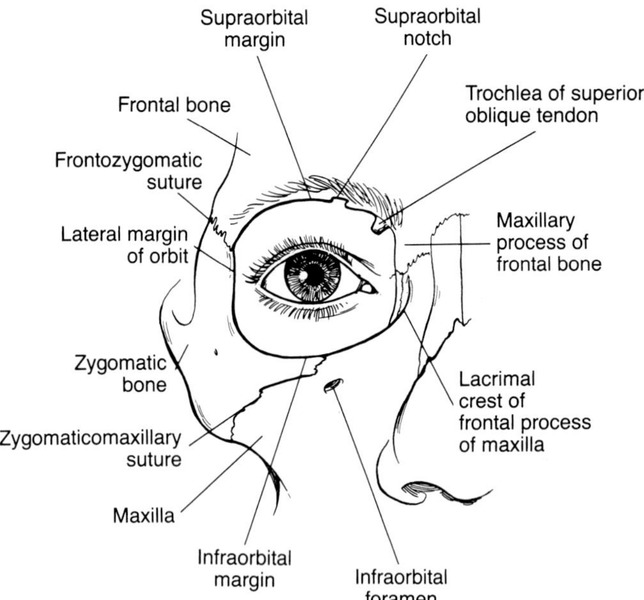

FIGURE 6–1 **Orbital anatomy.** External landmarks of the bony orbit.

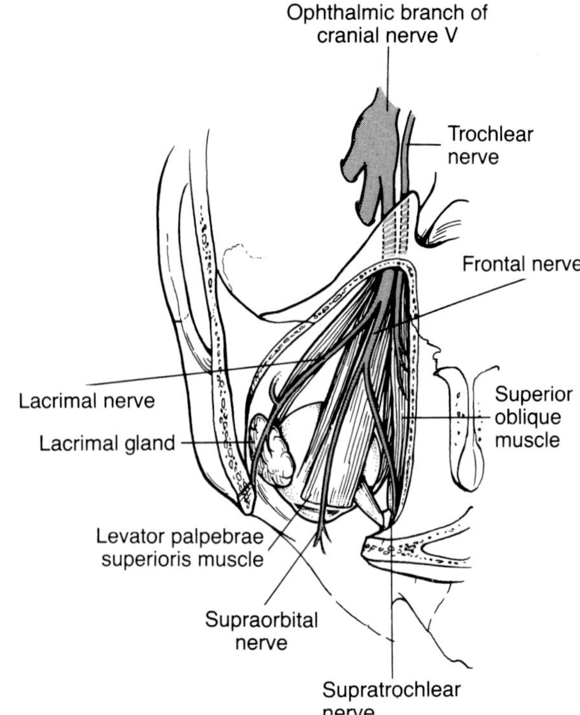

FIGURE 6–3 **Orbital anatomy.** Superior branches of the ophthalmic division of cranial nerve V and the trochlear nerve (cranial nerve IV).

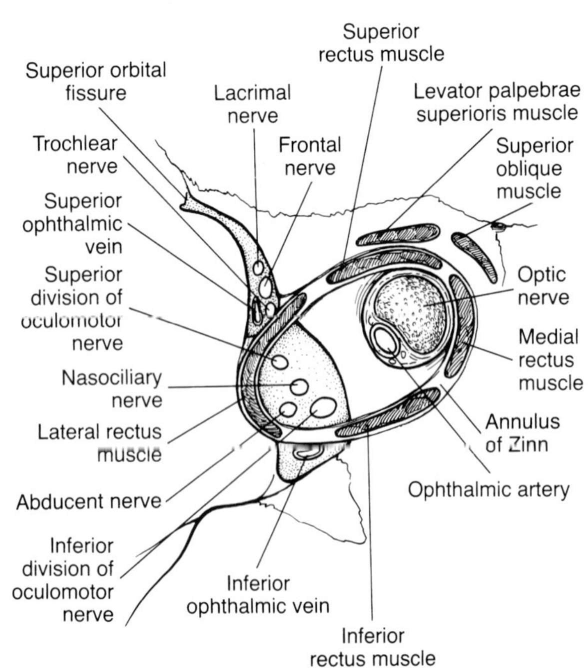

FIGURE 6–2 **Orbital anatomy.** Posterior orbit: the annulus of Zinn.

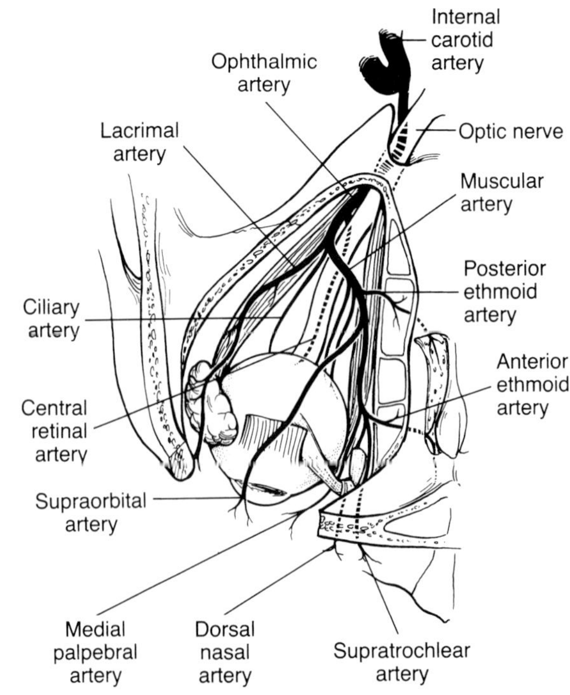

FIGURE 6–4 **Orbital anatomy.** The ophthalmic artery and its branches.

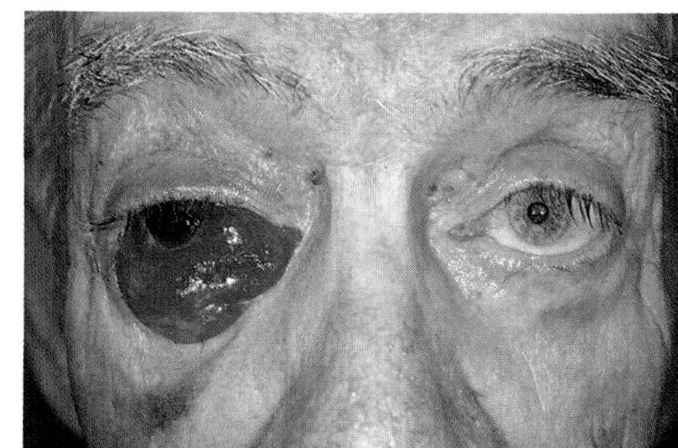

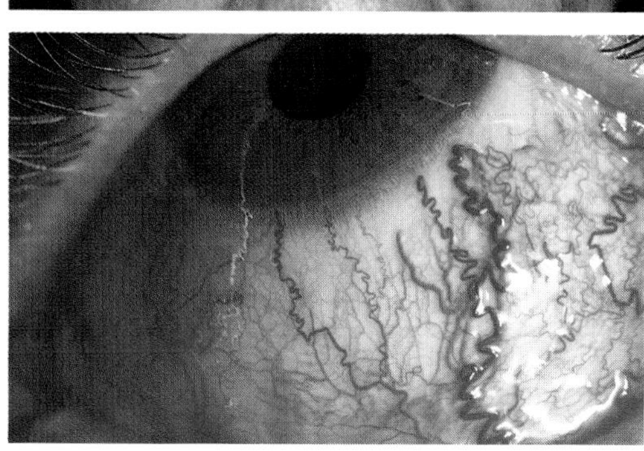

FIGURE 6–5 **Arteriovenous fistulas affecting the orbit.** *A*, High-flow carotid-cavernous fistula with acute congestion and cranial nerve palsies. *B*, Low-flow dural shunt with congestion of conjunctival vessels but minimal orbital signs except for mild exophthalmos.

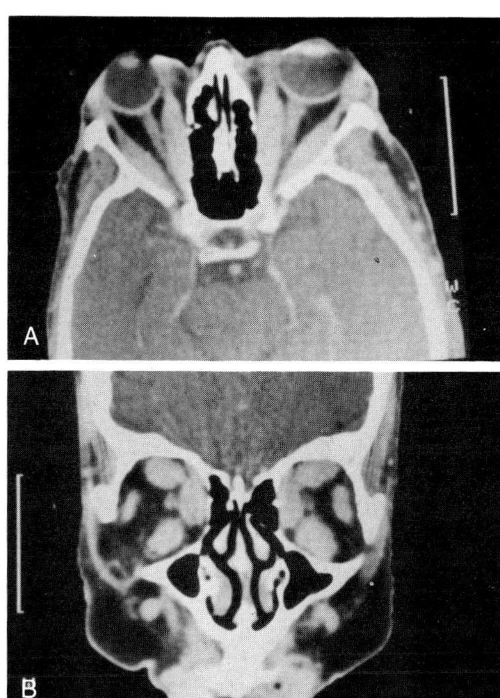

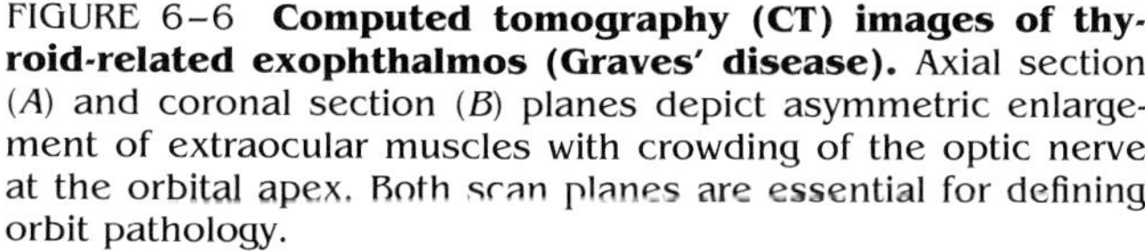

FIGURE 6–6 **Computed tomography (CT) images of thyroid-related exophthalmos (Graves' disease).** Axial section (*A*) and coronal section (*B*) planes depict asymmetric enlargement of extraocular muscles with crowding of the optic nerve at the orbital apex. Both scan planes are essential for defining orbit pathology.

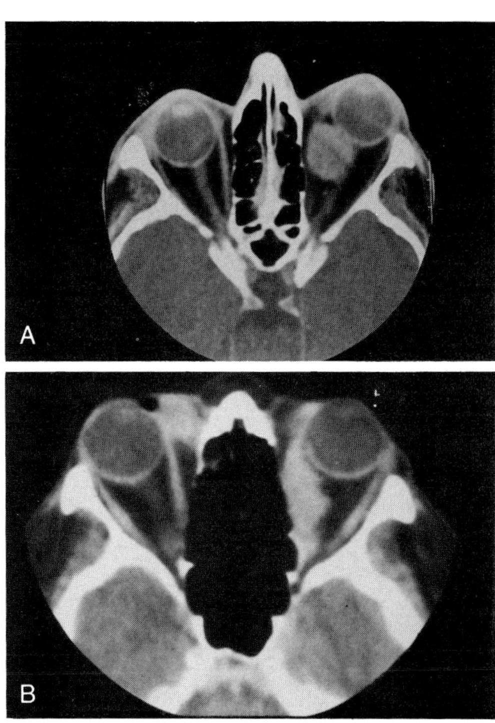

FIGURE 6–7 **CT images of orbit tumors.** *A*, Circumscribed mass posterior to the globe and displacing normal structures, characteristic of a benign tumor (hemangioma). *B*, Irregular mass extending deeply into the orbit, indicating an infiltrative neoplasm (lymphoma).

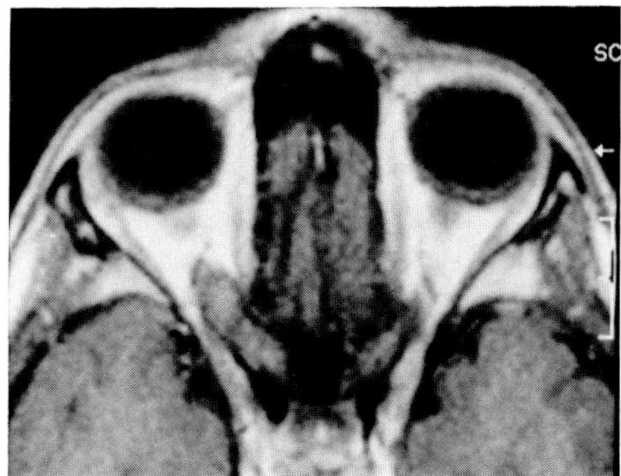

FIGURE 6-8 Magnetic resonance imaging scan of an orbital apex tumor extending through the optic canal and into the optic chiasm intracranially (glioma).

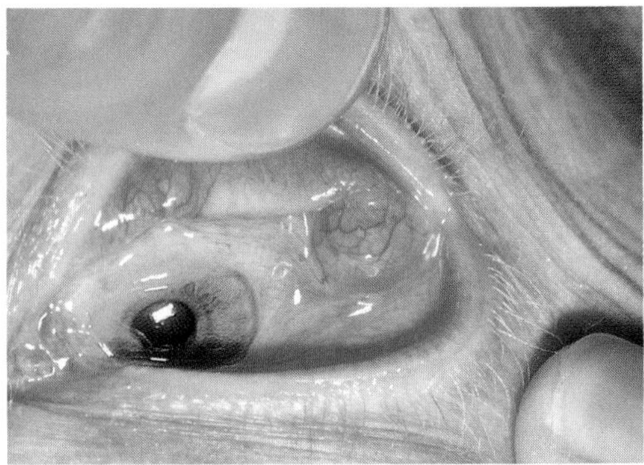

FIGURE 6-9 **Ductal cyst of the lacrimal gland.** Example of a typical ductal cyst. With the lid everted, the cyst can usually be directly viewed as it extends into the superior fornix and is easily seen. Occasionally the cyst extends into the orbital portion of the lacrimal gland.

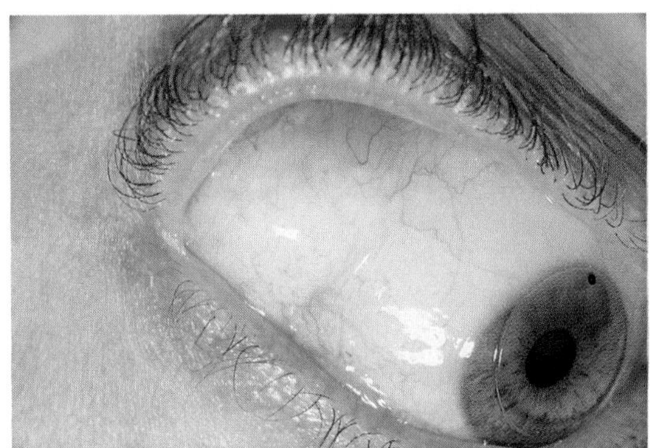

FIGURE 6-10 **Appearance of a typical lipodermoid.** This lesion usually occurs on the superior temporal epibulbar region and is often covered by fatty globules under conjunctiva. These lesions can occur occasionally in other positions on the globe and are sometimes associated with Goldenhar's syndrome. Because of the infiltrating nature and poor clinical response to surgical excision, these lesions should not be excised. In contrast to epidermoid and dermoid tumors, lipodermoids are not cystic.

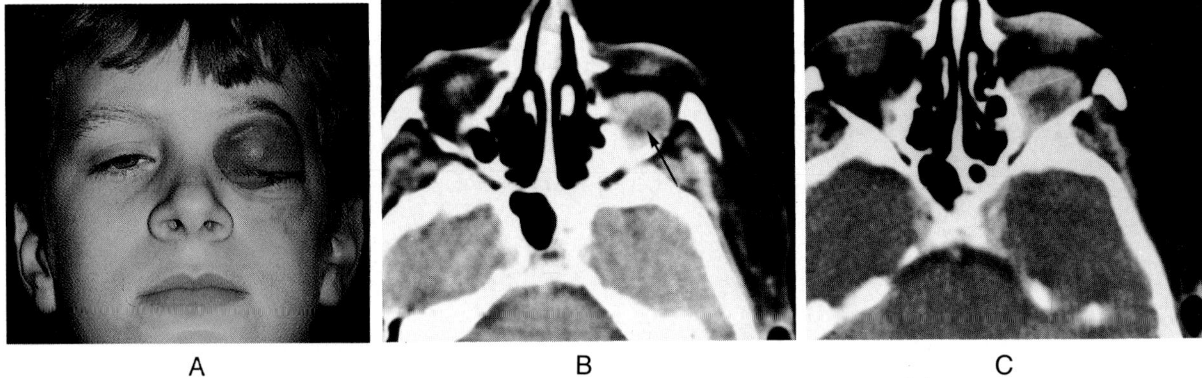

FIGURE 6-11 **Lymphangioma.** *A*, A spontaneous hemorrhage is shown here in an 8-year-old boy. Surgical extirpation revealed large fluid-filled cystic lesions. The histologic diagnosis was lymphangioma of the orbit. *B* and *C*, Lymphangiomas occur in children and usually present as an orbital mass. The lesions, which usually tend to appear solid on a CT evaluation usually can, however, occasionally have a somewhat cystic appearance on CT scan, as demonstrated here. (The *arrow* points to the area of low attenuation in the central portion of the lesion.)

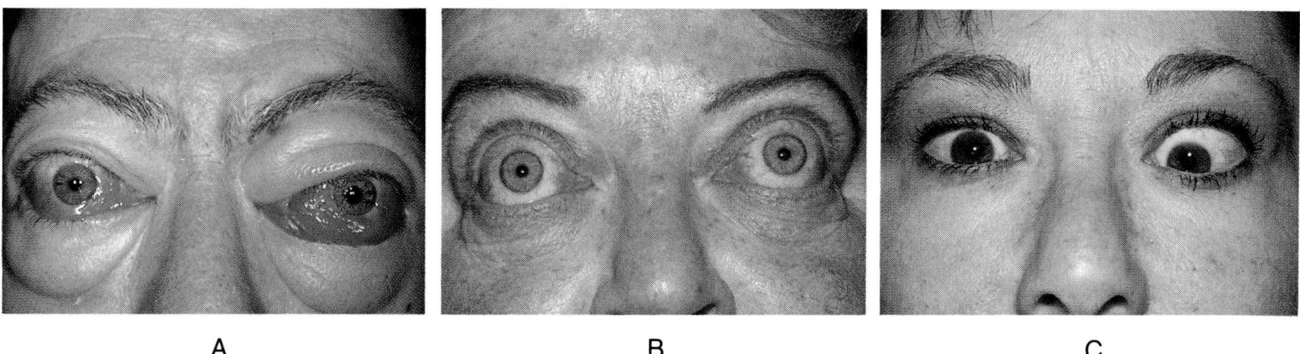

FIGURE 6–12 **Graves' disease.** Clinical appearance of orbitopathy of Graves' disease. *A,* Acute inflammatory and congestive phase with marked bilateral eyelid retraction, conjunctival chemosis, exophthalmos, and optic nerve compromise. *B,* Chronic stable phase with eyeball retraction and edema and firm exophthalmos. *C,* Chronic phase with marked strabismus from restrictive myopathy, resembling hypotropia and esotropia deviations and corresponding diplopia.

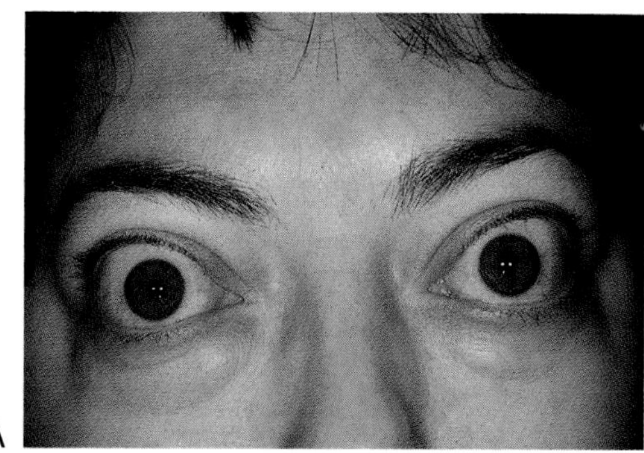

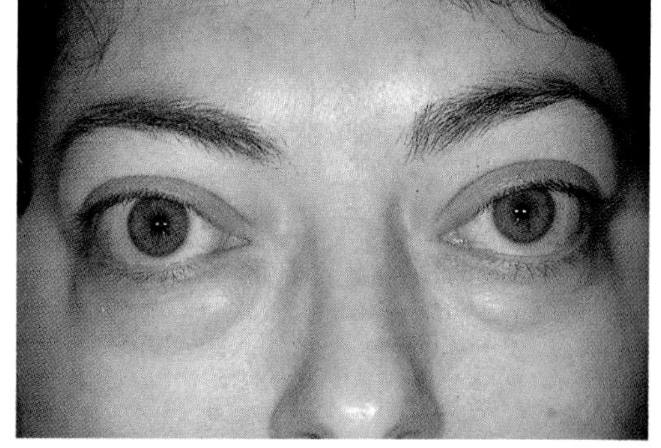

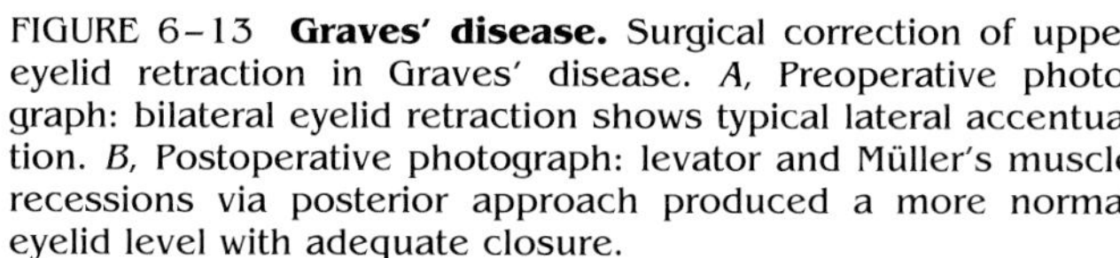

FIGURE 6–13 **Graves' disease.** Surgical correction of upper eyelid retraction in Graves' disease. *A,* Preoperative photograph: bilateral eyelid retraction shows typical lateral accentuation. *B,* Postoperative photograph: levator and Müller's muscle recessions via posterior approach produced a more normal eyelid level with adequate closure.

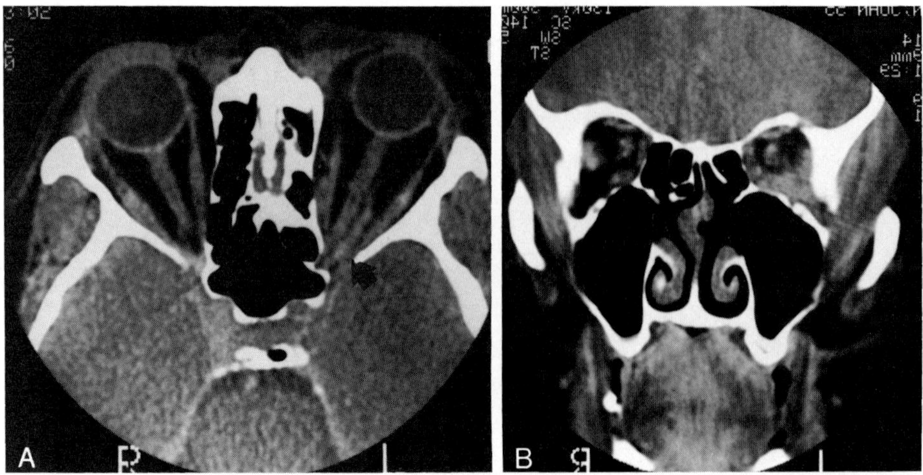

FIGURE 6–14 **Idiopathic orbital inflammation.** A 55-year-old man with progressive painless proptosis of the left eye and diplopia of 6 months' duration. Examination was significant for proptosis and increased resistance to ballottement of the globe. *A*, Contrast-enhanced axial CT scan of the orbit shows an infiltrating lesion in the posterior orbit of the left eye. *B*, Coronal CT scan demonstrates an infiltrating lesion of the inferolateral posterior orbit. Biopsy showed nonspecific idiopathic orbital inflammation. Recurring symptoms after discontinuation of corticosteroids necessitated the use of low-dose radiation for control.

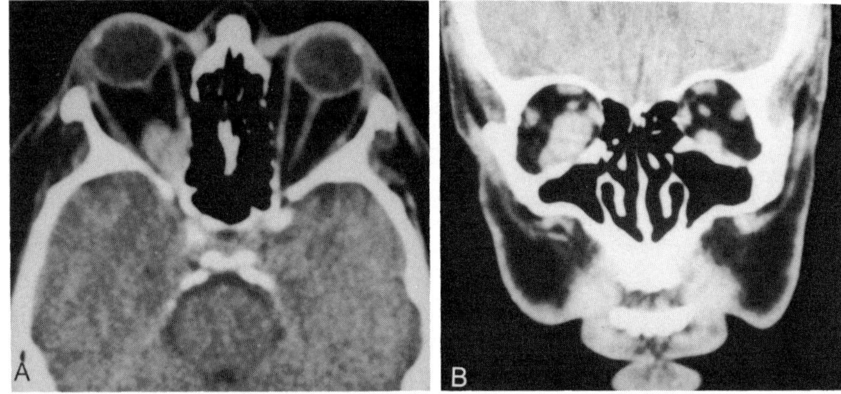

FIGURE 6–15 **Idiopathic orbital inflammation.** A 47-year-old man with a history of Graves' orbitopathy complained of increasing proptosis of the right eye and worsening diplopia. *A*, Contrast-enhanced axial CT scan of the orbit shows a lesion in the apex. *B*, Coronal CT scan demonstrates the mass displacing the inferior rectus and optic nerve. Results of the biopsy were consistent with nonspecific idiopathic orbital inflammation. The lesion responded poorly to corticosteroids, but radiation therapy was successful.

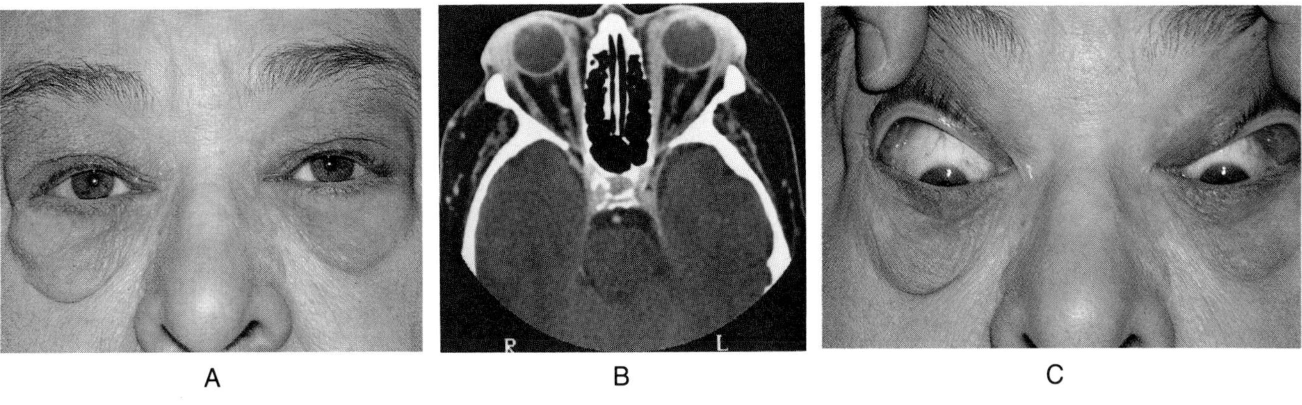

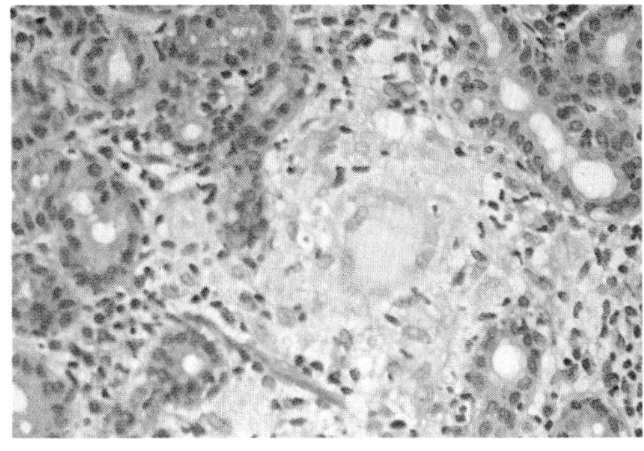

FIGURE 6–16 **Sarcoidosis.** *A,* A 67-year-old white woman complained of puffiness of the eyelids and pressure sensation around the eyes that lasted for 6 weeks. Examination was significant for visual acuity of 20/50 in both eyes, intraocular pressures of 40 mmHg in both eyes, mild exophthalmos, lacrimal gland enlargement, and conjunctival injection and chemosis. *B,* Contrast-enhanced axial CT scan demonstrates anterior orbital infiltrate involving the lacrimal gland and the medial rectus muscles bilaterally. *C,* Bilateral enlargement of the palpebral lobe of the lacrimal gland. *D,* Lacrimal gland biopsy specimen with noncaseating granulomas consistent with sarcoidosis. Positive lacrimal gland biopsy obviated the need for a more invasive procedure for pulmonary lesion biopsy. Oral corticosteroid therapy resulted in rapid resolution of signs and symptoms.

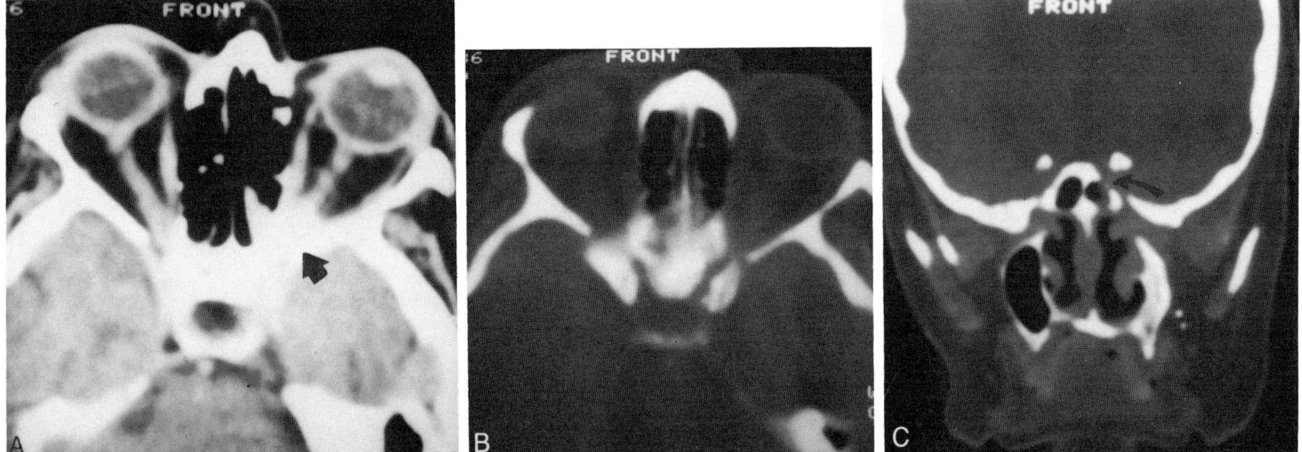

FIGURE 6–17 **Wegener's granulomatosis.** A 69-year-old woman complained of malaise, left-sided facial pain, and decreased vision of the left eye, which lasted for 6 months. *A,* Contrast-enhanced axial CT scan of the orbits demonstrates an infiltrative lesion involving the left orbital apex and adjacent paranasal sinuses. *B,* Axial CT scan, bone window technique. *C,* Coronal CT scan, bone window technique, demonstrates bony erosion in the wall of the spheroidal sinus. Ethmoidal biopsy revealed necrotizing granulomatous inflammation and vasculitis consistent with the diagnosis of Wegener's granulomatosis.

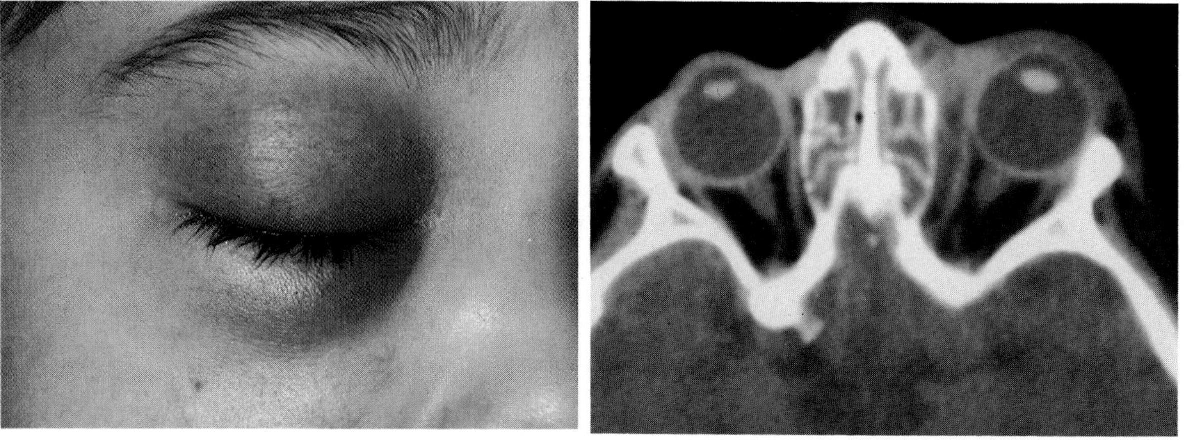

FIGURE 6–18 **Pediatric bacterial infections.** *A,* Presentation of a 3-year-old child with pain, local heat, redness, and edema of the periorbital tissues is typical of bacterial infection. Decreased ocular motility was suggestive of orbital involvement. Note the sharp demarcation line corresponding to the origin of the orbital septum, the arcus marginalis. This finding is frequently seen in postseptal infection. *B,* The CT scan demonstrates ethmoidal sinusitis with extension of the infectious process through the lamina papyracea into the medial orbit. There is no evidence of abscess formation. The child responded to antibiotics given intravenously.

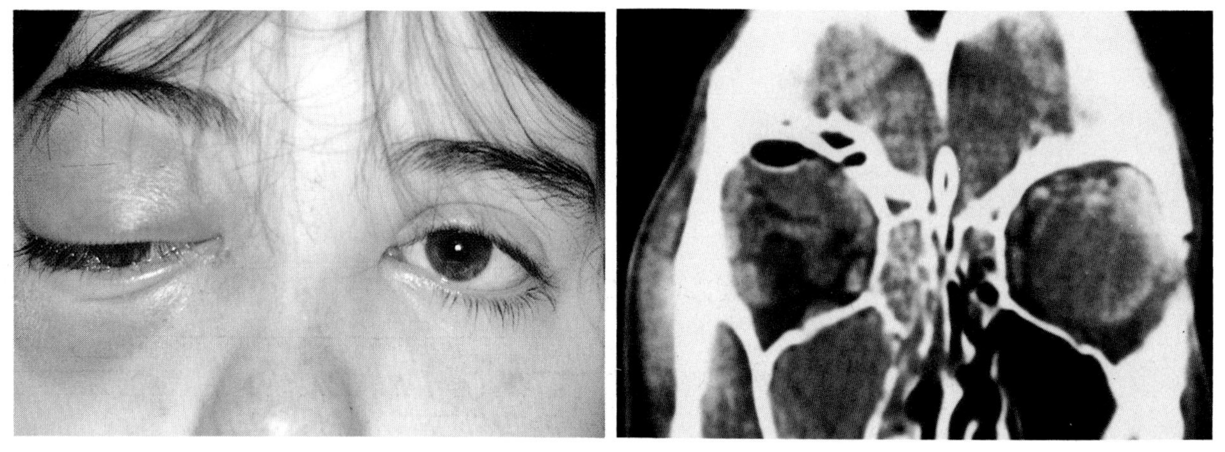

FIGURE 6–19 **Pediatric bacterial infections.** *A,* Marked proptosis, ptosis, ophthalmoplegia, and decreased visual acuity were presenting findings in a child with pansinusitis and an abscess in the superior orbit. *B,* CT scan shows maxillary and ethmoid sinus opacification as well as orbital inflammation and abscesses. Prompt surgical drainage of the orbital abscesses, anterior ethmoidectomy, and maxillary antrostomy followed by a prolonged course of antibiotics were necessary for resolving this life-threatening infection.

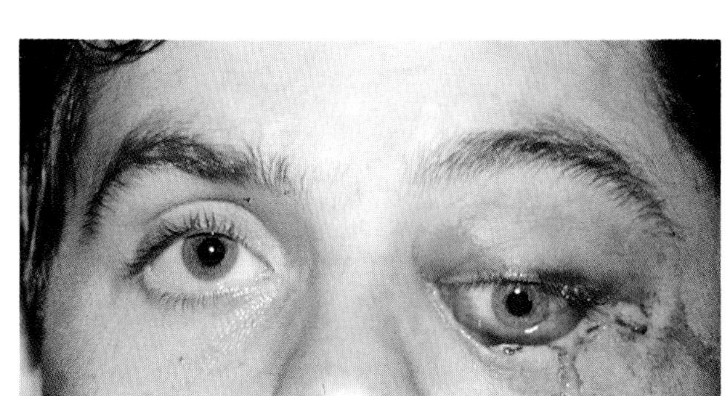

A

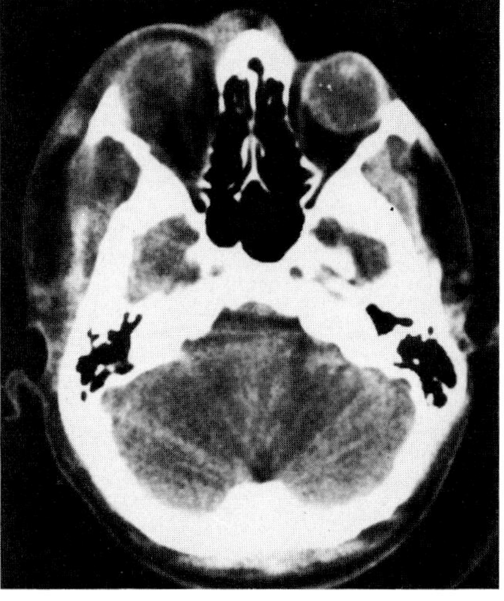

B

FIGURE 6–20 **Adult bacterial infections.** *A,* Surgical repair of a zygomatic fracture preceded the development of subperiosteal orbital abscess. Note the depression of the globe secondary to mass effect. *B,* Extension of the infectious process from the temporal fossa is evident on the CT scan. Prompt surgical drainage followed by a prolonged course of antibiotics led to resolution without functional sequelae.

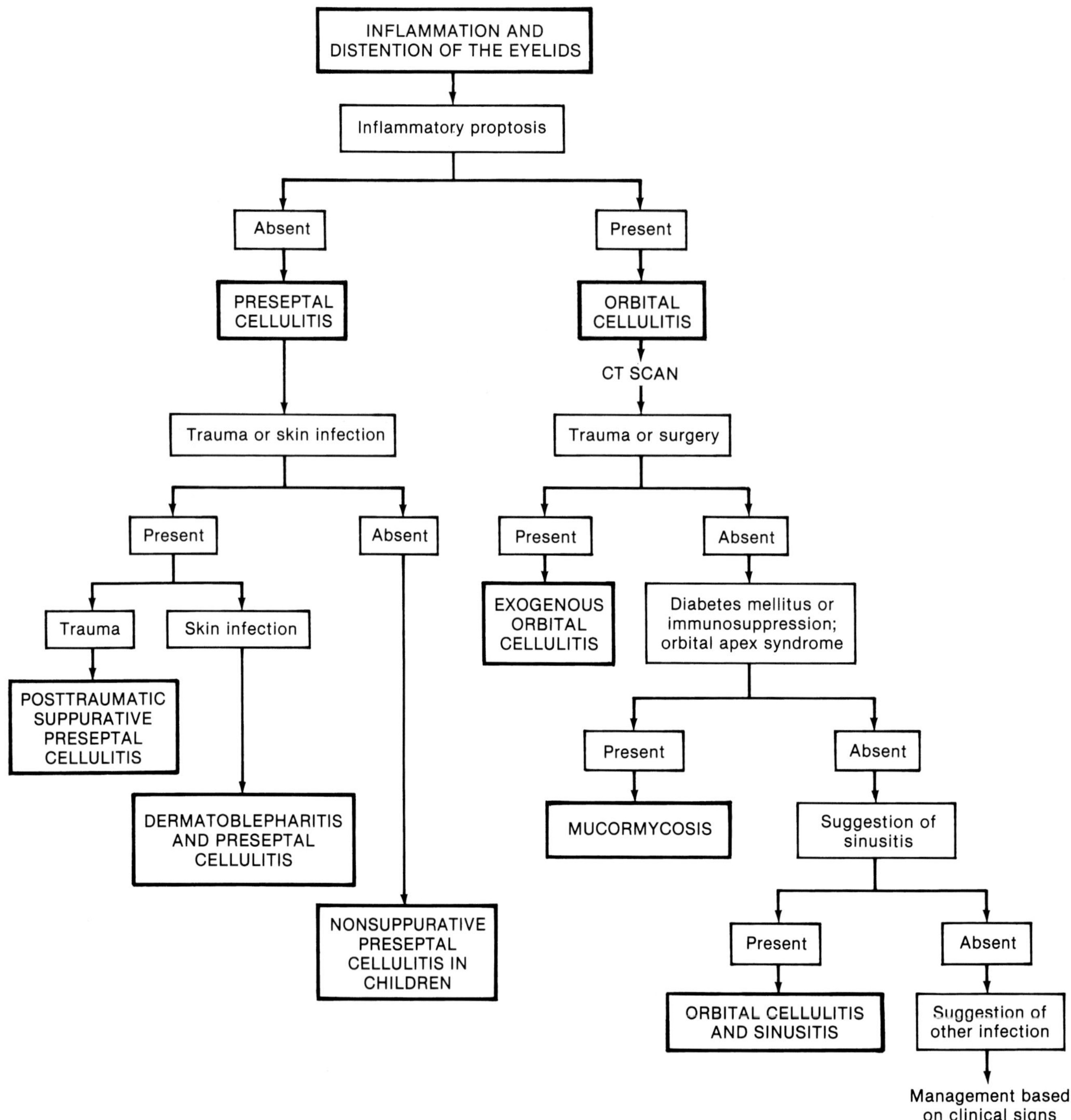

FIGURE 6–21 Algorithm for the evaluation of orbital infection. (From Jones DB, Steinkuller PG: Strategies for the initial management of acute preseptal and orbital cellulitis. Trans Am Ophthalmol Soc 86:94–112, 1988.)

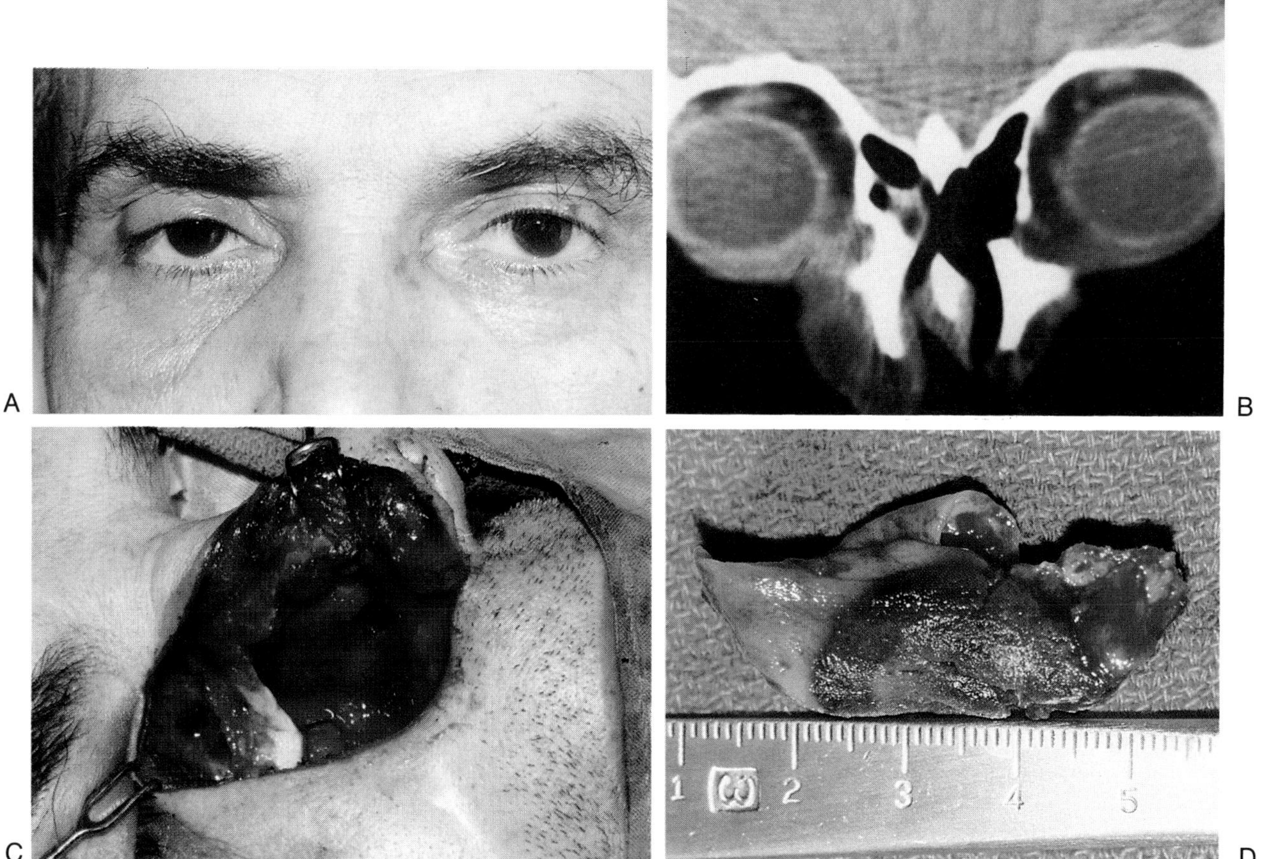

FIGURE 6–22 **Orbital infection due to *Aspergillus*.** *A*, Localized swelling of the nasolabial and infraorbital regions associated with mild ptosis and a minimal motility disturbance was caused by aspergillosis in a 68-year-old patient with leukemia. *B*, Coronal CT scan demonstrates soft tissue inflammation and mucosal thickening. *C*, Wide surgical débridement required resection of the nasal septum. *D*, The resected specimen. Note the area of necrosis.

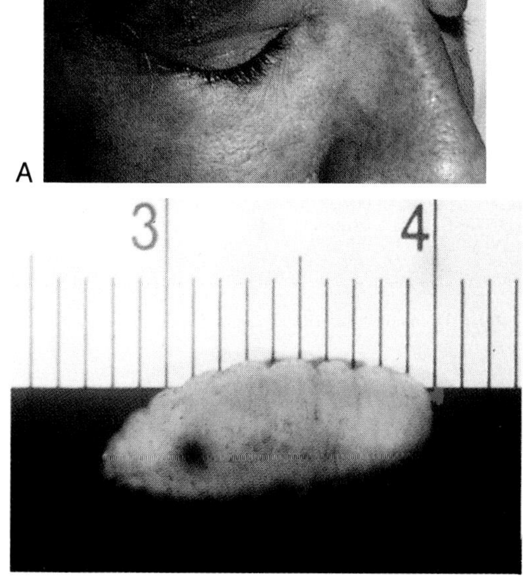

FIGURE 6–23 **Myiasis.** *A*, Multiple pruritic papular skin lesions in a middle-aged man 2 weeks after a visit to West Africa. Each lesion represented the larval stage of the Tumbu fly. Topical application of petroleum jelly forces the larva to the surface, enabling mechanical extraction. *B*, Extracted larva. (*A* and *B*, Courtesy of Monte Mills, M.D.)

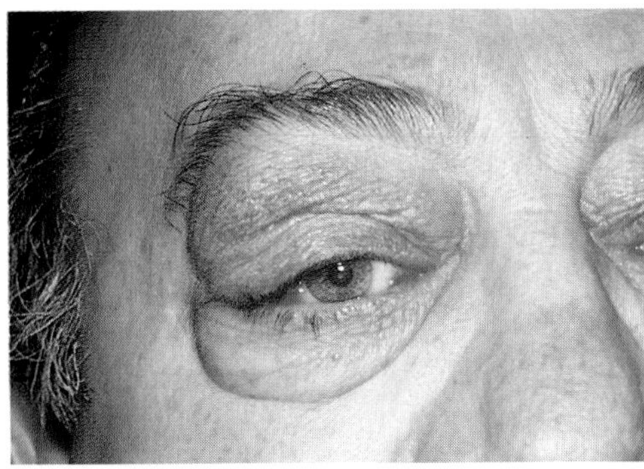

FIGURE 6–24 **Signs of lesions of the lacrimal fossa.** The normal contour of the upper eyelid is deformed into an S shape with enlargement of a mass in the lacrimal gland fossa.

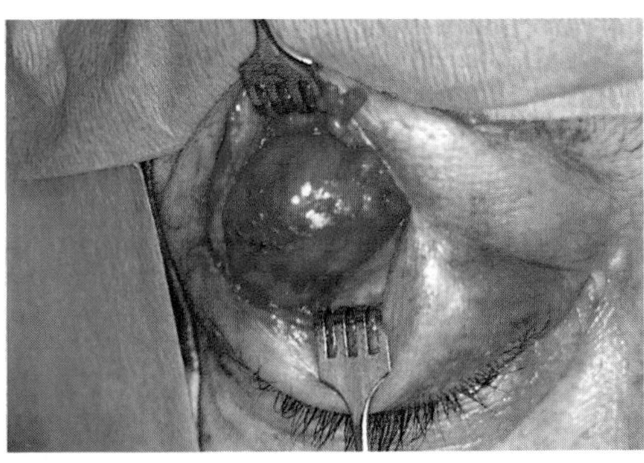

FIGURE 6–26 **Lymphoma.** Intraoperative photograph showing enlarged lacrimal gland.

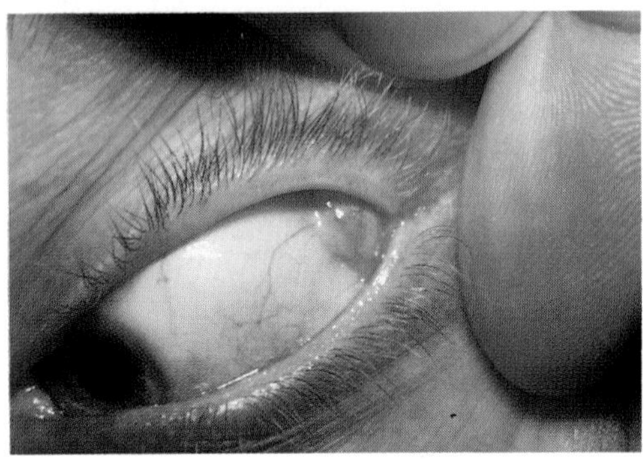

FIGURE 6–25 **Dacryoadenitis.** Dacryops following dacryoadenitis.

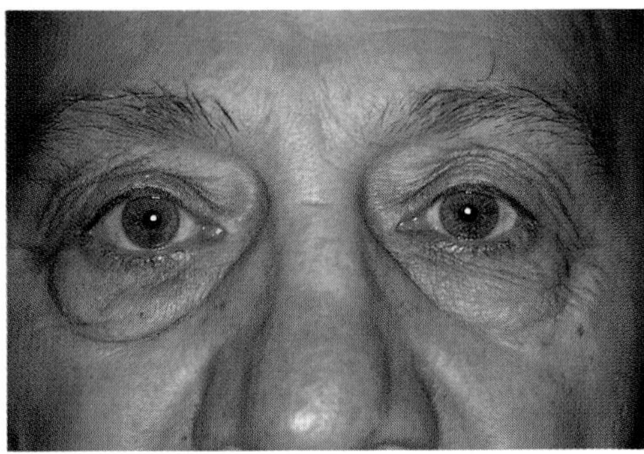

FIGURE 6–27 **Lymphoma.** Patient after chemotherapy for systemic lymphoma.

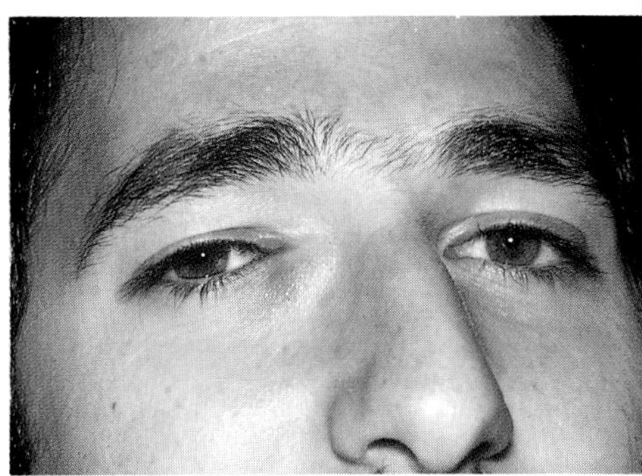

FIGURE 6–28 **Mucocele.** A patient with recurrent "blue cyst" in a corner of his right eye. The patient could massage the cyst to reduce it. When he performed this maneuver, he sensed a foul taste in his throat.

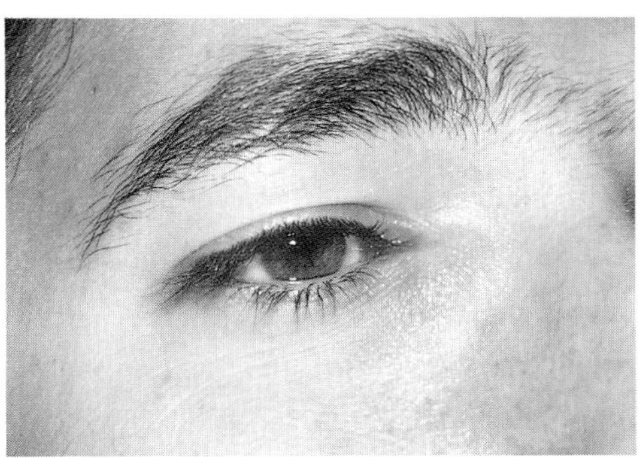

FIGURE 6–29 **Mucocele.** Close-up of blue cyst.

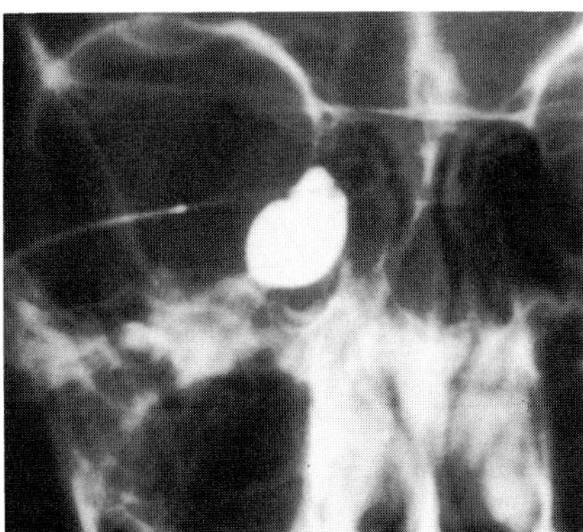

FIGURE 6–30 **Mucocele.** Dacryocystogram of the patient in Figure 6–28.

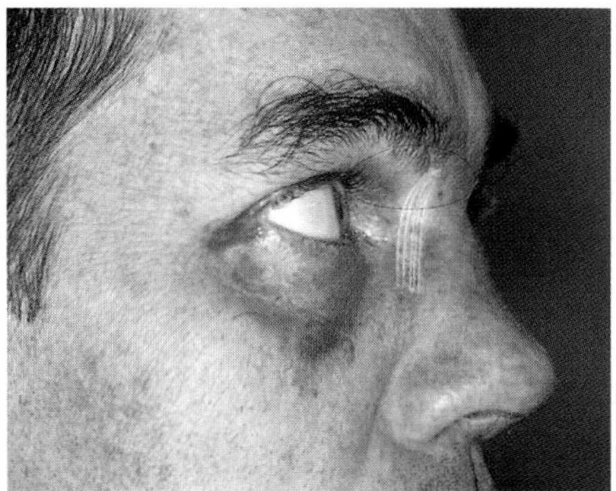

FIGURE 6–31 **Wegener's granulomatosis.** Profile showing the saddle deformity of Wegener's granulomatosis.

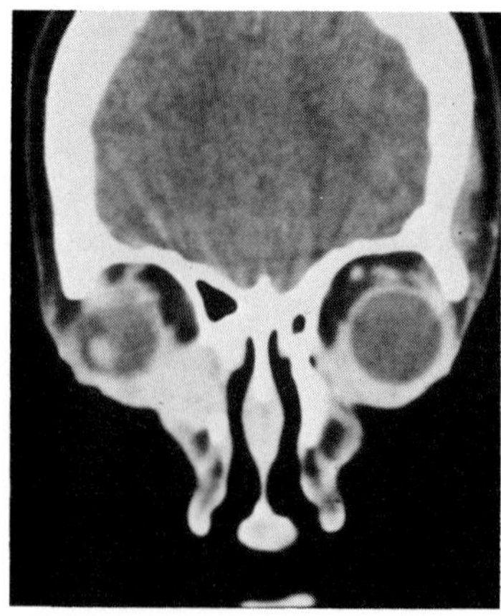

FIGURE 6–33 **Neurilemmoma.** CT scan revealed a mass in the vicinity of the nasolacrimal duct.

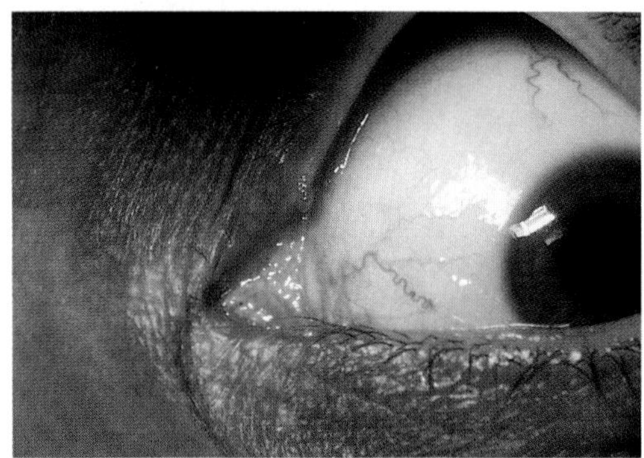

FIGURE 6–32 **Epithelial tumors.** The appearance of a papilloma extending from the punctum. This patient had multiple excisions of papillomas at this site with rapid recurrences.

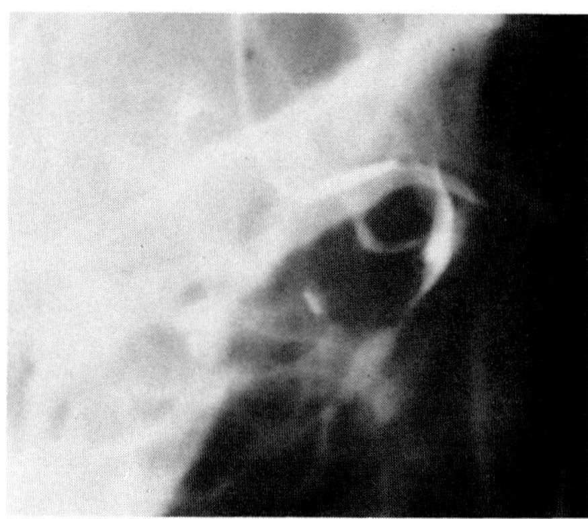

FIGURE 6–34 **Neurilemmoma.** A dacryocystogram shows an external indentation on the nasolacrimal sac–duct junction.

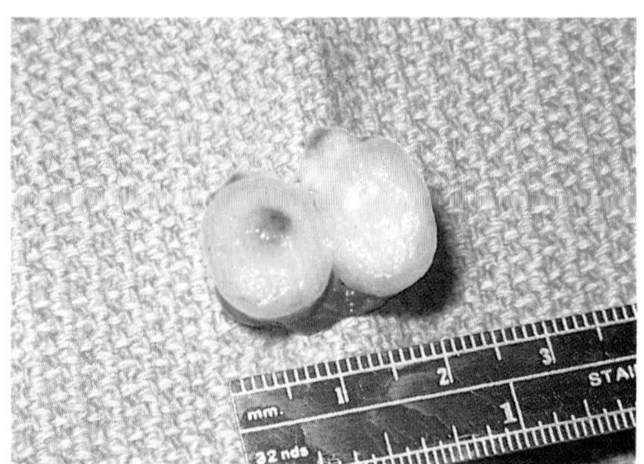

FIGURE 6–35 **Neurilemmoma.** An intraoperative photograph showing the bisected schwannoma.

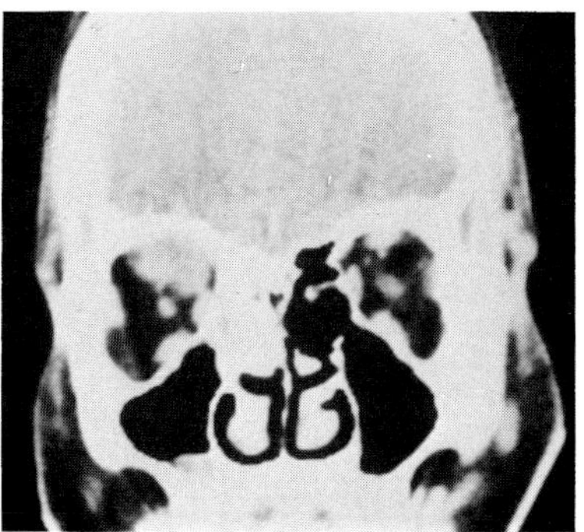

FIGURE 6–36 **Osteoma.** An osteoma arising from the ethmoidal sinus, causing secondary nasolacrimal duct obstruction.

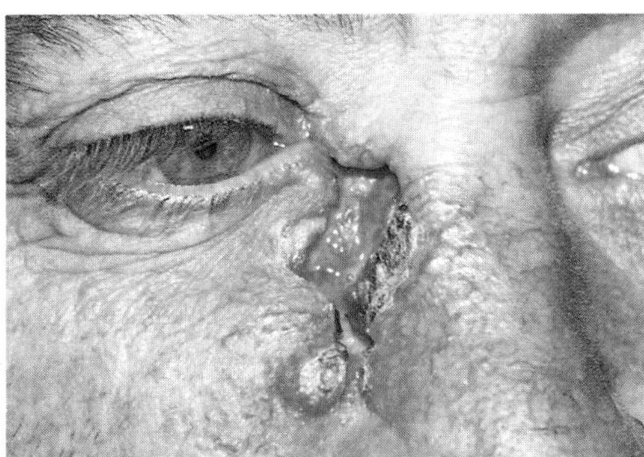

FIGURE 6–37 **Recurrent basal cell carcinoma.** Invasion of the nasolacrimal duct and sac area can occur secondary to the spread of cutaneous tumors such as this recurrent basal cell carcinoma.

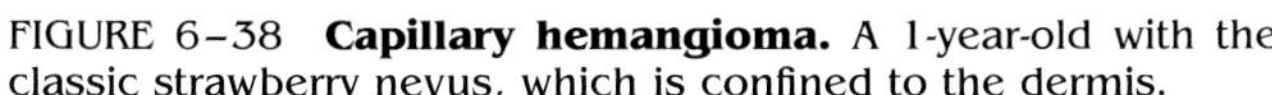

FIGURE 6–38 **Capillary hemangioma.** A 1-year-old with the classic strawberry nevus, which is confined to the dermis.

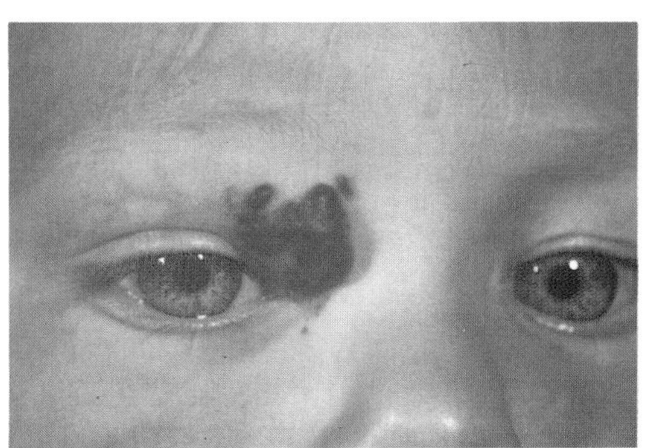

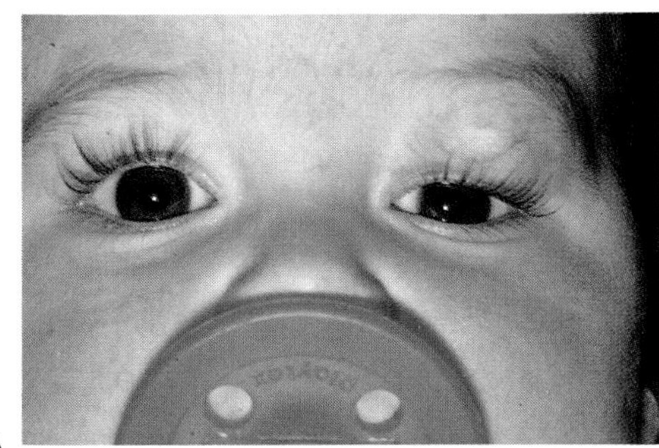

A

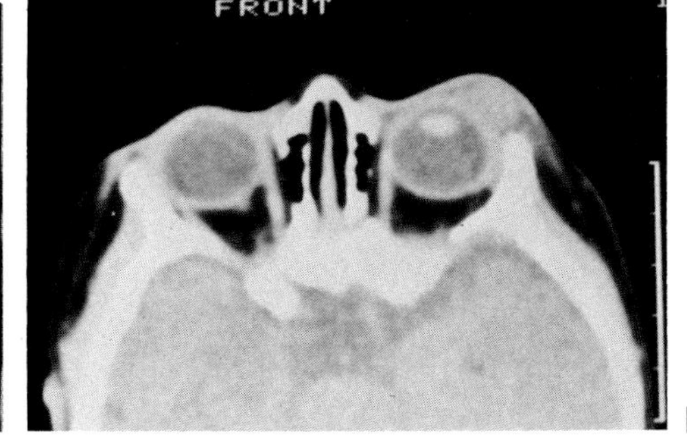

B

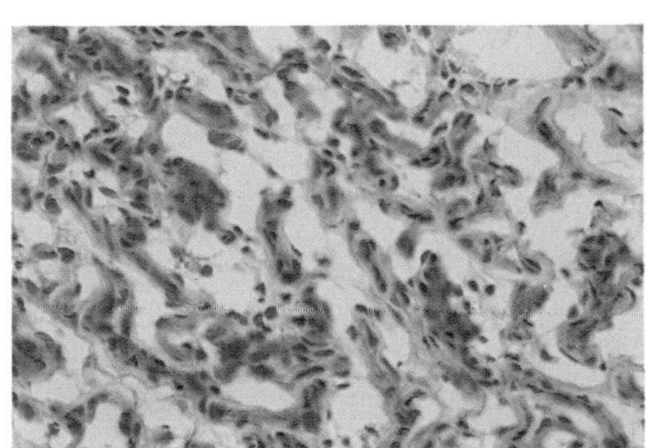

C

FIGURE 6–39 **Capillary hemangioma.** *A,* This 10-month-old infant was first noted to have a left upper eyelid mass at 4 weeks of age. The violaceous-colored lesion rapidly enlarged over a 20-week period. Retinoscopy disclosed 4 diopters of astigmatism. *B,* Axial CT scan demonstrates a smooth-contoured upper eyelid/anterior orbit mass. *C,* The lesion did not involute with intralesional steroids. Because of the high astigmatism, the tumor was excised. Fine endothelium-lined channels are apparent on tissue stained with H&E.

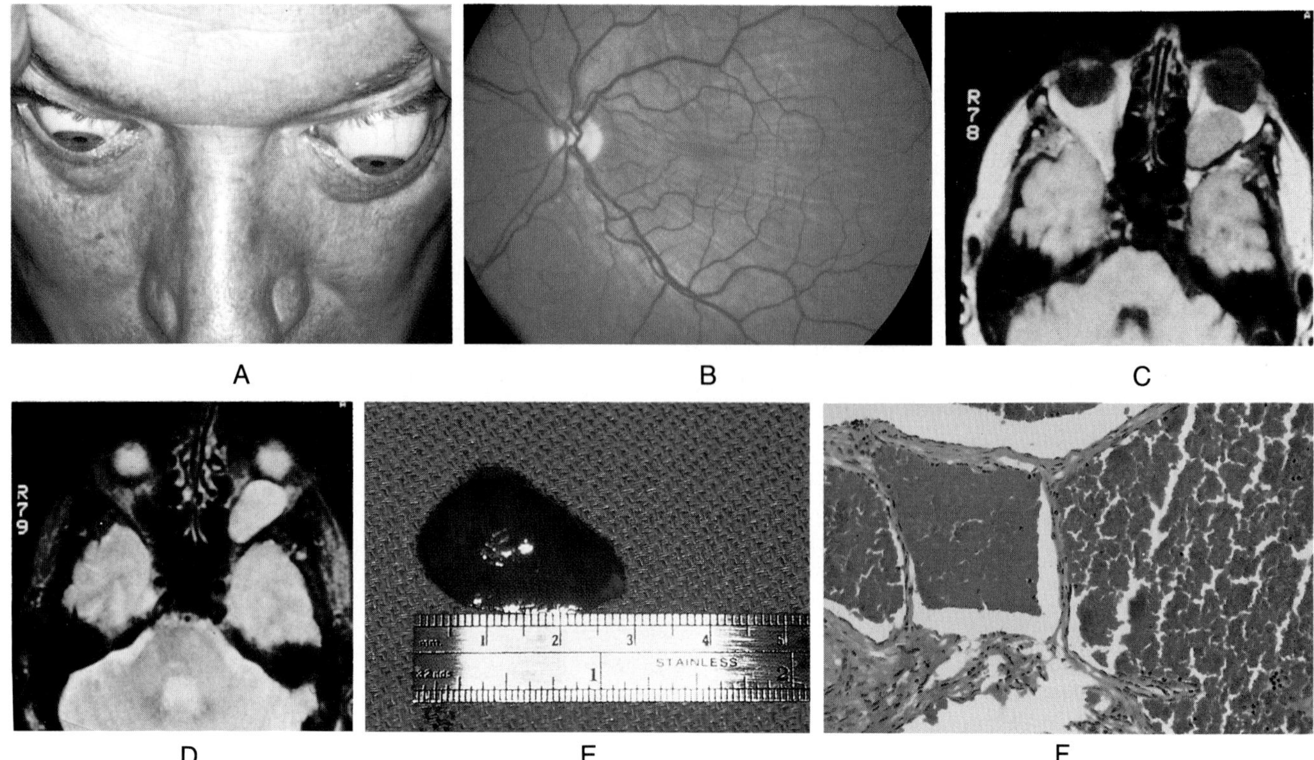

FIGURE 6–40 **Cavernous hemangioma.** *A,* This 42-year-old man had a 5-year history of gradually increasing axial proptosis. Neither the eyelids nor the globe is inflamed. *B,* The tumor's indentation on the globe produced hyperopia and choroidal striae. *C,* Magnetic resonance imaging depicts an ovoid, intraconal mass. On T_1-weighted images (TR = 800, TE = 20), the tumor is hypointense to fat. *D,* On T_2-weighted images (TR = 2000, TE = 80), the hemangioma is hyperintense to fat and relatively isointense to vitreous. *E,* The tumor was excised via a lateral orbitotomy. Its violaceous hue results from the stagnant and poorly oxygenated blood within it. *F,* Large vascular spaces 500 μ to 1 mm in size are lined by a flattened monolayer of endothelial cells. H&E, ×140.

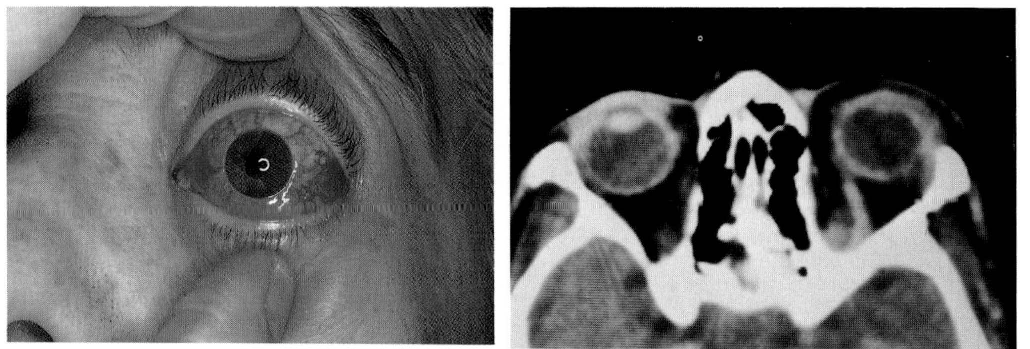

FIGURE 6–41 **Dural shunts.** *A,* Epibulbar vascular congestion, conjunctival chemosis, and a prominent globe may be mistaken for orbital inflammatory disease, but these signs typify arteriovenous communications. *B,* The right superior ophthalmic vein is dilated in this patient with a dural shunt.

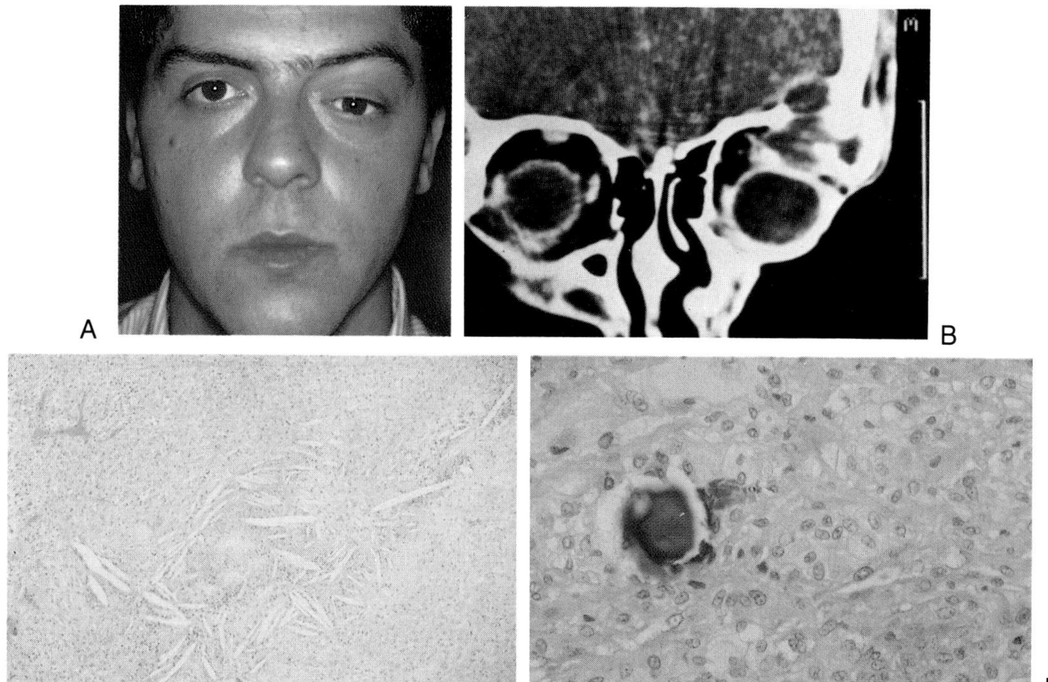

FIGURE 6–42 **Cholesterol granuloma.** *A,* This 32-year-old man complained of facial asymmetry. Visual acuity was 20/20 OS, but the globe was displaced inferiorly. A fullness was appreciated in the superior orbit. *B,* Axial CT scan reveals a cystic-appearing superior orbital mass with erosion of the orbital roof. *C,* The classic cholesterol clefts, inflammatory cell infiltrate, and erythrocytes of cholesterol granulomas. H&E, ×40. *D,* High-power magnification using H&E reveals calcium deposits and mononuclear cell infiltrate.

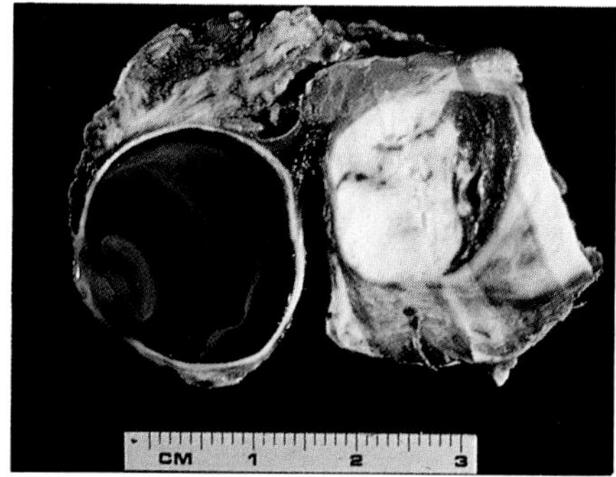

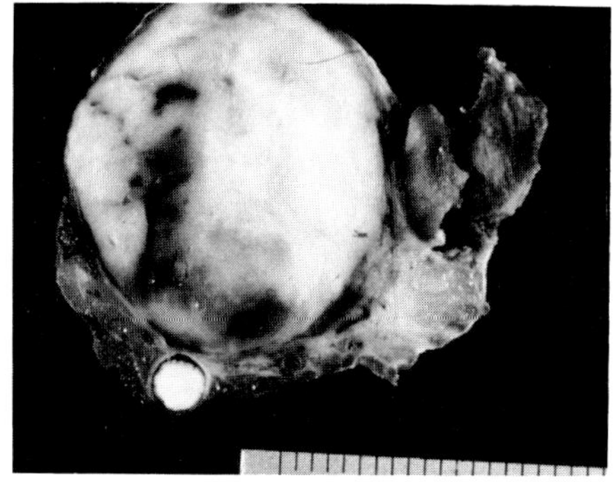

FIGURE 6–43 **Schwannoma.** *A,* Recurrent orbital schwannoma that was misinterpreted as a malignant lesion, leading to an unnecessary exenteration. Note that the mass is extremely well circumscribed, but it has an area of internal hemorrhagic cyst formation. *B,* The variegated cut surface of the lesion exhibits areas of yellow xanthomatous transformation, brown-black areas of hemorrhage, and at the periphery an attenuated perineural capsule. The optic nerve is present below. (*A* and *B,* Courtesy of Elise Torczynski, M.D.)

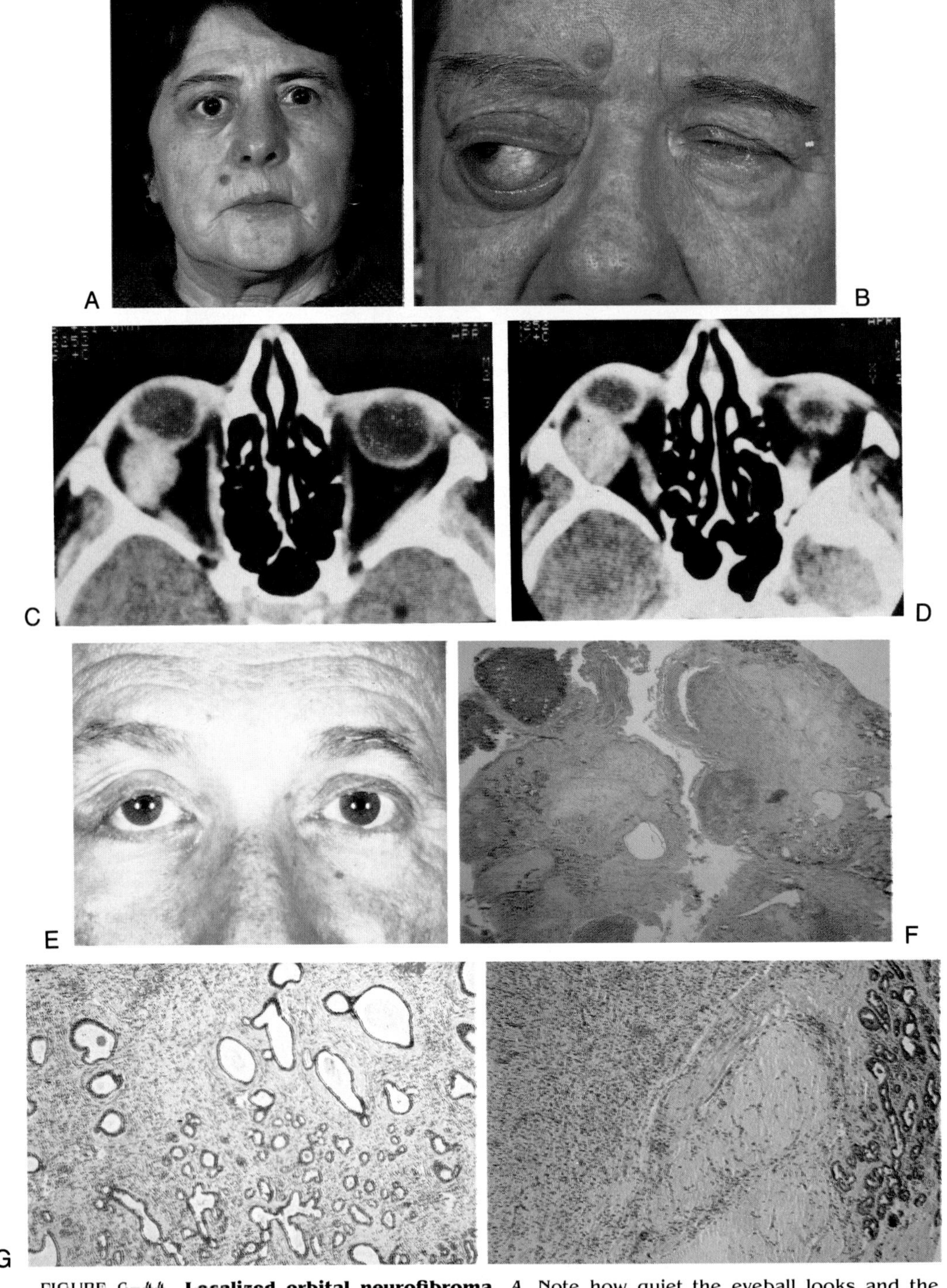

FIGURE 6–44 Localized orbital neurofibroma. *A,* Note how quiet the eyeball looks and the overall configuration of the eyelids, with 6 mm of well-tolerated proptosis. *B,* A 40-year history of a neglected right orbital neurofibroma has led to stretching of the eyelids with minimal congestion of the surface of the globe and absence of corneal exposure. The eyelids were able voluntarily to close completely on the globe. *C* and *D,* Two axial CT scans in somewhat different planes of a localized and isolated neurofibroma exhibiting slight irregularities in outline of the lesion, which is not as elegantly well encapsulated as the typical schwannoma (a lesion delineated by the perineurium of the nerve of origin, whereas the neurofibroma acquires a fibrous compression pseudocapsule). *E,* An unusual neurofibroma of the lacrimal gland producing a lateral ptosis of the right upper eyelid. *F,* The excised specimen obtained from the patient shown in *E* is a myxoid lesion that has infiltrated the parenchyma of the lacrimal gland, relatively undisturbed portions of which are shown toward the upper left, but islands of ductular tissue are also scattered throughout. *G,* Ectatic ductules of the lacrimal gland are separated by myxoid neurofibromatous tissue. Such an appearance might easily be confused with that of a benign mixed tumor (pleomorphic adenoma). The ductular units lack the characteristic splaying off of an outer myoepithelial layer, as seen in benign mixed tumors. *H,* Watery myxoid tissue is shown immediately to the left of surviving ducts of the preexistent lacrimal gland on the right. A somewhat more cellular but still loose proliferation of spindle cells is present on the far left.

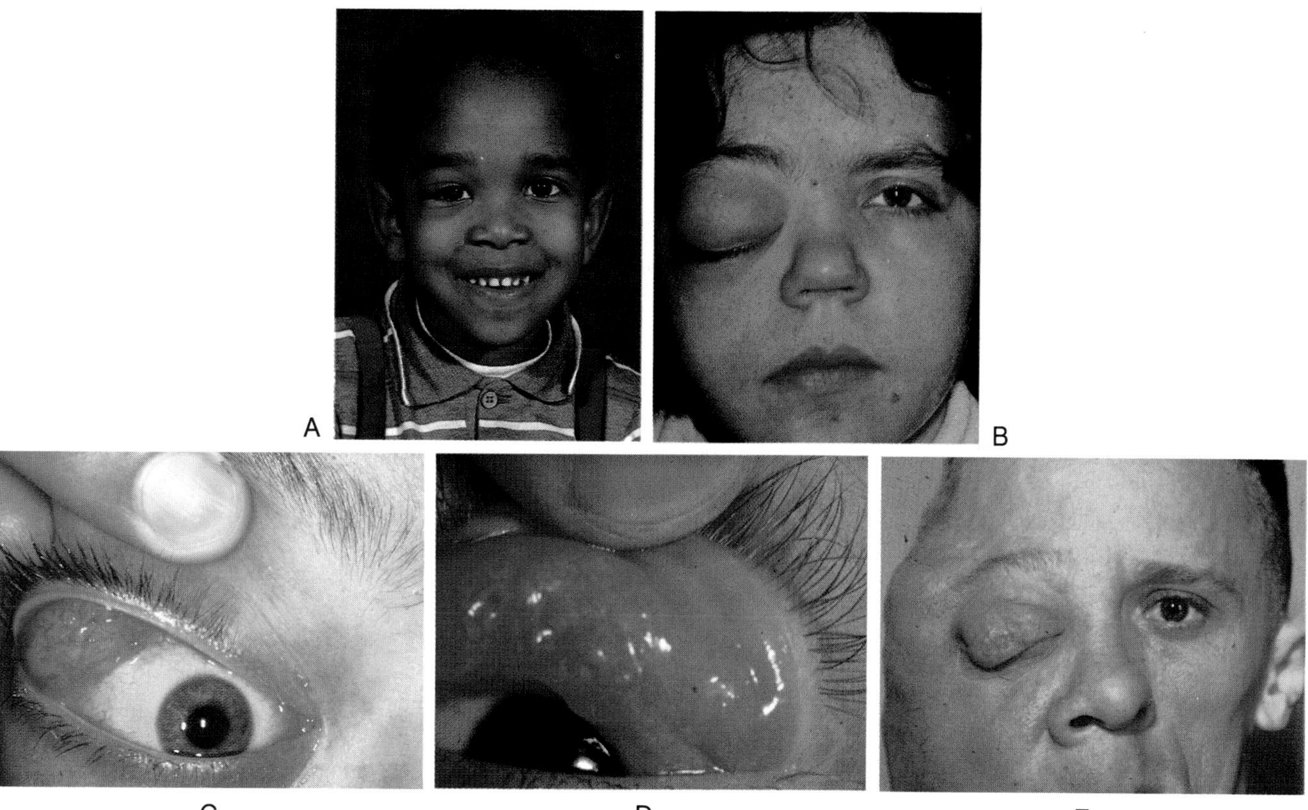

FIGURE 6–45 **Plexiform orbital and eyelid neurofibromas in neurofibromatosis type 1 (NF1).** *A,* Minimal degree of right orbital involvement with a plexiform neurofibroma has caused infiltration of the lacrimal gland and the lateral aspect of the right upper lid. *B,* More extensive eyelid and orbital infiltration. *C,* Eversion of the upper eyelid reveals massive enlargement of the palpebral lobe of the lacrimal gland from infiltration by plexiform neurofibroma. (*C,* Courtesy of Frederick Blodi, M.D.) *D,* Eversion reveals multiple small translucent submucosal neurofibromatous units of the superior tarsal and forniceal conjunctiva. *E,* This adult had massive facial deformity resulting from an extensive plexiform neurofibroma involving the eyelid and orbit. (*B* and *E,* Courtesy of Martha Farber, M.D., and Morton Smith, M.D.)

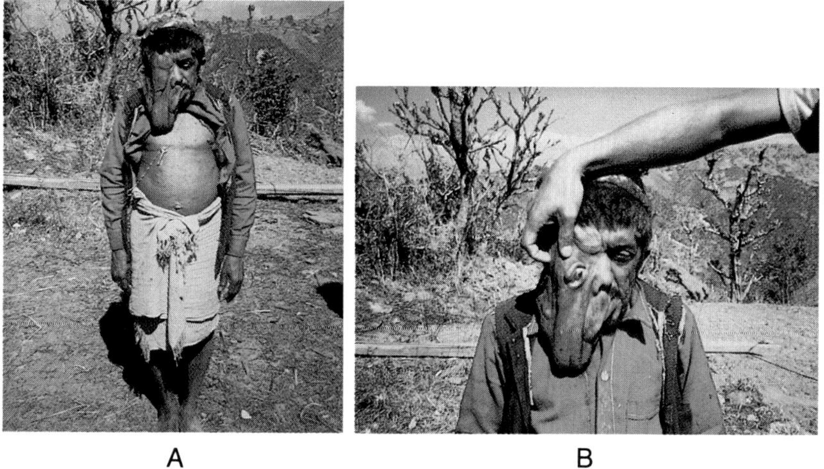

FIGURE 6–46 **Elephantiasis neuromatosa of the face in NF1.** *A,* A pendulous mass obscures the eyeball and also involves the right hemifacial structures. *B,* By elevating the redundant skin of the upper eyelid, a nonfunctioning globe is revealed. (*A* and *B,* Courtesy of William N. Hawks, M.D.)

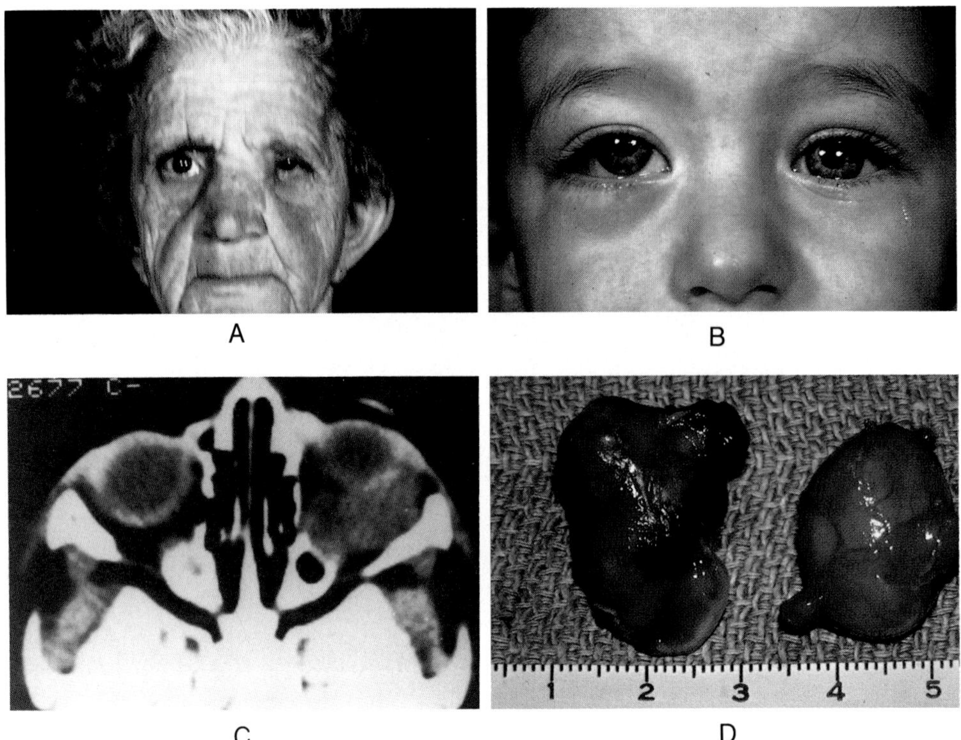

FIGURE 6–47 **Malignant peripheral nerve sheath tumors (malignant schwannoma).** *A*, An elderly patient had a left superonasal orbital mass that had produced hypesthesia in the distribution of the supraorbital nerve. *B*, A 5-year-old boy presented with a rapidly developing right orbital mass, presumed clinically to be a rhabdomyosarcoma. *C*, Axial CT scan of the patient shown in *B* revealed a bilobed lesion; the lobe in the more nasal and posterior orbit had a looser texture, whereas the more lateral and larger unit in this projection appeared to be solid. *D*, At the time of surgery, the bilobed tumor consisted of a myxoid neurofibroma, shown on the left, and a more solid malignant schwannoma, shown on the right. Nine years after local excision, the patient had a functioning globe, no orbital recurrence, and no distant metastases. (*B–D*, Courtesy of Albert Hornblass, M.D.)

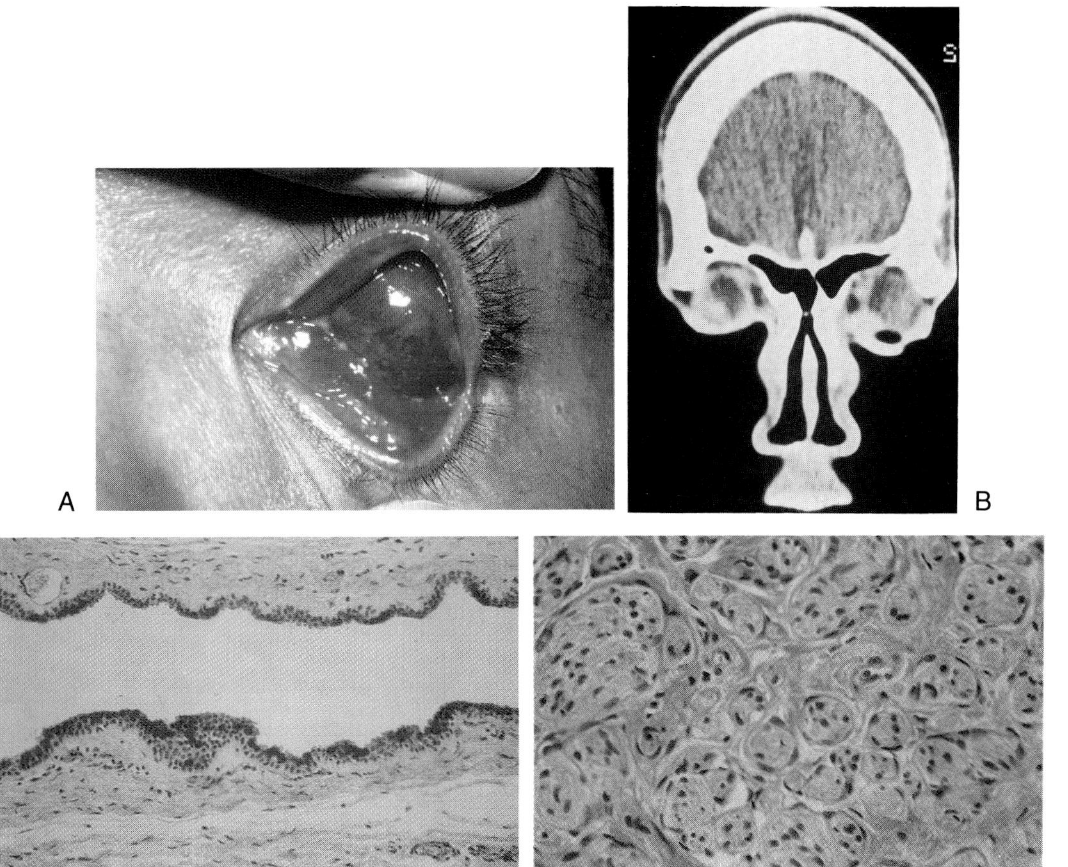

FIGURE 6–48 **Postamputation orbital neuroma.** *A,* Twenty-five years after removal of a phthisical eye, a transilluminable cystic lesion is present in the orbit. *B,* Coronal CT scan reveals a cystic lesion in the orbit with an adjacent round density at its inferonasal border. *C,* The excised cyst is lined by nonkeratinizing squamous epithelium containing mucus-producing goblet cells. *D,* In the inferonasal solid nodule, there is a proliferation of neuromatous tissue. An indistinct perineurium surrounds each unit and fuses with a fibrotic stroma. (*A–D,* From Messmer EP, Camara J, Boniuk M, Font R: Amputation neuroma of the orbit. A report of two cases and review of the literature. Ophthalmology 91:1420–1423, 1984.)

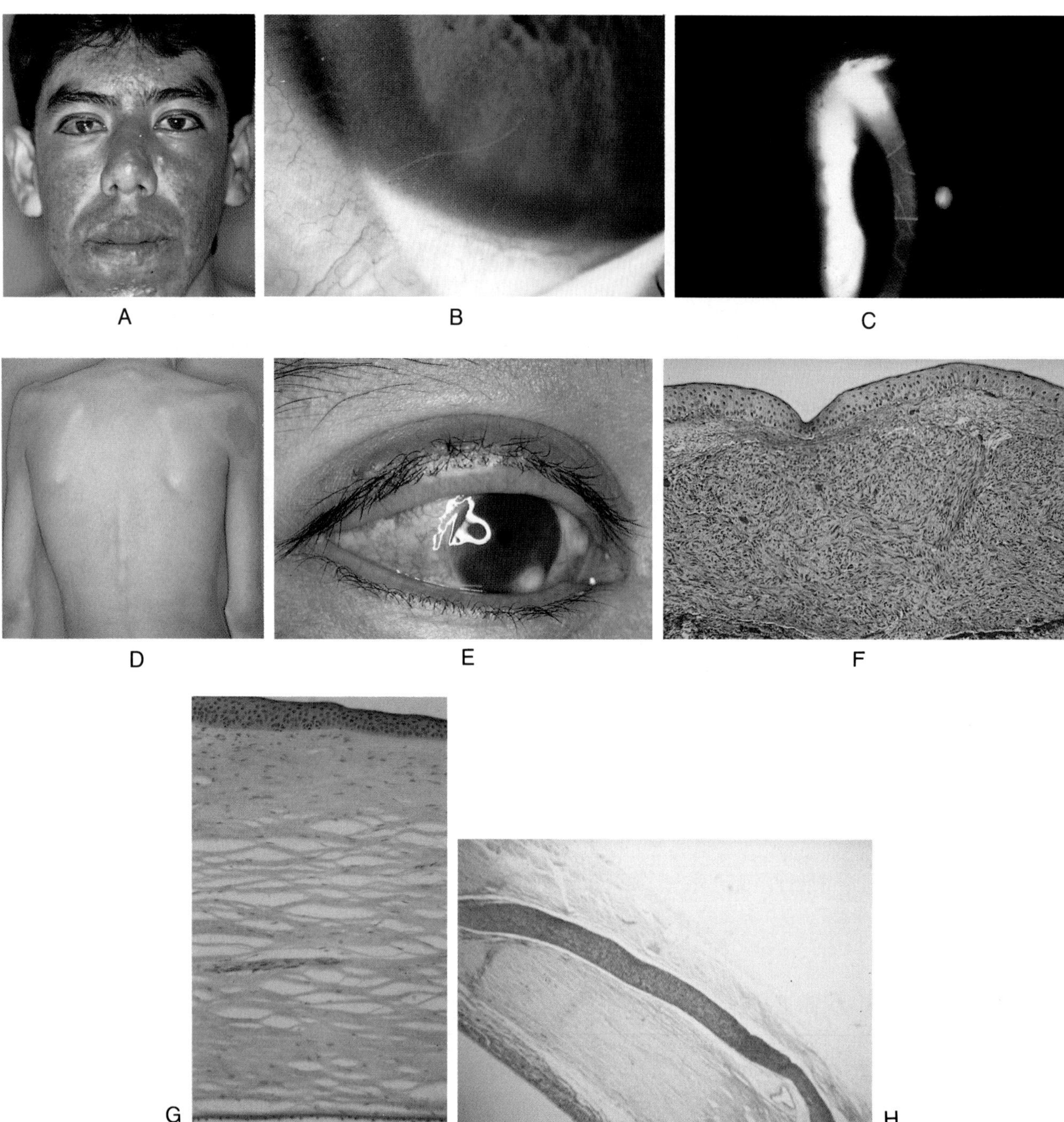

FIGURE 6–49 **Multiple endocrine neoplasia syndrome (MEN IIb).** *A,* Typical facies of a patient with MEN IIb, showing thickened lips and evidence of ocular irritation, particularly on the right. *B,* Several thickened corneal nerves are entering toward the bottom left. *C,* Slit-lamp view of criss-crossing thickened nerves in the paraxial cornea. *D,* The patient has a marfanoid habitus, with a café-au-lait spot in the right periaxillary deltoid region. *E,* Conjunctival irritation, along with a white peripheral conjunctival-corneal neurofibroma. Note the thickening of the eyelid margin and the rostral displacement of the eyelashes into several rows. *F,* A biopsy specimen of the white corneal lesion displays wavy bundles of neurofibromatous tissue beneath the nonkeratinizing conjunctival squamous epithelium. (*A, B, D–F,* Courtesy of Narsing Rao, M.D.) *G,* A thickened corneal nerve is shown in the lower third of the corneal button. Electron microscopy reveals that the nerves are not myelinated. (*C* and *G,* Courtesy of Gordon Klintworth, M.D.) *H,* A massively thickened long posterior ciliary nerve in a scleral canal. (*H,* Courtesy of Alan Friedman, M.D.)

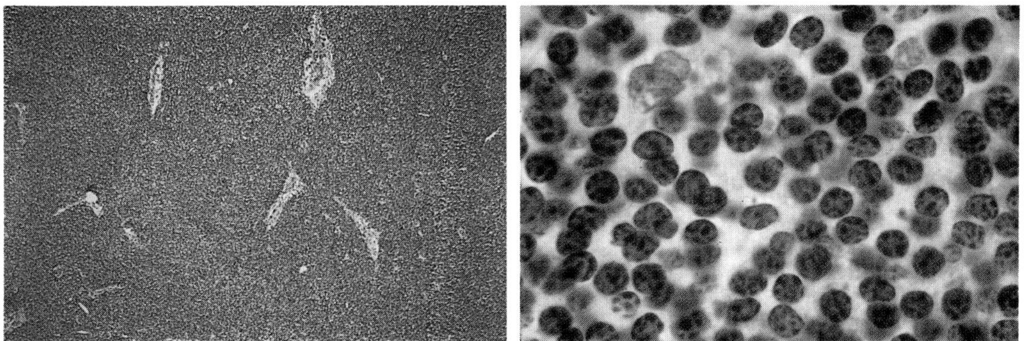

FIGURE 6–50 **Lymphoid tumors.** *A,* Low-power histopathology of a diffuse proliferation of lymphocytes. In contrast to the case with pseudotumors, there is scant interstitial stroma. *B,* A high-power view reveals a tightly packed array of well-differentiated lymphocytes.

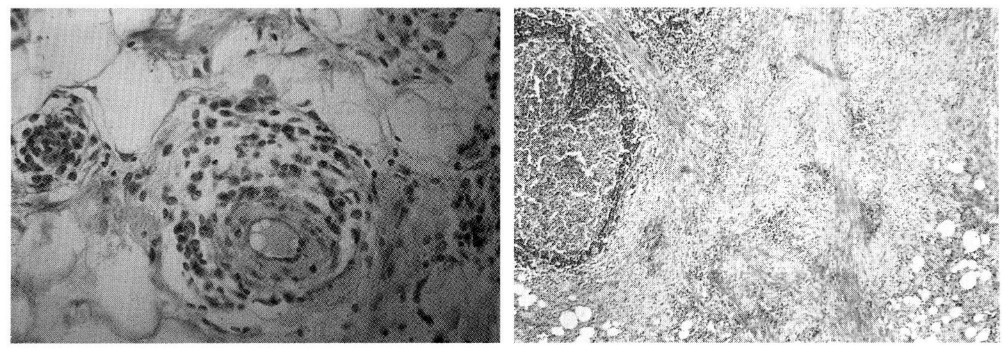

FIGURE 6–51 **Pseudotumor histopathology.** *A,* The infiltrate is relatively hypocellular. In the perivascular region, there is a characteristic polymorphous infiltrate, including eosinophils, plasma cells, and lymphocytes. *B,* A more advanced pseudotumor demonstrates fibrous replacement of orbital fat. There is a light interspersal of inflammatory cells in the fibrous tissue and a germinal center on the left.

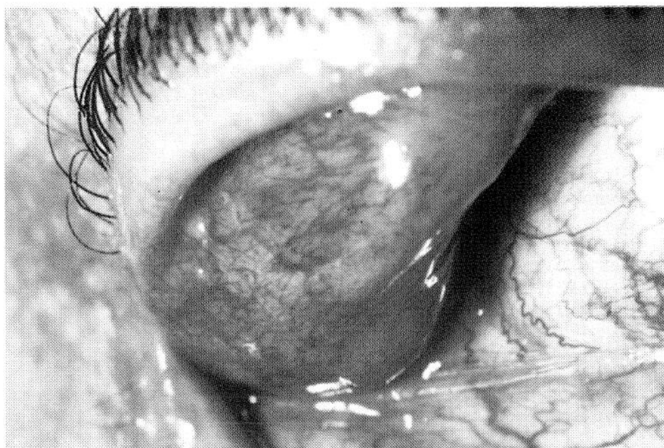

FIGURE 6–52 **Lymphoid infiltrate.** Lymphoid infiltrate of the lacrimal gland resulting in diffuse, uniform oblong enlargement of the lacrimal gland. The enlarged portion of the palpebral lobe is readily visualized in the superior fornix.

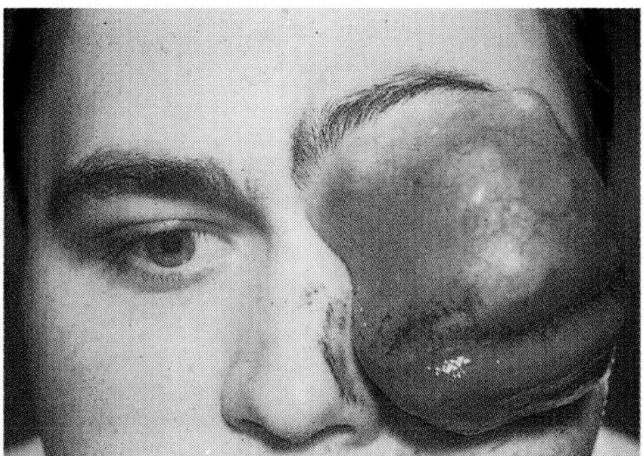

FIGURE 6–53 **Anaplastic lymphoma.** Systemically advanced anaplastic lymphoma with extensive orbital involvement. The patient succumbed to the systemic disease shortly after this picture was taken.

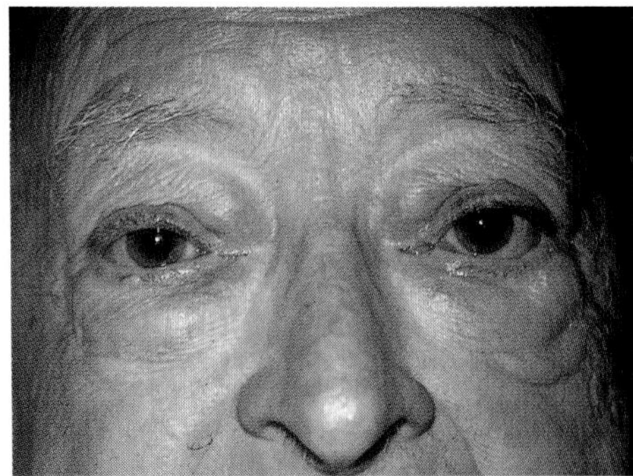
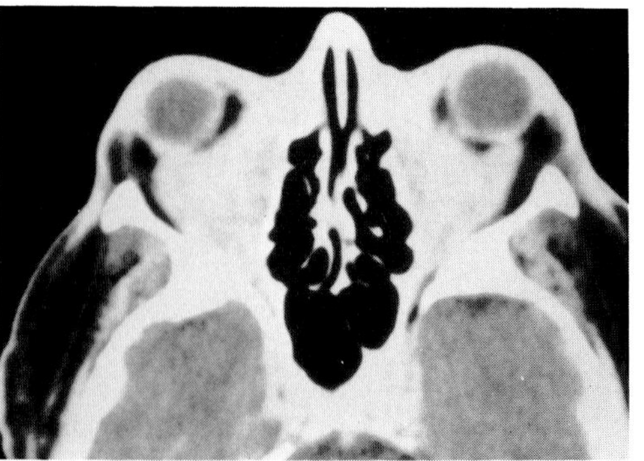

FIGURE 6–54 **Bilateral orbital lymphoma.** *A*, The clinical appearance of this patient is consistent with involutionary dermatochalasis, yet palpation of the lids demonstrated firm rubbery masses, not consistent with herniated orbital fat. *B*, The CT scan of this orbital lymphoma demonstrates bilateral symmetric soft tissue masses with exquisite molding to the globe.

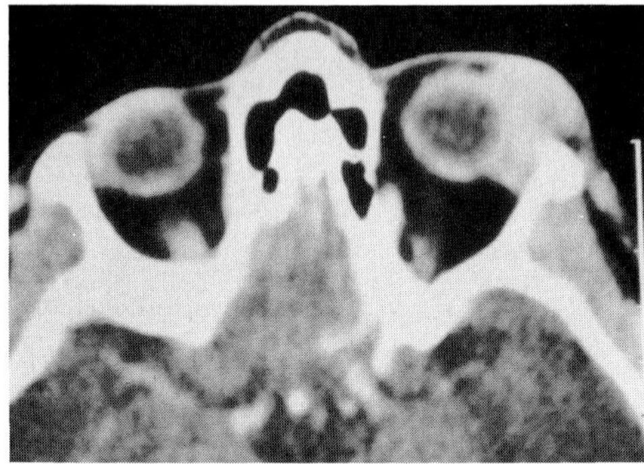

FIGURE 6–55 **Lymphoma.** An axial CT scan of a lymphoma primarily within the lacrimal gland. The origin of this lesion within the lacrimal fossa with a perpendicular take-off posteriorly without bone erosion, involvement of both the palpebral and orbital lobes of the lacrimal gland, and the fine serrations at the interface with the surrounding orbital fat are all characteristic of lymphocytic infiltrates of the lacrimal gland.

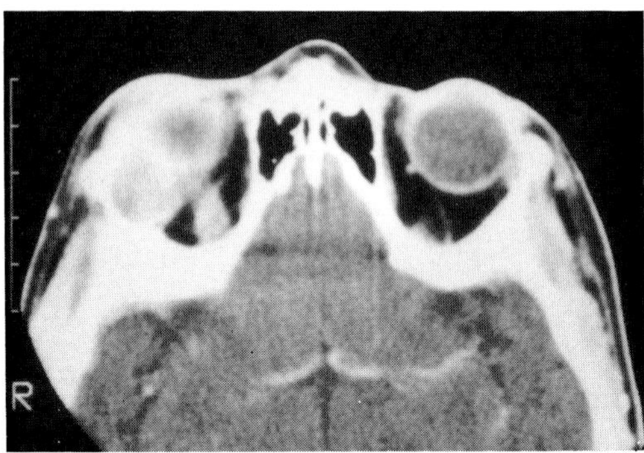

FIGURE 6–56 **Pleomorphic adenoma.** An axial CT scan of a pleomorphic adenoma of the lacrimal gland. In contrast to the lymphoid infiltrate of the lacrimal gland, this lesion is situated primarily posteriorly within the orbital lobe of the lacrimal gland, and bone erosion with fossa formation is present.

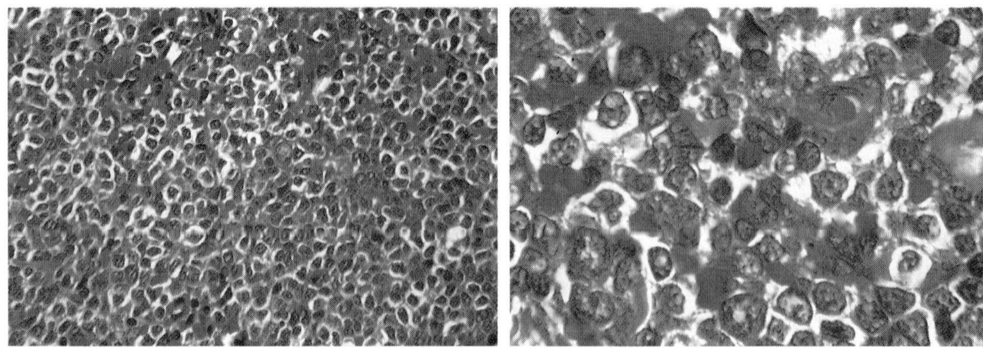

FIGURE 6–57 **Malignant lymphoma.** *A*, Low-power and, *B*, high-power histopathology. The high-power view (*B*) clearly demonstrates the high-grade nature of this lesion with its large, irregularly round anaplastic cells.

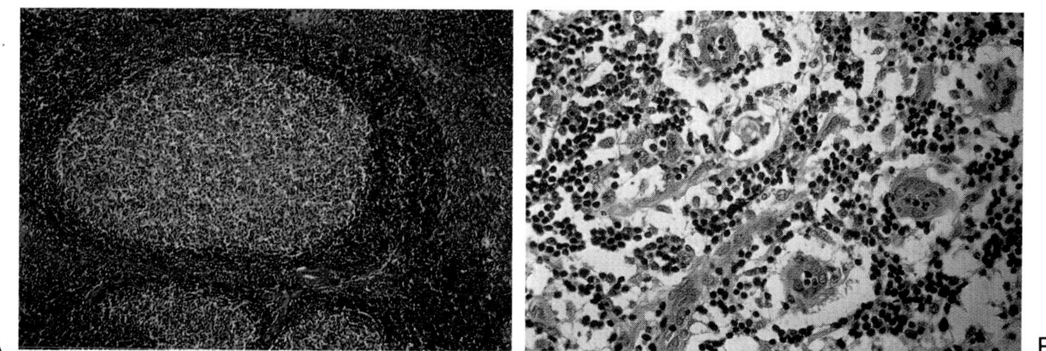

FIGURE 6–58 **Reactive hyperplasia or pseudolymphoma.** *A,* Well-defined germinal center with a clear mantle zone. Such lesions are typically polyclonal with a T-cell predominance. *B,* Capillary endothelial proliferation, typical of pseudolymphoma.

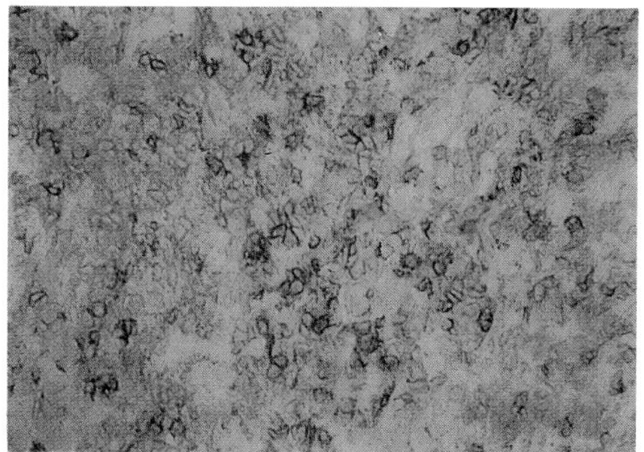

FIGURE 6–59 **B cell lymphoma.** Immunoperoxidase stain for kappa light chain establishes the diagnosis of B-cell monoclonal proliferation.

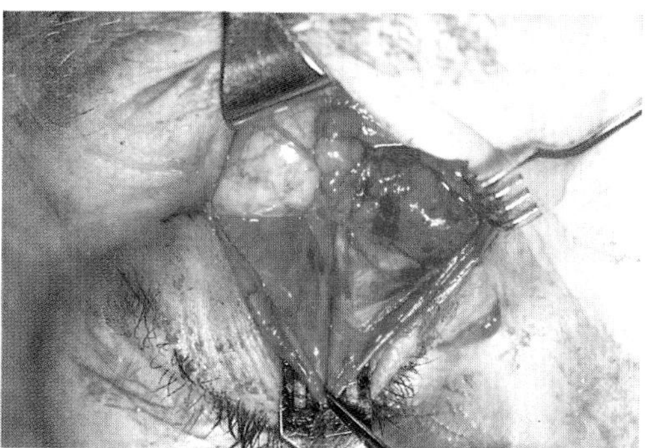

FIGURE 6–61 **Lid crease approach to anterior orbitotomy.** The normal orbital fat *(left)* is seen juxtapositioned to an orbital lymphoid infiltrate *(right).*

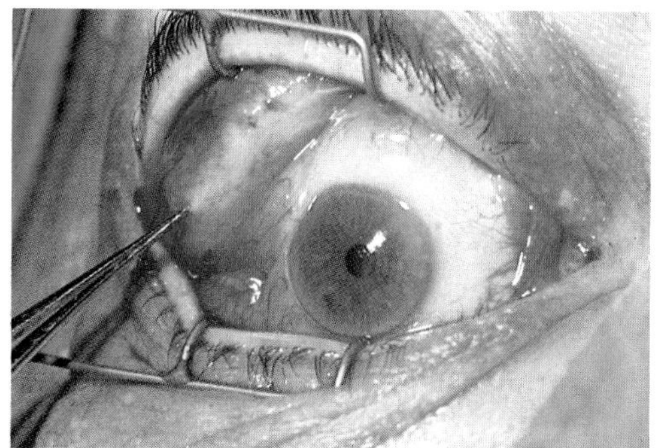

FIGURE 6–60 **Biopsy of lacrimal gland.** The specimen can usually be obtained transconjunctivally in lesions that are clinically and radiographically suggestive of a lymphoid process.

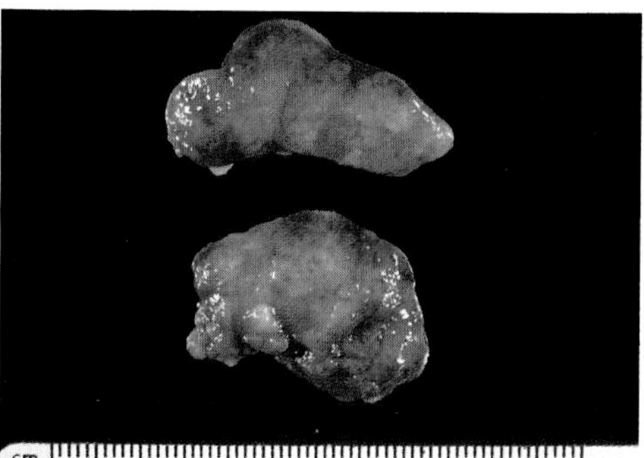

FIGURE 6–62 **Lacrimal gland tumor.** Gross fresh appearance of lacrimal gland tumor, demonstrating the fish-flesh character of lymphoid proliferation.

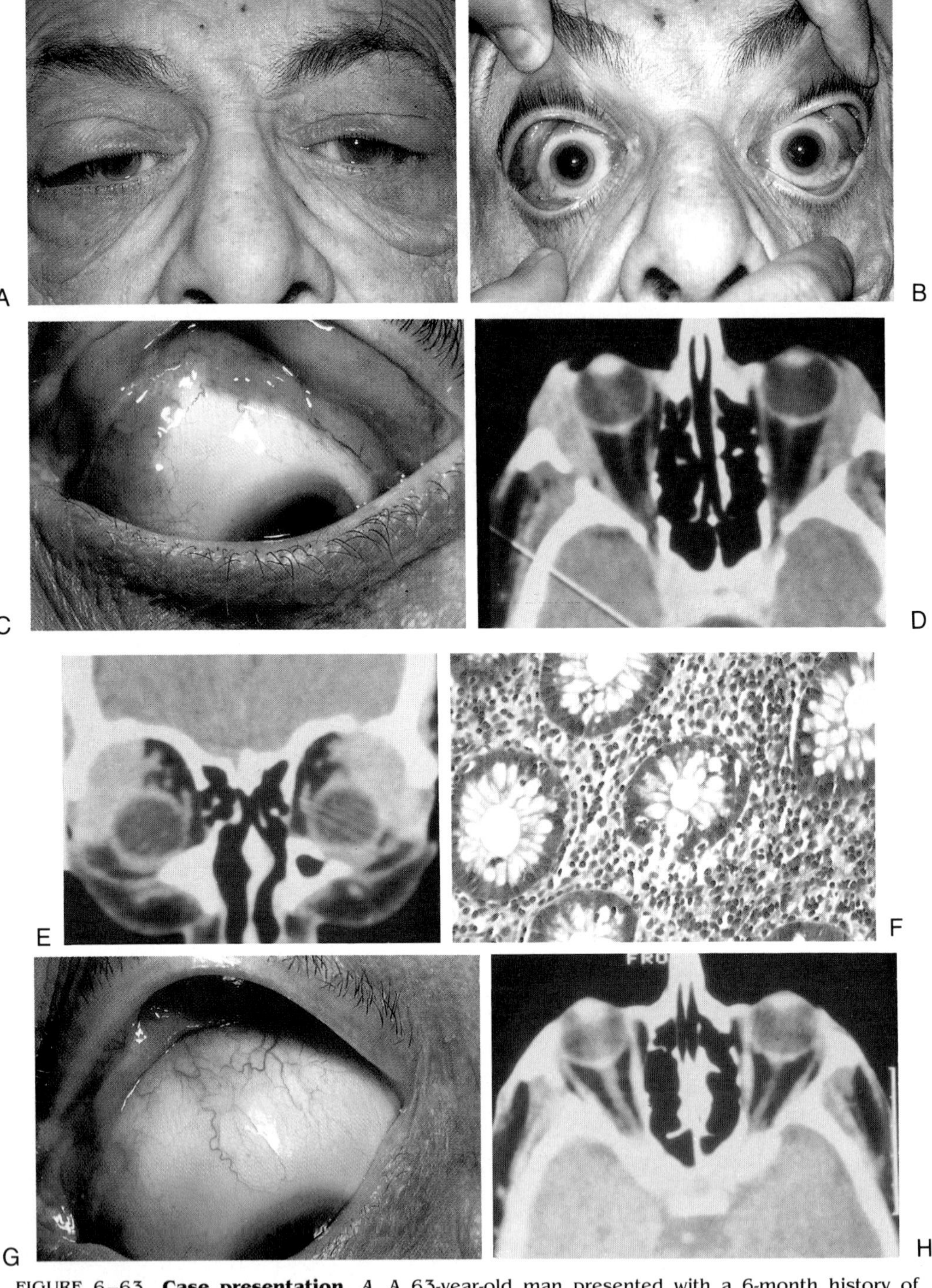

FIGURE 6–63 **Case presentation.** *A,* A 63-year-old man presented with a 6-month history of gradual ptosis bilaterally. *B,* Retraction of the upper eyelids revealed diffusely enlarged, tan-colored lacrimal glands. *C,* The superior epibulbar surface possessed a salmon-colored, fleshy mobile mass, classic for a lymphoid proliferation. *D,* The axial CT scan and, *E,* the coronal CT scan demonstrated exquisitely symmetric enlargement of the lacrimal glands. A biopsy of the lesion confirmed the diagnosis of a lymphoid tumor. *F,* The systemic work-up uncovered a lymphoid infiltration in the proximal gastrointestinal tract. A gastrointestinal biopsy specimen demonstrates the interstitial proliferation of lymphocytes. The disruption of the secretory acini *(center),* termed a lymphoepithelial lesion, is more commonly associated with monoclonal proliferations. Because the patient was found to have systemic disease and non–vision-threatening orbital disease, he was treated only with systemic chemotherapy. *G,* Clinically, there was complete regression of the conjunctival and lacrimal masses following the chemotherapy. *H,* The follow-up CT scan also highlights the impressive regression of the deeper orbital components.

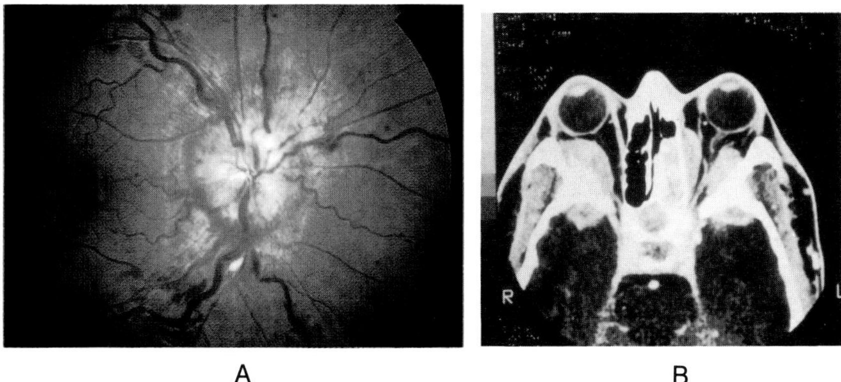

FIGURE 6–64 **Multiple myeloma.** *A*, Fundus photograph of a patient with multiple myeloma. The retinal venous tortuosity and optic nerve swelling are reflective of the hyperviscosity encountered in this disorder. Additionally the large orbital masses (*B*) cause orbital apical compression and contribute to the fundus findings. *B*, The CT scan shows extensive bilateral orbital involvement. Following systemic chemotherapy, there was marked resolution of the orbital masses. (Courtesy of Mark Balles, M.D.)

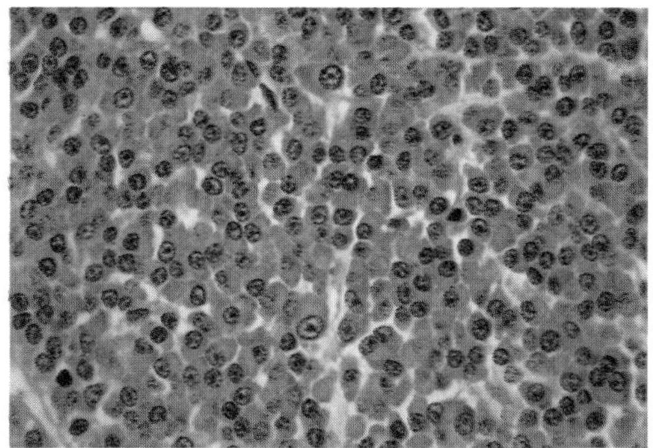

FIGURE 6–65 **Plasmacytic lesions.** Plasmacytoid features in a reasonably well-differentiated myelomatous deposit.

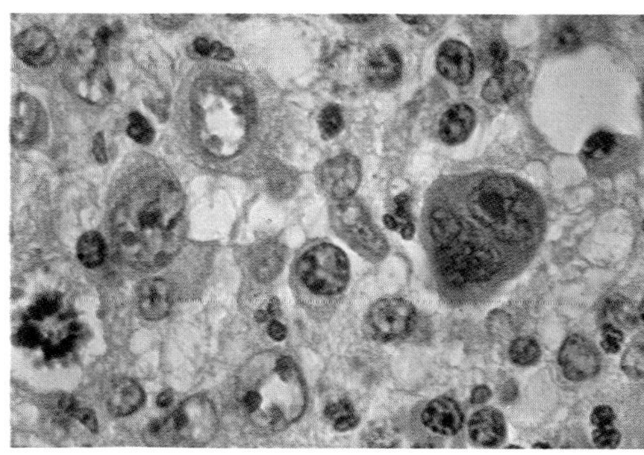

FIGURE 6–66 **Hodgkin's lymphoma and its histopathology.** A diagnostic Reed-Sternberg cell is present in the center of the field. An atypical star-burst mitotic figure is shown on the left.

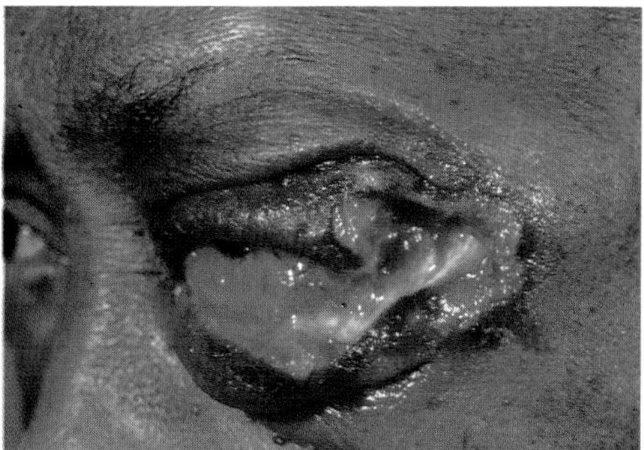

FIGURE 6–67 **Hodgkin's lymphoma.** Eyelid involvement and tissue necrosis in Hodgkin's lymphoma.

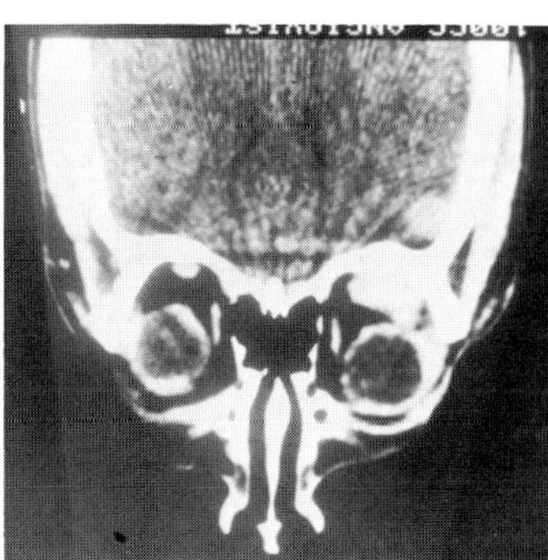

FIGURE 6–68 **Hodgkin's lymphoma.** A coronal CT scan of Hodgkin's lymphoma with intracranial involvement extending through the orbital roof. (From Case Records of the Massachusetts General Hospital (case 7-1989). New Engl J Med 320:447–457, 1989.)

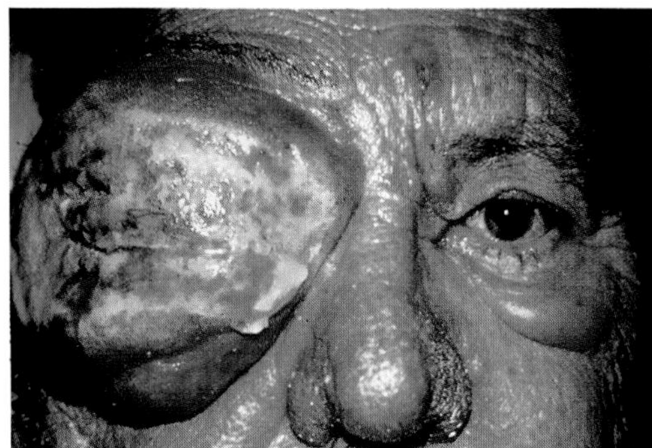

FIGURE 6–69 **Mycosis fungoides.** Mycosis fungoides with universal erythroderma. (Courtesy of Alan Proia, M.D.)

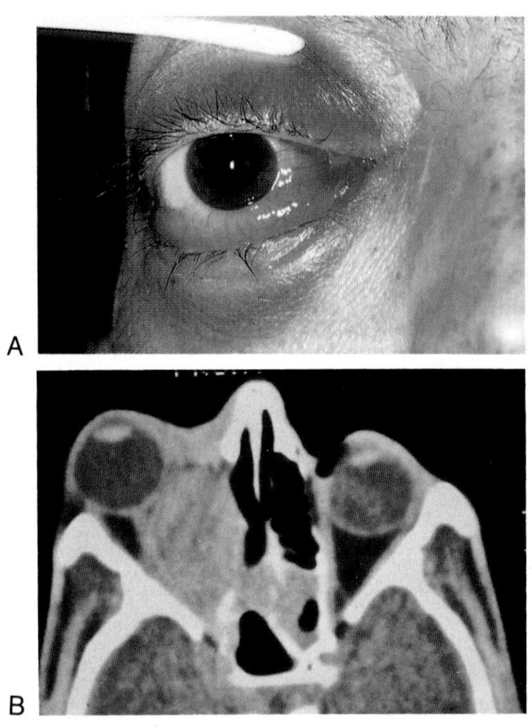

FIGURE 6–70 **B-cell lymphoma.** Orbital B-cell lymphoma in a patient with known acquired immunodeficiency syndrome (AIDS). *A*, This patient presented with painless proptosis and anterior orbital congestion. *B*, The CT scan demonstrated an infiltrating orbital soft tissue mass that was consistent with a neoplastic or opportunistic infectious mass. An orbital biopsy and cell surface marker studies established the diagnosis of an orbital lymphoma.

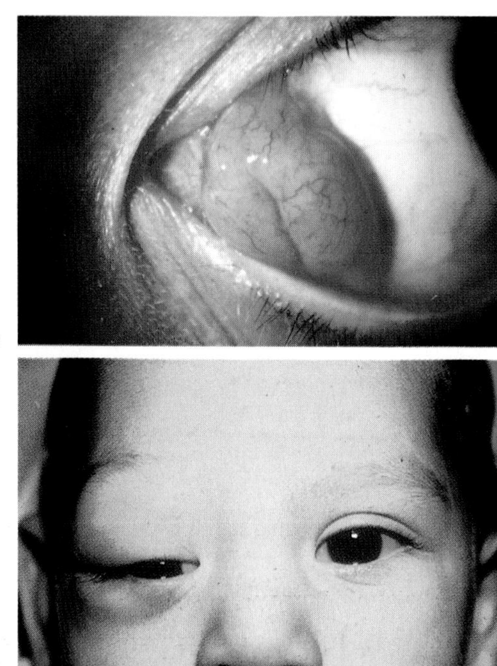

FIGURE 6–71 **Nonendemic Burkitt's lymphoma.** Unusual clinical presentations may include the following: *A*, Salmon-colored caruncular mass. (Courtesy of Barbara Streeten, M.D.) *B*, Rapidly growing orbital mass in the absence of bone destruction. (Courtesy of Charles Lee, M.D.)

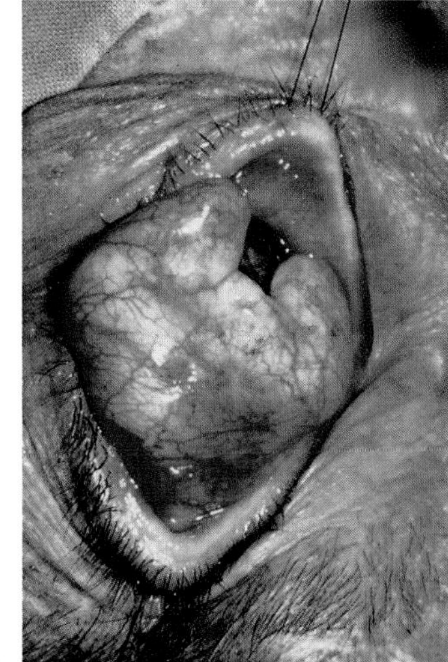

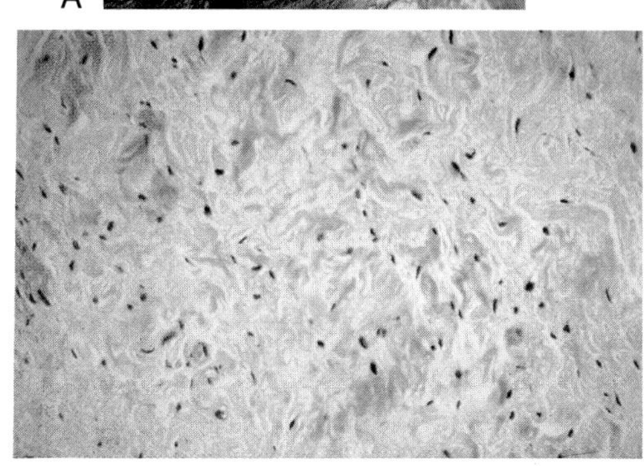

FIGURE 6–72 **Fibroma.** *A,* A multilobular white mass protrudes from the superior fornix. The surface epithelium is glistening and undisturbed, suggesting that the lesion is subepithelial. The white appearance is due to the copious presence of collagen. (*A,* Courtesy of Dr. Albert Hornblass.) *B,* The biopsy specimen reveals a sparse proliferation of fibroblasts, which are widely separated by keloid-like collagen.

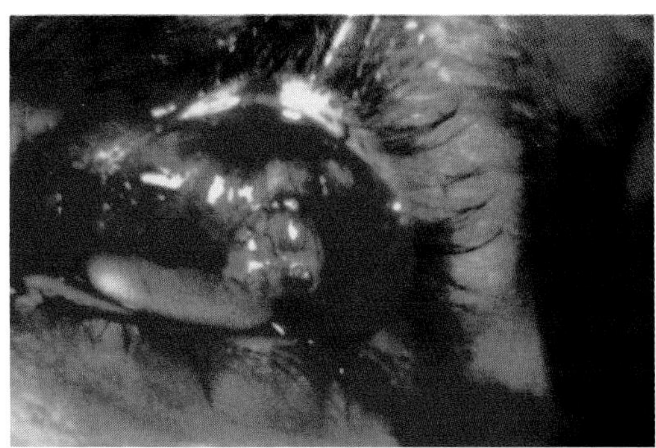

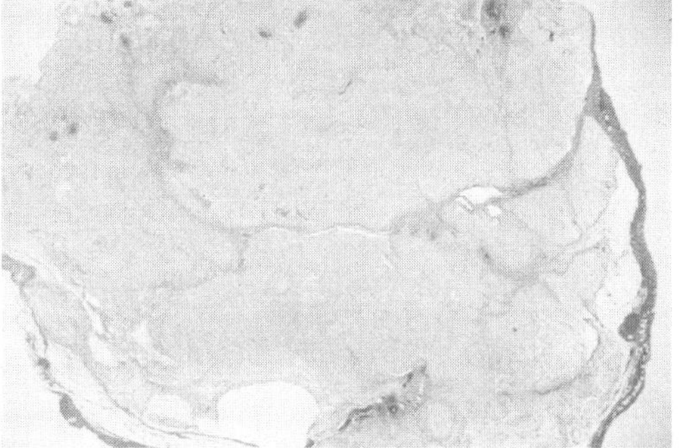

FIGURE 6–73 **Myxoma in Carney's complex.** *A,* A fluctuant upper eyelid myxoma protrudes from the tarsal conjunctiva. The tumor recurred and subsequently invaded the anterior orbit. *B,* The excised specimen is composed of an eosinophilic amorphous mass of myxoid material that is Alcian blue positive and represents hyaluronic acid synthesized by the scattered fibroblasts. In this syndrome, there can be many associated findings, such as bilateral caruncular pigmentation, freckles of the eyelids and cheeks, pituitary and adrenocortical dysfunction, potentially fatal cardiac myxomas, and non–germ cell (Leydig and Sertoli) tumors of the testes. (*A* and *B,* Courtesy of Drs. Joseph Flanagan and Ralph Eagle.)

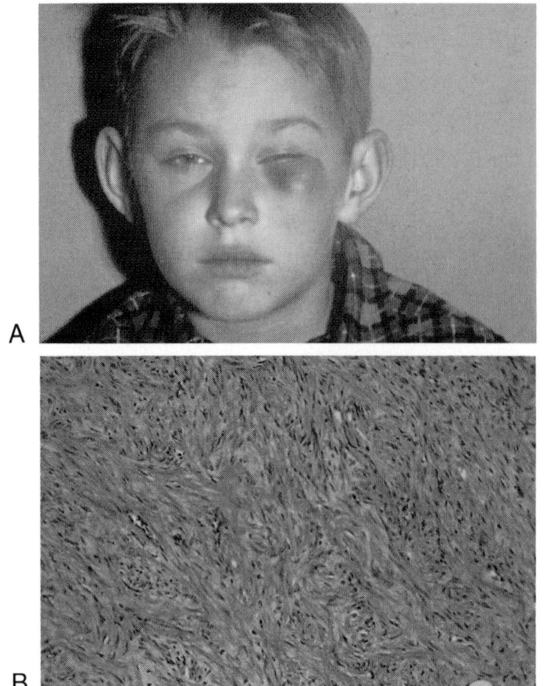

FIGURE 6–74 **Fibromatosis.** *A,* An inferior orbital tumor in a child has caused some overlying erythema of the skin of the eyelid. *B,* A somewhat lobular and fascicular orientation of the tumor cells in this lesion might invite the mistaken diagnosis of a leiomyoma. The nuclei are separated by collagen, and the lesion is less hypercellular than a fibrosarcoma. This tumor is locally aggressive but nonmetastasizing and is treated by wide local excision.

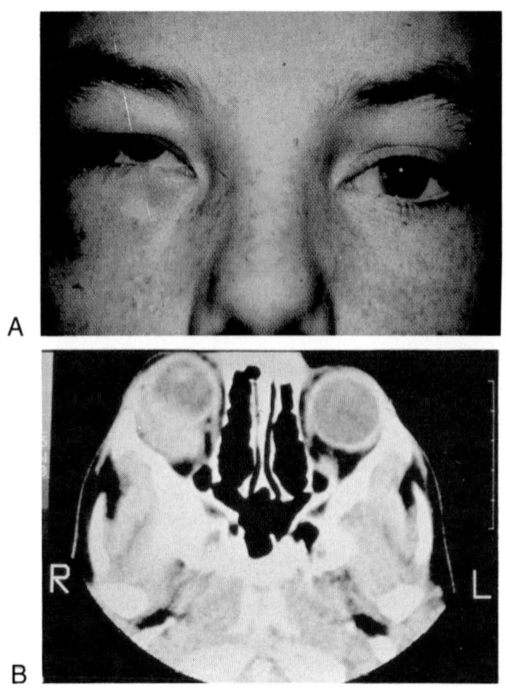

FIGURE 6–75 **Fibrosarcoma.** *A,* A juvenile example of orbital fibrosarcoma. *B,* The left inferior orbital tumor is circumscribed but not encapsulated (note slightly irregular margins) in this axial CT scan. This tumor is managed by wide local excision. (*A* and *B,* Courtesy of Dr. Ahmed Hidayat.)

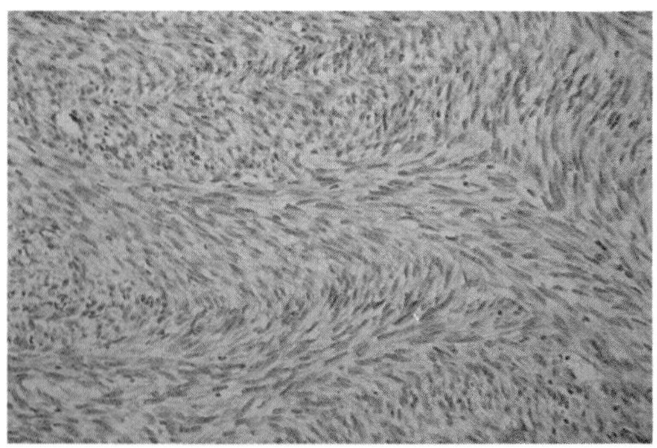

FIGURE 6–76 **Histopathologic features of fibrosarcoma.** The tumor cells are arranged in elongated fascicles that laterally interdigitate, creating what is called a herringbone pattern. The nuclei are closely packed owing to scant cytoplasm and collagen. This tumor is capable of metastasis and typically manifests mitotic figures.

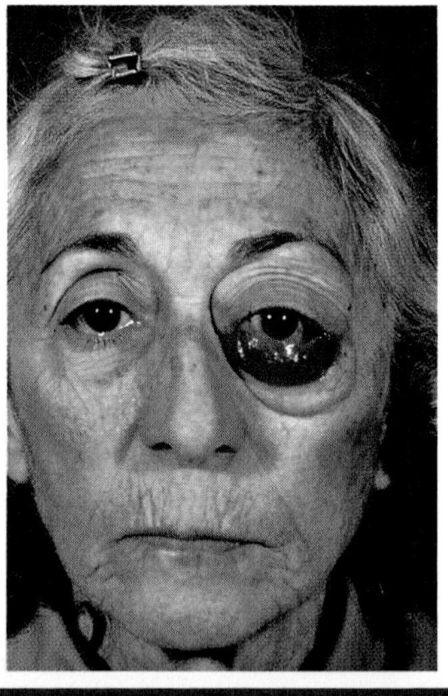

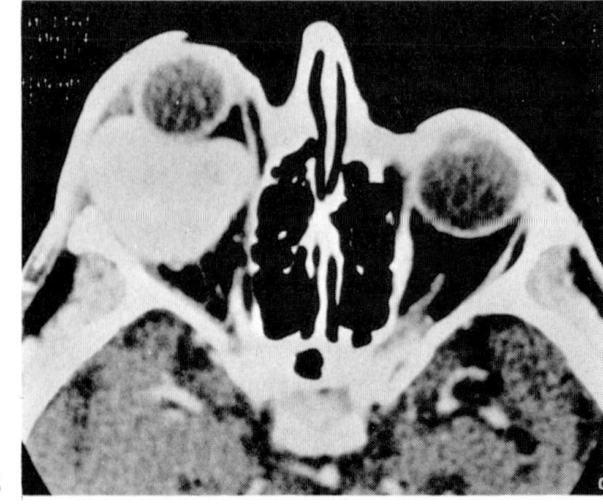

FIGURE 6–77 **Benign fibrous histiocytoma.** *A,* Axial proptosis with massive prolapse of chemotic conjunctiva. This is the most common orbital mesenchymal tumor of adults. Cavernous hemangioma and peripheral nerve tumors tend not to produce this degree of chemosis. *B,* Axial CT scan of a circumscribed tumor that has produced over 10 mm of proptosis and extends from the medial to the lateral orbital walls.

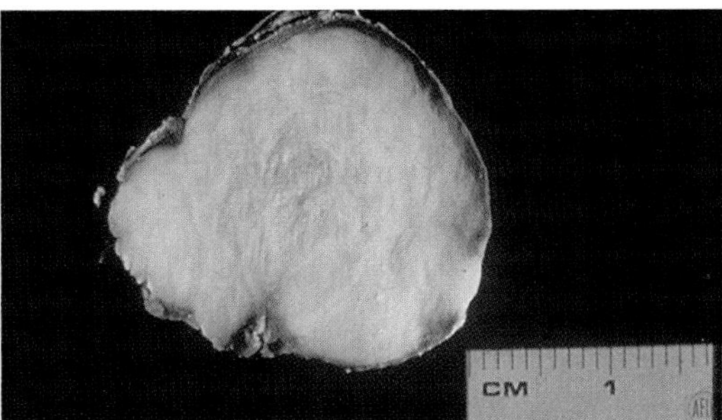

FIGURE 6–78 **Gross appearance of orbital fibrous histiocytoma.** Cut surface of a lesion retrieved from formalin shows a white trabeculation due to the presence of collagen as well as a clearly defined condensation pseudocapsule. Although cytologically benign, fibrous histiocytoma recurs if incompletely excised.

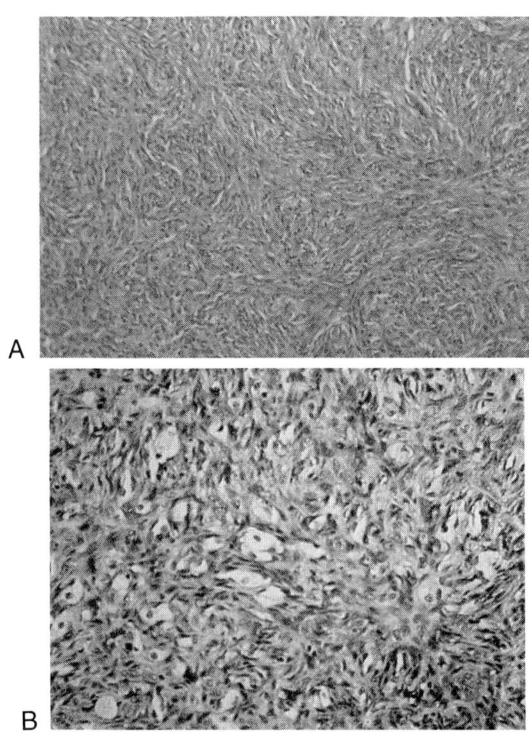

FIGURE 6–79 **Histopathologic features of benign fibrous histiocytoma.** *A*, The diagnostic pattern of a fibrous histiocytoma is called storiform, in which small bundles of cells twist in a cartwheel or spiral-nebular arrangement. *B*, Mononuclear xanthoma (lipid-containing) histiocytic cells are arranged in the midst of fibroblasts in a twisted configuration. This biphasic cell population is responsible for the name of the tumor. (*A* and *B*, Courtesy of Dr. Ahmed Hidayat.)

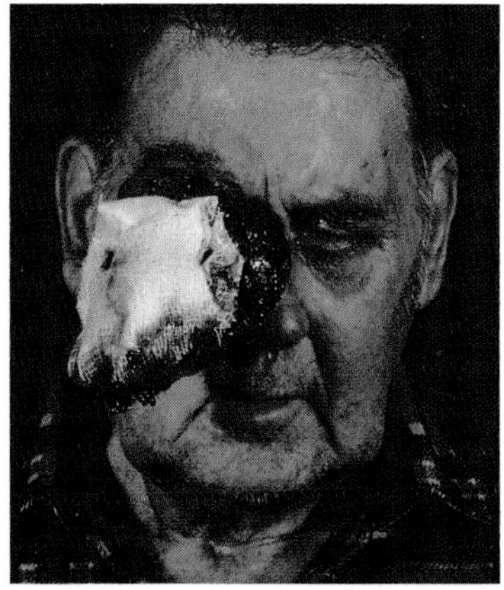

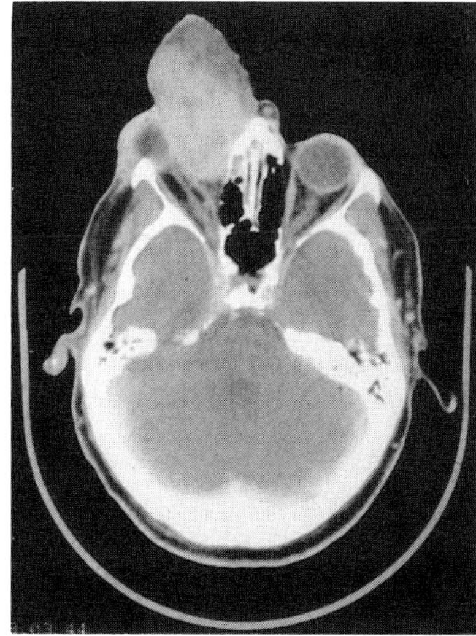

FIGURE 6–80 **Malignant fibrous histiocytoma.** *A*, A neglected massive orbital tumor is partially necrotic and covered by a gauze pad because of spontaneous drainage. *B*, Axial CT scan demonstrates the lesion's anterior location and that it has displaced the globe laterally beyond the orbital rim. As with most orbital sarcomas, the tumor was treated by orbital exenteration. (*A* and *B*, Courtesy of Dr. Albert Hornblass.)

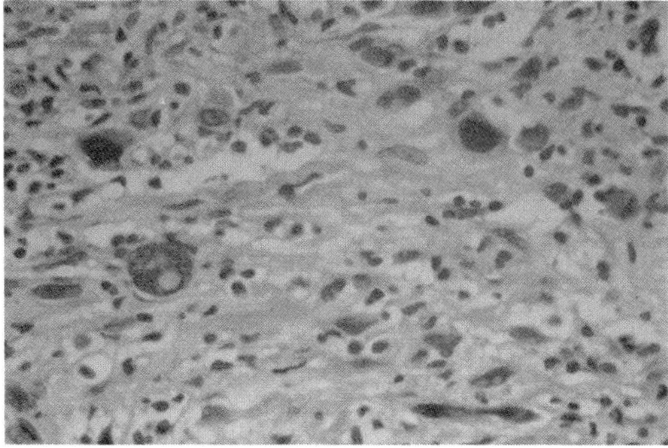

FIGURE 6–81 **Histopathology of malignant fibrous histiocytoma.** Tumor giant cells in a malignant fibrous histiocytoma are capable of collagen production. In addition to pleomorphism, necrosis and high mitotic activity are seen in malignancies.

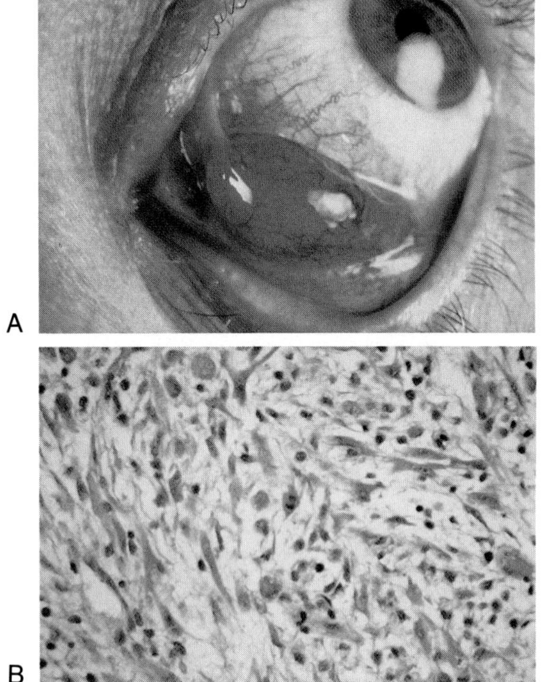

FIGURE 6–82 **Nodular fasciitis.** *A,* A benign but rapidly developing reddish tumor of the inferior fornix. *B,* The salient features include a watery matrix and a tissue culture appearance of the stimulated and reactive fibroblasts. Note the scattering of small dark lymphocytes. The tumor was managed by local excision. (*A* and *B,* Courtesy of Dr. Andrew Ferry.)

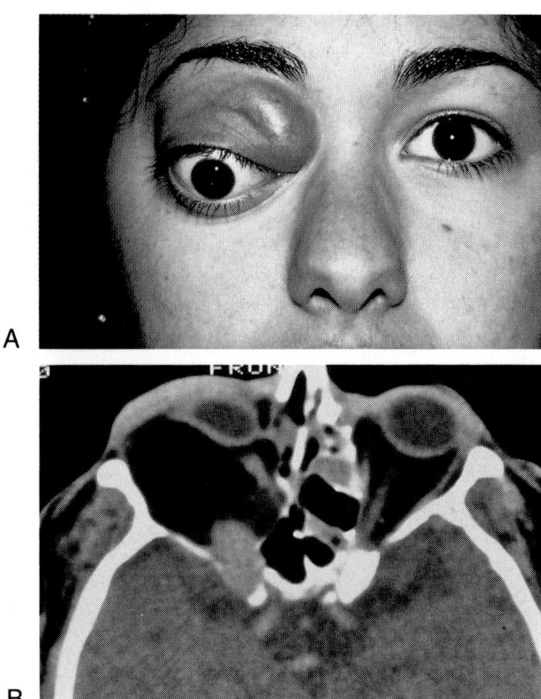

FIGURE 6–83 **Orbital liposarcoma.** *A,* Recurrent superonasal orbital liposarcoma that has produced high-grade proptosis and downward and outward displacement of the eye. The lesion felt rubbery but not rock hard. Most orbital liposarcomas are differentiated, slowly growing, and infiltrating tumors that locally recur and invade but metastasize late. *B,* Axial CT scan in another case shows nasal displacement of the globe. The orbit is enlarged because of the long duration of the tumor, which appears "cystic" because the tumor tissue has the same density as normal orbital fat. The comparatively solid component of the lesion at the orbital apex represented a more cellular region. (*B,* Courtesy of Dr. Richard Dallow.)

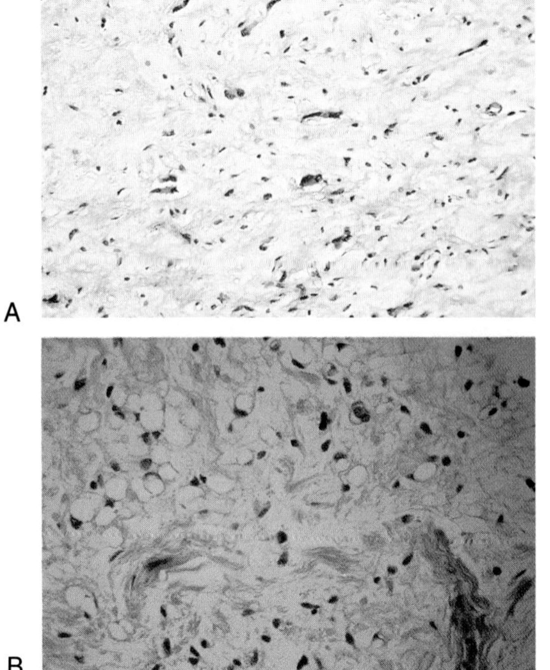

FIGURE 6–84 **Histopathologic features of orbital liposarcoma.** *A,* In lightly collagenized tissue, there are hyperchromatic cells. *B,* Myriad signet-ring univacuolar lipoblasts in a liposarcoma.

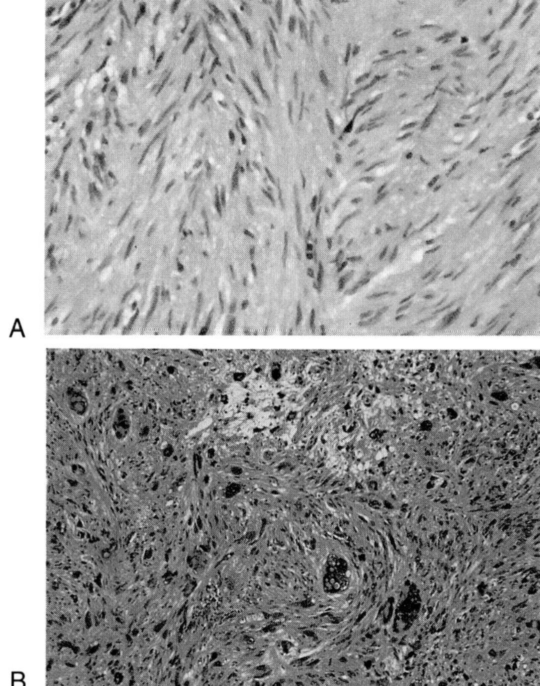

FIGURE 6–85 **Leiomyoma and leiomyosarcoma.** *A,* In this leiomyoma, the tumor cells have compact eosinophilic cytoplasm, and there is a tendency toward nuclear palisading. The tumor presents with slowly evolving proptosis and is encapsulated. The Masson trichrome stain reveals longitudinal cytoplasmic filaments, which can be further characterized with immunohistochemical reactions for muscle-specific actin. Because of nuclear palisading, leiomyoma can be confused with schwannoma except that the latter is S100 positive, whereas the former is not. Leiomyoma can arise deep in the orbit from vascular smooth muscle or more anteriorly from Müller's smooth muscle attached to the tarsal plates. *B,* A postradiation leiomyosarcoma with striking nuclear pleomorphism and tumor giant cells. This tumor is capable of metastasis.

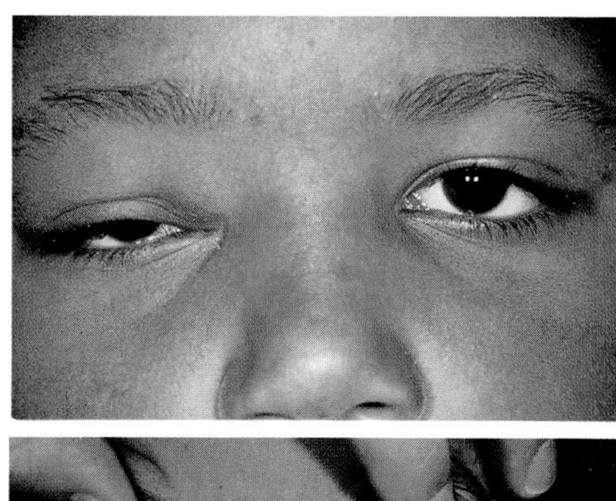

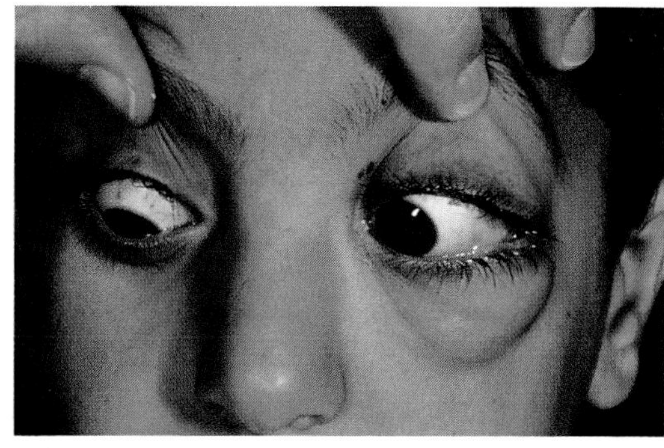

FIGURE 6–86 **Rhabdomyosarcoma.** *A,* Quiet, nonerythemic proptosis from a rapidly developing superonasal mass. This is the most common primary orbital malignancy of childhood and usually displays evidence of striated muscle differentiation. *B,* A less typical inferior orbital location, in which the tumor interferes with downward motility of the left globe. The alveolar variant has a propensity for this location. Rhabdomyosarcoma is a potentially metastasizing tumor that is treated by orbital radiotherapy and adjunctive chemotherapy after a biopsy establishes the diagnosis. (*A,* Courtesy of Dr. Richard Anderson.)

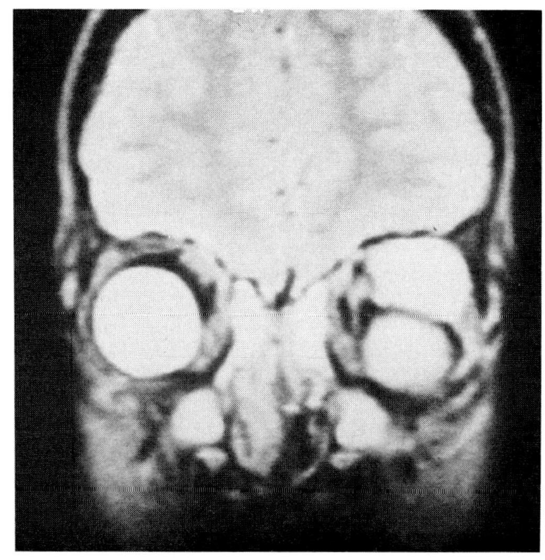

FIGURE 6–87 **Imaging study of orbital rhabdomyosarcoma.** A coronal magnetic resonance imaging study in a T_2-weighted image displays increased signal intensity of a well-circumscribed, superior orbital rhabdomyosarcoma, which is the most frequent location. The T_1 image was hypointense, as are most orbital tumors (with the exception of those containing lipid, melanin, mucus, or blood breakdown products).

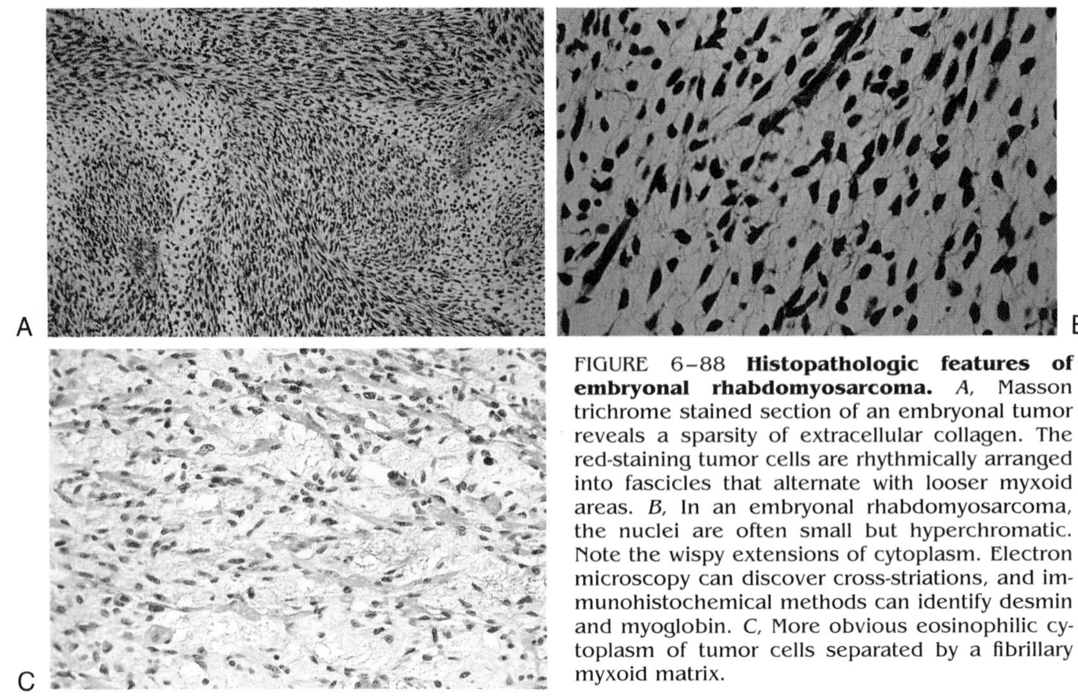

FIGURE 6–88 **Histopathologic features of embryonal rhabdomyosarcoma.** *A,* Masson trichrome stained section of an embryonal tumor reveals a sparsity of extracellular collagen. The red-staining tumor cells are rhythmically arranged into fascicles that alternate with looser myxoid areas. *B,* In an embryonal rhabdomyosarcoma, the nuclei are often small but hyperchromatic. Note the wispy extensions of cytoplasm. Electron microscopy can discover cross-striations, and immunohistochemical methods can identify desmin and myoglobin. *C,* More obvious eosinophilic cytoplasm of tumor cells separated by a fibrillary myxoid matrix.

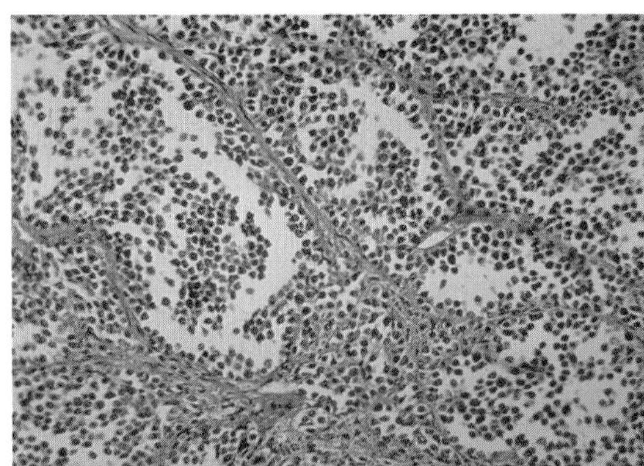

FIGURE 6–89 **Alveolar rhabdomyosarcoma.** Delicate fibrovascular septa subdivide the tumor, and rounded rhabdomyoblasts swim dyscohesively in the centers of the alveolar units. The variant is considered to be more malignant than the embryonal form.

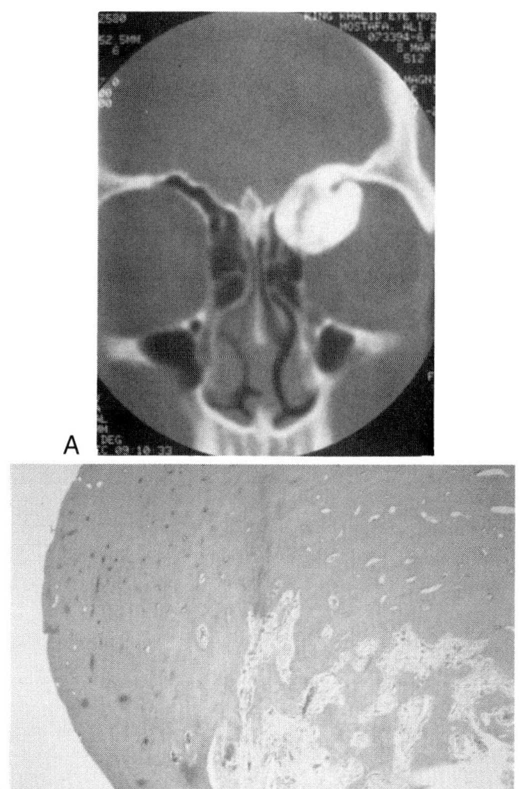

FIGURE 6–90 **Osteoma.** *A*, A coronal CT scan obtained by the bone window technique shows the density of the lesion, which involves the superomedial orbit and the contiguous sinus. *B*, Highly dense mature lamellar bone with few haversian canals is shown above and to the left, while toward the bottom right there is more reactive, looser bony tissue.

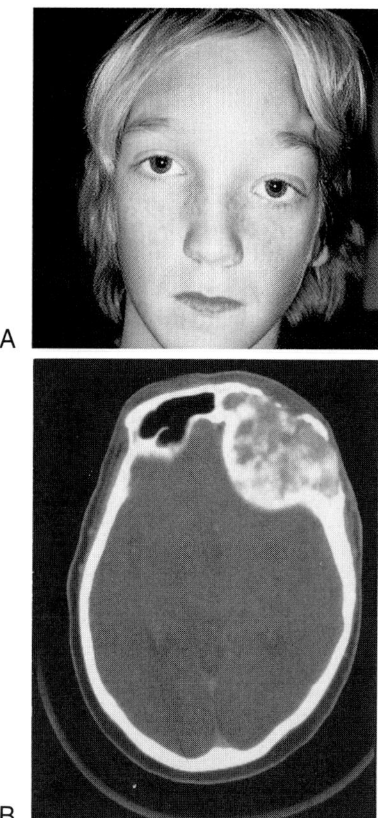

FIGURE 6–91 **Fibrous dysplasia.** *A*, A 12-year-old boy had over many years experienced widening of the central face and downward displacement of the entire orbital contents (dystopia). The extraocular motility was full, and the patient did not have any diplopia. Visual acuity is threatened when there is encroachment on the optic canal. *B*, Another case with involvement of the frontal bone and sinus with focus of fibrous dysplasia displaying a variegated internal radiodensity. (*A*, Courtesy of Dr. Robert Petersen.)

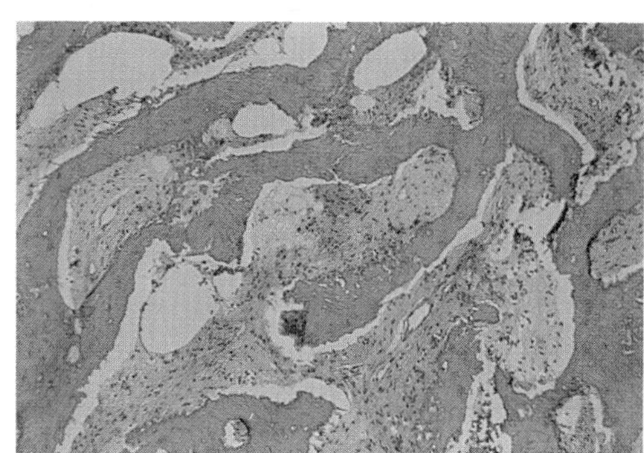

FIGURE 6–92 **Histopathology of fibrous dysplasia.** The stroma between the trabeculae of woven bone (with no rimming osteoblasts and with no internal lines demonstrable by polarizing microscopy) is variably vascularized and fibrotic.

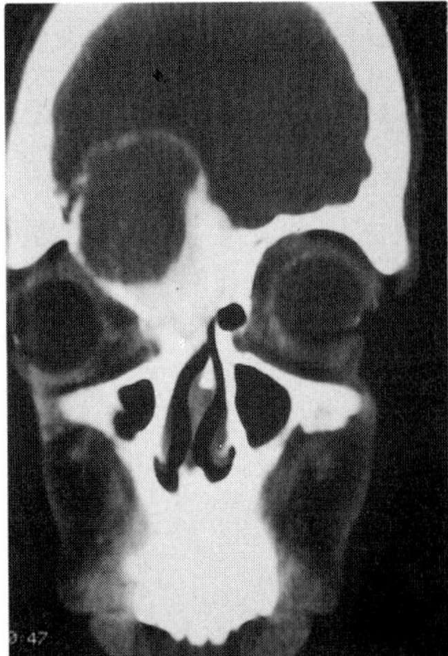

FIGURE 6–93 **Ossifying (juvenile psammomatoid) fibroma.** The coronal CT scan manifests an eggshell perimeter at the superior portion of the lesion, with a more solid radiodensity at its inferonasal margin. This lesion develops more rapidly and is more locally aggressive than fibrous dysplasia. (Courtesy of Dr. Curtis Margo.)

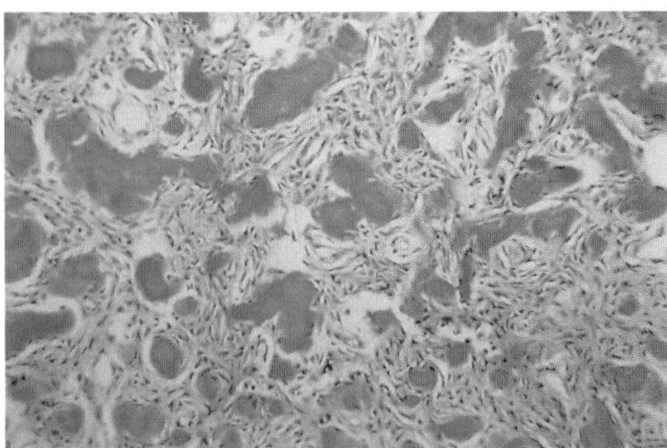

FIGURE 6–94 **Histopathology of ossifying fibroma.** Some of the trabeculae of lamellar bone (spicules may display rimming osteoblasts and internal lines with polarizing microscopy) are small and resemble psammoma bodies. In a childhood lesion, a frozen section of an ossifying fibroma can be misinterpreted as a meningioma. (Courtesy of Dr. Curtis Margo.)

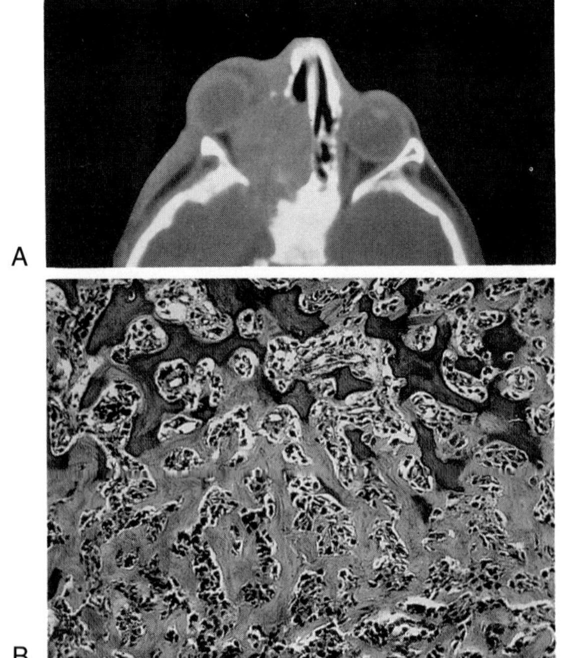

FIGURE 6–95 **Osteogenic sarcoma.** *A,* The majority of this tumor invading the orbit from the adjacent sinus and nose displays surprisingly little internal radiodensity. Besides local destructive growth, this tumor is capable of distant metastasis. *B,* Osteoid material that is poorly mineralized is present below and is being produced by hyperchromatic osteogenic sarcoma cells. The trabeculae of tumor-associated bone above are more intensely calcified. (*A,* Courtesy of Dr. Robert Petersen; *B,* courtesy of Dr. Lorenz E. Zimmerman.)

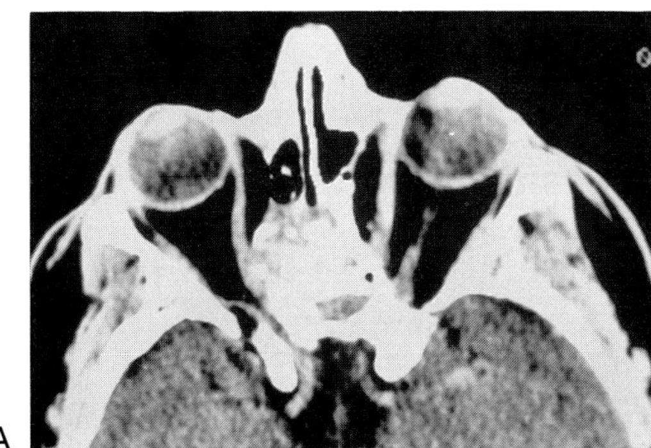
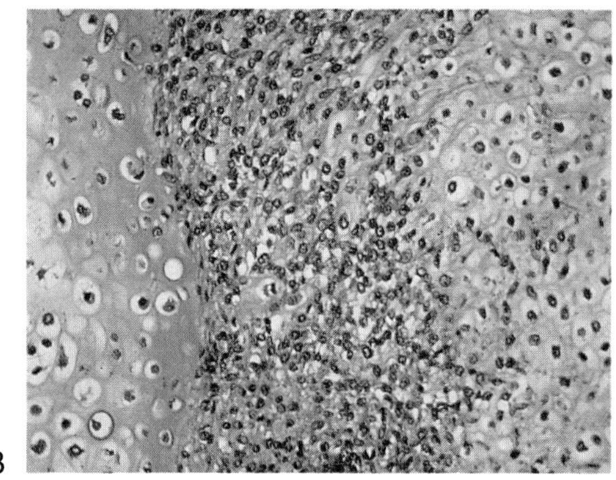

FIGURE 6–96 **Chondrosarcoma.** *A,* Axial CT scan of a sinus chondrosarcoma that has bilaterally involved the orbits. Note that the lesion shows more internal radiodensity than the preceding osteogenic sarcoma. Radiographically the two lesions cannot be distinguished. Periorbital chondrosarcoma tends to grow slower and metastasizes much later than osteogenic sarcoma. *B,* Hyperchromatic tumor cells are present vertically in the center of the field and merge on either side into clear-cut cartilage with hyperchromatic tumor cells exhibiting matrix formation. (*A,* Courtesy of Dr. Robert Petersen; *B,* courtesy of Dr. Lorenz E. Zimmerman.)

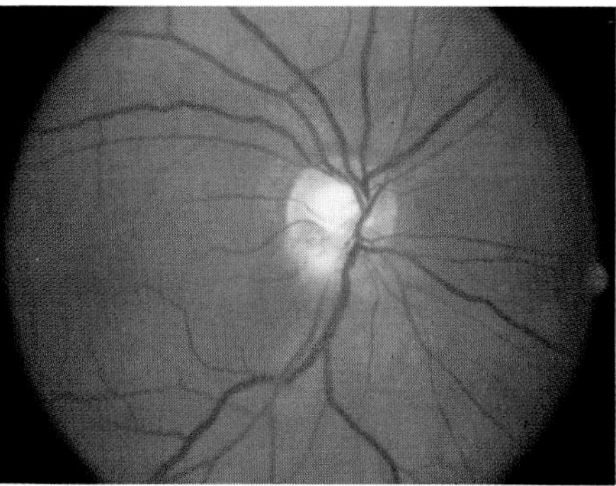

FIGURE 6–98 **Metastatic adrenal cell carcinoma.** Metastatic adrenal cell carcinoma involving the inferior pole of the optic nerve. (Courtesy of S. Lessell, M.D.)

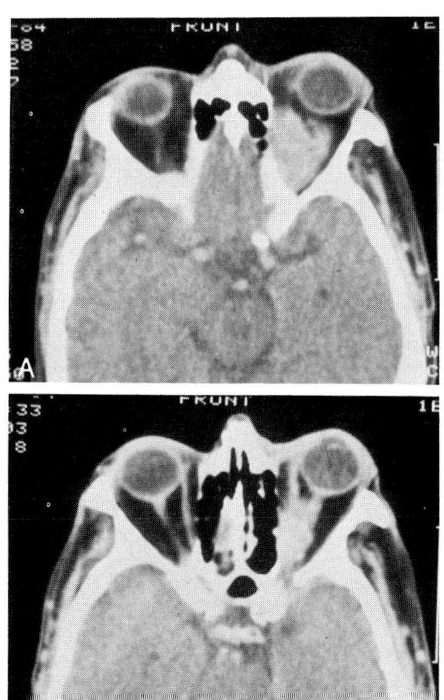

FIGURE 6–97 **Metastatic adenocarcinoma.** *A* and *B,* Axial CT scans showing diffuse involvement of orbital tissues by metastatic adenocarcinoma.

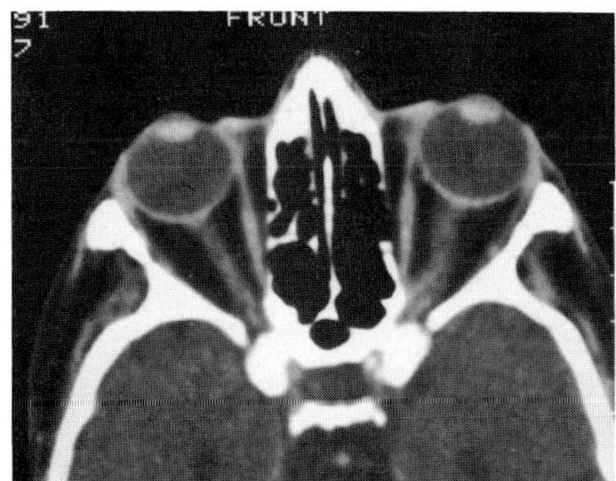

FIGURE 6–99 **Metastatic oat cell carcinoma.** CT scan appearance of diffuse thickening of the left optic nerve secondary to meningeal involvement by metastatic oat cell carcinoma.

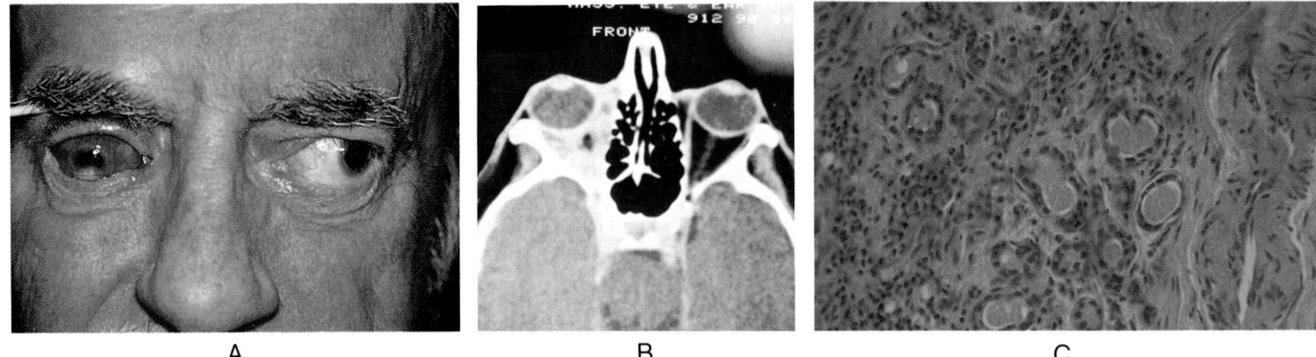

FIGURE 6–100 **Metastatic squamous cell carcinoma.** *A*, A 60-year-old man presented with proptosis of acute onset, frozen globe, and exposure keratitis resulting in a corneal ulceration. *B*, The CT scan shows diffuse involvement of orbital tissue. *C*, The biopsy specimen shows metastatic squamous cell carcinoma. The primary source of the tumor was unknown. (Courtesy of J. Shore, M.D.)

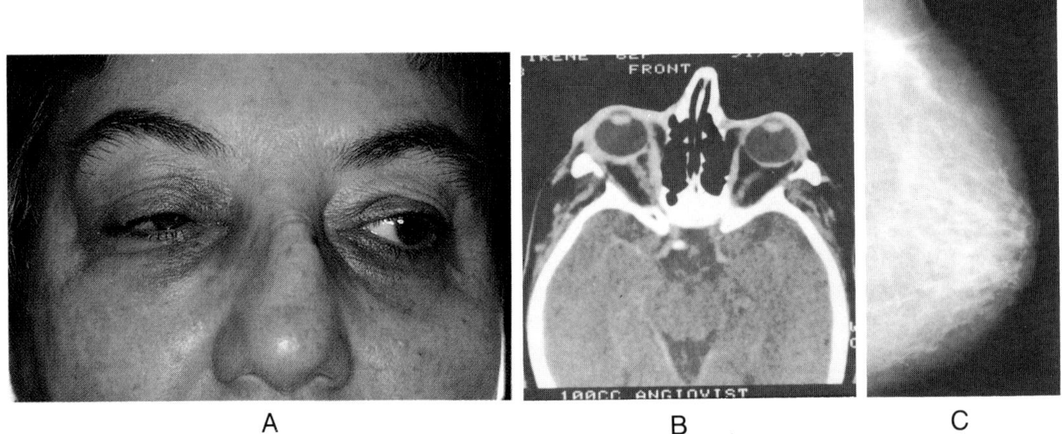

FIGURE 6–101 **Metastatic breast carcinoma.** *A*, A 50-year-old woman presented with an inflamed orbit, enophthalmos, and restricted motility. *B*, The CT scan shows irregular enlargement of the right medial rectus muscle and diffuse infiltration of the anterior orbital tissues. *C*, Mammography disclosed a calcified breast mass. (*A–C*, Courtesy of J. Shore, M.D.)

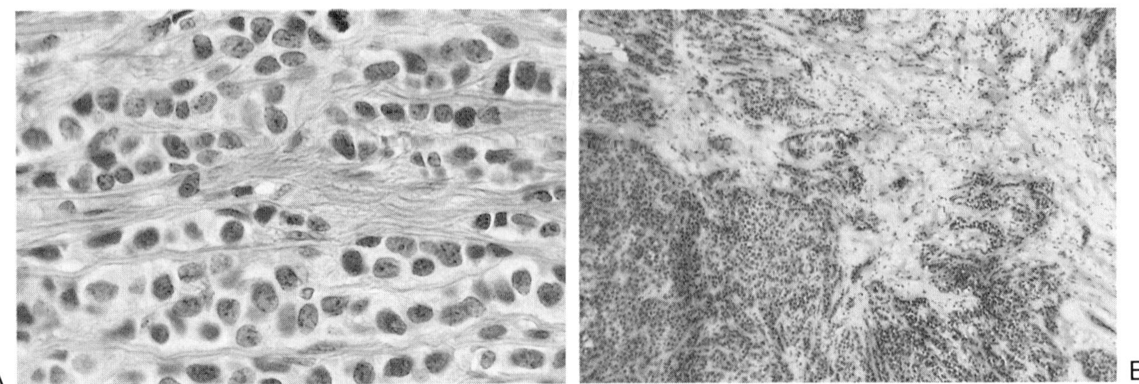

FIGURE 6–102 **Metastatic breast carcinoma.** Histopathology of specimen from the patient in Figure 6–101 shows typical "Indian file" organization of metastatic breast carcinoma cells (*A*) and scirrhous changes (*B*) responsible for enophthalmos. (*A* and *B*, Courtesy of J. Shore, M.D.)

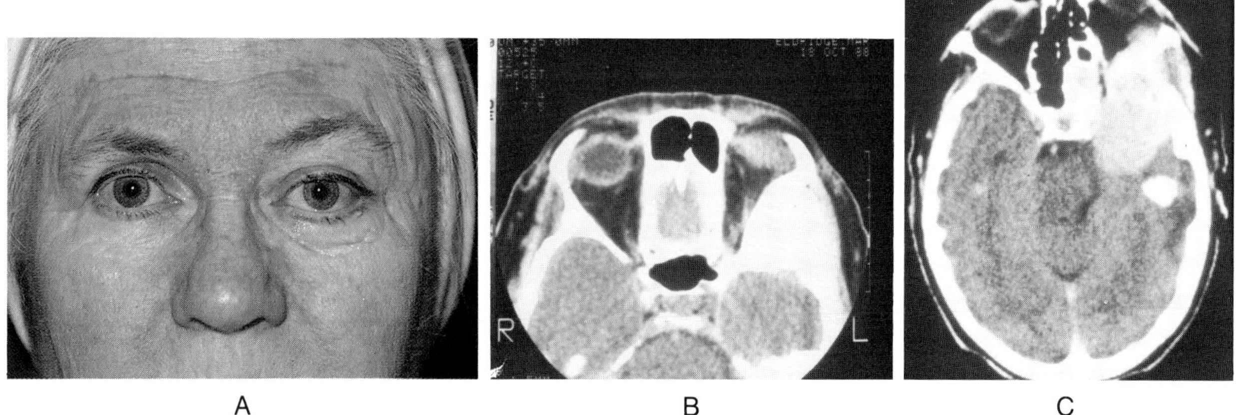

A B C

FIGURE 6–103 **Metastatic breast carcinoma.** *A*, A 58-year-old woman with a history of breast carcinoma presented with the gradual onset of proptosis. *B*, The CT scan appearance was consistent with left sphenoid wing meningioma. Note the hyperostosis of the lateral orbit wall. *C*, The CT scan of a different patient shows the typical appearance of breast carcinoma metastatic to the sphenoid wing with bony destruction. (Courtesy of J. Shore, M.D.)

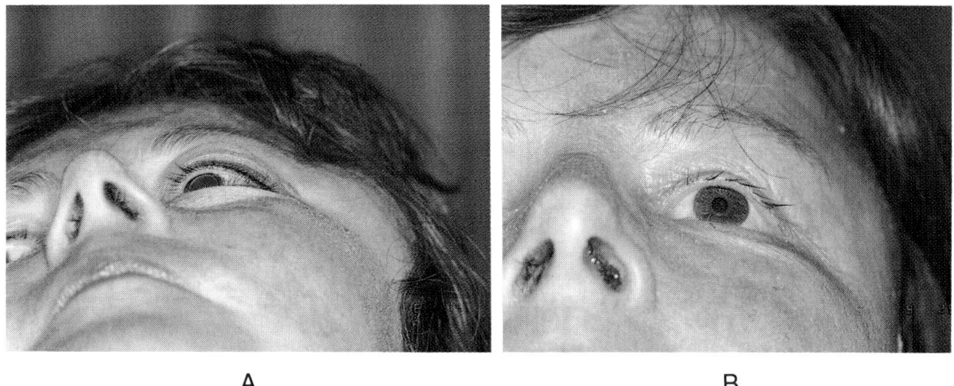

A B

FIGURE 6–104 **Metastatic breast carcinoma.** Preradiation (*A*) and postradiation (*B*) photographs of metastatic breast carcinoma to the left zygoma and orbit. Mass effect and proptosis were dramatically reduced.

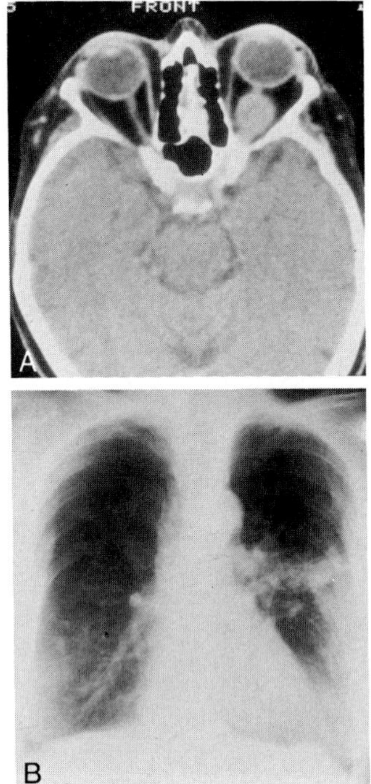

FIGURE 6–105 **Metastatic lung carcinoma.** An elderly man presented with proptosis of the left eye. *A*, The CT scan appearance was possibly consistent with a cavernous hemangioma. The orbital biopsy and chest x-ray (*B*) were diagnostic for metastatic lung carcinoma to the orbit.

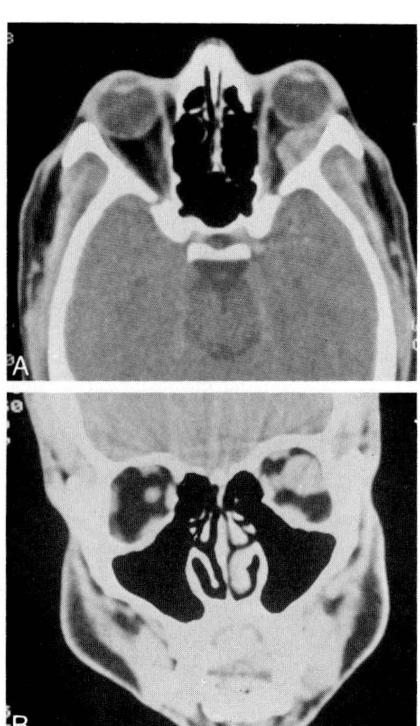

FIGURE 6–107 **Metastatic carcinoid tumor of the lung.** *A* and *B*, CT scan appearance of a solitary metastatic lesion to the orbit in a patient with carcinoid tumor of the lung. Occasionally the metastasis is isolated and discrete, and resection for cure can be attempted.

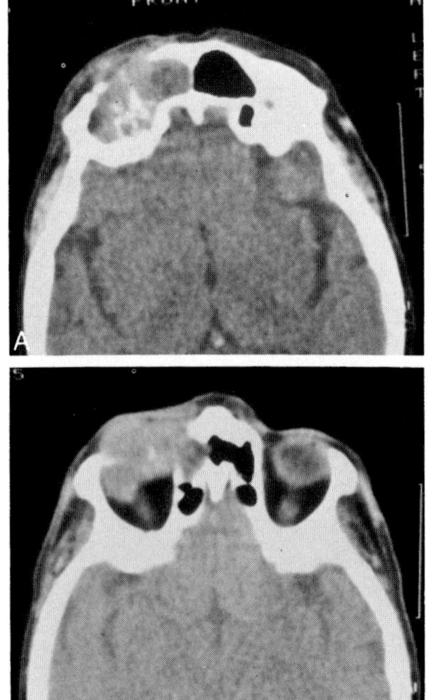

FIGURE 6–106 **Metastatic renal carcinoma.** *A* and *B*, CT scan appearance of massive bone destruction of the superior and medial orbit secondary to metastatic renal cell carcinoma. (Courtesy of A. Weber, M.D.)

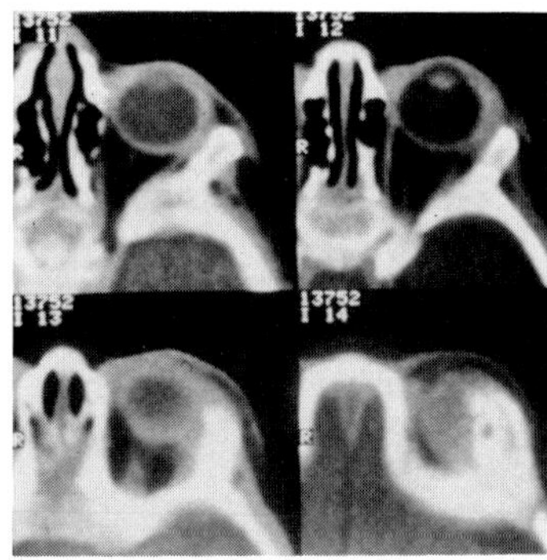

FIGURE 6–108 **Metastatic neuroblastoma.** CT scan shows a lytic bone lesion of the temporal orbit. (Courtesy of J. Woog, M.D.)

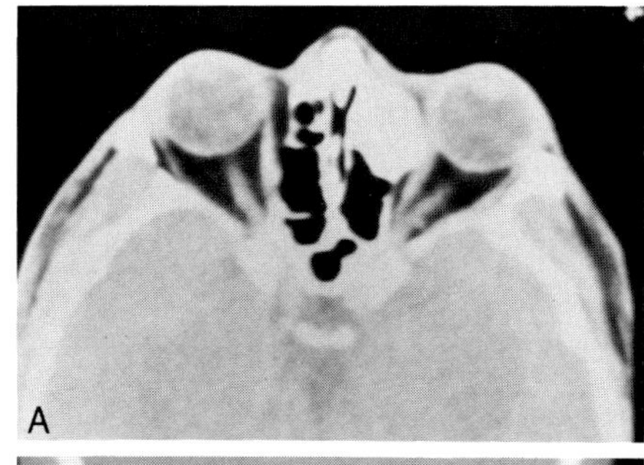

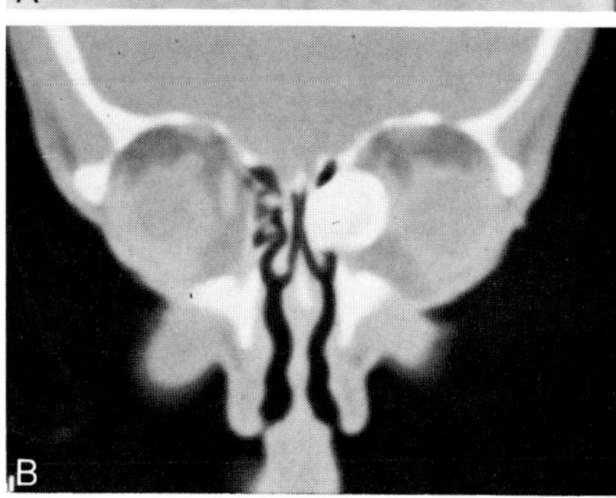

FIGURE 6–109 **Osteoma.** *A* and *B*, CT scan appearance of osteoma with extension into the left orbit. Bone windows (*A*) show compact bone. (Courtesy of M. Joseph, M.D.)

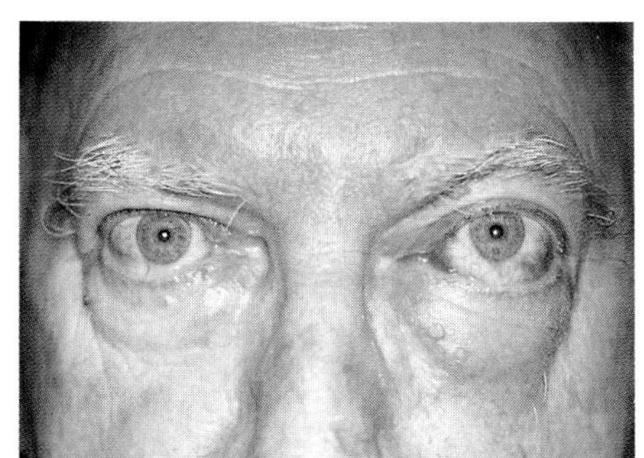

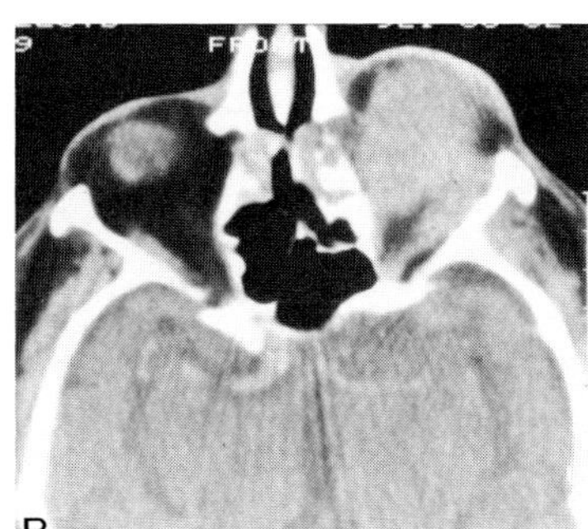

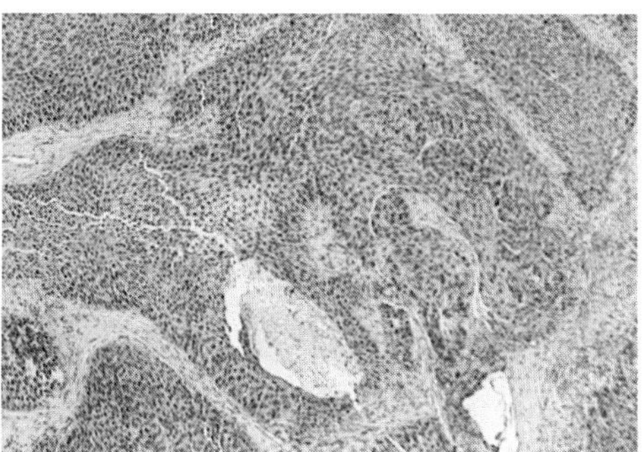

FIGURE 6–110 **Squamous cell carcinoma.** *A*, Upward displacement of the left globe secondary to antral carcinoma. *B*, The CT scan shows extension of the tumor into the inferior orbit. *C*, The biopsy specimen revealed nonkeratinizing squamous cell carcinoma. (Courtesy of P. Rubin, M.D.)

FIGURE 6–111 **Squamous cell carcinoma.** CT scan of a patient who presented with acute loss of vision secondary to optic neuropathy, showing squamous cell carcinoma of the right ethmoid extending into the orbital apex. (Courtesy of M. Joseph, M.D.)

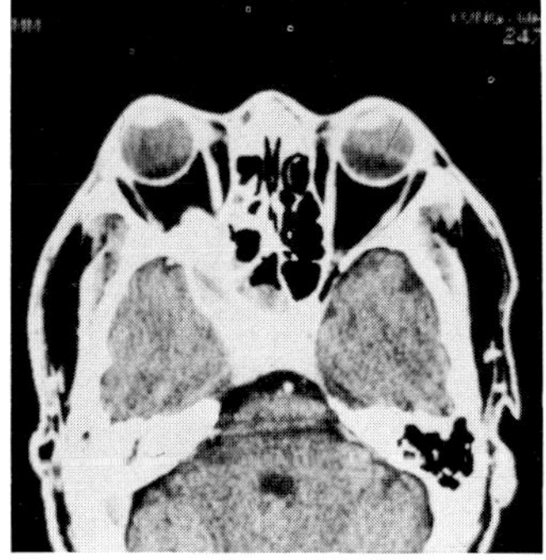

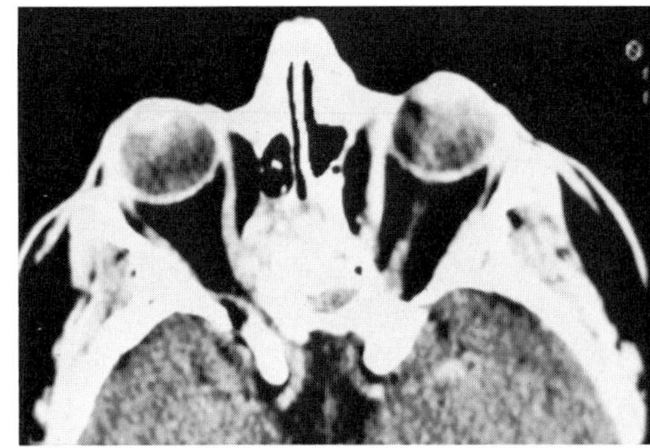
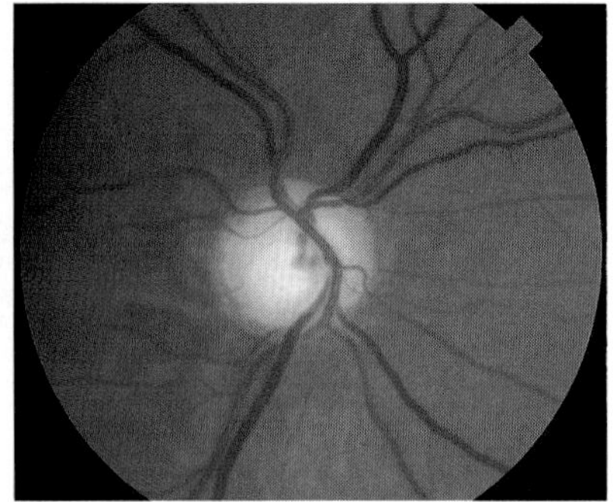

FIGURE 6-112 **Chondrosarcoma.** Chondrosarcoma of the right ethmoid sinus. The CT scan (*A*) shows extension into the orbit with resultant compressive optic neuropathy (*B*).

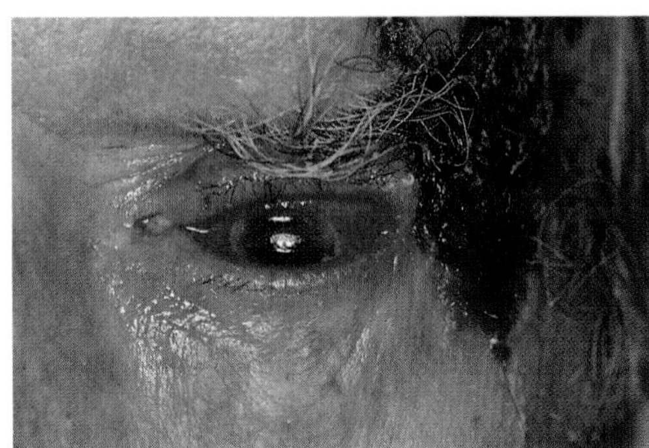

FIGURE 6-113 **Basal cell carcinoma.** Basal cell carcinoma of the left temporal fossa with invasion of the superior orbit, causing cicatrization and fixation to the bone of the left upper lid. This resulted in exposure and a sterile corneal melt. The patient had had the lesion for at least 9 years and had undergone three prior resections.

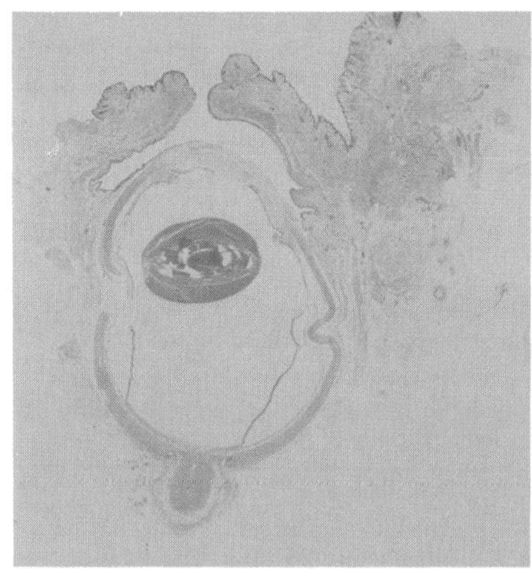
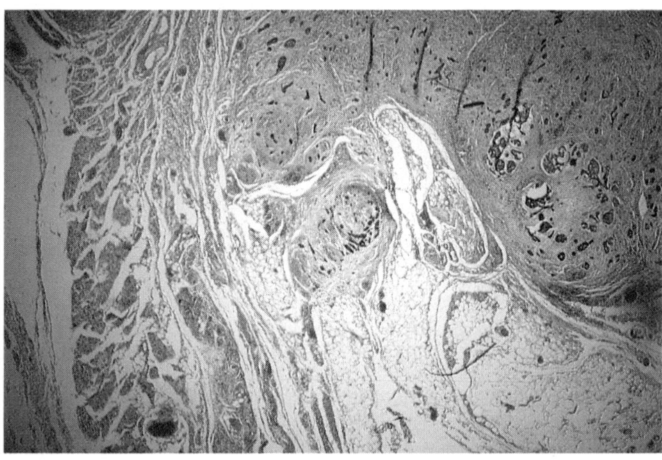

FIGURE 6-114 **Basal cell carcinoma.** *A*, Low-power view of an exenteration specimen from the patient in Figure 6-113. The upper right part of the field shows the invasion of the anterior orbit. *B*, A higher-power view shows foci of morpheaform basal cell carcinoma extending into the orbital fat.

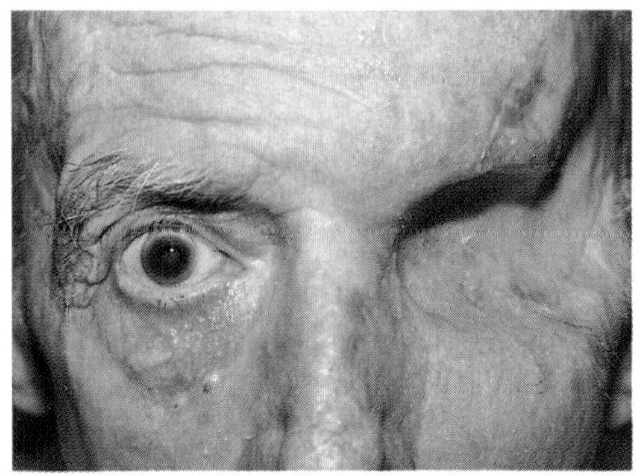

FIGURE 6-115 **Basal cell carcinoma.** The same patient as in Figures 6-113 and 6-114 is free of disease after exenteration and skin graft.

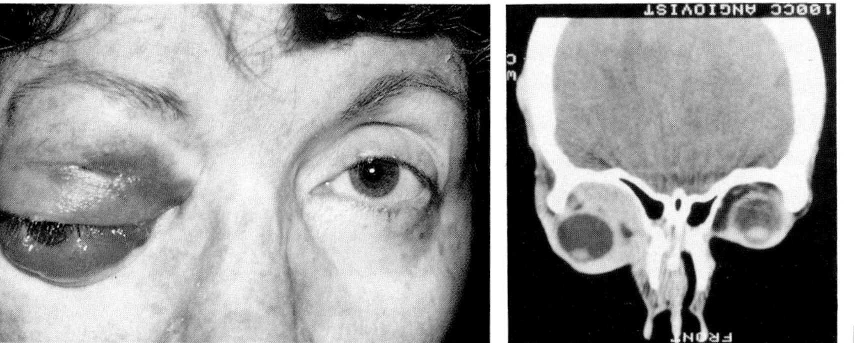

FIGURE 6–116 **Glioblastoma.** Clinical (*A*) and CT scan (*B*) appearance of chemosis and orbital congestion secondary to invasion of the orbital by glioblastoma. (Courtesy of P. Rubin, M.D.)

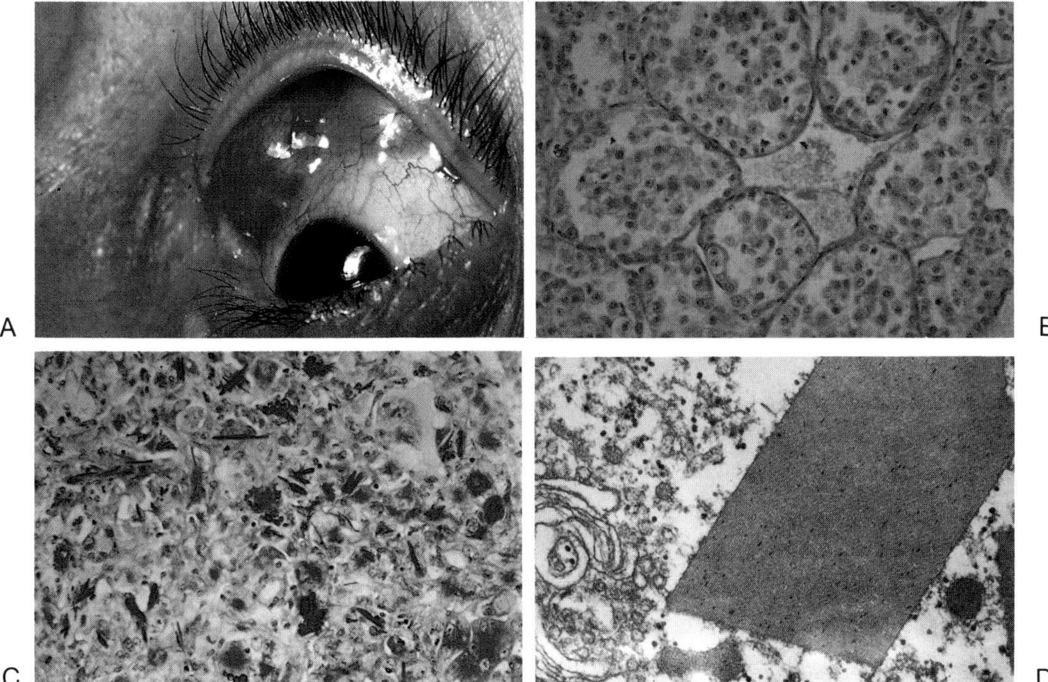

FIGURE 6–117 **Alveolar soft part sarcoma of the orbit.** *A,* Clinical photograph of the left eye of a 54-year-old woman with proptosis and tearing of several months' duration. A bilobed and yellowish red subconjunctival mass was present supranasally. The patient had an excisional biopsy performed followed by exenteration and was alive and well 5 years and 2 months after surgery. *B,* The tumor cells show a distinctive pseudoalveolar or organoid pattern, with nests of polyhedral cells separated by thin fibrovascular septa. The tumor cells in the center of the pseudoalveolar cavities or "soft part" may be loosely cohesive or degenerating. These cells may have granular acidophilic cytoplasm and eccentric paracentral nuclei, many of which contain a prominent single nucleolus. *C,* Many of the tumor cells contain the characteristic crystalline material positive for periodic acid–Schiff stain in the cytoplasm. These crystals are resistant to diastase predigestion (periodic acid–Schiff stain). *D,* Electron micrograph shows a crystalline inclusion with a regular periodicity of 8 to 10 nm. Well-developed Golgi lamellae are present on the left, and many small, round, electron-dense glycogen granules are present, especially in the upper left.

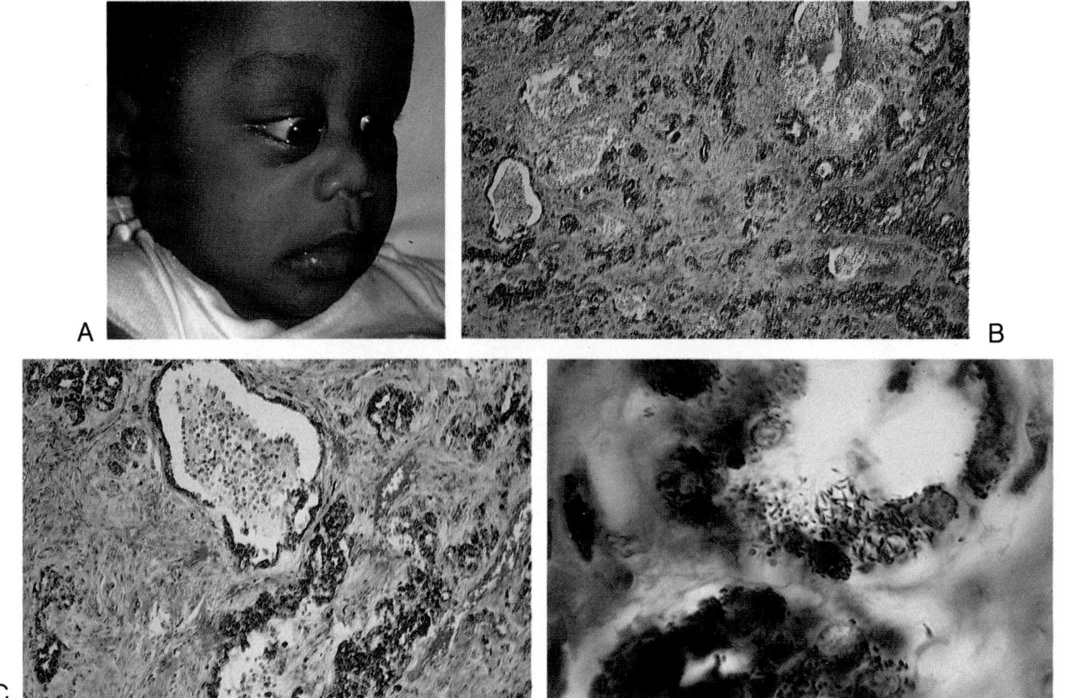

FIGURE 6–118 **Pigmented retinal choristoma.** *A,* A 4-month-old boy with right exophthalmos caused by orbital pigmented choristoma (retinal anlage tumor). (*A,* From Lamping KA, Albert DM, Lack E, et al: Melanocytic neuroectodermal tumor of infancy (retinal anlage tumor). Ophthalmology 92:144, 1985). *B,* Vascularized fibrous stroma contains numerous nests and cords of cells and irregular slitlike alveolar spaces (H&E). *C,* The alveolar spaces contain two cell types: large pigmented cuboidal cells, which line the alveolar spaces, and basophilic cells with scanty cytoplasm, filling the cavities of large spaces (H&E). *D,* Higher magnification of the pigmented cells shows large vesicular nuclei and abundant cytoplasm containing varying amounts of elongated pigment granules (H&E). (*B–D,* Courtesy of Lorenz E. Zimmerman, M.D.)

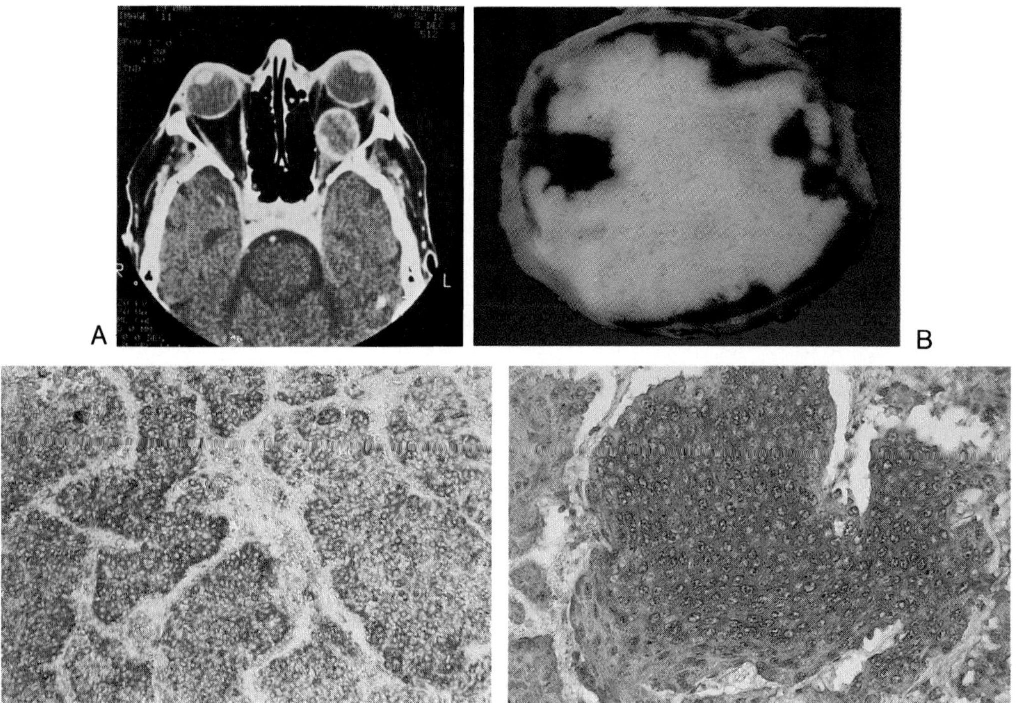

FIGURE 6–119 **Orbital carcinoid tumor.** A 71-year-old woman with metastatic carcinoid tumor of unknown primary site acquired proptosis and cranial nerve III palsy on the left side. *A,* CT scan shows a well-circumscribed intraconal mass in the left orbit. *B,* Gross specimen shows pale yellow central area of ischemic necrosis surrounded by rim of viable reddish brown tissue. *C,* Tumor cells show immunoreactivity for chromogranin A (×64). *D,* Tumor cells demonstrate immunoreactivity for synaptophysin (×100). (From Shetlar DJ, Font RL, Ordonex N, et al: A clinicopathologic study of three carcinoid tumors metastatic to the orbit. Ophthalmology 97:260, 1990.)

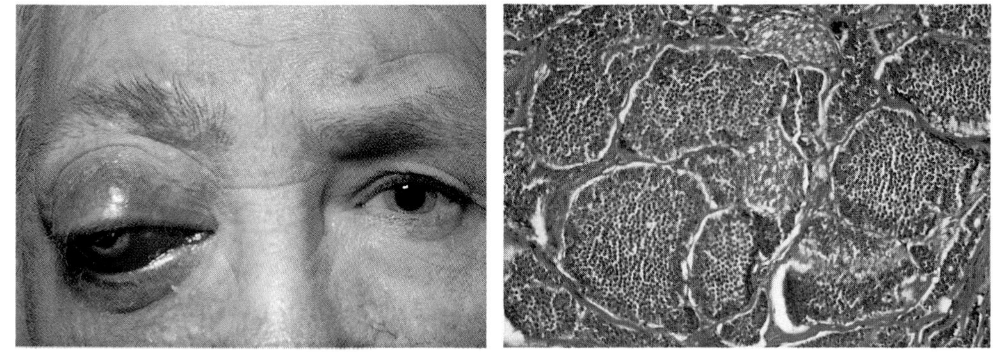

FIGURE 6–120 **Primary orbital carcinoid tumor.** *A,* A 71-year-old woman presented with slowly progressive proptosis of 11 years' duration. *B,* Low-power magnification shows lobules of basaloid tumor cells. The large tumor cells have eccentric nuclei displaying stippling of nuclear chromatin (H&E, ×60). (Courtesy of Lorenz E. Zimmerman, M.D., Armed Forces Institute of Pathology, Washington, DC.)

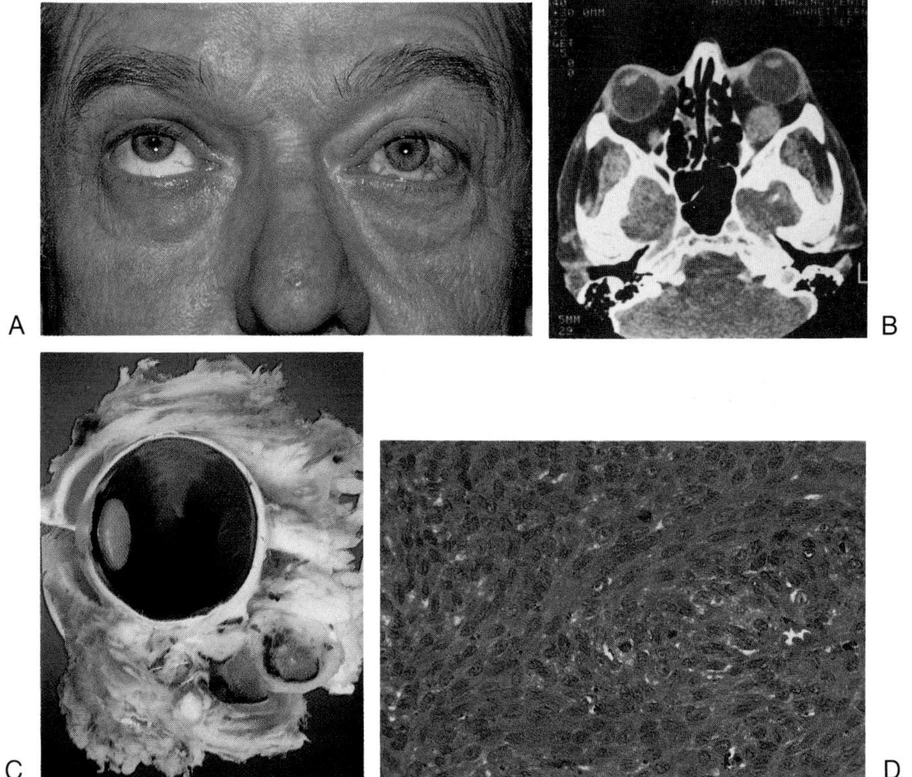

FIGURE 6–121 **Primary orbital melanoma.** *A,* A 50-year-old man with a restrictive myopathy of the left inferior rectus muscle. *B,* CT scan shows the tumor involving the left inferior rectus muscle. (*B,* Courtesy of R. Wilkins, M.D.) *C,* Examination of exenterated orbital contents shows the tumor associated with the inferior rectus muscle, which has several variably pigmented solid areas. *D,* This melanoma was composed predominantly of spindle cells (H&E, ×100).

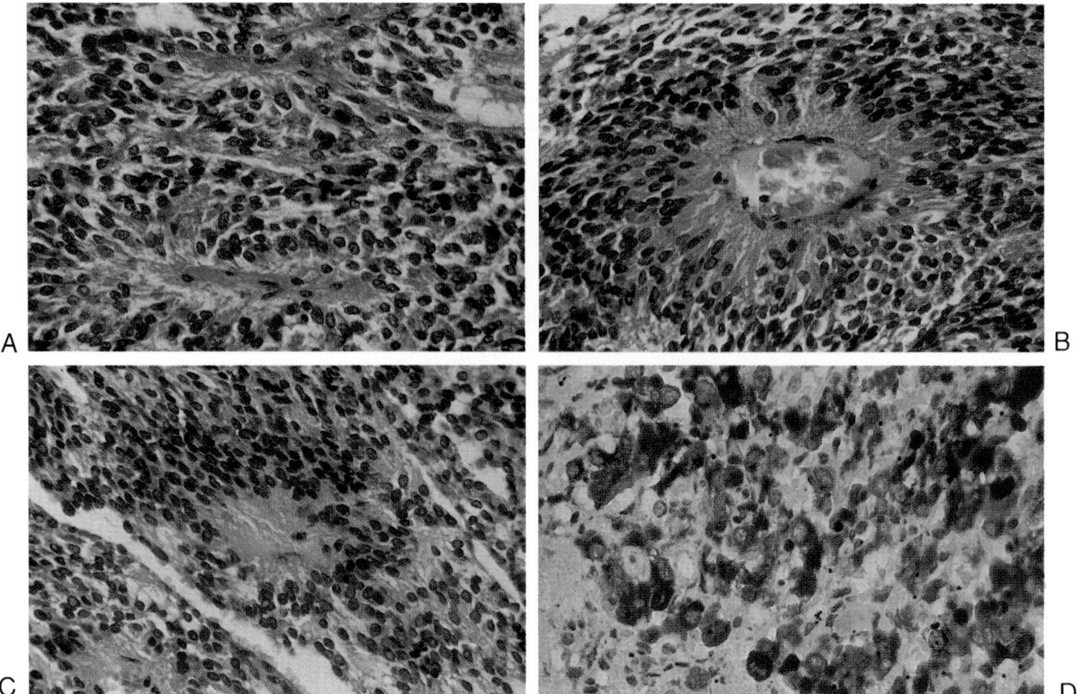

FIGURE 6–122 **Primary orbital neuroblastoma.** *A,* Tumor cells have orthochromatic nuclei and extend delicate eosinophilic processes to form a neutrophil background (H&E, original magnification ×320). *B,* Perivascular rosette with interwoven cytoplasmic processes directed perpendicularly to the wall of the capillary (H&E, original magnification ×320). *C,* A Wright rosette composed of centrally directed cellular processes (neurites) with a surrounding annulus of nuclei (H&E, original magnification ×320). *D,* Immunohistochemical staining for neuron-specific enolase is positive as indicated by cytoplasmic brown reaction product (immunoperoxidase reaction, original magnification ×320). (Published courtesy of Jakobiec FA, Klepach GL, Crissman JD, et al: Primary differentiated neuroblastoma of the orbit. Ophthalmology 94:255–266, 1987.)

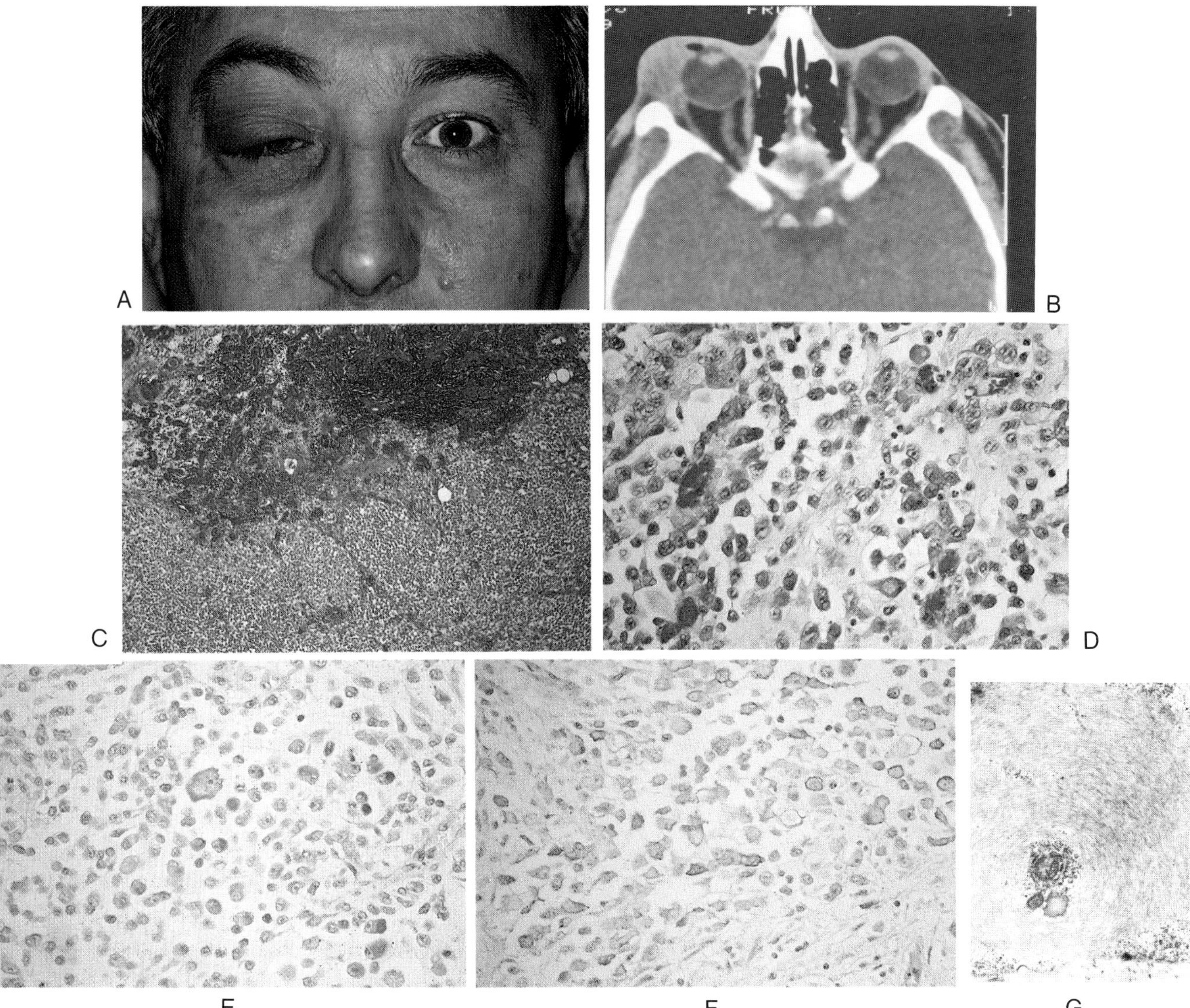

FIGURE 6–123 **Malignant rhabdoid tumor.** *A,* A 50-year-old man presented with a 1-month history of erythema and swelling of the right eyelids and proptosis. *B,* Axial CT scan shows a rounded mass lateral to the globe projecting anterior to the orbital rim. *C,* Microscopically, most of the tumor contained sheets of dyscohesive tumor cells. In the upper area of this photomicrograph, tumor cells infiltrate preexisting elements of the lacrimal gland (H&E, ×60). *D,* Higher-power magnification shows dyscohesive epithelioid or globoid cells with occasional prominent cytoplasmic eosinophilic inclusions (H&E, ×240). *E,* Immunohistochemical staining of tumor cells shows positive staining for cytoplasmic vimentin filaments (immunoperoxidase reaction, ×220). *F,* Cell membranes of tumor cells stain positively for epithelial membrane antigen (immunoperoxidase reaction, ×220). *G,* Transmission electron microscopy demonstrates whorls of cytoplasmic intermediate filaments (×41,000). (From Niffenegger JH, Jakobiec FA, Shore JW et al: Adult extrarenal rhabdoid tumor of the lacrimal gland. Ophthalmology 99:568, 570, 573, 1992.)

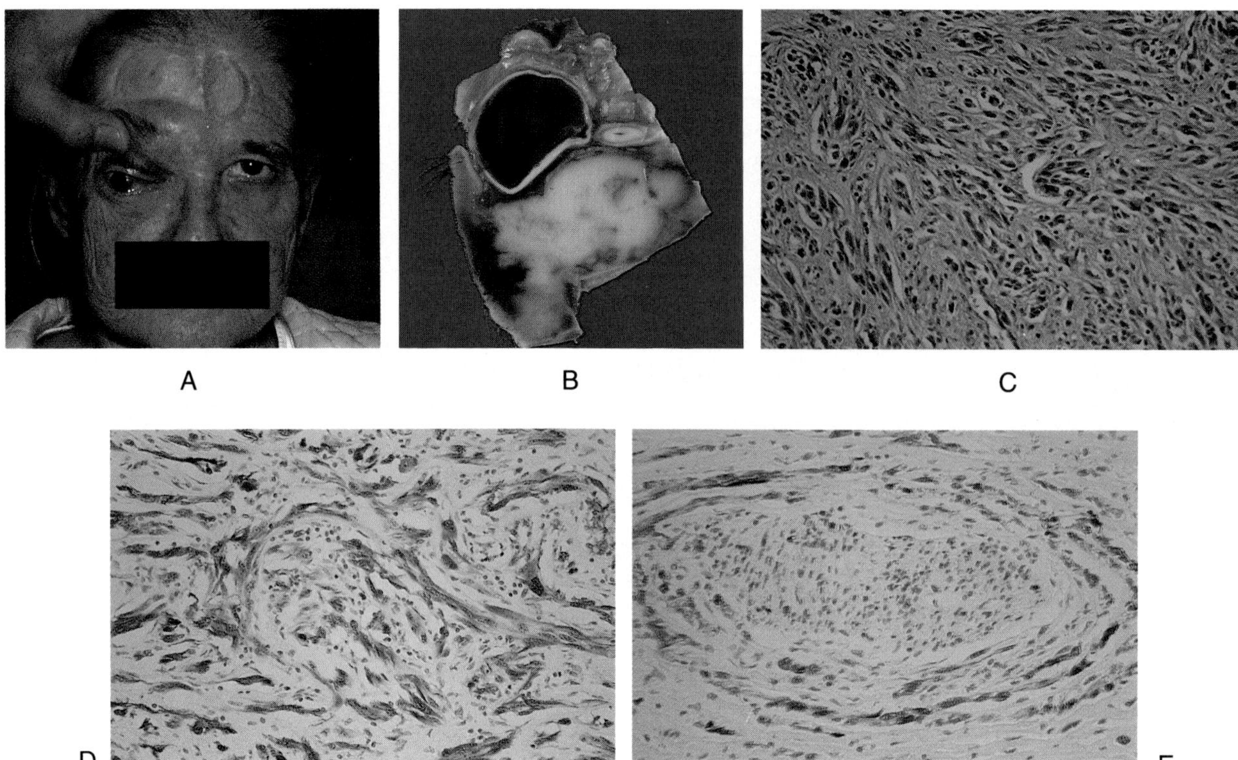

FIGURE 6–124 **Malignant peripheral nerve sheath tumor.** *A,* A 79-year-old woman had three recurrences of mass located in the periorbital region supranasally. She subsequently underwent orbital exenteration with resection of the frontal bone but acquired intracranial invasion of the tumor and died approximately 1 year later. *B,* Examination of exenterated orbital contents shows a tumor involving the superior orbit. *C,* The tumor is composed of interlacing fascicles of spindle-shaped cells intermixed with scattered plumper epithelioid cells (H&E, ×51). *D,* Immunohistochemical staining for S100 protein demonstrates positive staining of the tumor cells (immunoperoxidase reaction, ×51). *E,* Tumor cells extending along nerve (perineural invasion) show positive staining for S100 protein (immunoperoxidase reaction, ×64).

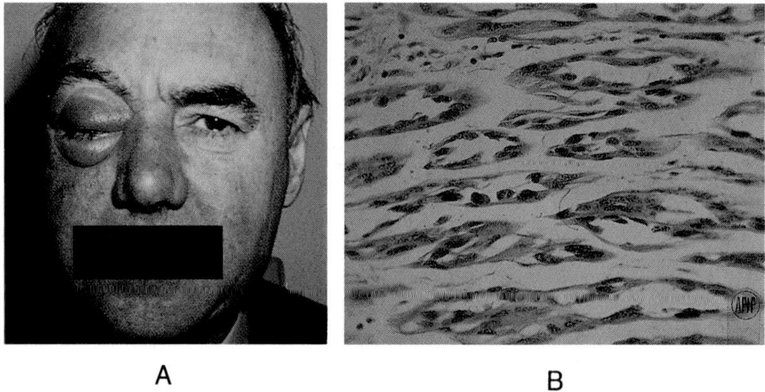

FIGURE 6–125 **Malignant peripheral nerve sheath tumor.** *A,* A 50-year-old man presented with swollen eyelids 1 year after removal of a supranasal subcutaneous lesion misinterpreted as a sweat gland carcinoma. The patient had diminished sensation in the distribution of the ophthalmic division of the trigeminal nerve because of involvement with tumor. *B,* An area of tumor showing a neurotubular pattern composed of plump spindle cells lining elongated pseudolumens. There were no axon cylinders in this area (H&E, ×220).

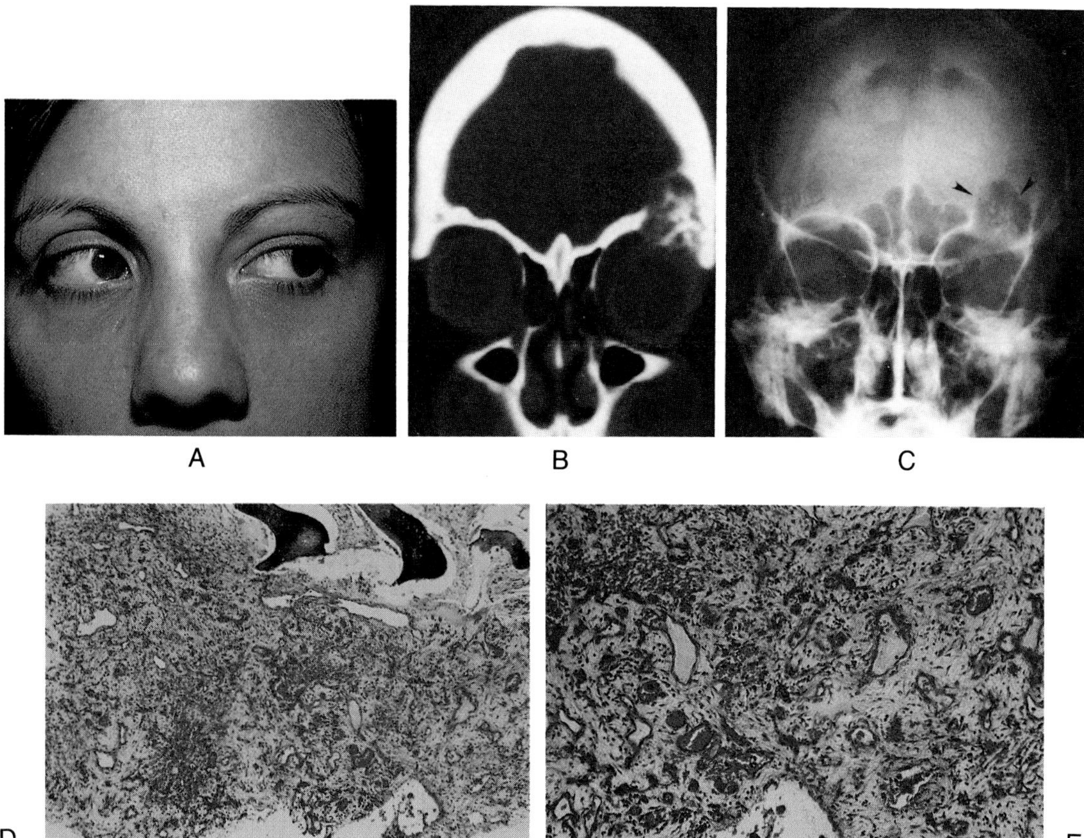

FIGURE 6–126 **Primary intraosseous capillary hemangioma.** *A,* A 31-year-old woman presented with an 18-month history of slowly progressive blepharoptosis of the left eye. The clinical photograph shows mild blepharoptosis of the left eyelid and subtle fullness between the superior eyelid sulcus and the eyebrow. Results of the motility examination were normal. *B,* Plain x-ray film of the skull shows a well-circumscribed lytic lesion with fine radiating reticulated pattern *(arrowheads). C,* CT scan displays a lytic lesion with coarse, internal bone reticulations. *D,* There is a loose stroma with prominent capillary proliferation and extravasation of erythrocytes resembling granulation tissue. In the upper right, several blue-stained bony trabeculae are present (Masson's trichrome, ×20). *E,* The tumor shows a proliferation of capillaries that display variable caliber of their lumens. These vascular lumens are lined by low cuboidal endothelium–like cells (Masson's trichrome, ×40).

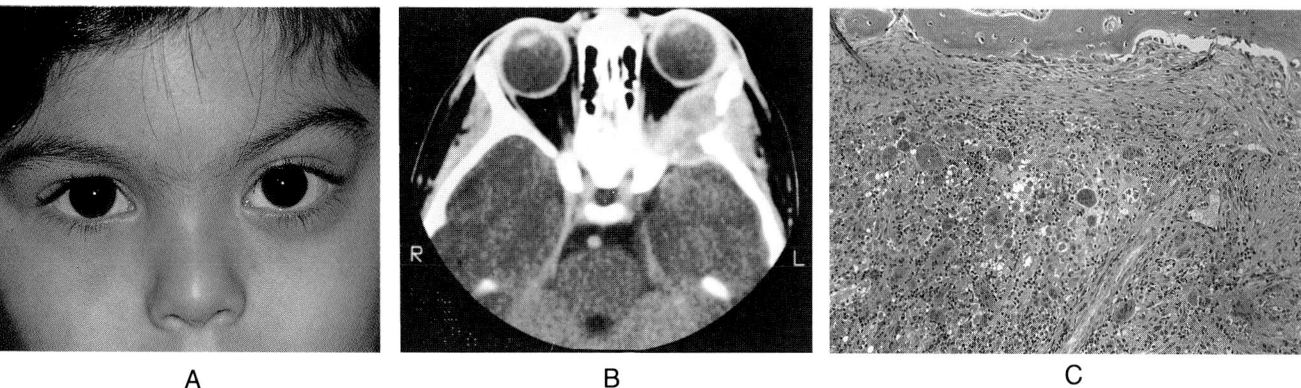

FIGURE 6–127 **Histiocytosis X.** *A,* A 4-year-old boy presented with a 3-week history of swelling and ptosis of the left upper eyelid and 3-day history of proptosis of the left eye. *B,* CT scan shows a lytic lesion with irregular borders involving the superotemporal orbit. *C,* Microscopic examination shows multinucleated giant cells with a background of histiocytes, eosinophils, and lymphocytes (H&E, ×40). (*A–C,* Courtesy of J. A. Shields, M.D., Wills Eye Hospital.)

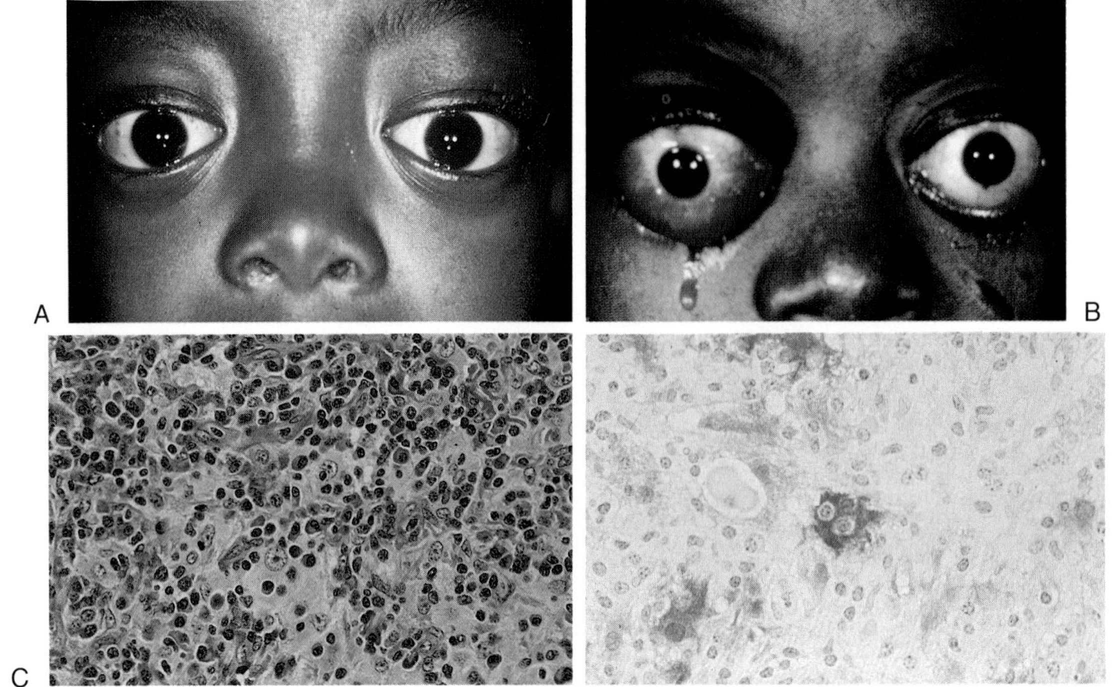

FIGURE 6–128 **Sinus histiocytosis with massive lymphadenopathy.** *A*, A 4-year-old boy with bilateral symmetric proptosis. (*A*, Courtesy of David S. Friendly, M.D.) *B*, Bilateral proptosis with visible subconjunctival mass in the right eye. Microscopically the orbital lesions are composed of lobules of histiocytes admixed with mononuclear inflammatory cells separated by dense bands of connective tissue. (*B*, Courtesy of Pierre Dhermy, M.D.) *C*, High-power view shows polymorphic infiltrate of histiocytes, lymphocytes, and plasma cells. The cytoplasm of the histiocytes may contain lymphocytes, erythrocytes, or plasma cells, as demonstrated in this photomicrograph (H&E, ×128). *D*, The histiocytes stain positively for S100 antigen (immunoperoxidase stain).

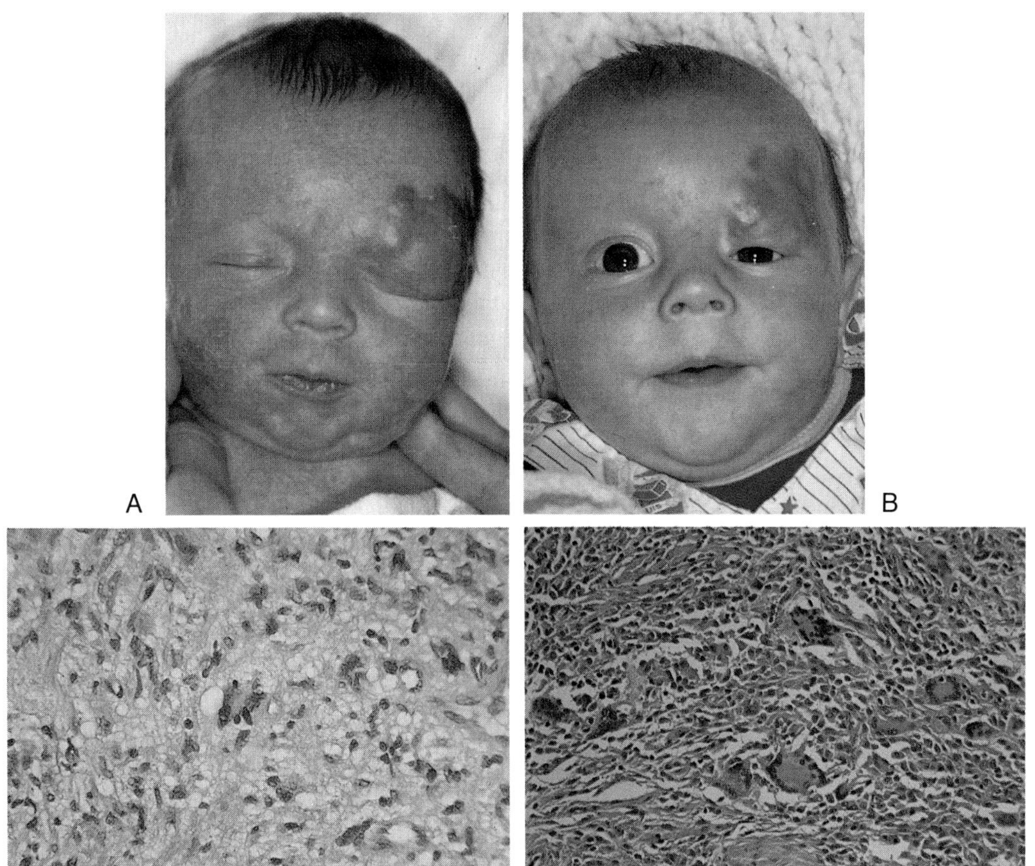

FIGURE 6–129 **Juvenile xanthogranuloma.** A full-term male infant with a congenital upper eyelid lesion. Biopsy of the yellowish red nodule showed juvenile xanthogranuloma. *A*, Complete ptosis of the left upper eyelid before therapy. *B*, Two weeks after intralesional corticosteroid injection, the lesion had significantly regressed and the eyelid is elevated above the pupil. The lesion continued to improve and nearly completely disappeared 1 year after treatment. *C*, Microscopic examination shows vacuolated histiocytes with a Touton giant cell in the center of the field (H&E, ×100). (*A–C*, from Schwartz TL, Carter KD, Judisch GF, et al: Congenital macronodular juvenile xanthogranuloma of the eyelid. Ophthalmology 98:1230, 1991.) *D*, Photomicrograph of another orbital lesion shows sheets of benign-appearing histiocytes with occasional Touton giant cells. (*D*, Courtesy of C. L. Shields, Wills Eye Hospital.)

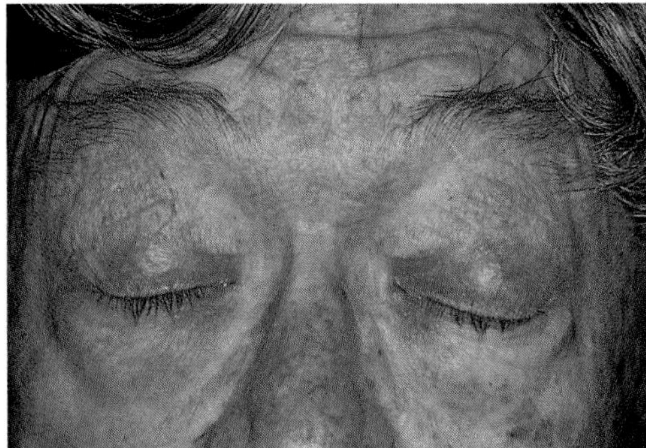

FIGURE 6–130 **Erdheim-Chester disease.** Firm yellow lesions of the eyelid in a patient with Erdheim-Chester disease. Although they superficially resemble xanthelasma, these lid lesions are more indurated than ordinary xanthelasma. (Courtesy of J. A. Shields, Ocular Oncology Service, Wills Eye Hospital.)

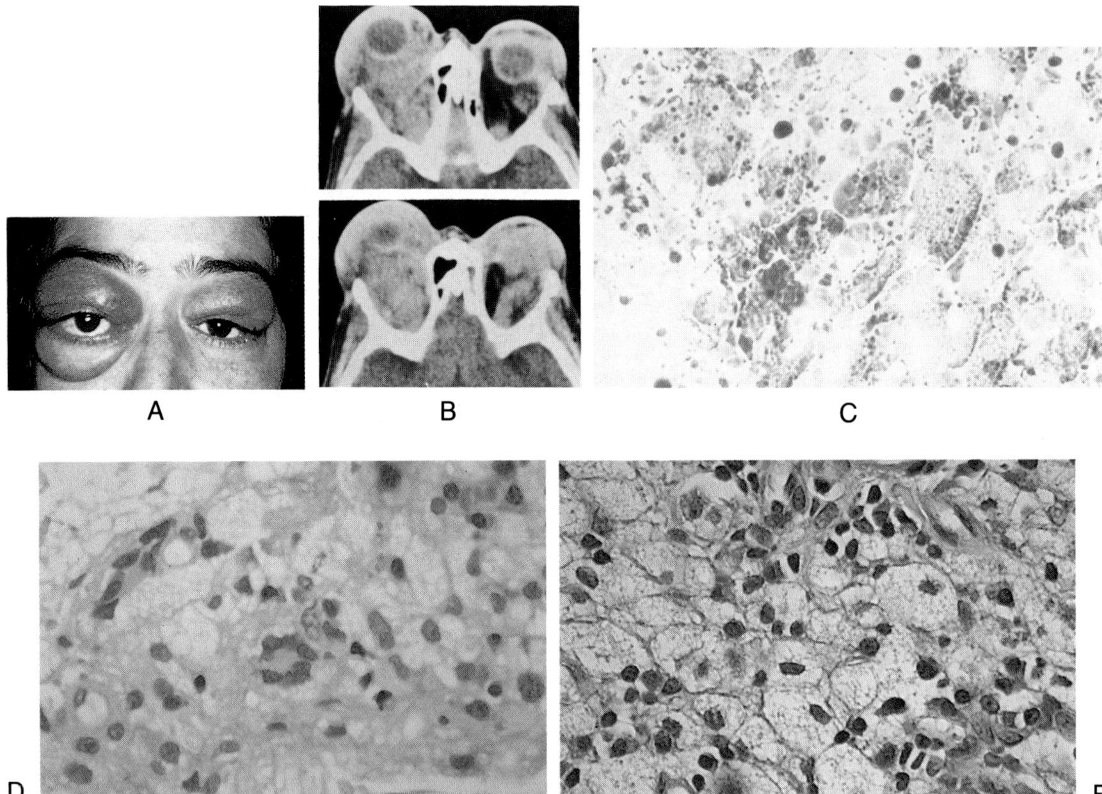

FIGURE 6–131 **Adult orbital xanthogranuloma.** *A,* Patient with severe bilateral proptosis and swollen eyelids; the right side is more severely affected than the left. Systemic evaluation shows no involvement of bones or other organs. *B,* Axial CT scan showing dense bilateral soft tissue mass lesions; the right orbit is more severely affected than the left. *C,* Frozen section of xanthoma cells containing intracytoplasmic lipid, which is stained red (oil red O, ×350). *D,* Touton giant cell is present centrally, with a background of mononucleated xanthoma cells. *E,* Xanthoma cells with foamy vacuolated, pale cytoplasm and small nuclei. (*A–C,* Courtesy of A. Hidayat, Armed Forces Institute of Pathology.)

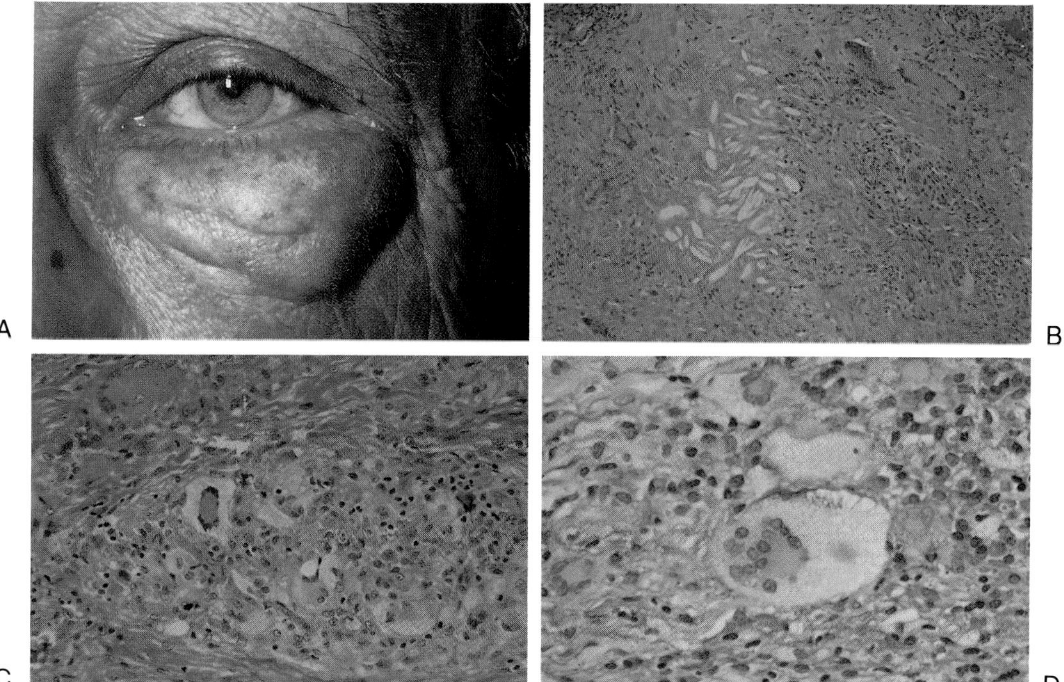

FIGURE 6–132 **Necrobiotic xanthogranuloma.** *A,* Yellowish mass in the left lower lid. *B,* An area of eosinophilic collagen degeneration (necrobiosis) is surrounded by histiocytes, giant cells, and lymphocytes. *C,* Areas of xanthomatous histiocytes, lymphocytes, and multinucleated giant cells (Touton and foreign body types) are separated by bands of hyaline necrobiosis. *D,* Higher-power micrograph of a Touton giant cell with a background of xanthoma cells.

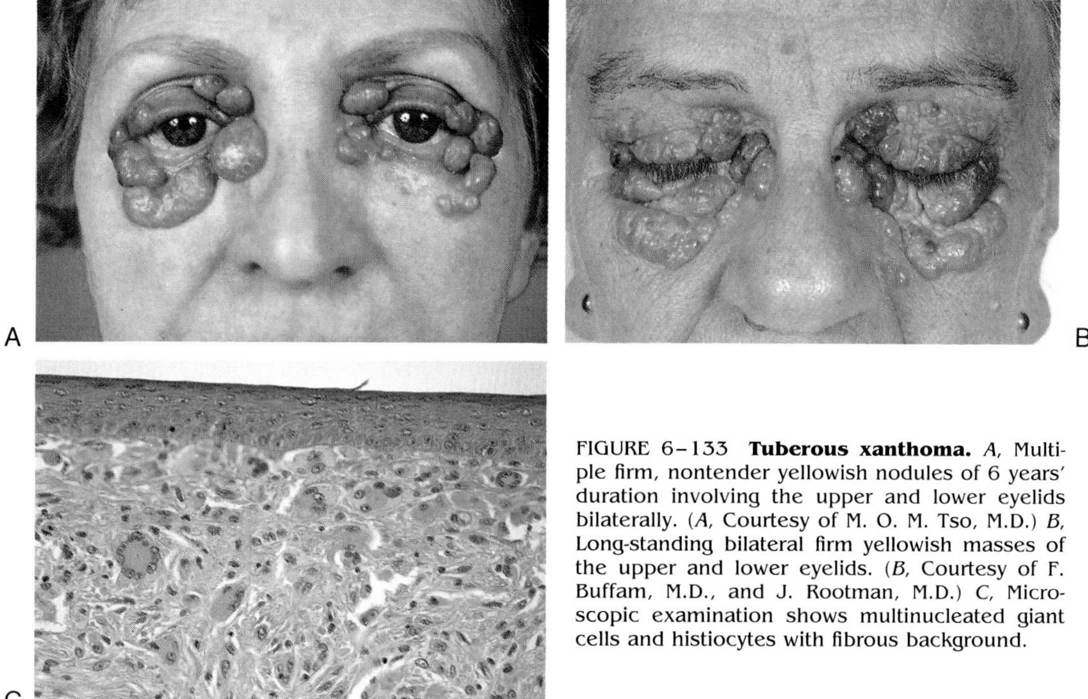

FIGURE 6–133 **Tuberous xanthoma.** *A,* Multiple firm, nontender yellowish nodules of 6 years' duration involving the upper and lower eyelids bilaterally. (*A,* Courtesy of M. O. M. Tso, M.D.) *B,* Long-standing bilateral firm yellowish masses of the upper and lower eyelids. (*B,* Courtesy of F. Buffam, M.D., and J. Rootman, M.D.) *C,* Microscopic examination shows multinucleated giant cells and histiocytes with fibrous background.

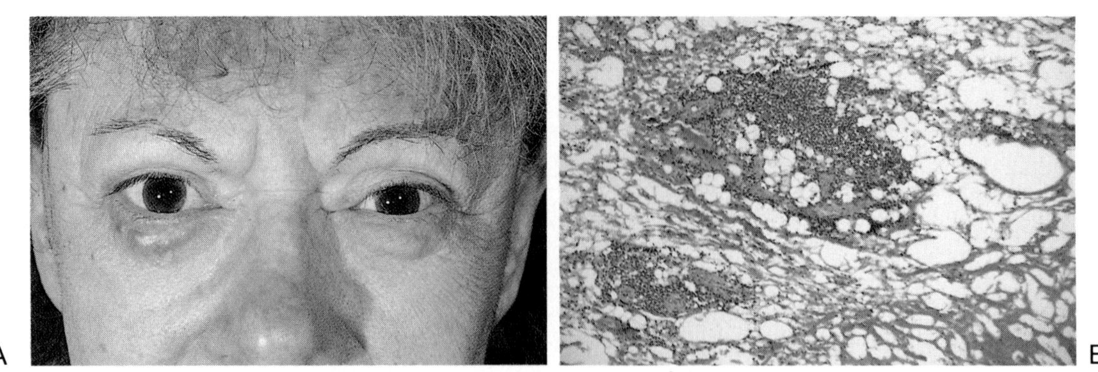

FIGURE 6–134 **Lipogranuloma.** *A*, Chronic bilateral eyelid masses following cosmetic silicone injections. *B*, Histologically, spaces of various sizes are surrounded by collagen and mononuclear inflammatory cells with few remaining histiocytes. The clear spaces contained silicone removed during tissue processing. (*A* and *B*, Courtesy of E. H. Sacks, M.D.)

SECTION 7

Neuroophthalmology

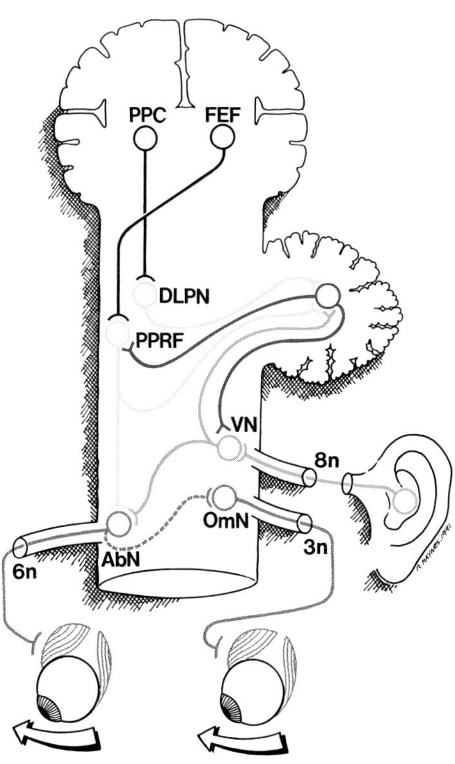

FIGURE 7–1 **Schematic representation of the hierarchical organization of the ocular motor system.** The example shown is the organization of rightward eye movements. *Level 1 (black):* A supranuclear or "upper" ocular motoneuron for rightward saccades projects from the frontal eye fields (FEF) of the left cerebral hemisphere to a pre-motor neuron (*shown in blue*) in the paramedian reticular formation of the right pons (PPRF). A supranuclear ocular motoneuron for rightward smooth pursuit projects from the posterior parietal cortex (PPC) to a pre-motoneuron to the dorsolateral nucleus of the right pons (DLPN). *Level 2 (blue):* A pre-motor neuron for rightward saccadic eye movements and a pre-motoneuron for rightward smooth pursuit project from the right PPRF and the right DLPN to "lower" ocular motoneurons *(shown in brown)* in the right abducens nucleus (AbN) (abducens motoneuron) and in the left oculomotor nucleus (OmN) (medial rectus motoneuron). *Level 3 (brown):* The motoneurons project to the extraocular muscles *(level 6 (brown))* through the abducens (6n) and oculomotor (3n) nerves. An abducens interneuron is shown by the interrupted brown line. Brain stem pre-motoneurons also project to cerebellar neurons *(level 4 (purple)),* which project back to the pre-motoneurons. *Level 5 (yellow):* A primary vestibular neuron from the left labyrinth projects to a second vestibular neuron in the left vestibular nucleus (VN) via the left vestibular nerve (8n). These neurons represent the afferent limb of the vestibuloocular reflex arc. The secondary vestibular neuron projects to the "lower" ocular motoneurons in the right abducens nucleus to produce a rightward eye movement response to the leftward head rotation stimulus.

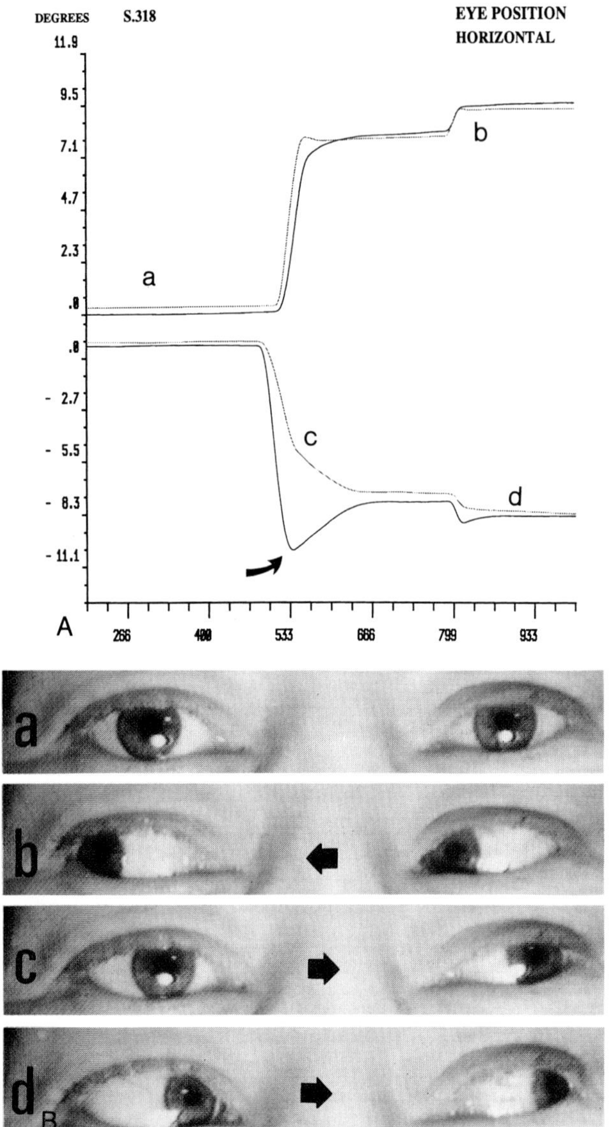

FIGURE 7–2 **Left internuclear ophthalmoplegia.** *A,* Binocular search coil recordings of horizontal eye movements. Upward deflections indicate leftward eye movements. Movements of the right eye are shown in interrupted lines; movements of the left eye, in continuous lines. An attempted 10-degree leftward saccade reveals low adduction of the right eye (peak velocity = 148 degrees/sec, in contrast to 400 degrees/sec for left eye adduction). There is also the characteristic abduction overshoot of the left eye (*arrow*). The mild slowing of the left eye adduction and the slight right eye abduction during the rightward saccade could be normal. (a, b, c, and d refer to video frames in *B.*) *B,* Single frames from a video recording of the patient with the left internuclear ophthalmoplegia whose oculographic recordings are shown in *A.* There was no abnormality in the primary position (a). There was no limitation of the amplitude of adduction in the right eye and therefore no exotropia on holding gaze to the left *after* the leftward saccade (d); however, because of the delay in adduction of the right eye, there was in fact a marked exotropia *during* the leftward saccade (c). There was no delay in adduction of the left eye during a rightward saccade (b). The patient did experience momentary diplopia when looking to the left.

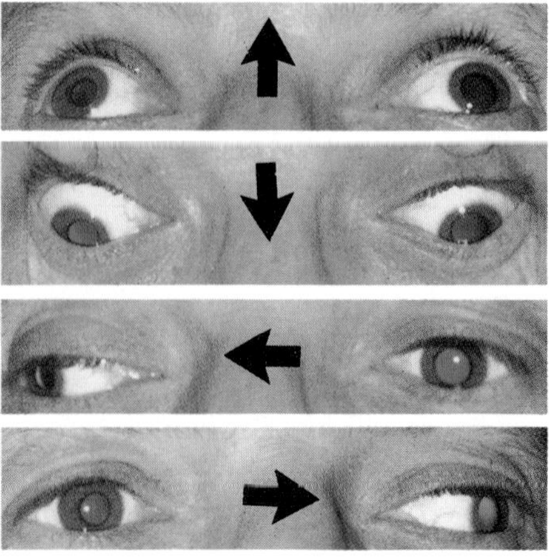

FIGURE 7–3 **"Wall-eyed" bilateral internuclear ophthalmoplegia (WEBINO syndrome).** The patient not only had an advanced bilateral internuclear ophthalmoplegia with inability to adduct either eye past the midline, but also he had a bilateral exotropia with alternating fixation. Although vertical saccades were normal, he had, as expected, a severe vertical vestibular palsy that produced vertical oscillopsia during head movement. Convergence was absent in this patient; however, it is preserved in some patients with the WEBINO syndrome.

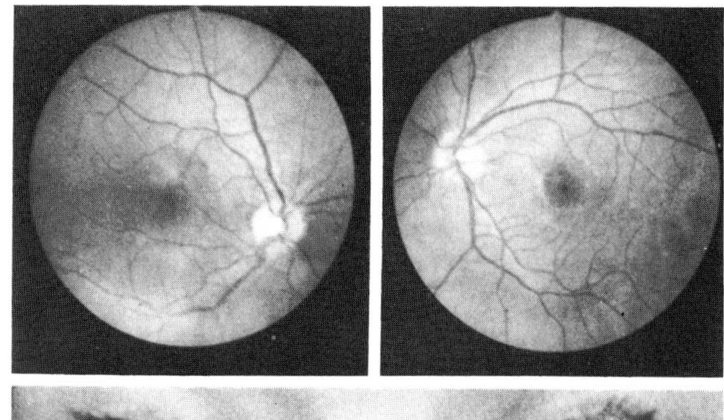

FIGURE 7–4 **Tonic contraversive ocular tilt reaction caused by a unilateral midbrain-thalamic lesion.** *A,* The patient had a leftward ocular tilt reaction consisting of a leftward head tilt, left hyperopia, and leftward torsion of each eye as shown in the fundus photographs. *B,* The lesion, a hemorrhage caused by a right (R) midbrain-thalamic arteriovenous malformation, is shown on T_1-weighted parasagittal magnetic resonance imaging (MRI). (From Halmagyi GM, Brandt T, Dieterich M, et al: Tonic contraversive ocular tilt reaction due to unilateral mesodiencephalic lesion. Neurology 40:1503, 1990.)

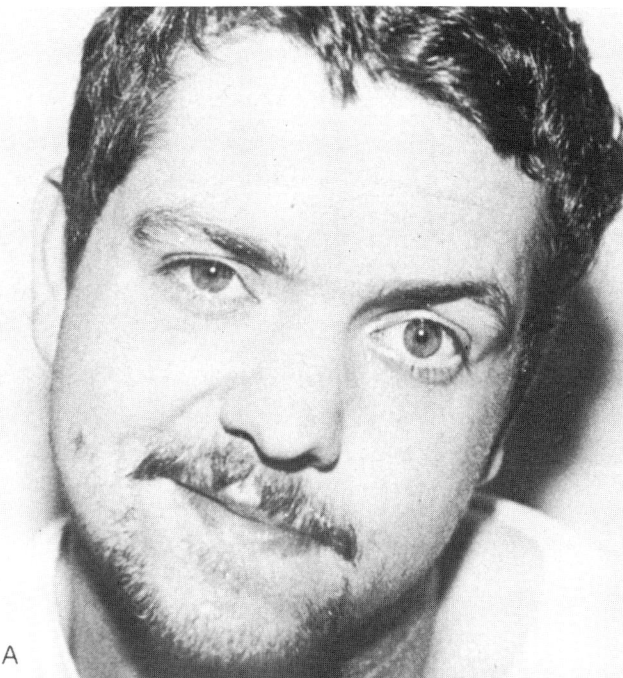

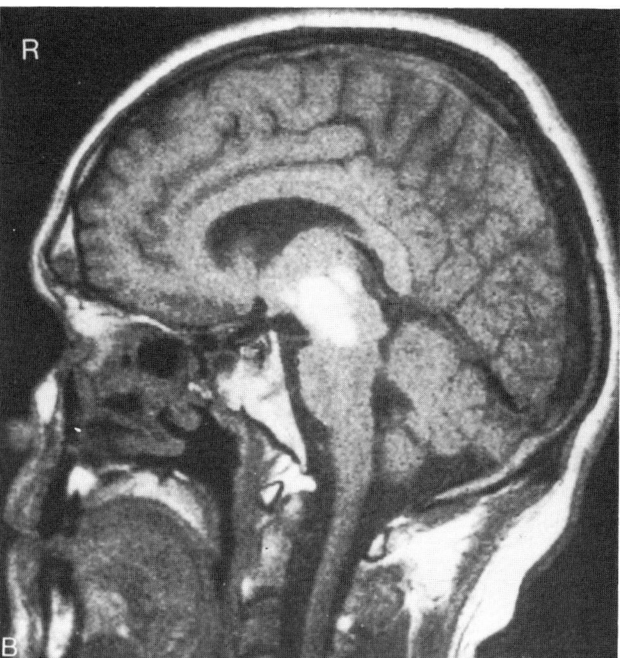

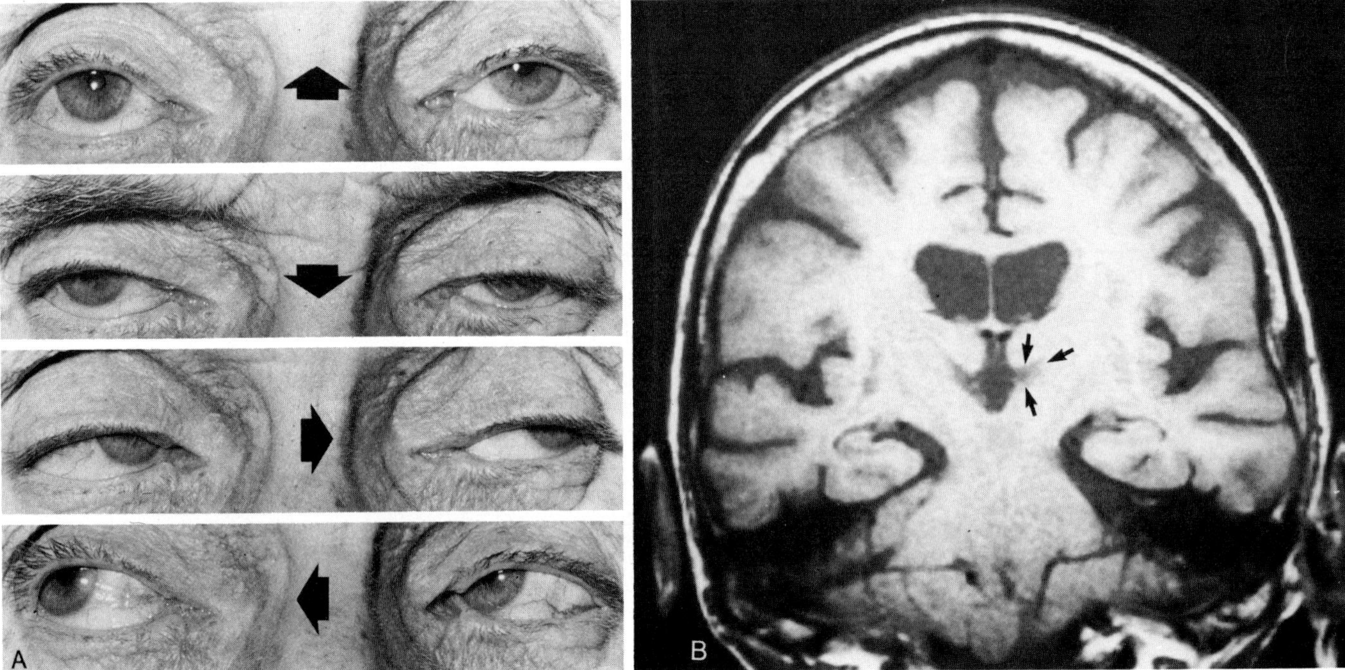

FIGURE 7–5 **Total downgaze palsy.** *A,* The patient could make no eye movements at all below the horizontal meridian. Downward saccades to the vertical meridian were slightly restricted, but this is not necessarily abnormal at the age of 83 years, since upward saccades were of normal velocity. There was also bilateral asymmetric ptosis. *B,* T_1-weighted MRI showed bilateral symmetric lesions at the midbrain-thalamic junction in the region of the rostral interstitial nucleus of the medial longitudinal fasciculus; three *arrows* show the lesion on the left. The patient had mitral stenosis with atrial fibrillation and had presented 15 years previously with transient confusion and permanent downgaze palsy. She had presumably suffered a "top-of-the-basilar" syndrome caused by embolic occlusion of the posterior thalamic-subthalamic artery.

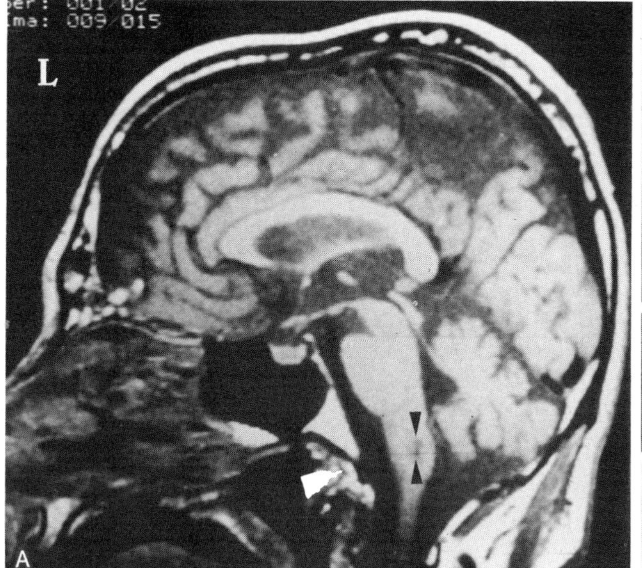

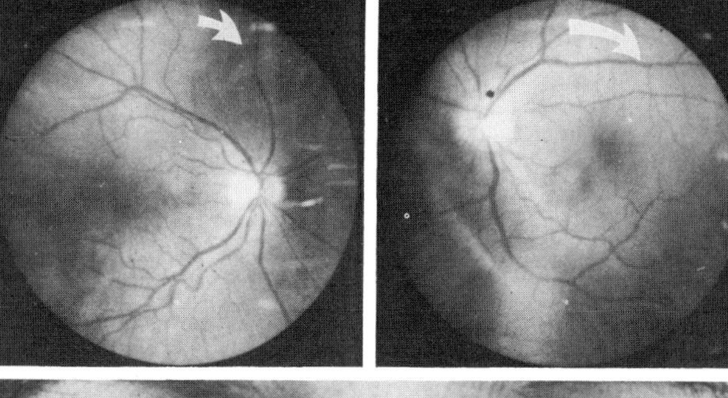

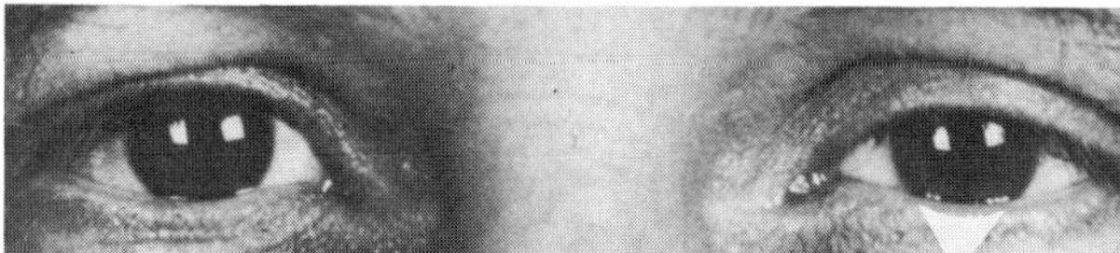

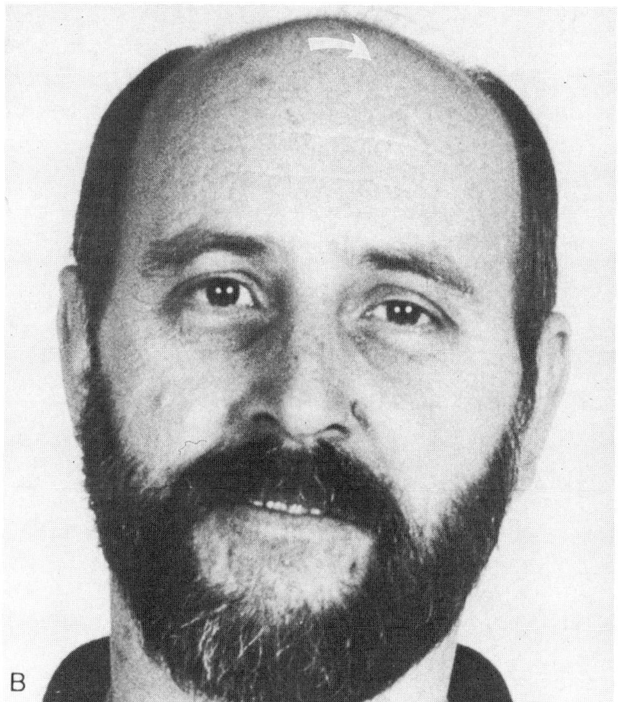

FIGURE 7–6 **Medullary lesion with eye movement disorder.** *A,* Left (L) lateral medullary infarct *(arrowheads)* involving the left vestibular nucleus, shown by parasagittal T_1-weighted MRI. *B,* The patient had Horner's syndrome and a leftward ocular tilt reaction with left hypotropia, leftward head tilt, and dysconjugate leftward ocular torsion, about 20 degrees (excyclotropia) in the left eye but only about 5 degrees (incyclotropia) in the right eye. He also had loss of pain and temperature sensation on the left side of the face and on the right side of the body. (Courtesy of T. Brandt, M.D.)

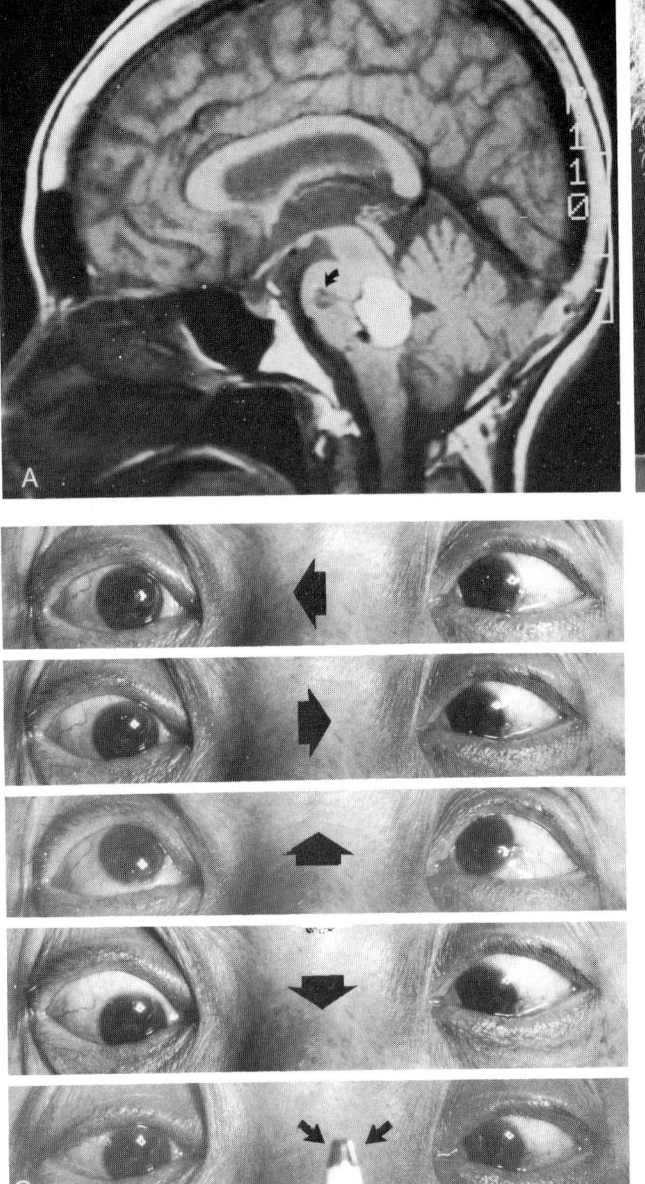

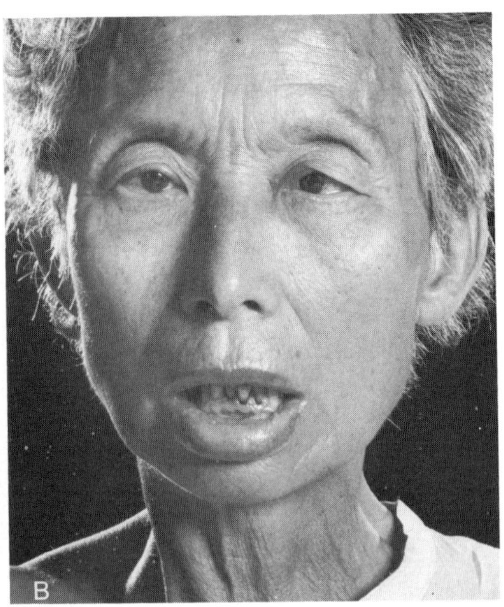

FIGURE 7–7 **Pontine lesion with eye movement disorder.** *A,* A large pontine tegmental hemorrhage, possibly caused by a capillary angioma, in the basis pontis *(arrow),* shown by T_1-weighted sagittal MRI. (R, right.) *B,* The patient was a 78-year-old woman who had an acquired "pseudo-Möbius" syndrome. *C,* Horizontal gaze was absent, but vertical saccades and convergence were intact. There was also primary position esotropia and bilateral total facial palsy, but no disturbance of consciousness and no long-tract signs.

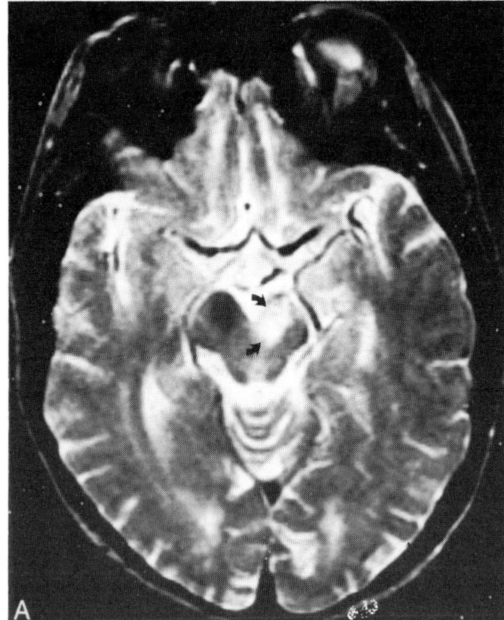

FIGURE 7–8 **Midbrain lesion with eye movement disorder.** *A,* An infarct in the ventral midbrain caused by a "top-of-the-basilar" embolus is shown on T_2-weighted MRI. The lesion *(arrows)* involves the left pyramidal tract and the emergent fibers on the left oculomotor nerve. *B, C,* On presentation, the patient had a pupil-sparing, but otherwise complete, left third-nerve palsy (shown here partly recovered) as well as right hemiparesis.

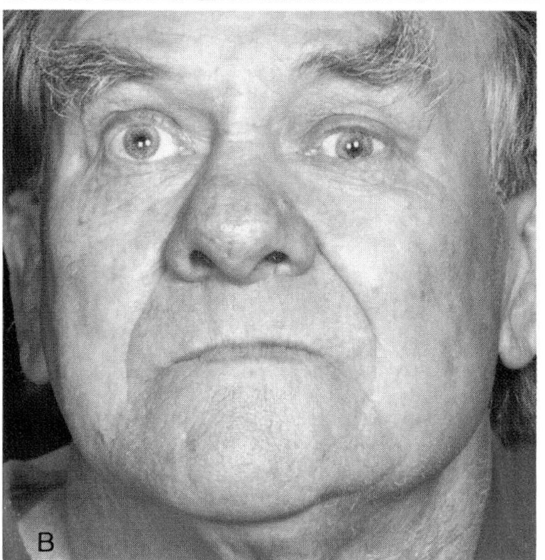

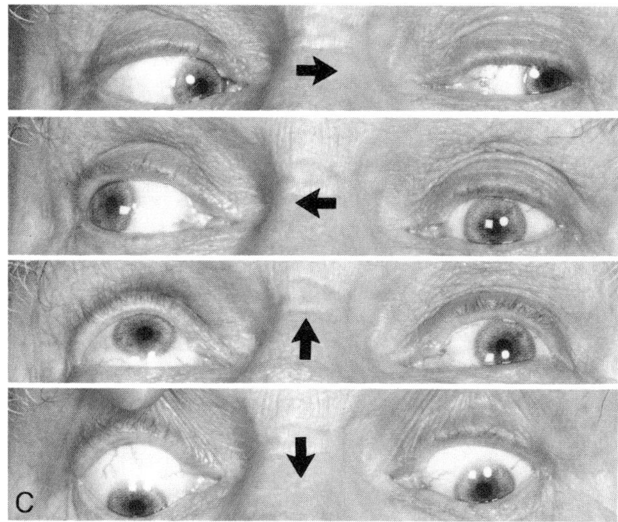

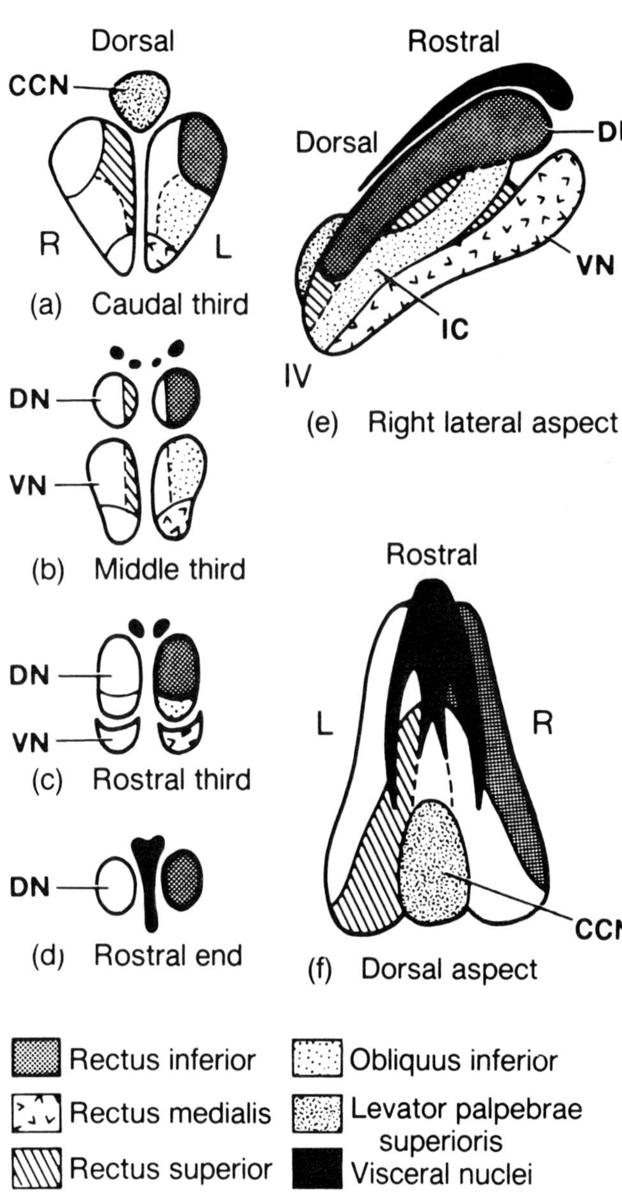

FIGURE 7–9 **Organization of the oculomotor nucleus.** Warwick's schema of topographic organization within the oculomotor nucleus. Note the caudal dorsal midline position of the motor pool for the levator palpebrae superioris. (CCN, caudal central nucleus.) The motor pool of the superior rectus is contralateral to the extraocular muscle that it innervates. (R, right; L, left; DN, dorsal nucleus; IC, intermediate column; IV, region of the trochlear nucleus; VN, ventral nucleus.) (From Miller NR: Walsh and Hoyt's Clinical Neuro-ophthalmology, 4th ed, vol 2, p. 569. Copyright 1985, the Williams & Wilkins Co., Baltimore. Redrawn from Warwick R: Representation of extraocular muscles in oculomotor nuclei of monkey. J Comp Neurol 98:449–503, 1953.)

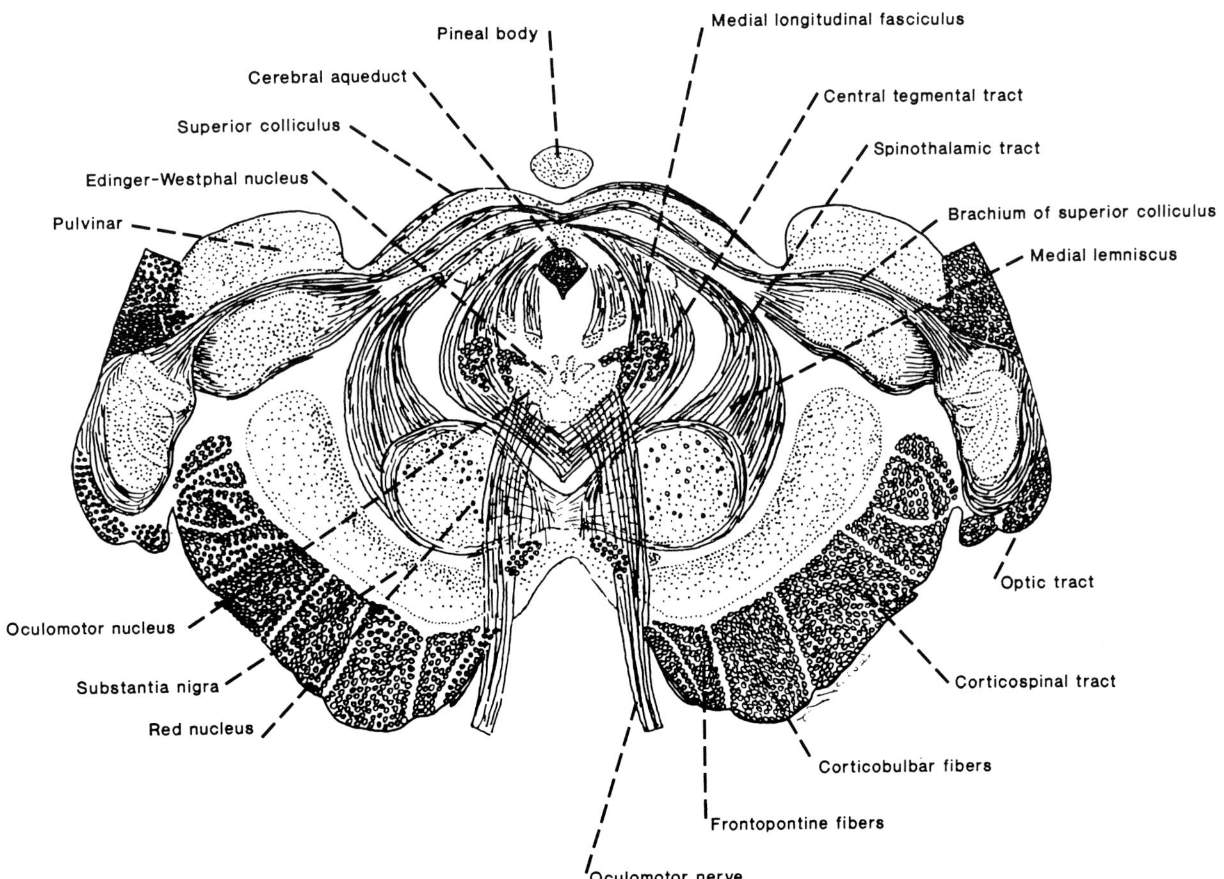

FIGURE 7–10 **Oculomotor nerves.** Cross section of the midbrain at the level of the superior colliculi and the oculomotor nerves. (Adapted from Ferner H (ed): Pernkopf Atlas der topographischen und angewandten Anatomie des Menchen, 3rd ed, vols 1 and 2. Baltimore-Munich, Urban & Schwarzenberg, 1987, p. 91.)

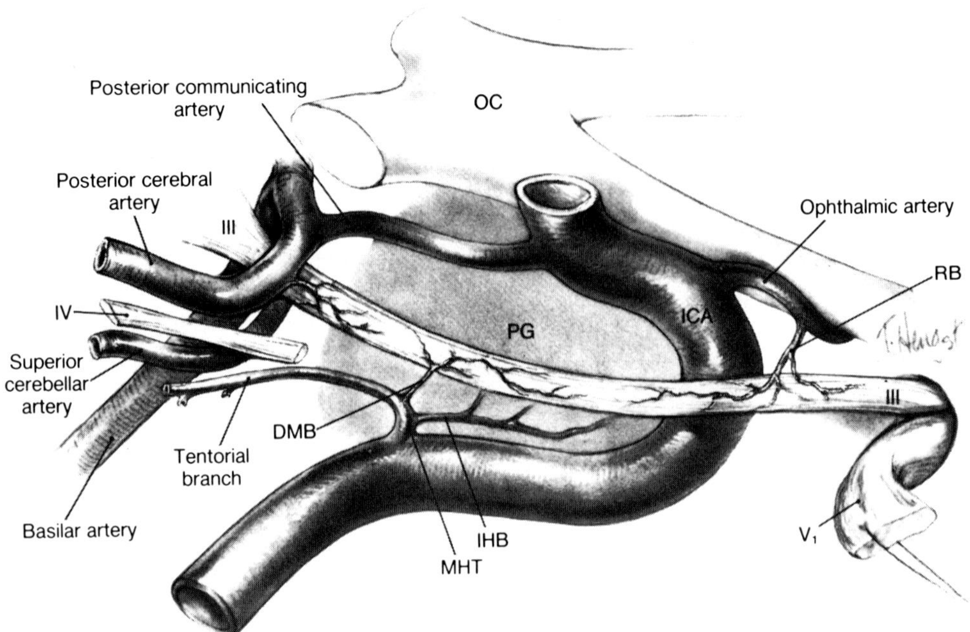

FIGURE 7–11 **Oculomotor nerves.** Lateral view of the subarachnoid and intracavernous portions of the oculomotor nerve (III) and its vascular supply. (DMB, dorsal meningeal branches; MHT, meningohypophyseal trunk; ICA, internal carotid artery; IHB, inferior hypophyseal branches; RB, recurrent collateral branches of the ophthalmic artery; IV, trochlear nerve; V_1, ophthalmic division of the trigeminal nerve; OC, optic chiasm; PG, pituitary gland. (From Miller NR: Walsh and Hoyt's Clinical Neuro-ophthalmology, 4th ed, vol 2, p. 577. Copyright 1985, the Williams & Wilkins Co., Baltimore. Redrawn from Nadeau SE, Trobe JD; Pupil sparing in oculomotor palsy: A brief review. Ann Neurol 13:143–148, 1983.)

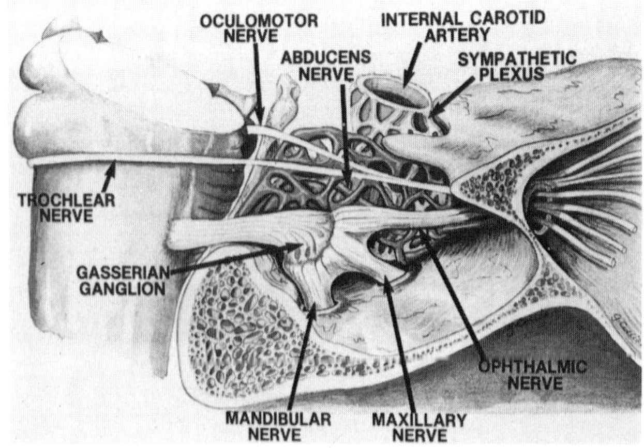

FIGURE 7–12 **Cavernous sinus.** A coronal section of the right cavernous sinus viewed anteriorly. (From Kline LB, Acker JD, Post MJD: Computed tomographic evaluation of the cavernous sinus. Ophthalmology 89:374–385, 1982.)

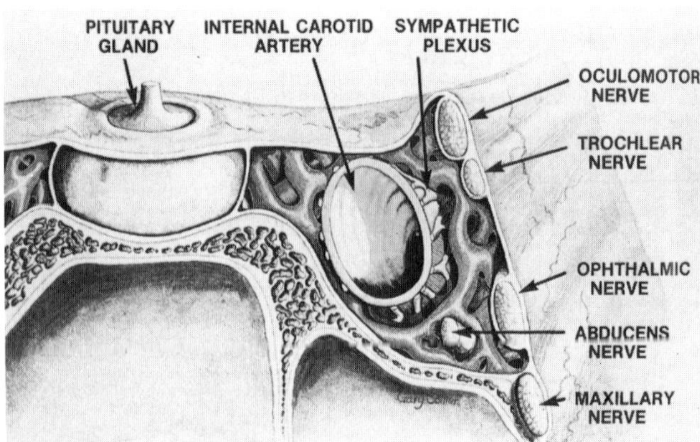

FIGURE 7–13 **Cavernous sinus.** The right cavernous sinus viewed laterally. (From Kline LB: The Tolosa-Hunt syndrome. Surv Ophthalmol 27:82, 1982.)

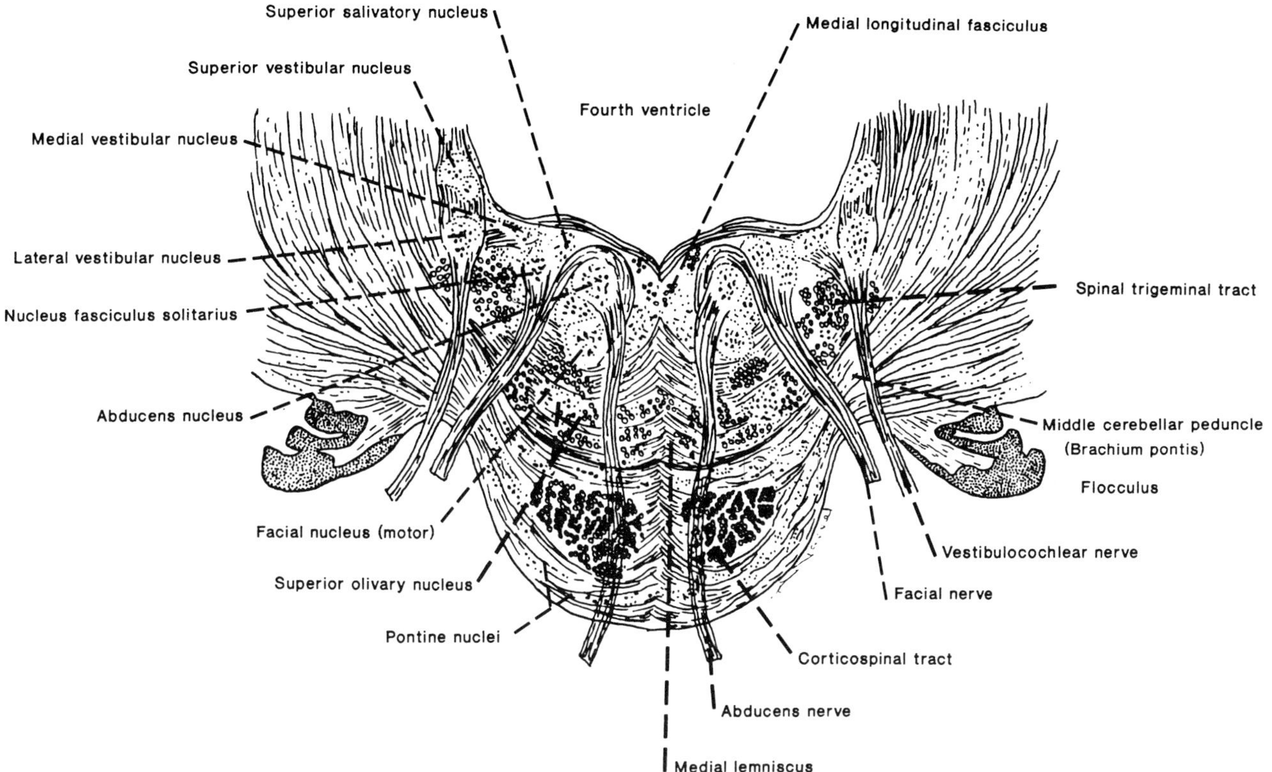

FIGURE 7–14 **Pons.** Cross section of the pons at the level of the abducens and the facial nerves. (Adapted from Ferner H (ed): Pernkopf Atlas der topographischen und angewandten Anatomie des Menchen, 3rd ed, vols 1 and 2. Baltimore-Munich, Urban & Schwarzenberg, 1987, p. 90.)

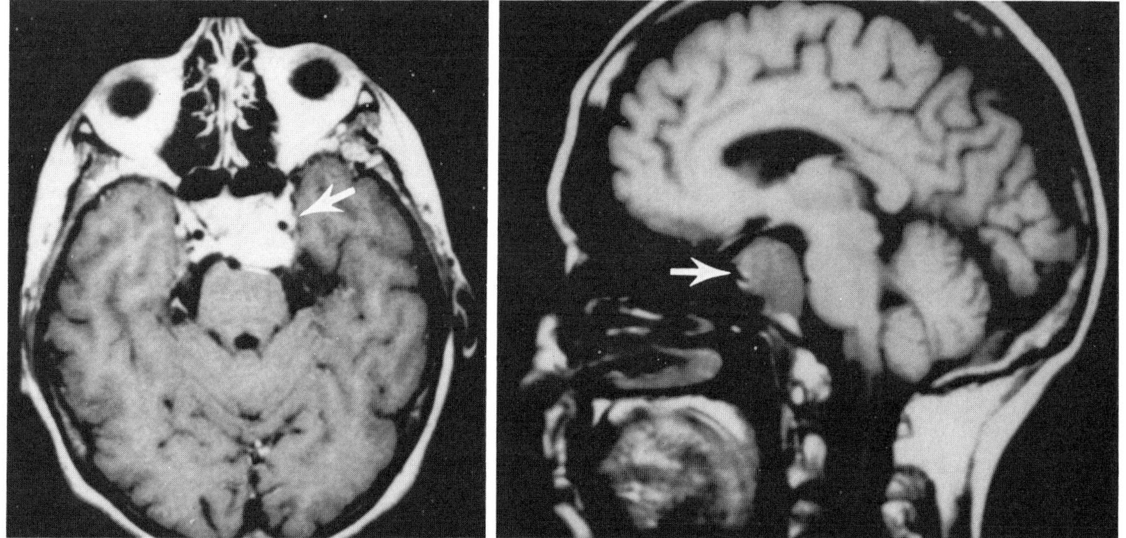

FIGURE 7–15 **Sixth nerve palsies.** Axial *(left)* and sagittal *(right)* MRI of the brain of a patient with bilateral sixth nerve palsies. A clivus chordoma *(arrows)* is demonstrated.

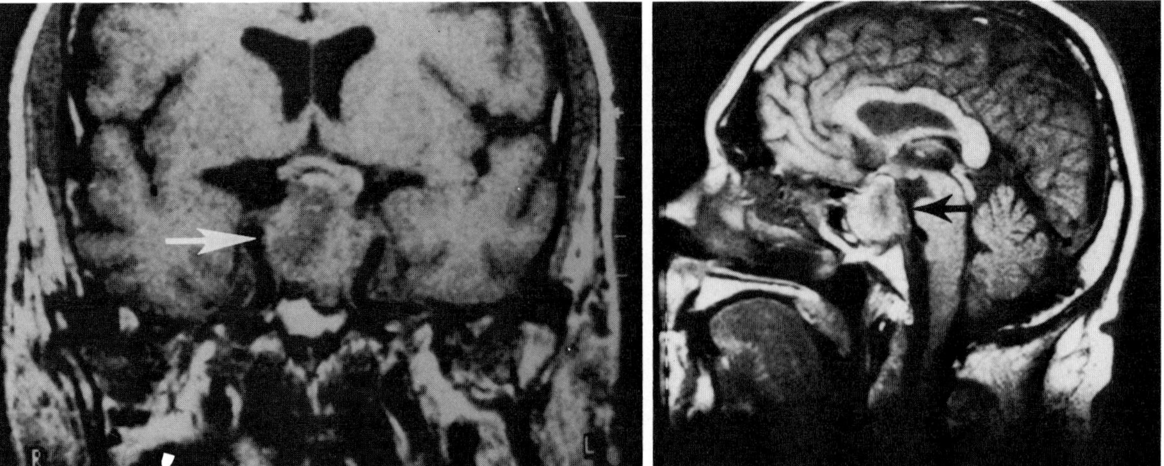

FIGURE 7–16 **Pituitary apoplexy.** Coronal *(left)* and sagittal *(right)* MRI of the brain of a patient with pituitary apoplexy. The patient presented with headache and a complete ptosis and ophthalmoplegia on the left. MRI revealed a large pituitary tumor with areas of inhomogeneous intensity that were suggestive of previous hemorrhage (*arrows*).

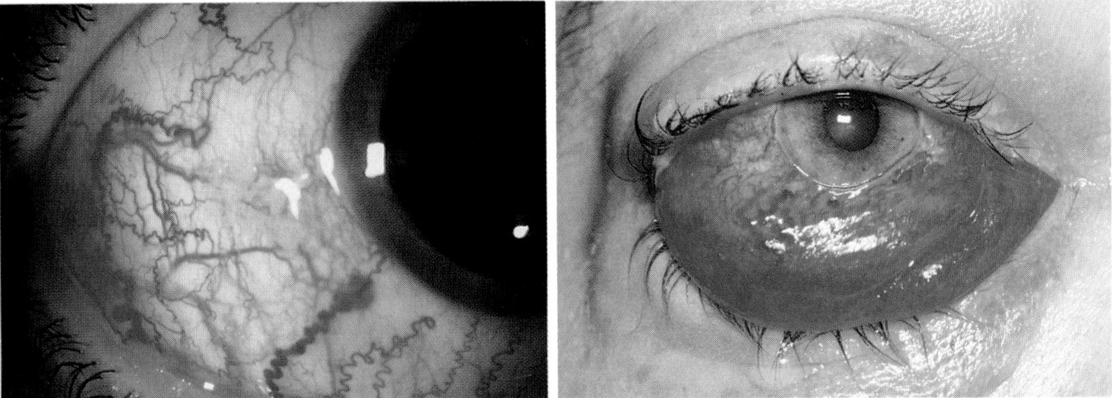

FIGURE 7–17 **Carotid cavernous fistulas.** Conjunctival appearance in patients with carotid-cavernous fistulas. The eye on the *left* illustrates the arterialization of the conjunctival vessels with the characteristic corkscrew appearance. The patient whose eye appears on the *right* had a traumatic fistula with resultant severe chemosis and proptosis.

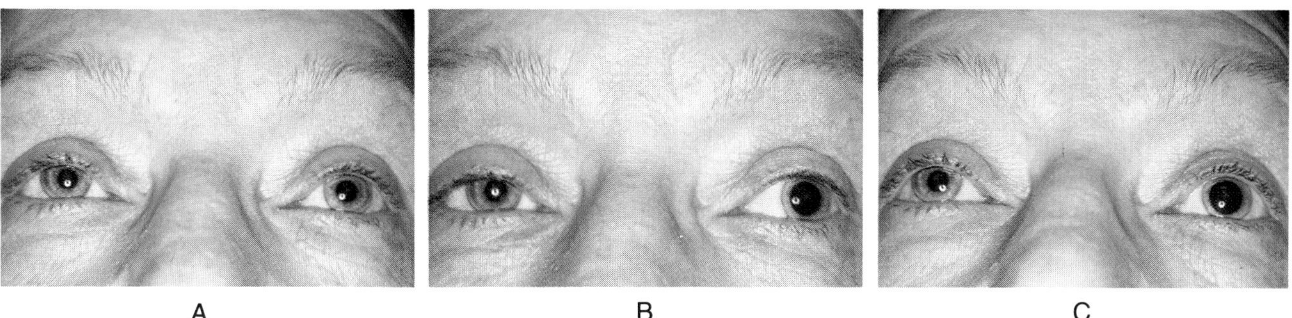

FIGURE 7–18 **Horner's syndrome.** An example of postganglionic Horner's syndrome. *A,* Right-sided Horner's syndrome. *B,* Only the left pupil dilates after cocaine 4 percent is instilled into both eyes. *C,* The left pupil dilates much better than the right pupil after OH-amphetamine 1 percent is instilled in both eyes.

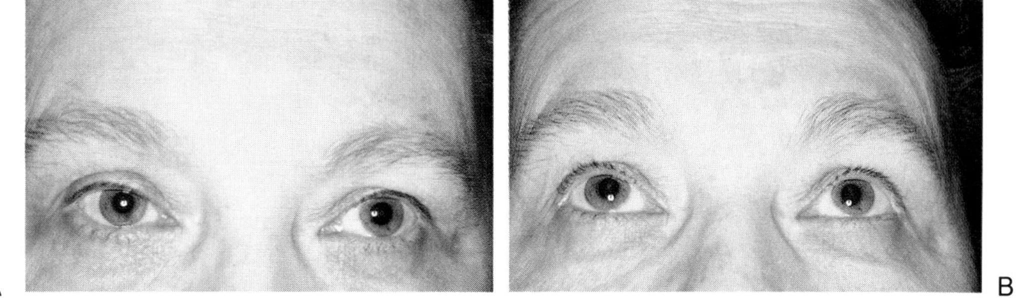

FIGURE 7–19 **Horner's pupil.** *A,* An example of a preganglionic Horner's pupil that appeared after chest surgery. *B,* Both pupils dilate after OH-amphetamine 1 percent is administered.

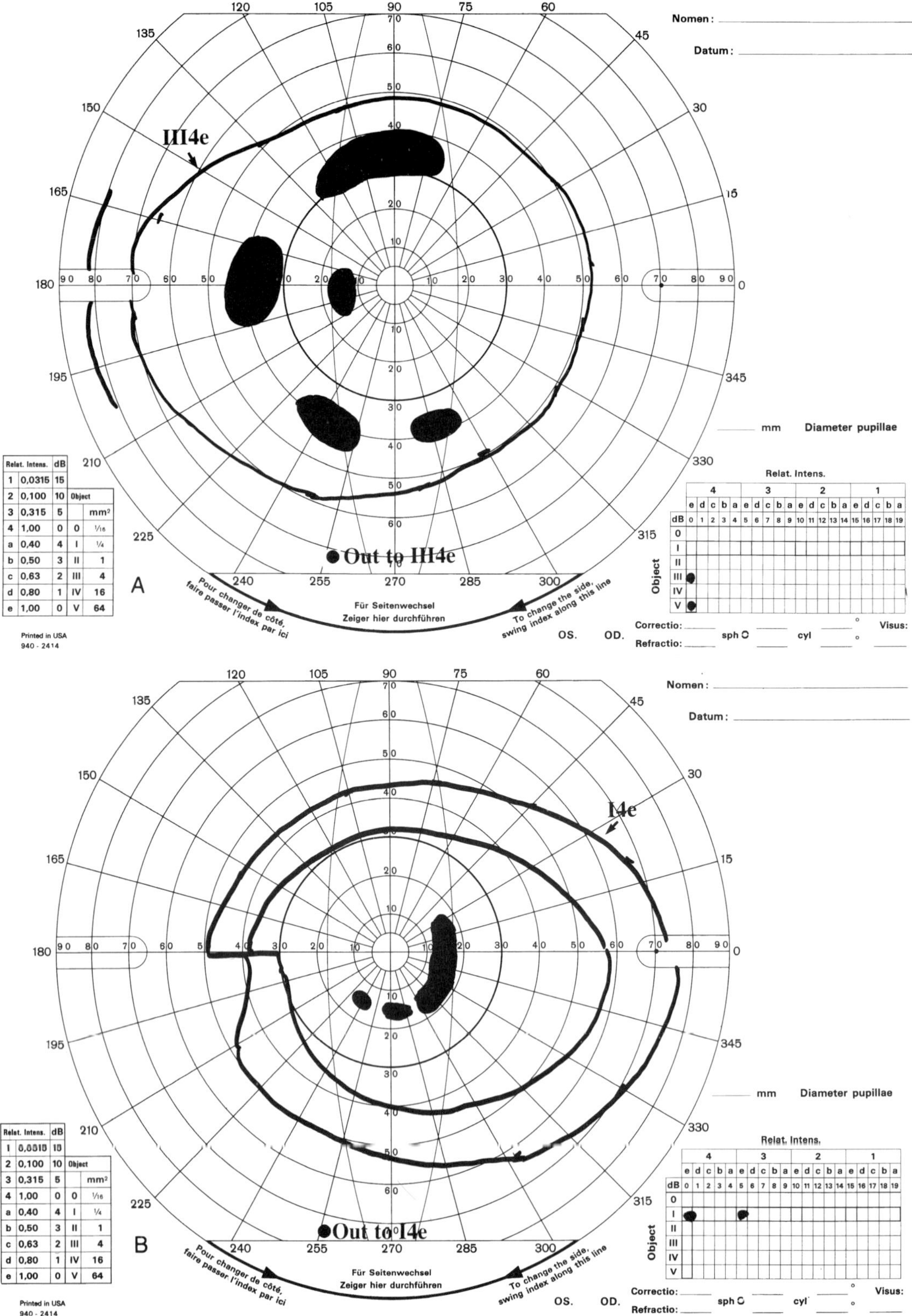

FIGURE 7–20 **Visual field defects in retinal disease.** Common patterns of visual field defects associated with disease of the retina (*A*) and optic nerve (*B*). *A*, Degenerative retinal disease often produces midperipheral scotomata that cross the vertical meridian. This field also shows generalized constriction. *B*, The visual field defects that respect the horizontal meridian are characteristic of optic nerve disease. The nasal step shown here has this characteristic. This field also shows nerve fiber bundle defects that are manifested by arcuate (Bjerrum's) scotomata and elongation of the blind spot.

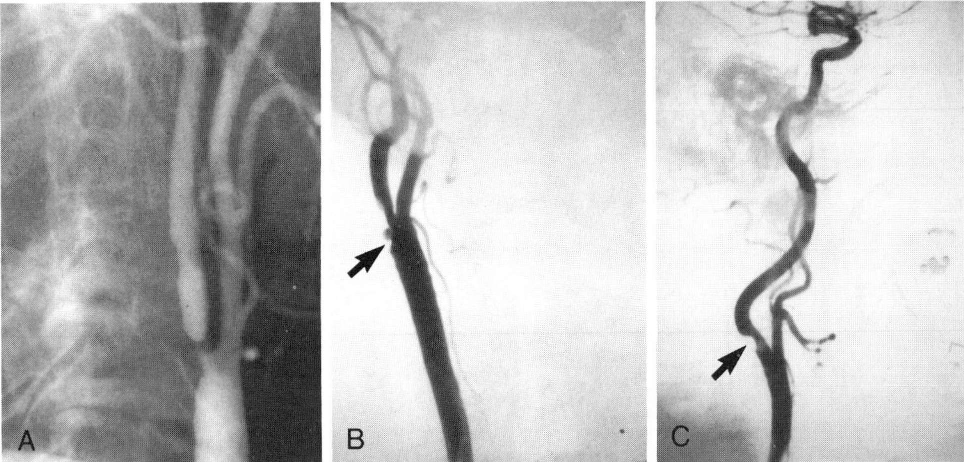

FIGURE 7–21 **Atherosclerotic disease.** Carotid artery angiograms showing classic features of atherosclerotic disease. *A,* Lumen of the internal carotid artery is markedly narrowed. *B,* An area of ulceration *(large arrow)* can be identified by the concave pooling of the angiographic dye. *C,* An atherosclerotic plaque *(small arrow)* protrudes into the lumen of the artery.

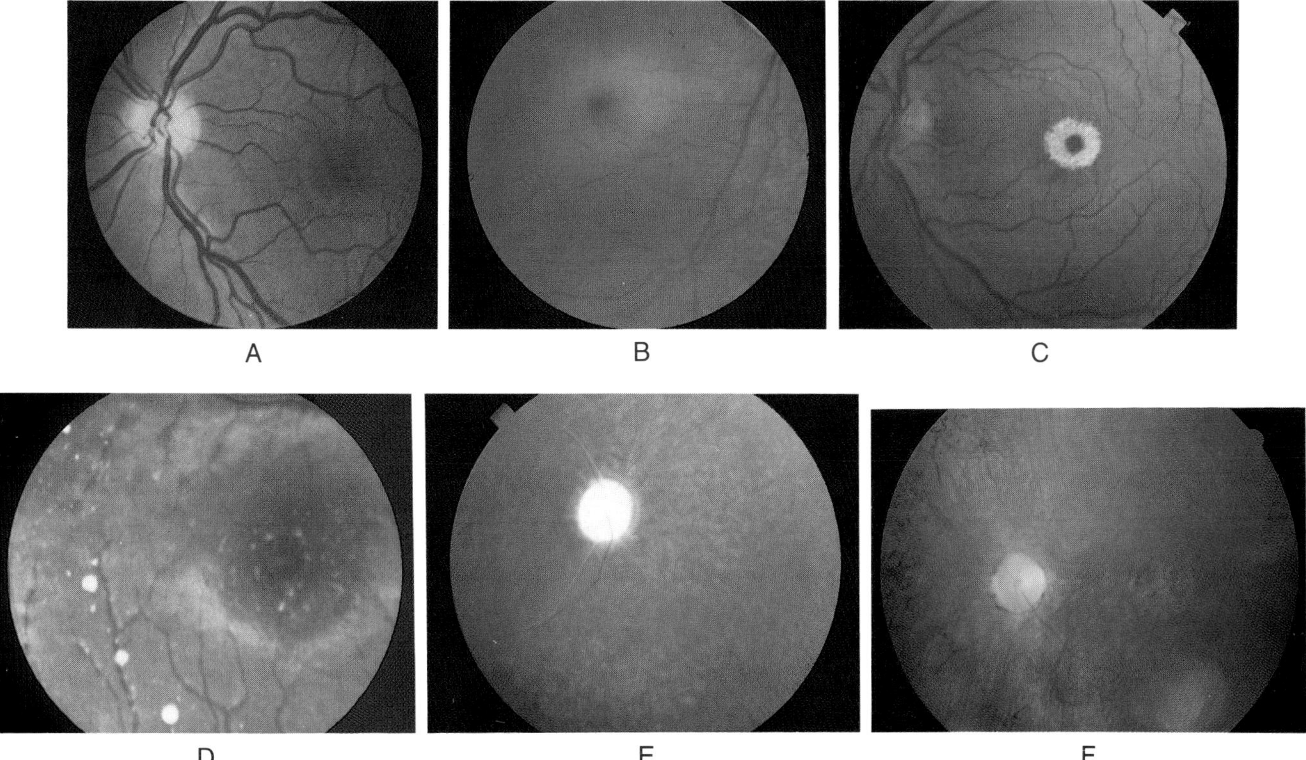

FIGURE 7–22 **Neurodegenerative diseases involving the retina.** Funduscopic features of some neurodegenerative diseases that involve the retina. Examples of three major categories of retinal pathology are shown. *A,* Marked atrophy of the optic nerve indicating the widespread loss of retinal ganglion cells in the Riley-Day syndrome. *B,* Cherry-red spot associated with Tay-Sachs disease, an example of deposition of storage material within the retina. The hexaminidase B enzyme defect results in abnormal accumulation of sphingolipids within neurons. *C,* White annulus ("macular halo") surrounding the fovea in Niemann-Pick disease. *D,* White spots in the retina in a patient with Niemann-Pick disease. *E,* Marked optic atrophy and thinning of retinal arterioles with alteration in retinal pigment in a patient with neuronal ceroid lipofuscinosis. *F,* Pigmentary degeneration of the retina (best seen near the nasal border of the photograph) in a patient with Laurence-Moon-Bardet-Biedl syndrome. Thinning of retinal arterioles and optic atrophy are also present. (*B* and *D,* Courtesy of Dr. David Cogan.)

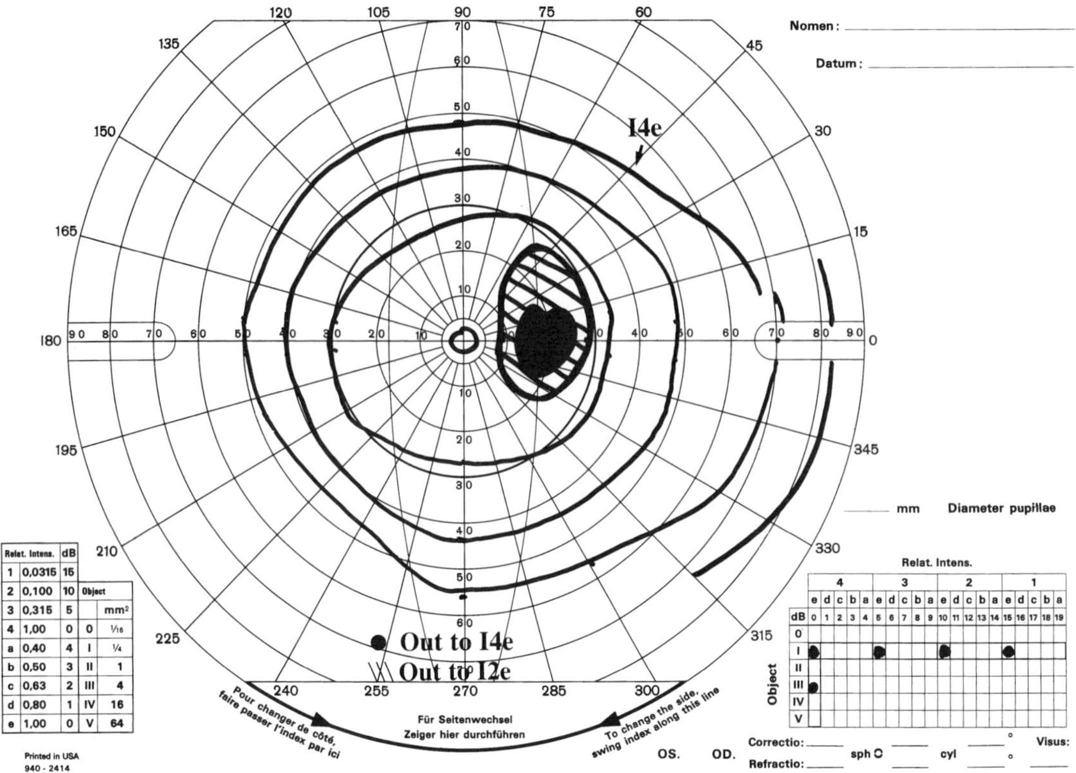

FIGURE 7–23 **Big blind spot syndrome.** Visual field of a patient with the big blind spot syndrome. A large and dense scotoma is present around the blind spot.

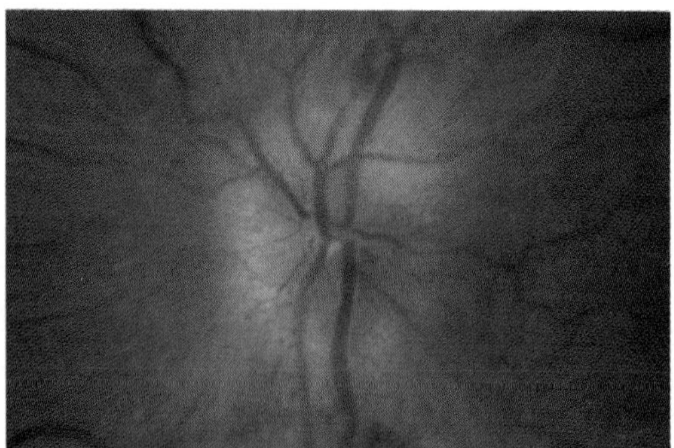

FIGURE 7–24 **Papilledema in pseudotumor cerebri.** Chronic and resolving optic disc edema in an obese 15-year-old boy with pseudotumor cerebri. The intracranial pressure of 520 mm of water at diagnosis was brought down to under 200 mm for 10 days, leading to the partial resolution of this previously fulminate disc edema.

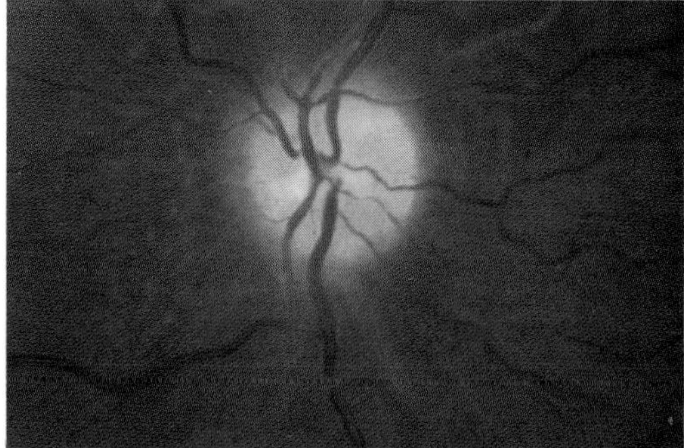

FIGURE 7–25 **Papilledema in pseudotumor cerebri.** The same optic disc depicted in Figure 7–24, 2 months after the intracranial pressure had been brought down to normal levels. The disc edema has resolved, leaving behind secondary optic atrophy. The changes associated with secondary optic atrophy can be fairly subtle. Despite the absence of severe disc pallor, visual restriction in this eye was extremely severe.

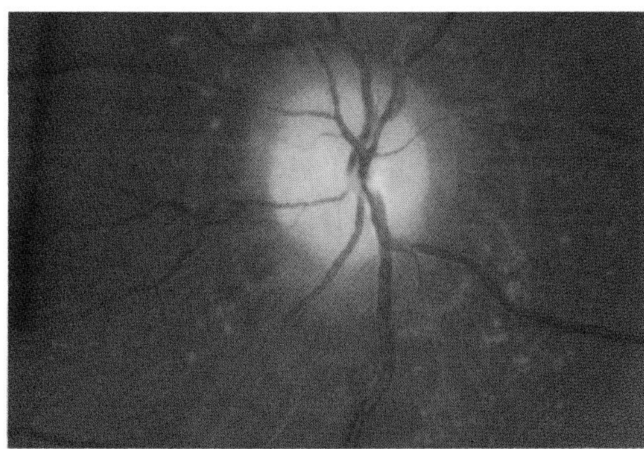

FIGURE 7–26 **Papilledema in pseudotumor cerebri.** The other eye of the patient described in Figure 7–24 is seen in a slightly more severe form. Note the hazy, grayish margins. The patient's visual field was reduced to a central 5-degree island.

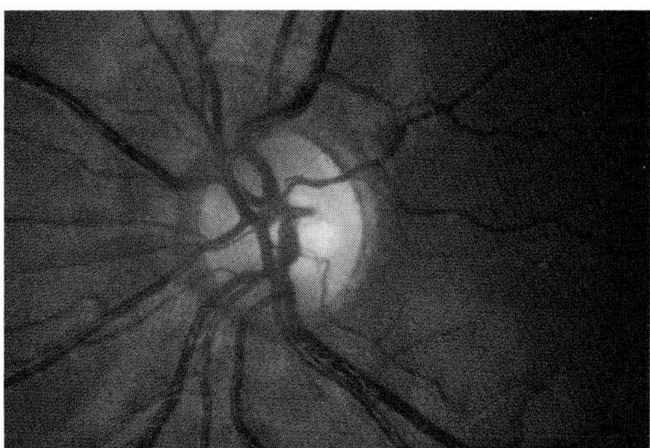

FIGURE 7–28 **Optic atrophy.** Left optic disc of patient in Figure 7–27. The patient had sustained complete transsection of the optic nerve at the level of the canal 22 days earlier. Note temporal pallor.

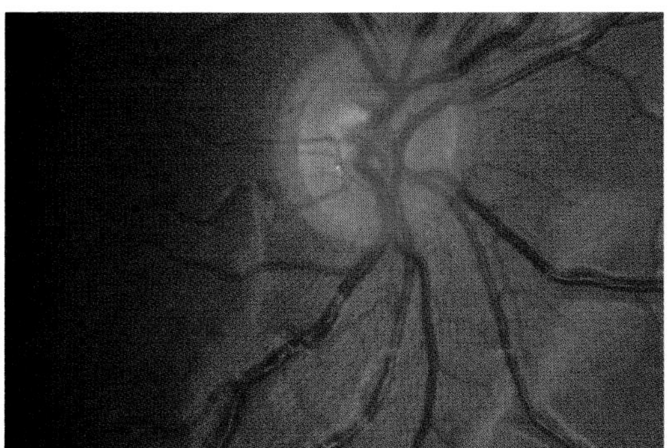

FIGURE 7–27 **Normal right optic disc.** Note pink coloration.

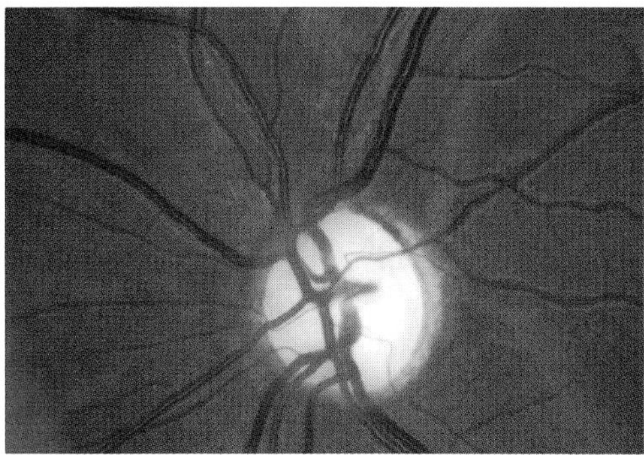

FIGURE 7–29 **Optic atrophy.** Same optic disc as in Figure 7–28. Note severe optic atrophy 2 months after traumatic transsection of the optic nerve.

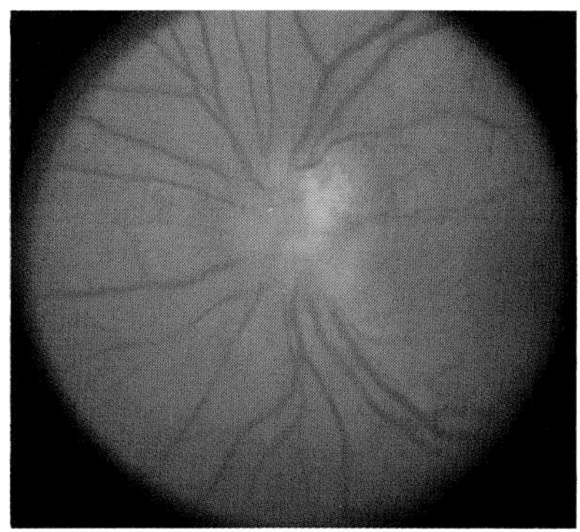

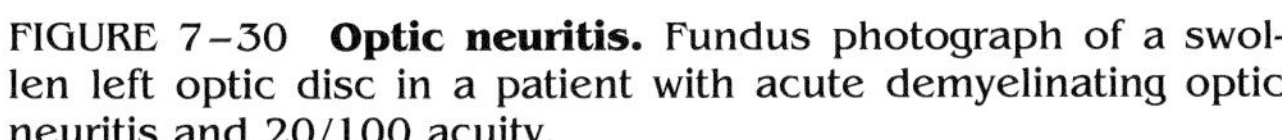

FIGURE 7–30 **Optic neuritis.** Fundus photograph of a swollen left optic disc in a patient with acute demyelinating optic neuritis and 20/100 acuity.

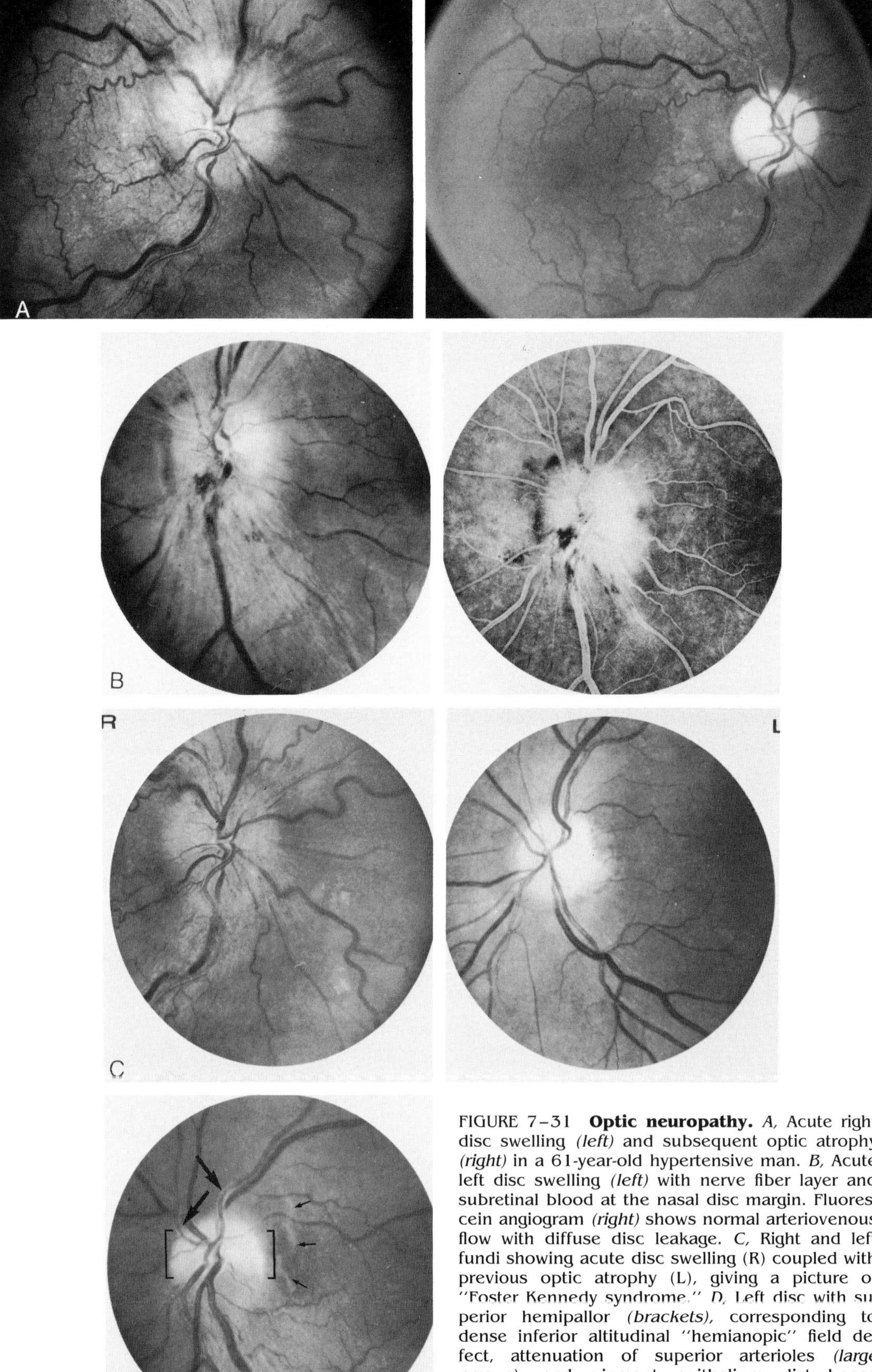

FIGURE 7–31 **Optic neuropathy.** *A,* Acute right disc swelling *(left)* and subsequent optic atrophy *(right)* in a 61-year-old hypertensive man. *B,* Acute left disc swelling *(left)* with nerve fiber layer and subretinal blood at the nasal disc margin. Fluorescein angiogram *(right)* shows normal arteriovenous flow with diffuse disc leakage. *C,* Right and left fundi showing acute disc swelling (R) coupled with previous optic atrophy (L), giving a picture of "Foster Kennedy syndrome." *D,* Left disc with superior hemipallor *(brackets),* corresponding to dense inferior altitudinal "hemianopic" field defect, attenuation of superior arterioles *(large arrows),* and pigment epithelium disturbance *(small arrows)* forming a "high-water line" as evidence of previous edema.

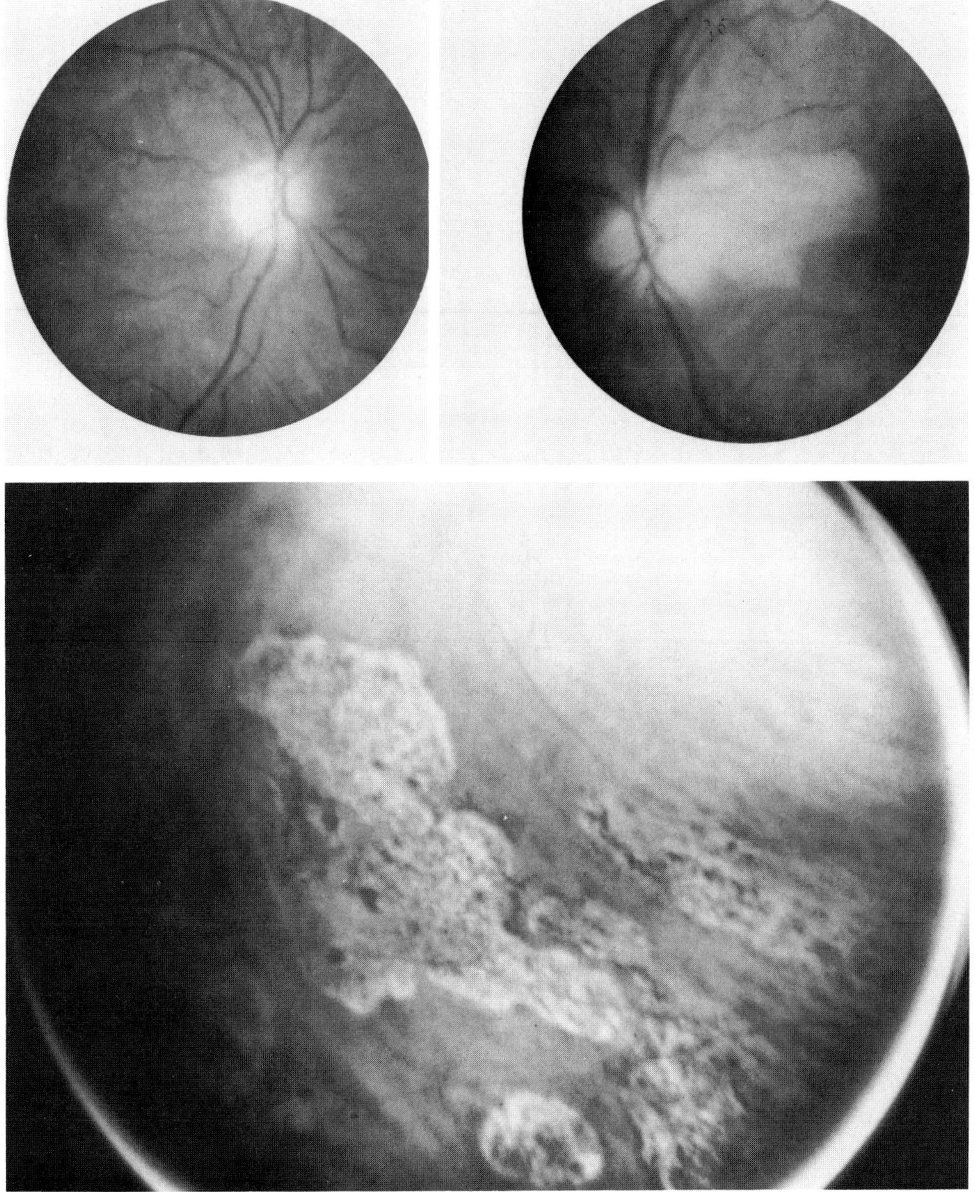

FIGURE 7-32 **Arteritic ischemic neuropathy.** *Top left,* Milky pale disc edema. *Top right,* Pale disc edema with infarction extending into the macular portion of the retina. *Bottom,* Choroidal infarcts.

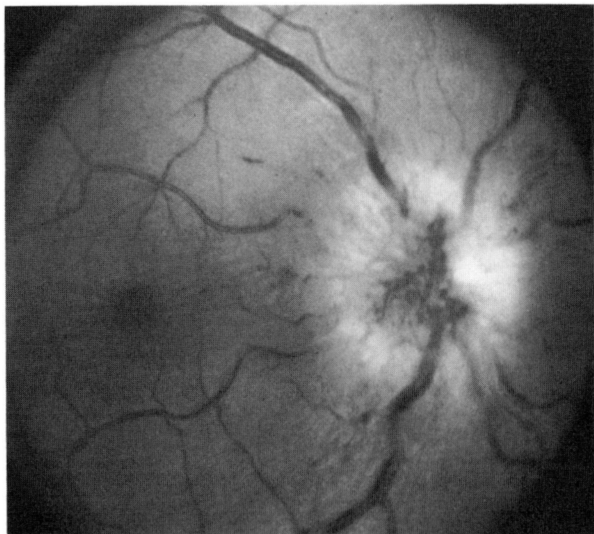

FIGURE 7–33 **Papillopathy in juvenile diabetes.** Note the florid capillary hyperemia on the disc surface and minimal background retinopathy. In this case, there is a small foveal edema cyst that reduced acuity.

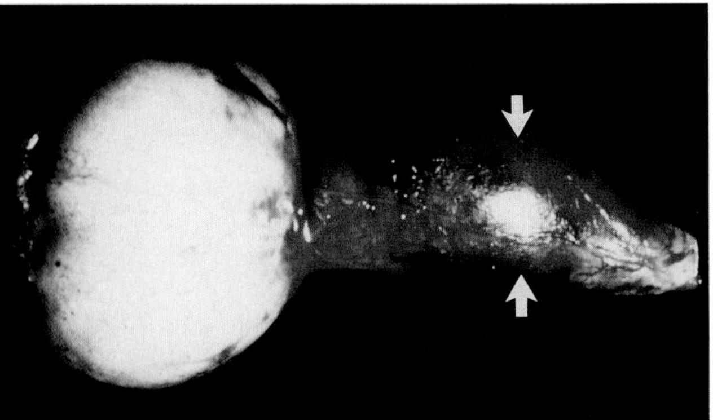

FIGURE 7–34 **Glioma.** En bloc resection of intraorbital optic nerve glioma demonstrates fusiform enlargement of the optic nerve without disruption of the dural sheath.

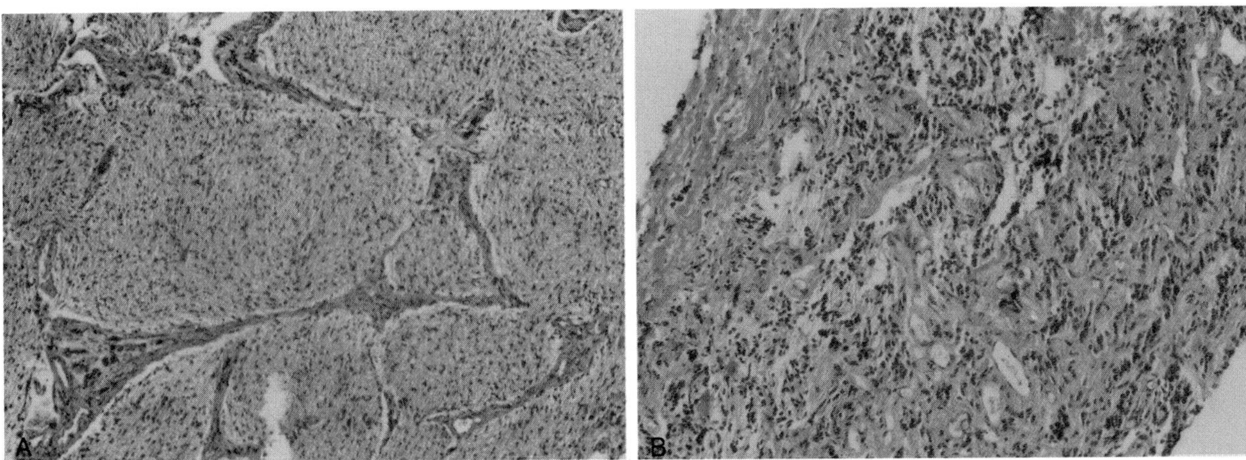

FIGURE 7–35 **Glioma.** Histopathologic appearance of resected optic nerve glioma confined by radiologic criteria to the orbit; however, the proximal end of the specimen just anterior to the chiasm demonstrated microscopic invasion with tumor. *A,* Benign astrocytic infiltration spreading between septa of the intraorbital optic nerve. *B,* Distal section of same tumor at higher magnification demonstrated marked cellular atypia, which is consistent with malignant degeneration.

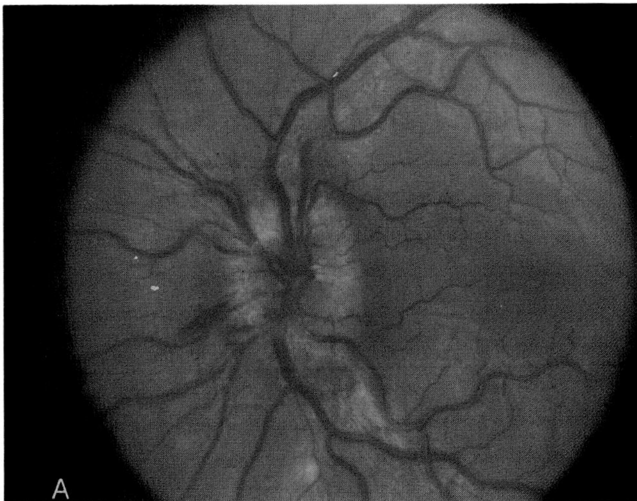

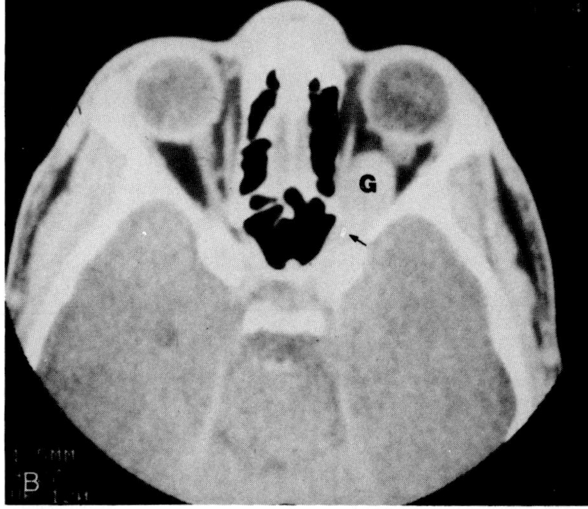

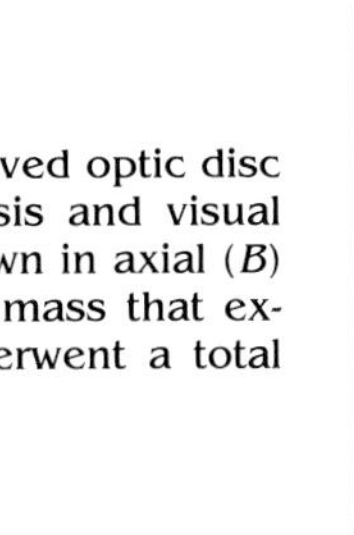

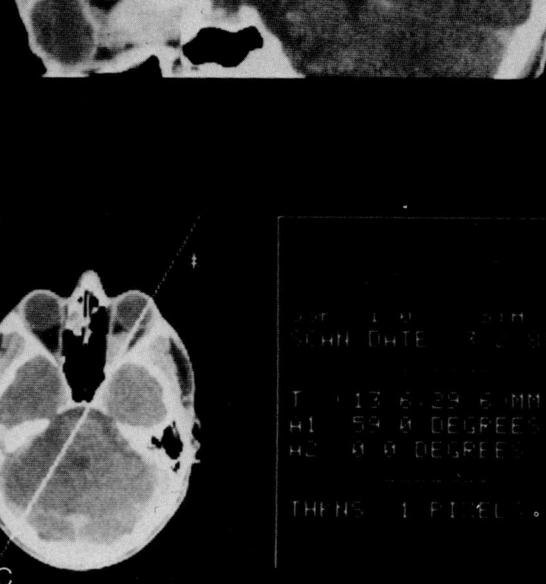

FIGURE 7-36 **Glioma.** Marked swelling of involved optic disc (*A*) in a 20-year-old man with unilateral proptosis and visual loss. Enhanced computed tomography scan, shown in axial (*B*) and sagittal (*C*) planes, demonstrates an apical mass that extends into optic canal *(arrow)*. The patient underwent a total surgical resection of the lesion.

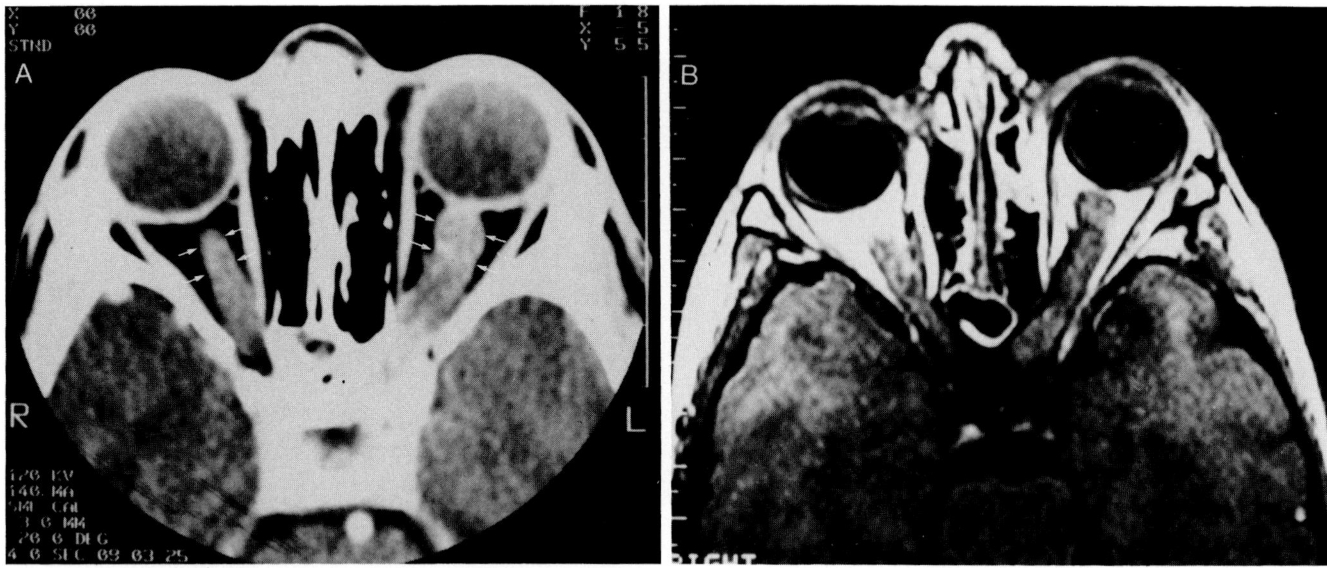

FIGURE 7–37 **Neurofibromatosis.** A 5-year-old boy with no stigmata or family history of neurofibromatosis presented with primary left-sided proptosis and visual loss. Both computed tomography scan (*A*) and T_1-weighted MRI scan (*B*) demonstrate bilateral asymmetric widening of the optic nerves *(arrows)* extending from the globe through the optic canals. Higher sections (not shown) document thickening of the optic chiasm as well. Optic disc, visual acuity, and visual fields in the right eye have remained normal over 3 years, without treatment.

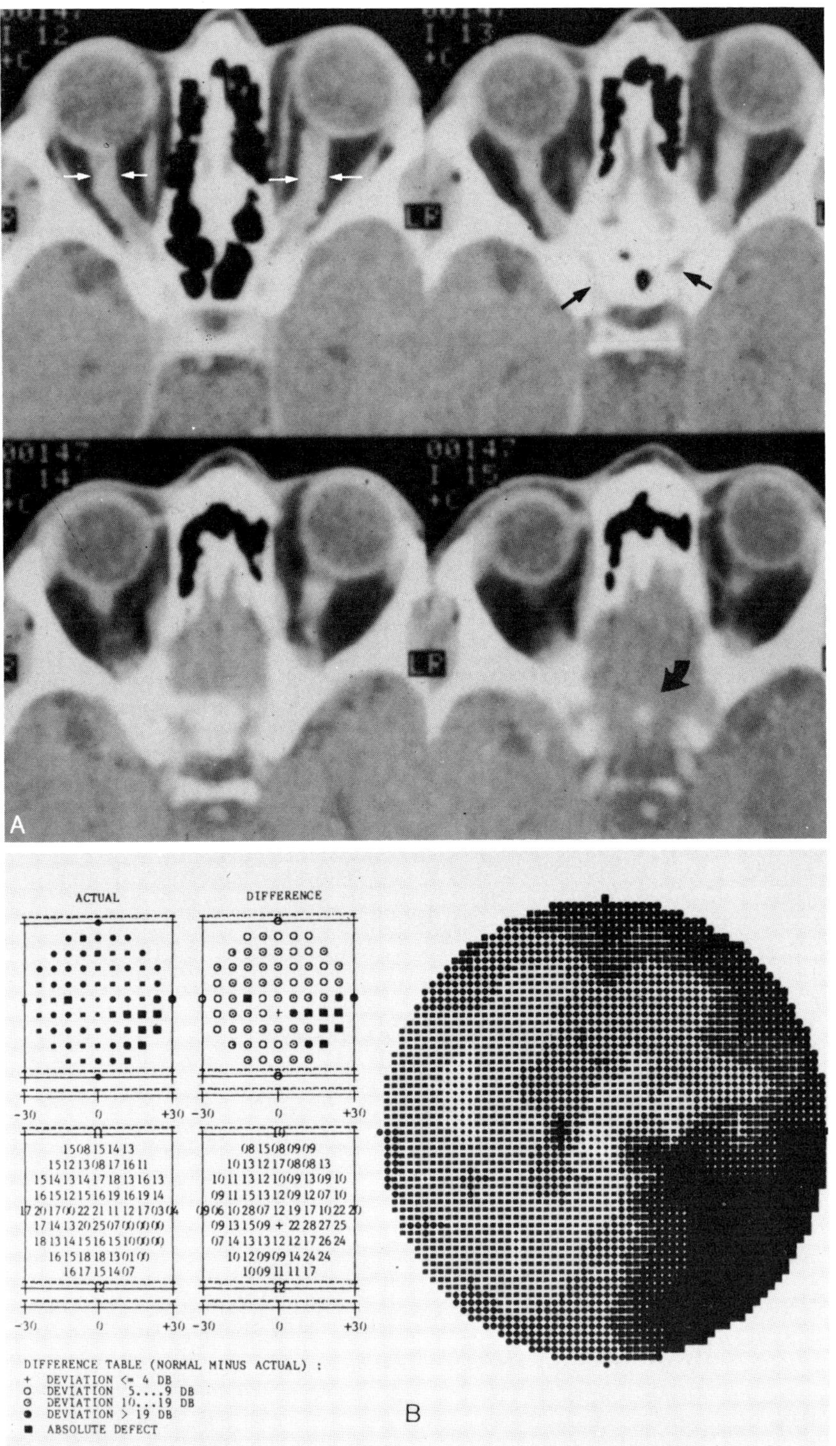

FIGURE 7–38 **Meningioma.** *A,* Four axial sections from the enhanced computed tomography scan from a middle-aged woman with progressive visual loss in the left eye show bilateral thickening of the optic nerve sheaths *(white arrows).* The low density of the optic nerve parenchyma results in the "railroad tracks" characteristic of meningiomas. The bony orbit canals do not appear widened *(black arrows),* and there is no evidence of a common intracranial component *(curved black arrow). B,* The 30-degree central field of the patient's left eye, demonstrating an inferior nasal step superimposed on overall field depression. The visual field of the patient's right eye was normal.

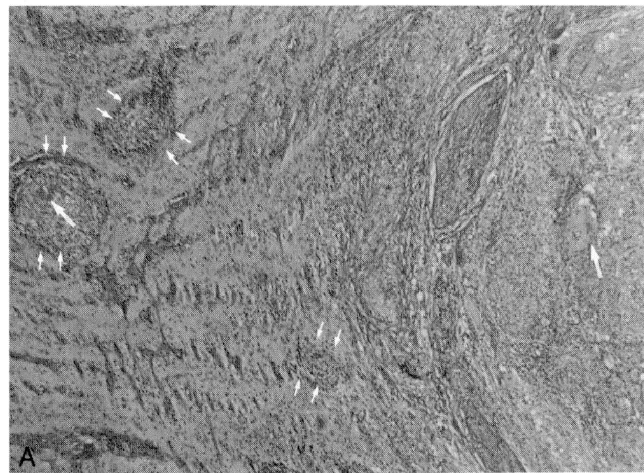

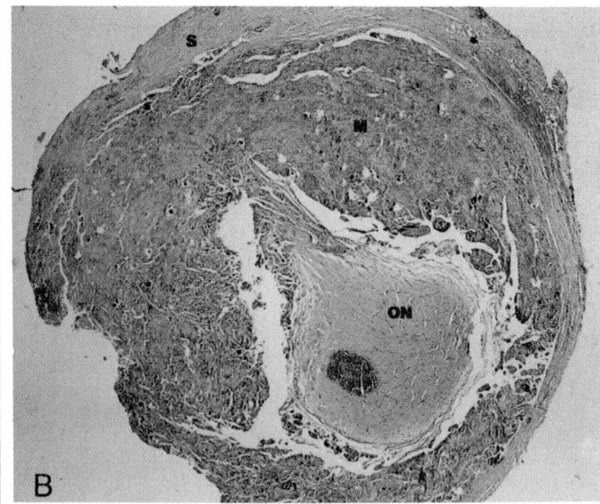

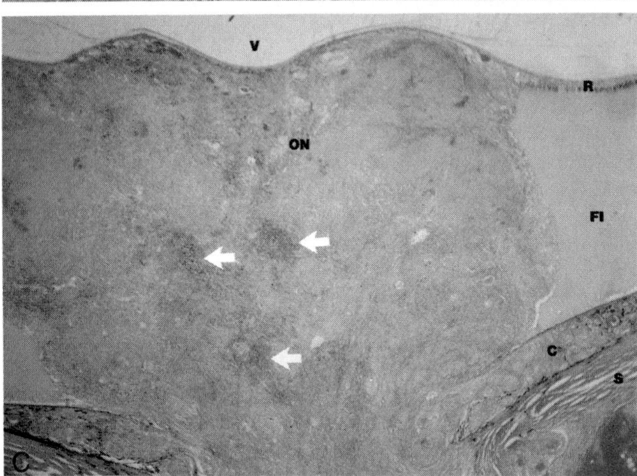

FIGURE 7–39 **Meningioma.** *A,* Meningioma may invade optic nerve substance, producing characteristic whorls *(small arrows)* and psammoma bodies *(large arrows)*. *B,* Meningioma (M) may also expand between the optic nerve sheath (S) and the optic nerve (ON) as a circumferential growth. *C,* In some cases, elevation of the optic disc (ON) may be caused by direct infiltration of the meningioma. In this case, whorls of tumor cells with psammoma bodies *(arrows)* can be seen producing marked expansion of the optic nerve head into the vitreous cavity (V). There is juxtapapillary detachment of the sensory retina (R) and accumulation of subretinal fluid (Fl). Even the juxtapapillary choroid (C) is slightly infiltrated by meningioma.

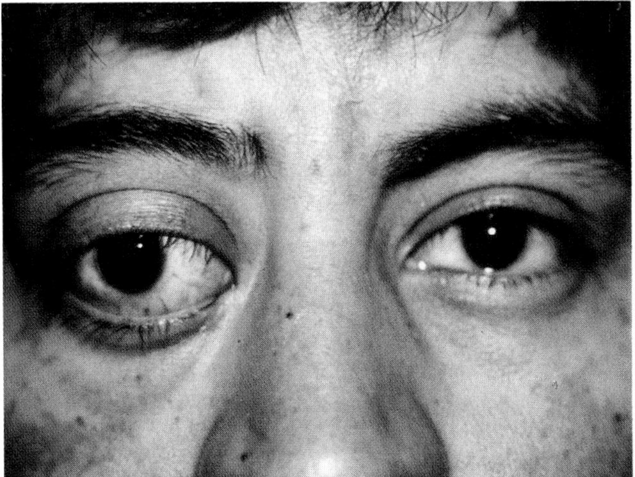

FIGURE 7–40 **Meningioma.** A patient with optic nerve meningioma and proptosis of the right eye.

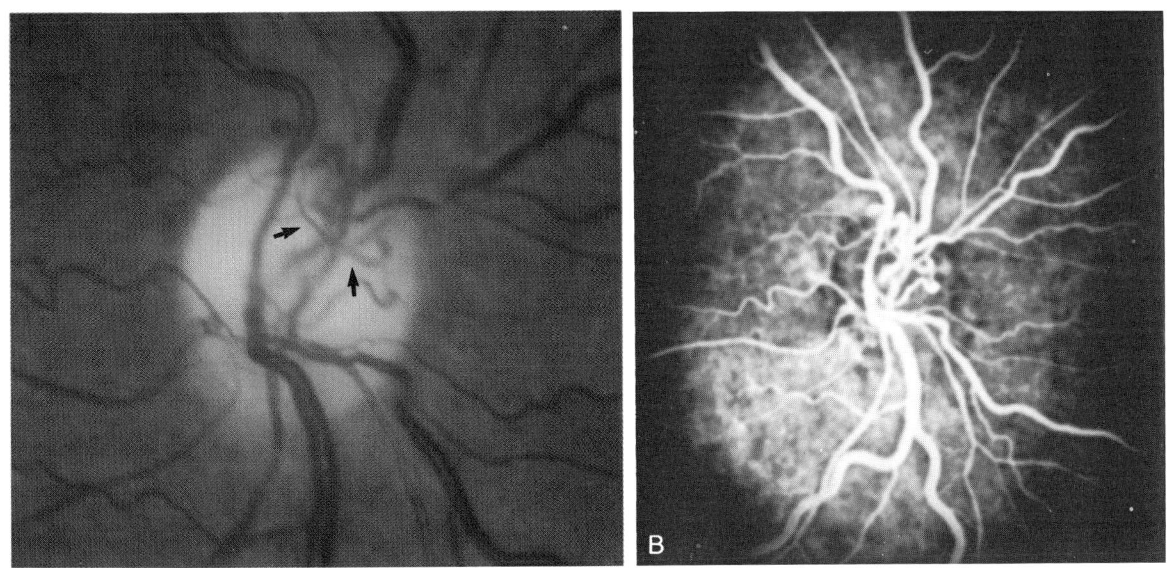

FIGURE 7–41 **Meningioma.** Disc photograph (*A*) and fluorescein angiogram (*B*) from a patient with optic nerve meningioma demonstrates pallor, blurred disc margins, and multiple optociliary shunt vessels *(arrows)*.

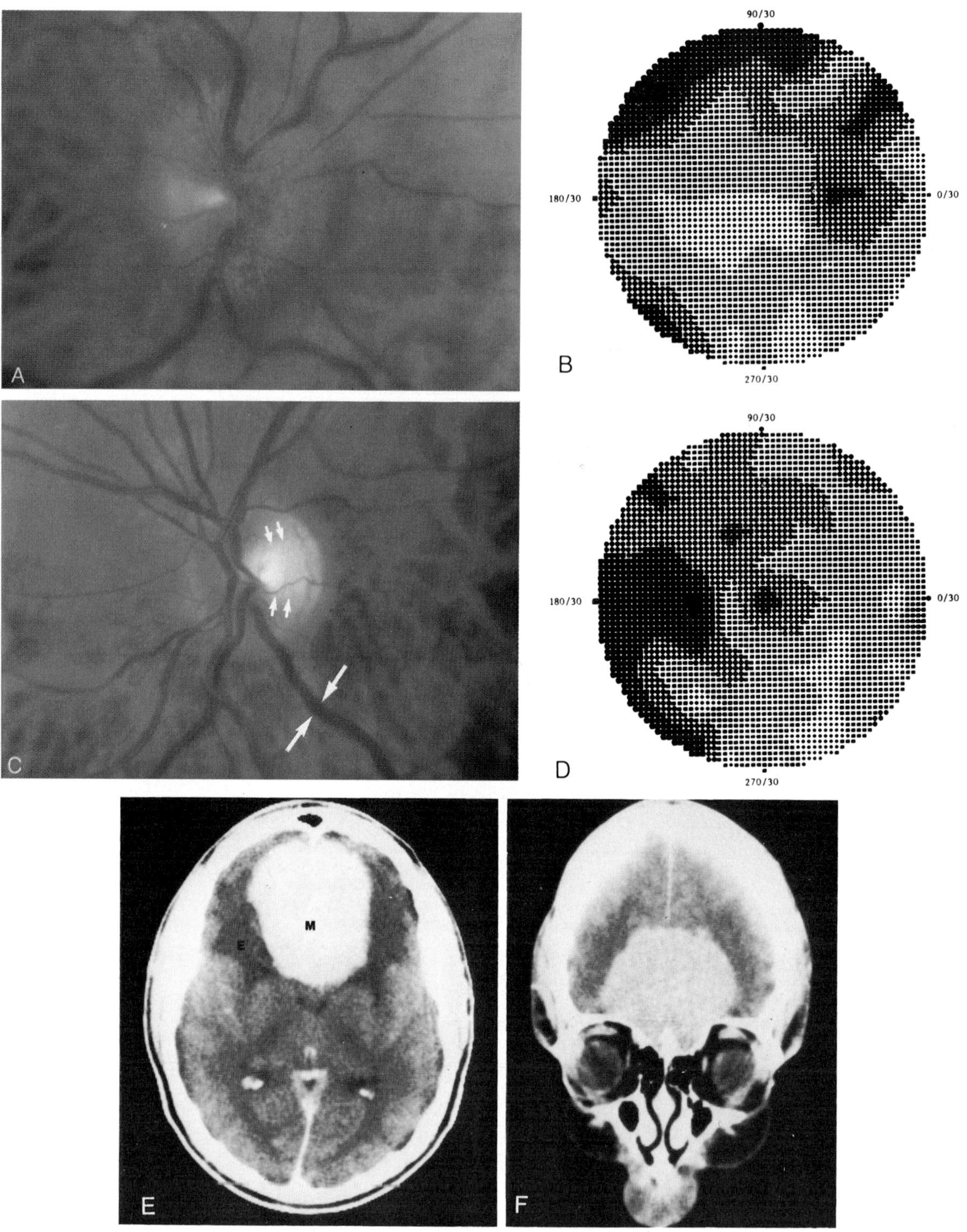

FIGURE 7–42 **Foster Kennedy syndrome.** A middle-aged man with a 5-year history of anosmia and mild alteration of personality complained of decreased vision in the left eye. On ophthalmoscopy of the right eye (*A*), the optic disc was edematous and there was dilatation of the retinal veins. Automated perimetry of the right eye (*B*) documented an enlarged blind spot and a possible early superior arcuate field defect. On ophthalmoscopy of the left eye (*C*), the optic disc was mildly blurred nasally and showed marked temporal pallor *(small arrows)*. Dilated veins are apparent *(large arrows)* even in the absence of obvious disc edema. Automated perimetry of the left eye (*D*) documented an enlarged blind spot, a central scotoma, and superior field depression. A large subfrontal mass (M) with surrounding edema (E) was noted on enhanced axial computed tomography scan (*E*). Coronal computed tomography scan (*F*) shows the involvement extending to the olfactory groove. Sections obtained more posteriorly (not shown) suggested involvement of the prechiasmal portion of the optic nerves, especially on the left side. Histologic appearance of the tumor was typical of meningioma. Anosmia, unilateral optic nerve swelling, and contralateral optic atrophy caused by subfrontal masses are components of the Foster Kennedy syndrome. (From Jarus GD, Feldon SE: Clinical and computed tomographic findings in the Foster Kennedy syndrome. Am J Ophthalmol 93:317–322, 1982. Published with permission from the American Journal of Ophthalmology. Copyright by The Ophthalmic Publishing Company.)

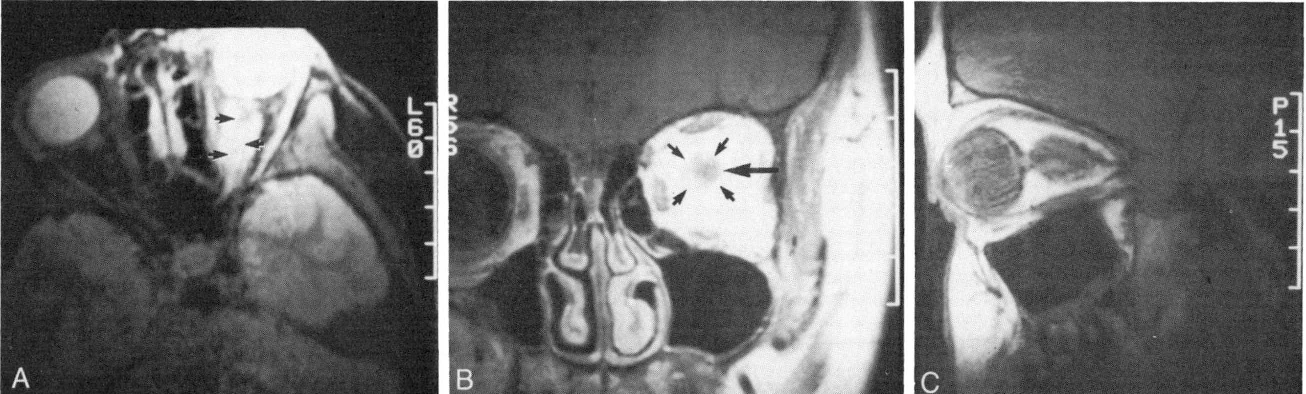

FIGURE 7–43 **Meningioma.** MRI scan from an 11-year-old girl with biopsy-proven unilateral optic nerve meningioma. Axial scan (*A*) using inversion recovery technique demonstrates the nerve (*arrows*) traversing through the tumor. T_1-weighted coronal scan (*B*) shows the tumor (*small arrows*) to be of different intensity from the optic nerve substance (*large arrow*). T_1-weighted sagittal scan (*C*) documents typical fusiform thickening of the optic nerve.

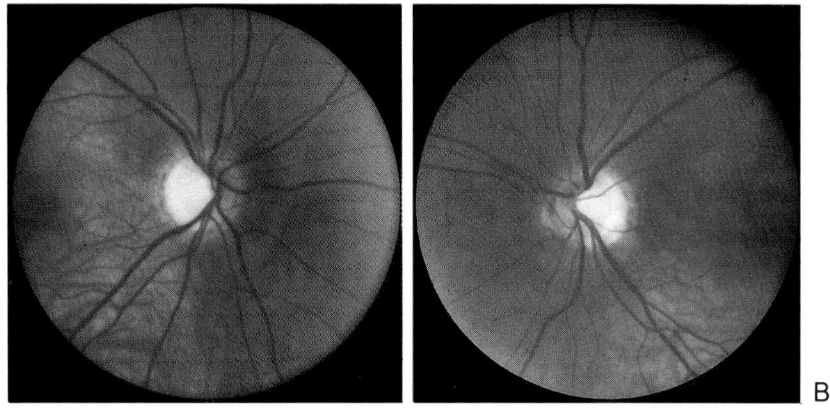

FIGURE 7–44 **Optic atrophy.** Typical appearance of optic nerve pallor affecting the temporal aspect of disc with associated temporal excavation. *A,* O.D. *B,* O.S.

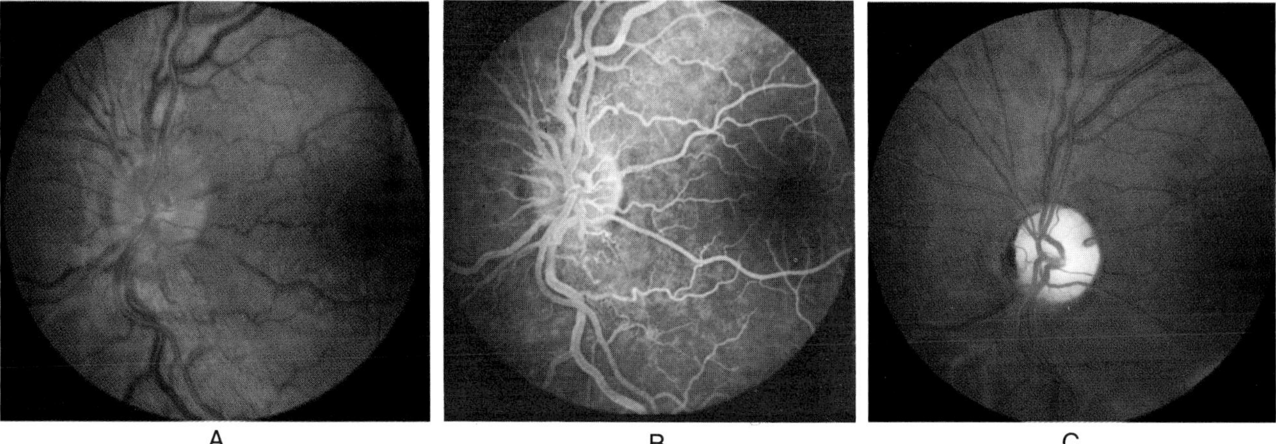

FIGURE 7–45 **Leber's optic neuropathy.** *A,* Typical appearance of optic nerve head during acute phase of Leber's optic neuropathy. Disc is edematous and hyperemic with circumpapillary telangiectatic microangiopathy characterized by prominent vascular tortuosity of vessels on and just off the surface of the disc. *B,* Fluorescein angiogram in the same patient during acute phase, demonstrating fine arteriovenous shuntlike vessels within peripapillary retina and absence of leakage from the disc itself despite presence of disc edema. *C,* Late atrophic phase of same nerve head, demonstrating loss of many of the previously visible telangiectatic vessels and diffuse pallor with nerve fiber layer loss. (Courtesy of Eeva Nikoskelainen, M.D.)

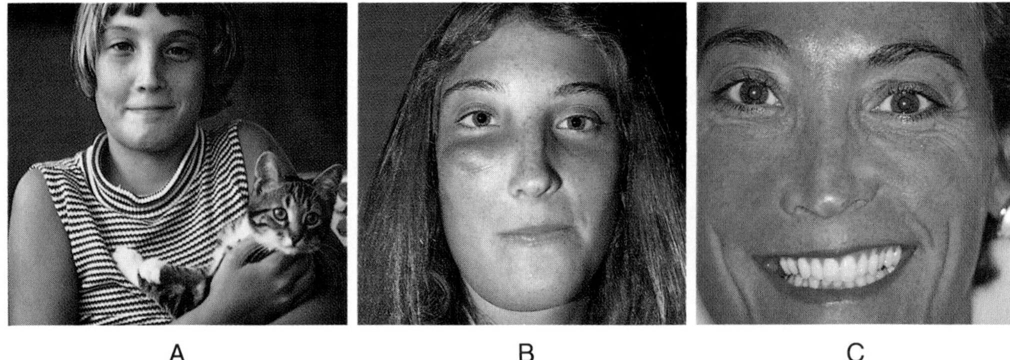

FIGURE 7–46 **Progressive fibrous dysplasia.** Progressive fibrous dysplasia at ages 12 (with cat, "Mittens"), 19, and 29 years. Facial asymmetry was first noted at approximately 7 years of age.

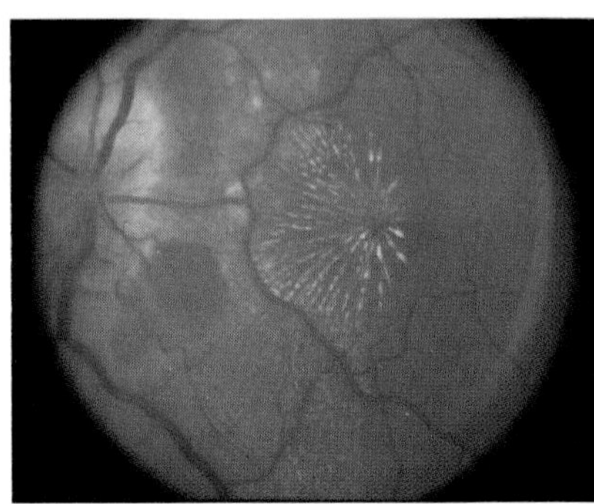

FIGURE 7–47 **Neuroretinopathy.** Characteristic fundus appearance in neuroretinitis.

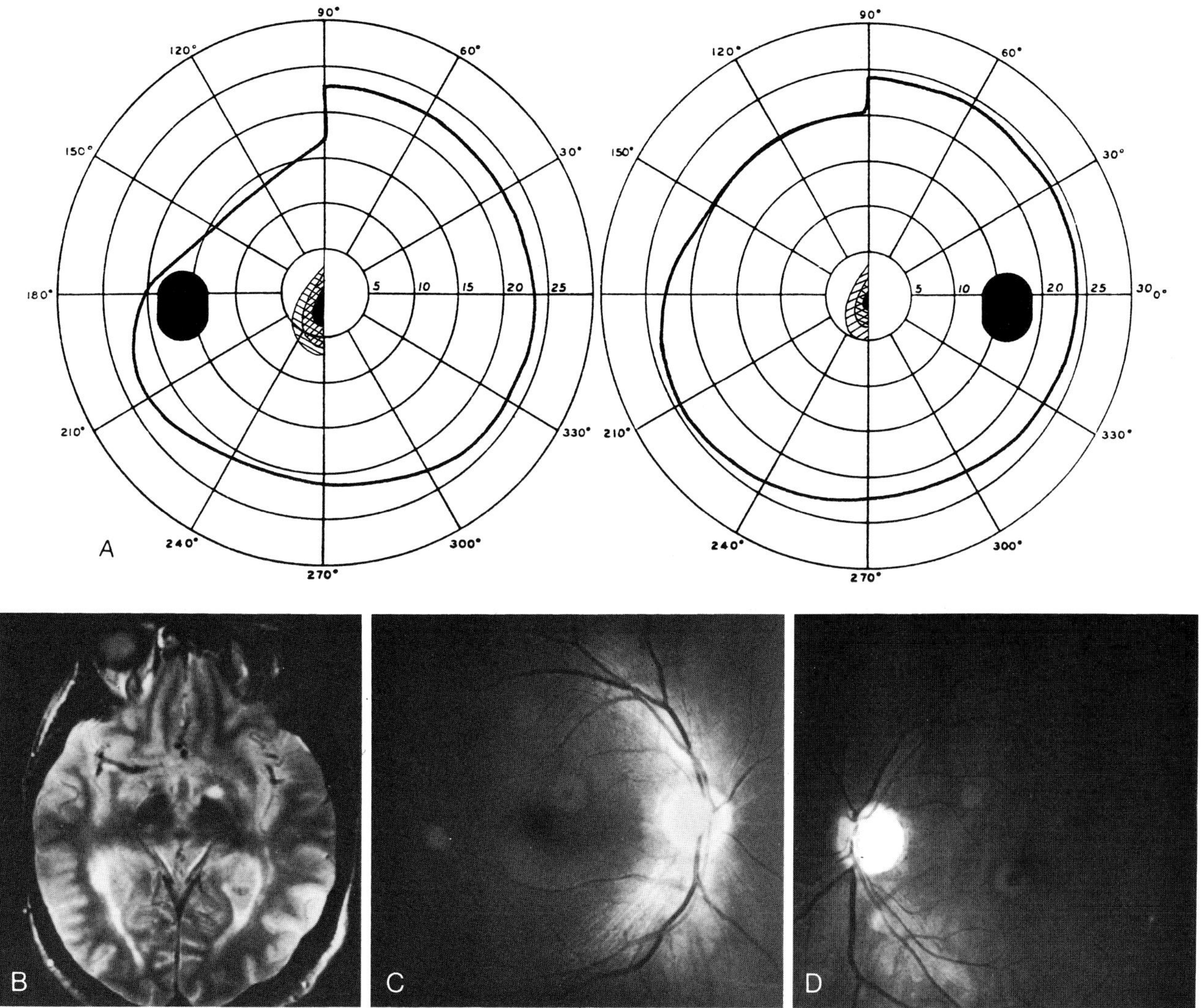

FIGURE 7–48 **Retrochiasmal lesions.** *A,* Incongruous, left, hemianopic scotomas that split fixation, owing to demyelinating lesion of the contralateral tract shown on MRI (*B*). *C* and *D,* Red-free nerve fiber–layer photograph of a patient with a complete left hemianopia due to an optic tract lesion. The contralateral eye (*C*) shows drop-out of nerve fibers temporal and nasal to the optic disc with preservation of the superior and inferior nerve fibers. The nerve fiber layer in the left eye (*D*) is diffusely affected.

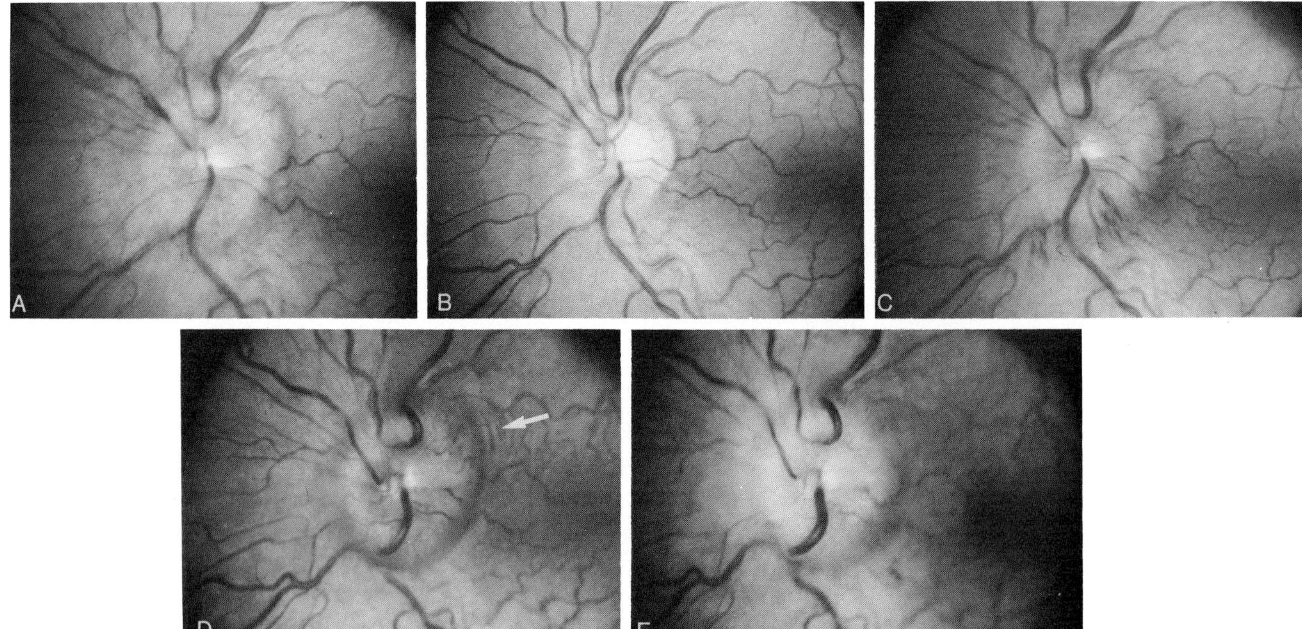

FIGURE 7–49 **Pseudotumor cerebri.** *A,* Obese 25-year-old woman with headaches and transient visual obscurations. Intracranial pressure never measured less than 550 mm H_2O. Patient was treated with dexamethasone and acetazolamide with rapid resolution of headache and papilledema. *B,* Enlarged cup, preserved neuroretinal rim, and slight residual peripapillary swelling. *C,* With the patient off the steroids and acetazolamide a month, papilledema returns. Steroids were restarted but not acetazolamide because of gastrointestinal upset. *D,* Intraocular pressure rises to 26 to 28 mmHg; on repeated examination, visual field begins to constrict inferiorly and superiorly. The visual field was previously full. Peripapillary folds, which may be observed in instances of chronic swelling of the optic nerve head, are subtly visible. *E,* Within 2 months of restarting treatment, disc pallor denotes ischemic and compressive changes. Visual field is strikingly and permanently constricted.

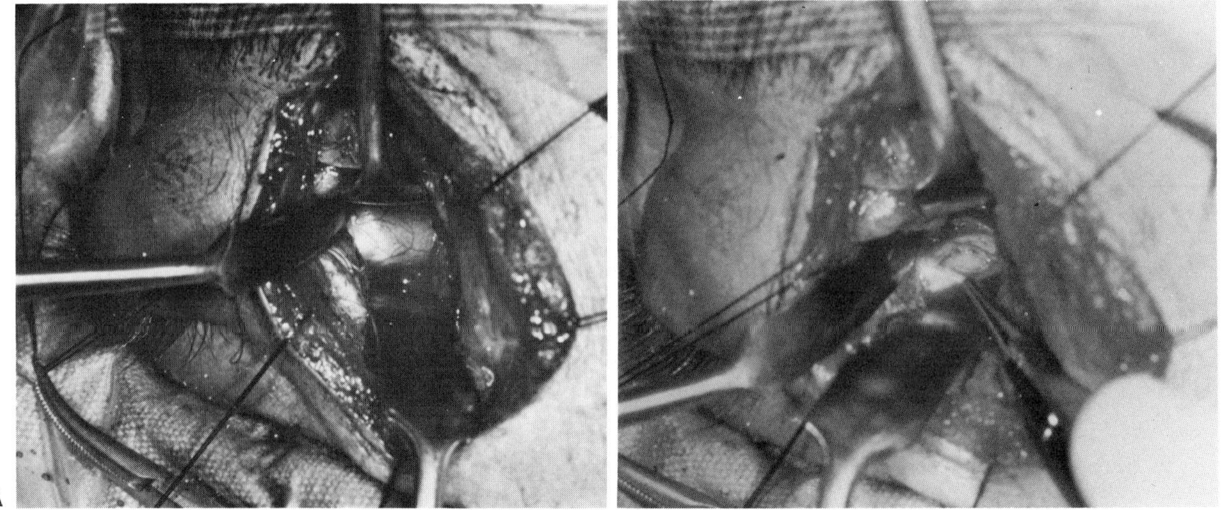

FIGURE 7–50 **Pseudotumor cerebri.** *A,* Optic nerve sheath visualized through a lateral orbitotomy. Before fenestration. *B,* Optic nerve sheath after 5 × 5-mm excision of dura and arachnoid. (Courtesy of Jeff Nerad, M.D.)

SECTION 8

Pediatric Ophthalmology

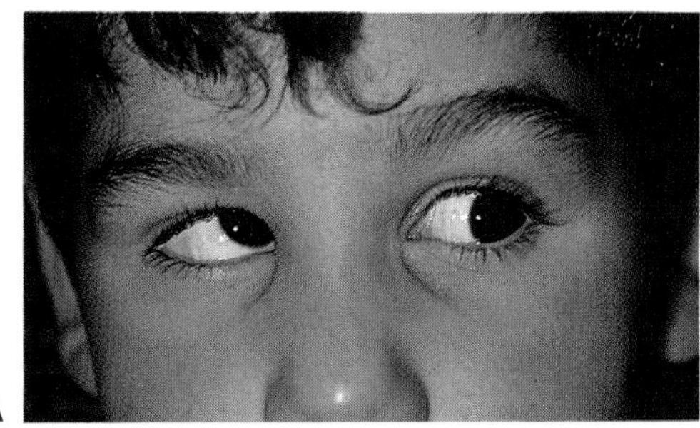

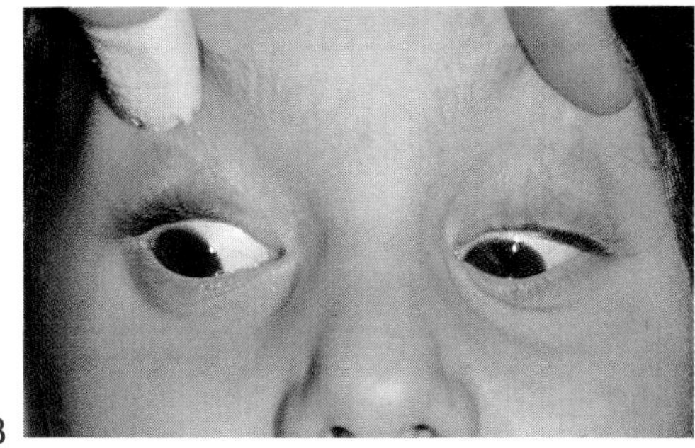

FIGURE 8–1 **Childhood strabismus.** *A,* Child with overaction of the right inferior oblique muscle, which causes an upward drift in adduction. *B,* Child with overaction of the left superior oblique muscle, which causes downward deviation in adduction.

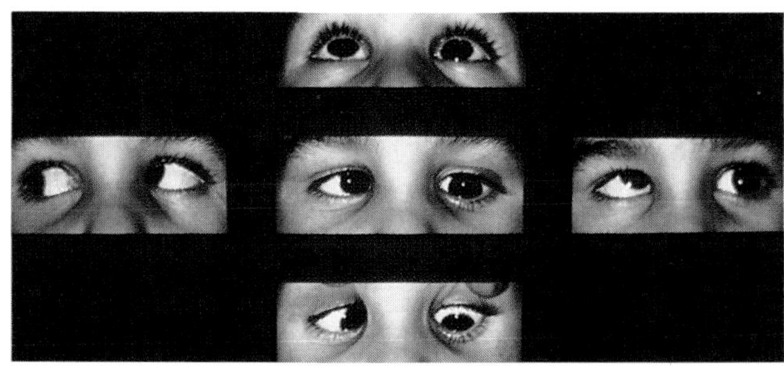

FIGURE 8–2 **Patient with V-pattern esotropia.** The deviation is more pronounced in downgaze than in upgaze. On lateral gaze, overaction of both inferior oblique muscles is evident.

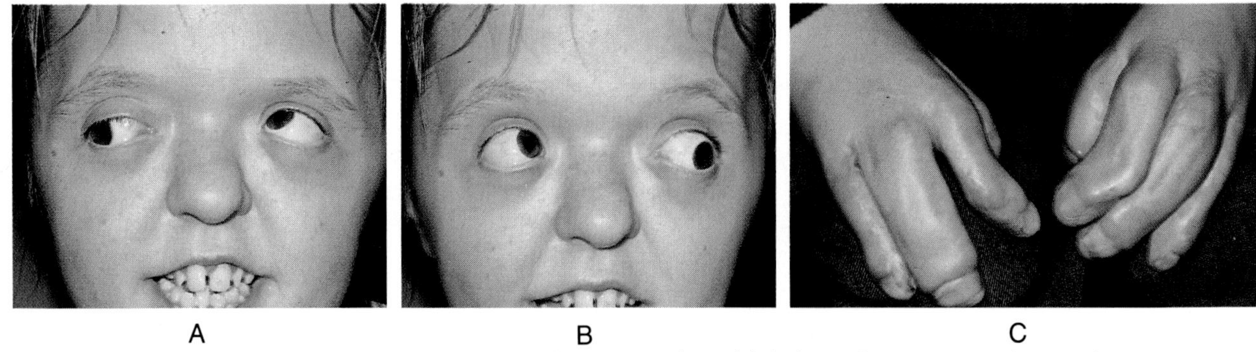

FIGURE 8–3 **Apert's syndrome.** *A* and *B,* Overaction of inferior oblique muscles in a patient with Apert's syndrome, a variety of craniofacial dysostosis that is associated with syndactyly *(C).*

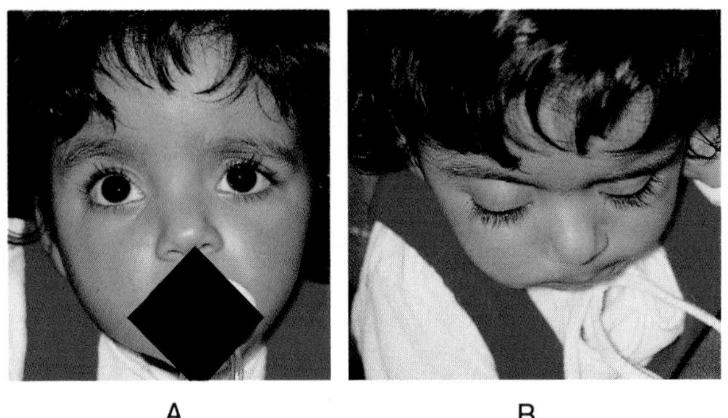

FIGURE 8–4 **Coronal synostosis.** *A,* Right hyperopia in a patient with right coronal synostosis. *B,* View of the same patient from above, showing flattening of the right superior orbital rim and frontal bone.

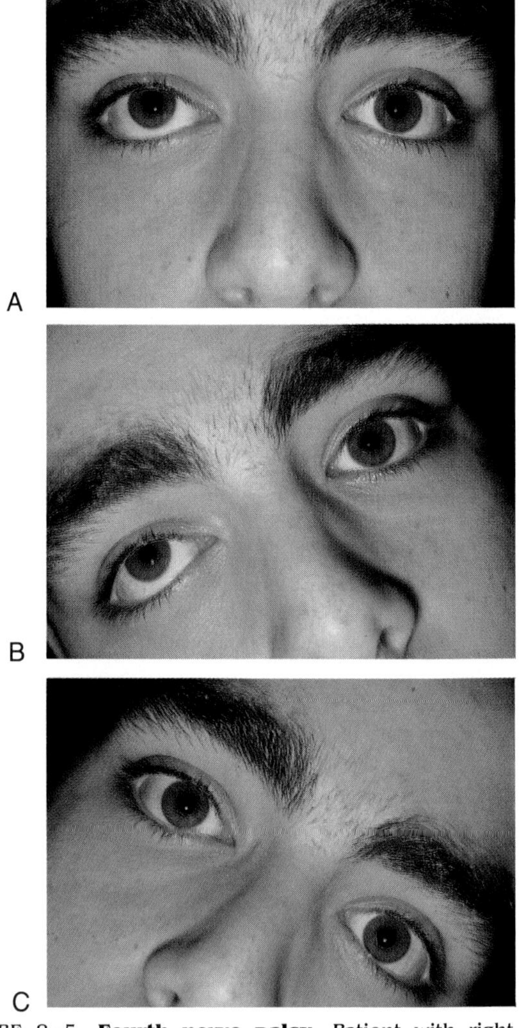

FIGURE 8–5 **Fourth nerve palsy.** Patient with right fourth nerve palsy causing right hypertropia in the primary position *(A).* The Bielschowsky head tilt test reveals that the right hypertropia is increased on head tilt to the right *(B)* and decreased on tilt to the left *(C),* consistent with paresis of the right superior oblique muscle.

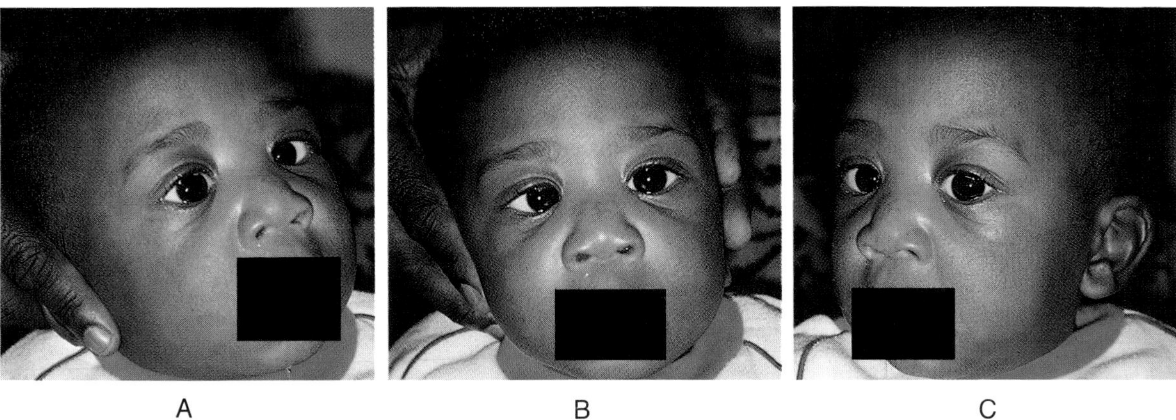

FIGURE 8–6 **Gradenigo's syndrome.** *A–C,* Child with right sixth nerve palsy secondary to middle ear infection (Gradenigo's syndrome). The right esotropia was associated with poor abduction.

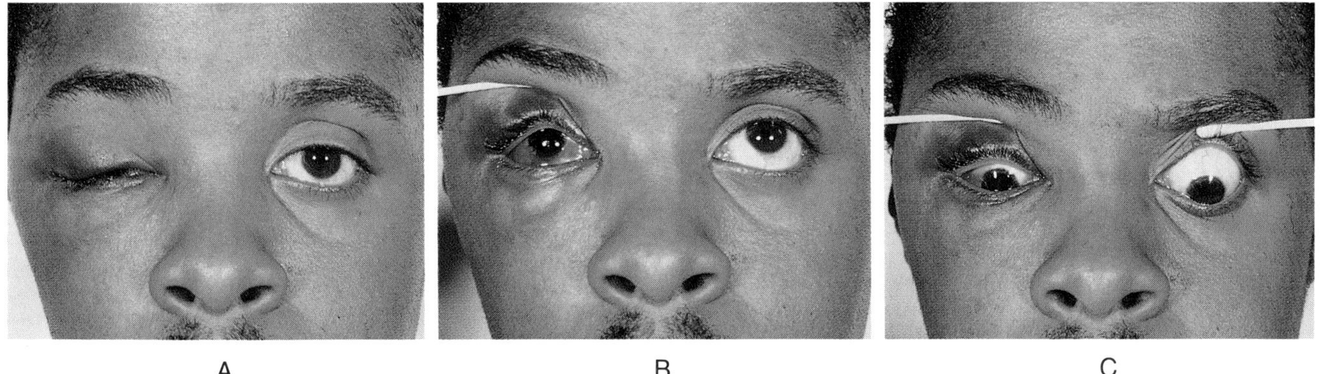

FIGURE 8–7 **Blowout fracture.** *A,* Patient with blowout fracture of the right orbital floor due to blunt trauma. *B,* The right eye exhibits restricted elevation because of entrapment of the inferior rectus muscle in the fracture line. Forced ductions would reveal a mechanical restriction of elevation in the eye. *C,* Downward movement of the right eye is also limited by the entrapment, but forced ductions would not show restricted movement in this direction.

FIGURE 8–8 **Graves' disease.** Patient with Graves' disease, exhibiting lid retraction, right hypotropia due to infiltration and restricted movement of right inferior rectus muscle, and injection over insertion of horizontal rectus muscles in both eyes.

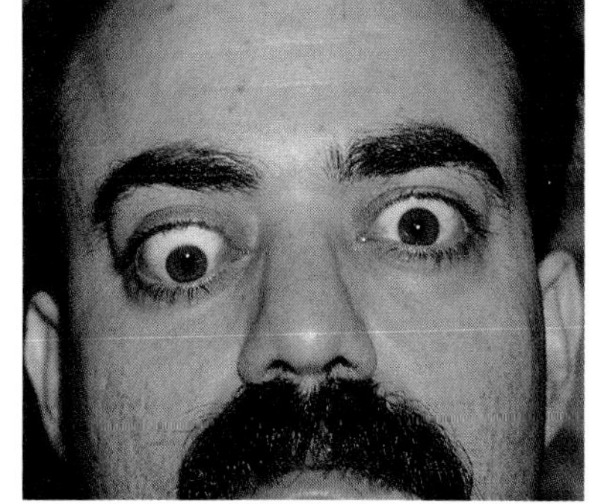

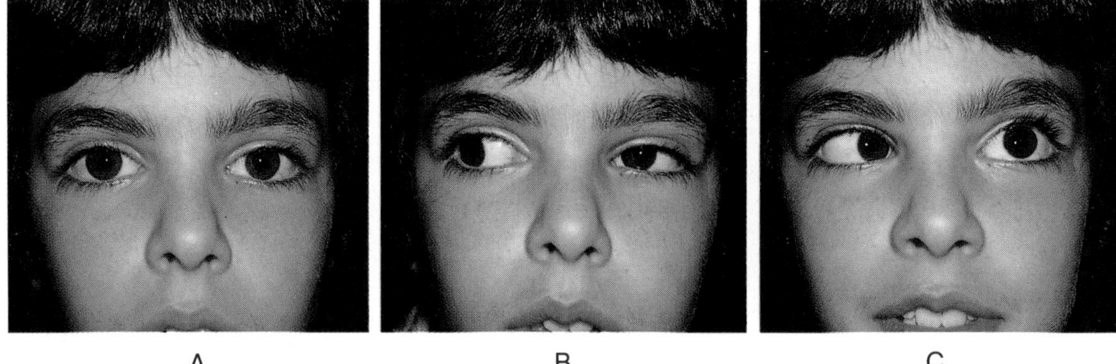

FIGURE 8–9 **Duane's retraction syndrome.** Patient with Duane's retraction syndrome in the left eye. The eyes are straight in the primary position *(A)*, but an esotropia develops in left gaze *(B)* owing to the restricted abduction of the left eye. In right gaze *(C)*, the left palpebral fissure narrows owing to co-contraction of the left medial and lateral rectus muscles, causing retraction of the globe.

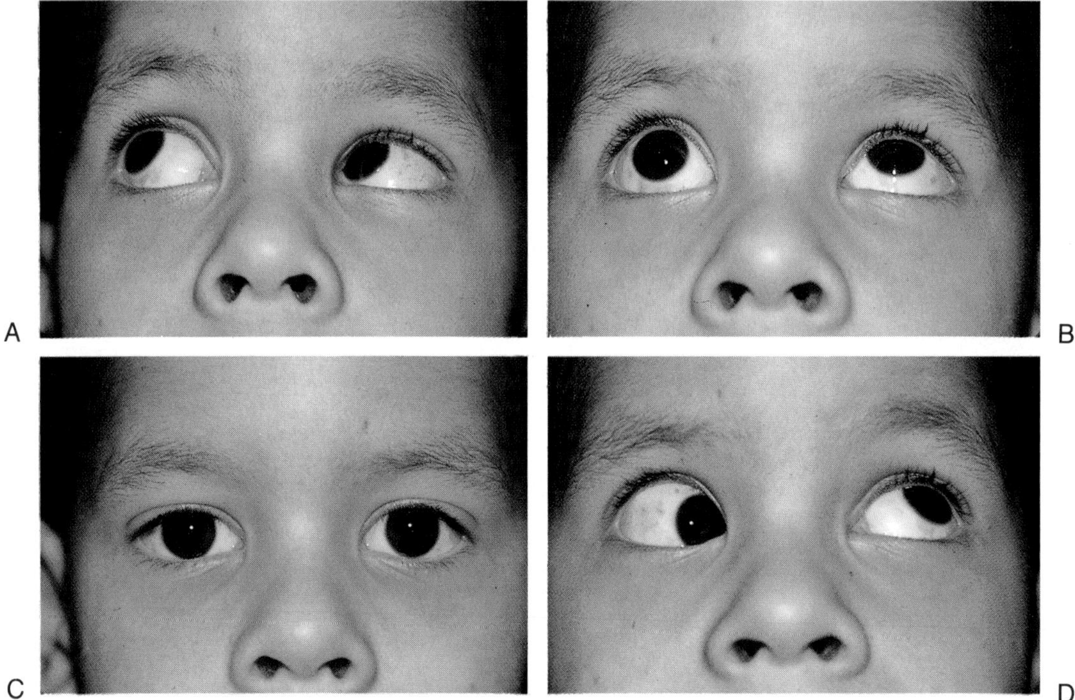

FIGURE 8–10 **Brown's syndrome.** *A*, Patient with Brown's syndrome involving right superior oblique tendon. The eyes are straight in the primary position *(B)*, but in upward gaze there is restriction of elevation in the adducted position *(C)*. In abduction *(D)*, the elevation is full.

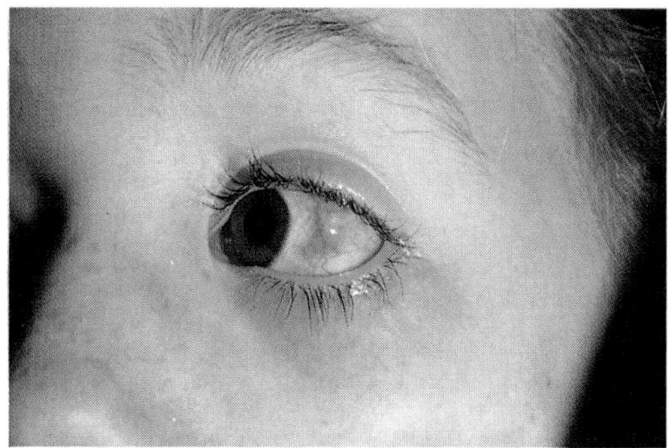

FIGURE 8–11 **Suture granuloma.** Suture granuloma at the site of reattachment of lateral rectus muscle 1 month after strabismus surgery in which gut sutures were used.

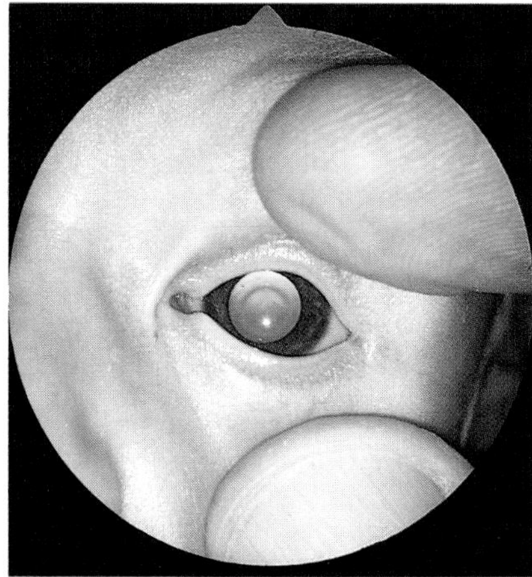

FIGURE 8–12 **Galactosemia cataract.** Oil droplet lens opacity in newborn infant with galactosemia due to galactose-1-phosphate transferase deficiency. Such an opacity would be expected to disappear when lactose was removed from the infant's diet.

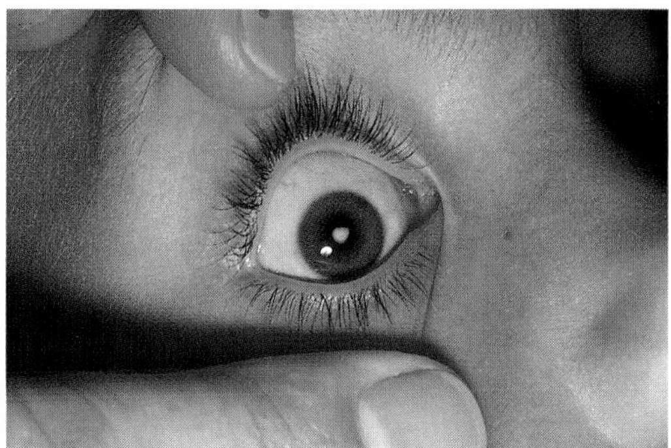

FIGURE 8–13 **Anterior polar cataract.** Anterior polar cataract located centrally in the pupillary space and evident on diffuse external transillumination.

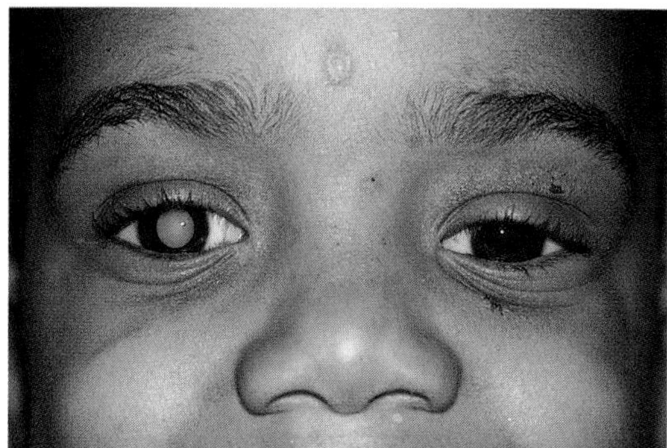

FIGURE 8–14 **Cataract.** A mature cataract in this patient's right eye is visible with diffuse external illumination.

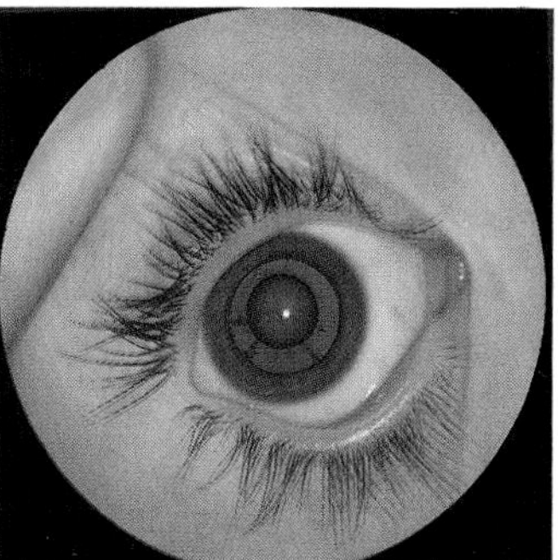

FIGURE 8–15 **Lamellar cataract.** A lamellar cataract with several peripheral spoke opacities can be seen against fundus reflex as it would be with light from a direct ophthalmoscope.

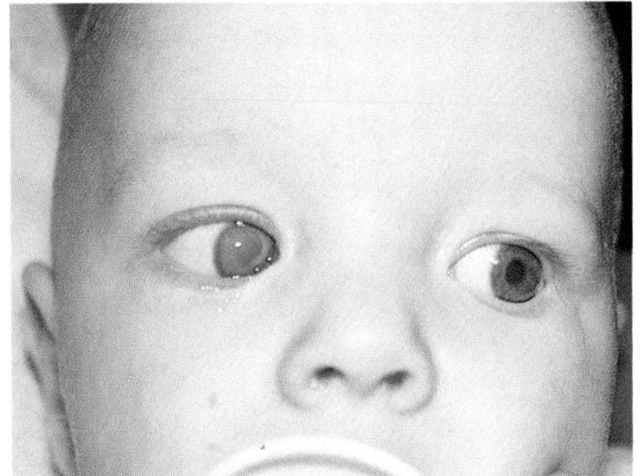

FIGURE 8–16 **Infantile glaucoma.** Acute, advanced corneal opacification in the right eye of this child with infantile glaucoma. Bilateral corneal enlargement and opacification with a pressure of 38 mmHg were found in each eye; breaks in Descemet's membrane were present only on the right side.

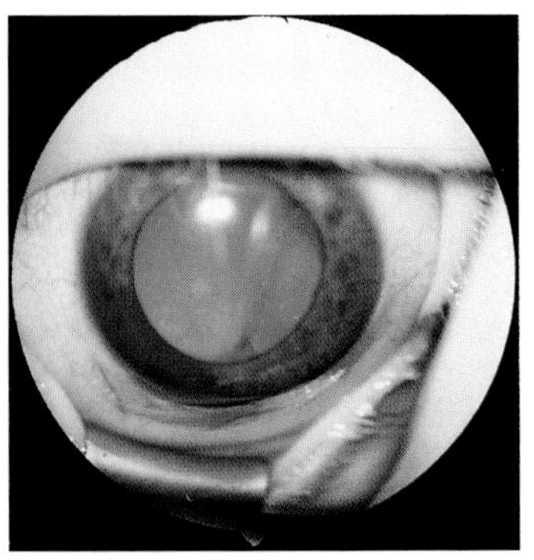

FIGURE 8–17 **Secondary glaucoma.** In this left eye of a young boy, glaucoma occurred secondary to rubeosis, complicating a cystic medulloepithelioma seen displacing the lens nasally.

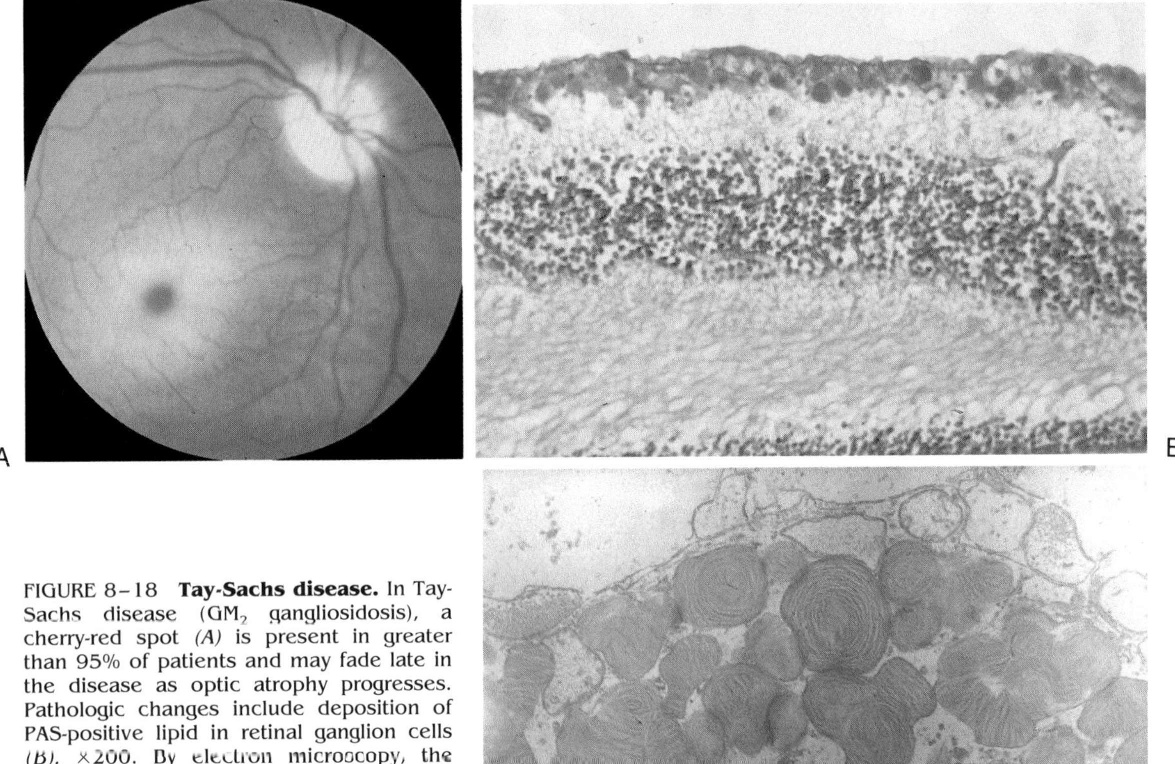

FIGURE 8–18 **Tay-Sachs disease.** In Tay-Sachs disease (GM_2 gangliosidosis), a cherry-red spot *(A)* is present in greater than 95% of patients and may fade late in the disease as optic atrophy progresses. Pathologic changes include deposition of PAS-positive lipid in retinal ganglion cells *(B)*. ×200. By electron microscopy, the lipid is found intracellularly in membrane-bound lamellar inclusions *(C)*. ×14,000.

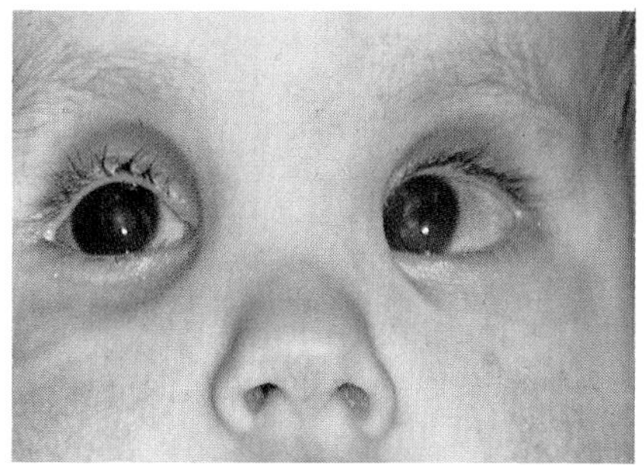

FIGURE 8–19 **Oculocerebrorenal syndrome of Lowe.** The oculocerebrorenal syndrome of Lowe is inherited in an X-linked manner. Affected males have cataracts, glaucoma, nystagmus, psychomotor retardation, aminoaciduria, and acidosis.

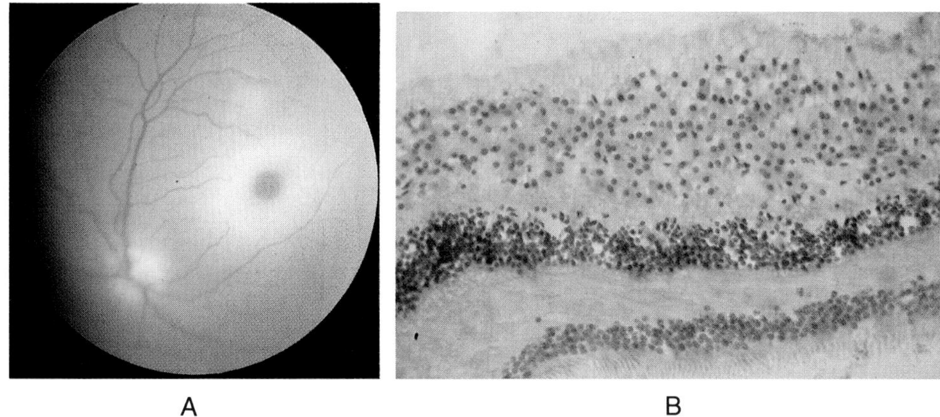

FIGURE 8–20 **Niemann-Pick disease.** Niemann-Pick disease (type A or infantile form) is rapidly fatal with progressive loss of developmental milestones. A macular cherry-red spot *(A)* is characteristic, as are large, foamy lipid-laden retinal ganglion cells *(B)* stained here with oil red O. ×250.

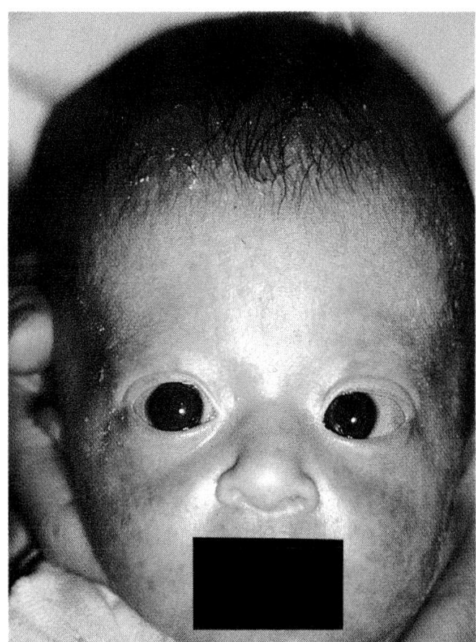

FIGURE 8–21 **Zellweger's syndrome.** The facial features of cerebrohepatorenal syndrome (Zellweger's syndrome) include a long narrow head, a high forehead, and shallow supraorbital ridges.

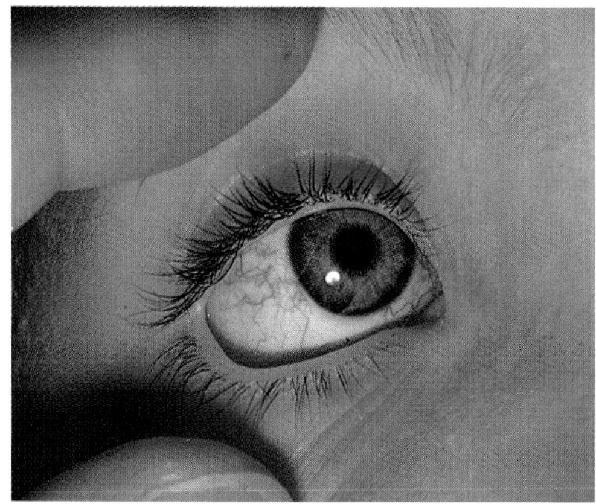

FIGURE 8–22 **Ataxia telangiectasia.** Ataxia telangiectasia is a disease of abnormal DNA repair culminating in lymphatic malignancy. Tortuous conjunctival vessels are characteristic.

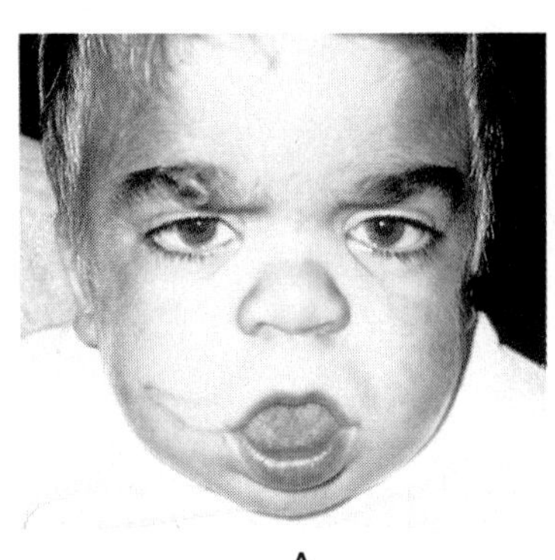

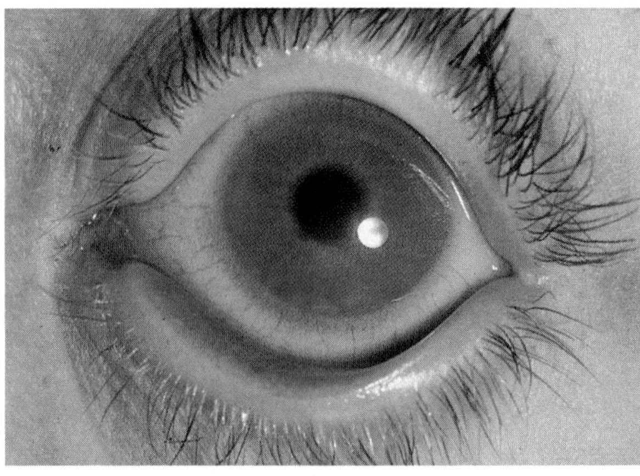

A B

FIGURE 8–23 **Hurler's syndrome.** Hurler's syndrome (MPS I-H, or iduronidase deficiency, Hurler type) is the prototype of mucopolysaccharidoses. Patients are clinically normal at birth and deteriorate progressively, with dwarfism, coarse facial features *(A)*, hepatosplenomegaly, mental retardation, stiff joints, and corneal clouding *(B)* increasing until death.

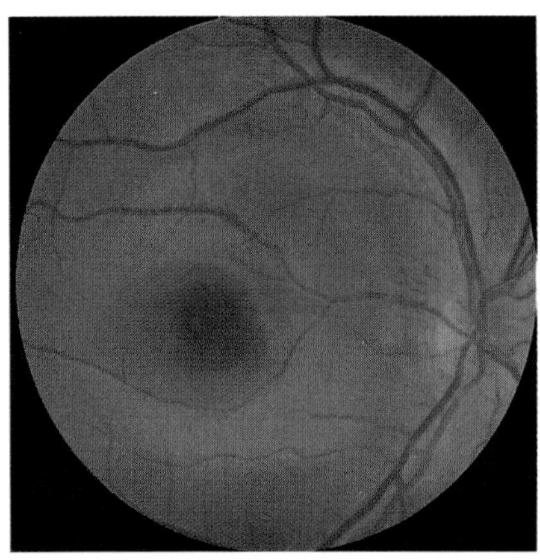

FIGURE 8–24 **Batten's disease.** Batten's disease may have pigmentary macular changes as illustrated. These are different from a cherry-red spot because there is no gross deposition of lipid in the ganglion cells. The electroretinogram response is severely attenuated in Batten's disease.

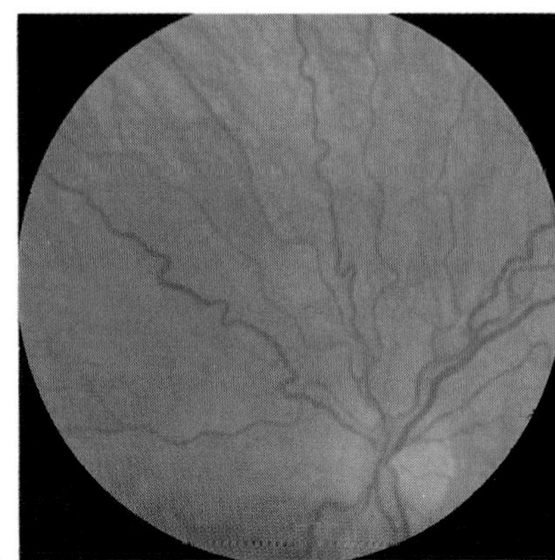

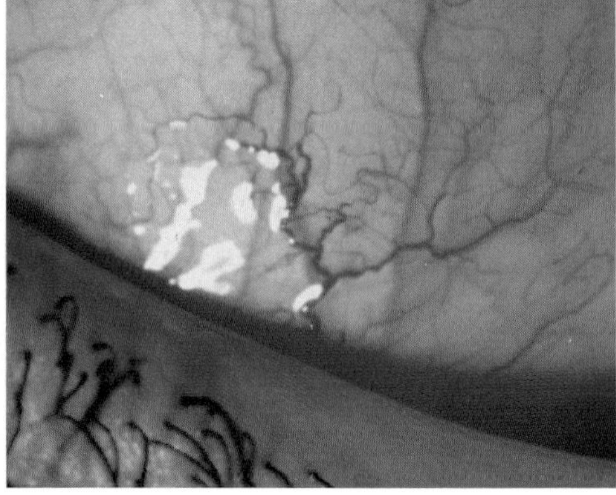

A B

FIGURE 8–25 **Farber's disease.** Galactosidase A deficiency or Farber's disease leads to systemic deposition of glycosphingolipids in viscera and in vascular endothelium. This results in pain in the extremities and vascular ectasia (angiokeratomas) as well as vascular tortuosity in retina *(A)* and conjunctiva *(B)*. Subtle corneal opacities occur in a whorl pattern, and spokelike posterior lens opacities are characteristic.

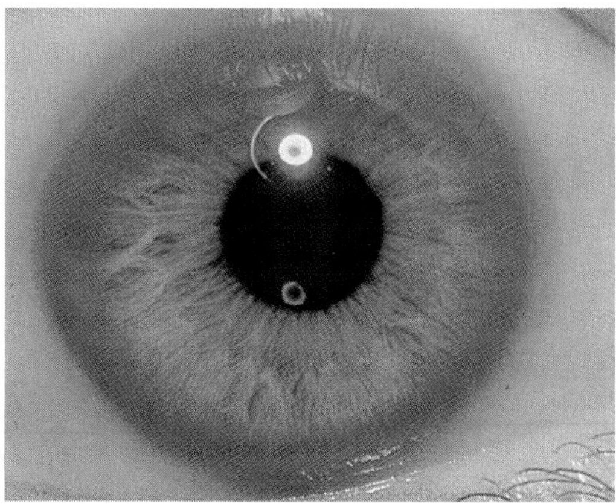

FIGURE 8–26 **Wilson's disease.** In Wilson's disease, abnormal copper metabolism results in accumulation of copper in the liver and other tissues. The copper deposition in Descemet's membrane in the peripheral cornea results in the classic Kayser-Fleischer ring, seen most densely at the upper and lower poles.

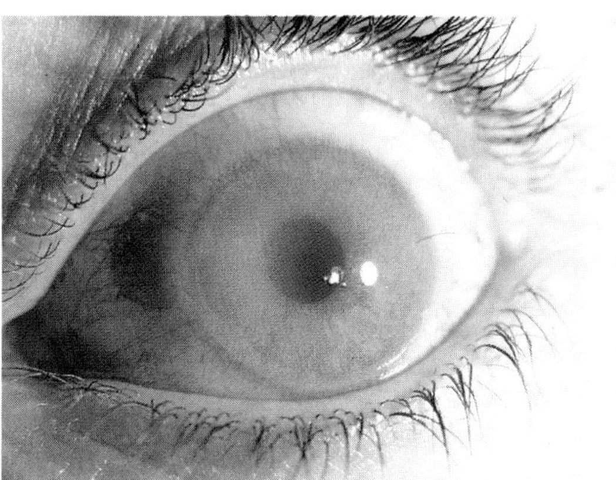

FIGURE 8–27 **Scheie's syndrome.** Scheie's syndrome (MPS I-S) is characterized by severe corneal clouding but normal intelligence and stature (in contrast to Hurler's syndrome, despite the same deficiency of α-iduronidase).

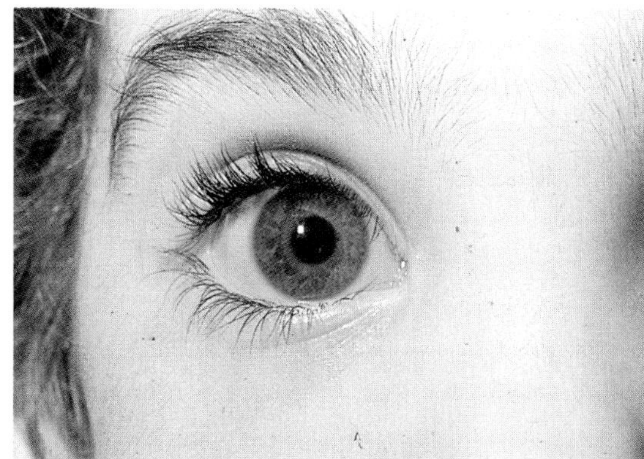

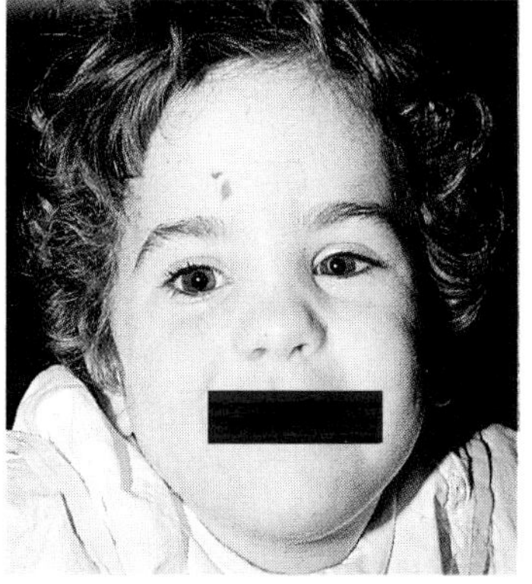

FIGURE 8–28 **Morquio's syndrome.** Morquio's syndrome (MPS IV) results from galactosamine-6-sulfate sulfatase deficiency (MPS IV-A) or β-galactosidase deficiency (MPS IV-B). The most prominent features are severe skeletal dysplasia, progressive deafness, mild late corneal clouding *(A)*, and normal intelligence *(B)*.

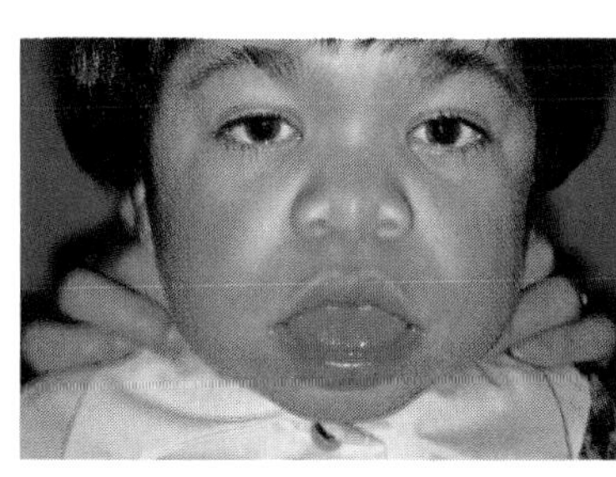

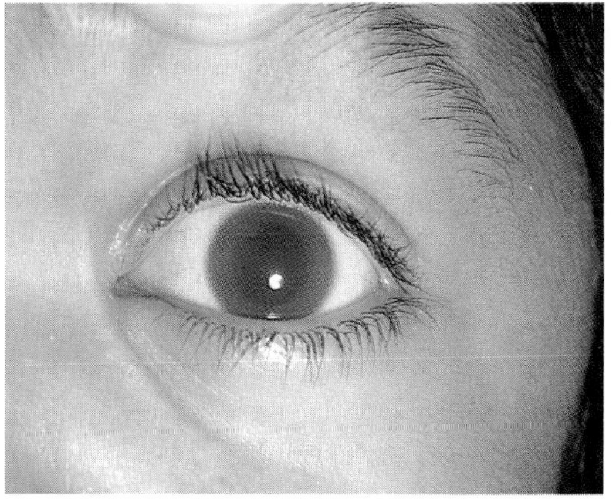

FIGURE 8–29 **Maroteaux-Lamy syndrome.** MPS VI or Maroteaux-Lamy syndrome is characterized by progressive dwarfism, coarse facial features *(A)*, severe corneal clouding *(B)*, and normal intelligence. It is a result of *N*-acetylgalactosamine-4-sulfatase (arylsulfatase B) deficiency.

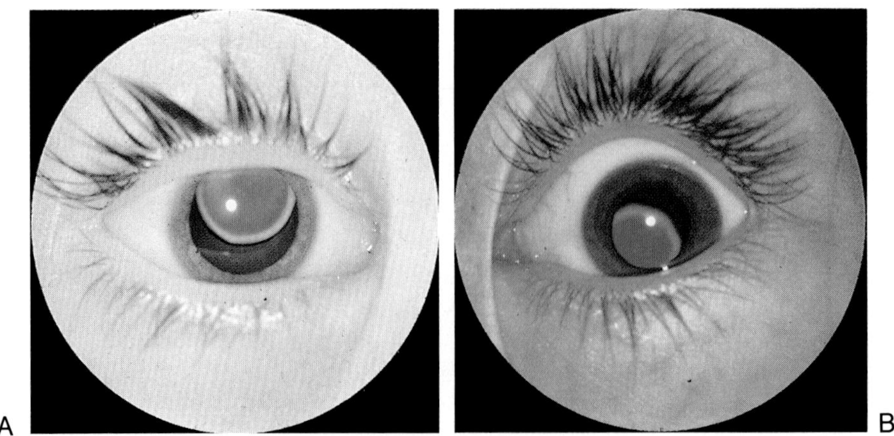

FIGURE 8–30 **Ectopia lentis.** Ectopia lentis with superior displacement is more characteristic of Marfan's syndrome, which is also associated with arachnodactyly, cardiac abnormalities, and high myopia *(A)*. Ectopia lentis with inferior displacement is more characteristic of homocystinuria *(B)*.

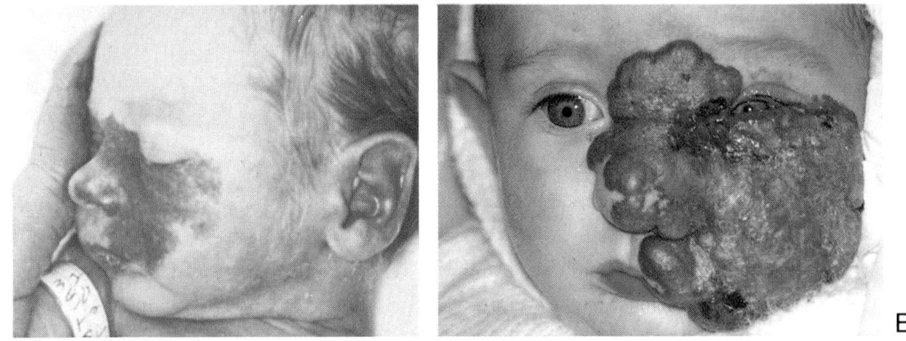

FIGURE 8–31 **Hemangioma.** *A,* Newborn infant with flat hemangioma in left maxillary area and bridge of the nose, *B,* Same infant at 8 months of age showing exuberant growth of the hemangioma and involvement of the entire left lower lid.

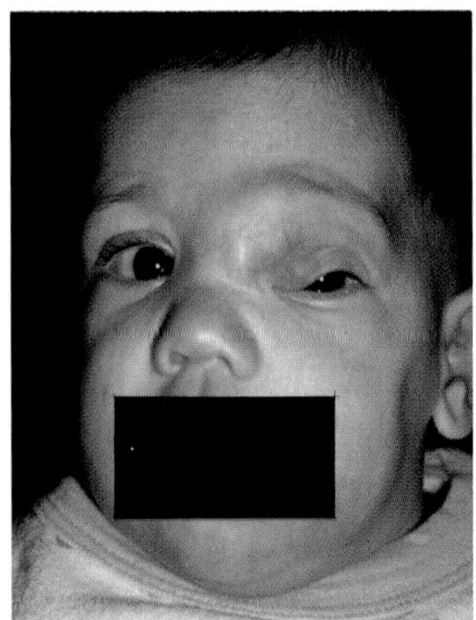

FIGURE 8–32 **Hemangioma.** Five-month-old infant with hemangioma at inner aspect of left upper lid and brow. Lesions in this location are particularly apt to induce oblique astigmatism because of pressure on the cornea.

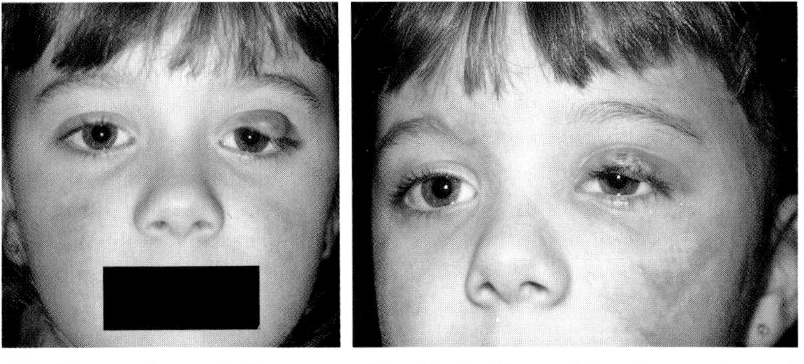

FIGURE 8–33 **Hemangioma.** *A,* Three-year-old patient with pendulous hemangioma of left upper lid that was amenable to local excision after its active growth had stopped. *B,* Same patient 2 days after partial excision of hemangioma.

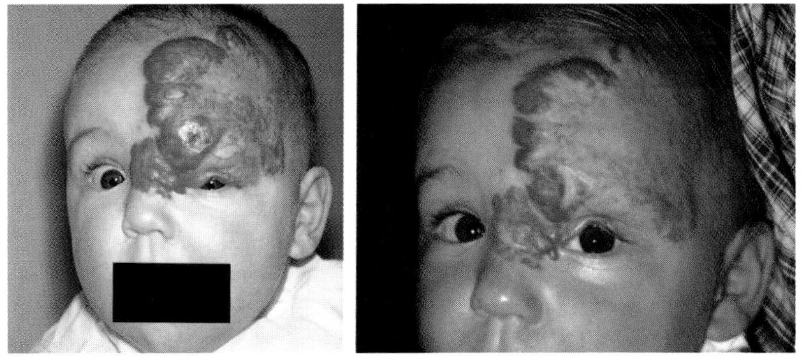

FIGURE 8–34 **Hemangioma.** *A,* Five-month-old infant with hemangioma of left upper lid, brow, and forehead. Corticosteroids were injected into the upper lid and brow. *B,* Patient 6 months after local steroid injection.

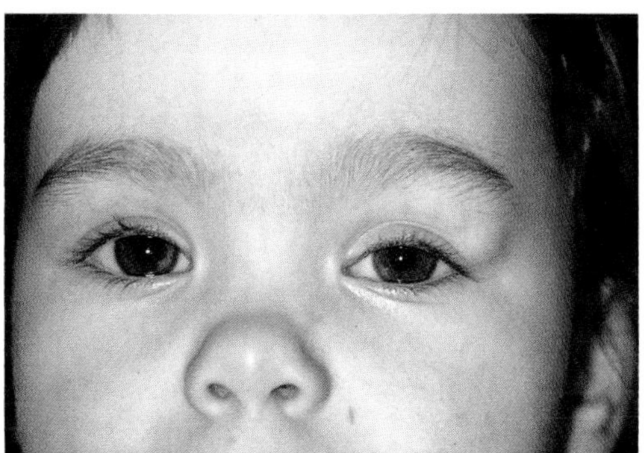

FIGURE 8–35 **Dermoid cyst.** Child with dermoid cyst at temporal aspect of left upper lid near orbital margin.

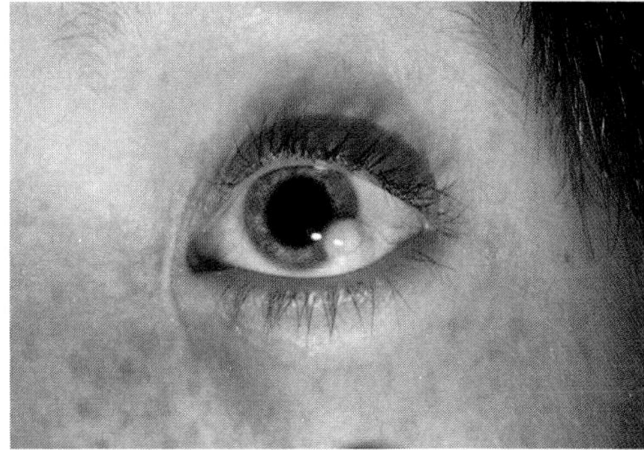

FIGURE 8–36 **Dermoid cyst.** Epibulbar dermoid at inferotemporal limbus, at which 76% of such lesions occur.

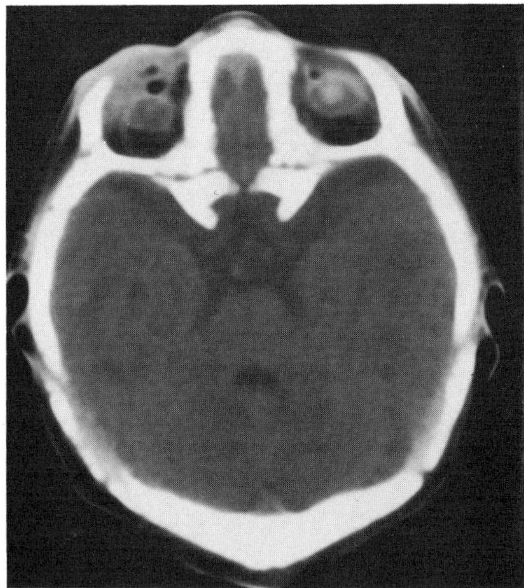

FIGURE 8–37 **Microphthalmia.** Computed tomography scan of the orbits of an infant with severe microphthalmia. Small globes containing lenses can be found on each side.

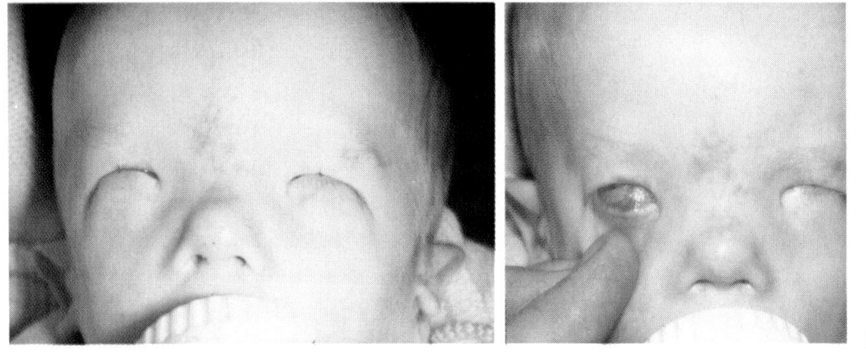

FIGURE 8–38 **Bilateral microphthalmia.** *A,* Patient with bilateral microphthalmia with cyst. *B,* The cyst extends forward into the lower eyelid, obscuring the rudimentary globe behind it.

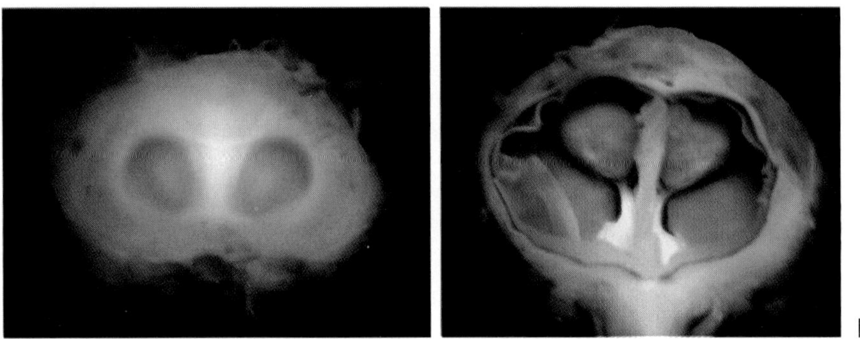

FIGURE 8–39 **Enucleated synophthalmic eye.** *A,* Two corneas can be seen, but the globes are fused medially. *B,* Same eye viewed from above after superior calotte has been removed. Two lenses and a medial partition can be seen.

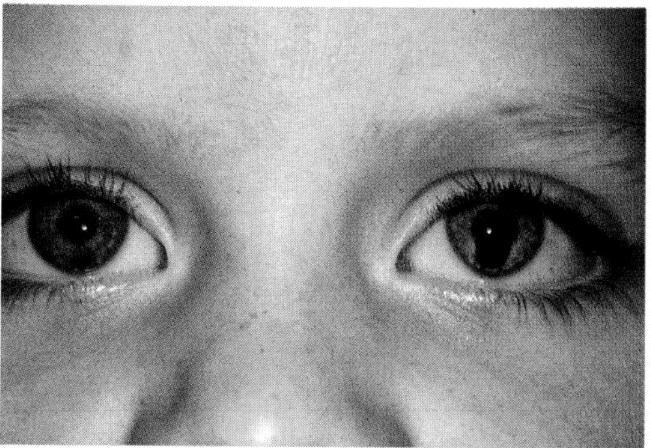

FIGURE 8-40 **Coloboma.** Patient with inferonasal iris coloboma in left eye.

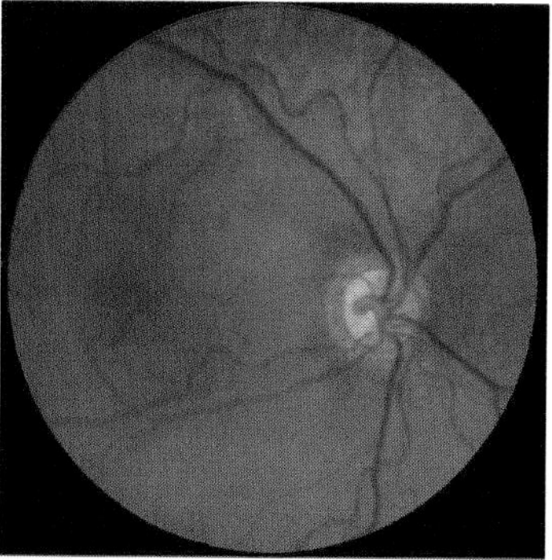

FIGURE 8-42 **Optic nerve hypoplasia.** Note small size of optic disc and irregular termination of retinal pigment epithelium at disc margin.

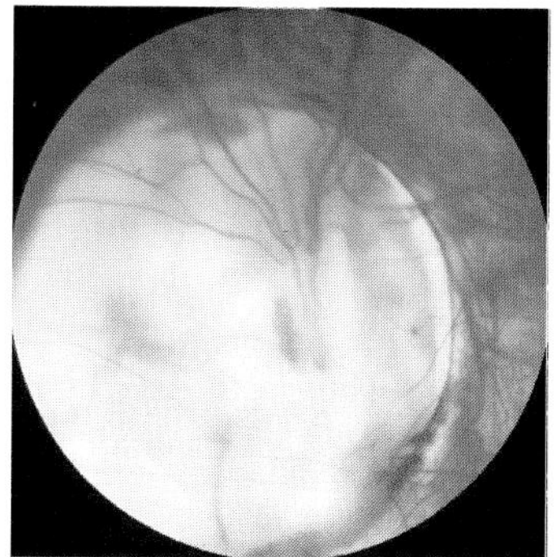

FIGURE 8-41 **Coloboma of the optic disc.** Retinal vessels can be seen coursing over the upper aspect of the coloboma.

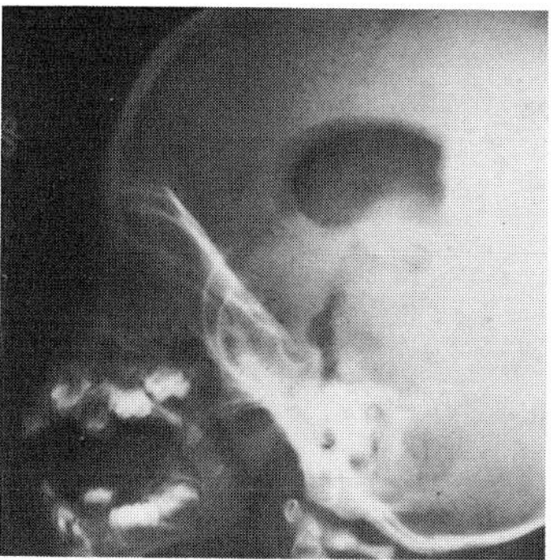

FIGURE 8-43 **Bilateral optic nerve hypoplasia.** Pneumoencephalogram of patient with bilateral optic nerve hypoplasia showing lack of septum pellucidum, an anatomic defect without known functional significance.

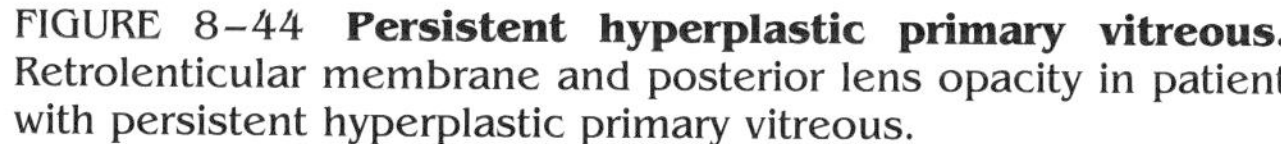

FIGURE 8-44 **Persistent hyperplastic primary vitreous.** Retrolenticular membrane and posterior lens opacity in patient with persistent hyperplastic primary vitreous.

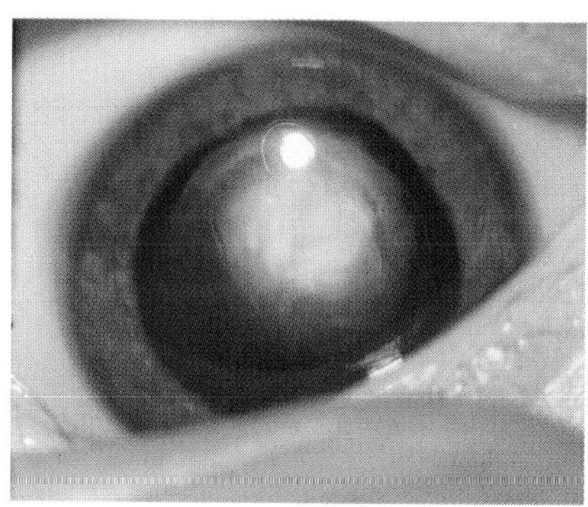

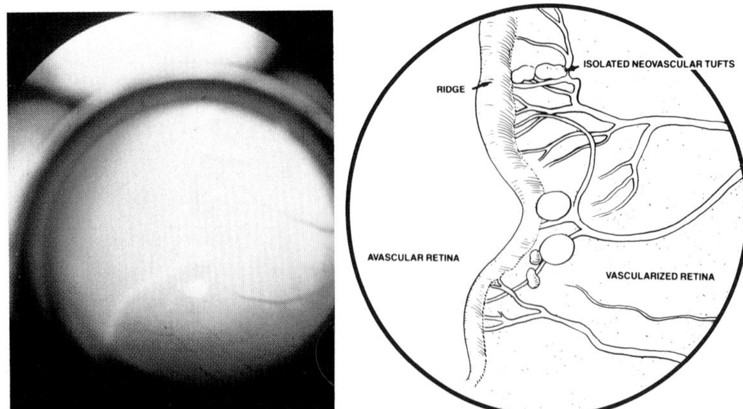

FIGURE 8–45 **Retinopathy of prematurity.** Stage 2 retinopathy of prematurity. (From The Committee for Classification of Retinopathy of Prematurity: An international classification of retinopathy of prematurity. Arch Ophthalmol 102:1131, 1984. Copyright 1984, American Medical Association.)

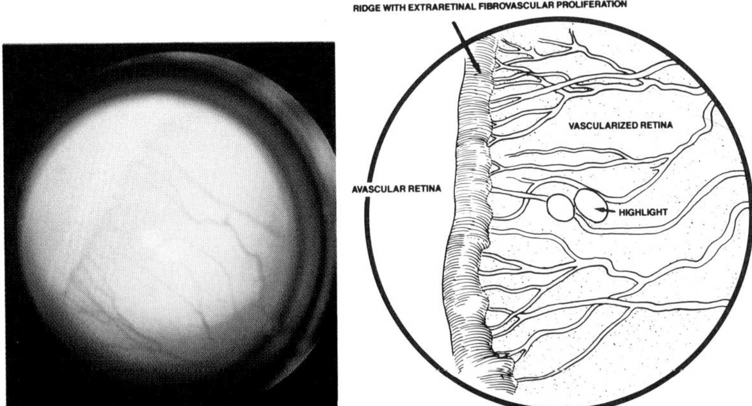

FIGURE 8–46 **Retinopathy of prematurity.** Stage 3 retinopathy of prematurity. (From The Committee for Classification of Retinopathy of Prematurity: An international classification of retinopathy of prematurity. Arch Ophthalmol 102:1131, 1984. Copyright 1984, American Medical Association.)

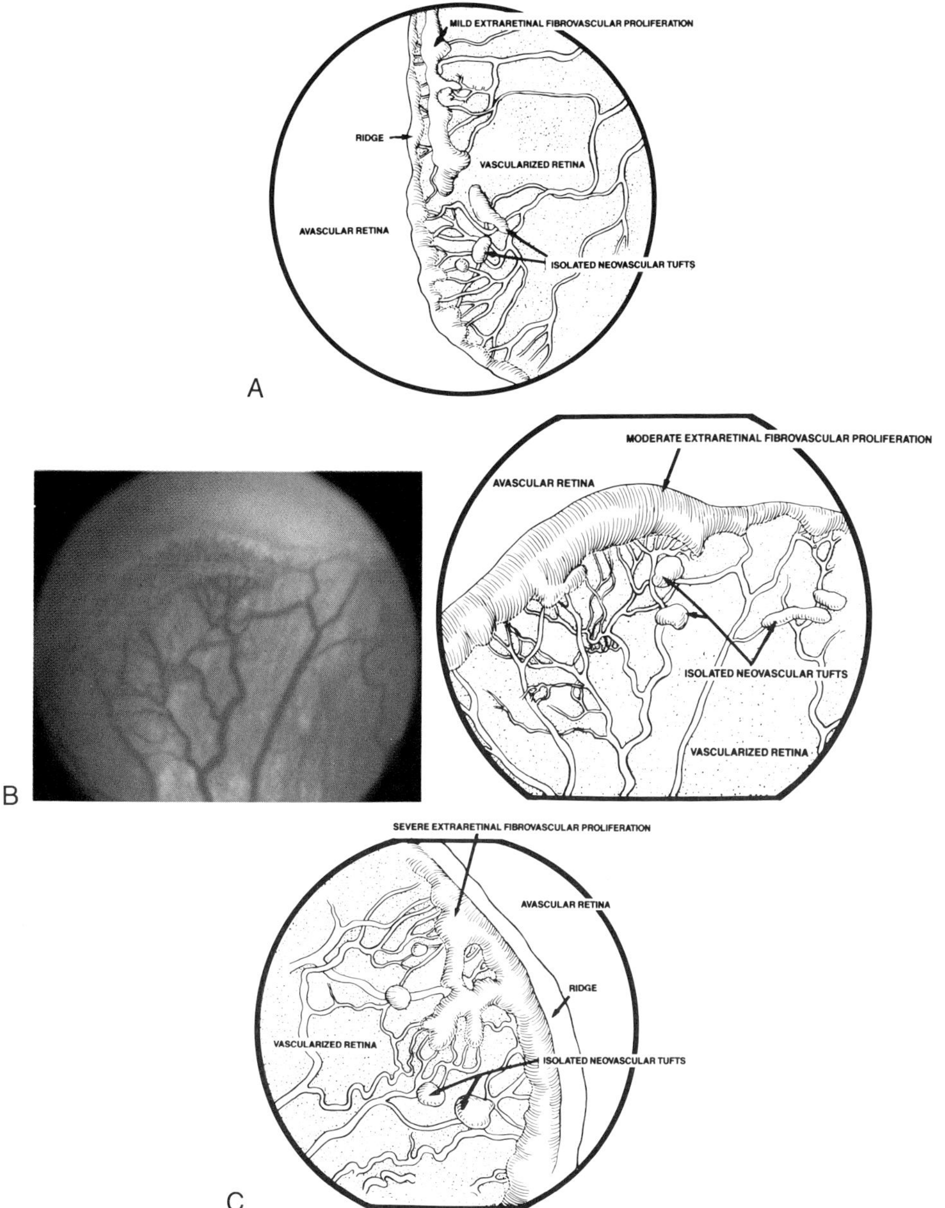

FIGURE 8–47 **Retinopathy of prematurity.** Severities of stage 3 retinopathy: *A,* Mild; *B,* moderate; *C,* severe. (From The Committee for Classification of Retinopathy of Prematurity: An international classification of retinopathy of prematurity. Arch Ophthalmol 102:1131, 1984. Copyright 1984, American Medical Association.)

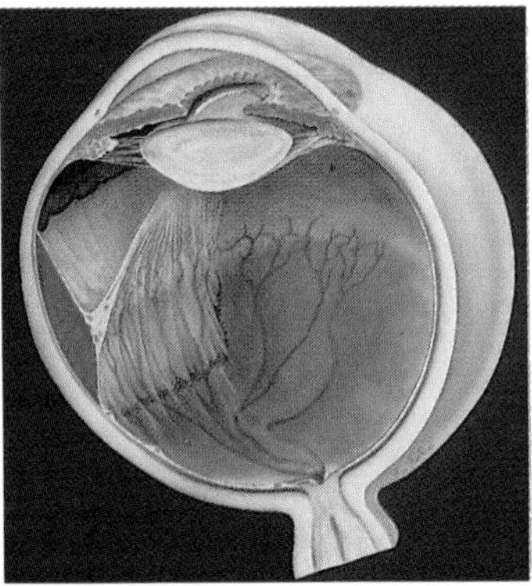

FIGURE 8-48 **Retinopathy of prematurity.** Peripheral retinal detachment in stage 4A retinopathy of prematurity. (From The International Committee for Classification of Late Stages of Retinopathy of Prematurity: An international classification of retinopathy of prematurity. II. The classification of retinal detachment. Arch Ophthalmol 105:906–912, 1987. Copyright 1987, American Medical Association.)

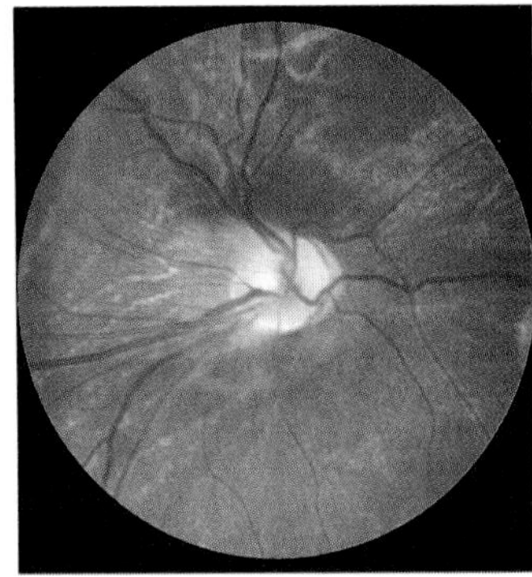

FIGURE 8-49 **Retinopathy of prematurity.** Temporal traction of the retina in cicatricial retinopathy of prematurity.

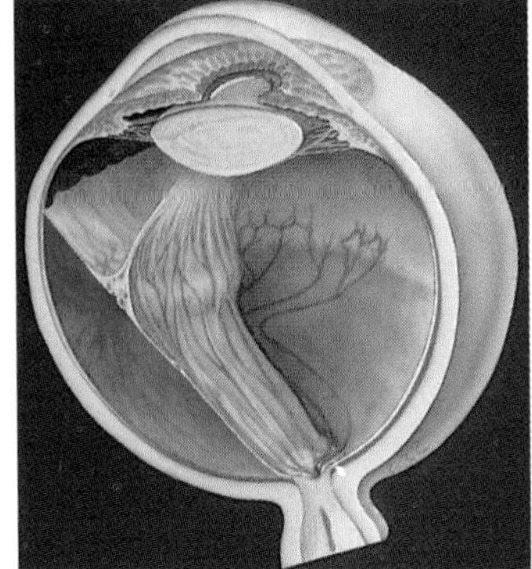

FIGURE 8-50 **Retinopathy of prematurity.** Partial retinal detachment involving the macula in stage 4B retinopathy of prematurity. (From The International Committee for Classification of Late Stages of Retinopathy of Prematurity: An international classification of retinopathy of prematurity. II. The classification of retinal detachment. Arch Ophthalmol 105:906–912, 1987. Copyright 1987, American Medical Association.)

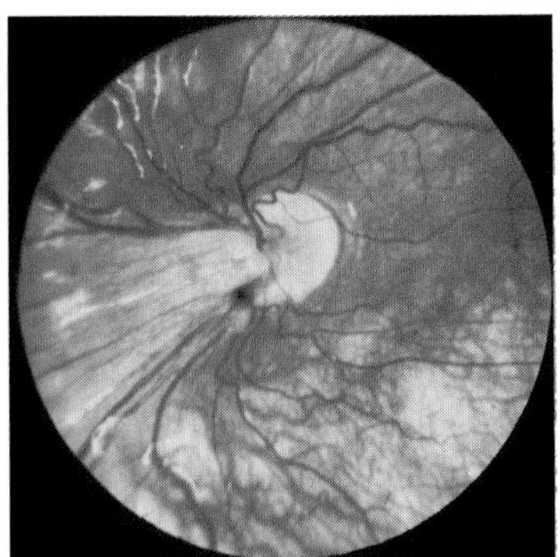

FIGURE 8-51 **Retinopathy of prematurity.** Cicatricial stage 4B of retinopathy of prematurity. Fixed fold of detached retina in cicatricial stage 4B of retinopathy of prematurity.

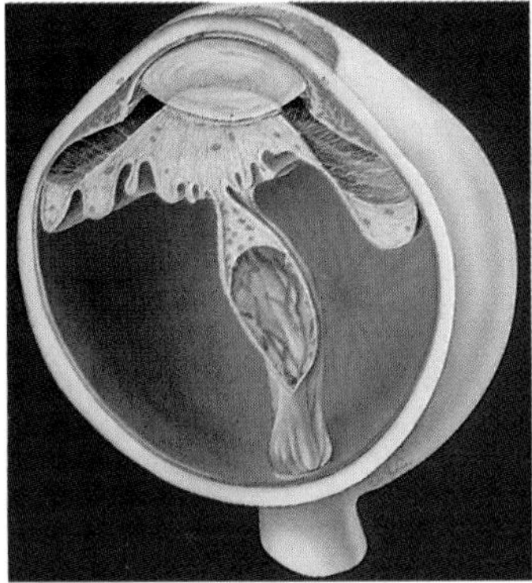

FIGURE 8-52 **Retinopathy of prematurity.** Stage 5 retinopathy of prematurity: closed funnel. (From Machemer R: Description and pathogenesis of late stage of retinopathy of prematurity. *In* Flynn JT, Phelps DL (eds): Retinopathy of Prematurity: Problem and Challenge. New York, Alan R. Liss, Inc, 1988, pp. 275–280.)

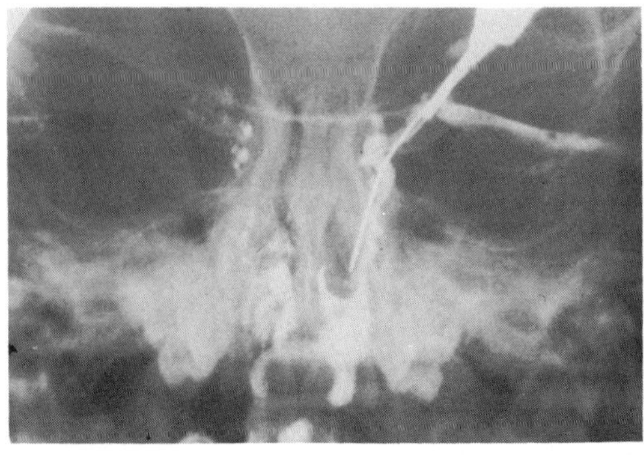

FIGURE 8-53 **Congenital nasolacrimal duct obstruction.** The probe is in a false passage. The dacryocystogram was performed by injecting contrast material through the lower canaliculus while the metallic probe was in place through the upper canaliculus. (From Jazbi BU, Cibis GW: Nasolacrimal duct probing in infants. Ophthalmology 86:1488–1491, 1979.)

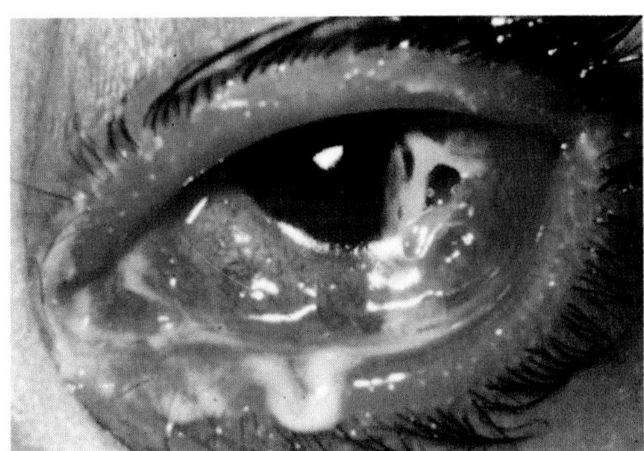

FIGURE 8–54 **Gonorrhea.** Hyperacute conjunctivitis of *Neisseria gonorrhoeae.* Note the marked purulence and conjunctival chemosis.

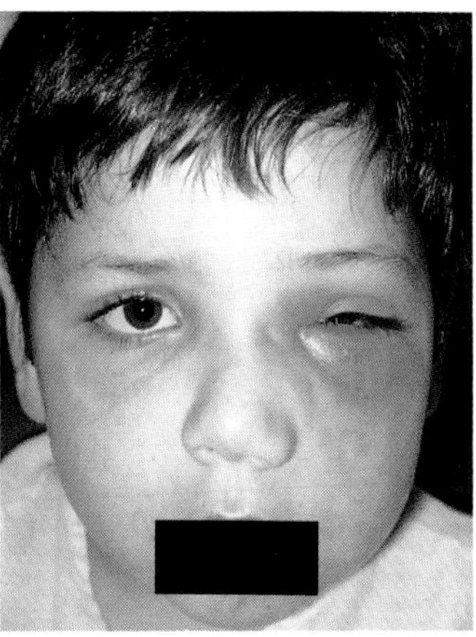

FIGURE 8–57 **Preseptal cellulitis.** There is edema and erythema of the eyelids without proptosis.

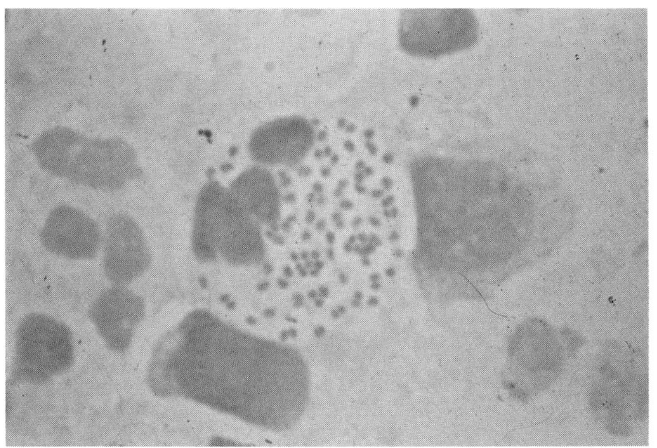

FIGURE 8–55 **Gonorrhea.** Gram stain showing intracellular gram-negative diplococci characteristic of *N. gonorrhoeae* infection.

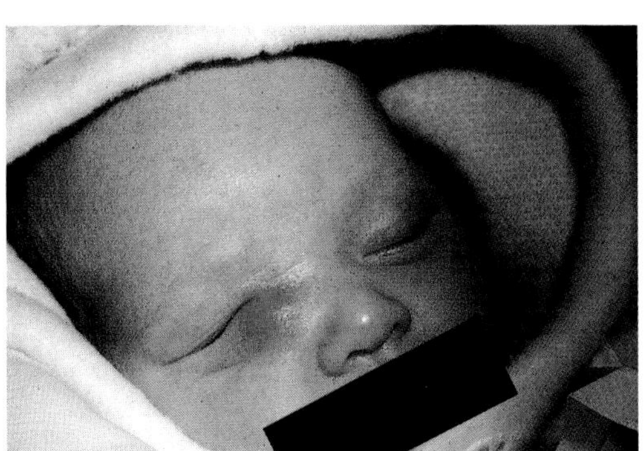

FIGURE 8–58 **Dacryocystitis.** Infection in the nasolacrimal sac is a common cause of suppurative preseptal cellulitis in infancy.

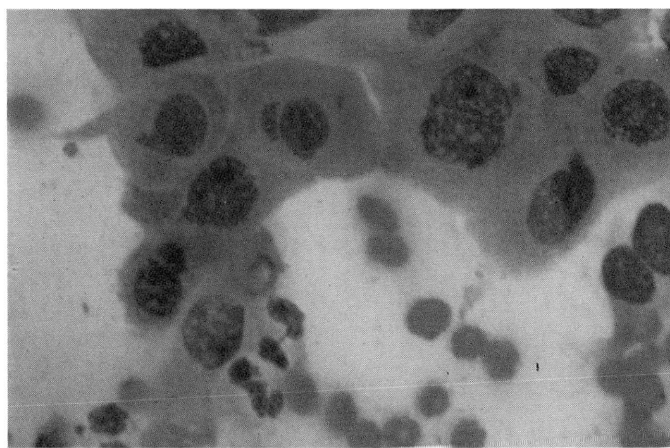

FIGURE 8–56 **Trachoma.** Giemsa stain showing basophilic cytoplasmic inclusion bodies characteristic of *Chlamydia trachomatis.*

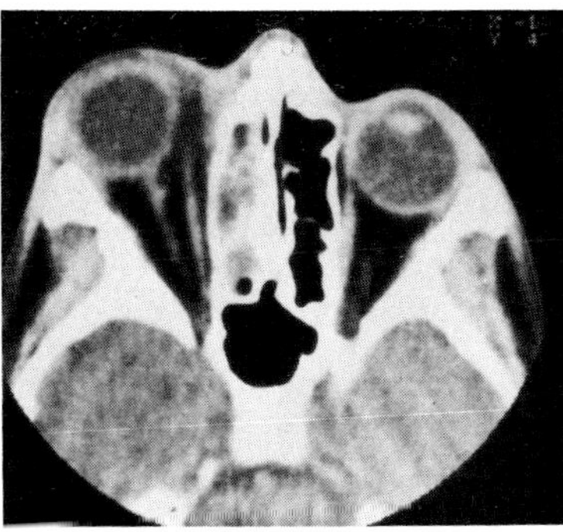

FIGURE 8–59 **Cellulitis.** Computed tomography scan of the orbits demonstrates ethmoid cellulitis with spread into the orbit. The medial rectus is displaced, and the anterior orbit is opacified. Note the marked proptosis.

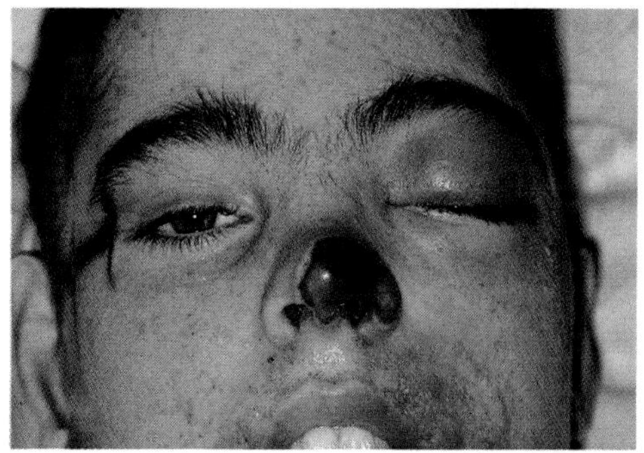

FIGURE 8–60 **Mucormycosis.** Mucormycosis of the orbit with ischemic necrosis of the nose.

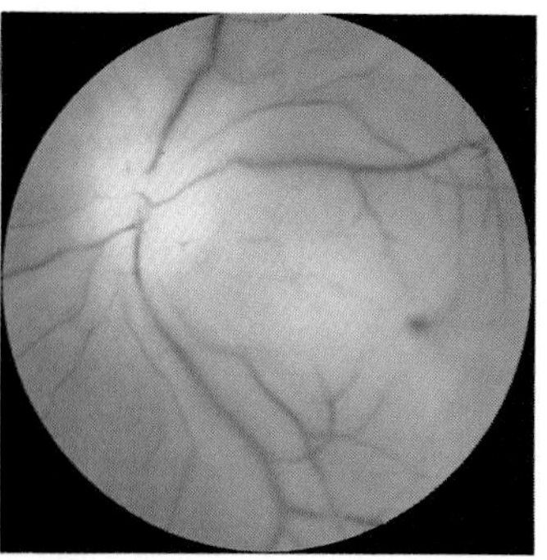

FIGURE 8–61 **Mucormycosis.** Same patient as in Figure 8–60. Central retinal artery occlusion secondary to mucormycosis of the orbit.

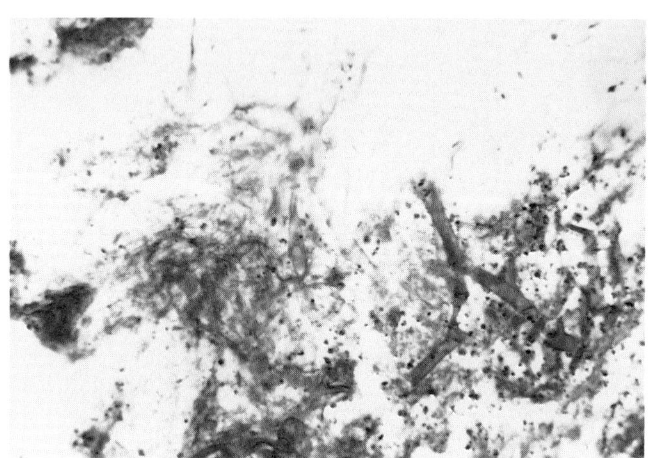

FIGURE 8–62 H&E stain of orbital tissue infected by *Zygomyces.* Note the branching, nonseptate hyphae.

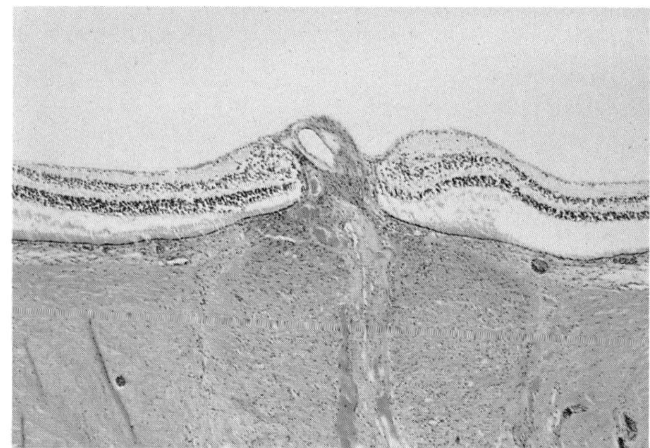

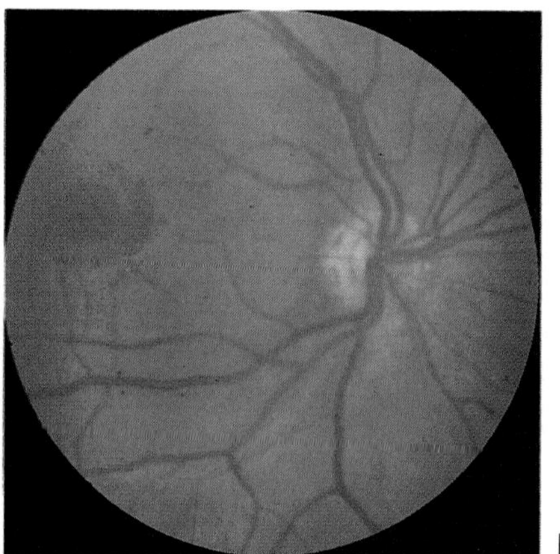

FIGURE 8–63 **Optic nerve hypoplasia.** *A* and *B,* An eye with marked optic nerve hypoplasia such as shown here is not expected to see well. Note that this small optic nerve lies within a hypopigmented annulus. Other features of the fundus, including the caliber and distribution of the retinal vasculature and the foveal reflex, are normal.

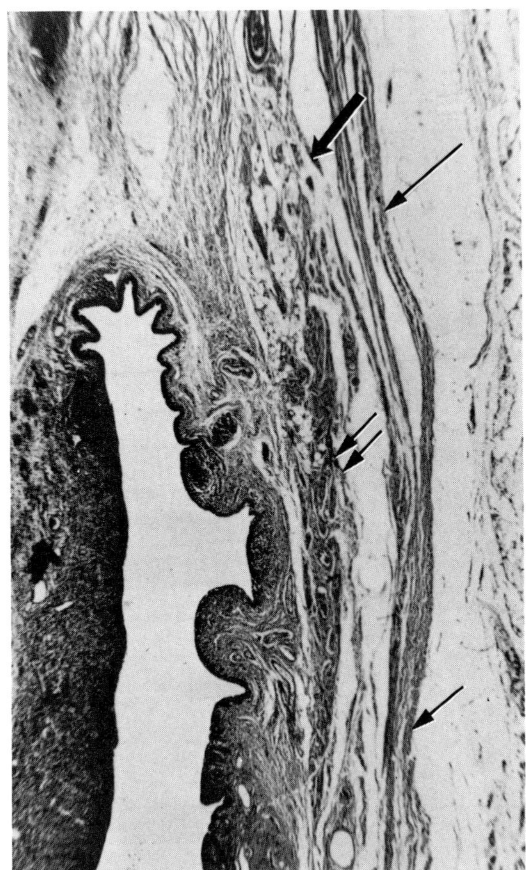

FIGURE 8–64 **The upper inner portion of the human upper eyelid.** The posterior portion of the levator muscle ends abruptly *(thick arrow)* and changes into Müller's smooth muscle *(double arrows)*. The frontal half of the levator muscle becomes the aponeurosis, which extends toward the lid *(thin arrows)*. This connective tissue does not attach to the tarsus but fans out into the orbicularis muscle. Celloidin section (H&E; original magnification ×32). (From Kuwabara T, Cogan DG, Johnson CC: Structure of the muscles of the upper eyelid. Arch Ophthalmol 93:1189, 1975. Copyright 1975, American Medical Association.)

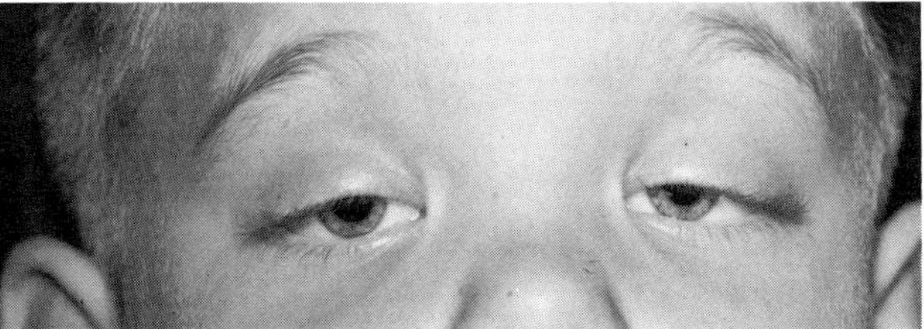

FIGURE 8–65 **Epicanthus palpebralis.** (From Johnson CC: Epicanthus and epiblepharon. Arch Ophthalmol 96:1031, 1978. Copyright 1978, American Medical Association.)

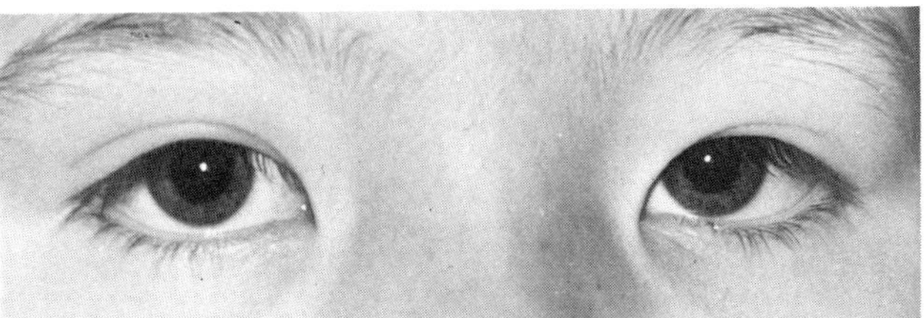

FIGURE 8–66 **Epicanthus tarsalis.** (From Johnson CC: Epicanthus and epiblepharon. Arch Ophthalmol 96:1031, 1978. Copyright 1978, American Medical Association.)

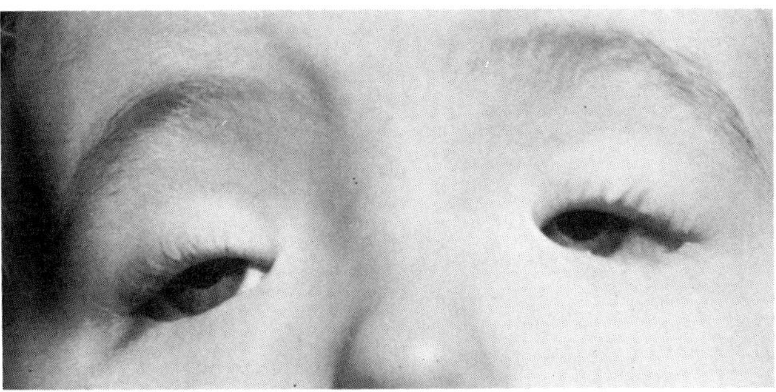

FIGURE 8–67 **Epicanthus inversus.** (From Johnson CC: Epicanthus. Am J Ophthalmol 66:939, 1968. Published with permission from the American Journal of Ophthalmology. Copyright by the Ophthalmic Publishing Company.)

SECTION 9

The Eye and Systemic Disease

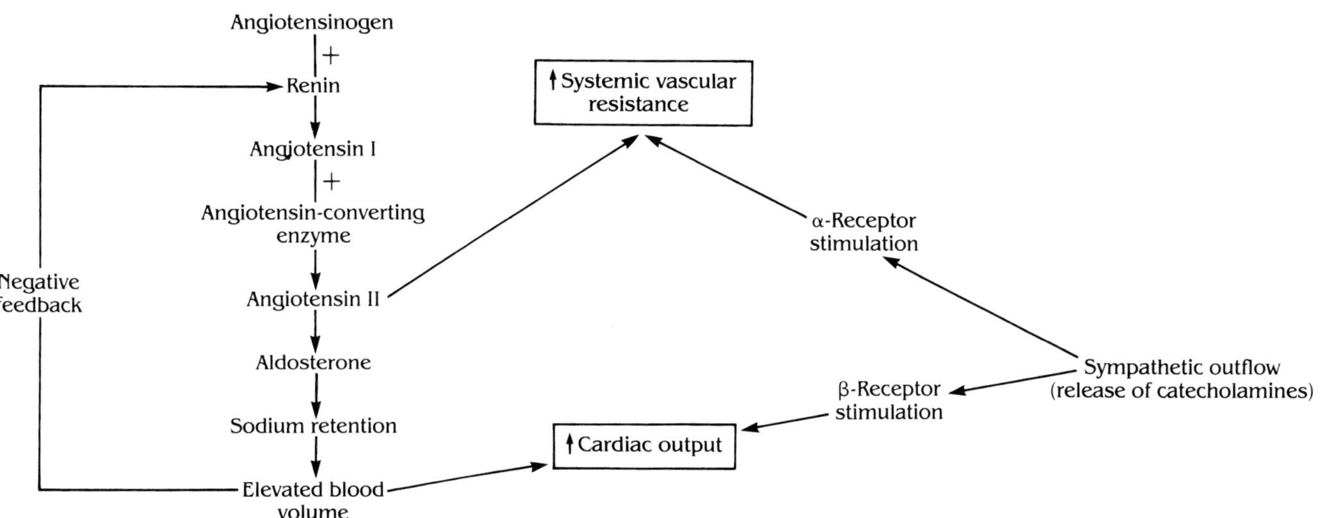

FIGURE 9–1 **Renin-angiotensin-aldosterone pathways.** Pathways through which the renin-angiotensin-aldosterone system and the sympathetic nervous system cause vasoconstriction and an elevated cardiac output.

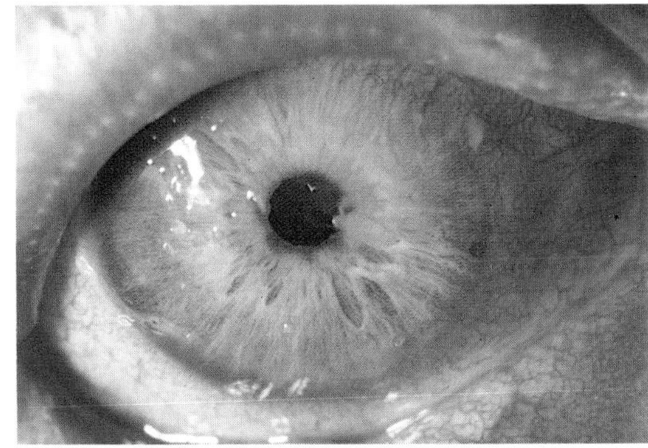

FIGURE 9–2 **Filamentary keratitis in rheumatoid arthritis.** Filamentary keratitis in a patient with rheumatoid arthritis and Sjögren's syndrome with dry eyes.

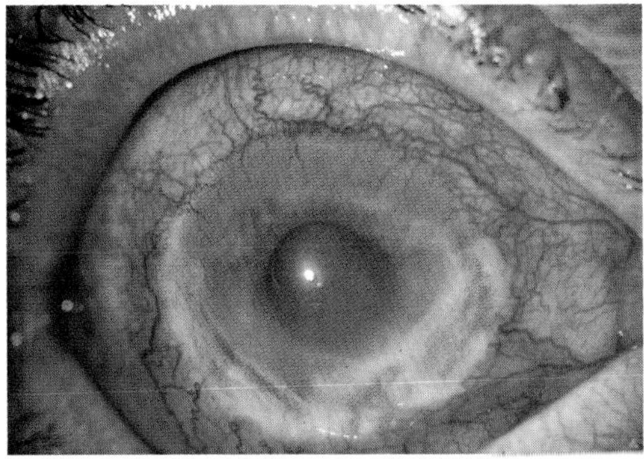

FIGURE 9–3 **Peripheral ulcerative keratitis in rheumatoid arthritis.** Peripheral ulcerative keratitis in a patient with rheumatoid arthritis. Notice the peripheral location of the lesion, its ulcerative nature with loss of stromal substance, and the inflammatory characteristics with white cell infiltrates in the corneal stroma.

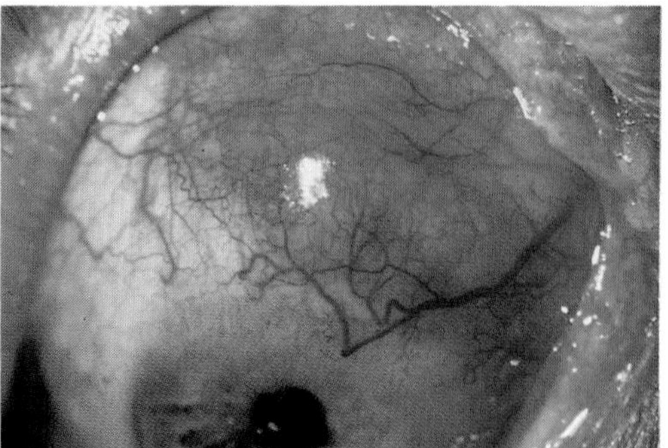

FIGURE 9–4 **Nodular scleritis in rheumatoid arthritis.** Note not only the area of scleral inflammation with nodule formation, but also the area anterior to the nodule of mild "uveal show," showing the loss of sclera from an area of previous inflammation.

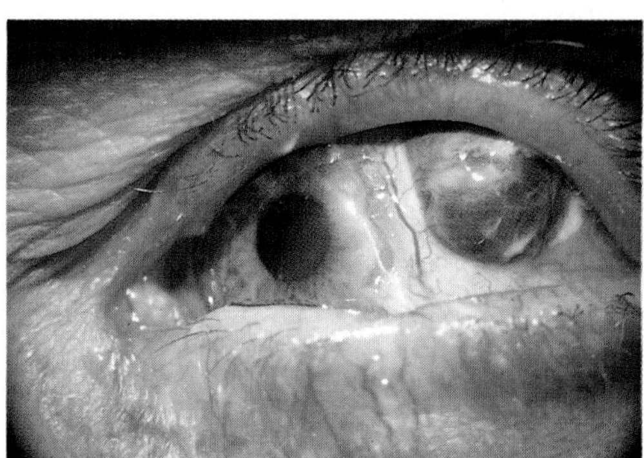

FIGURE 9–5 **Rheumatoid arthritis.** Scleromalacia perforans.

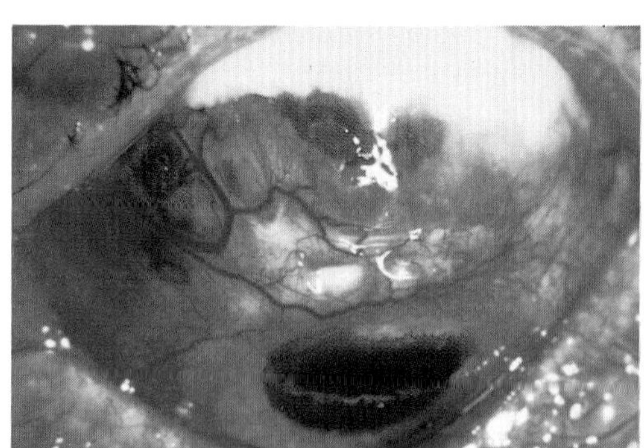

FIGURE 9–6 **Necrotizing scleritis in a patient with rheumatoid arthritis.** Note scleral loss, the uveal show, and the inflamed tissue surrounding the uveal show.

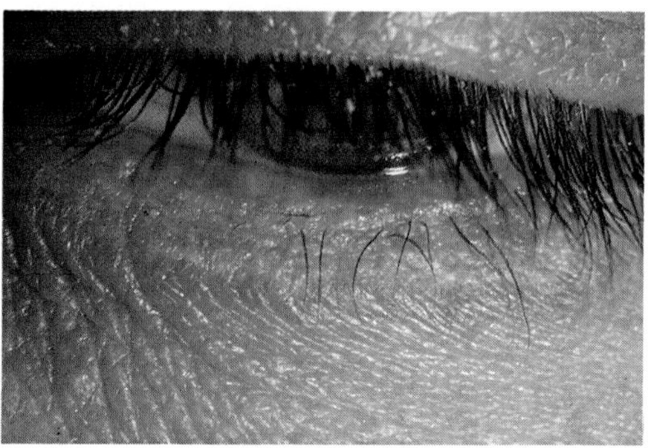

FIGURE 9–7 **Discoid systemic lupus erythematosus.** Discoid systemic lupus erythematosus, lower eyelid skin. Note the erythematous, raised, scaly dermatitis with madarosis and thick, erythematous lid margins.

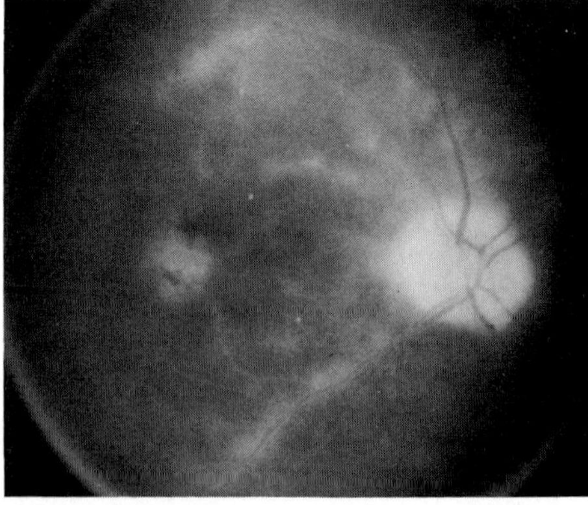

FIGURE 9–8 **Lupus erythematosus retinopathy.** Fluorescein angiogram of systemic lupus erythematosus retinopathy. Note the late staining of retinal vessels, particularly the arterioles, with areas of nonperfusion.

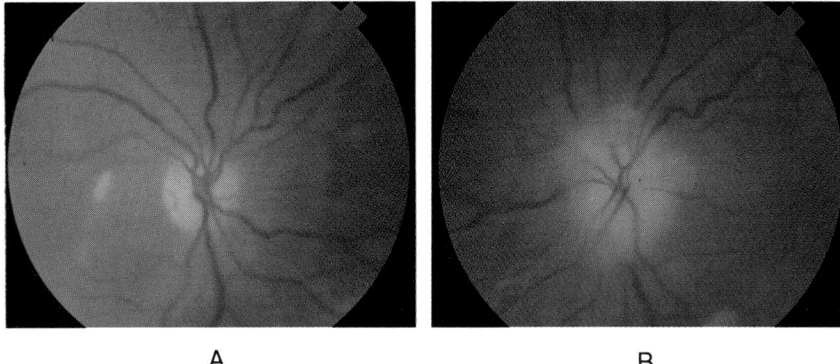

FIGURE 9–9 **Temporal arteritis.** Fundus photographs of the right (*A*) and left (*B*) optic discs of a 69-year-old woman with temporal arteritis. Photographs were taken 1 day after presentation. The patient complained of severe bilateral temporal and frontal headache and "a cold" for several weeks, 10-day history of vision loss OD, and a 1-day history of vision loss OS. The erythrocyte sedimentation rate was greater than 169.5 mm/hour. Visual acuity was "no light perception" OD and "light perception" OS. The right fundus shows a pale, slightly edematous disc; a cotton-wool spot; and venous congestion, consistent with recent arthritic anterior ischemic optic neuropathy (AION). The left fundus shows a chalky, pale, markedly edematous disc; no hemorrhage; and a cotton-wool spot, all typical of acute arthritic AION.

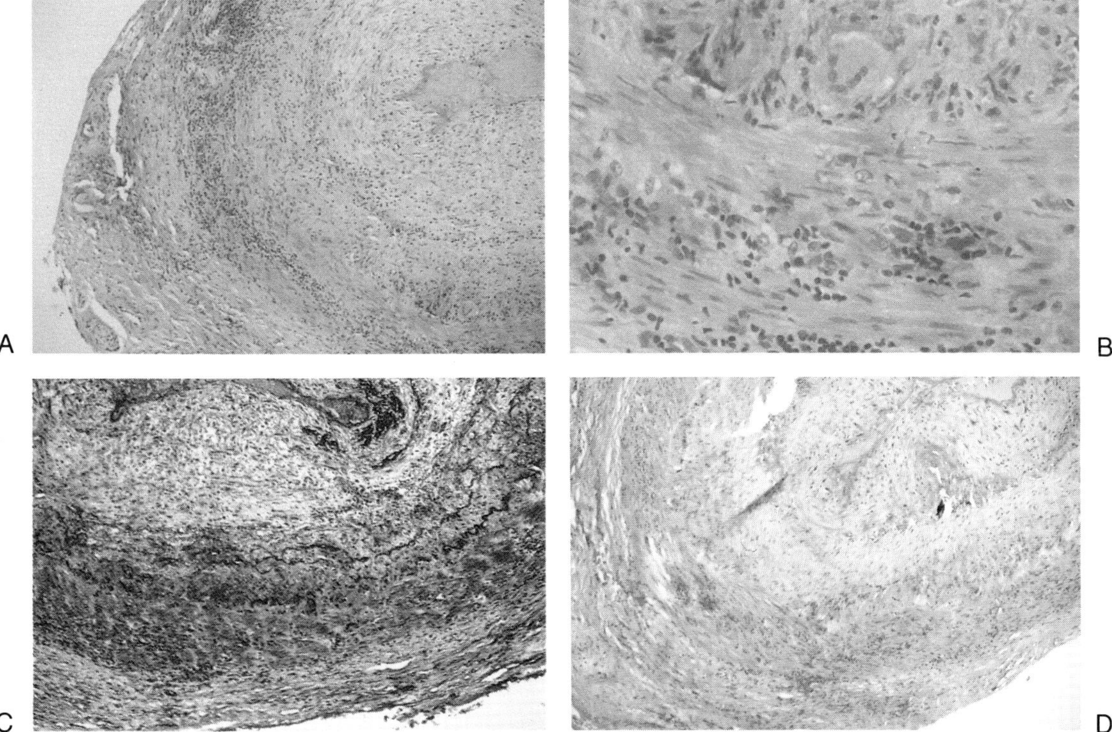

FIGURE 9–10 **Temporal artery biopsy.** Photomicrographs of abnormal temporal artery biopsy specimen from the patient whose fundus photographs were presented in Figure 9–9. *A,* A low-power view of the temporal artery showing thrombosis, intimal hyperplasia, and inflammatory infiltration of the muscular layers of the arterial wall. At the lower right-hand corner of the photograph, a multinucleated giant cell is present just internal to the muscularis, at the level of the internal elasticum, which cannot be discerned with this stain. H & E. *B,* A high-power view of this multinucleated giant cell. This micrograph also shows the mononuclear inflammatory infiltration of the muscularis seen in *A. C,* A low-power view of a section similar to *A* showing disruption and reduplication of the elastic laminae (Verhoeff's modified elastic stain). *D,* A photomicrograph of another region from this same temporal artery biopsy specimen, demonstrating virtually no arteritic involvement. The existence of skip areas such as this one mandates the microscopic examination of biopsied arteries at several points along their length so as not to miss the diagnosis.

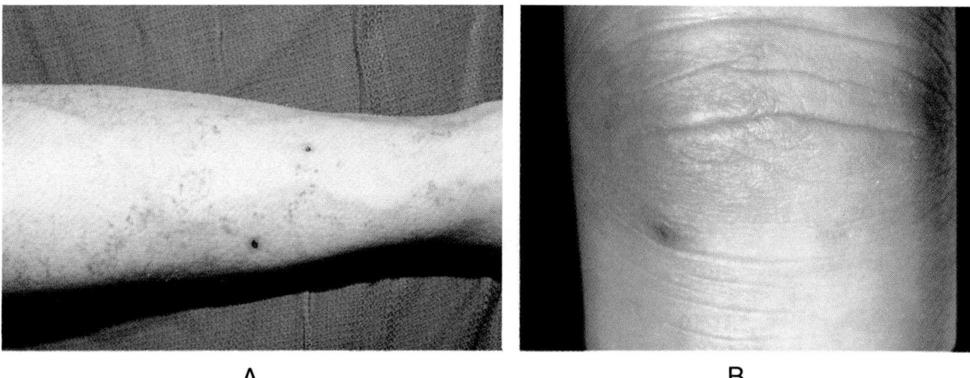

FIGURE 9–11 **Wegener's granulomatosis.** *A,* Ulcers and palpable purpura in a patient with Wegener's granulomatosis. *B,* Purpuric vesicle in another patient with active generalized Wegener's granulomatosis.

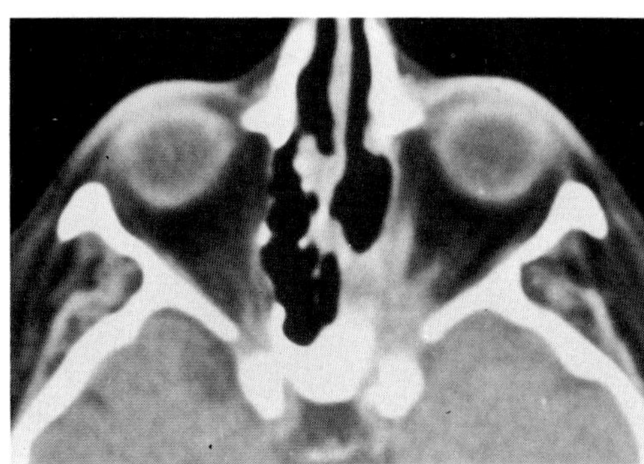

FIGURE 9–12 **Wegener's granulomatosis.** Computed tomography scan showing a mass at the left orbital apex in a 69-year-old woman who presented with progressive left-sided proptosis, ophthalmoplegia, optic neuropathy, and malaise. The mass extended to the cavernous sinus, and there was opacification of the sphenoid sinus. The patient developed *Klebsiella* meningitis. Exploration of the sinuses to localize the cerebrospinal fluid leak revealed inflammatory tissue suggestive of Wegener's granulomatosis. Biopsy of this tissue confirmed the diagnosis.

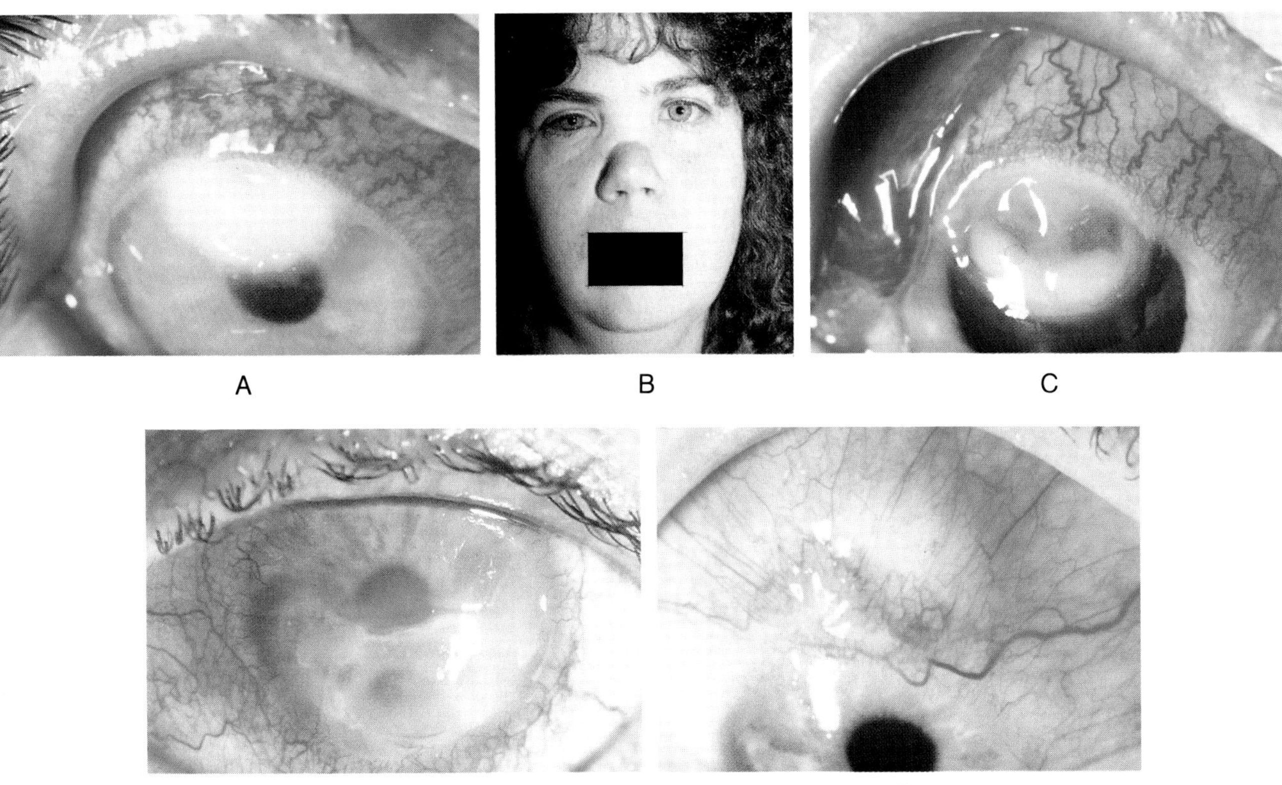

FIGURE 9–13 **Wegener's granulomatosis.** *A,* Focal ophthalmic involvement in the form of superinfected peripheral ulcerative keratitis as a localized recurrence in a 32-year-old woman with a history of Wegener's granulomatosis. The patient had a history of scleritis and renal, sinus, and central nervous system involvement but had been in remission for 8 years after cyclophosphamide therapy. *B,* Photograph of patient's face showing saddle nose deformity seen in some patients with Wegener's granulomatosis. *C,* Progressive melting of the cornea after pneumococcal superinfection was eradicated, despite the use of topical medroxyprogesterone as a collagenase inhibitor. At the time of therapeutic conjunctival resection, necrotizing scleritis was noted. Tissue adhesive and bandage contact lens were applied. Systemic cyclophosphamide therapy was initiated for this sight-threatening process. *D,* Peripheral ulcerative keratitis in another patient with Wegener's granulomatosis. *E,* Nodular scleritis in another patient with Wegener's granulomatosis.

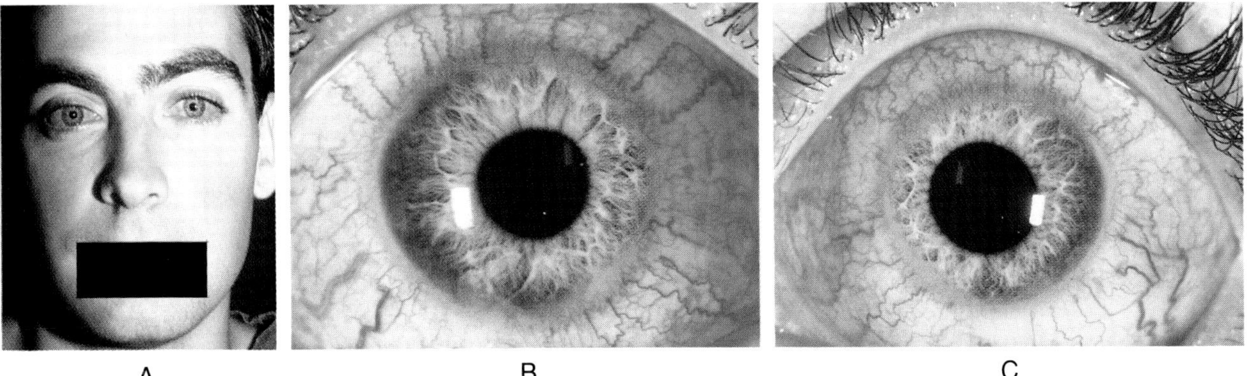

FIGURE 9–14 **Wegener's granulomatosis.** *A,* A 22-year-old man with a 6-week history of "red eyes" unresponsive to topical antibiotic and steroid therapy. There was no change in vision or discomfort of any kind. *B* and *C,* Higher magnification, showing diffuse bilateral episcleritis. Systemic work up was positive for C-antineutrophil cytoplasmic antibodies (ANCA), abnormal urinary sediment containing red blood cells and casts, and rising blood urea nitrogen and serum creatinine. Review of systems was significant for a 6-week history of epistaxis. Chest x-ray and sinus films were normal. The diagnosis of generalized Wegener's granulomatosis was made, and the patient received intravenous pulse therapy of cyclophosphamide followed by maintenance therapy.

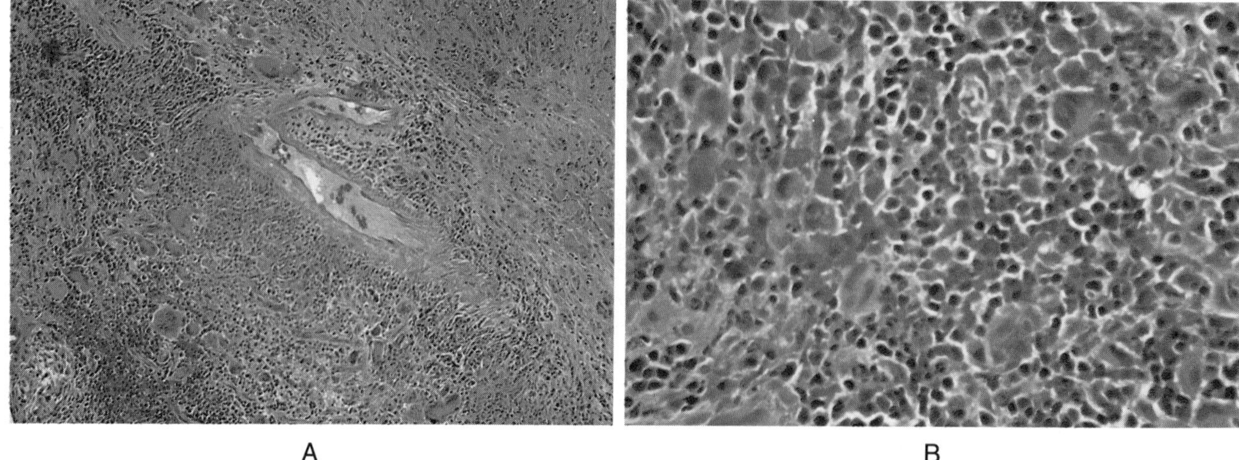

FIGURE 9–15 **Histopathology of Wegener's granulomatosis.** *A* and *B,* Photomicrographs of involved ocular and orbital tissue from patients with positive ANCA titers, showing granulomatous foci, collagen necrosis, perivascular infiltration, and infiltration with neutrophils.

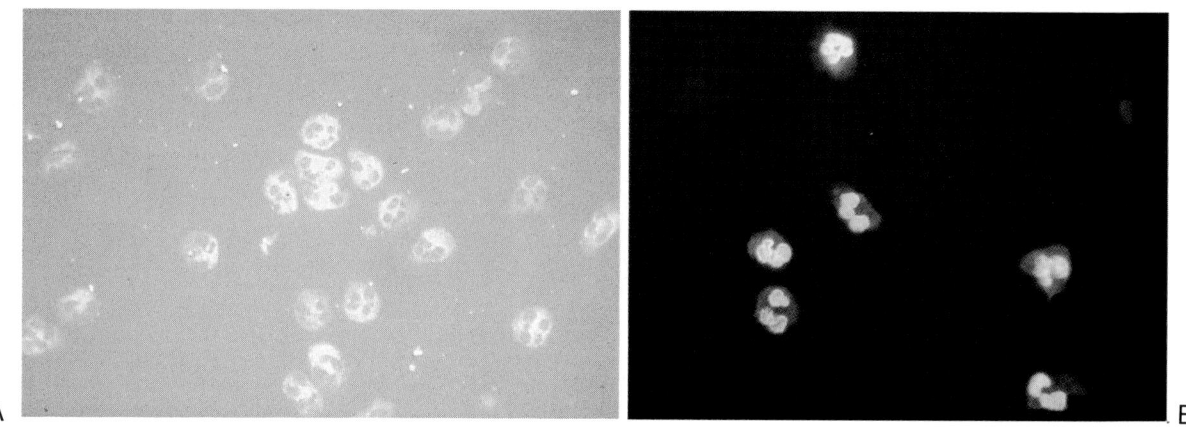

FIGURE 9–16 **Histopathology of Wegener's granulomatosis.** *A,* Photomicrograph showing the positive ANCA pattern of staining by indirect immunofluorescence technique. This micrograph reveals the presence of ANCA in the cytoplasmic staining characteristic of Wegener's granulomatosis. *B,* This micrograph reveals the presence of ANCA in the parameter (P) or P-ANCA pattern of staining, which is more characteristic of polyarteritis nodosa and crescentic and idiopathic glomerulonephritis. (Photomicrographs courtesy of John Niles, M.D., Departments of Nephrology and Immunopathology, Massachusetts General Hospital, Boston.)

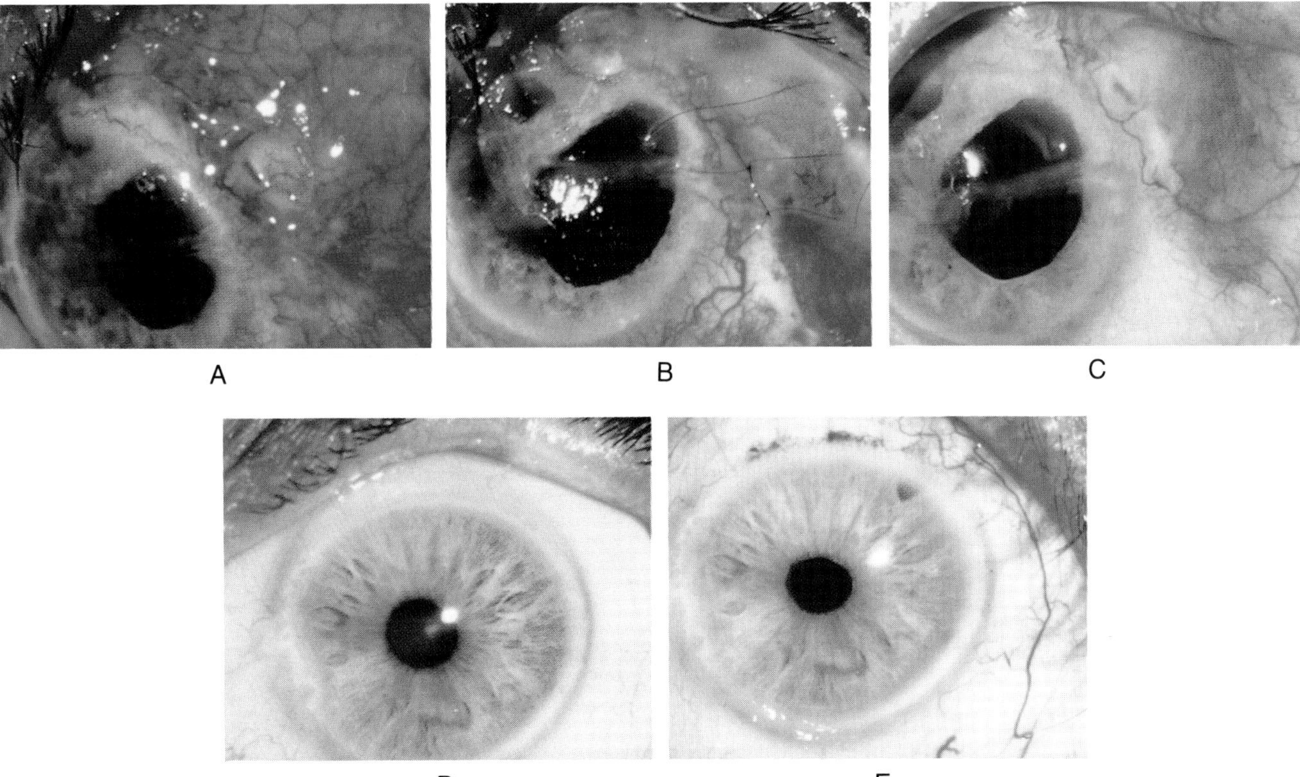

FIGURE 9-17 **Wegener's granulomatosis.** *A,* Postsurgical necrotizing scleritis at the wound in a patient with treated Wegener's granulomatosis who underwent routine cataract extraction while in remission and off cyclophosphamide. *B,* Progression of necrotizing process despite conjunctival resection and tectonic grafting, with melting and loss of the graft. *C,* Reduction of inflammation and halting of necrosis after induction of remission with a second course of cyclophosphamide. The prominent staphyloma remained stable until the patient's death many years later from alcoholic liver disease. *D,* Preoperative and, *E,* postoperative photographs from this same patient, who subsequently underwent cataract extraction in the other eye while on maintenance therapy of cyclophosphamide and prednisone. No unusual inflammation occurred.

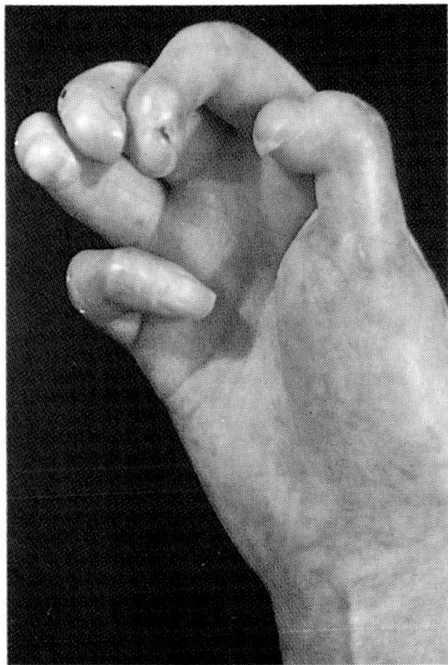

FIGURE 9-18 **CREST syndrome.** Note the calcinosis at the tips of the fingers, the obvious sclerodactyly, and even the presence of a nail-bed infarct on the middle finger.

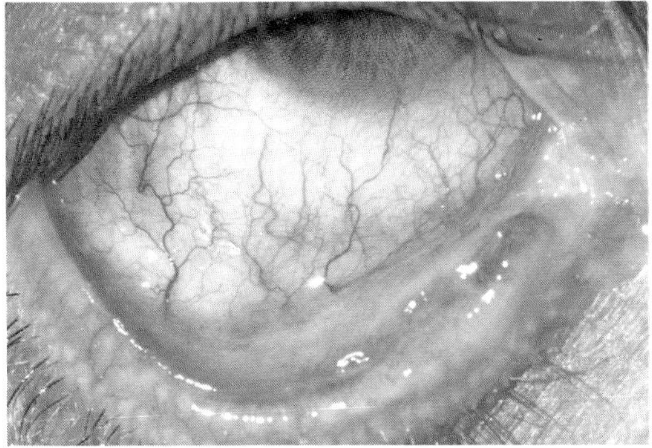

FIGURE 9-19 **Conjunctival subepithelial fibrosis in a patient with progressive systemic scleroderma.** Note the fornix foreshortening and the white fibrosis under the tarsal and fornix conjunctival epithelium. No frank symblepharon exists.

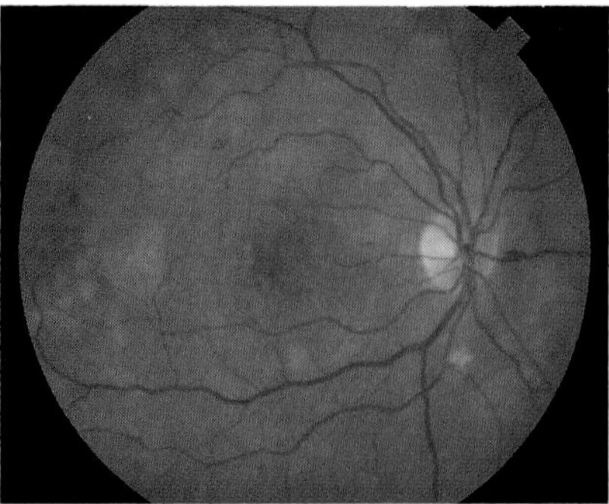

FIGURE 9–20 **Progressive systemic sclerodermic retinopathy.** Note the scattered intraretinal exudates, hemorrhages, and the multifocal choroidal infarcts.

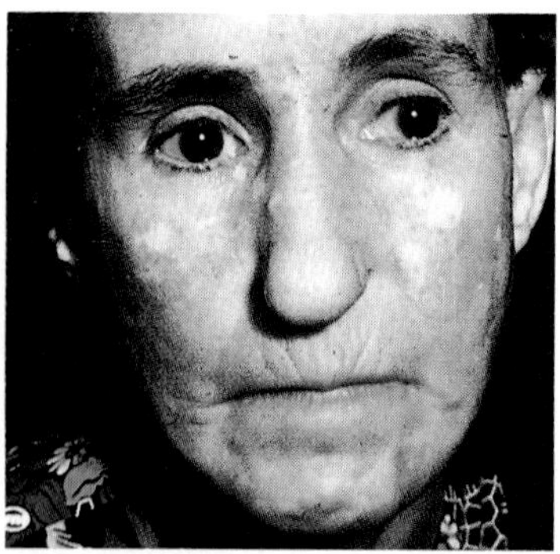

FIGURE 9–22 **Moderately advanced progressive systemic scleroderma.** Typical blepharophimosis and pursed lip appearance of a patient with progressive systemic scleroderma, moderately advanced.

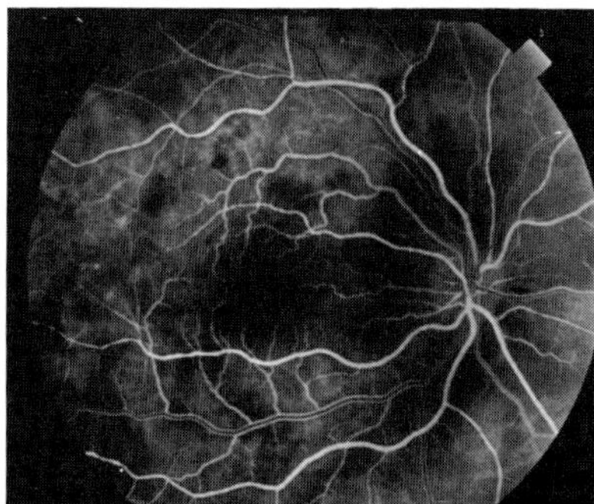

FIGURE 9–21 **Progressive systemic sclerodermic retinopathy.** Same patient as in Figure 9–20, fluorescein angiogram, early transient. Note especially the fluorescein angiographic pattern in the choroid, with the focal nonperfusion and patchy distribution of areas of nonfilling of the choroidal vasculature.

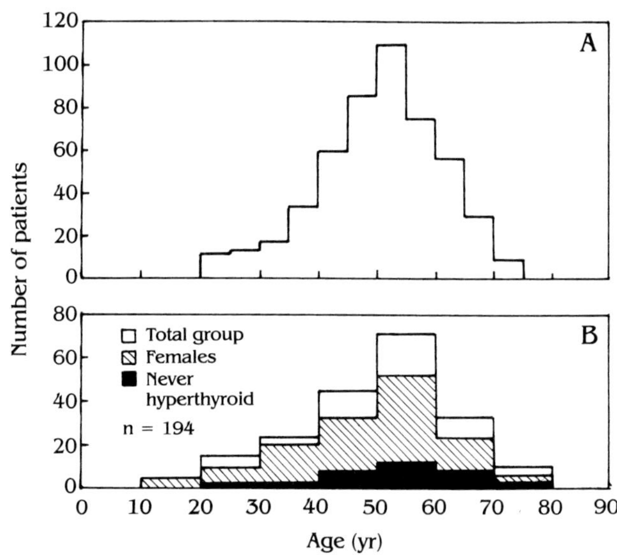

FIGURE 9–23 **Age distribution of hyperthyroidism.** Age distribution of 500 patients with hyperthyroidism (*A*) compared with that of 194 patients who underwent orbital decompression for severe orbitopathy (*B*). (From Jacobson DH, Gorman CA: Endocrine ophthalmopathy: Current ideas concerning etiology, pathogenesis, and treatment. Endocr Rev 5:202, 1984. Copyright by the Endocrine Society.)

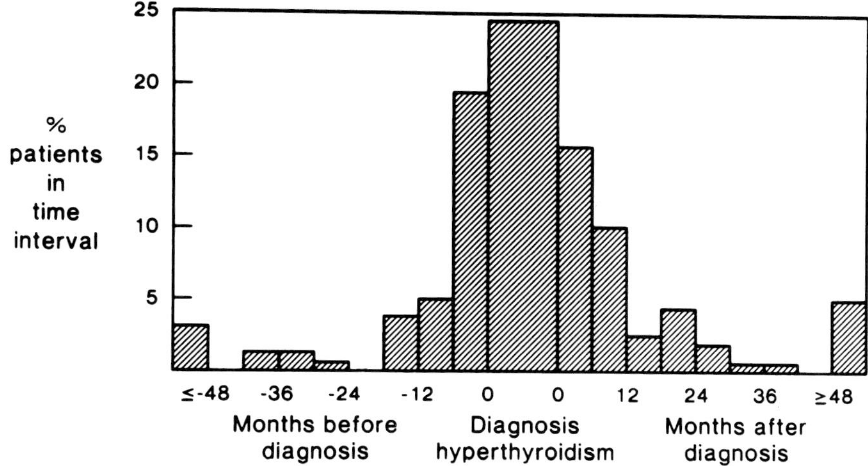

FIGURE 9–24 **Hyperthyroidism and Graves' disease.** Temporal relationship between the onset of hyperthyroidism and the onset of Graves' ophthalmopathy. The time of diagnosis of hyperthyroidism is zero on the horizontal axis. The number of patients who first experienced eye symptoms within a given 6-month period is expressed as a percentage of the entire group. (From Gorman CA: Temporal relationship between the onset of Graves' ophthalmopathy and diagnosis of thyrotoxicosis. Mayo Clin Proc 58:517, 1983.)

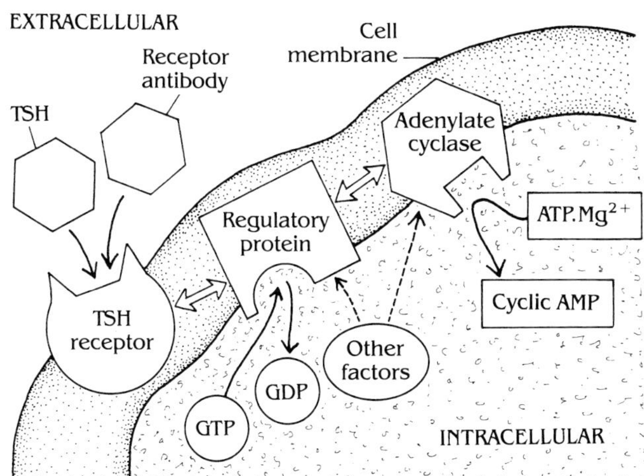

FIGURE 9–25 **Mechanism of thyrotropin (TSH) and TSH receptor antibody.** TSH receptor, activating the adenylate cyclase–cyclic AMP second messenger system, increases the production of thyroid hormone. (Modified from Baxter JD, Funder JW: Hormone receptors. N Engl J Med 301:1153, 1980.)

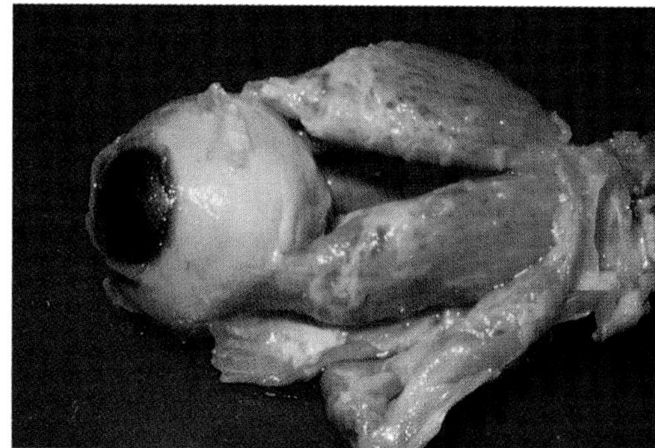

FIGURE 9–26 **Enlarged extraocular muscles in thyroid ophthalmopathy.** The specimen is from the exenterated orbital contents of a patient with Graves' ophthalmopathy. The orbital fat has been dissected away to show the massively swollen extraocular muscles. (From Hufnagel TJ, Hickey WF, Cobbs WH, et al: Immunohistochemical and ultrastructural studies on the exenterated orbital tissues of a patient with Graves' disease. Ophthalmology 91:1411–1419, 1984.)

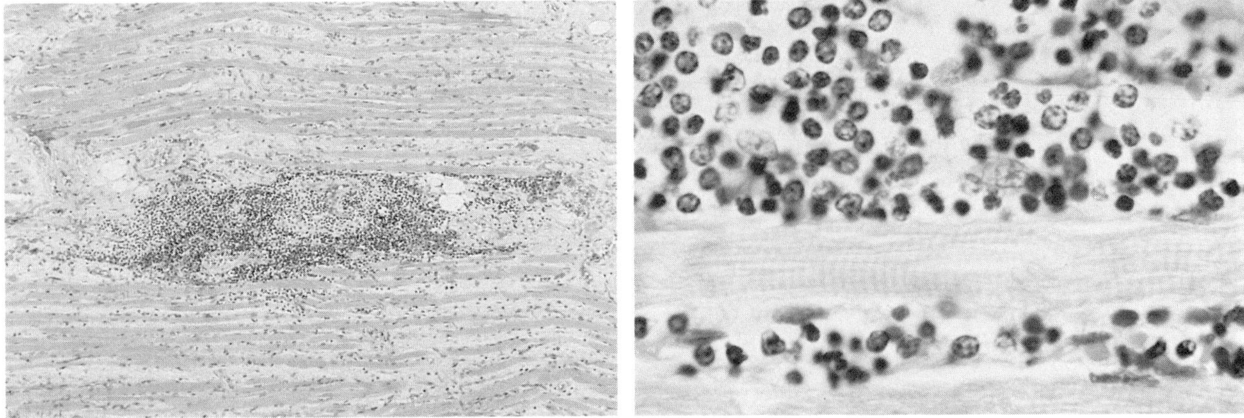

FIGURE 9–27 **Pathologic changes early in the course of thyroid ophthalmopathy.** In the acute phase, there is a lymphocytic inflammatory infiltrate. *A,* Lymphoid infiltrates may be focal and can initially involve the endomysial connective tissue. H&E stain. *B,* At higher magnification, note the dense lymphoid infiltrate and increased intracellular fluid content. H&E stain. (From Jakobiec FA, Font RL: Orbit. *In* Spencer WH (ed): Ophthalmic Pathology, 3rd ed, Vol. 3. Philadelphia, WB Saunders, 1986.)

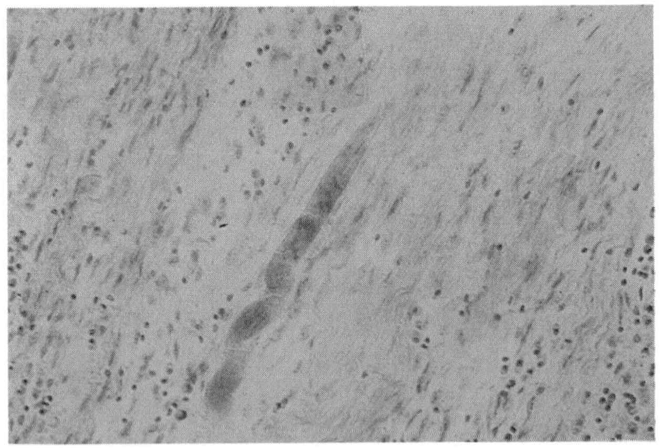

FIGURE 9–28 **Pathologic changes late in the course of thyroid ophthalmopathy.** In thyroid ophthalmopathy, there is progressive fibrosis of extraocular muscles. Note that the entire muscle has been replaced by fibrosis with a scattering of mononuclear inflammatory cells. H&E stain.

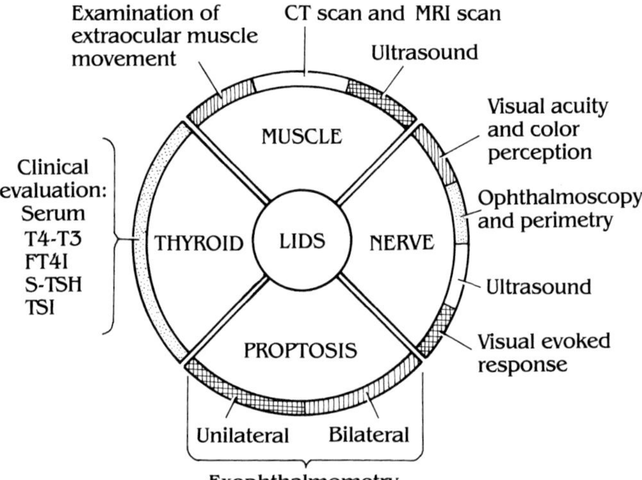

FIGURE 9–29 **Clinical and laboratory findings associated with thyroid ophthalmopathy.** When all features are present, the diagnosis is certain. The diagnosis is likely when all features in a single quadrant are present. Isolated eyelid, muscle, or nerve involvement is uncommon in thyroid ophthalmopathy. (Modified from Gorman CA: Extrathyroidal manifestations of Graves' disease. *In* Ingbar SH, Braverman LE (eds): The Thyroid. Philadelphia, JB Lippincott, 1984, p. 1021.)

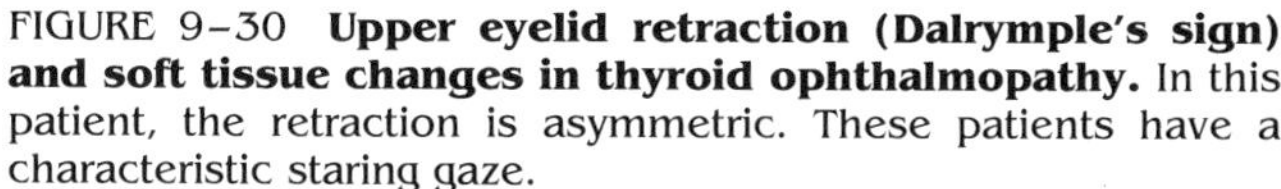

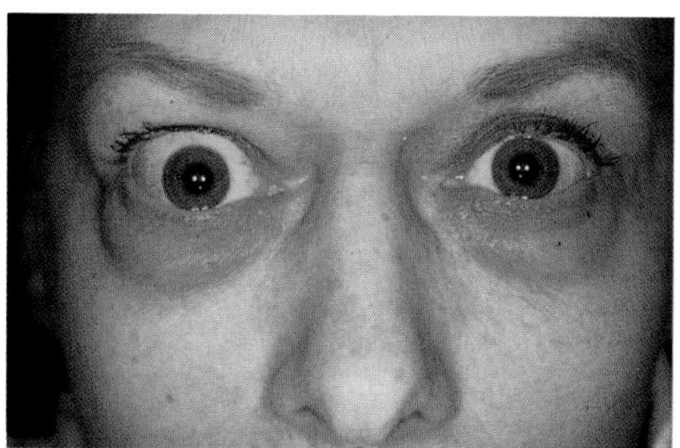

FIGURE 9-30 **Upper eyelid retraction (Dalrymple's sign) and soft tissue changes in thyroid ophthalmopathy.** In this patient, the retraction is asymmetric. These patients have a characteristic staring gaze.

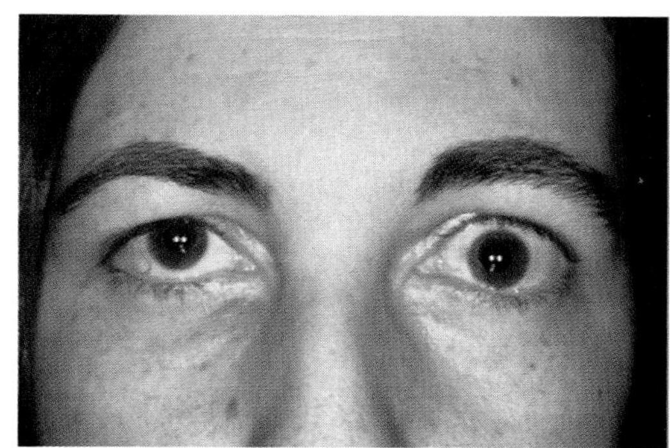

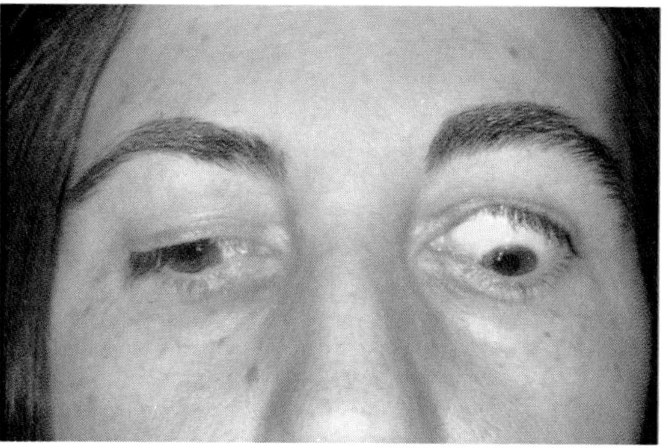

FIGURE 9-31 **Von Graefe's sign in thyroid ophthalmopathy.** *A,* Left upper eyelid retraction and, *B,* upper eyelid lag on downgaze (von Graefe's sign) in a patient with thyroid ophthalmopathy.

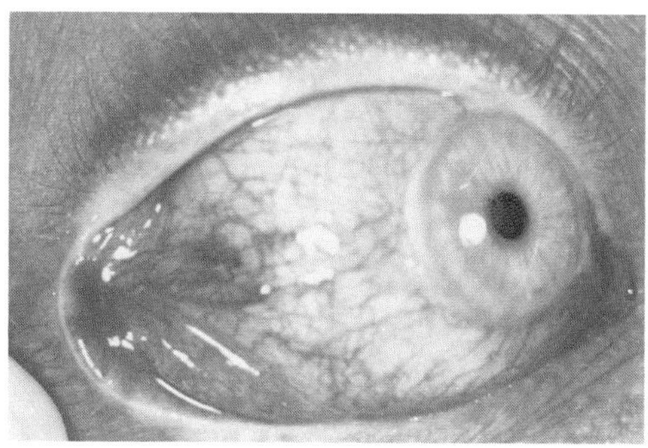

FIGURE 9-32 **Goldzieher's sign in thyroid ophthalmopathy.** Deep injection of temporal conjunctival vessels (Goldzieher's sign).

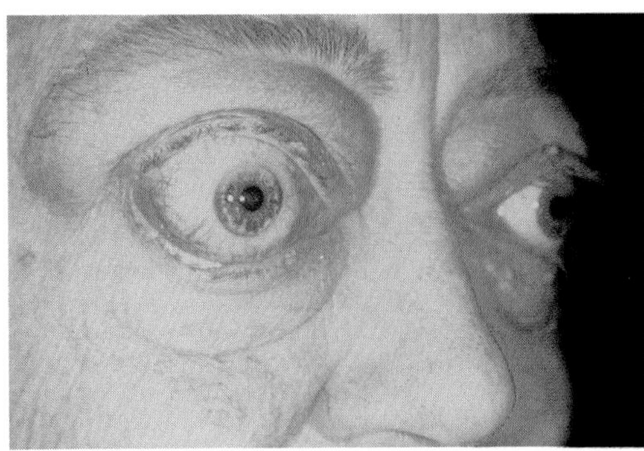

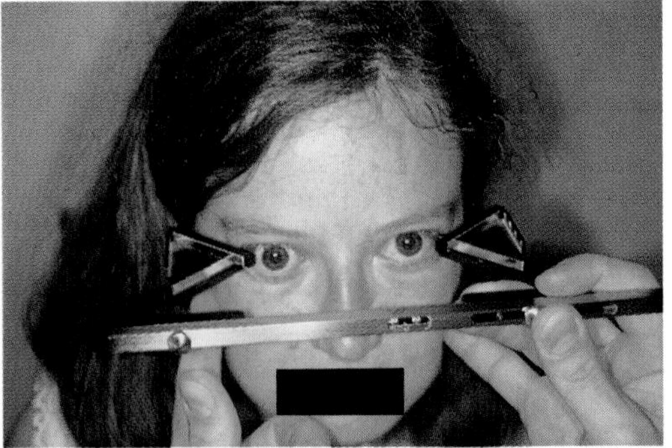

FIGURE 9–33 **Thyroid ophthalmopathy.** *A,* Marked proptosis in thyroid ophthalmopathy associated with upper and lower eyelid retraction. *B,* Measurement of exophthalmos with exophthalmometer.

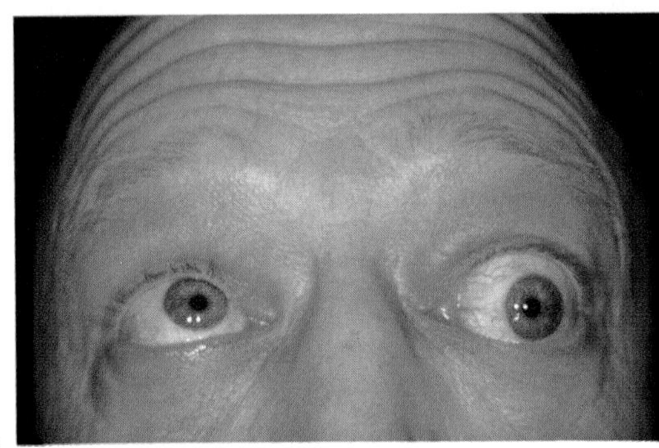

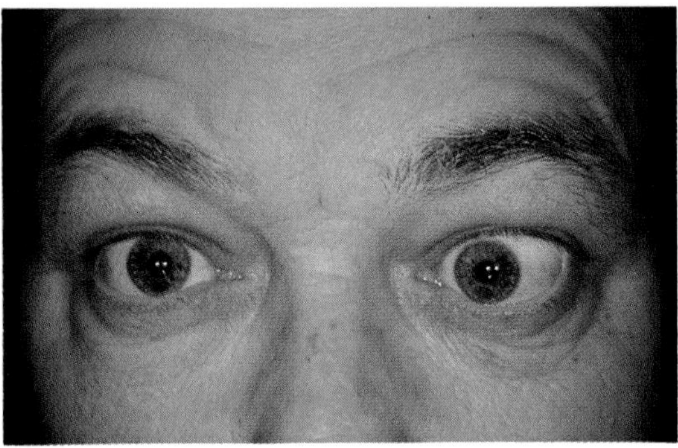

FIGURE 9–34 **Thyroid ophthalmopathy.** *A,* Limitation of upgaze of the left eye due to restrictive myopathy of the left inferior rectus muscle. *B,* Left esodeviation due to a tethered left medial rectus muscle.

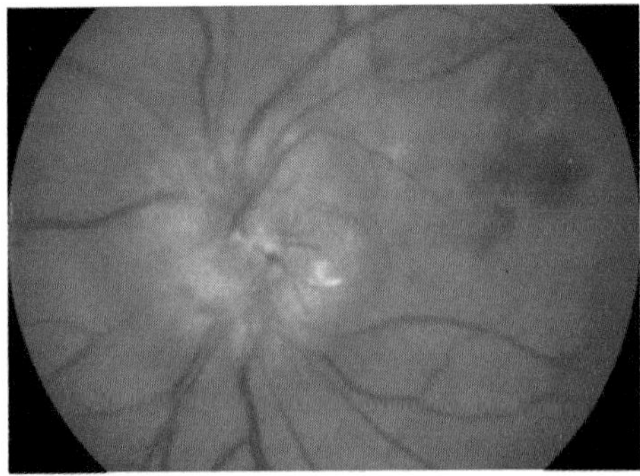

FIGURE 9–35 Optic nerve swelling in a patient with thyroid ophthalmopathy. Most patients with optic neuropathy do not have optic nerve changes on ophthalmoscopy.

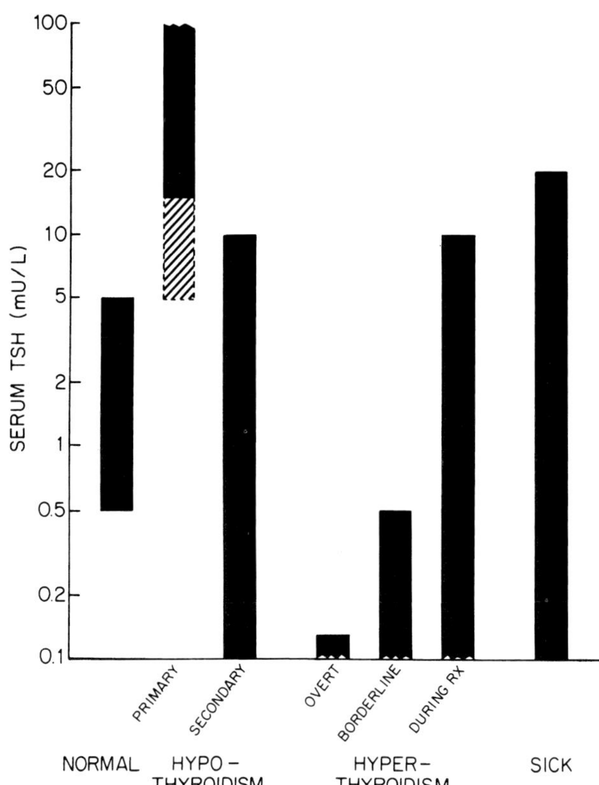

FIGURE 9–36 The range of values of sensitive TSH assay (S-TSH) for normal individuals and patients with hypothyroidism, hyperthyroidism, and acute nonthyroidal illness. (From Larsen PR, Ingbar S: The thyroid gland. *In* Williams RH (ed): Textbook of Endocrinology, 8th ed. Philadelphia, WB Saunders, 1992.)

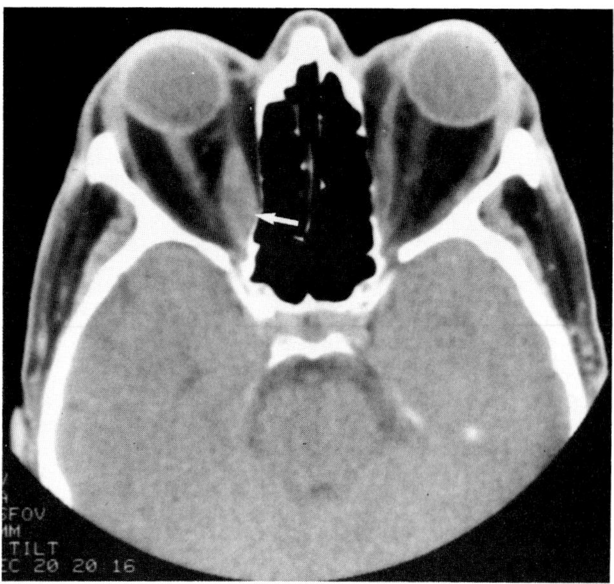

FIGURE 9–37 **Muscle changes in thyroid ophthalmopathy.** Axial computed tomography image of a patient with enlargement of the nontendinous portion of extraocular muscles. The equator of the globe is anterior to the lateral orbital rim, indicating proptosis. The right medial rectus muscle *(arrow)* is markedly abnormal.

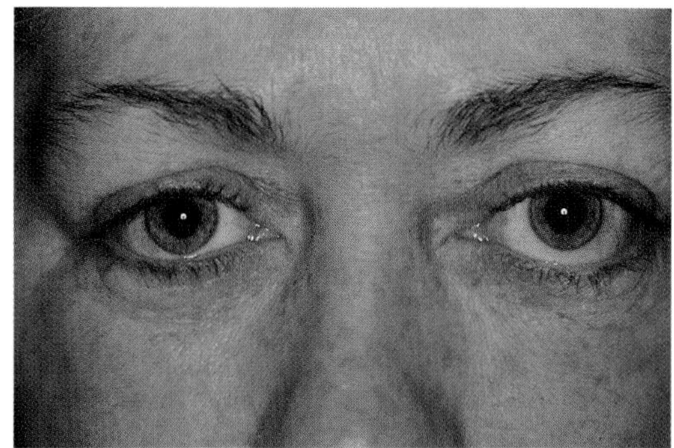

A

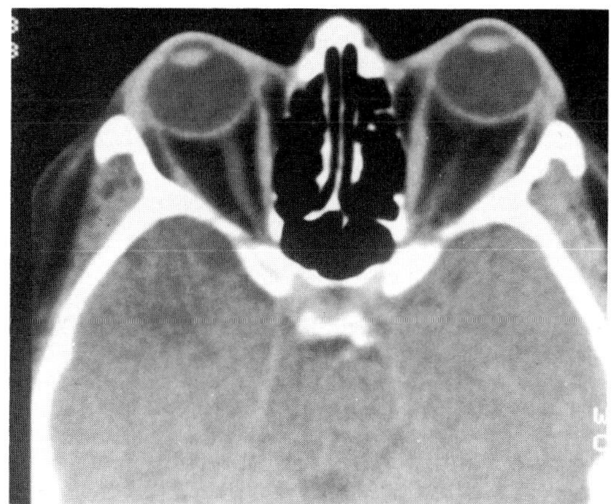

B

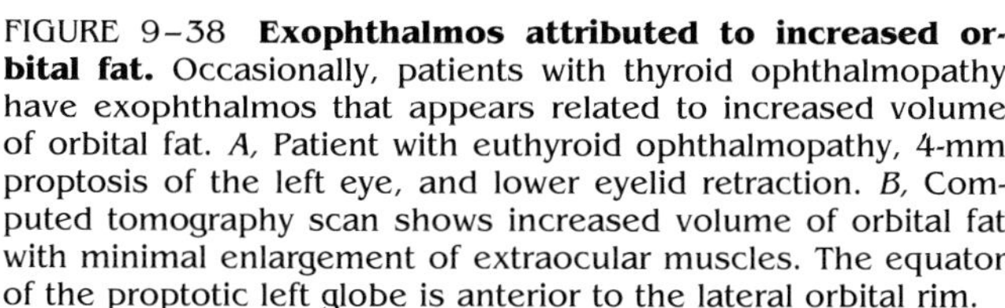

FIGURE 9–38 **Exophthalmos attributed to increased orbital fat.** Occasionally, patients with thyroid ophthalmopathy have exophthalmos that appears related to increased volume of orbital fat. *A,* Patient with euthyroid ophthalmopathy, 4-mm proptosis of the left eye, and lower eyelid retraction. *B,* Computed tomography scan shows increased volume of orbital fat with minimal enlargement of extraocular muscles. The equator of the proptotic left globe is anterior to the lateral orbital rim.

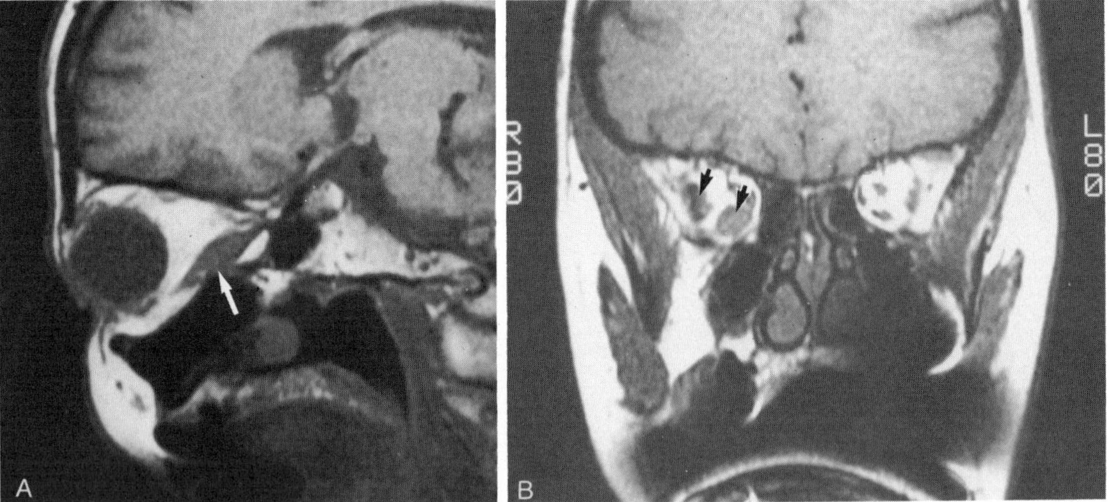

FIGURE 9–39 **Magnetic resonance imaging of patient with thyroid ophthalmopathy.** *A,* Parasagittal image shows enlargement of the nontendinous portion of the right inferior rectus muscle *(arrow)*. *B,* Coronal image demonstrates enlargement of the right inferior and lateral rectus muscles *(arrows)*.

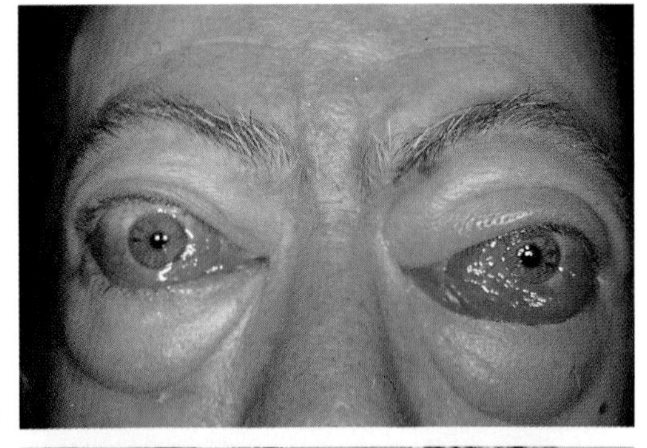
A

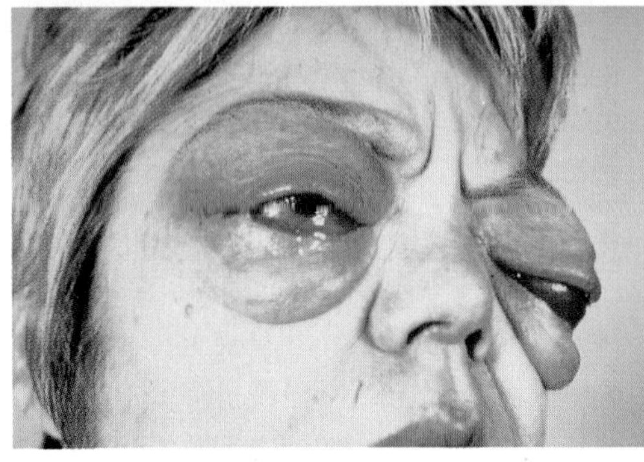
B

FIGURE 9–40 **Malignant exophthalmos.** *A,* A patient with characteristic findings of severe acute thyroid ophthalmopathy (so-called malignant exophthalmos), including hyperthyroidism, soft tissue inflammation and congestion, exophthalmos, and visual loss due to optic neuropathy. The majority of patients present with more subtle findings of thyroid eye disease. *B,* Another patient with fulminating thyroid ophthalmopathy who has marked lid swelling and secondary ptosis, rather than the more typical eyelid retraction. (*B,* Courtesy of G. H. Daniels, M.D., Thyroid Unit, Massachusetts General Hospital, Boston.)

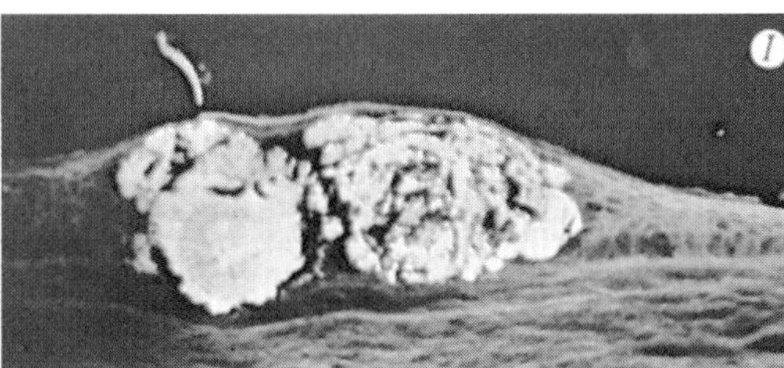

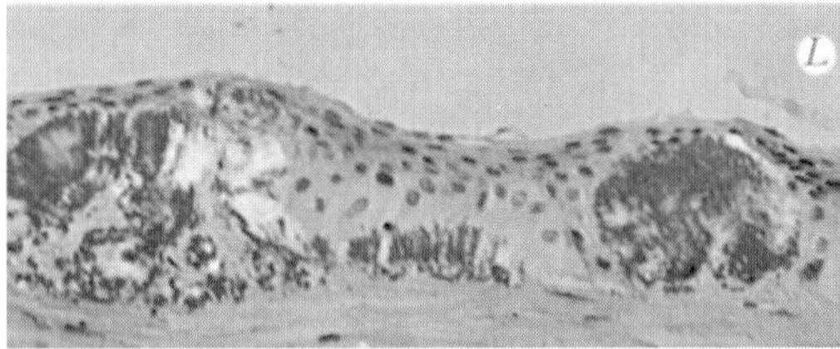

FIGURE 9–41 **Histopathology of amyloid.** *Top,* Congo red preparation of amyloid deposit, showing birefringence. *Bottom,* Congo red preparation of amyloid deposit, showing red-green dichroism. (From Smith M, Zimmerman LE: Amyloidosis of the eyelid and conjunctiva. Arch Ophthalmol 75(1):51, 1966. Copyright 1966, American Medical Association.)

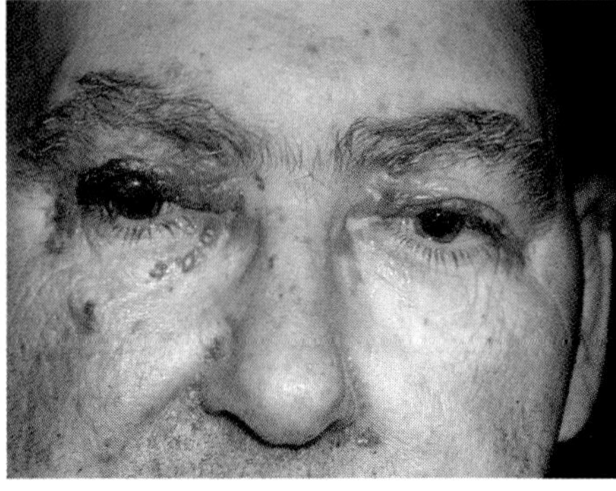

FIGURE 9–42 **Primary systemic amyloidosis.** Eyelid and facial skin involvement in primary systemic amyloidosis.

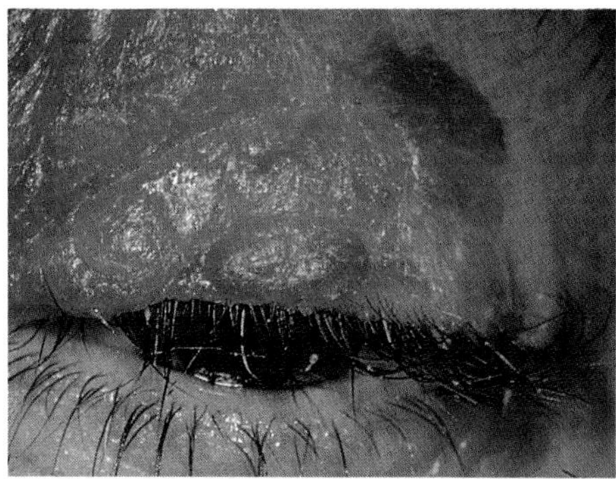

FIGURE 9–43 **Eyelid involvement in amyloidosis.** Close-up of waxy, hemorrhagic papules in eyelid amyloid deposits.

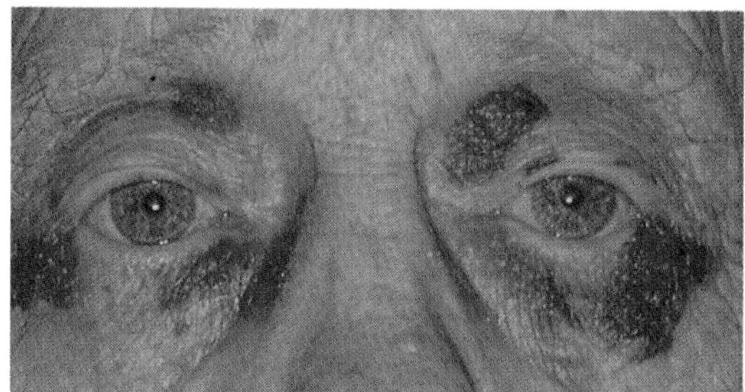

FIGURE 9–44 **Periorbital purpura.** Postproctoscopic periorbital purpura in previously unrecognized systemic amyloidosis. (From Slagel GA, Lupton GP: Postprotoscopic periorbital purpura. Arch Dermatol 122(4):464, 1986. Copyright 1986, American Medical Association.)

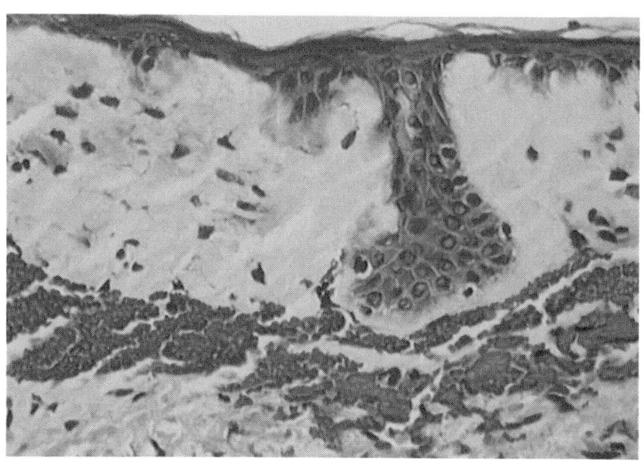

FIGURE 9–45 Dermal biopsy from patient shown in Figure 9–44. Note amyloid deposits in dermis with overlying epidermal atrophy and underlying hermorrhage (From Slagel GA, Lupton GP: Postprotoscopic periorbital purpura. Arch Dermatol 122(4):464, 1986. Copyright 1986, American Medical Association.)

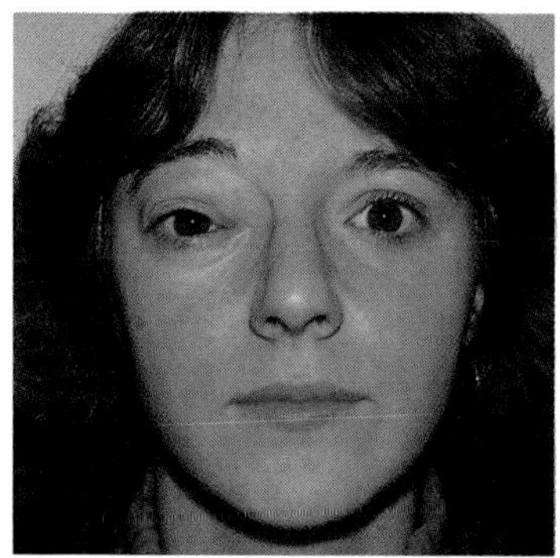

A

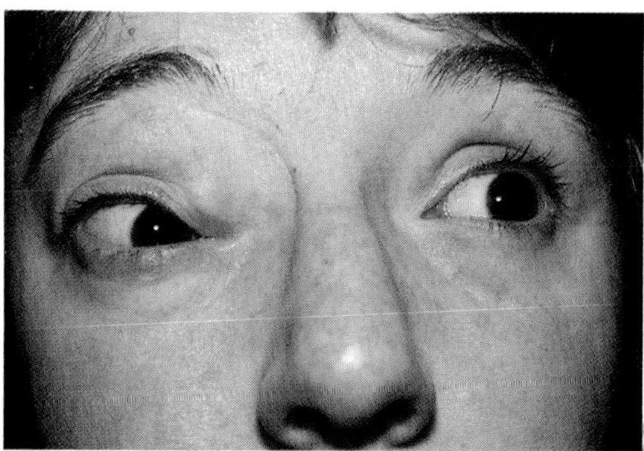

B

FIGURE 9–46 **Orbital amyloid tumor.** *A* and *B,* Orbital amyloid tumor. (Courtesy of Simmons Lessell, M.D.)

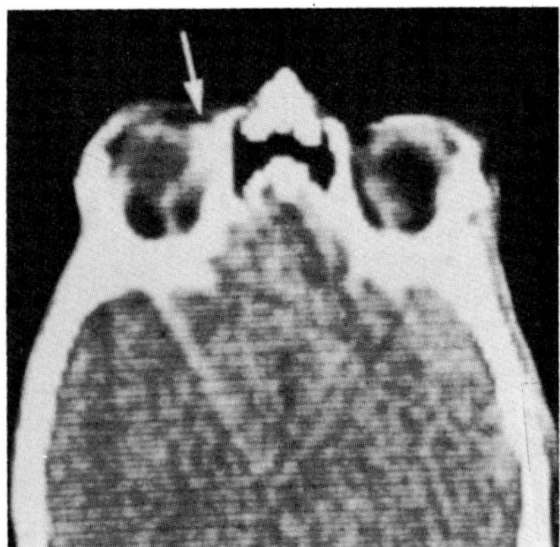

FIGURE 9–47 **Orbital amyloid tumor.** Computed tomography from patient depicted in Figure 9–46. (From Cohen AS, Lessell S: Amyloid tumor of the orbit. Neuroradiology 18:158, 1989.)

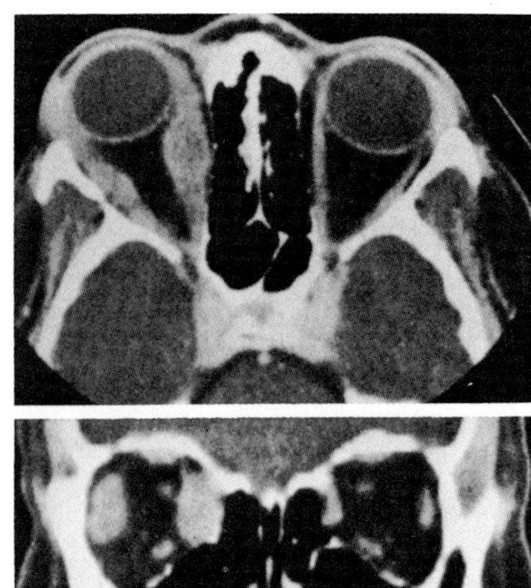

FIGURE 9–48 **Infiltration of extraocular muscles by amyloid.** Computed tomography depicting selective infiltration of extraocular muscles by amyloid. (From Erie JC, Garrity JA, Norman ME: Orbital amyloidosis involving the extraocular muscles. Arch Ophthalmol 107(10):1429, 1989. Copyright 1989, American Medical Association.)

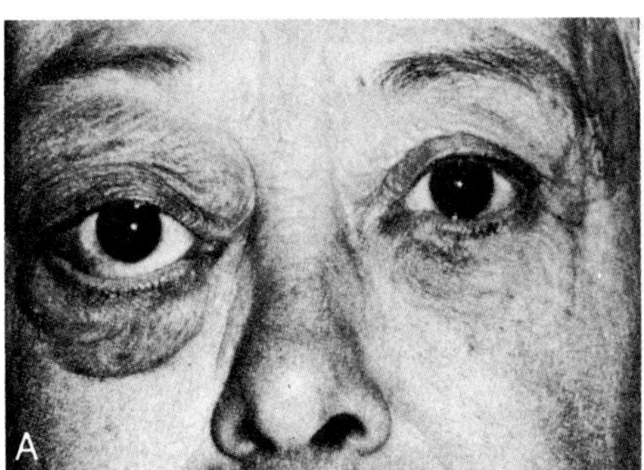

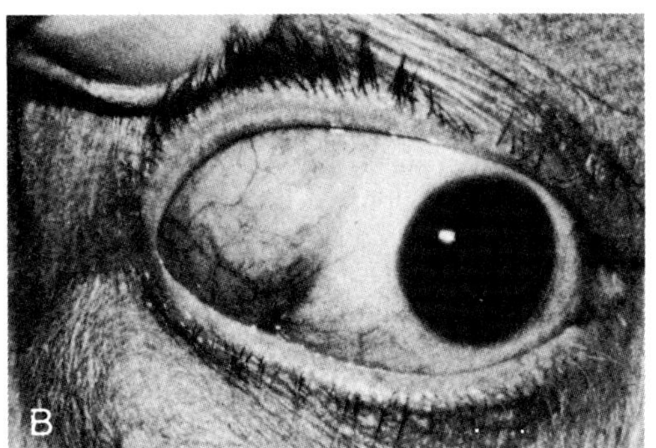

FIGURE 9–49 **Lacrimal gland amyloidosis.** *A* and *B*, Lacrimal gland amyloidosis simulating neoplasm. (From Levine MR, Buckman G: Primary localized amyloidosis. Ann Ophthalmol 18:166, 1986.)

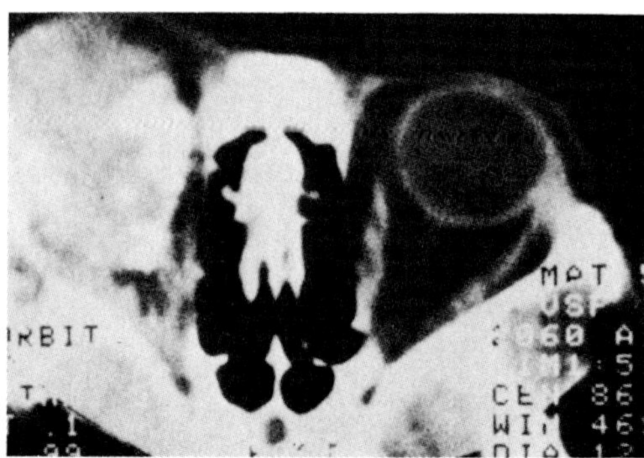

FIGURE 9–50 **Lacrimal gland amyloidosis.** Computed tomography from the patient depicted in Figure 9–49. (From Levine MR, Buckman G: Primary localized amyloidosis. Ann Ophthalmol 18:166, 1986.)

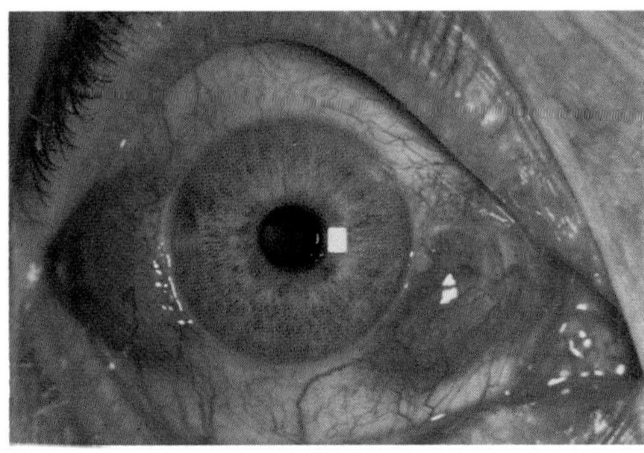

FIGURE 9–51 **Conjunctival amyloidosis.** Tumefactive conjunctival amyloidosis.

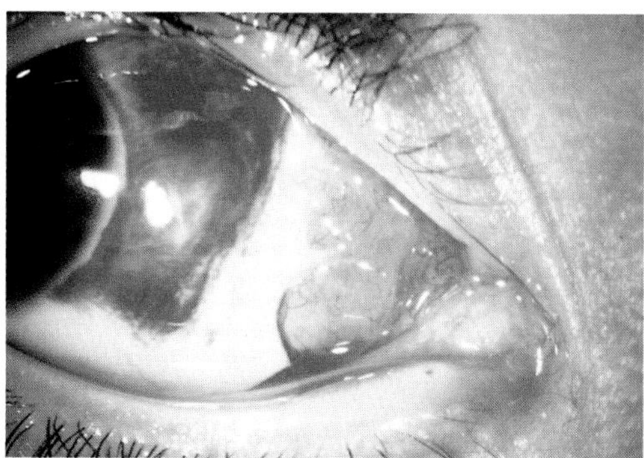

FIGURE 9–52 **Amyloid infiltration of the conjunctiva.** Nodular amyloid infiltration of the conjunctiva with spontaneous hemorrhage.

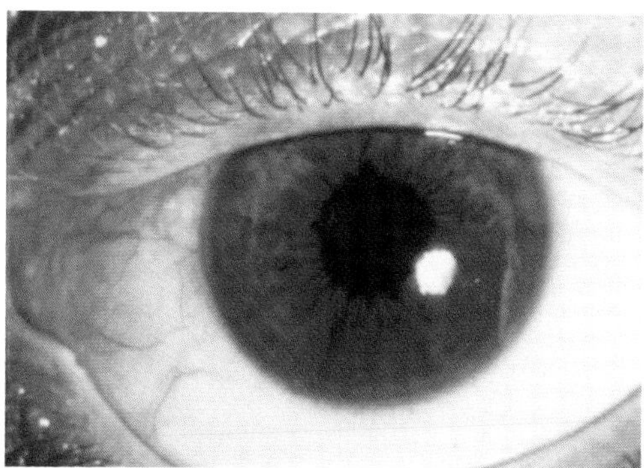

FIGURE 9–55 **Amyloidosis.** Scalloped pupil seen in heredofamilial neuropathic amyloidoses. (From Lessell S, Wolf PA, Benson MD, Cohen AS: Scalloped pupils in familial amyloidosis. N Engl J Med 293:914–915, 1975.)

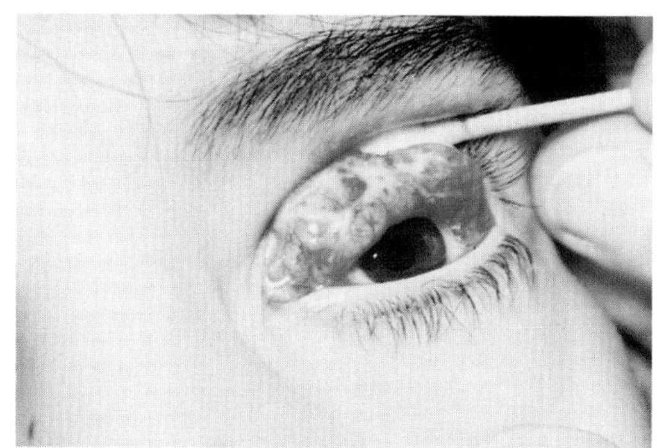

FIGURE 9–53 **Amyloid infiltration of the conjunctiva.** Diffuse amyloid infiltration of the palpebral conjunctiva.

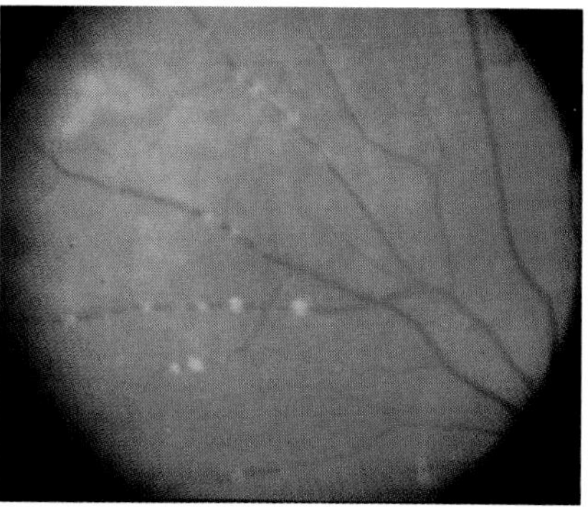

FIGURE 9–56 **Amyloidosis.** Amyloid deposits within retinal circulation. (From Schwartz MF, Green WR, Michels RG, et al: An unusual case of ocular involvement in primary systemic nonfamilial amyloidosis. Ophthalmology 89:394–401, 1982.)

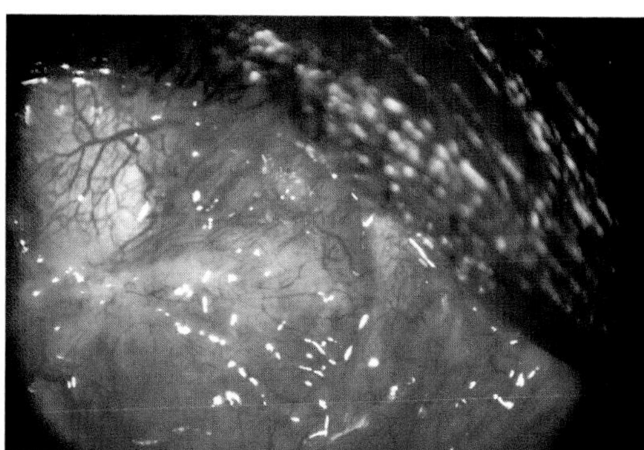

FIGURE 9–54 **Conjunctival amyloidosis.** Diffuse amyloid infiltration of the bulbar conjunctiva.

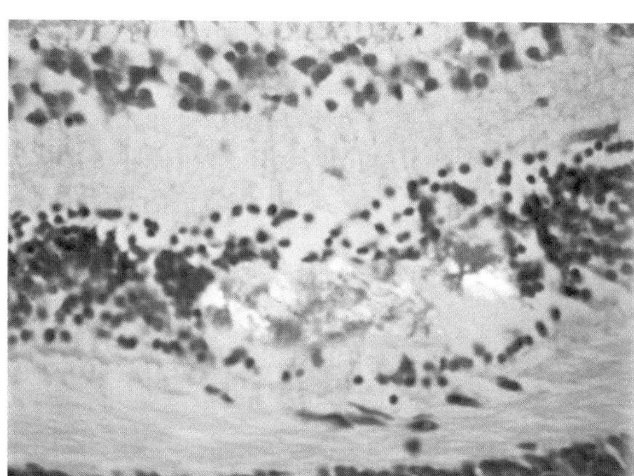

FIGURE 9–57 **Amyloidosis.** Congo red preparation of retina. Note dichroic deposit within retinal vessel. (From Schwartz MF, Green WR, Michels RG, et al: An unusual case of ocular involvement in primary systemic nonfamilial amyloidosis. Ophthalmology 89:394–401, 1982.)

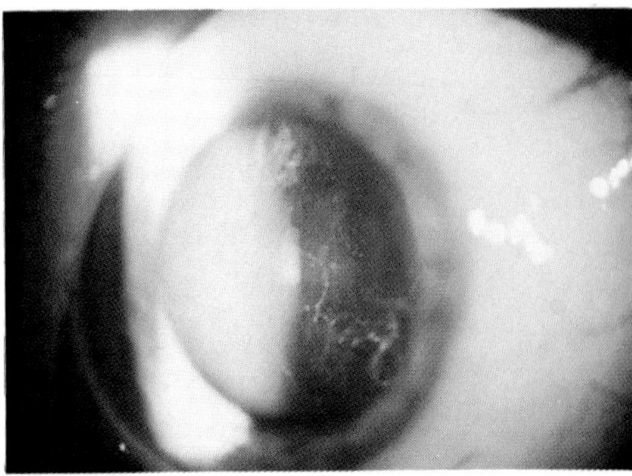

FIGURE 9–58 **Amyloidosis.** Magnified view of vitreous opacification. (From Schwartz MF, Green WR, Michels RG, et al: An unusual case of ocular involvement in primary systemic nonfamilial amyloidosis. Ophthalmology 89:394–401, 1982.)

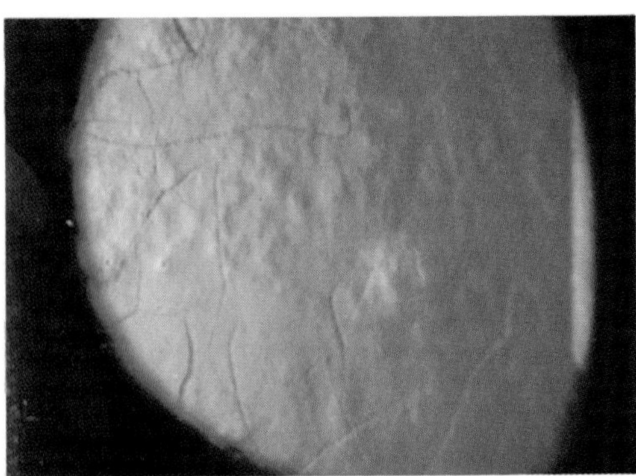

FIGURE 9–61 **Meretoja's syndrome.** Corneal deposits of Meretoja's syndrome (lattice type II, familial amyloidotic polyneuropathy type IV). Note the location along the course of corneal nerves. (From Purcell JJ Jr, Rodrigues M, Chishti MI, et al: Lattice corneal dystrophy associated with familial systemic amyloidosis. Ophthalmology 90:1512–1517, 1983.)

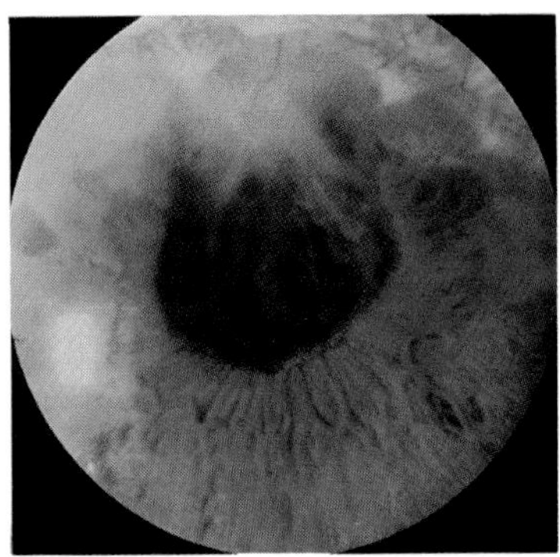

FIGURE 9–59 **Amyloidosis.** Vitreous amyloidosis simulating endophthalmitis in aphakic eye. (Courtesy of Robert Brockhurst, M.D.)

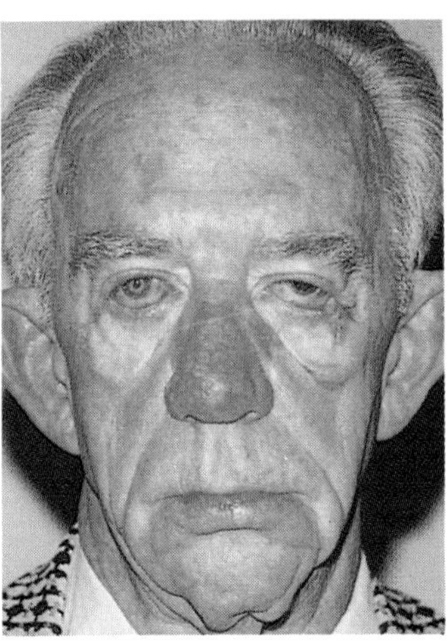

FIGURE 9–62 **Meretoja's syndrome.** Typical bloodhound facies of Meretoja's syndrome. (From Purcell JJ Jr, Rodrigues M, Chishti MI, et al: Lattice corneal dystrophy associated with familial systemic amyloidosis. Ophthalmology 90:1512–1517, 1983.)

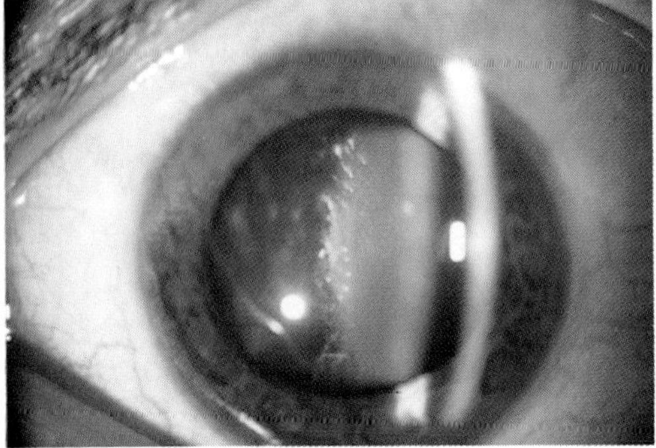

FIGURE 9–60 **Amyloidosis.** Typical lens "footplates" seen in advanced vitreous amyloidosis (deposits aligning themselves on posterior lens capsule). (From Doft BH, Machemer R, Skinner M, et al: Pars plana vitrectomy for vitreous amyloidosis. Ophthalmology 94:307–611, 1987.)

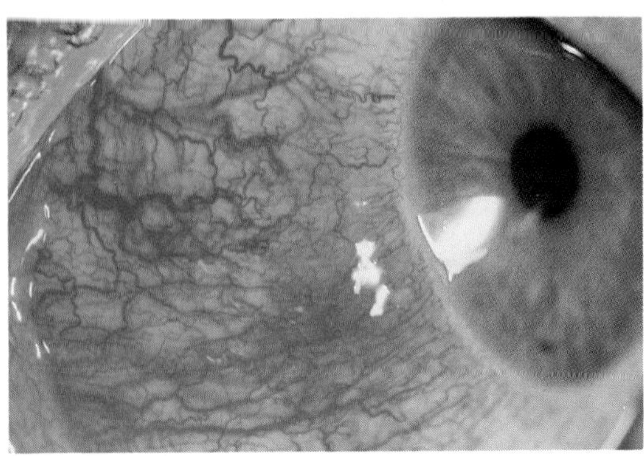

FIGURE 9–63 **Ulcerative colitis.** Nodular scleritis in a patient with ulcerative colitis.

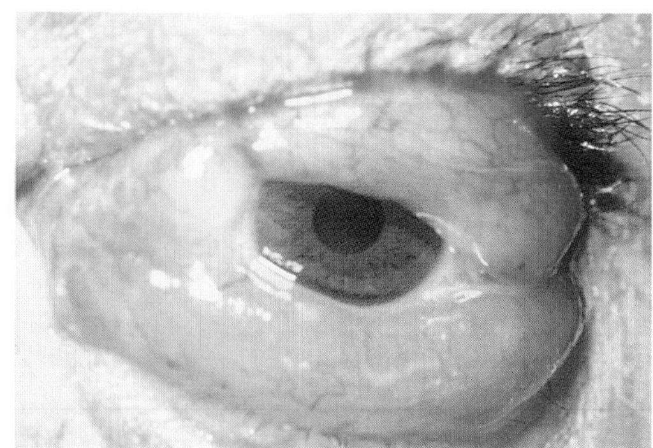

FIGURE 9–64 **Crohn's disease.** Recurrent, bilateral orbital inflammation in a patient with Crohn's disease. (Courtesy of Lisa McHam, M.D.)

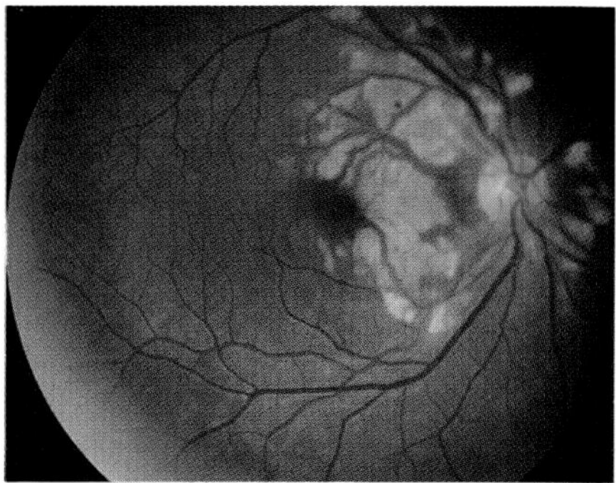

FIGURE 9–66 **Alcoholic pancreatitis.** Ischemic retinopathy in a patient with alcoholic pancreatitis. (Courtesy of David Guyer, M.D.)

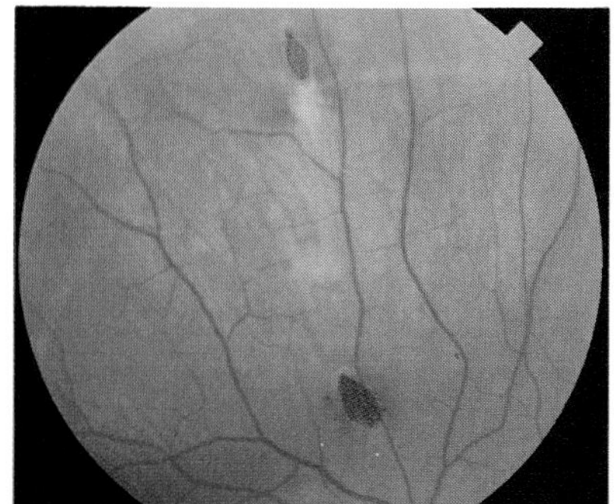

FIGURE 9–65 **Familial adenomatous polyposis.** Two areas of congenital hypertrophy of the retinal pigment epithelium in a patient with familial adenomatous polyposis.

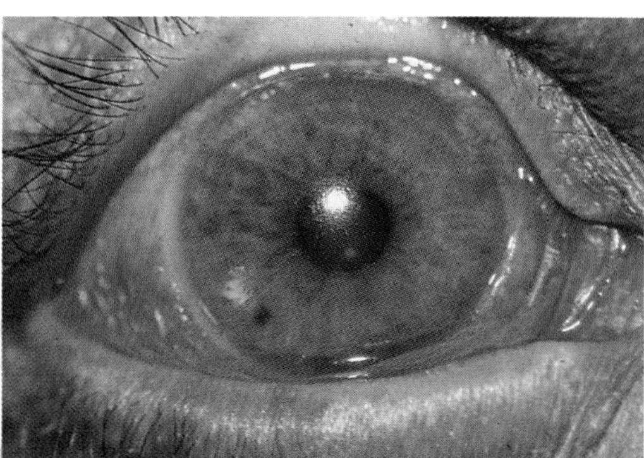

FIGURE 9–67 **Alcoholism.** A patient with malnutrition, liver failure, and vitamin A deficiency secondary to alcoholism. Note lack of corneal luster despite an ample tear meniscus. The conjunctiva is thickened with moderate injection. (Courtesy of Claes Dohlman, M.D.)

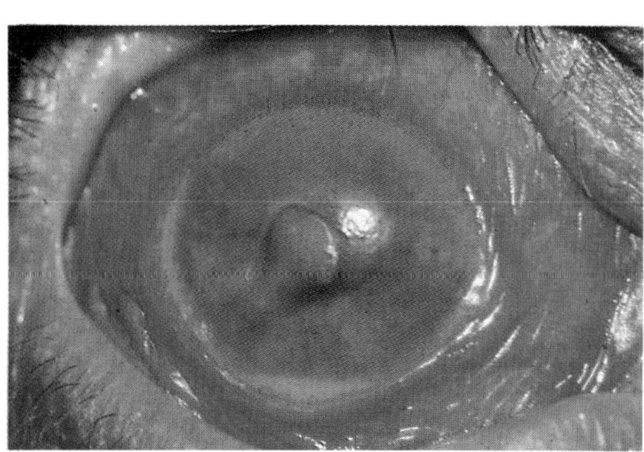

FIGURE 9–68 **Alcoholism.** Central circumscribed bacterial ulcer with an infiltrate and small hypopyon in vitamin A deficiency secondary to alcoholism. Note the "dry" appearance of the injected conjunctiva. (Courtesy of Claes Dohlman, M.D.)

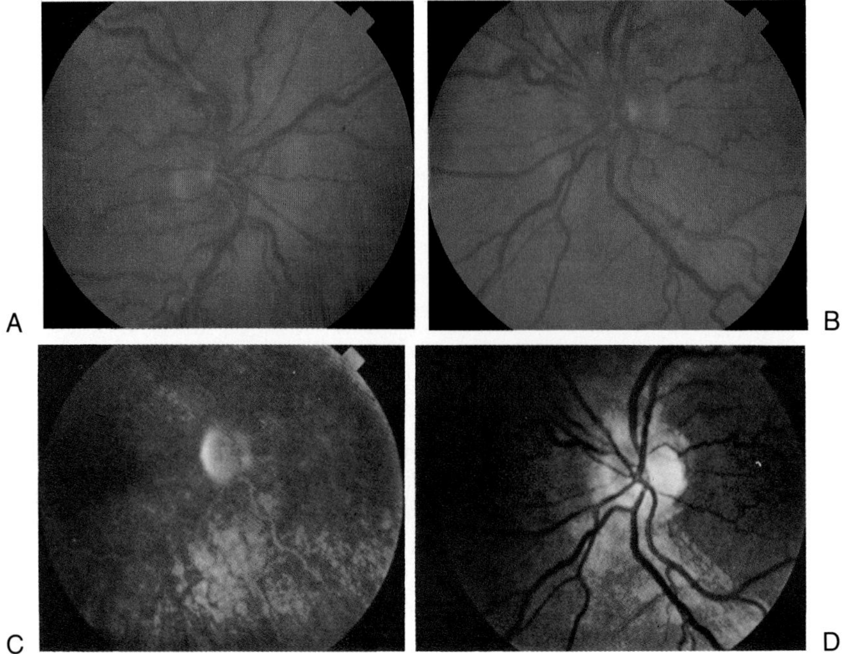

FIGURE 9–69 **Crohn's disease.** *A, B,* Bilateral optic neuropathy in a patient with vitamin B_{12} deficiency secondary to an ileal resection for Crohn's disease. Note peripapillary vessel tortuosity, microangiopathy, and pseudodisc edema; these findings are similar to those found in Leber's hereditary optic neuropathy. *C, D,* Late views of fluorescein angiography show absence of optic disc staining (edema). (Courtesy of Joseph Rizzo, M.D.)

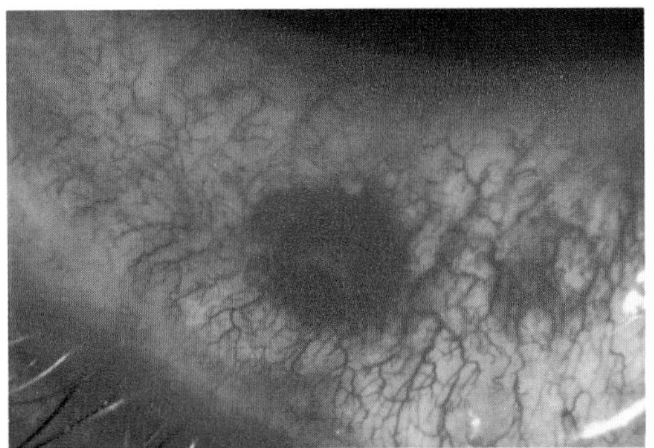

FIGURE 9–70 **Bacterial endocarditis.** Subconjunctival petechiae associated with a case of *Streptococcus aureus* endocarditis.

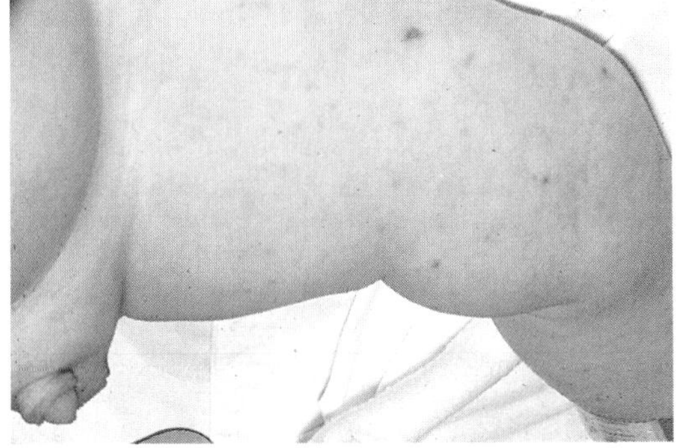

FIGURE 9–71 **Meningococcemia.** Petechial skin lesions in a child with meningococcemia.

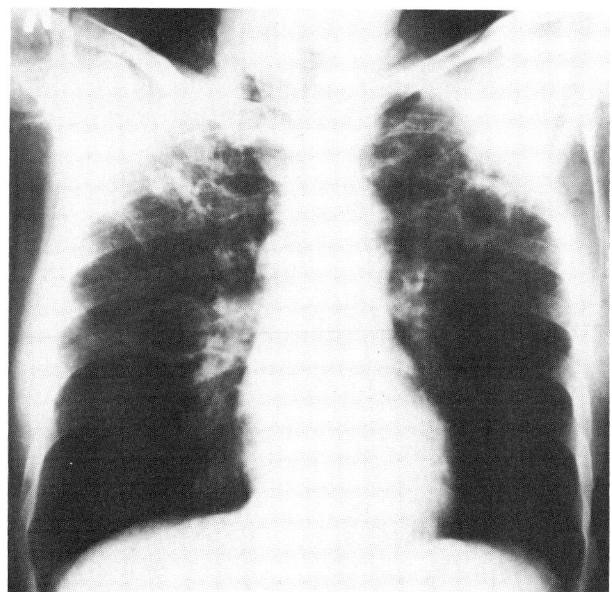

FIGURE 9–72 **Tuberculosis.** Chest radiograph of an adult patient with reactivation tuberculosis, demonstrating typical apical infiltrates with cavities. (Courtesy of Reginald Greene, M.D.)

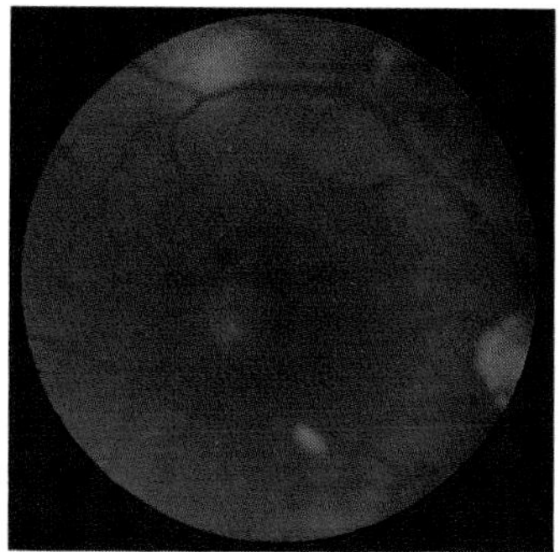

FIGURE 9–73 **Miliary tuberculosis.** Choroidal tubercles in a patient with miliary tuberculosis. (Courtesy of David Donaldson, M.D.)

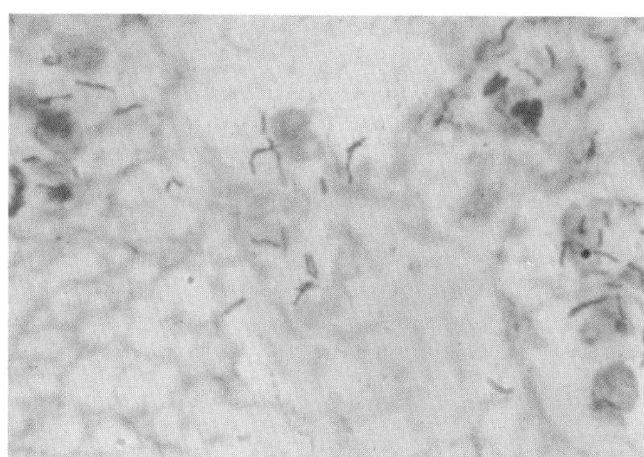

FIGURE 9–74 **Tuberculosis.** Acid-fast stain of sputum sample showing numerous acid-fast bacilli in a patient with cavitary pulmonary tuberculosis. (Courtesy of Harriet Provine, M.S.)

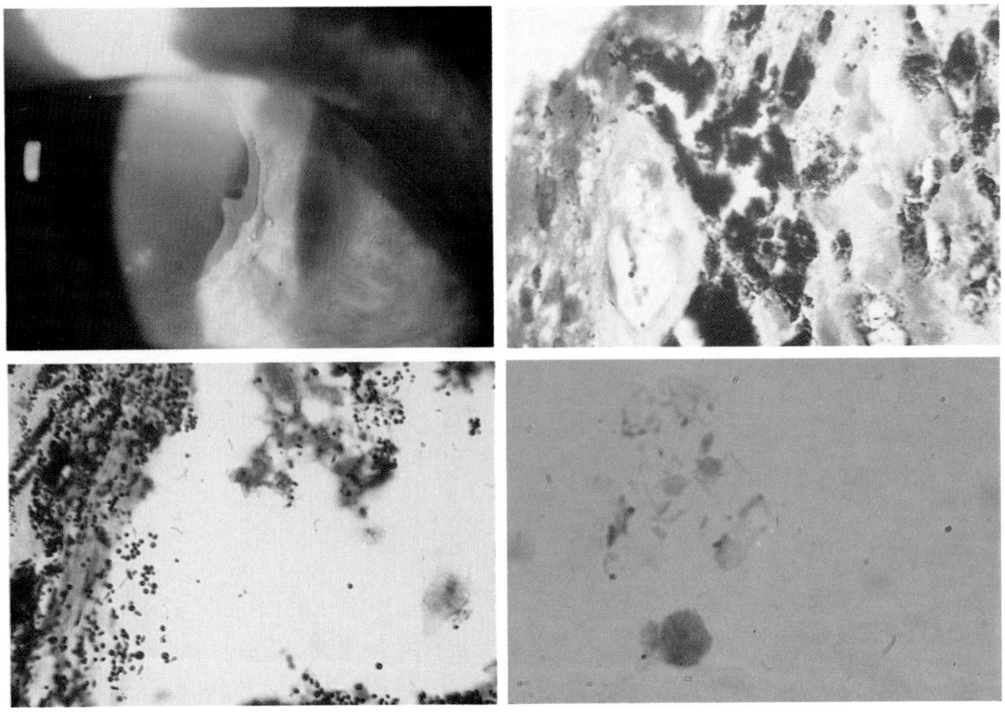

FIGURE 9–75 **Lepromatous leprosy.** Photographs from a patient with lepromatous leprosy. *A,* Slit-lamp photograph of iris granulomas and posterior synechiae. Iris nodule (granuloma) is present at the pupillary margin. (Courtesy of Michael Raizman, M.D.) *B* and *C,* Light micrographs of a biopsy of the iris granuloma. *Arrow* indicates numerous rod-shaped bacteria consistent with *Mycobacterium leprae.* There are multiple pigment granules within the iris stroma (Fite's stain). *D,* Acid-fast stain of the anterior chamber tap demonstrating numerous acid-fast bacilli. *E,* Disfigurement of hands secondary to cutaneous nodules and peripheral nerve damage. (D and E, Courtesy of Noreen Hynes, M.D.)

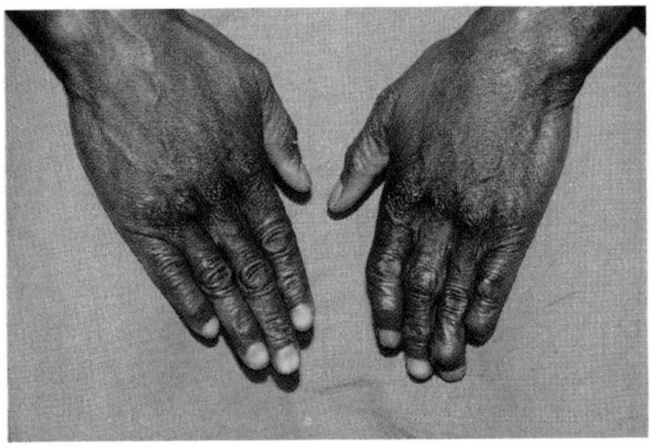

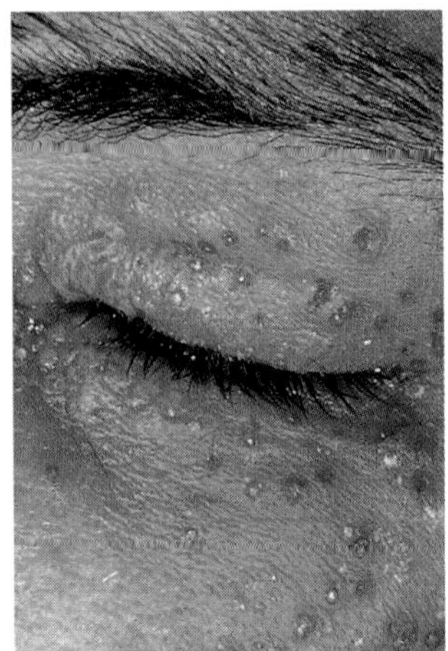

FIGURE 9–76 **Herpes simplex.** Herpes simplex involving the face and eyelids (varicelliform eruption of Kaposi).

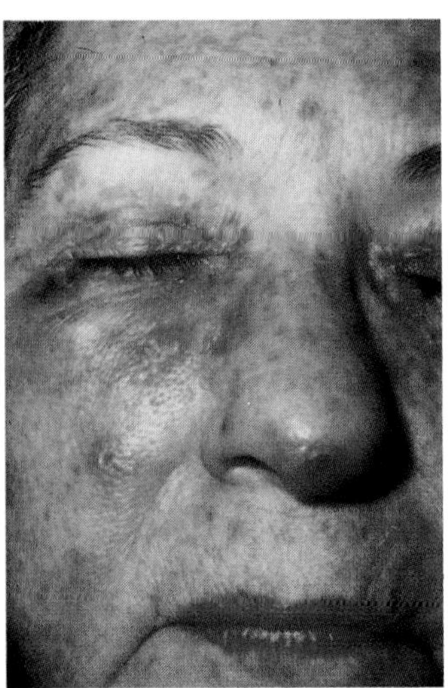

FIGURE 9–77 **Herpes zoster ophthalmicus.** Note the vesicle involving the tip of the nose. (Courtesy of Dr. T. Hutchinson.)

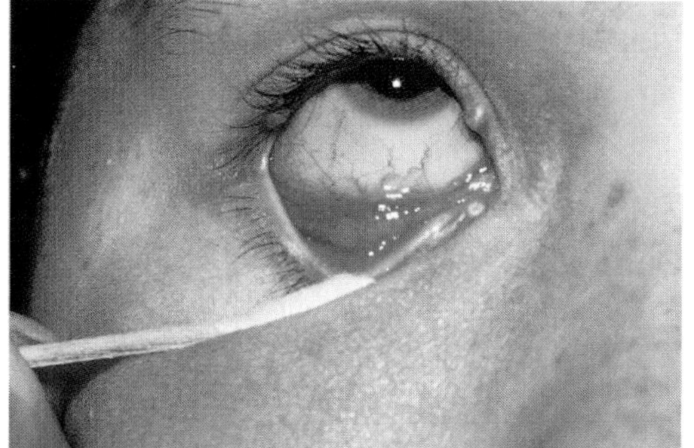

FIGURE 9–78 **Molluscum contagiosum.** Molluscum contagiosum involving conjunctiva and eyelids. (Courtesy of the American Academy of Ophthalmology.)

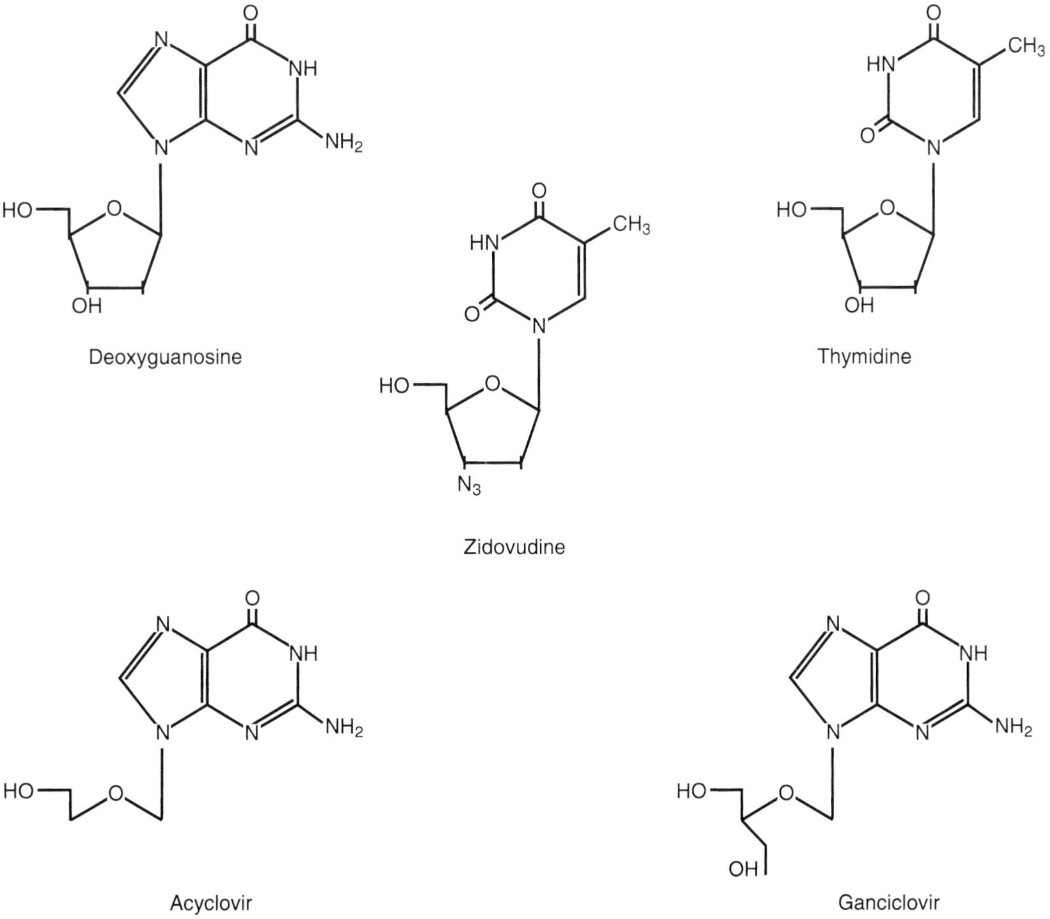

Deoxyguanosine

Zidovudine

Thymidine

Acyclovir

Ganciclovir

FIGURE 9–79 Nucleoside analogs and the corresponding nucleosides. Acyclovir and ganciclovir are analogs of deoxyguanosine, and zidovudine is an analog of thymidine.

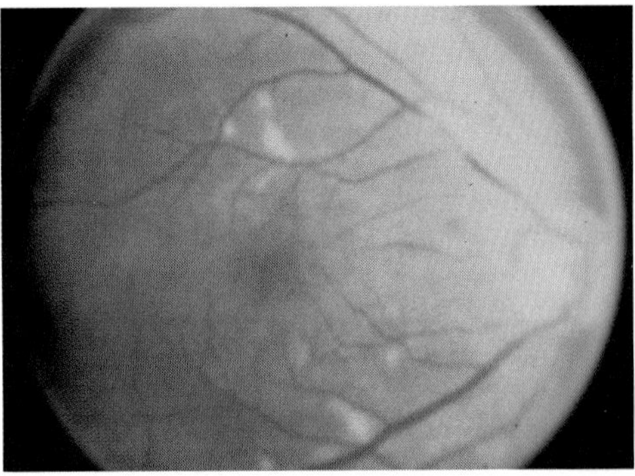

FIGURE 9–80 ***Candida* endophthalmitis.** Immunocompromised patient with endogenous *Candida* endophthalmitis with retinal infiltrates. (Courtesy of D. J. D'Amico, M.D., and A. S. Baker, M.D.)

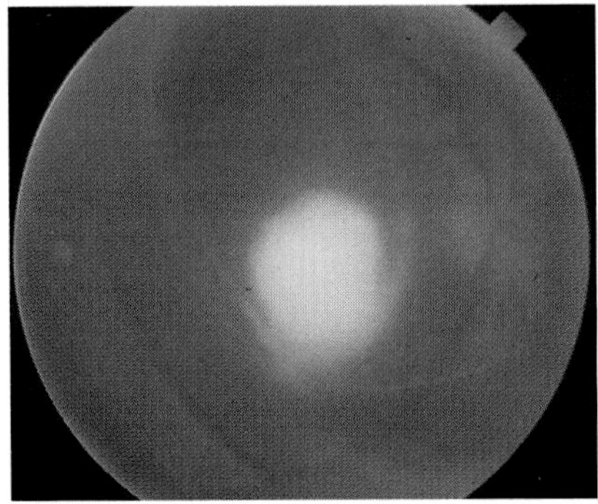

FIGURE 9–81 ***Candida* endophthalmitis.** Endogenous *Candida* endophthalmitis O.D. with vitreous infiltrate ("headlight in the fog"). (Courtesy of S. Foster, M.D., and A. S. Baker, M.D.)

A

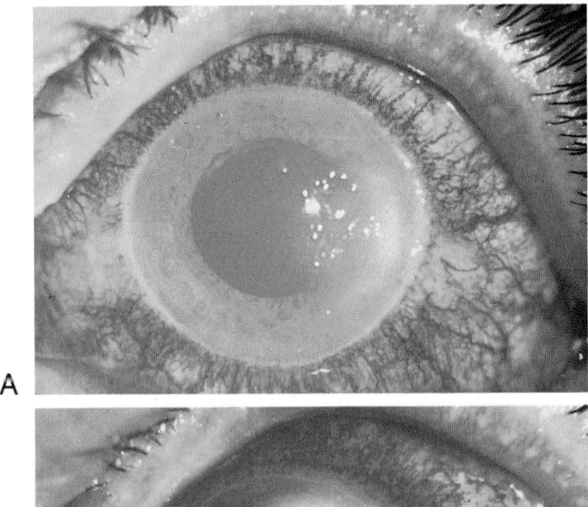

B

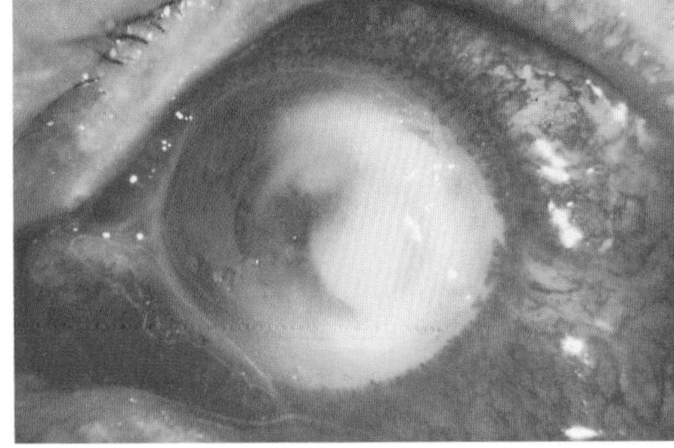

FIGURE 9–82 ***Aspergillus.*** *A,* Early corneal infiltrate with *Aspergillus. B,* Progressive corneal infiltrate with *Aspergillus.* (Courtesy of K. Kenyon, M.D., and A. S. Baker, M.D.)

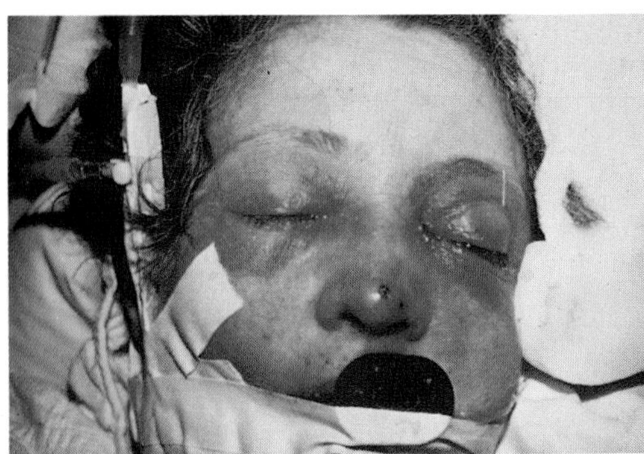

FIGURE 9–83 ***Rhizopus.*** Patient with diabetic ketoacidosis with *Rhizopus* rhinocerebral mucormycosis and cavernous sinus thrombosis. (Courtesy of A. W. Karchmer, M.D., and A. S. Baker, M.D.)

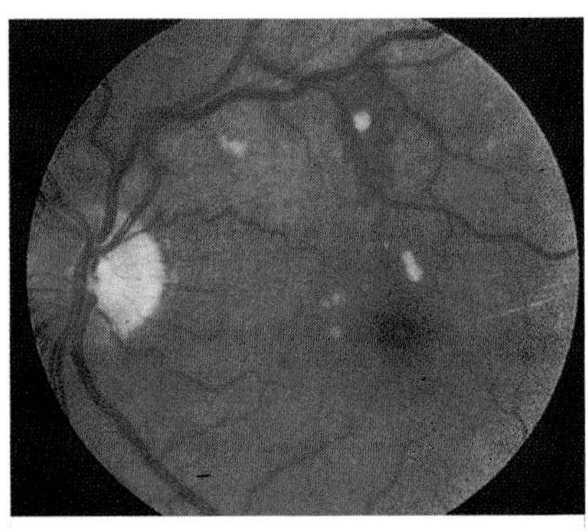

FIGURE 9–84 **Histoplasmosis.** Histoplasmosis retinal infiltrates and hemorrhage in the left eye. (From Specht CS, Mitchell KT, Bauman AE, et al: Ocular histoplasmosis with retinitis in a patient with AIDS. Ophthalmology 98:1357, 1991.)

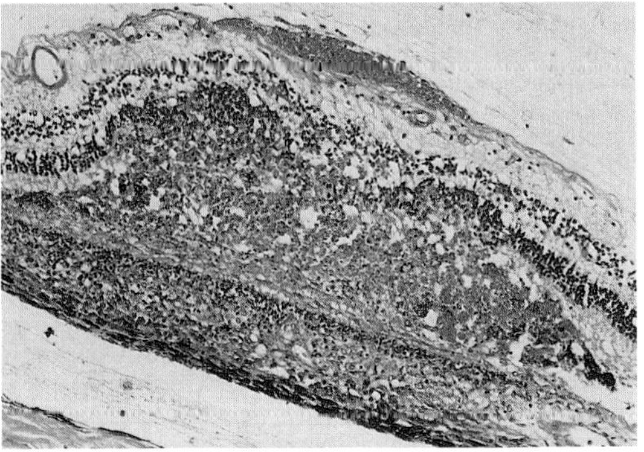

FIGURE 9–85 **Histoplasmosis.** Histoplasmic retinitis in the right eye, involving all retinal layers and associated with choroiditis. PAS stain (×40). (From Specht CS, Mitchell KT, Bauman AE, et al: Ocular histoplasmosis with retinitis in a patient with AIDS. Ophthalmology 98:1357, 1991.)

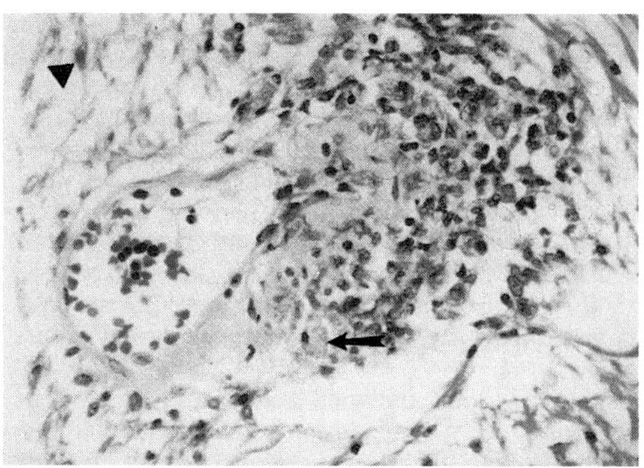

FIGURE 9–86 **Histoplasmosis.** Left retina with intracellular *Histoplasma* in a perivascular lymphohistiocytic inflammatory infiltrate. H&E stain (×100). (From Specht CS, Mitchell KT, Bauman AE, et al: Ocular histoplasmosis with retinitis in a patient with AIDS. Ophthalmology 98:1357, 1991.)

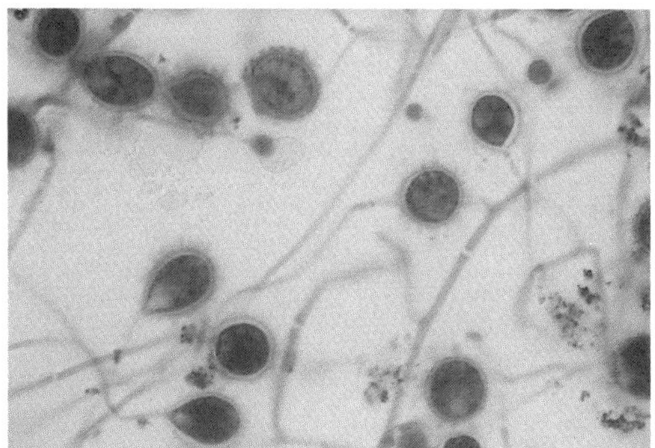

FIGURE 9–87 **Histoplasmosis.** Lactophenol cotton blue stain of *Histoplasma capsulatum* (×40). (Courtesy of the Department of Bacteriology. Massachusetts General Hospital, Boston.)

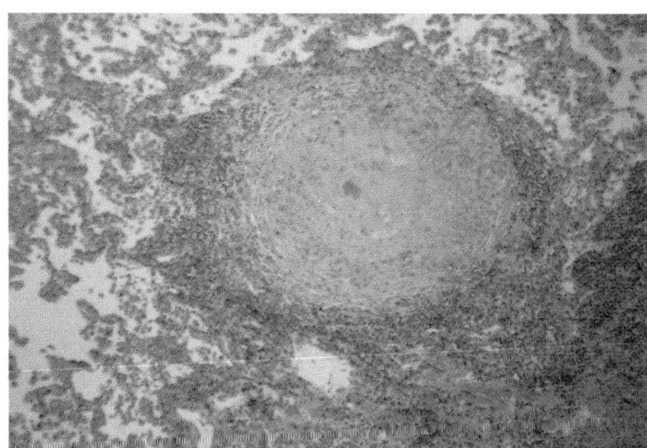

FIGURE 9–88 **Histoplasmosis.** H&E of histoplasmoma from a lung biopsy (×4). (Courtesy of H. Provine, M.S., and the Department of Bacteriology, Massachusetts General Hospital, Boston.)

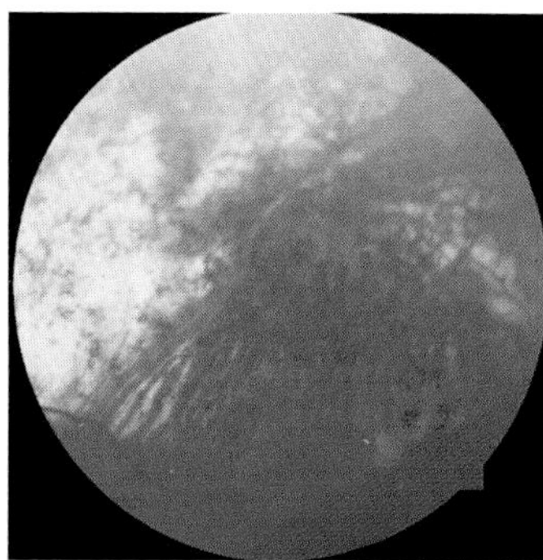

FIGURE 9–89 **Syphilis.** Resolution of inflammation shown in syphilitic infection following treatment with penicillin. Note the chorioretinal scarring.

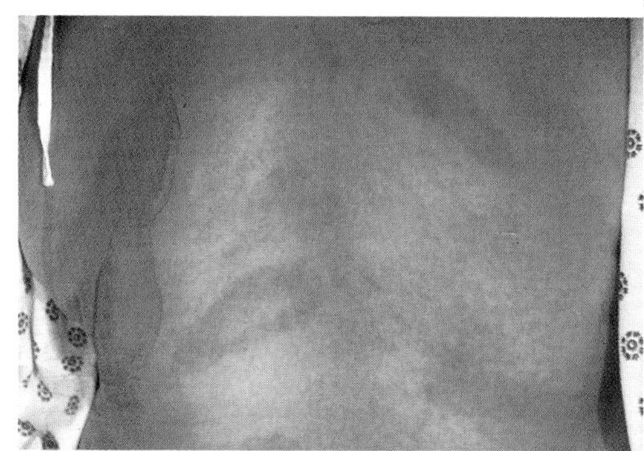

FIGURE 9–90 **Lyme disease.** Characteristic lesions of erythema migrans associated with Lyme disease.

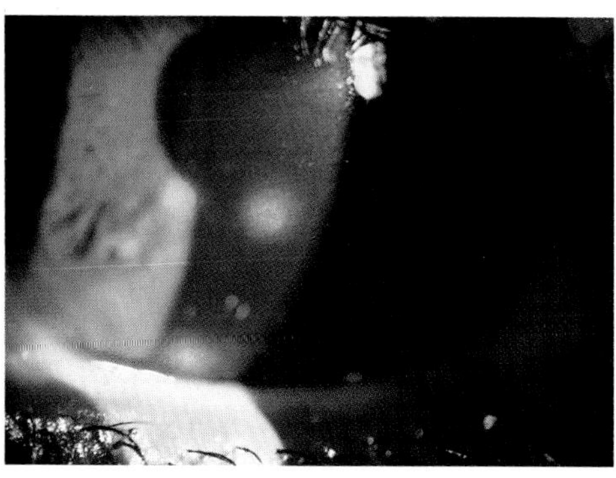

FIGURE 9–91 **Lyme disease.** Multiple intrastromal lesions of Lyme keratitis. (Courtesy of Ernest Kornmehl, M.D.).

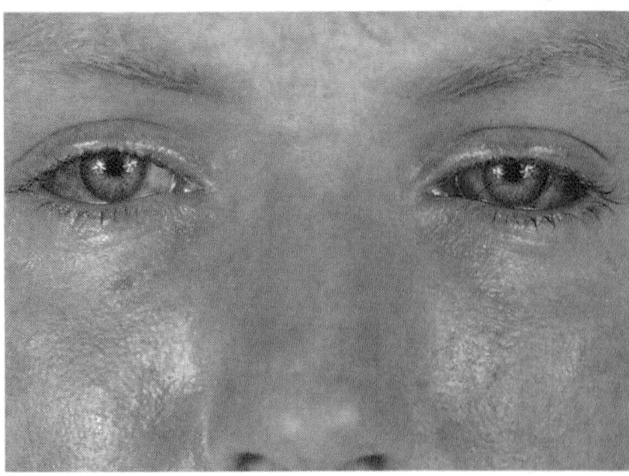

FIGURE 9–92 **Reiter's syndrome with conjunctivitis.** Bilateral conjunctivitis associated with anterior uveitis. (From Fitzpatrick TB, et al: Color Atlas and Synopsis of Clinical Dermatology, 2nd ed. New York, McGraw-Hill, 1983, pp. 276–278.)

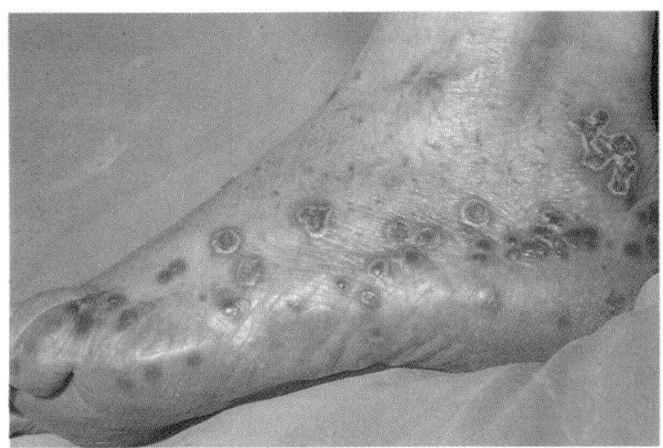

FIGURE 9–93 **Reiter's syndrome with keratoderma blennorrhagicum.** Red-to-brown papules, vesicles, pustules, with central erosion and confluence of lesions on the foot. (From Fitzpatrick TB, et al: Color Atlas and Synopsis of Clinical Dermatology, 2nd ed. New York, McGraw-Hill, 1983, pp. 276–278.)

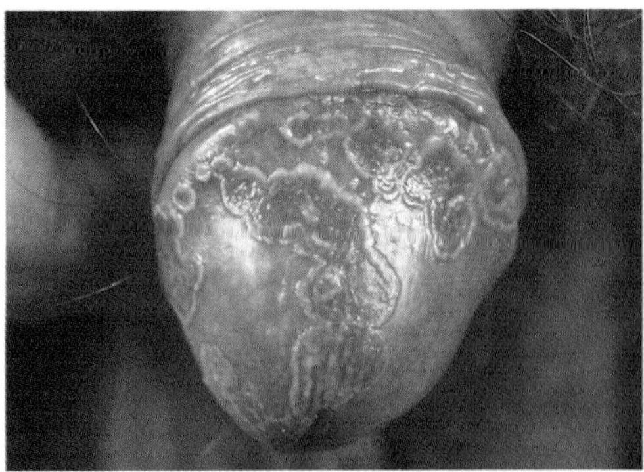

FIGURE 9–94 **Reiter's syndrome with balanitis circinata.** Circinata balanitis with moist, well-demarcated erosions with slightly raised border. (From Fitzpatrick TB, et al: Color Atlas and Synopsis of Clinical Dermatology, 2nd ed. New York, McGraw-Hill, 1983, pp. 276–278.)

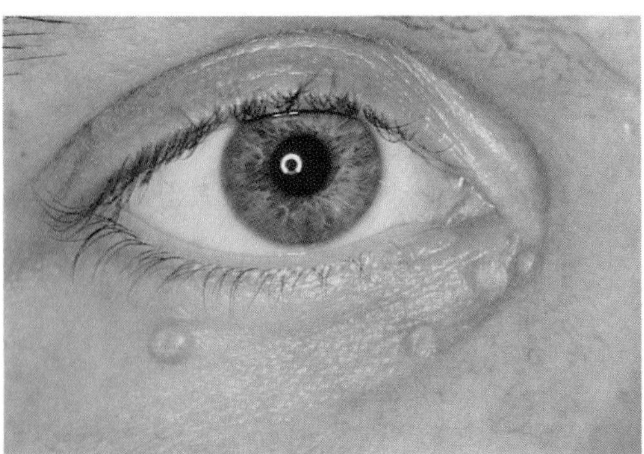

FIGURE 9–95 **Molluscum contagiosum.** Lesions of molluscum contagiosum on the lower lid of a patient with acquired immunodeficiency syndrome (AIDS). (Courtesy of Shizuo Mukai, M.D.)

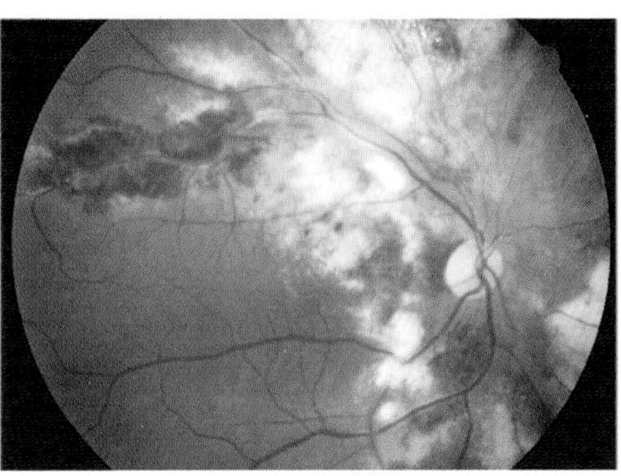

FIGURE 9–96 **Cytomegalovirus retinitis.** Hemorrhagic form of cytomegalovirus retinitis in a patient with AIDS.

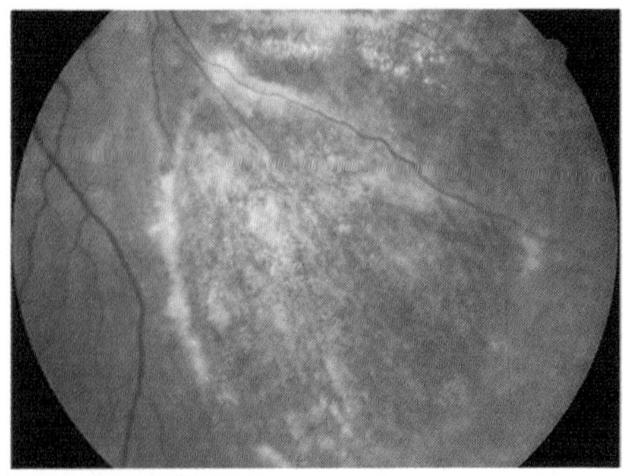

FIGURE 9–97 **Cytomegalovirus retinitis.** Cytomegalovirus retinitis exhibiting a brush-fire pattern in an AIDS patient.

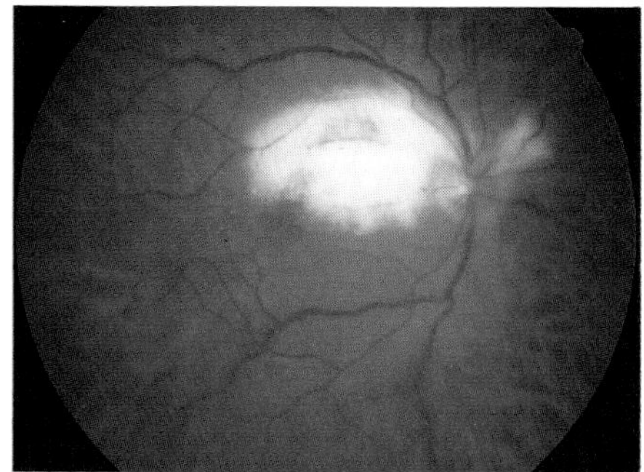

FIGURE 9-98 ***Toxoplasma* retinitis in a patient with AIDS.** Note the lack of vitritis that is common in the AIDS patient.

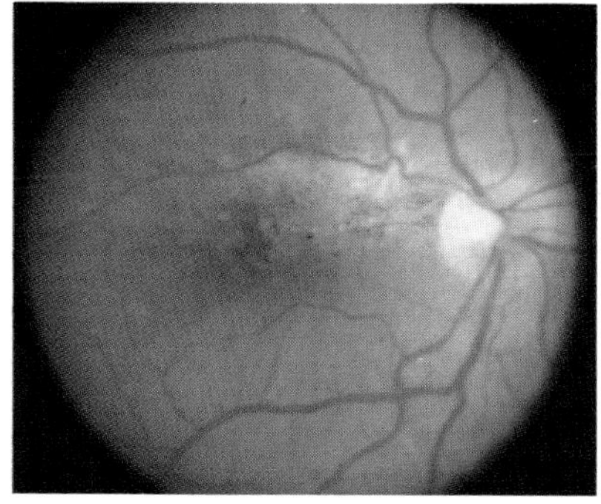

FIGURE 9-99 ***Toxoplasma* retinitis.** Inactivation of the *Toxoplasma* lesion seen in Figure 9-98 after treatment.

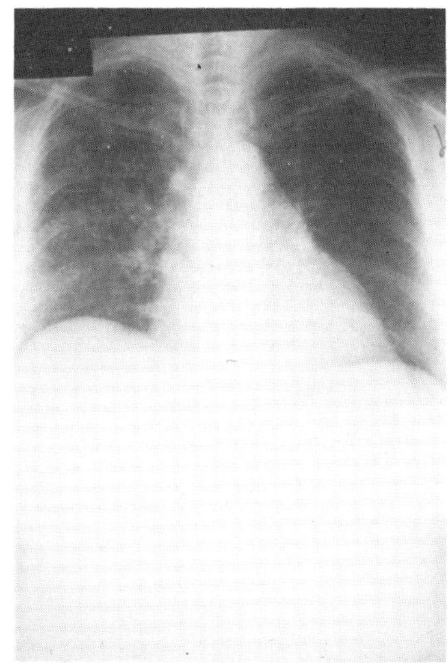

FIGURE 9-100 ***Pneumocystis carinii.*** Chest radiograph showing bilateral infiltrates of *Pneumocystis carinii.* (In this patient, the infiltrates were most prominent in the right lower and middle lobe.)

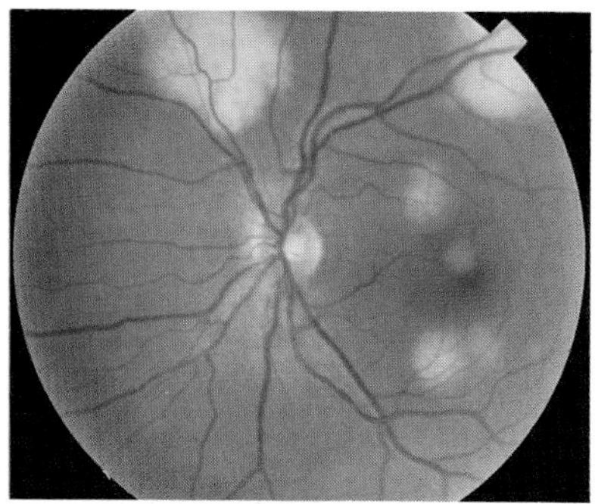

FIGURE 9-101 ***Pneumocystis carinii* choroiditis.** *Pneumocystis carinii* choroiditis in a patient with AIDS on aerosolized pentamidine prophylactic therapy.

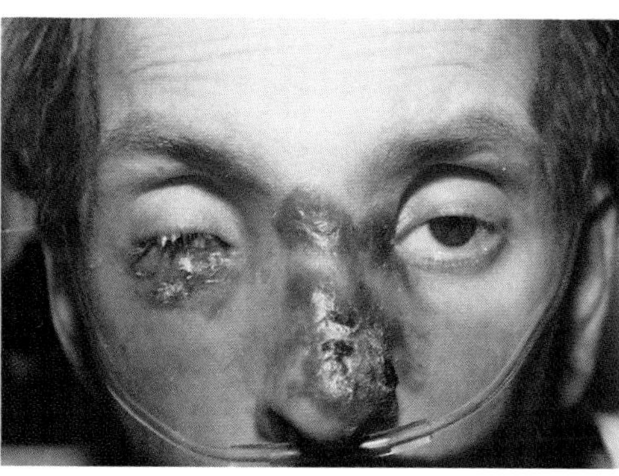

FIGURE 9-102 **Kaposi's sarcoma.** Advanced Kaposi's sarcoma involving the face and lids of a patient with AIDS.

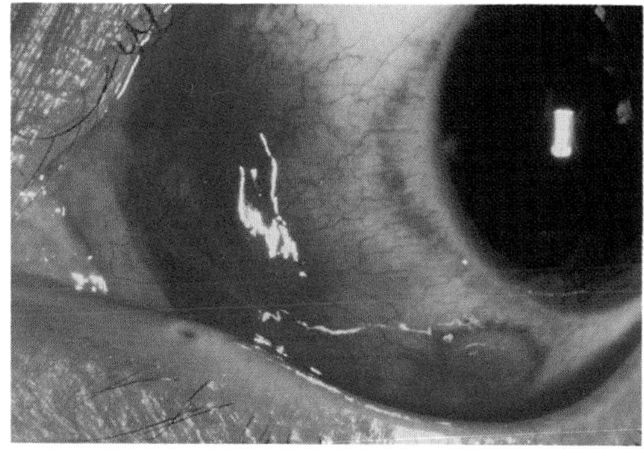

FIGURE 9-103 **Kaposi's sarcoma.** Conjunctival involvement with Kaposi's sarcoma. This lesion was asymptomatic and required no specific treatment.

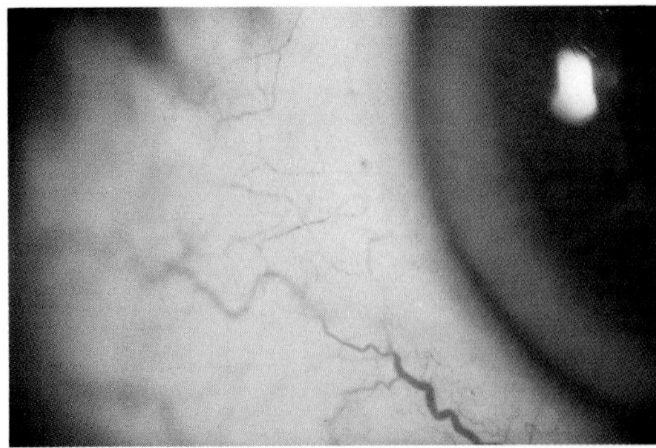

FIGURE 9–104 **The conjunctiva of a patient with human immunodeficiency virus (HIV) infection.** Note the granularity of the blood column seen in several of the smaller vessels.

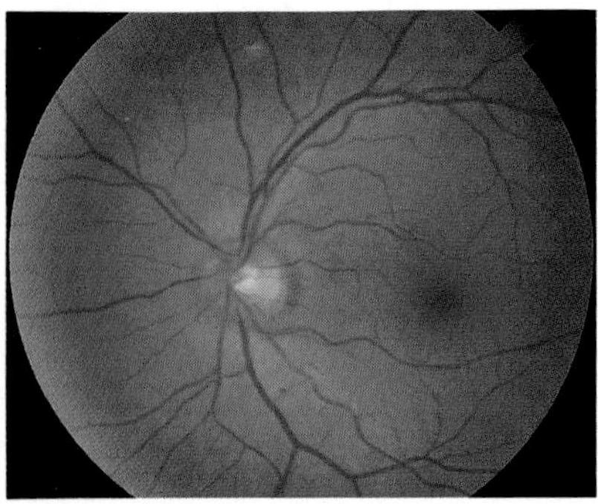

FIGURE 9–106 Appearance of the fundus 2 months after the photograph in Figure 9–105, showing resolution of the cotton-wool spots.

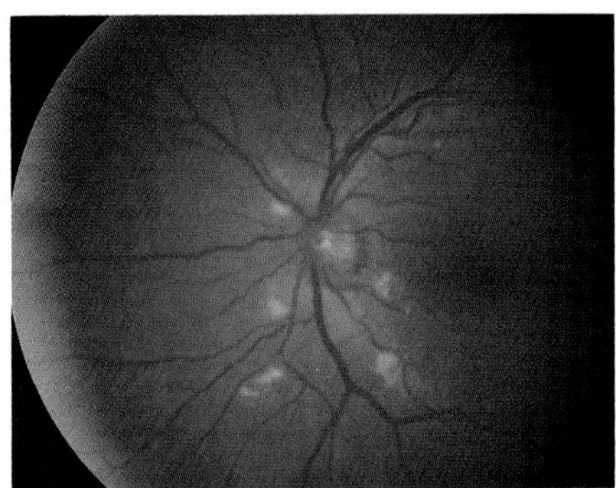

FIGURE 9–105 **Cotton-wool spots in the fundus of a patient with AIDS.** Note their typical distribution near the optic nerve.

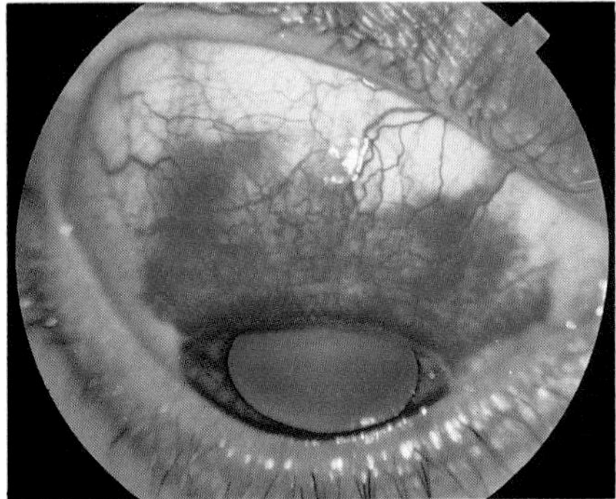

FIGURE 9–107 **Kaposi's sarcoma.** Presumed subconjunctival hemorrhage that did not resolve with time. Biopsy revealed Kaposi's sarcoma. (Courtesy of D. Fong, M.D.)

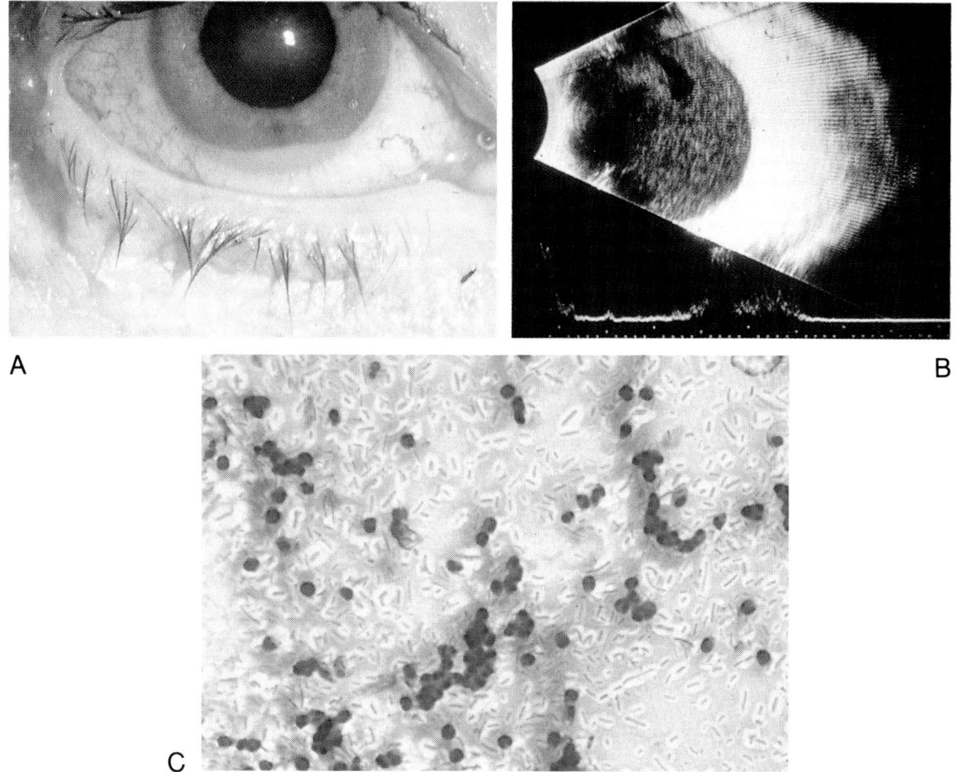

FIGURE 9–108 **Endogenous endophthalmitis.** *A,* Endogenous endophthalmitis due to *Klebsiella* sepsis with hypopyon, loss of red reflex, and minimal conjunctival reaction. *B,* Ultrasound examination discloses anterior and posterior echoes as well as mild thickening of the retinochoroid layer. *C,* Gram stain of the vitreous biopsy reveals abundant gram-negative rods.

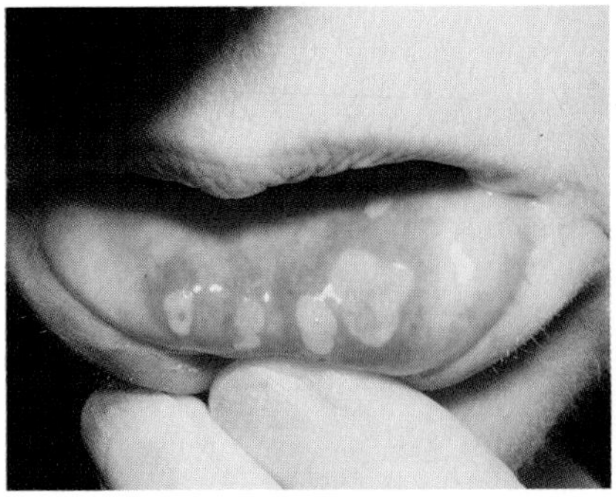

A 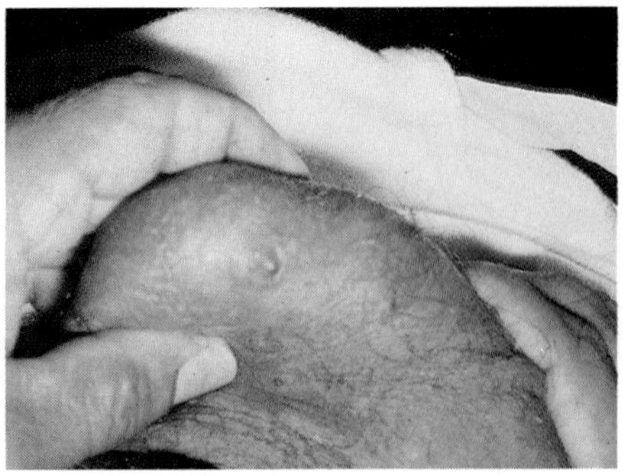 B 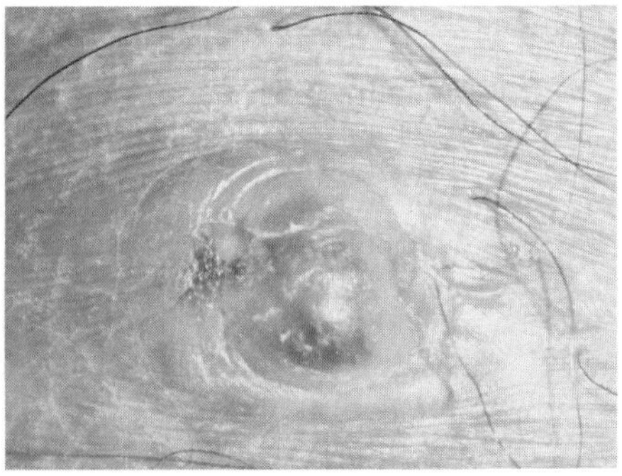 C

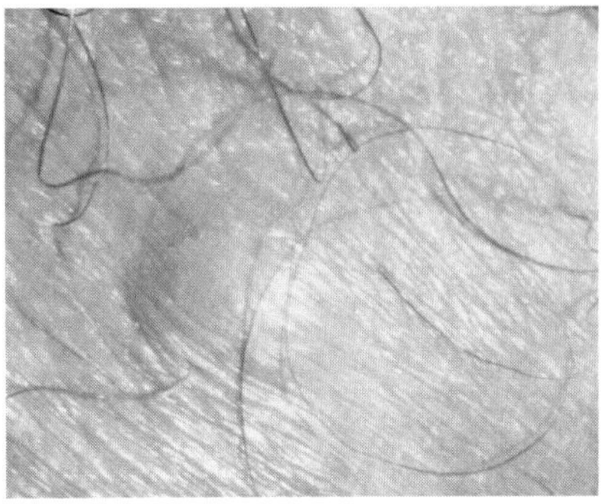

D 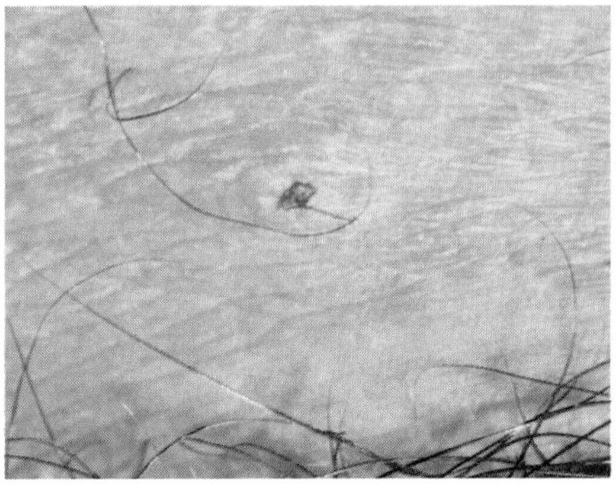 E 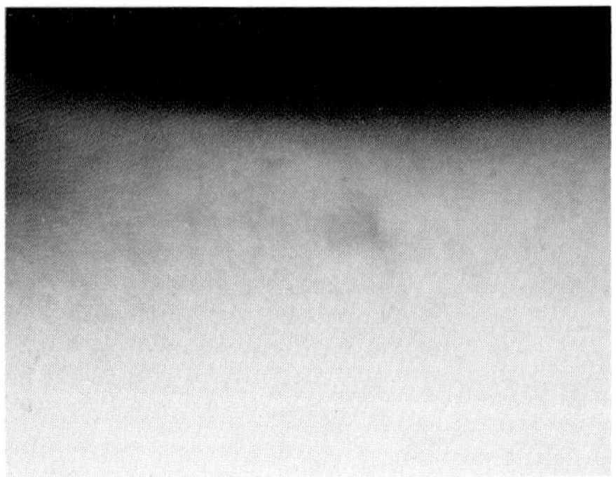 F

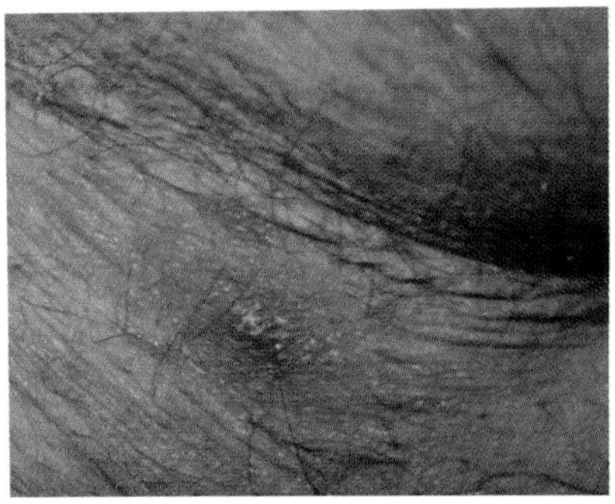

G

FIGURE 9–109 **Dermatologic lesions of Behçet's disease.** *A,* Typical oral ulceration. Mucosal genital ulceration is similar in appearance. *B–E,* Nonmucosal genital ulceration. These ulcerating nodular lesions are on the scrotum. *F,* Erythema nodosum lesion of the skin at the ankle. *G,* Pseudofolliculitis lesion of the skin.

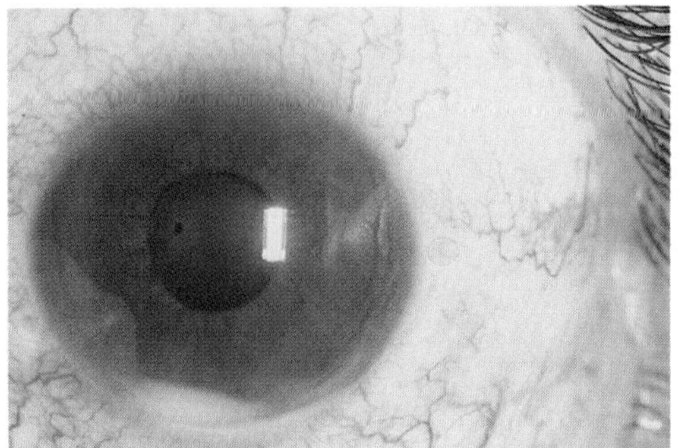

FIGURE 9–110 **Sterile hypopyon typical of Behçet's disease.** This patient also had the genital lesions depicted in Figure 9-109, *B–E.*

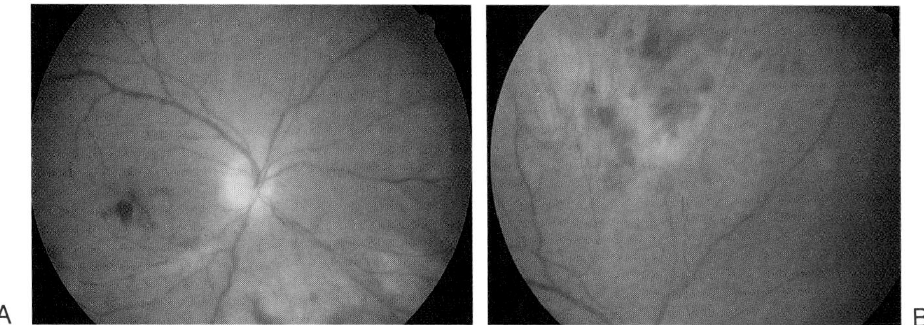

FIGURE 9–111 **Fundus findings typical of Behçet's disease.** These photographs, centered on *A,* the disc, and *B,* superior periphery of the right eye of a patient with Behçet's disease, illustrate the multifocal pattern of hemorrhage and infarction. In *A,* perivascular exudate, arteriolar attenuation, and venous dilatation and tortuosity are seen.

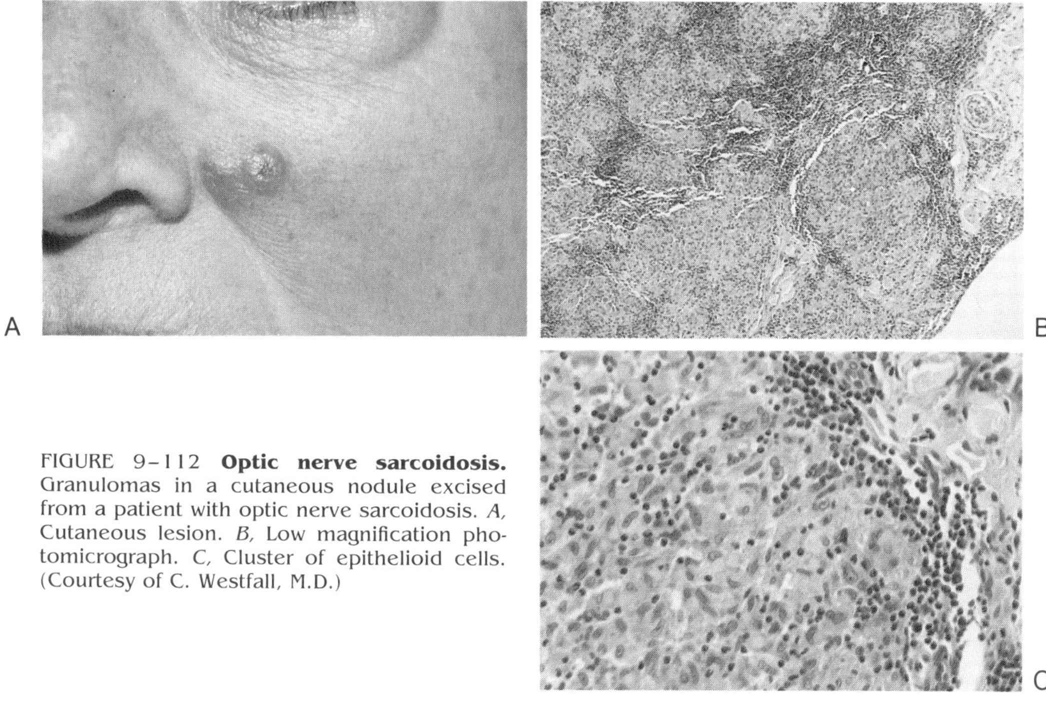

FIGURE 9–112 **Optic nerve sarcoidosis.** Granulomas in a cutaneous nodule excised from a patient with optic nerve sarcoidosis. *A,* Cutaneous lesion. *B,* Low magnification photomicrograph. *C,* Cluster of epithelioid cells. (Courtesy of C. Westfall, M.D.)

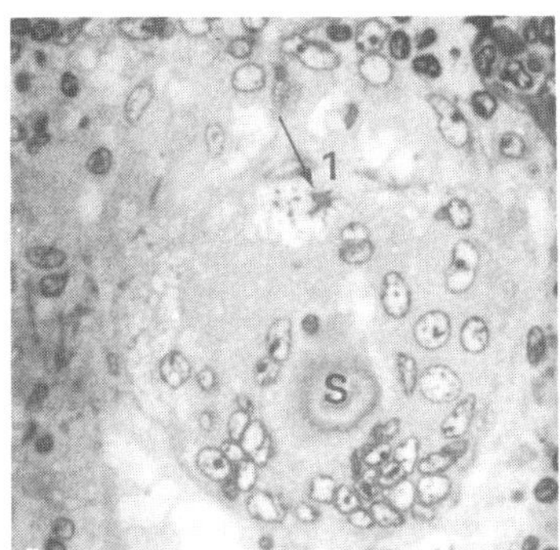

FIGURE 9–113 **Sarcoid granuloma.** Semithin section of giant cells in resin-embedded granulomas obtained from a 60-year old woman with sarcoidosis. An asteroid body *(arrow 1)* and a Schaumann body (S) are present within the cell. (From Kirkpatrick CJ, Curry A, Bisset DL: Light and electron microscopic studies on multinucleated giant cells in sarcoid granuloma: New aspects of asteroid and Schaumann bodies. Ultrastruc Path 12:584, 1988.)

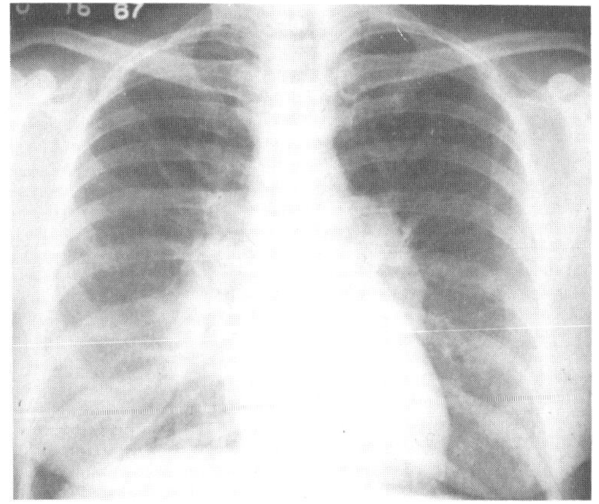

FIGURE 9–114 **Hilar adenopathy.** Characteristic hilar adenopathy in a patient with sarcoidosis. (Courtesy of A. Weinberg, M.D.)

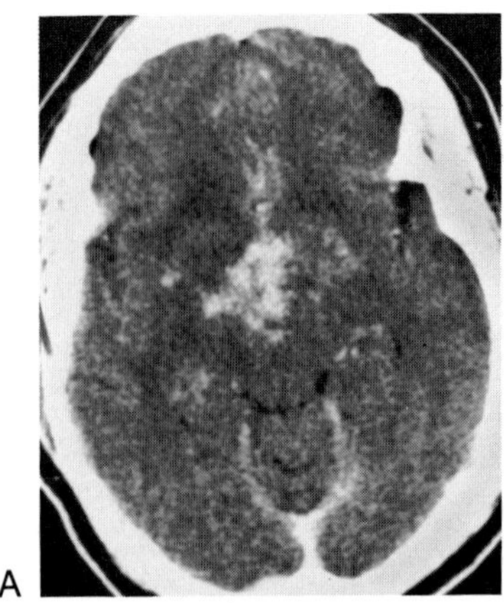

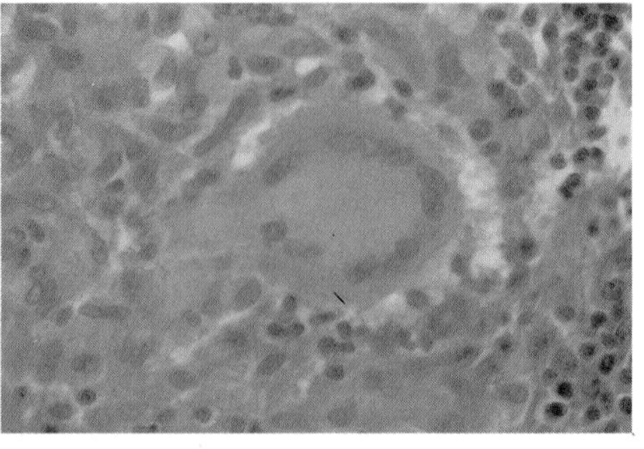

FIGURE 9–115 **Sarcoidosis.** Cranial computed tomography scan of a 30-year-old man who presented to the Massachusetts Eye and Ear Infirmary complaining of visual loss. History revealed somnolence, behavioral abnormalities, and polydipsia. He had optic atrophy and an abnormal chest x-ray. *A,* An enhancing, irregular, infiltrating mass was present in a contrast-enhanced computed tomography scan of the head. *B,* Multinucleated giant cells, were observed in the mediastinal lymph node biopsy, which revealed numerous sarcoid granulomas. (*A,* From Case records of the Massachusetts General Hospital: Case 10, 1991. N Engl J Med 324:679, 1991.)

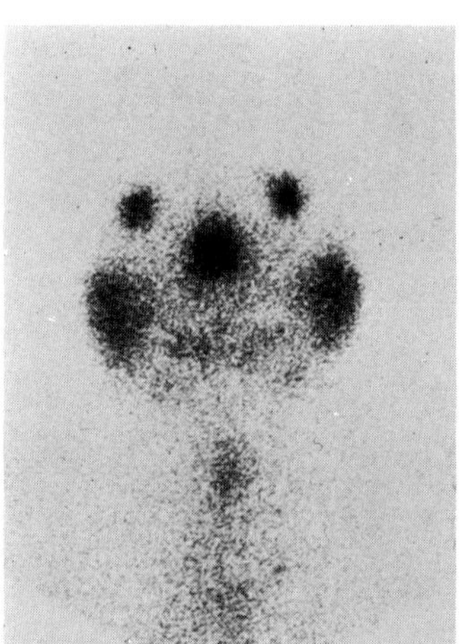

FIGURE 9–116 **Gallium scan of a patient with sarcoidosis.** Note the involvement of lacrimal, parotid, and submandibular glands (Panda sign).

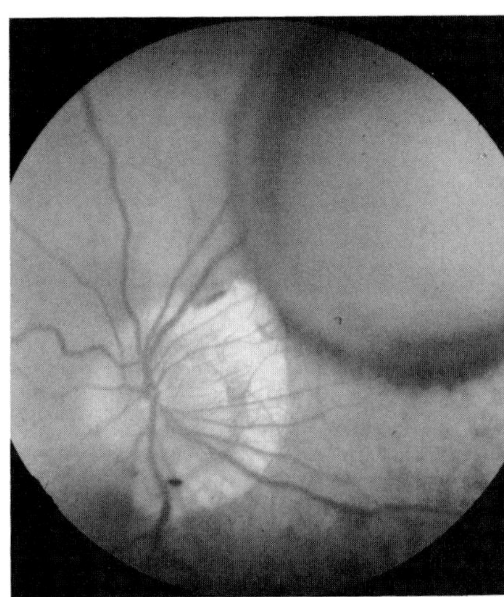

FIGURE 9–117 **Marfan's syndrome.** Dislocated lens resting on the retina of a patient with Marfan's syndrome. Note the myopic peripapillary changes.

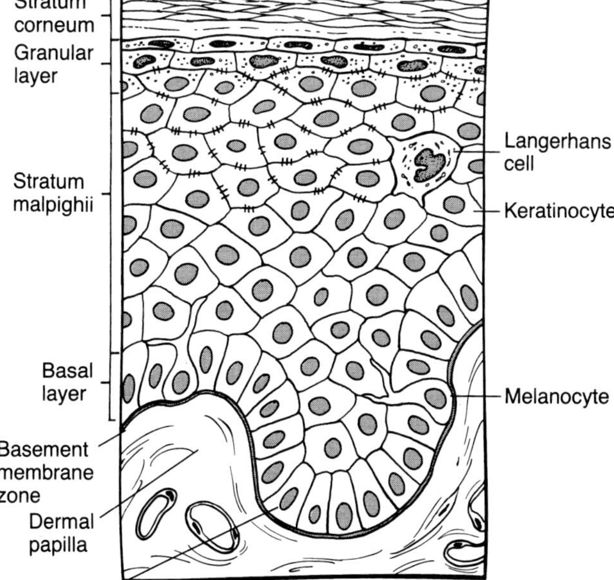

FIGURE 9–118 Diagram of the layers of the epidermis.

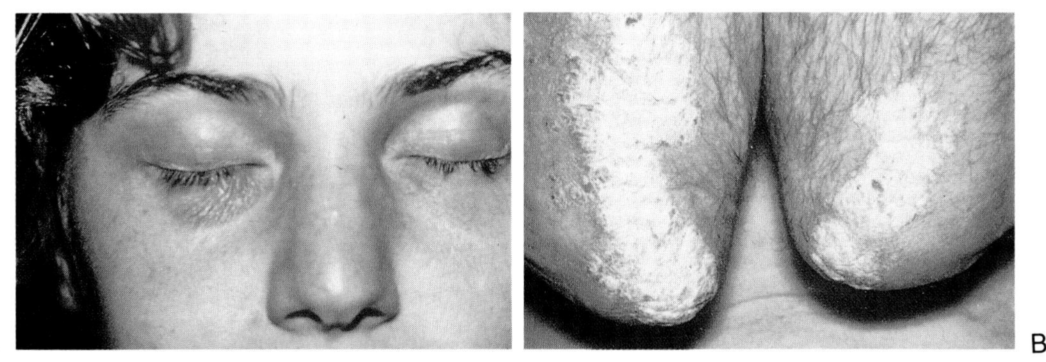

FIGURE 9–119 **Psoriasis.** Psoriasis affecting the periorbital areas (*A*) and the elbows (*B*). Note the micaceous scale on the elbow lesions. (*A,* Courtesy of Lynn Drake, M.D. *B,* From Fitzpatrick TB, Eisen AZ, Wolff K, et al. (eds): Dermatology in General Medicine, 3rd ed. Copyright 1987 by McGraw-Hill, Inc. Used by permission of McGraw-Hill Book Company.)

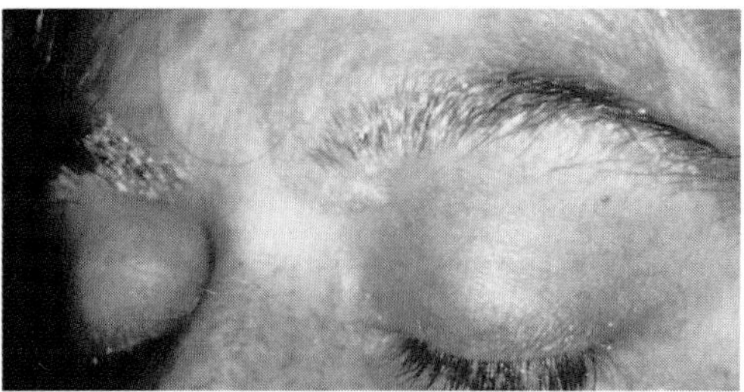

FIGURE 9–120 **Seborrheic dermatitis involving the eyebrows.** Note the prominent scale and some erythema. (Courtesy of Lynn Drake, M.D.)

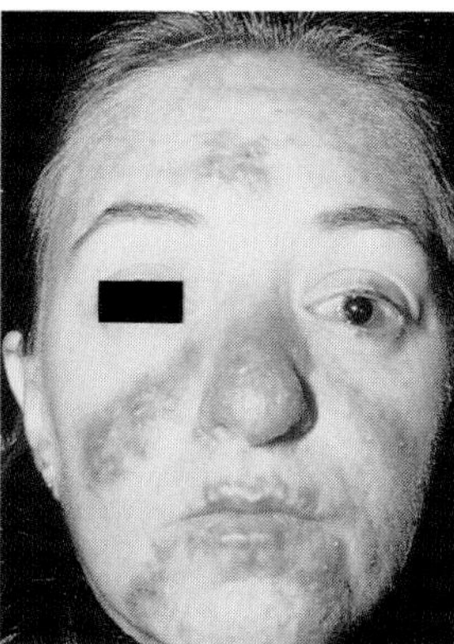

FIGURE 9–123 **Severe acne rosacea.** Note involvement of the left eye. (Courtesy of Lynn Drake, M.D.)

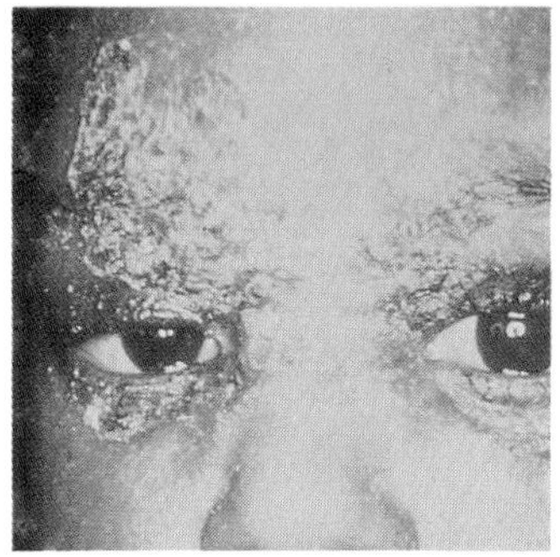

FIGURE 9–121 **Atopic dermatitis.** Severe atopic dermatitis involving the periorbital areas in a child. (Courtesy of Lynn Drake, M.D.)

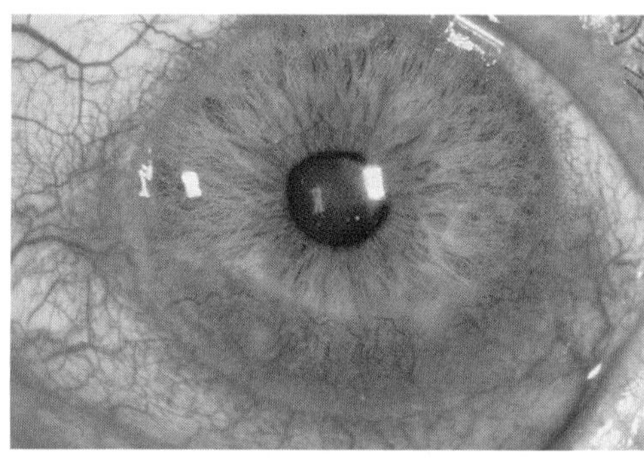

FIGURE 9–124 **Ocular involvement with acne rosacea.** Note conjunctivitis and keratitis with vascularization of the cornea. (Courtesy of Lynn Drake, M.D.)

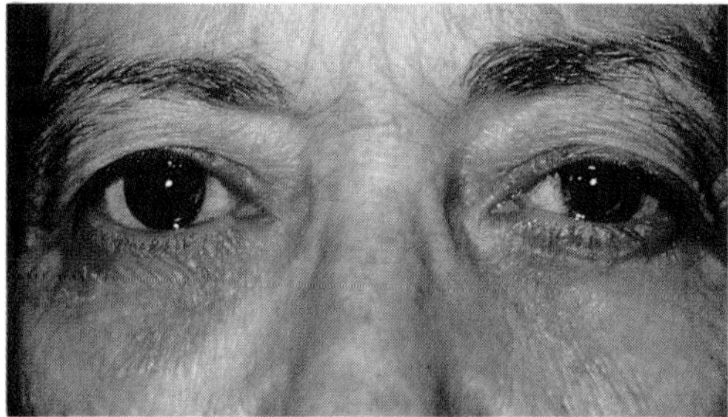

FIGURE 9–122 **Allergic contact dermatitis.** Allergic contact dermatitis in a periorbital distribution from a component of a hand cream. This is an example of the ability of an offending agent applied to the hands to be carried to the periorbital region. (Courtesy of Lynn Drake, M.D.)

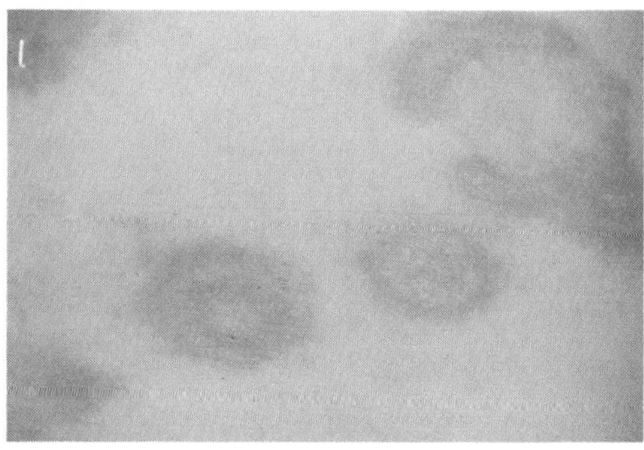

FIGURE 9–125 **Urticaria.** Typical lesions of urticaria.

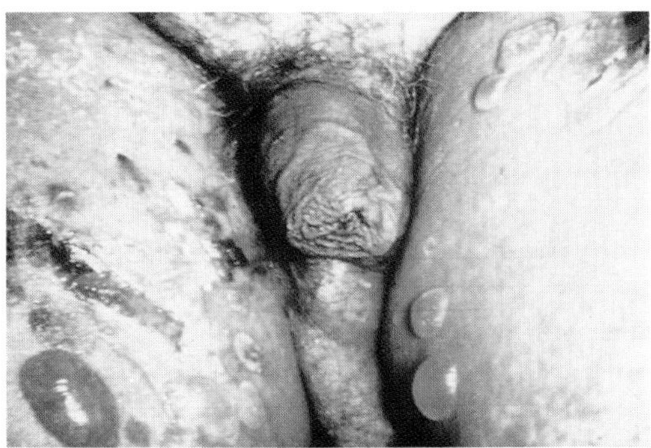

FIGURE 9–126 **Bullous pemphigoid.** Typical lesions of bullous pemphigoid. Note the tense bullae.

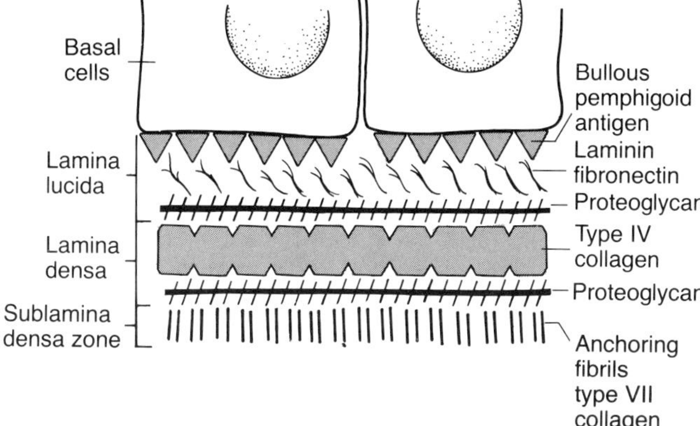

FIGURE 9–127 **Schematic drawing of the basement membrane zone.** The lamina lucida and the lamina densa are regions that are lucent and dense, respectively, by electron microscopy. (Modified from Katz SI: The epidermal basement membrane zone—structure, ontogeny, and the role in disease. J Am Acad Dermatol 11:1025–1037, 1984. Copyright 1984 with permission from Mosby-Year Book, Inc.)

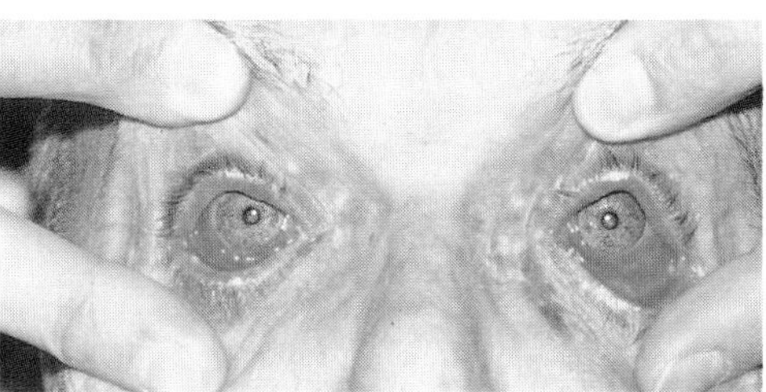

FIGURE 9–128 **Ocular cicatricial pemphigoid.** Note the severe conjunctival involvement. (Courtesy of Doyle Stulting, M.D.)

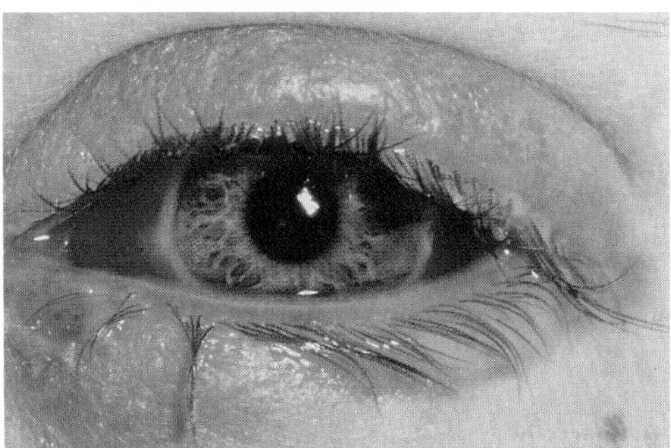

FIGURE 9–129 **Ocular involvement in toxic epidermal necrolysis.** Note prominent conjunctival involvement and purulent discharge. (Courtesy of Doyle Stulting, M.D.)

SECTION 10

Ocular Oncology

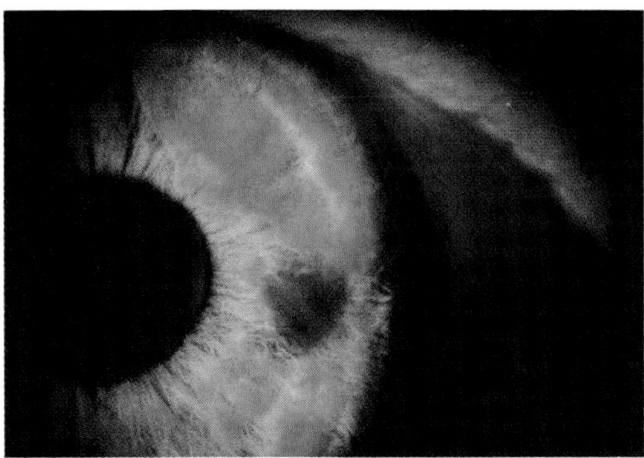

FIGURE 10–1 **Iris freckle.** An iris freckle represents an increase in pigmentation without focal clinical thickening in the iris stroma and may be due to either a minimal increase in the number of anterior border layer melanocytes or an increased number of melanin granules in normal numbers of stromal melanocytes.

A 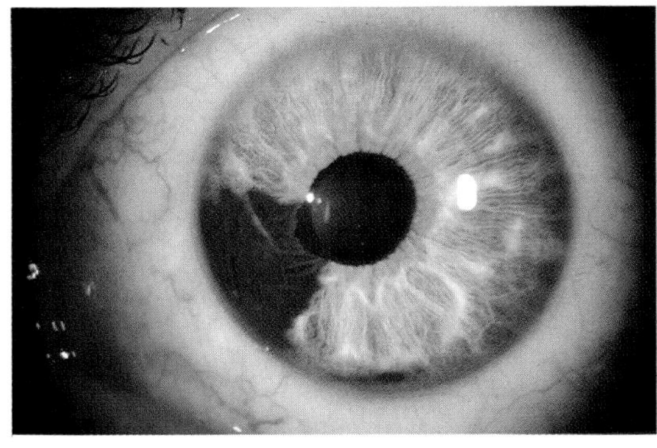

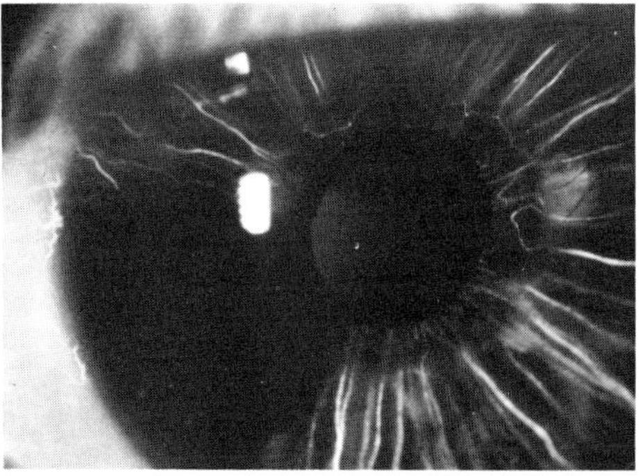 B

FIGURE 10–2 **Iris nevus.** *A,* A highly pigmented sectoral iris melanocytic nevus has caused minimal placoid thickening of the iris stroma and ectropion uvea. *B,* Fluorescein angiography discloses that the lesion has not induced a prominent neovasculature and blocks the normally occurring radial iris vessels in the quadrant involved. It is of interest that benign, highly pigmented melanocytic nevi in the iris tend to be hypovascularized or nonvascularized.

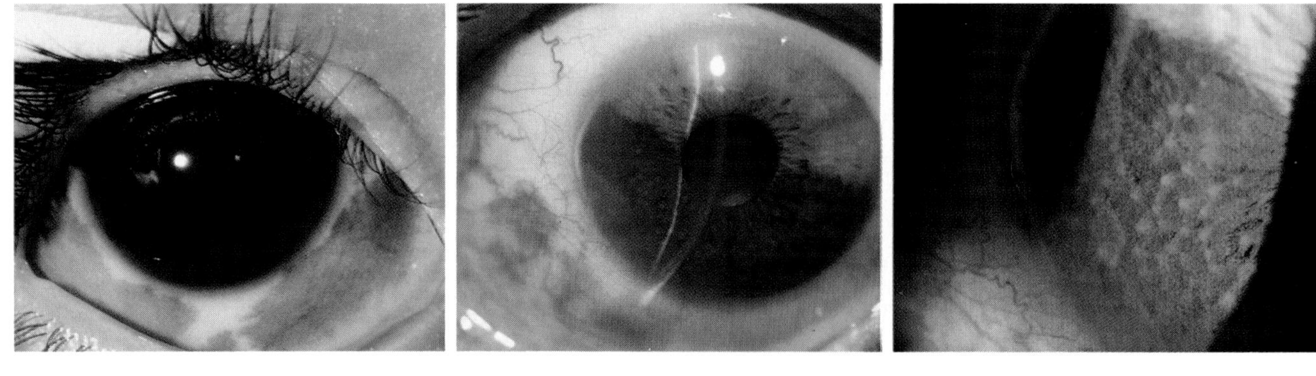

FIGURE 10–3 **Melanosis.** *A,* Epibulbar slate-gray pigmentation in Ota's nevus, which coexisted with intense pigmentation of the iris and the choroid. In such cases, there are increased numbers of heavily melaninized melanocytes in the uvea and episclera. *B,* Conjunctival, epibulbar, and iris melanocytosis. *C,* High-powered view of iris melanocytosis demonstrating micropebble architecture, typical of this lesion.

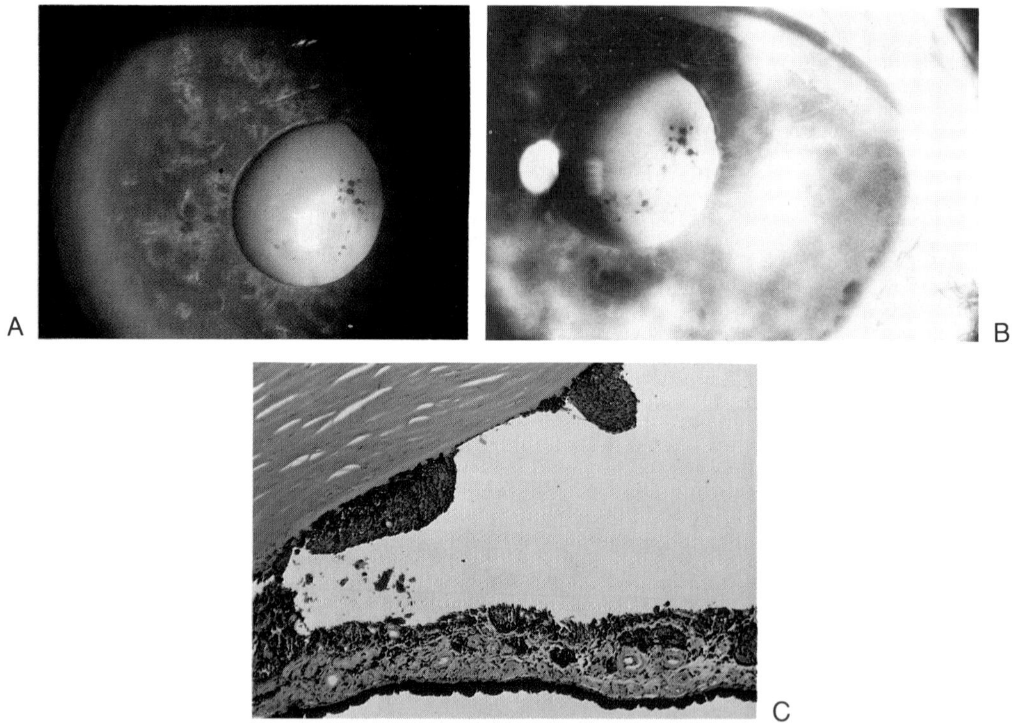

FIGURE 10–4 **Iris melanoma.** *A,* A diffusely pigmented iris melanoma causing glaucoma. Notice the heterogeneous and irregular character of the thickened iris stroma. There is pigment on the anterior capsule of the lens, which is rare in iris nevi. *B,* Iris fluorescein angiogram discloses leaky tumor-associated vessels that are small and indistinct as well as a few new large tumor feeder vessels. *C,* The anterior segment of the enucleated globe shows a diffuse and dyscohesive iris tumor, which has also involved the chamber angle and the posterior aspect of the cornea. Benign iris melanocytic proliferations tend to end at Schwalbe's line (H&E ×80).

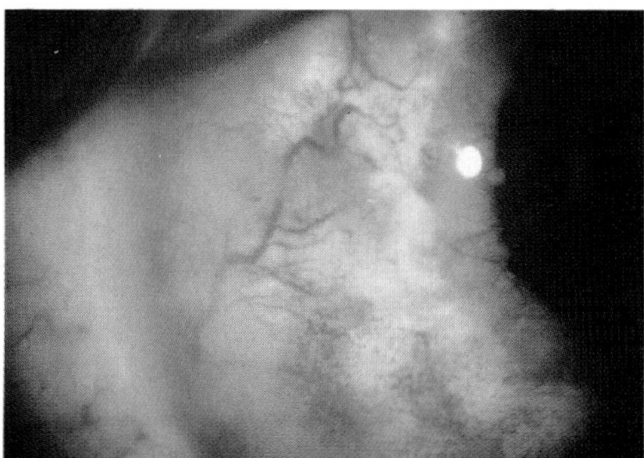

FIGURE 10–5 **Amelanotic melanoma.** A diffuse nonpigmented iris melanoma with large new tumor vessels that do not respect the radial pattern of the indigenous vessels of the iris. The other eye was blue, and the tumor consisted of epithelioid cells.

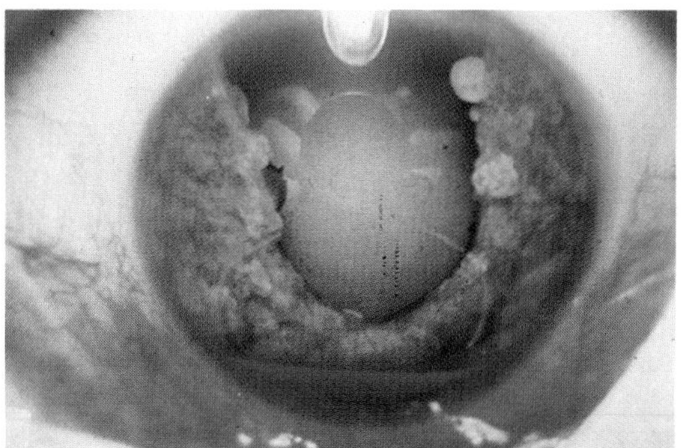

FIGURE 10–6 **Tapioca melanoma of iris.** Multinodular nonpigmented iris melanomas exhibiting a delicate vascularity have sometimes been referred to as tapioca-like in appearance. This lesion has bled spontaneously, which led to an iris biopsy, disclosing a mixed spindle and epithelioid cell melanoma with associated glaucoma.

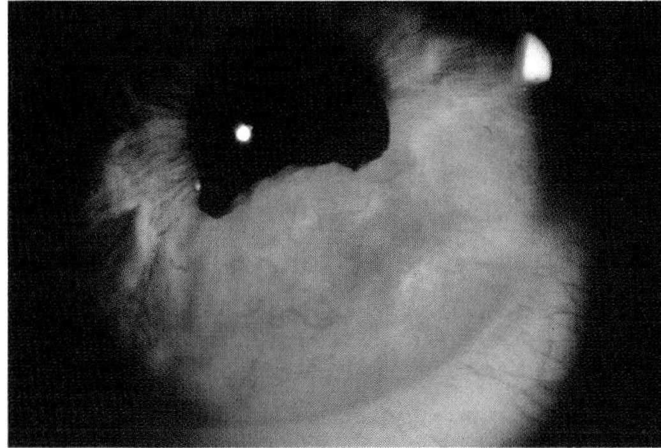

A

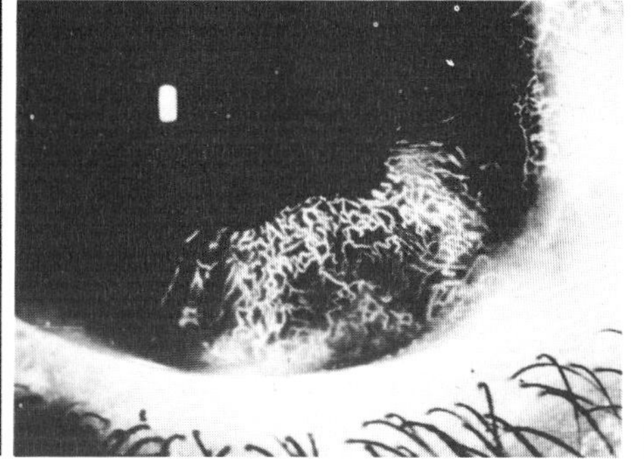

B

FIGURE 10–7 **Nonpigmented melanocytic nevus.** *A,* An elevated, sectoral, nonpigmented lesion of the iris that has not grown during a 15-year period of follow-up. Note the visible intrinsic vascularity to the lesion and that it is plastered to the peripheral cornea. *B,* An iris fluorescein angiogram discloses a luxuriant spaghetti-like collection of visible tumor-associated vessels that leaked later in the angiogram. Curiously, nonpigmented melanocytic nevi of the iris tend to engender the richest vascularity of all noninflammatory lesions of the iris.

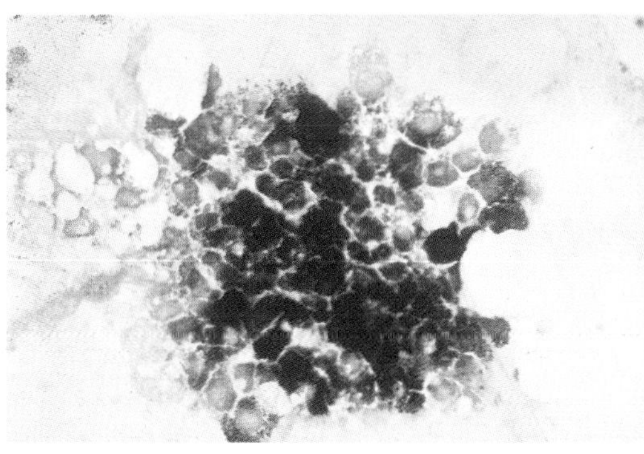

FIGURE 10–8 **Iris melanoma.** Needle biopsy from an anterior segment malignant melanoma shows a poorly cohesive pavement stone collection of pigmented epithelioid cells.

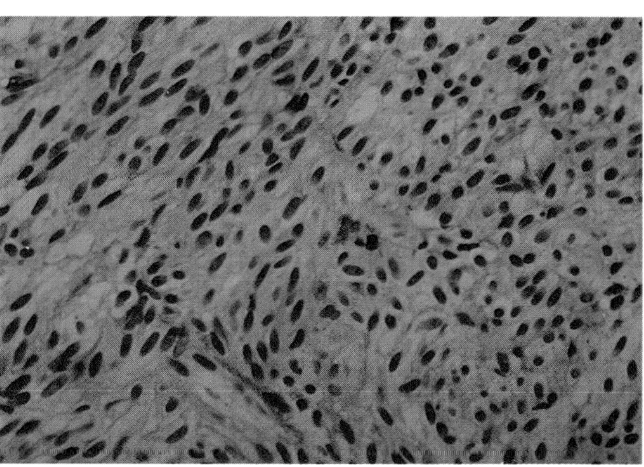

FIGURE 10–9 **Melanocytic nevi.** The majority of pigmented and nonpigmented melanocytic nevi of the iris are composed of banal spindle cells, some of which have in the past been called spindle A cells. Note the small nuclei, the low nuclear-to-cytoplasmic ratio, and the absence of mitotic figures (H&E ×140).

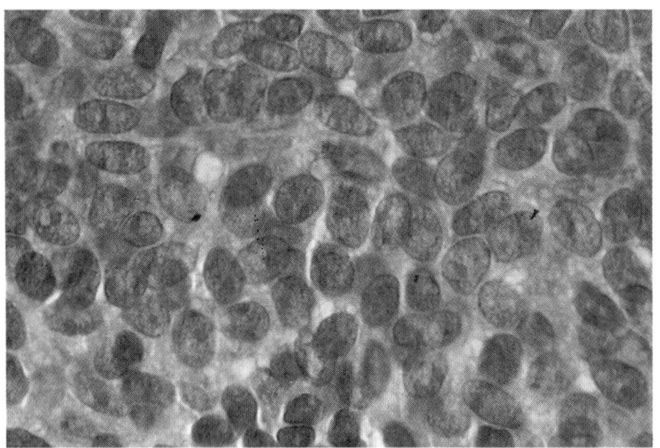

FIGURE 10–10 **Iris melanoma.** A field from a malignant melanoma in the iris composed of plump spindle B cells with distinct nucleoli (H&E ×210).

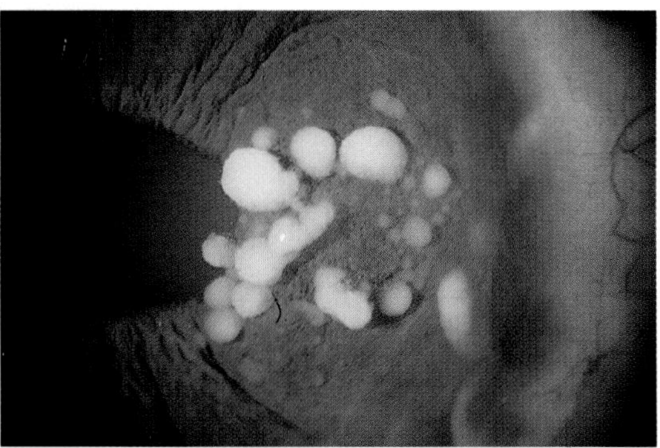

FIGURE 10–12 **Metastases to the iris.** Multiple nodules of metastatic carcinoma of the iris. The lesion appears to resemble sarcoid nodules, but there were no keratic precipitates.

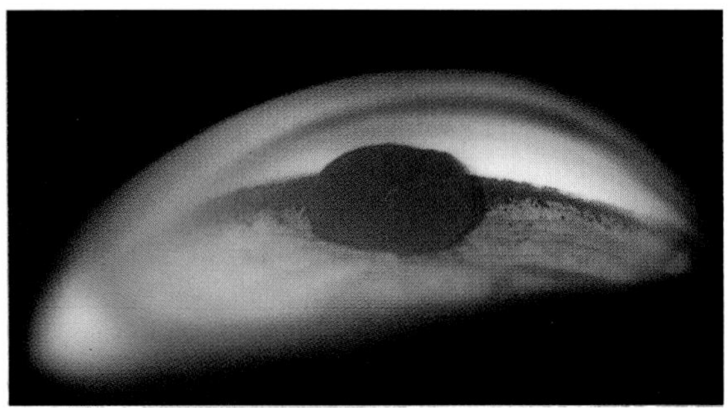

FIGURE 10–11 **Extension of ciliary body melanoma.** A peripheral iris nodule with flangelike extension of solid tissue in the chamber angle. Transillumination of the globe revealed a contiguous ciliary body mass.

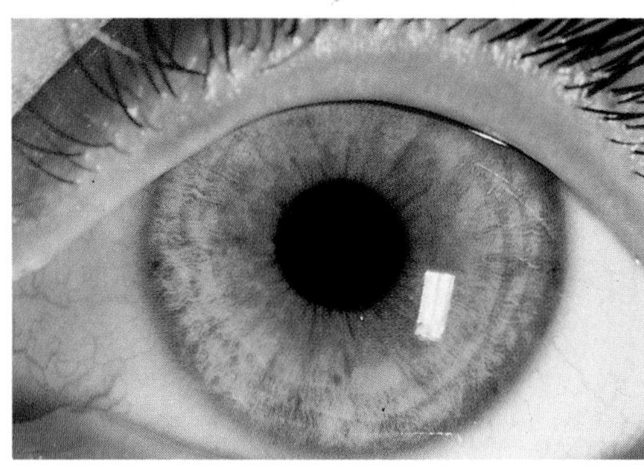

FIGURE 10–13 **Lisch nodules.** Lisch nodules in a patient with neurofibromatosis type 1.

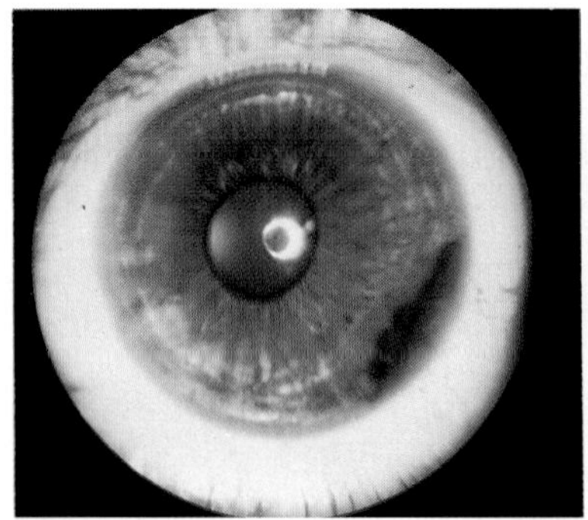

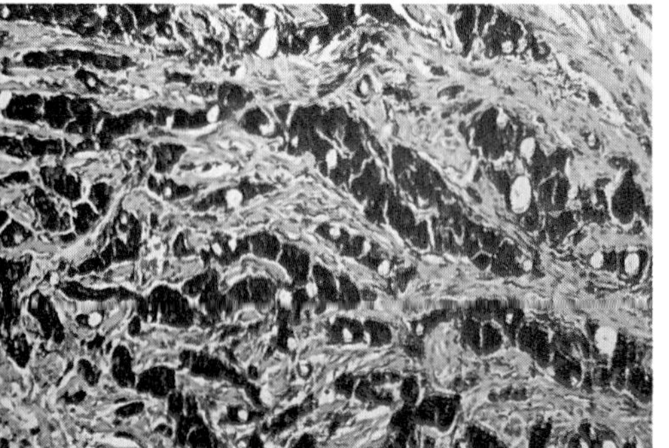

FIGURE 10–14 **Adenoma of the iris pigment epithelium.** *A,* Clinical photograph of multinodular, pigmented lesion in the peripheral iris of an 11-year-old boy. *B,* Photomicrograph of the adenoma of the iris pigment epithelium showing cords of pigmented cells, intracytoplasmic vesicles, and connective tissue septae. (From Shields JA, Augsburger JJ, Sandborn GE, Klein RM: Adenoma of the iris-pigment epithelium. Ophthalmology 90:735–739, 1983.)

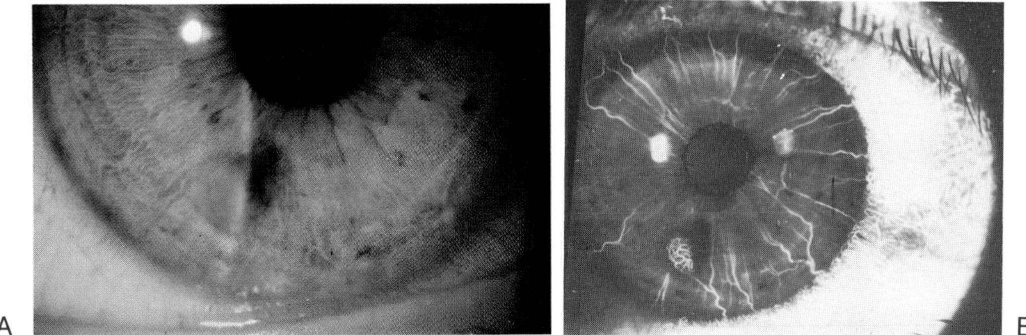

FIGURE 10–15 **Iris nevus.** *A,* A static iris nevus that is part pigmented and part nonpigmented. *B,* The iris fluorescein angiogram shows that the nonpigmented portion possesses a distinct skein of new, tumor-associated vessels, whereas the heavily pigmented area is devoid of vessels and blocks the fluorescence of the normally occurring radial iris vessels.

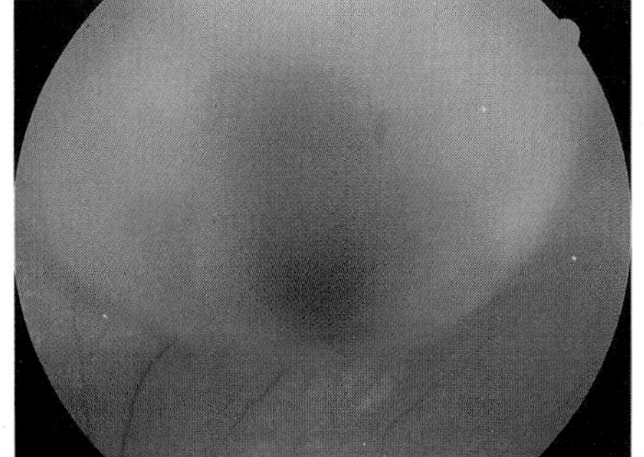

FIGURE 10–16 **Choroidal melanoma.** Fundus photograph of a large, highly pigmented, choroidal melanoma that has broken through Bruch's membrane.

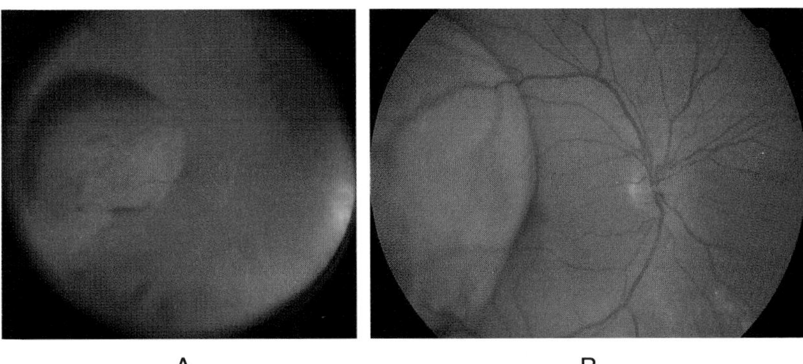

FIGURE 10–17 **Choroidal melanoma.** Equator-plus-fundus photograph *(A)* and a fundus photograph *(B)* of a moderately pigmented choroidal melanoma that has broken through Bruch's membrane and that involves the temporal macula.

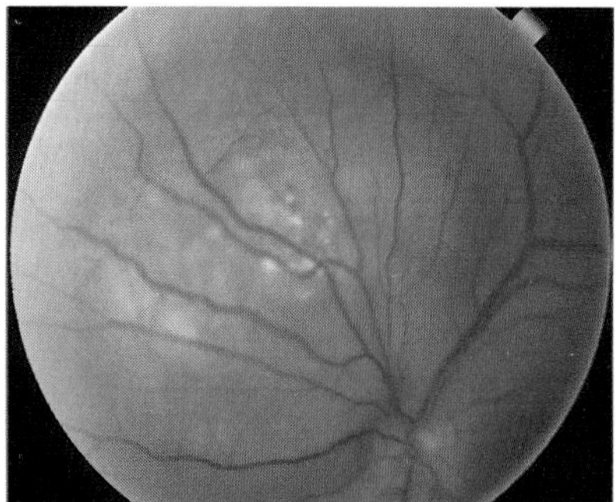

FIGURE 10–18 **Choroidal melanoma.** Large, dome-shaped choroidal melanoma with moderate pigmentation.

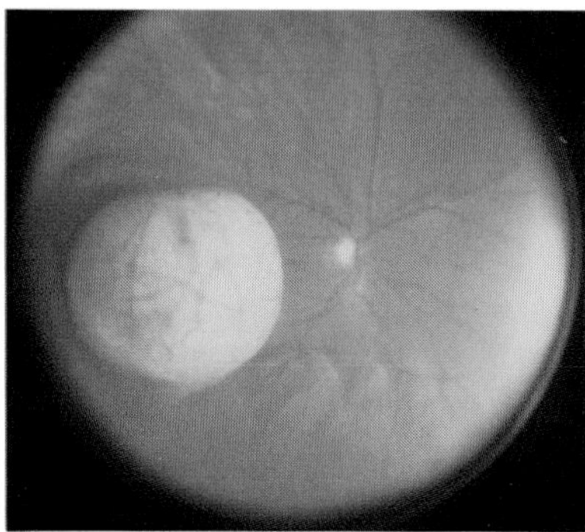

FIGURE 10–19 **Amelanotic choroidal melanoma.** Equator-plus-fundus photograph of a collar button–shaped amelanotic choroidal melanoma with inferior serous retinal detachment.

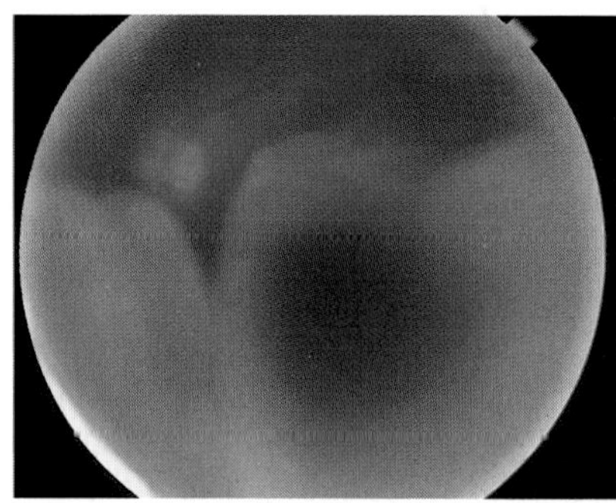

FIGURE 10–20 **Choroidal melanoma.** Large serous retinal detachment from a large choroidal melanoma.

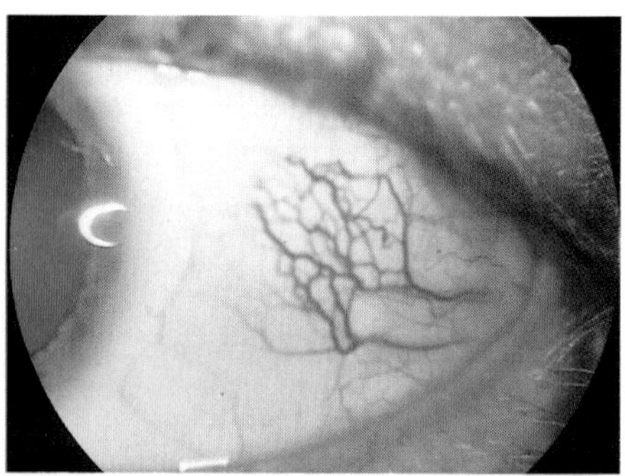

FIGURE 10–21 **Choroidal melanoma.** Sentinel vessels in a case of large choroidal melanoma.

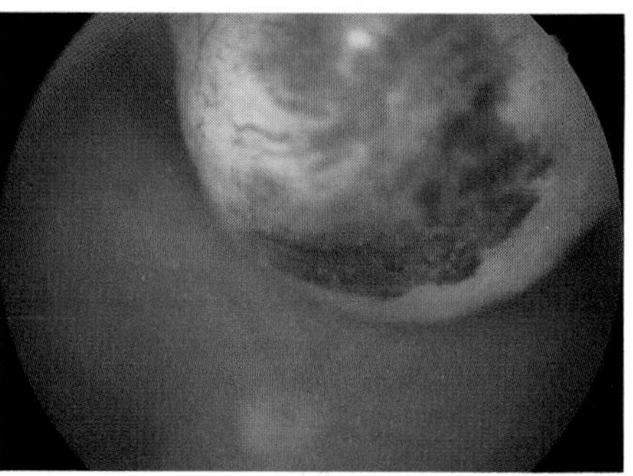

FIGURE 10–22 **Choroidal melanoma.** Hemorrhage overlying a large choroidal melanoma that has broken through Bruch's membrane.

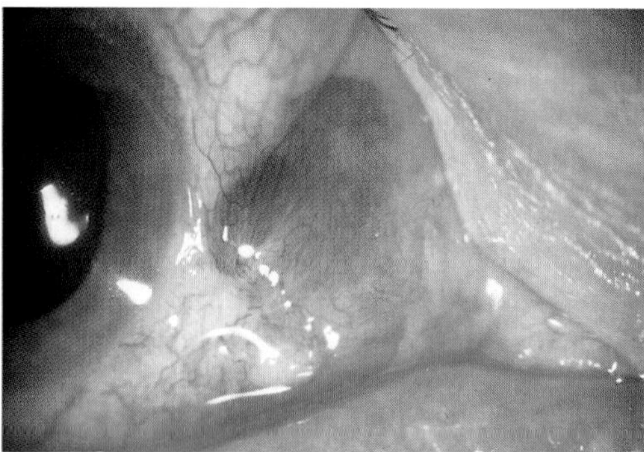

FIGURE 10–23 **Extrascleral extension of choroidal melanoma.** Extrascleral extension of large, highly pigmented, choroidal melanoma.

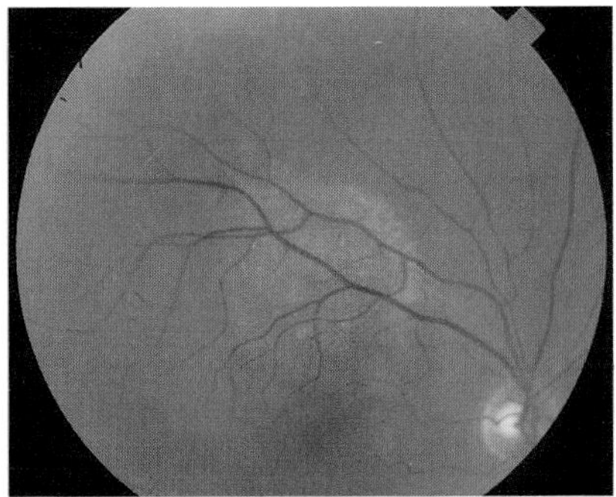

FIGURE 10–24 **Choroidal melanoma.** Intermediate elevated pigmented choroidal tumor that is 2 mm in height with drusen and hypopigmentation of the perimeter.

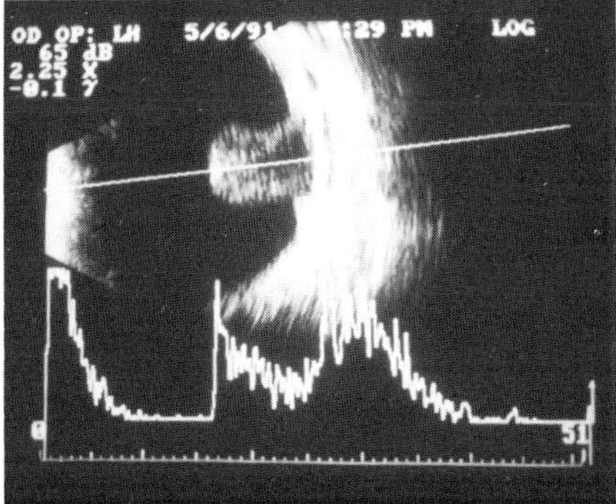

FIGURE 10–25 **Choroidal melanoma.** B-scan ultrasonography of a mushroom-shaped choroidal melanoma with a superimposed A-scan through the middle of the tumor. Note the smooth attenuation of the medium to low internal echoes. (Courtesy of Lois A. Hart, R.D.M.S.)

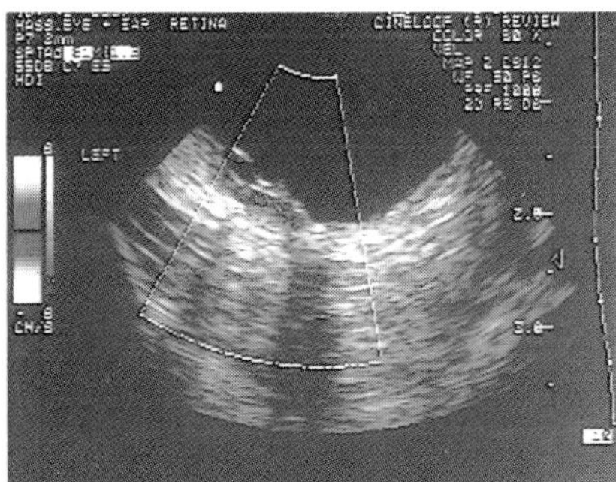

FIGURE 10–26 **Choroidal melanoma.** Doppler ultrasonography of choroidal melanoma. (Courtesy of Lois A. Hart, R.D.M.S.)

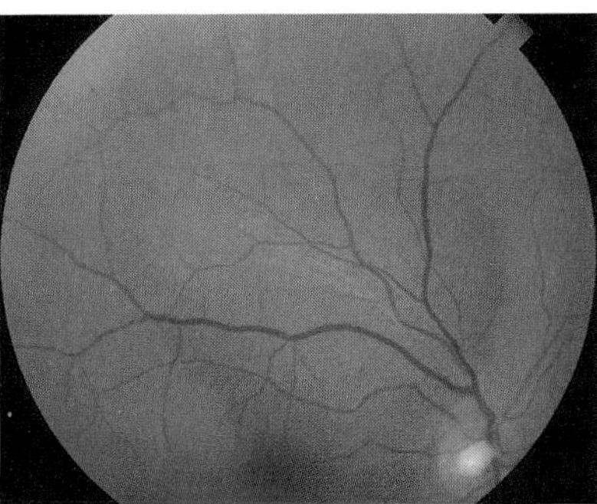

FIGURE 10–27 **Choroidal nevus.** Large, flat, pigmented choroidal nevus.

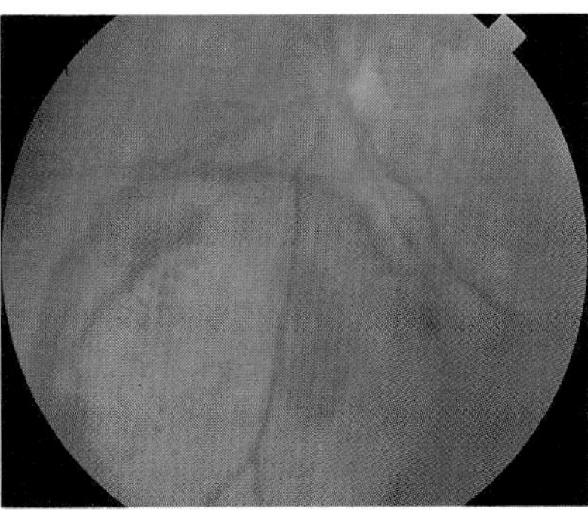

FIGURE 10–28 **Subretinal pigment epithelial hemorrhage.** Subretinal pigment epithelial hemorrhage that mimics a choroidal melanoma.

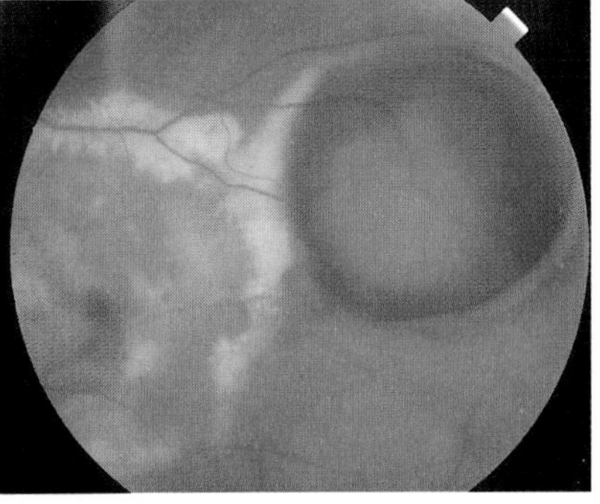

FIGURE 10–29 **Subretinal hemorrhage.** Subretinal hemorrhage associated with a disciform lesion in age-related maculopathy.

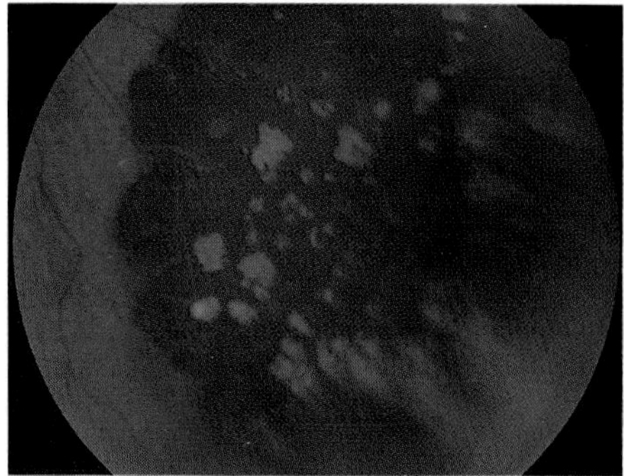

FIGURE 10–30 **Hypertrophy of the retinal pigment epithelium (RPE).** Congenital retinal pigment epithelial hypertrophy with scalloped margins and amelanotic lacunae.

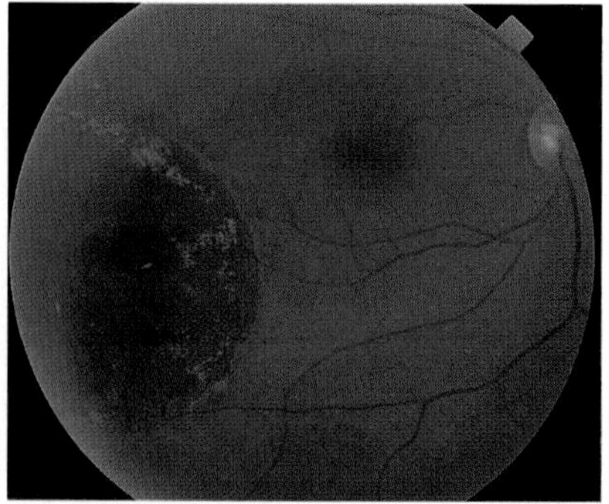

FIGURE 10–31 **Hypertrophy of the RPE.** Congenital hypertrophy of the RPE with small, amelanotic fenestrations.

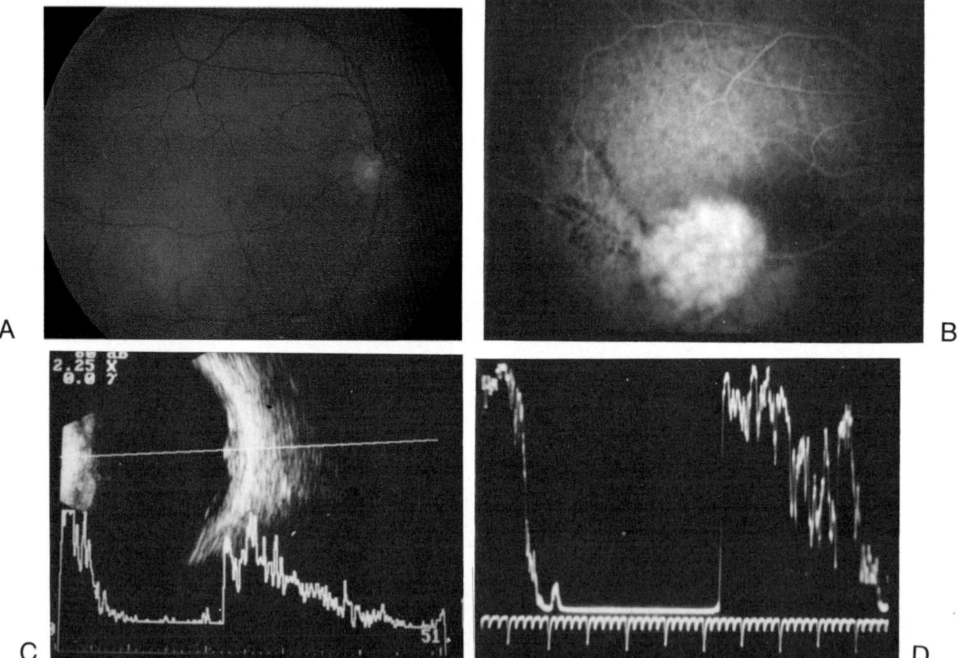

FIGURE 10–32 **Choroidal hemangioma.** *A,* Fundus photograph of a choroidal hemangioma. *B,* Fluorescein angiogram of the same lesion showing irregular hyperfluorescence. *C,* B-scan ultrasonography demonstrating the elevated nature of this choroidal lesion. *D,* A-scan through the tumor shows high internal reflectivity characteristic of a choroidal hemangioma.

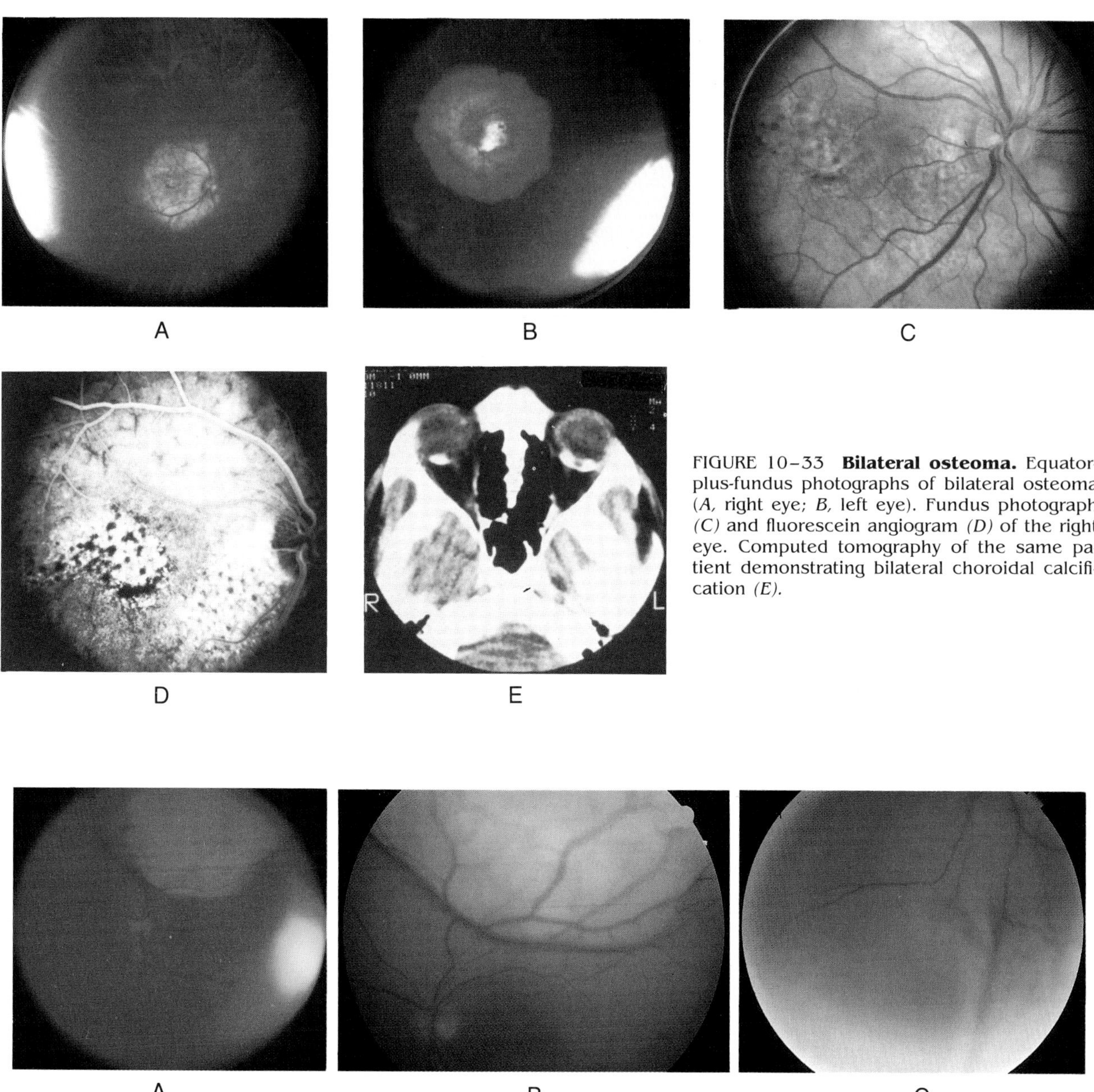

FIGURE 10–33 **Bilateral osteoma.** Equator-plus-fundus photographs of bilateral osteoma (*A*, right eye; *B*, left eye). Fundus photograph (*C*) and fluorescein angiogram (*D*) of the right eye. Computed tomography of the same patient demonstrating bilateral choroidal calcification (*E*).

FIGURE 10–34 **Metastatic carcinoma.** Equator-plus-fundus photograph (*A*) and fundus photographs (*B* and *C*) of a nonpigmented metastatic lesion from lung carcinoma. Note the prominent inferior serous retinal detachment.

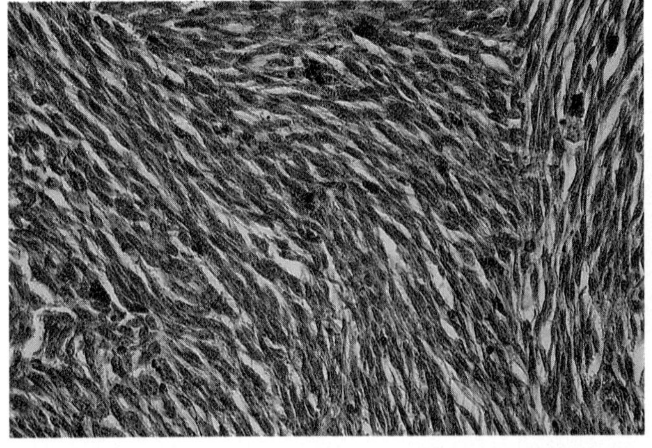

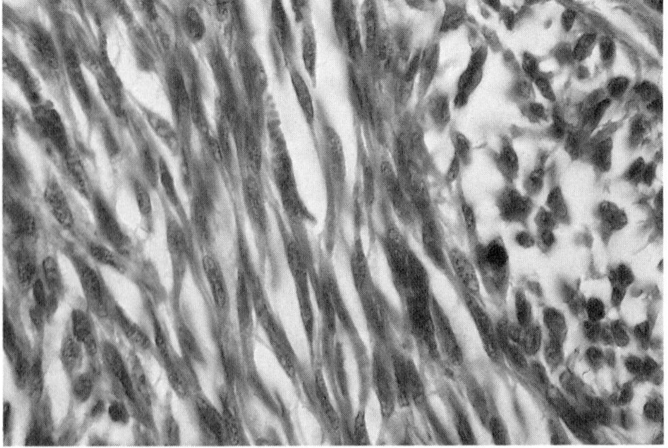

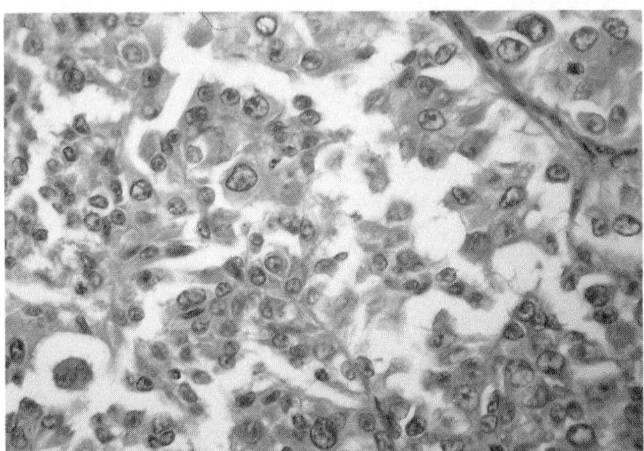

FIGURE 10–35 **Histopathology of choroidal melanoma.** *A,* In spindle cell melanomas of the choroid, the cells are usually organized into loose bundles or fascicles, three of which are shown in this photomicrograph running in various directions. When highly regimented with nuclear palisading, such spindle lesions are referred to as fascicular (only 6 percent of all spindle cell tumors). *B,* A spindle melanoma is composed of cells with bipolar elongated cytoplasm containing varying amounts of melanin. Some of the spindle cells on the right have been cut in cross-section, whereas most of the others have been sectioned longitudinally. Almost 50 percent of choroidal melanomas are composed of spindle cells. *C,* Epithelioid cells grow dyscohesively (frequently breaking away from each other owing to the absence of intercellular desmosomes) and feature abundant eosinophilic cytoplasm. The nuclei are large, with prominent and frequently eosinophilic nucleoli. Only 3 percent of choroidal melanomas are entirely composed of epithelioid cells, whereas approximately 45 percent of tumors are composed of some mixture of spindle and epithelioid cells. The greater the number of epithelioid cells present, the higher the risk for metastasis.

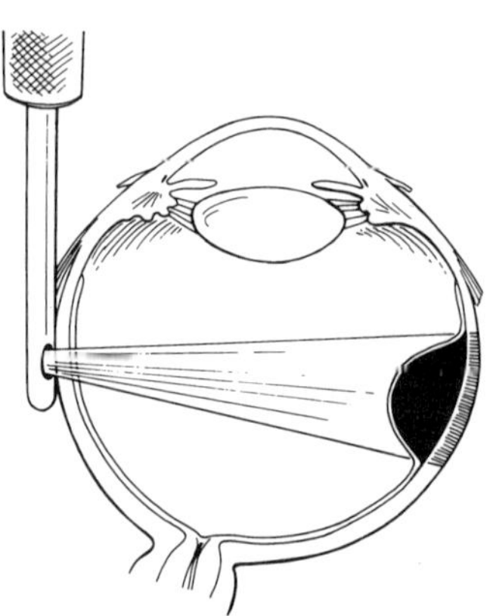

FIGURE 10–36 **Plaque treatment of choroidal melanoma.** Transillumination of a tumor to obtain the true base measurements. The probe is held 180 degrees from the tumor to avoid parallax of the tumor apex.

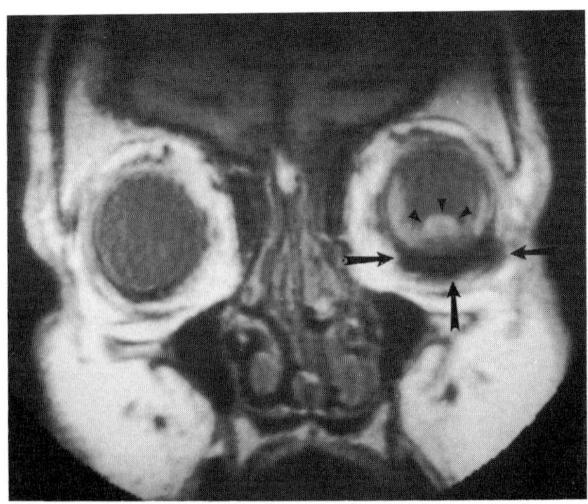

FIGURE 10–37 **Plaque treatment of choroidal melanoma.** Magnetic resonance imaging of plaque on scleral surface. *Arrowheads* outline the tumor, and *arrows* outline the radioactive plaque.

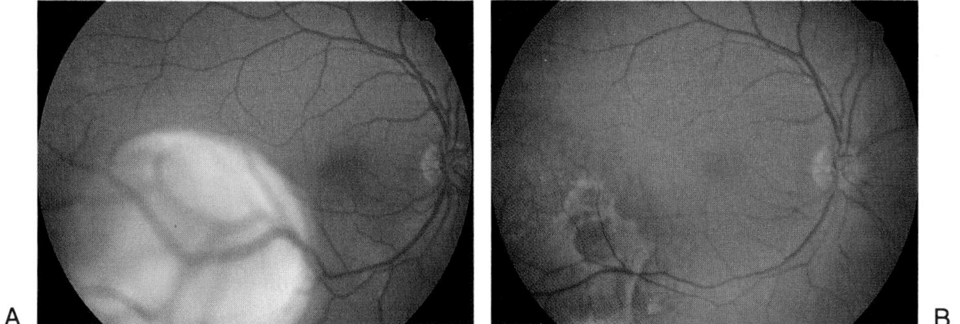

FIGURE 10–38 **Medium-sized choroidal melanoma.** *A,* Before irradiation. *B,* Three years after treatment.

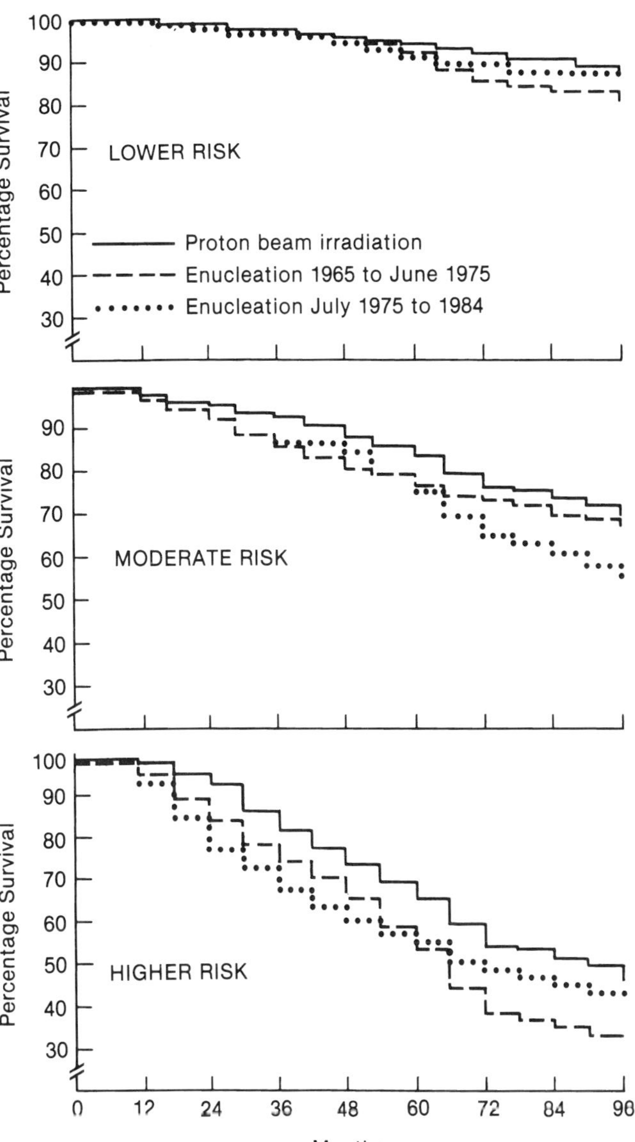

FIGURE 10–39 Survival probabilities for patients with uveal melanoma without extrascleral extension in alternative treatment groups, based on adjustment of prognostic factors in proportional hazards models fitted to 2-year intervals. Curves depict lower risk (50 years of age; posterior tumor; tumor diameter, 10 mm; tumor height, 5 mm), moderate risk (60 years of age; anterior tumor without ciliary body involvement; tumor diameter, 15 mm; tumor height, 8 mm), and higher risk (65 years of age; anterior tumor involving ciliary body; tumor diameter, 17 mm; tumor height, 10 mm) patients. (From Seddon JM, Gragoudas ES, Egan KM, et al: Relative survival rates after alternative therapies for uveal melanoma. Ophthalmology 97:769–777, 1990.)

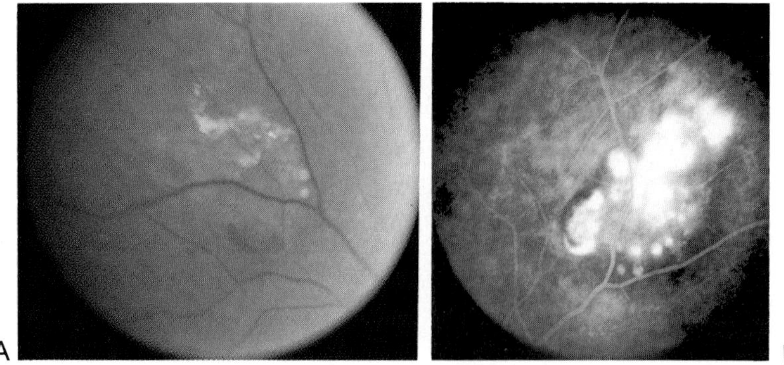

FIGURE 10–40 **Choroidal nevus.** Choroidal nevus with overlying drusen and orange pigment. *A,* Color retinography; *B,* fluorescein angiogram. (Courtesy of A. R. Frederick, M.D., Boston.)

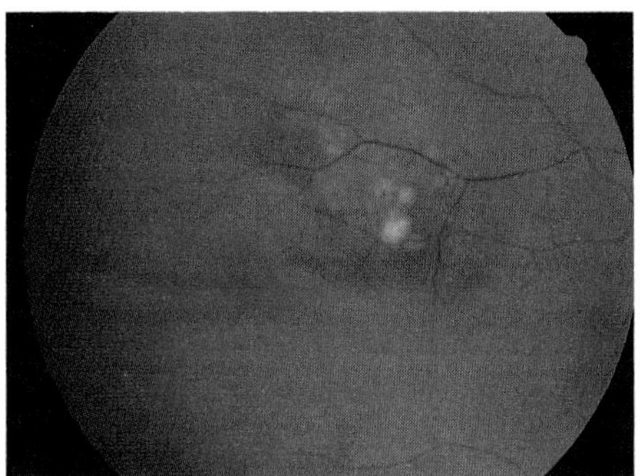

FIGURE 10–41 **Choroidal nevus.** Choroidal nevus with overlying pigment epithelial defects and drusen. (Courtesy of A. R. Frederick, M.D., Boston.)

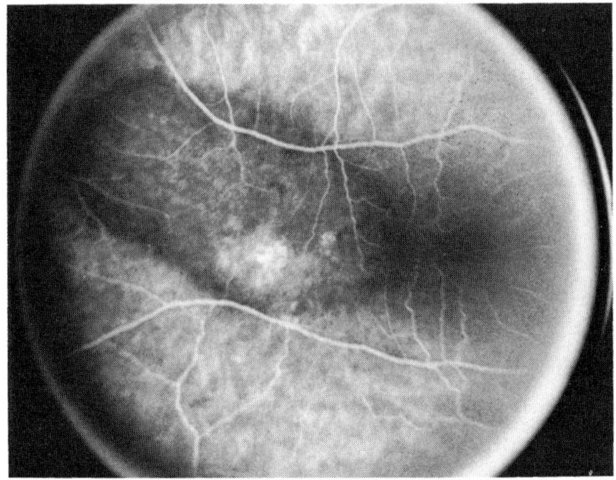

FIGURE 10–42 **Choroidal nevus: fluorescein angiography.** Retinal pigment epithelial defects overlying a long-standing nevus inducing localized hyperfluorescence. (Courtesy of A. R. Frederick, M.D., Boston.)

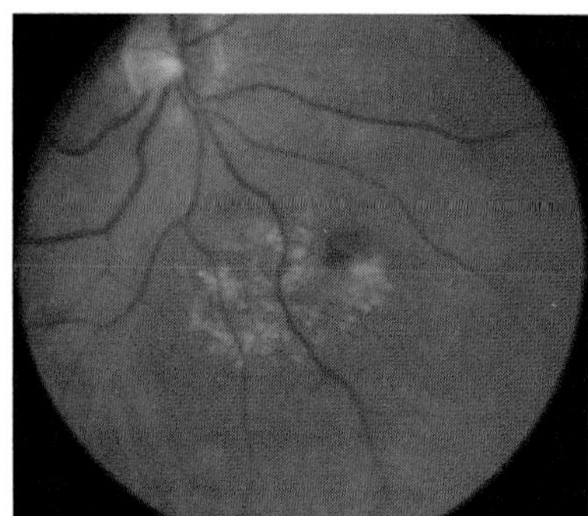

FIGURE 10–43 **Color retinography.** Hemorrhage complicating subretinal neovascularization in a choroidal nevus. (Courtesy of A. R. Frederick, M.D., Boston.)

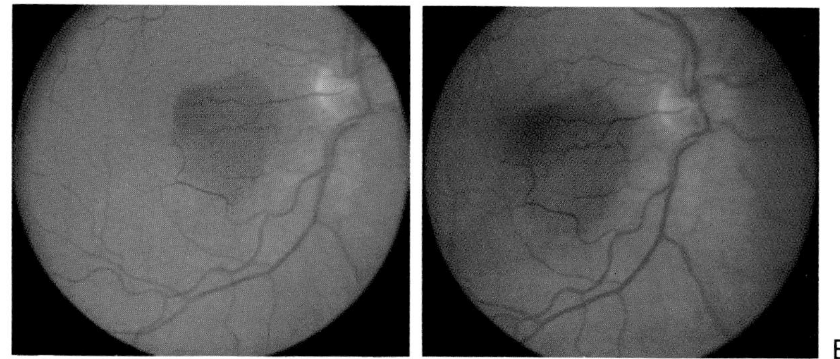

FIGURE 10–44 **Choroidal nevus.** A choroidal nevus followed over a 4-year period. *A*, April 1985; *B*, December 1989. (Courtesy of A. R. Frederick, M.D., Boston.)

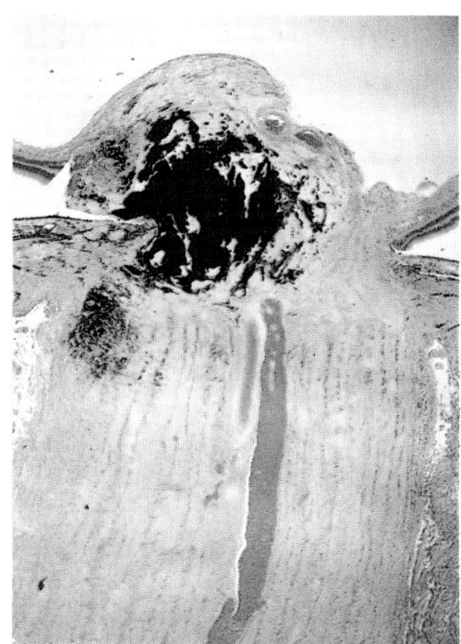

FIGURE 10–45 **Melanocytoma.** Usual histopathologic aspect under low power. The retrolaminar extension occurs frequently. (From Brini A, Dhermy P, Sahel J: Oncology of the Eye and Adnexa: Atlas of Clinical Pathology. Boston, Kluwer Academic Publishers, 1990.)

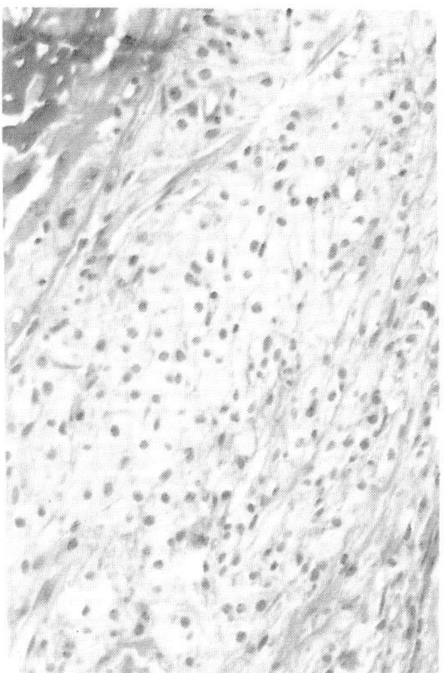

FIGURE 10–46 **Melanocytoma.** After depigmentation of a melanocytoma. Polyhedral regular cells with small nuclei and scanty nucleoli. (From Brini A, Dhermy P, Sahel J: Oncology of the Eye and Adnexa: Atlas of Clinical Pathology. Boston, Kluwer Academic Publishers, 1990.)

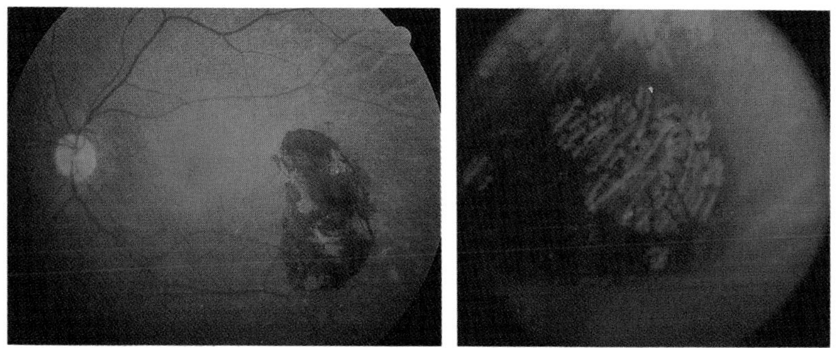

FIGURE 10–47 **Congenital hypertrophy of the RPE.** Note areas of depigmentation within each lesion (*A* and *B*). Progressive enlargement of the lacunae may eventually lead to totally depigmented lesions (*B*).

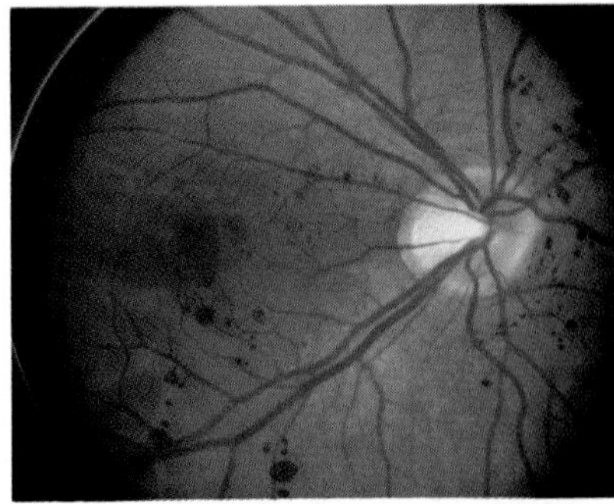

FIGURE 10–48 Clusters of hypertrophic RPE simulating bear tracks.

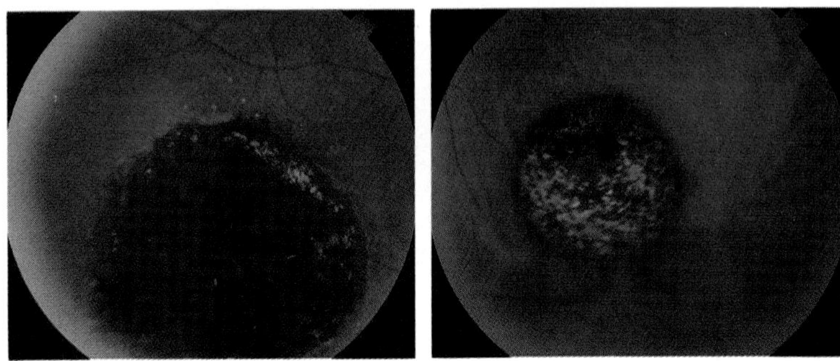

FIGURE 10–49 **Congenital hypertrophy of the RPE.** Peripheral lesions may appear elevated and may be confused with choroidal melanoma.

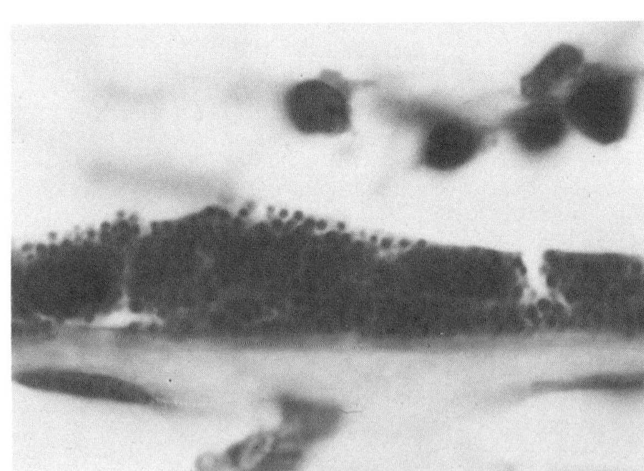

FIGURE 10–50 **Congenital hypertrophy of the RPE.** Note the presence of large pigment granules in the hypertrophied RPE cells (H&E, bleached). (Courtesy of W. Richard Green, M.D.)

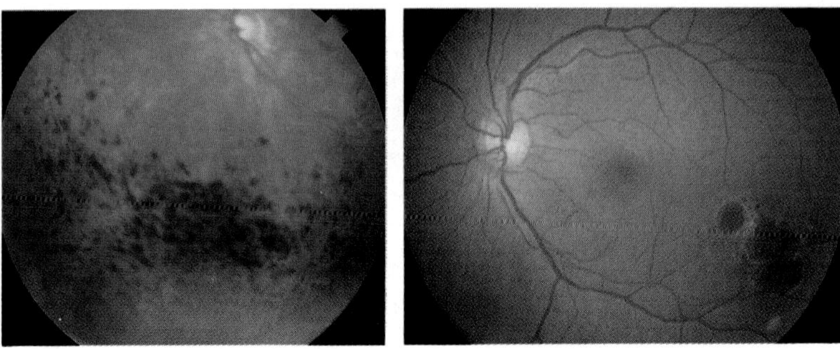

FIGURE 10–51 Reactive hyperplasia of the RPE following ocular trauma.

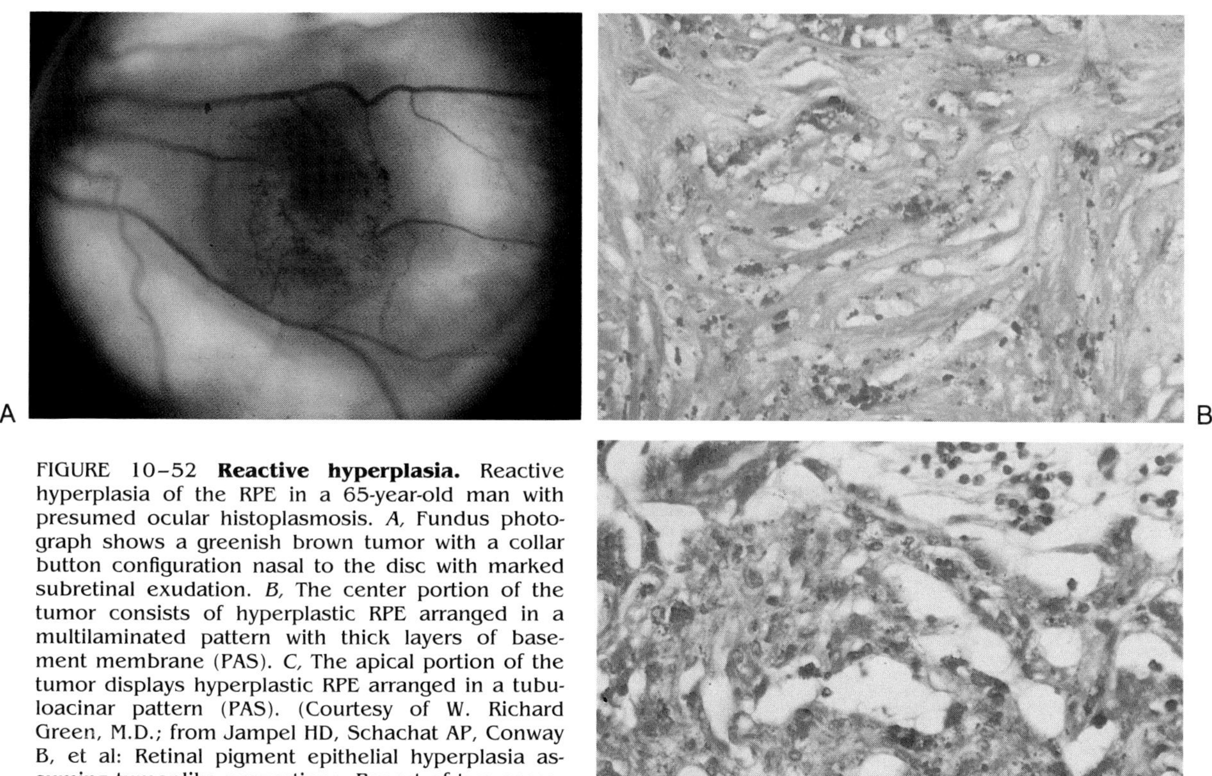

FIGURE 10–52 **Reactive hyperplasia.** Reactive hyperplasia of the RPE in a 65-year-old man with presumed ocular histoplasmosis. *A,* Fundus photograph shows a greenish brown tumor with a collar button configuration nasal to the disc with marked subretinal exudation. *B,* The center portion of the tumor consists of hyperplastic RPE arranged in a multilaminated pattern with thick layers of basement membrane (PAS). *C,* The apical portion of the tumor displays hyperplastic RPE arranged in a tubuloacinar pattern (PAS). (Courtesy of W. Richard Green, M.D.; from Jampel HD, Schachat AP, Conway B, et al: Retinal pigment epithelial hyperplasia assuming tumor-like proportions: Report of two cases. Retina 6:105–112, 1986.)

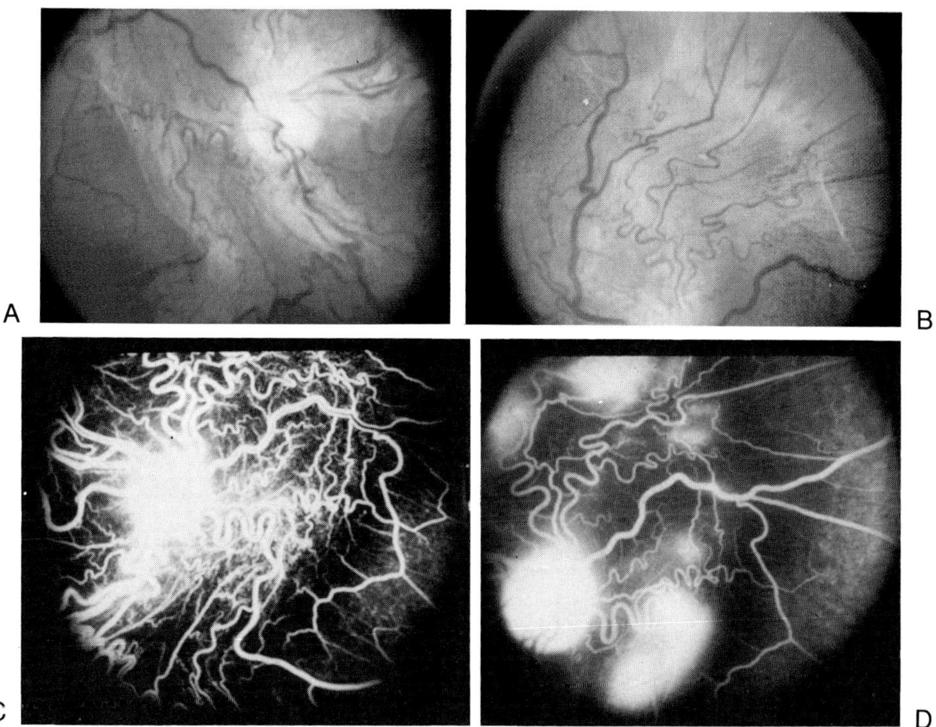

FIGURE 10–53 **Combined hamartoma of the retina and RPE.** Note extensive peripapillary vascular tortuosity and prominent vitreoretinal interface change *(A).* Superior and nasal to the disc, the lesion is elevated and pigmented *(B).* Fluorescein angiography shows leakage of dye from the abnormal vessels (*C* and *D*).

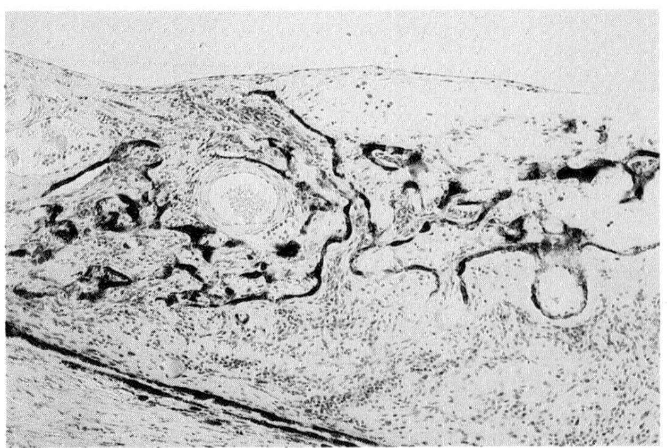

FIGURE 10–54 **Combined hamartoma of the retina and RPE.** Note disorganization of the retina and marked proliferation of the RPE along the inner retinal surface and blood vessels (H&E). (Courtesy of Lorenz E. Zimmerman, M.D.)

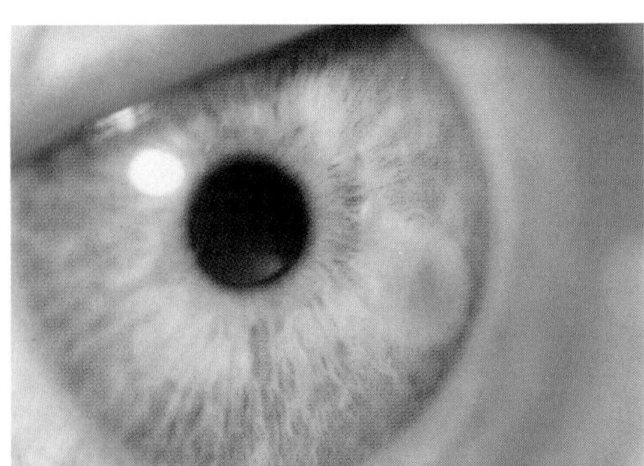

FIGURE 10–57 Metastatic iris lesion in an otherwise asymptomatic patient. The primary tumor was unknown.

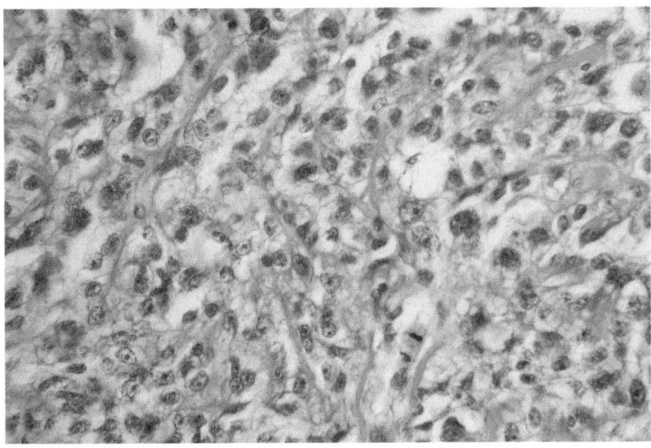

FIGURE 10–55 **Adenocarcinoma of the RPE.** The tumor consists of anaplastic cells with large and pleomorphic nuclei. Mitotic figures are present *(arrow)*. (Courtesy of Alec Garner, M.D.)

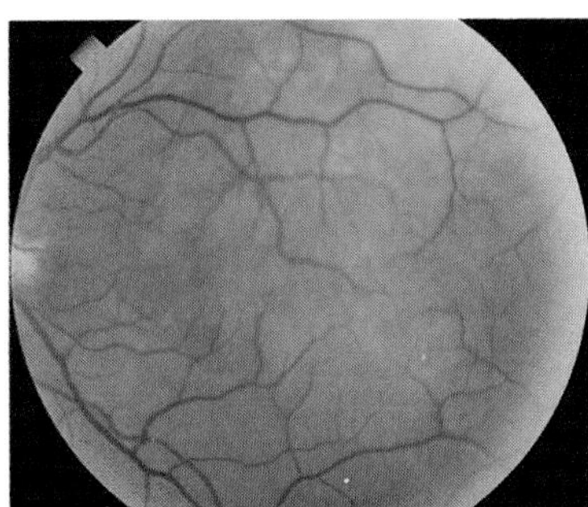

FIGURE 10–58 **Metastatic lung carcinoma.** This 54-year-old man with a history of heavy cigarette smoking presented with a central scotoma and 20/400 visual acuity. Submacular metastatic lung carcinoma to the choroid was diagnosed.

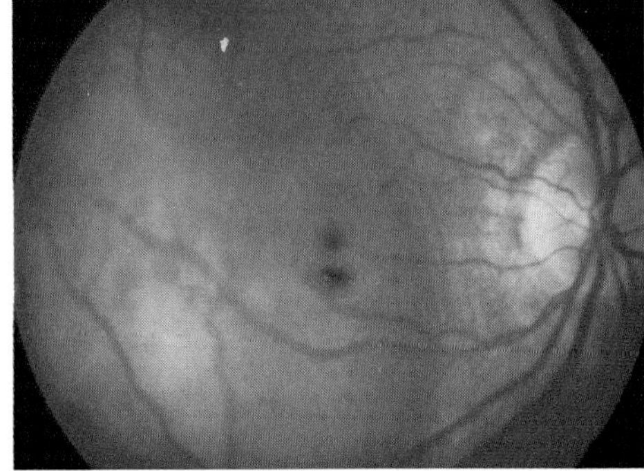

FIGURE 10–56 Breast carcinoma metastatic to the submacular choroid.

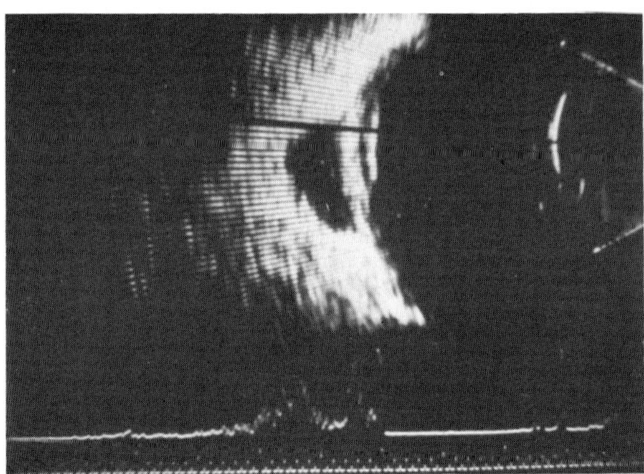

FIGURE 10–59 **Metastatic lung carcinoma.** B-scan ultrasonography of lung carcinoma metastatic to the choroid demonstrates elevation of the retina by a lesion of moderate-to-high reflectivity.

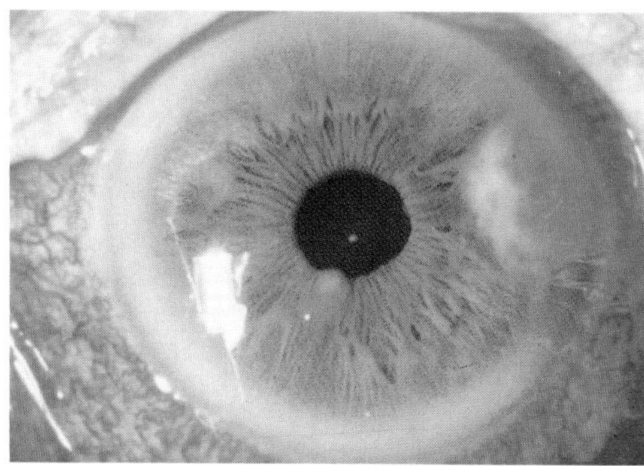

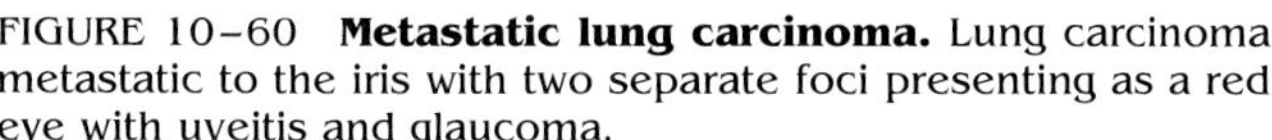

FIGURE 10–60 **Metastatic lung carcinoma.** Lung carcinoma metastatic to the iris with two separate foci presenting as a red eye with uveitis and glaucoma.

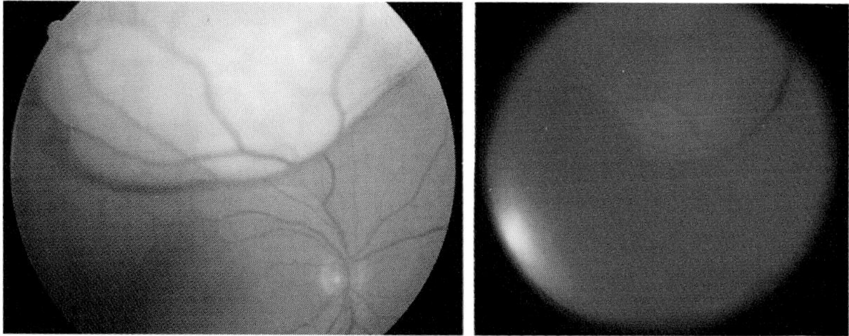

FIGURE 10–61 **Metastatic lung carcinoma.** Standard *(left)* and wide-angle *(right)* fundus photographs of a metastatic lung carcinoma. The solitary lesion appears markedly elevated and somewhat pigmented, making distinction from primary choroidal melanoma difficult. (Courtesy of E. Gragoudas, M.D.)

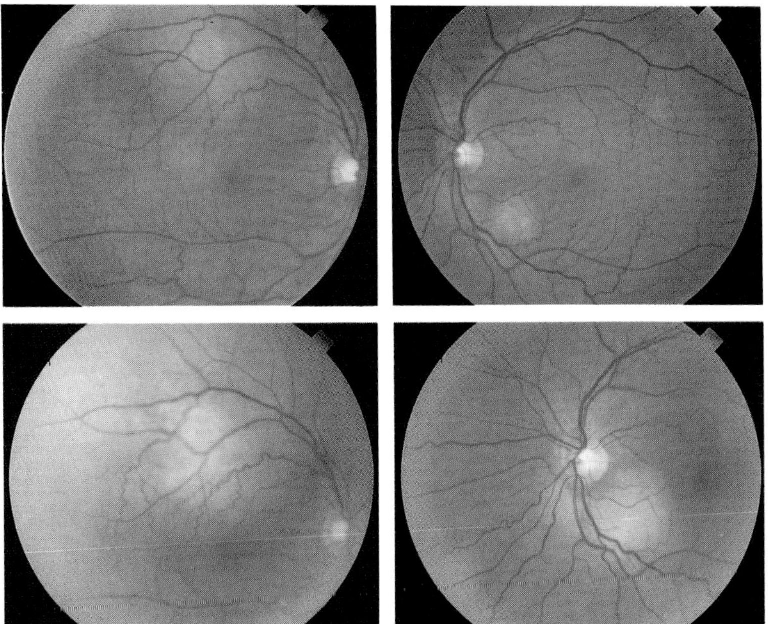

FIGURE 10–62 **Metastatic breast carcinoma.** *Upper panels,* Right and left eyes, revealing multiple metastases from breast carcinoma. Eight weeks later *(lower panels),* there is obvious growth of the lesions.

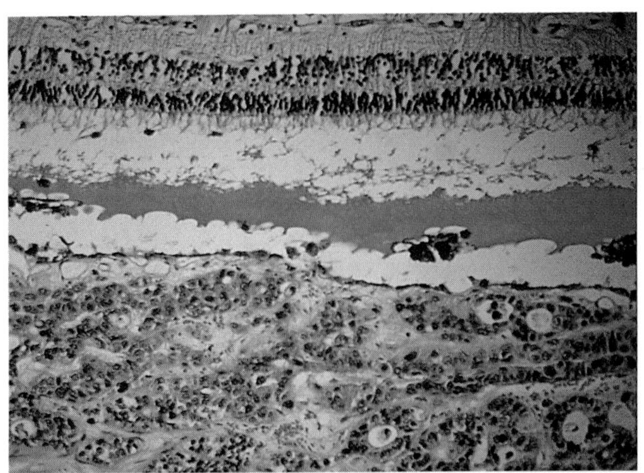

FIGURE 10–63 **Metastatic adenocarcinoma.** Enucleation specimen demonstrating acini formation in adenocarcinoma metastatic to the choroid. The location of the primary tumor could not be determined.

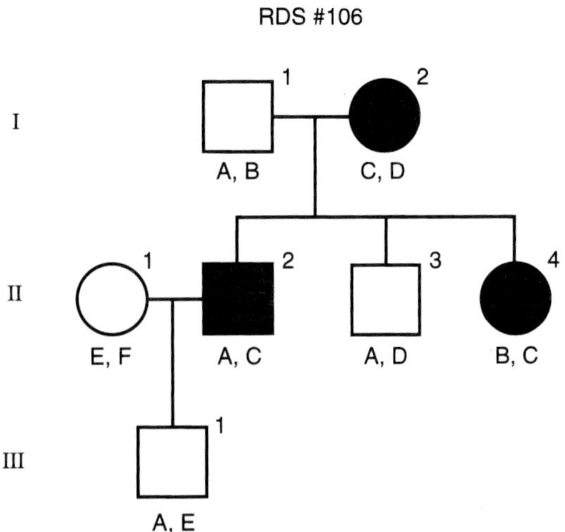

FIGURE 10–64 **Hereditary retinoblastoma.** Inheritance of copies of the retinoblastoma gene in a family (RDS #106) with hereditary retinoblastoma. As in all figures, darkened circles and squares denote females and males, respectively, who developed at least one retinoblastoma in childhood. Beneath each symbol are arbitrary letters designating allelic copies of the retinoblastoma gene. Each allele corresponds to a haplotype that was determined by analyzing up to five intragenic DNA polymorphisms. In this pedigree, the "C" haplotype correlates with the disease. (From Yandell DW, Dryja TP: Detection of DNA sequence polymorphisms by enzymatic amplification and direct genomic sequencing. Am J Hum Genet 45:547–555, 1989.)

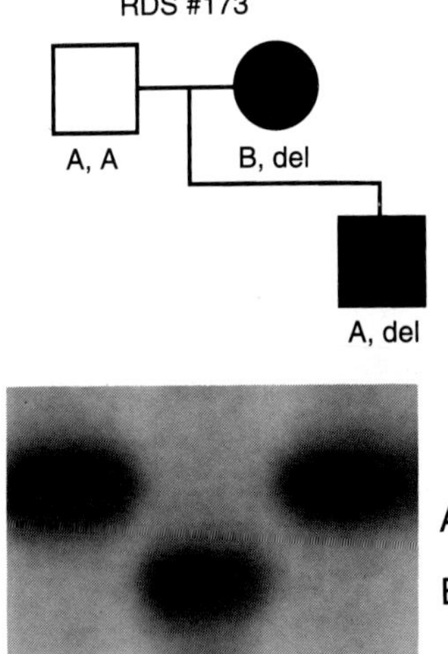

FIGURE 10–65 **Detection of a germline deletion of the retinoblastoma gene.** The autorad beneath the schematic pedigree shows the data derived from the intragenic polymorphisms detected by probe p68RS2.0. The father is homozygous for the band labeled *A*. The mother is hemizygous for the band labeled *B*. The presence of the deletion becomes obvious from the observation that the son does not appear to have an allele derived from his mother. In fact, he inherited the deleted (del) allele.

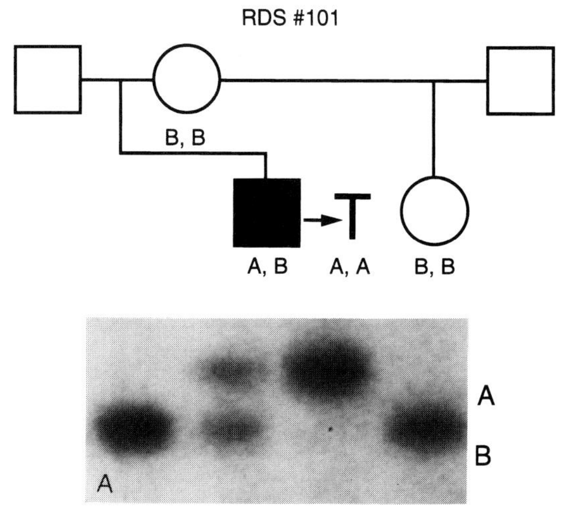

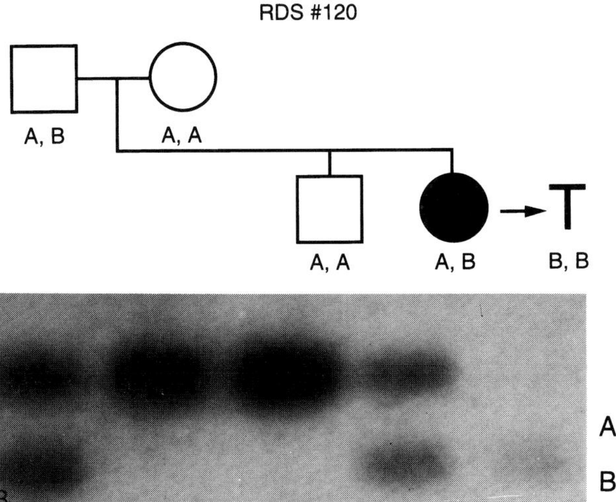

FIGURE 10–66 **Retinoblastoma.** Use of homozygosity in a tumor to reduce risk in siblings of the affected simplex retinoblastoma patient. *RDS #101,* The polymorphism shown in the autorad is detected by probe p35RO.6. One of the tumors from the bilaterally affected child is homozygous for the A allele. This allele must have the germline mutation. Because this allele is not present in the mother, it must have been derived from the father (who did not provide a blood sample). Therefore, the father is possibly an asymptomatic carrier; the mother is not. The second child, who has a different father, is at no increased risk. *RDS #120,* In this pedigree, a tumor from the bilaterally affected child is homozygous for the B allele, which is derived from the father. Only the father could possibly be an asymptomatic carrier of the germline mutation carried by the affected daughter. Because the son did not inherit this copy of the gene, he is at no increased risk for the disease. The polymorphism illustrated beneath this family pedigree is detected by probe #P68RS2.0.

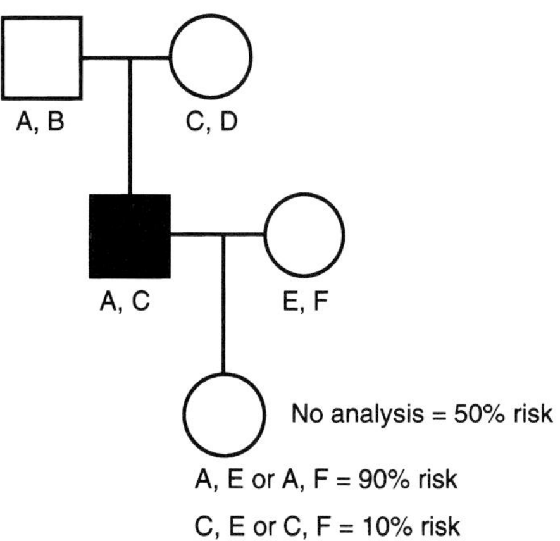

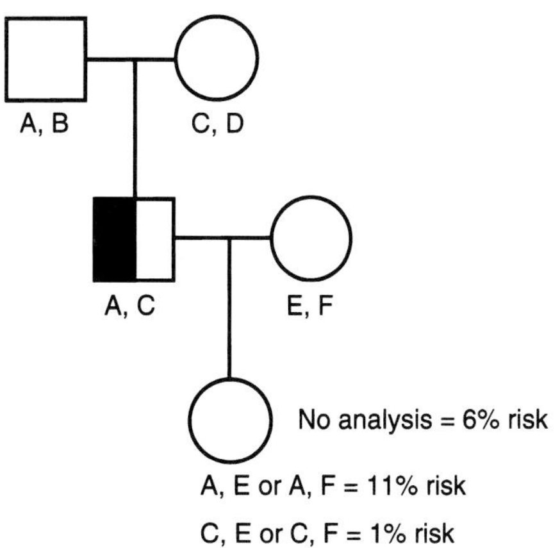

FIGURE 10–67 **Retinoblastoma.** Modification of risk based on grandparental origin of alleles. If the offspring of a simplex case inherits the grandpaternal copy of the retinoblastoma gene, the risk is approximately 10-fold higher than if the child inherits the grandmaternal copy.

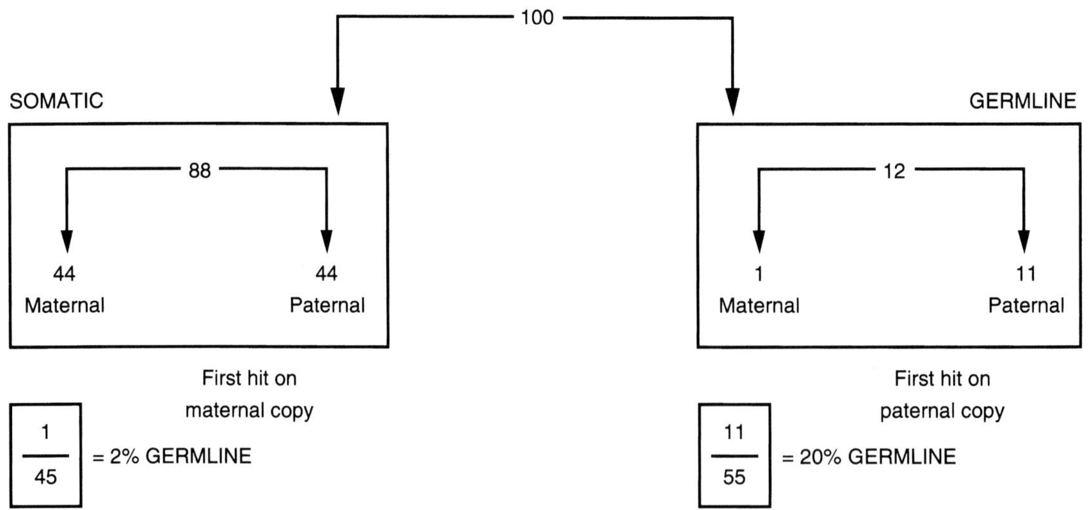

FIGURE 10–68 **Risk of germline mutation.** In unilateral simplex retinoblastoma, the risk of a germline mutation varies according to the parental origin of the allele that carries the initial mutation. The figure illustrates the calculation of those risks. Out of 100 such persons, one would expect 12 to have a new germline mutation. Of those 12, approximately 90%, or approximately 11 persons, would have that new germline mutation on the paternally derived copy of the gene. Of the 88 persons with a somatic, initial mutation, half would have the initial mutation on the paternal copy and half on the maternal copy. Therefore, of the 55% of persons with an initial mutation on the paternally derived copy, 11, or 20%, would have a new germline mutation. In contrast, of the 45% of patients with an initial mutation on the maternally derived copy, only 1, or approximately 2%, would have a new germline mutation.

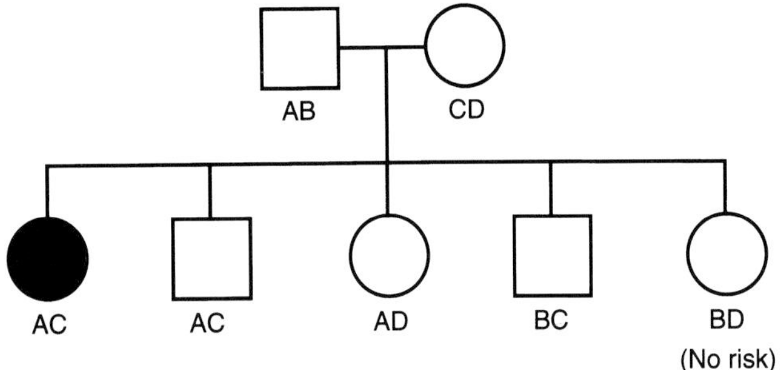

FIGURE 10–69 **Segregation of alleles in families with simplex retinoblastoma.** If a parent is an asymptomatic carrier, the mutant copy must be the one passed on to the affected child. In this family, only the A copy of the father or the C copy of the mother could possibly have carried a germline mutation that caused disease in the oldest child. Any child who inherits both the B and D alleles is at no increased risk. Such an analysis works whether the affected child had unifocal or multifocal disease.

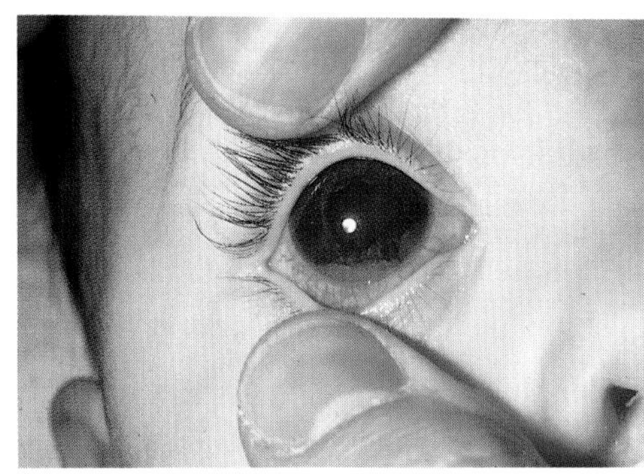

FIGURE 10–71 **Retinoblastoma.** Retinoblastoma cells in anterior chamber.

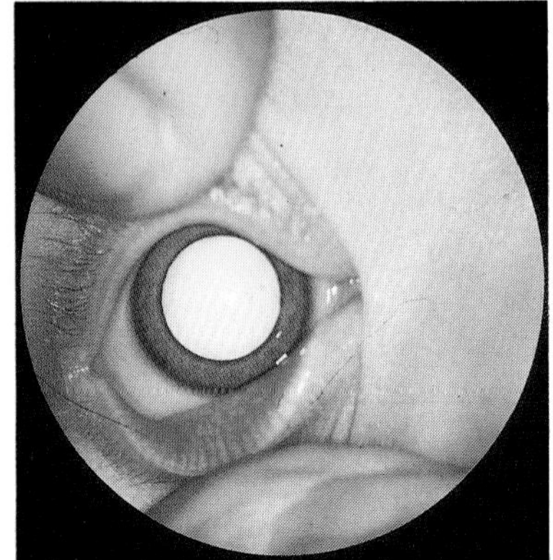

FIGURE 10–70 **Retinoblastoma.** Leukocoria in retinoblastoma.

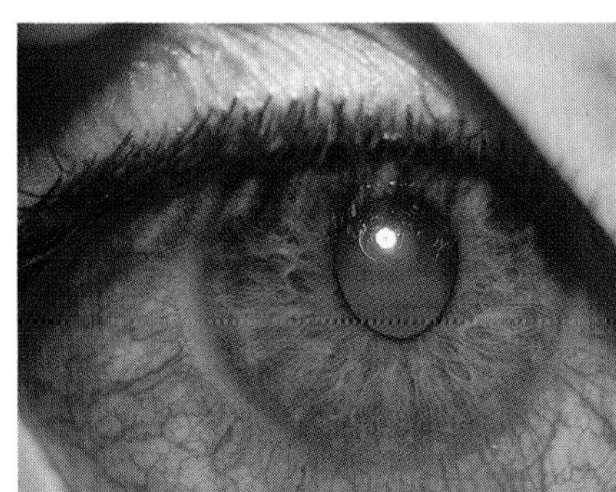

FIGURE 10–72 **Retinoblastoma.** Glaucoma from retinoblastoma.

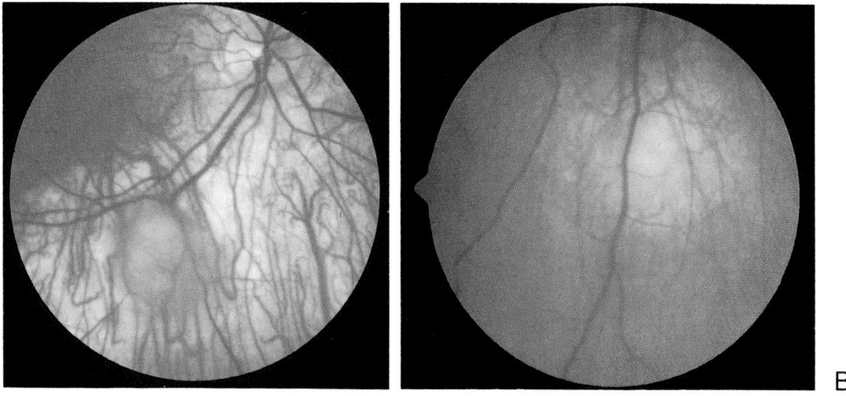

FIGURE 10–73 **Differential diagnosis.** *A,* Astrocytic hamartoma in tuberous sclerosis; *B,* small retinoblastoma.

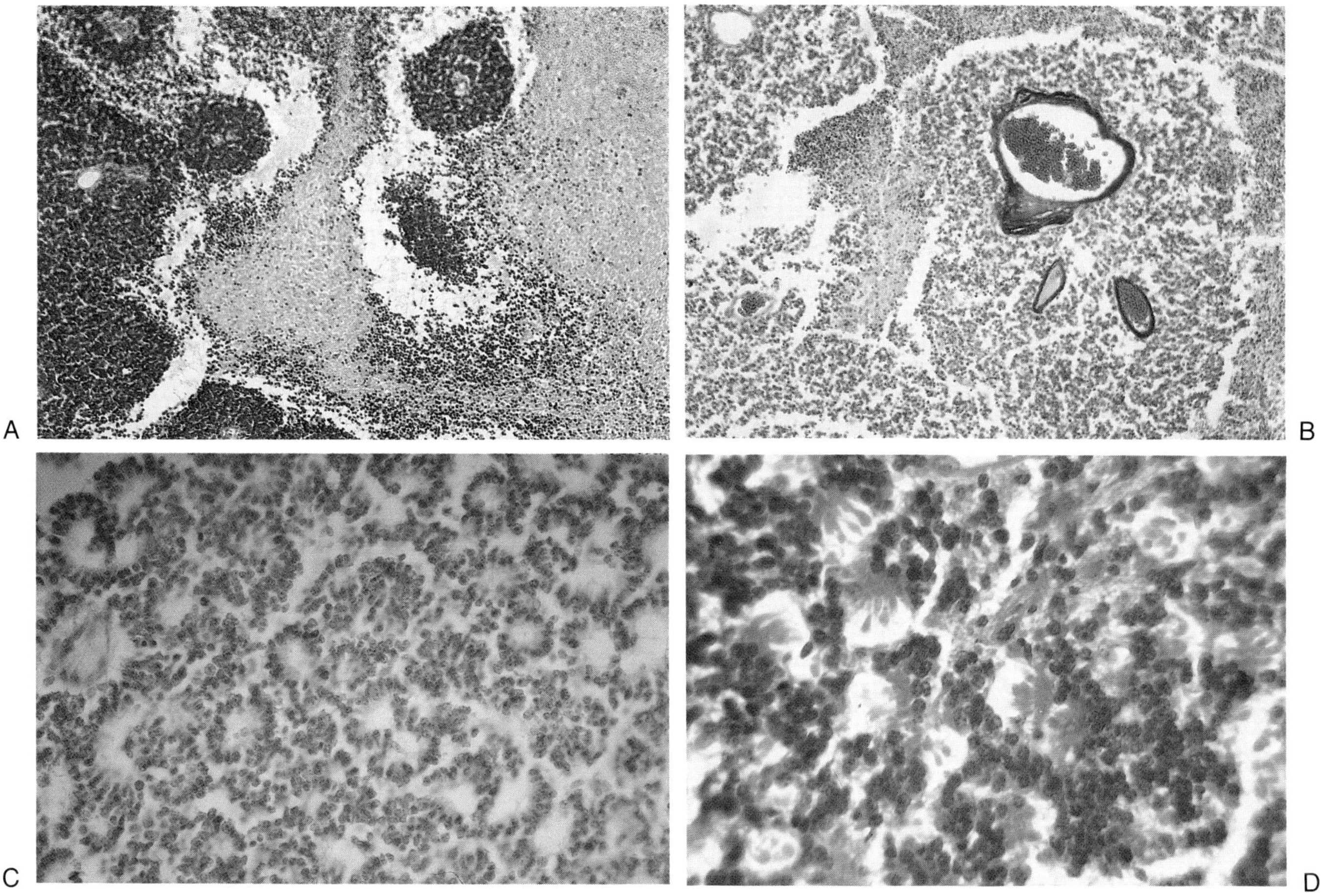

FIGURE 10–74 **Histopathology of retinoblastoma.** *A,* Cuffs of small basophilic, undifferentiated, neuroblastic cells surround a central blood vessel. The eosinophilic and granular areas represent foci of necrosis beyond the nutritive radius of the blood vessels. Such perivascular collections of viable tumor cells have also been referred to as pseudorosettes. *B,* An area of vastly necrotic retinoblastoma with eosinophilic granular cellular debris contains three variably-sized blood vessels with intense basophilic staining of the blood vessel wall, due to deposition of calcium-DNA complexes. *C,* Areas of retinoblastomas that are more differentiated frequently feature lumen-forming structures referred to as Flexner-Wintersteiner rosettes. *D,* In the most differentiated tumors there is evidence of photoreceptor morphology. Cell bouquets or fleurettes feature protrusions of bulbous cellular processes, which give evidence of outer and inner segment photoreceptor differentiation ultrastructurally and are joined as an external limiting membrane. Tumors that are mitotically quiet and composed of such photoreceptor elements, as well as of cells with an abundance of eosinophilic cytoplasm, have been referred to as retinocytomas or retinomas.

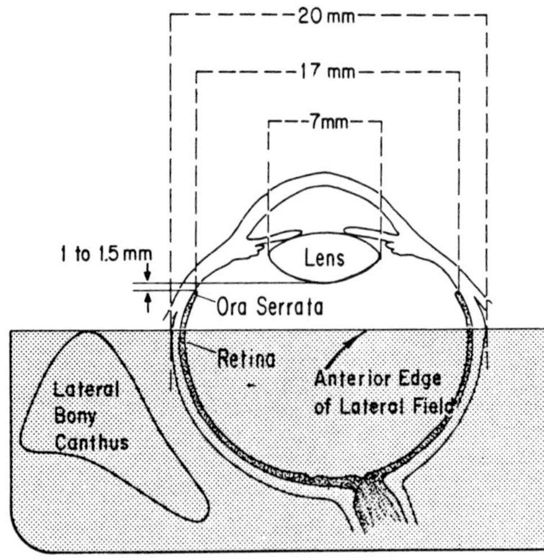

FIGURE 10–75 Schematic representation of an infant's eye, demonstrating the size of the globe and lens and positioning of the retina in relation to the lens and equator of the eye. (From Weiss DR, Cassady JR, Petersen R: Retinoblastoma: A modification in radiation therapy technique. Radiology 114:705–708, 1975. Courtesy of Radiological Society of North America.)

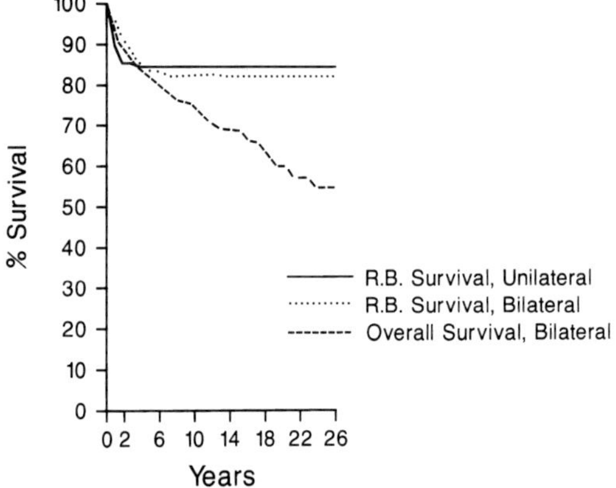

FIGURE 10–76 **Survival for unilateral and bilateral retinoblastoma.** Graph demonstrating equivalent survival from retinoblastoma for unilateral (largely nonirradiated) and bilateral (irradiated) patients. No adverse survival effect from irradiation of the tumor owing to failure to control retinoblastoma is demonstrated. A delayed, steadily decreasing overall survival of bilateral patients that is largely related to second, nonretinoblastic tumor formation, however, is shown. Some of these second tumors are caused by irradiation; some are not.

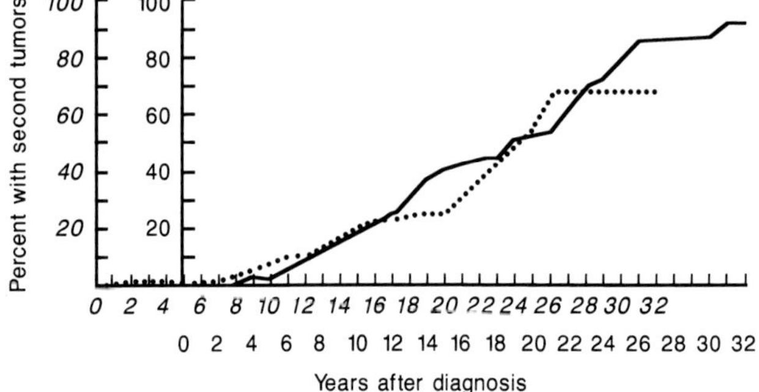

FIGURE 10–77 Actuarial development of second tumors in irradiated *(solid line)* and nonirradiated *(dotted line)* patients. Note the shorter latent period of approximately 5 years in the irradiated patients.

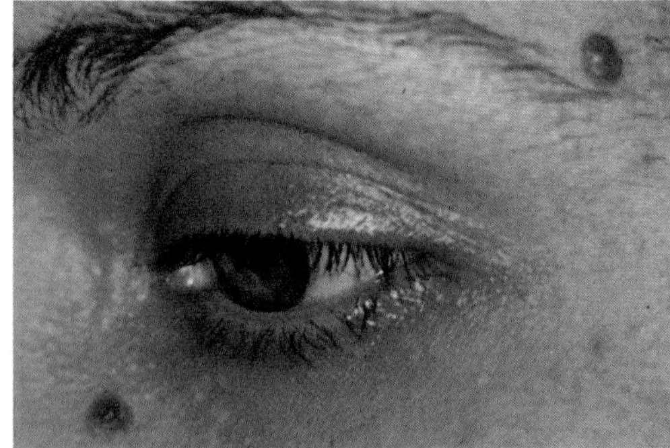

FIGURE 10–78 Neurofibromatosis. AFIP Acc. 776134.

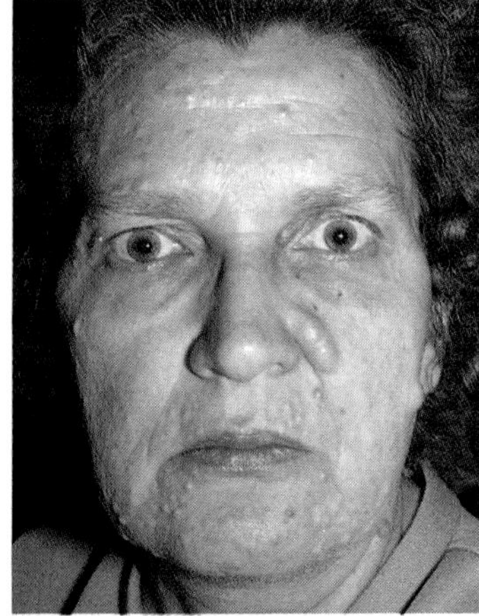

FIGURE 10–79 Larger cutaneous neurofibroma in affected patient.

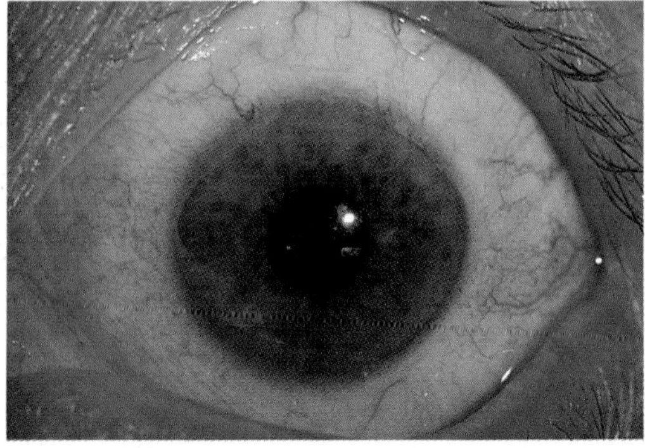

FIGURE 10–80 Iris lesions occurring in neurofibromatosis.

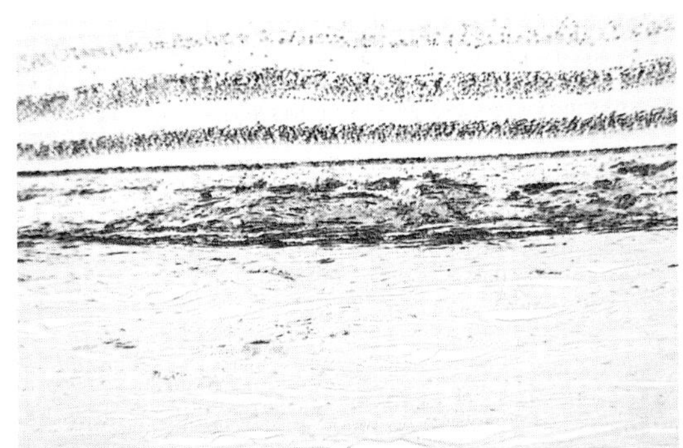

FIGURE 10–81 Area of thickened choroid and increased pigmentation in a patient with neurofibromatosis. AFIP Neg 60-6795.

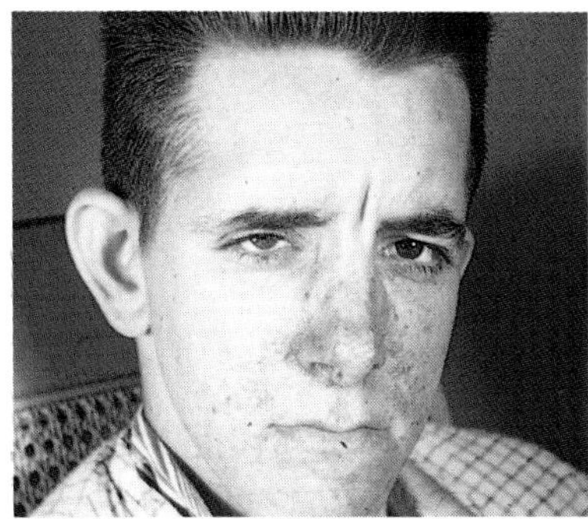

FIGURE 10–84 Typical lesions on skin of face (fibroangiomas) occurring in tuberous sclerosis and clinically referred to as adenoma sebaceum. AFIP Acc. 511046.

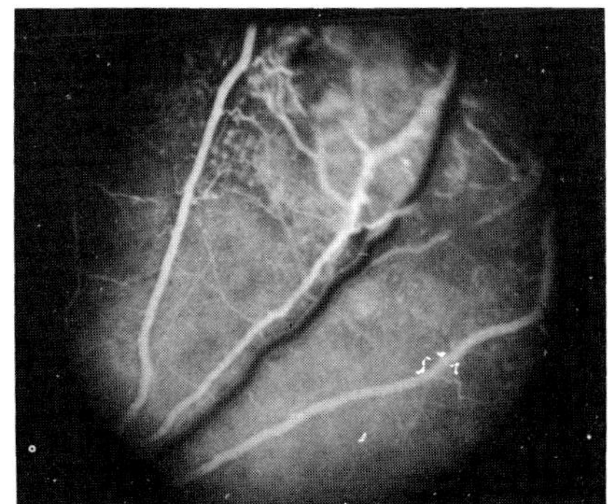

FIGURE 10–82 **Neurofibromatosis.** Fluorescein angiogram demonstrating vascularized retinal mass. (From Destro M, D'Amico DJ, Gragoudas ES, et al: Retinal manifestations of neurofibromatosis: Diagnosis and management. Arch Ophthalmol 109:662, 1991. Copyright 1991 American Medical Association.)

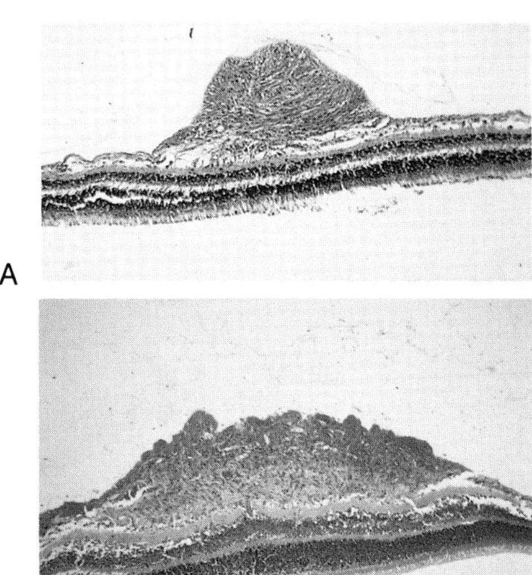

FIGURE 10–85 Examples of astrocytic hamartoma of retina occurring in tuberous sclerosis. Note that tumors arise from nerve fiber layer and do not disrupt deeper layers. *A,* H&E, ×48, ADIP Acc. 51-1048. *B,* H&E, ×36; AFIP Neg. 68-196.

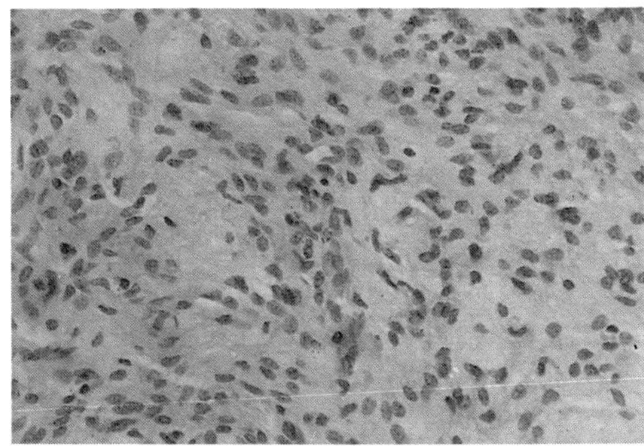

FIGURE 10–83 Light microscopic appearance of retinal biopsy of lesion in Figure 10–82 revealed an astrocytic hamartoma of the retina. (From Destro M, D'Amico DJ, Gragoudas ES, et al: Retinal manifestations of neurofibromatosis: Diagnosis and management. Arch Ophthalmol 109:662, 1991. Copyright 1991 American Medical Association.)

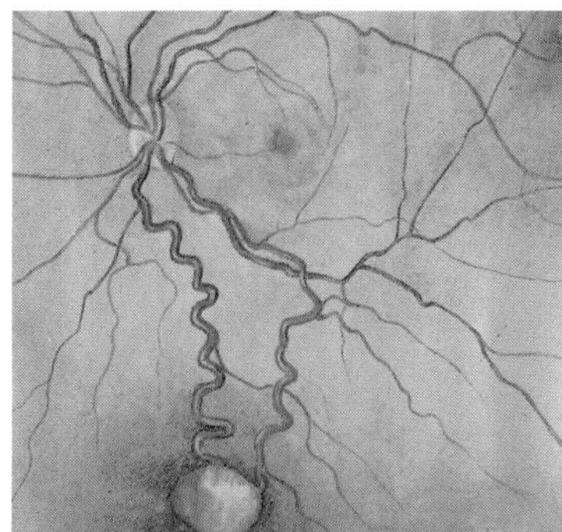
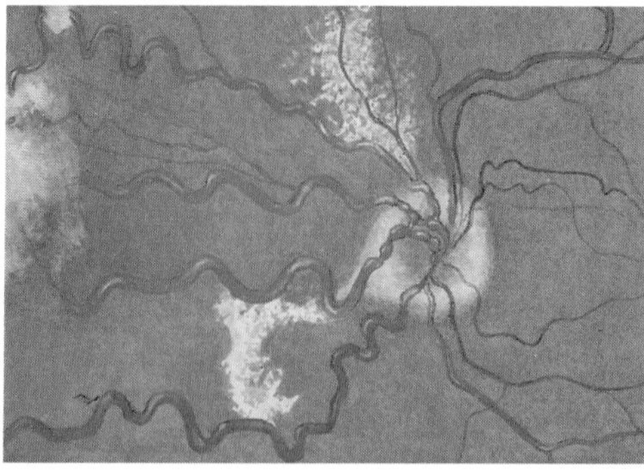

FIGURE 10–86 **Angiomatosis retinae.** *A,* Drawing of retinal angioma occurring in von Hippel–Lindau disease. Note the tortuous and enlarged feeder vessels. *B,* Angiomas occurring near disc with associated exudate. (*A* and *B,* From Brini A, Dhermy P, Sahel J: Oncology of the Eye and Adnexa: Atlas of Clinical Pathology. Dordrecht, Holland, Kluwer Academic Publishers, 1990.)

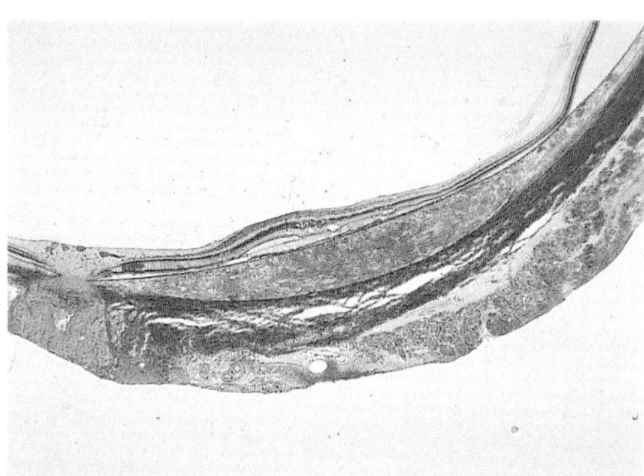

FIGURE 10–87 Juxtapapillary choroidal angioma occurring in Sturge-Weber disease. AFIP Acc. 171647.

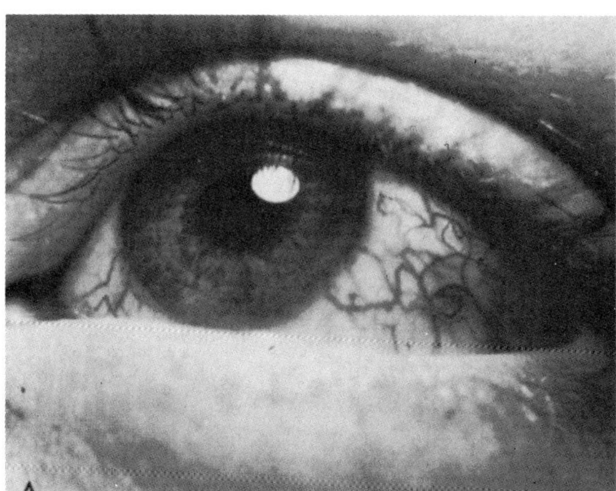
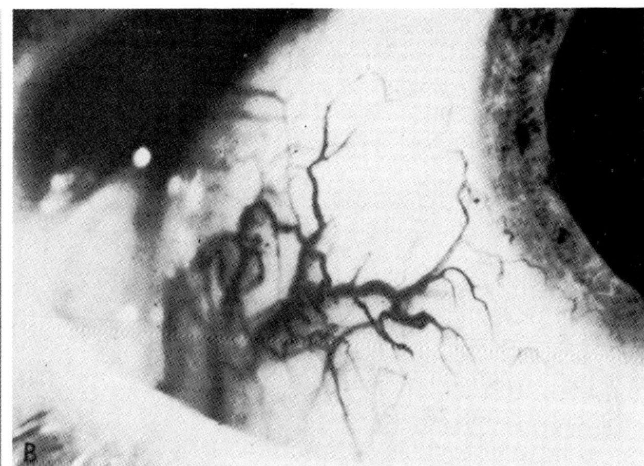
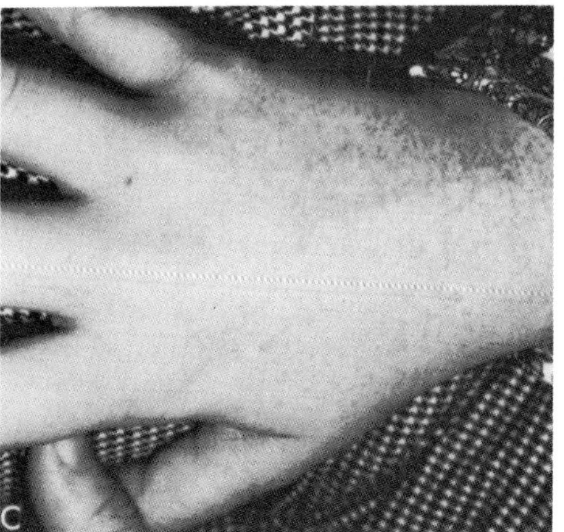

FIGURE 10–88 **Ataxia telangiectasia.** Clinical appearance of dilated, engorged, bulbar conjunctival vessels of a 7-year-old boy *(A)* and a 6-year-old girl *(B)* with progressive cerebellar dysfunction. *C,* Telangiectasia of the skin of the dorsum of the hand of patient depicted in *B.* (Courtesy of J. B. Crawford, M.D.)

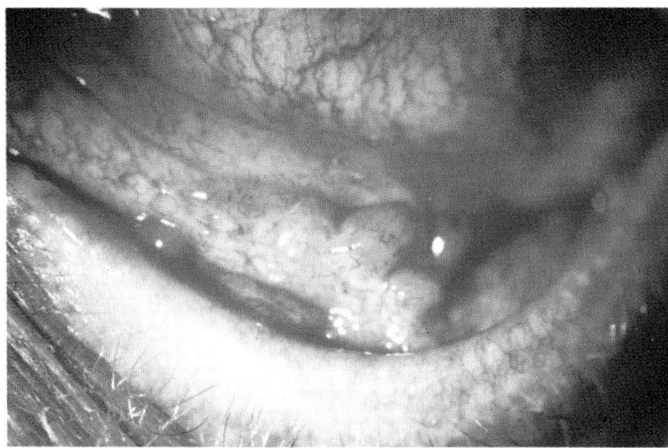

FIGURE 10–89 **Lymphoma.** Well-differentiated small lymphocytic lymphoma. Forniceal cluster of salmon-colored, moderately congested, subconjunctival nodules. (Courtesy of John J. Schietroma, M.D.)

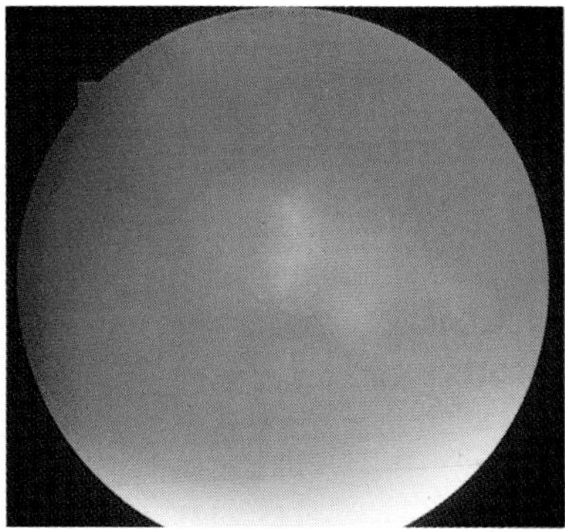

FIGURE 10–92 **Primary lymphoma of retina and vitreous.** Nearly complete opacification of the vitreous has occurred in 4 months. (Courtesy of James E. Memmen, M.D.)

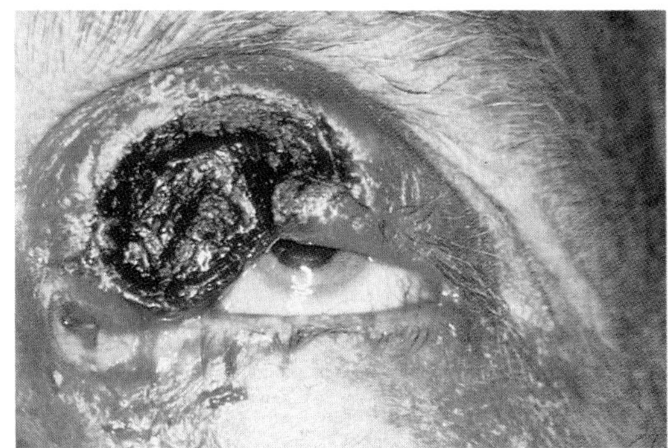

FIGURE 10–90 **Large-cell lymphoma, T cell.** A black, encrusted ulcer is present on the left upper eyelid. The ulcer is surrounded by swollen, erythematous tissue. (From Kirsch LS, Brownstein S, Codere F: Immunoblastic T-cell lymphoma presenting as an eyelid tumor. Ophthalmology 97:1352, 1990.)

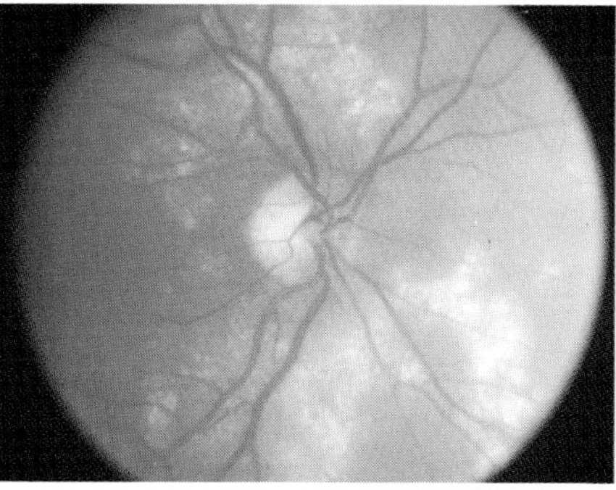

FIGURE 10–93 **Primary lymphoma of retina and vitreous.** In this case, pale yellow granular and confluent lesions lie at the level of the RPE. (Courtesy of David J. Wilson, M.D.)

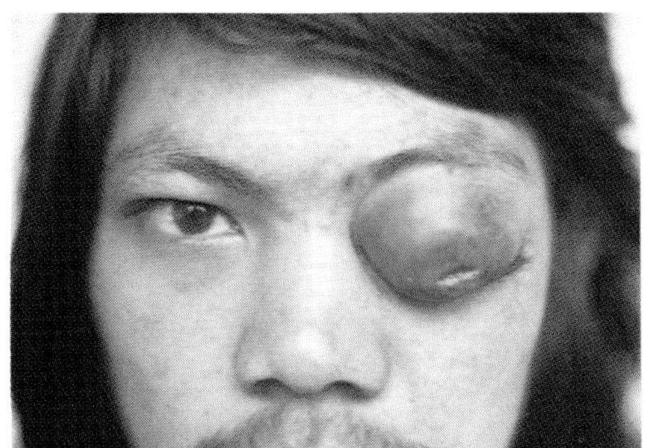

FIGURE 10–91 **Lymphoma.** Massive proptosis due to a high-grade orbital lymphoma. (Courtesy of Miguel N. Burnier, M.D., Ph.D.)

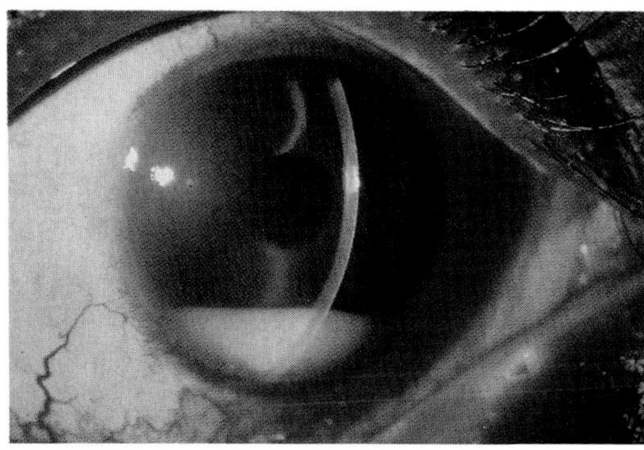

FIGURE 10–94 **Acute lymphocytic leukemia.** Child with pseudohypopyon. (Courtesy of Elise Torczynski, M.D.)

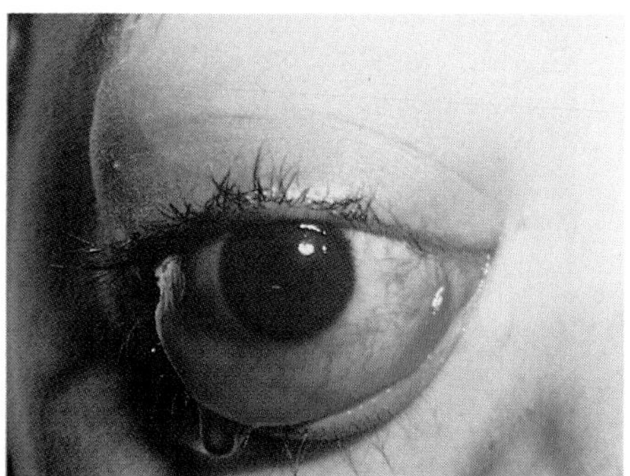

FIGURE 10–95 **Granulocytic sarcoma.** Proptosis due to orbital infiltrate. (Courtesy of Miguel N. Burnier, M.D., Ph.D.)

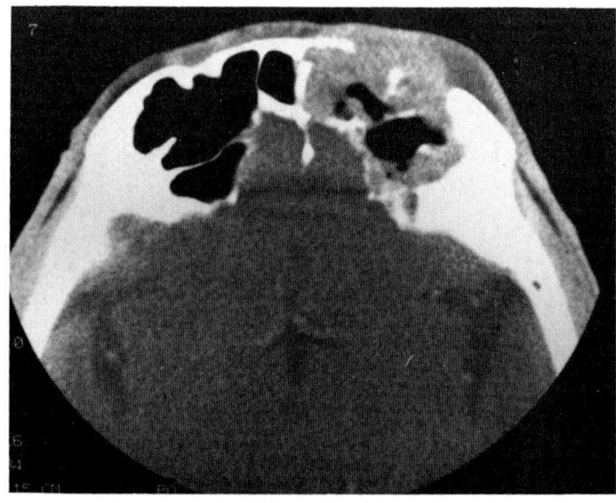

FIGURE 10–96 **Large cell lymphoma.** This enhancing tumor from the left frontal sinus has invaded the orbit and periocular subcutaneous tissue. A computed tomography (CT) scan with contrast. (Courtesy of Daniel P. Schaefer, M.D.)

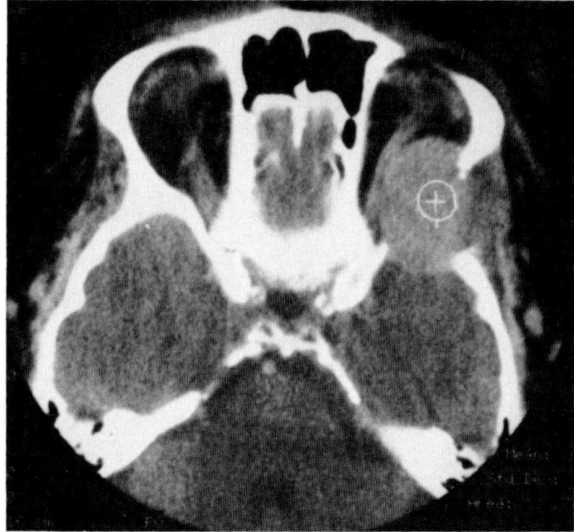

FIGURE 10–97 **Plasmacytoma.** This enhancing left orbital tumor has eroded through the posterior and lateral orbital walls to invade the temporalis muscle and brain. A CT scan with contrast. (Courtesy of Mark W. Scroggs, M.D.)

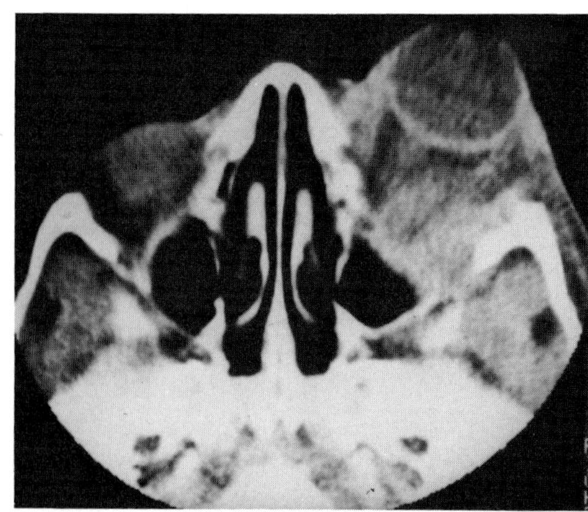

FIGURE 10–98 **Granulocytic sarcoma.** Massive infiltration of right orbit with marked proptosis. Although the pattern of the extraocular muscle cone and optic nerve is maintained, this enhancing tumor has caused extensive erosion of bone with intracranial invasion. A CT scan with contrast. (Courtesy of Miguel N. Burnier, M.D., Ph.D.)

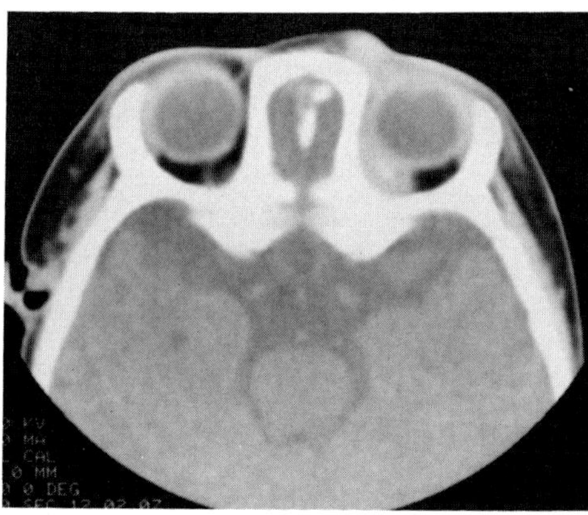

FIGURE 10–99 **Juvenile xanthogranuloma.** Enhancing subcutaneous mass over the inferior orbital rim, extending into the nasal orbit. Note sharp demarcation posteriorly within the orbit and lack of ocular compression or bone erosion. A CT scan with contrast. (From Shields CL, et al: Solitary orbital involvement with juvenile xanthogranuloma. Arch Ophthalmol 108:1587, 1990. Copyright 1990 American Medical Association.)

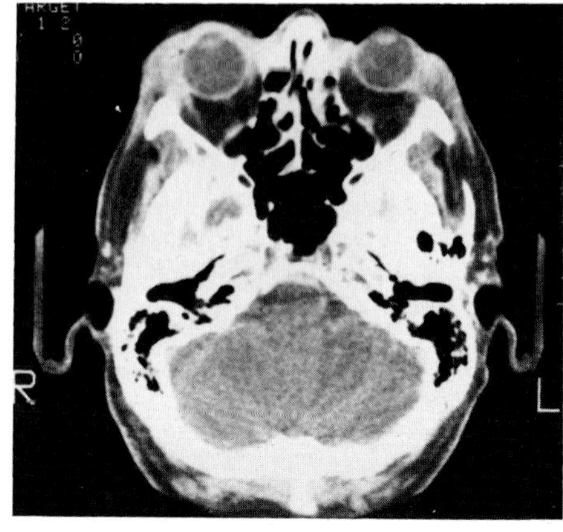

FIGURE 10–100 **Necrobiotic xanthogranuloma.** Bilateral enhancing masses in periocular subcutaneous tissue and anterior orbit. There is no bone erosion. A CT scan with contrast. (Courtesy of Robert W. Neuman, M.D.)

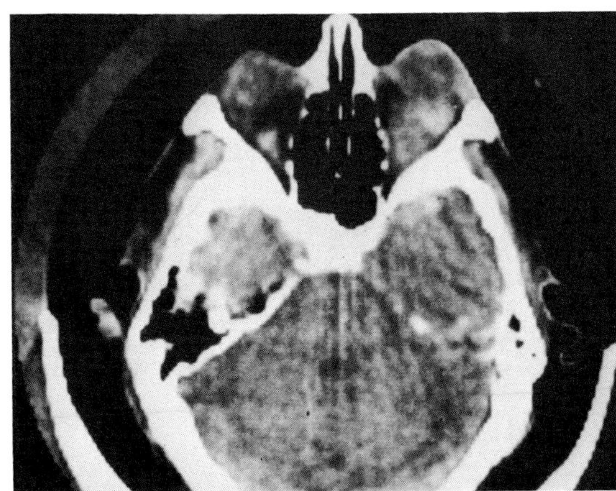

FIGURE 10–101 **Erdheim-Chester disease.** Variably enhancing mass of posterior left orbit, causing proptosis. Notice lack of bone erosion in this plane. A CT scan with contrast. (From Alper MG, Zimmerman LE, LaPiana FG: Orbital manifestations of Erdheim-Chester disease. Trans Am Ophthalmol Soc 81:64, 1983.)

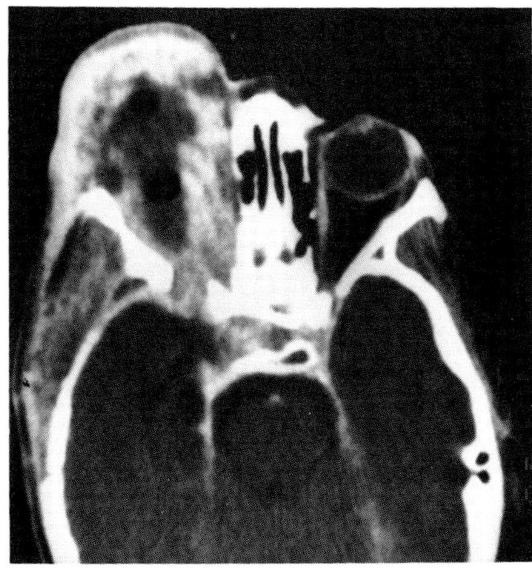

FIGURE 10–102 **Sinus histiocytosis.** This massive enhancing tumor obliterates orbital anatomy while invading the cavernous sinus and temporalis muscle. A CT scan with contrast. (Courtesy of Edward M. Burton, M.D.)

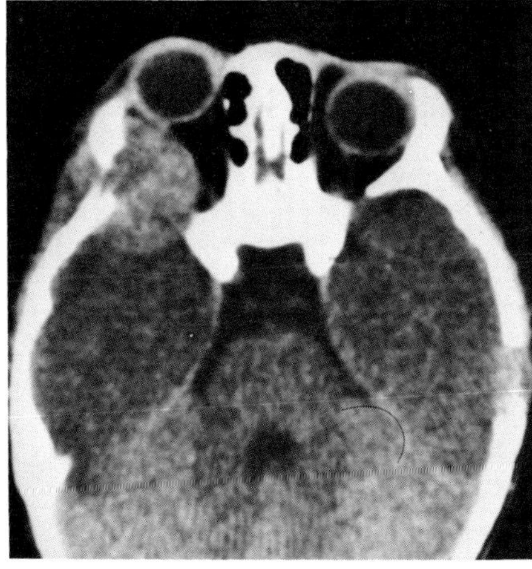

FIGURE 10–103 **Langerhans' cell histiocytosis.** This enhancing right orbital tumor has eroded through bone to invade the temporalis muscle and brain. A CT scan with contrast. (Courtesy of Elise Torczynski, M.D.)

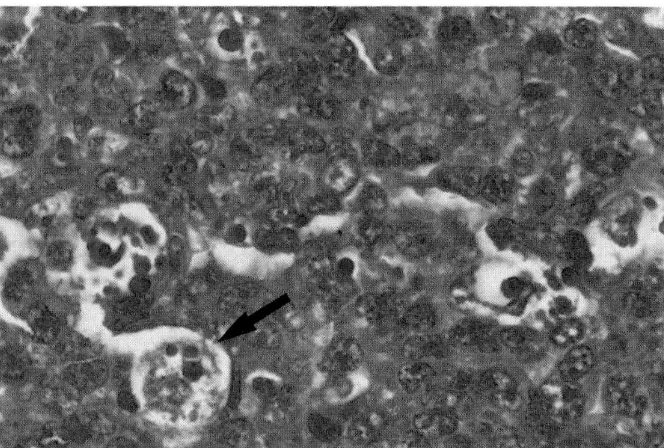

FIGURE 10–104 **Burkitt's lymphoma.** The malignant cells show rounded, moderately pleomorphic nuclei with coarse chromatin and prominent nucleoli. Tingible-body macrophages with nuclear debris are present *(arrow).* (H&E original magnification ×250.) AFIP-MIS #91-10139.

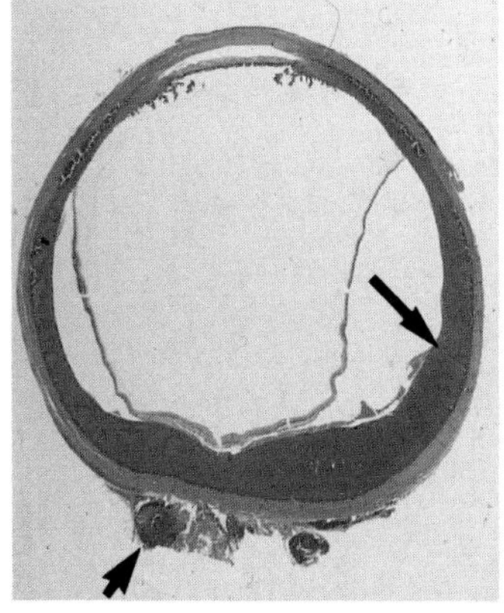

FIGURE 10–105 **Primary lymphoma of the uvea.** There is extensive thickening of the choroid and pars plana by a malignant lymphoid infiltrate containing scattered follicles *(arrow).* Note the episcleral extension posteriorly *(arrowhead).* AFIP-MIS #91-10142.

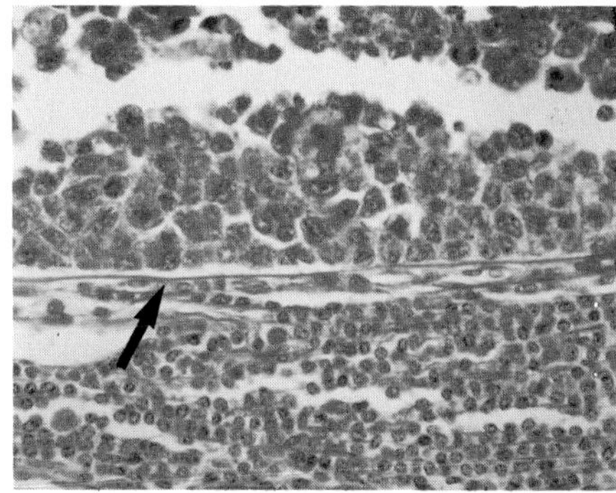

FIGURE 10–106 **Primary lymphoma of retina and vitreous.** Subretinal pigment epithelium infiltration by a large cell lymphoma with pleomorphic nuclei and mitotic activity. Bruch's membrane *(arrow)* separates the tumor from a reactive choroidal infiltrate of benign lymphocytes. (H&E, original magnification ×220.) AFIP-MIS #67-11087. (From Vogel MH, Font RL, Zimmerman LE, Levine RA: Reticulum cell sarcoma of the retina and uvea: Report of six cases and review of the literature. Am J Ophthalmol 66:205, 1968. Copyright by the Ophthalmic Publishing Company.)

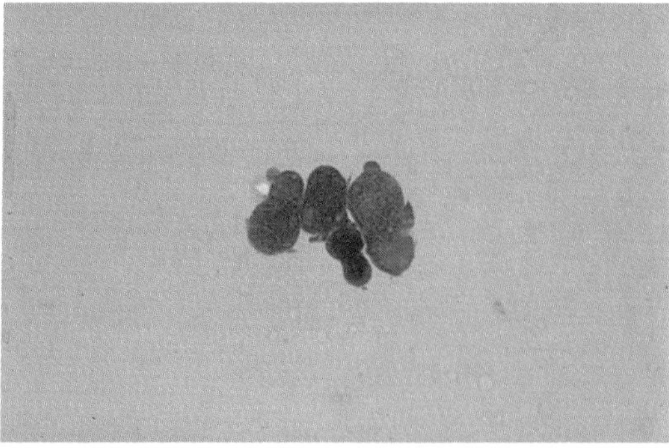

FIGURE 10–107 **Acute lymphocytic leukemia.** The tumor cells in this aqueous tap have rounded irregular nuclei and lack cytoplasmic granules. (Wright, original magnification ×330.) (Courtesy of Elise Torczynski, M.D.)

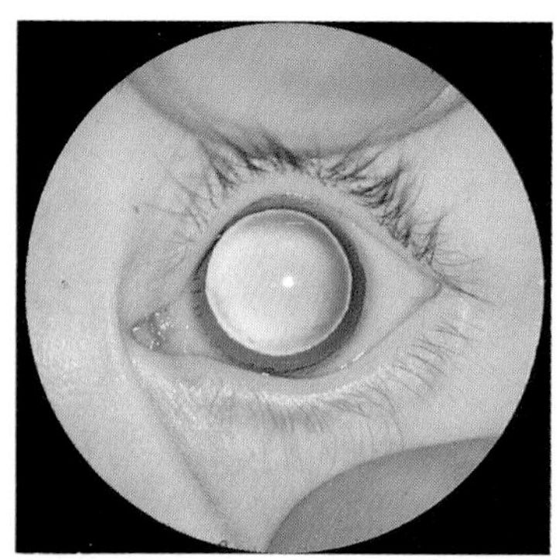

FIGURE 10–110 **Aniridia.** Photograph of a patient with aniridia showing the rudimentary iris stump. (Courtesy of R. Robb, M.D.)

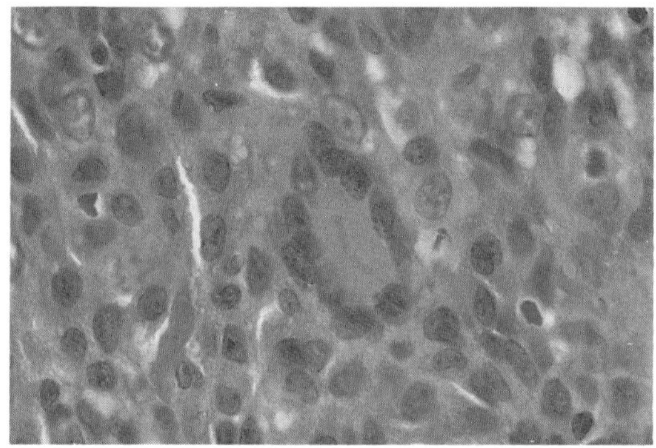

FIGURE 10–108 **Juvenile xanthogranuloma.** Touton giant cells with wreathlike nuclei in an orbital lesion. Other tumor cells show round to oval nuclei, typical of juvenile xanthogranuloma in connective tissue. (H&E original magnification ×250.) AFIP-MIS #91-10146.

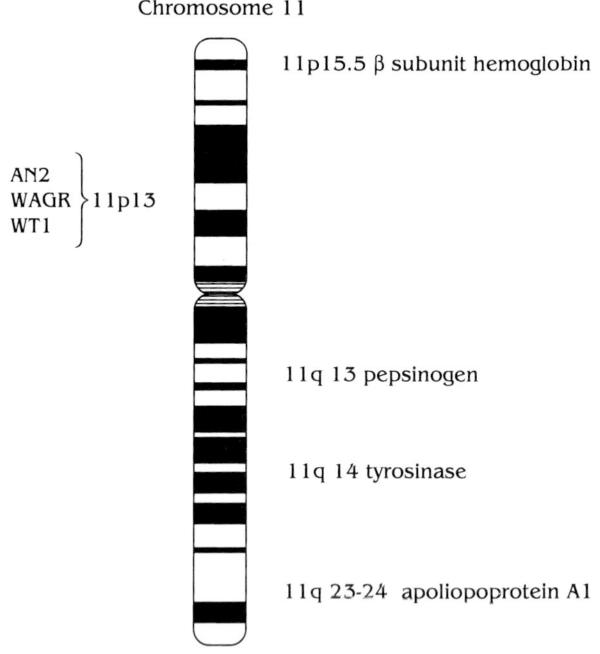

FIGURE 10–111 **Aniridia.** Genetic map of chromosome 11.

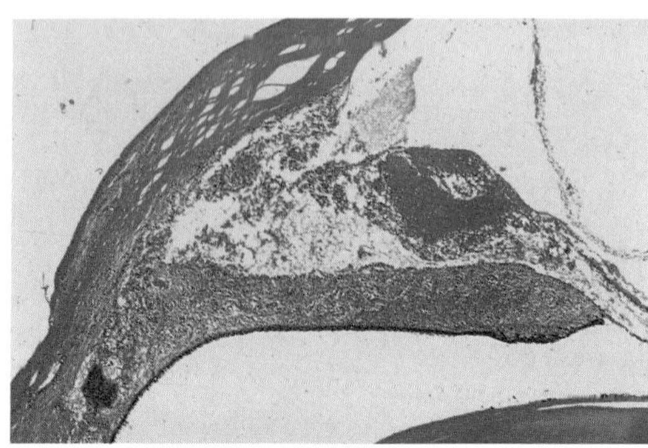

FIGURE 10–109 **Juvenile xanthogranuloma.** The tumor fills the iris stroma and extends into the anterior chamber, where it mingles with hyphema. (H&E, original magnification ×25.) AFIP-MIS #91-10147.

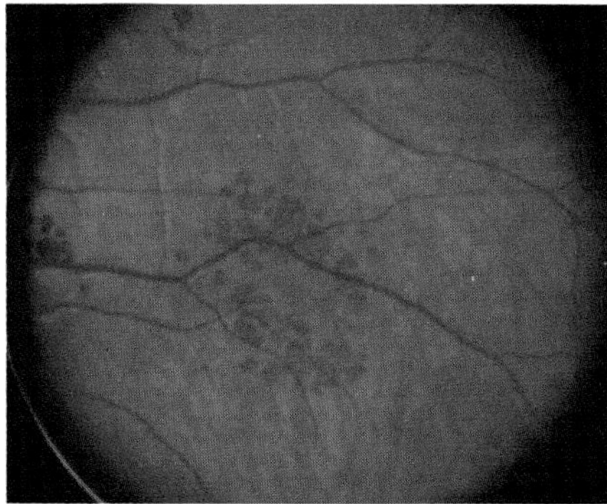

FIGURE 10–112 **Gardner's syndrome.** Color fundus photograph showing congenital RPE hypertrophy in a patient with Gardner's syndrome.

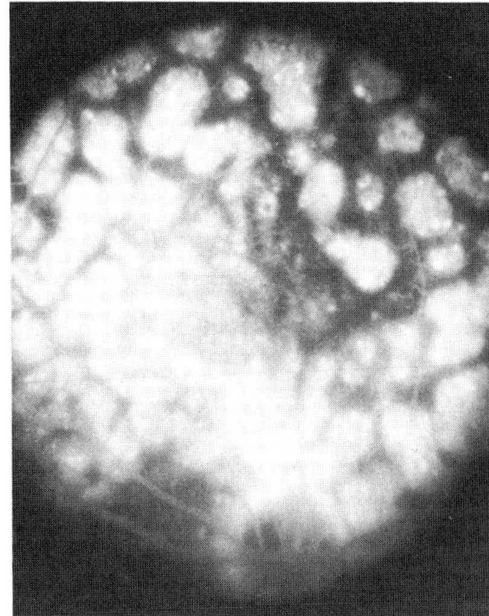

FIGURE 10–114 **Adenocarcinoma of the ovary.** Fluorescein angiography in a patient with diffuse uveal melanocytic tumors and adenocarcinoma of the ovary. (Courtesy of E. Gragoudas, M.D.)

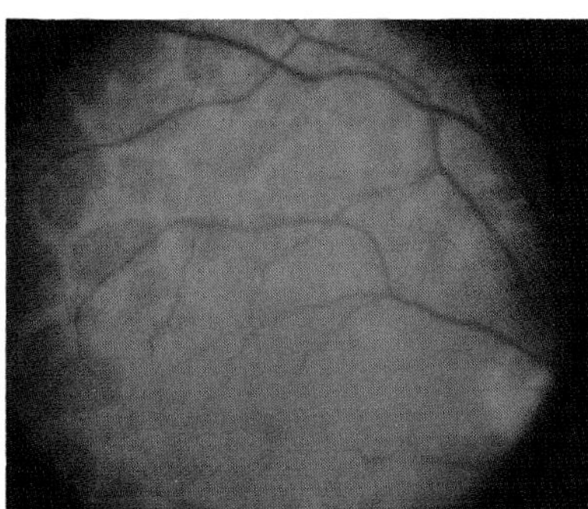

FIGURE 10–113 **Adenocarcinoma of the ovary.** Color fundus photograph showing diffuse uveal melanocytic tumors in a patient with adenocarcinoma of the ovary. (Courtesy of E. Gragoudas, M.D.)

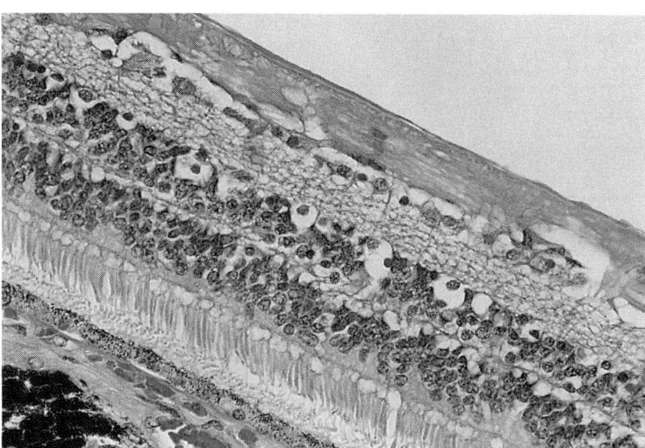

FIGURE 10–115 **Cancer-associated retinopathy (CAR) syndrome.** Adenocarcinoma of the ovary. Photomicrograph demonstrating loss of ganglion cells from the retina in a patient with the CAR syndrome.

SECTION 11

Trauma

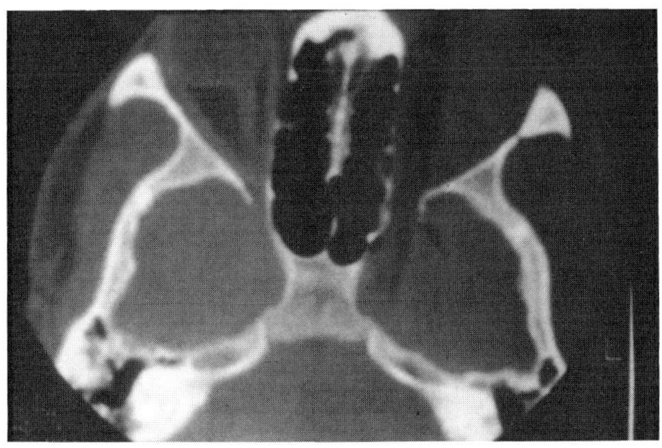

FIGURE 11–1 **Anterior segment trauma.** Computed tomography (CT) scan shows extension of stick through superior orbital fissure into the cranial cavity. (Courtesy of John Shore, M.D.)

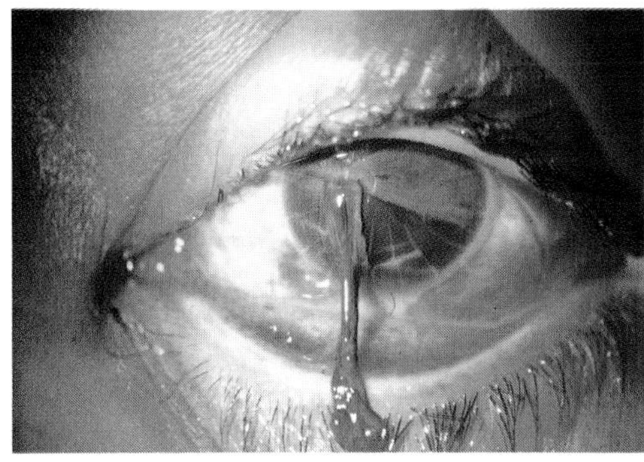

FIGURE 11–3 **Ruptured radial keratotomy wound.** This 24-year-old patient was hit in the eye with a fist, resulting in a ruptured radial keratotomy wound (6 years after radial keratotomy), with extensive iridodialysis and iris prolapse. (Courtesy of Nicholas Volpe, M.D.)

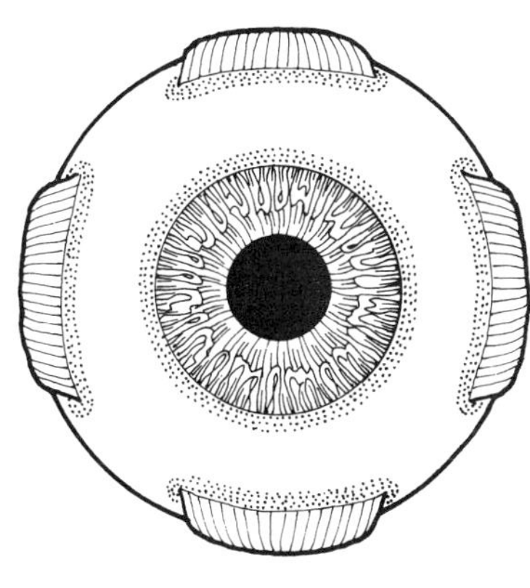

FIGURE 11–2 **Rupture sites.** The most common locations of globe rupture are at the limbus, at the insertions of the extraocular muscles, in the peripapillary region, and at the site of previous intraocular surgery.

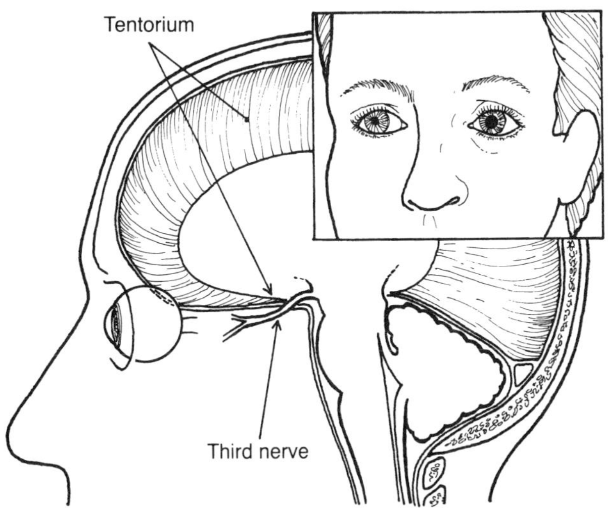

FIGURE 11–4 **Trauma and the pupil.** Increased intracranial pressure may lead to pressure on the oculomotor nerve at the tentorial edge, resulting in an ipsilateral dilated fixed pupil.

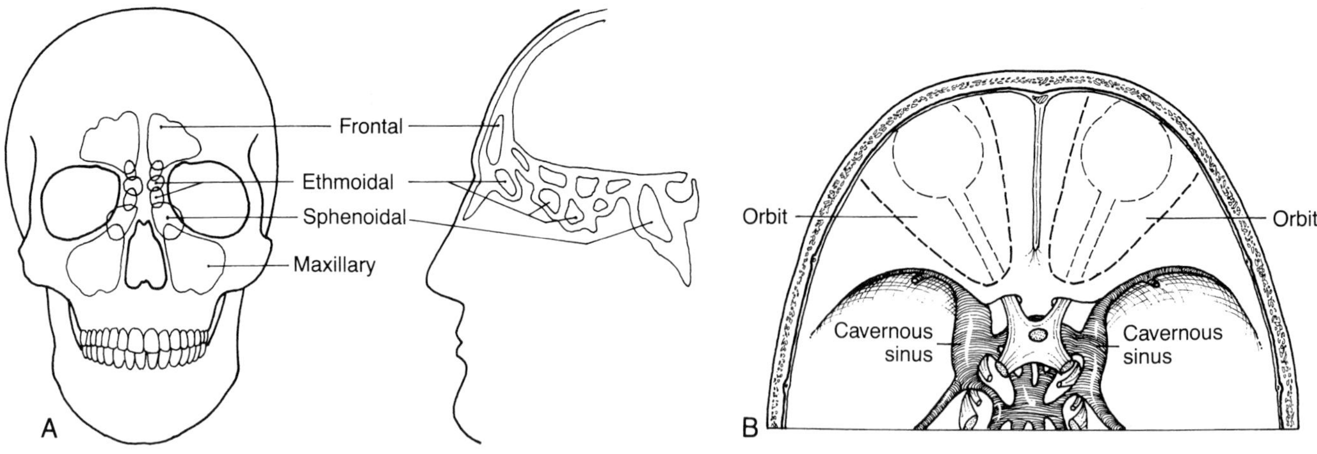

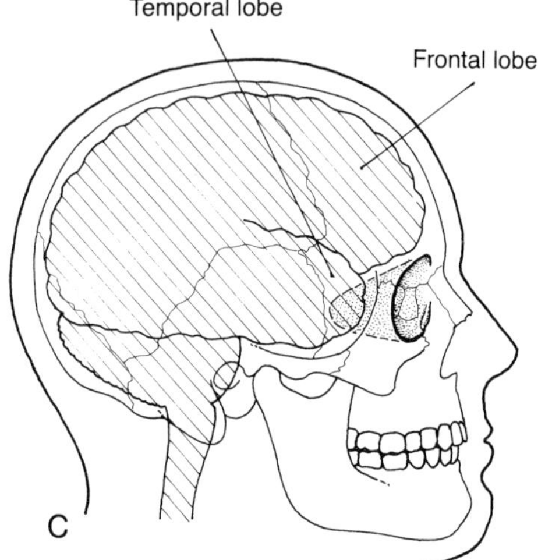

FIGURE 11–5 **Schematic anatomy of the orbit.** The orbit lies in close proximity to the paranasal sinuses *(A)*, the cavernous sinus *(B)*, and the cranial cavity *(C)*.

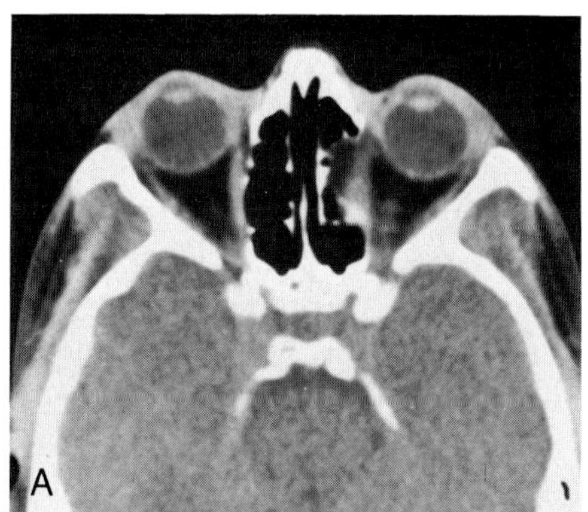

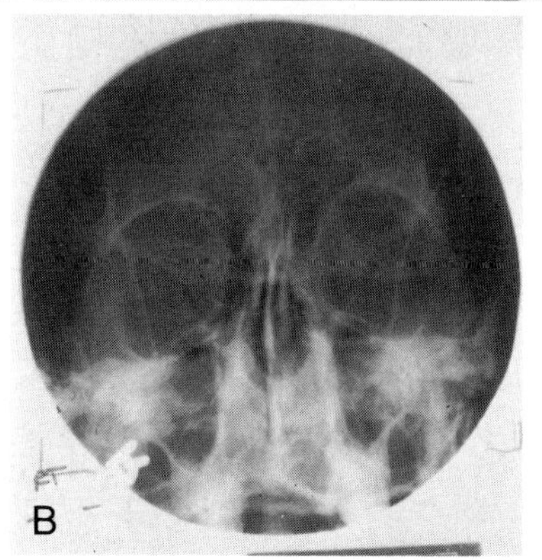

FIGURE 11–6 **Traumatic fracture of the orbital wall.** *A*, Axial CT scan of patient with traumatic left medial orbital wall (ethmoid) fracture. *B*, Caldwell projection of plain orbital films in the same patient. (Courtesy of Alfred Weber, M.D.)

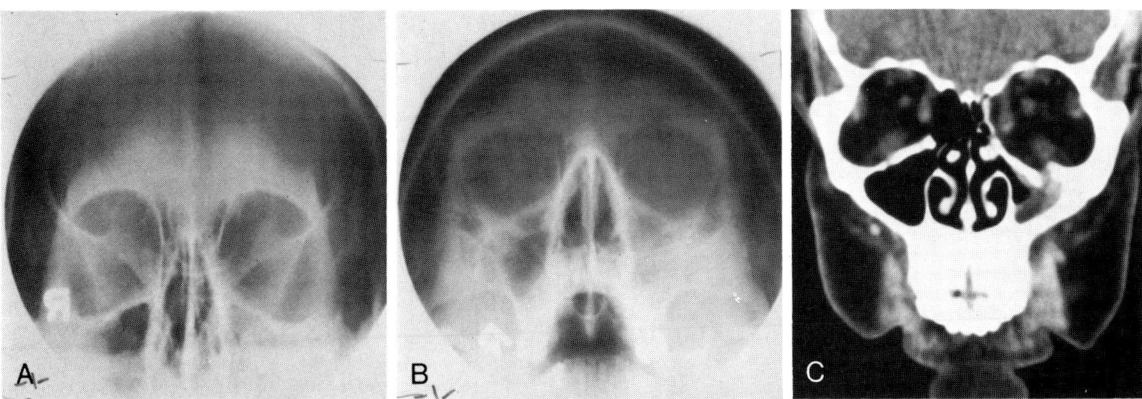

FIGURE 11–7 **Traumatic fracture of the floor of the orbit.** *A,* Left orbital floor fracture on Caldwell projection of plain orbital films. *B,* Left orbital floor fracture on Waters' view of plain orbital films. *C,* Left orbital floor fracture on coronal CT scan.

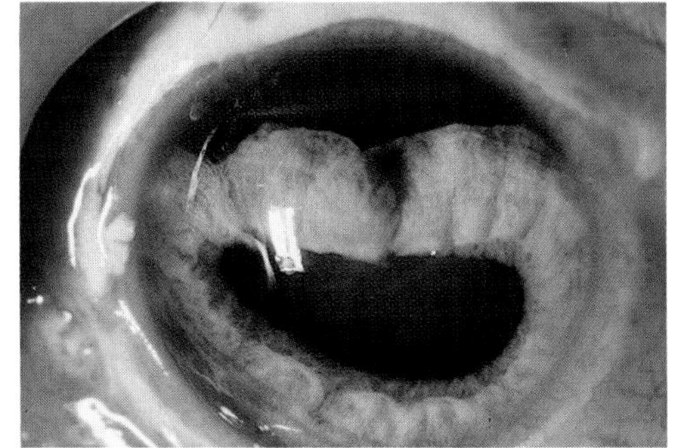

FIGURE 11–8 **Damage to the iris root.** Significant iridodialysis resulting in a D-shaped pupil.

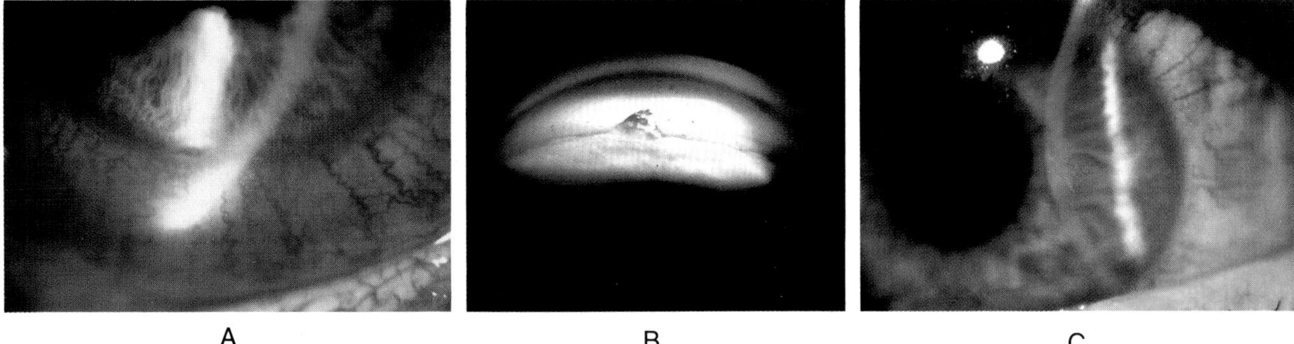

FIGURE 11–9 **Intraocular foreign body.** Clinical *(A)* and gonioscopic *(B)* views of anterior chamber metallic foreign body. Note the subtle corneal entry site *(C).*

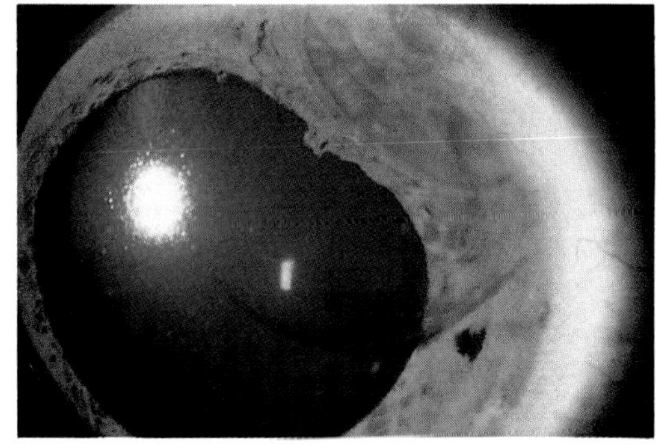

FIGURE 11–10 **Iridodialysis with vitreous prolapse.** Blunt trauma may result in iridodialysis along with vitreous prolapse into the anterior chamber; blood outlines the leading edge of prolapsed vitreous in this traumatized patient. (Courtesy of John Irvine, M.D.)

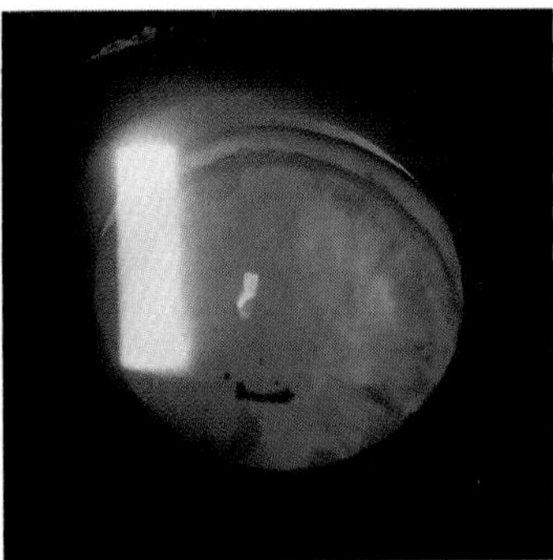

FIGURE 11–11 **Traumatic lens subluxation.** The lens zonules are visible on retroilluminated view with slit lamp and patient's pupils dilated. (Courtesy of Jeffrey Lamkin, M.D.)

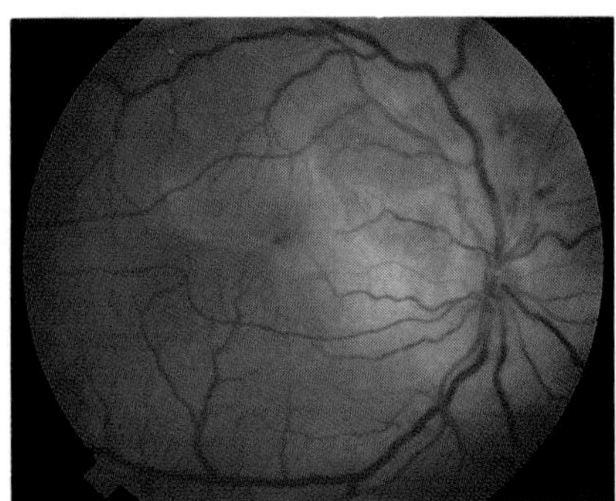

FIGURE 11–13 **Commotio retinae.** Extensive posterior pole commotio retinae in a patient with blunt ocular and orbital trauma.

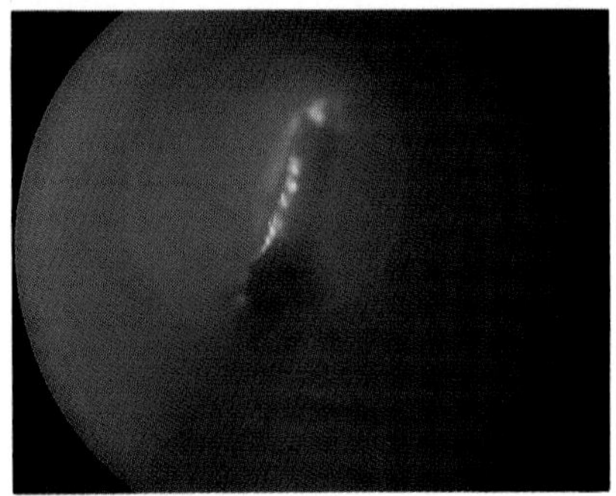

FIGURE 11–12 **Intraocular foreign body.** Intraocular foreign body surrounded by subretinal fluid and intraretinal hemorrhage.

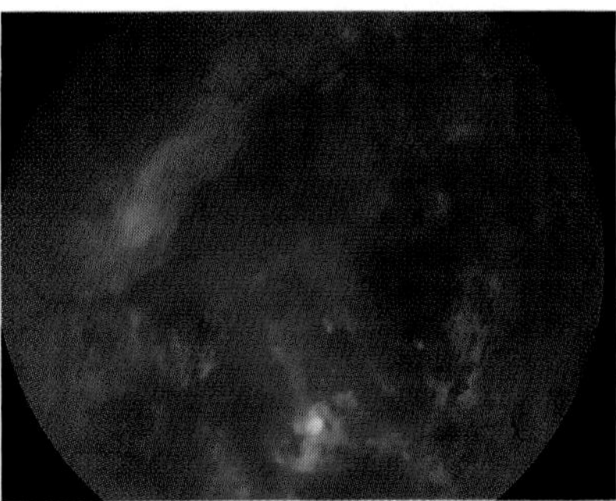

FIGURE 11–14 **Chorioretinitis sclopetaria.** Resulting from a pellet injury. Note the massive choroidal and retinal hemorrhage. (Courtesy of Eddy Anglade, M.D.)

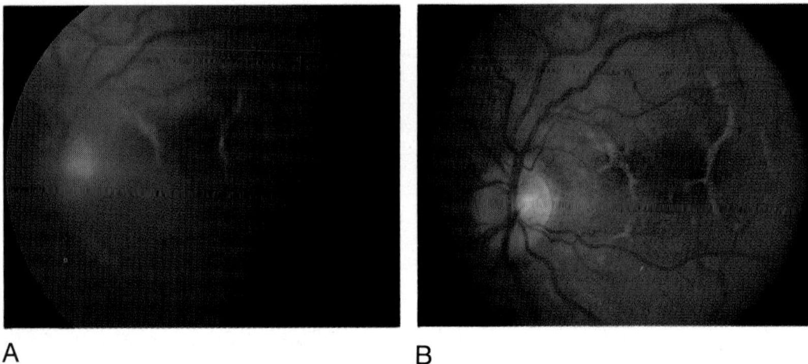

FIGURE 11–15 **Choroidal rupture.** *A,* Acute choroidal rupture in a typical location (concentric to optic disc) associated with hemorrhage. *B,* Same patient 3 months later. Note the surrounding pigmentary changes suggesting firm chorioretinal adhesion.

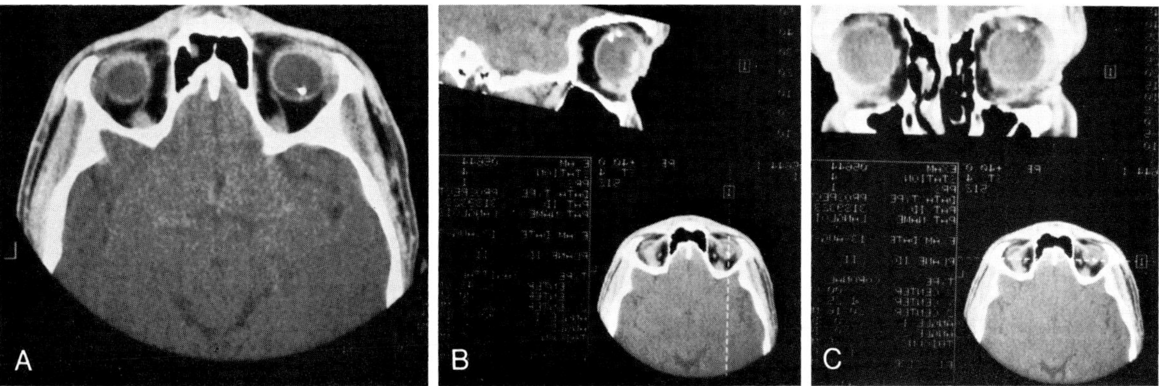

FIGURE 11–16 **Intraocular foreign body.** *A,* Axial view of CT scan of patient with history of hammering metal on metal. *B* and *C,* CT scan reconstruction techniques reveal the obvious intraocular location of the foreign body.

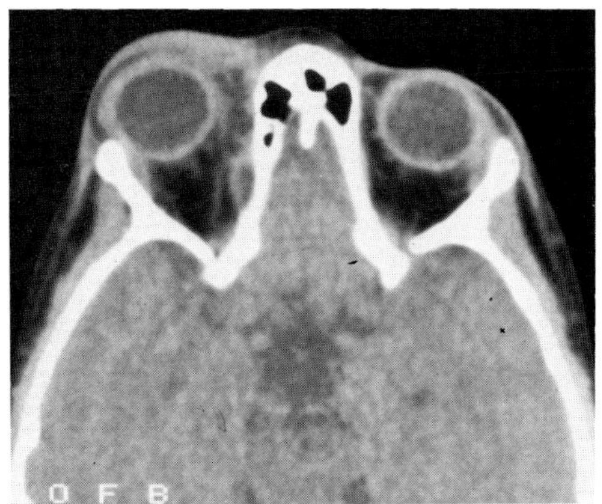

FIGURE 11–17 **Intraocular foreign body.** Axial CT scan of a patient with an intraorbital wooden foreign body located in the medial orbit. Note the poor delineation from surrounding orbital structures. (Courtesy of Alfred Weber, M.D.)

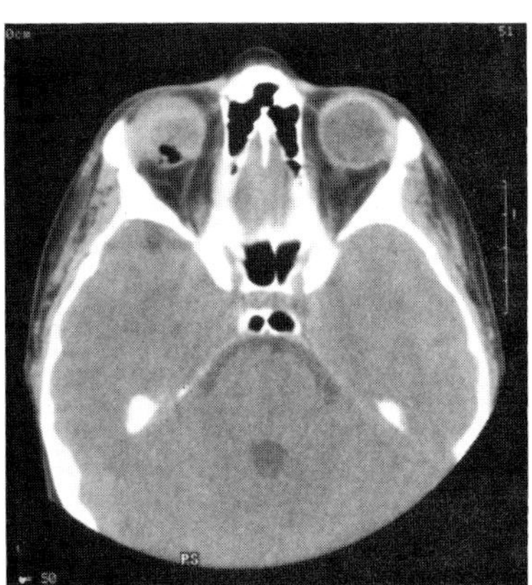

FIGURE 11–19 **Intraocular air.** Intraocular air is pathognomonic for ocular penetration.

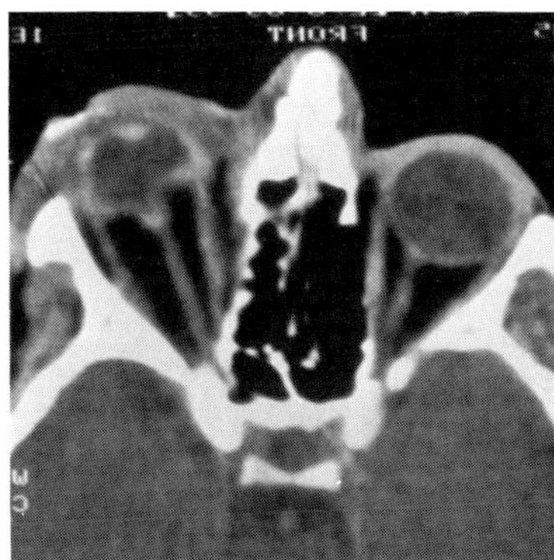

FIGURE 11–18 **Distortion of scleral contour following blunt trauma.** Note distortion of posterior scleral contour in this patient with significant blunt ocular trauma.

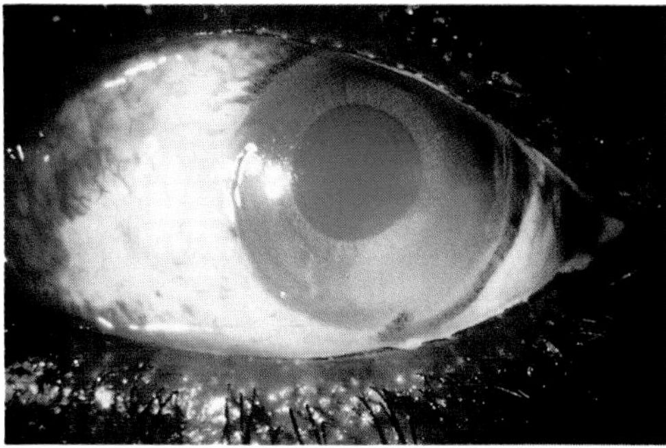

FIGURE 11–20 **Chemical injuries.** Note extensive limbal ischemia and necrosis in this ocular injury caused by an ammonia splash. Inferonasal corneal stromal opacification can also be seen.

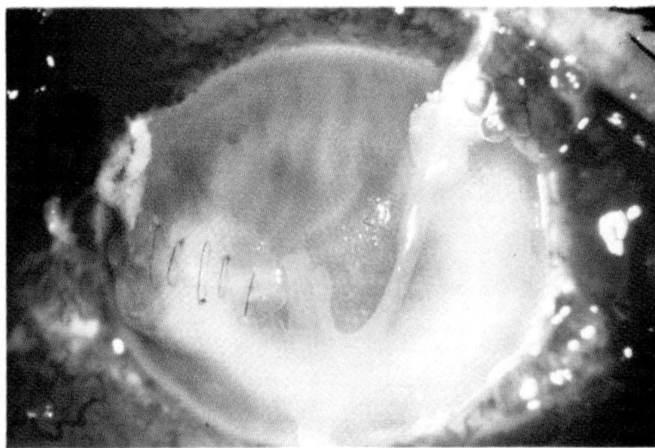

FIGURE 11–21 **Traumatic endophthalmitis.** Endophthalmitis with corneal infiltrate and hypopyon after corneal laceration repair. (Courtesy of Patrick Rubsamen, M.D.)

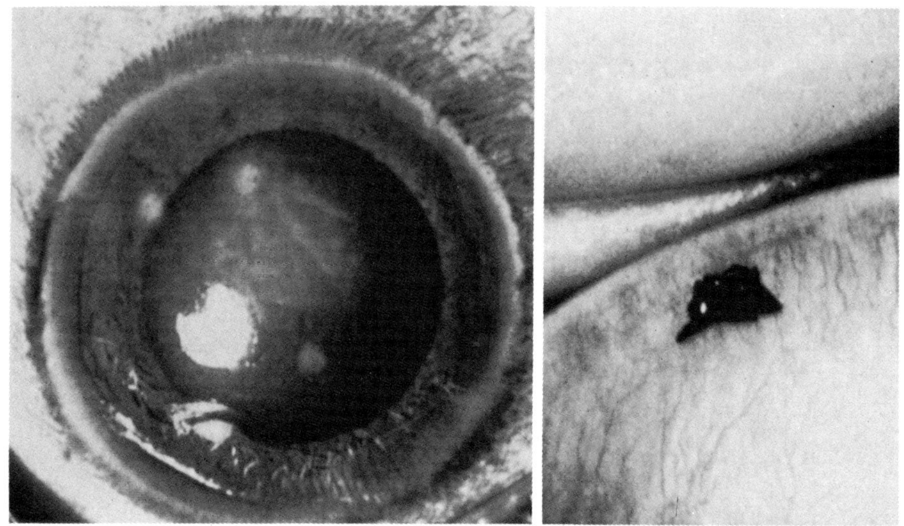

FIGURE 11–22 **Corneal foreign body.** Vertically oriented linear corneal abrasions *(left)* associated with a metal foreign body retained on the upper tarsal conjunctiva *(right).* Corneal foreign bodies and stromal edema are also evident. (From Shingleton BJ, Hersh PH, Kenyon KR [eds]: Eye Trauma. St. Louis, Mosby-Year Book, 1991, p. 64.)

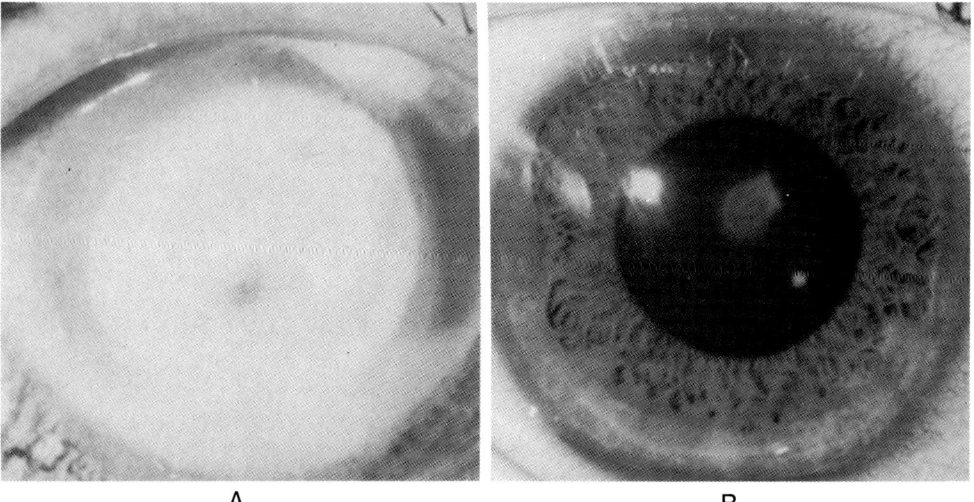

FIGURE 11–23 **Corneal abrasion.** *Pseudomonas* keratitis related to soft contact lens wear. *A,* Intense stromal infiltration and liquefaction. *B,* Small superficial ulcer is also *Pseudomonas* culture positive. (From Shingleton BJ, Hersh PH, Kenyon KR [eds]: Eye Trauma. St. Louis, Mosby-Year Book, 1991, p. 77.)

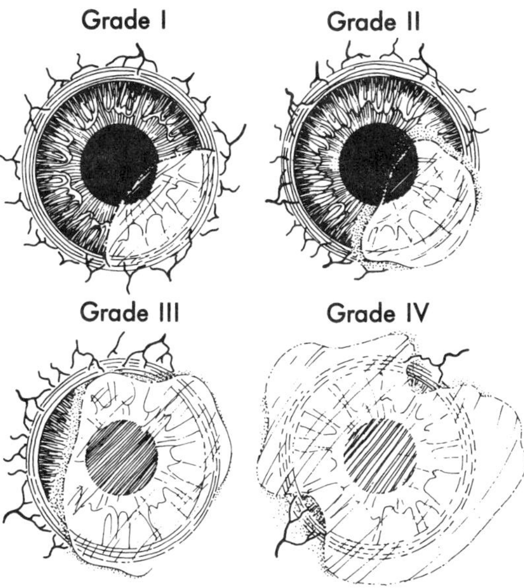

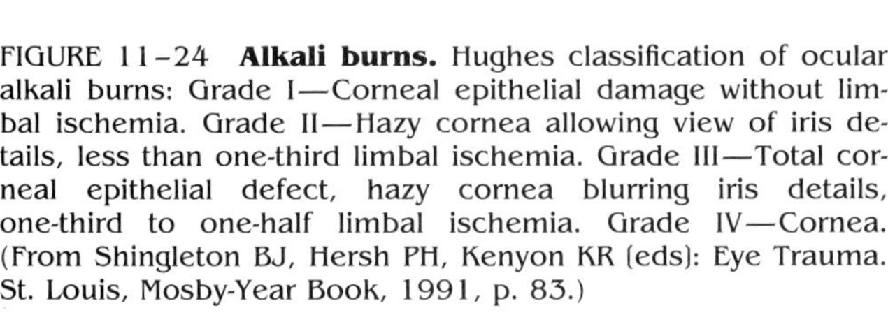

FIGURE 11–24 **Alkali burns.** Hughes classification of ocular alkali burns: Grade I—Corneal epithelial damage without limbal ischemia. Grade II—Hazy cornea allowing view of iris details, less than one-third limbal ischemia. Grade III—Total corneal epithelial defect, hazy cornea blurring iris details, one-third to one-half limbal ischemia. Grade IV—Cornea. (From Shingleton BJ, Hersh PH, Kenyon KR (eds): Eye Trauma. St. Louis, Mosby-Year Book, 1991, p. 83.)

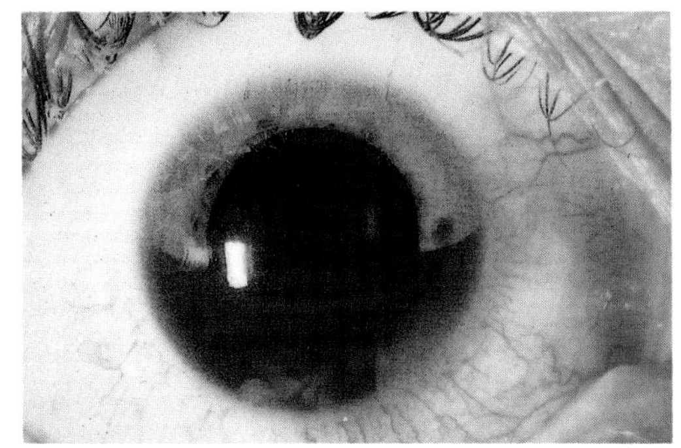

A

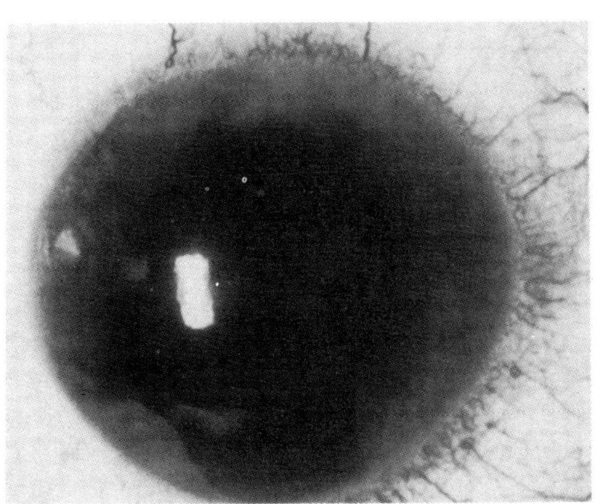

B

FIGURE 11–25 **Antifibrolytic agents in anterior segment trauma.** *A,* Five days after traumatic hyphema on aminocaproic acid treatment. Blood is layered, and anterior chamber is otherwise clear. Applanation tension = 16 mmHg. *B,* Twenty-four hours after discontinuation of aminocaproic acid. Note obscuration of iris details by free-floating red blood cells without evidence of rebleed. Applanation tension = 46 mmHg. (From Dieste MC, Hersh PS, Kylstra JA, et al: Intraocular pressure increase associated with epsilon-aminocaproic acid therapy for traumatic hyphema. Am J Ophthalmol 106:383, 1988. Copyright by the Ophthalmic Publishing Company.)

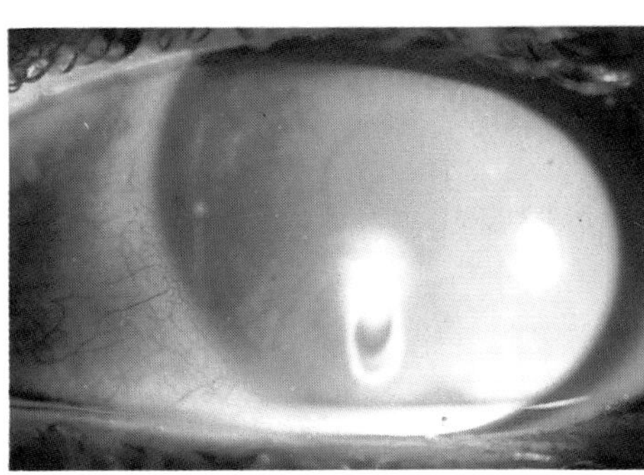

FIGURE 11–26 **Corneoscleral laceration.** Positive Seidel's test using 2% fluorescein after corneal puncture wound with a wire. (From Shingleton BJ, Hersh PH, Kenyon KR (eds): Eye Trauma. St. Louis, Mosby-Year Book, 1991, color plate 13–1.)

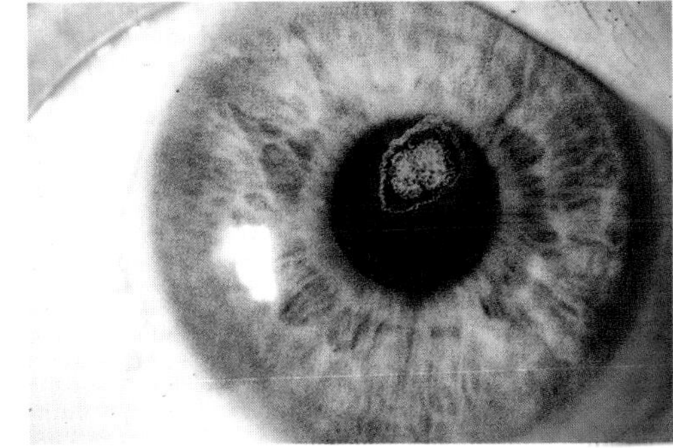

FIGURE 11–27 **Simple full-thickness corneal laceration.** Small puncture wound sealed with cyanoacrylate tissue adhesive. (From Shingleton BJ, Hersh PH, Kenyon KR (eds): Eye Trauma. St. Louis, Mosby-Year Book, 1991, color plate 13–2.)

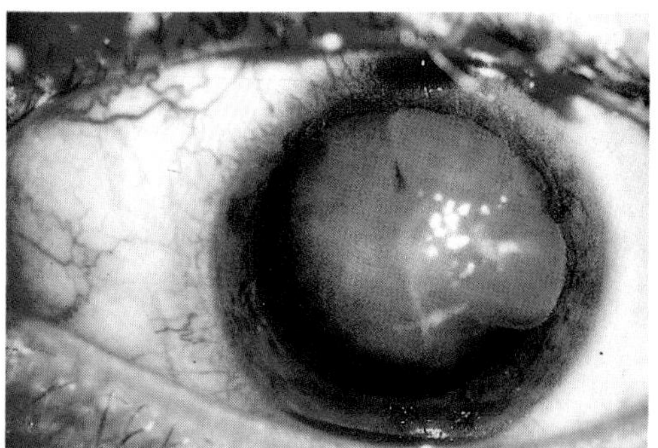

FIGURE 11–28 **Corneal laceration with lens involvement.** Corneal laceration with rupture of anterior lens capsule. The flocculent lens material was aspirated with preservation of the posterior capsule during primary repair. (From Shingleton BJ, Hersh PH, Kenyon KR (eds): Eye Trauma. St. Louis, Mosby-Year Book, 1991, color plate 13–5.)

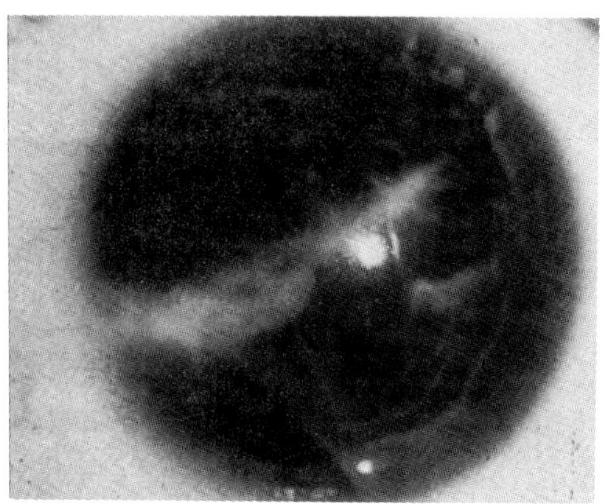

A

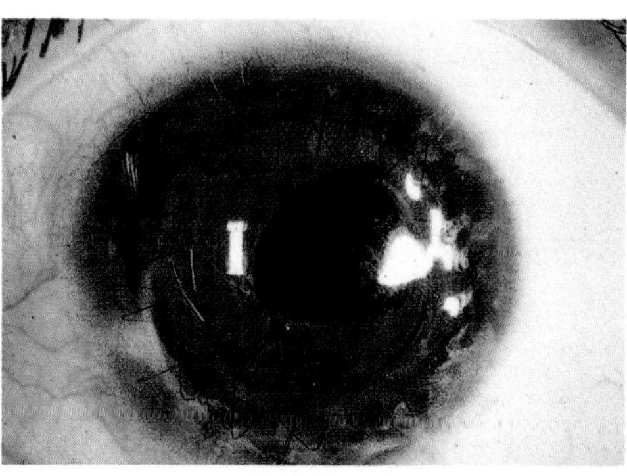

B

FIGURE 11–29 **Anterior segment reconstruction.** *A,* Pupil secluded by adherent leukoma after penetrating injury with a knife. A large iridodialysis is present. *B,* After penetrating keratoplasty, goniosynechialysis, iris resuspension and iridoplasty, removal of cataract remnants and anterior vitrectomy, and implantation of anterior chamber lens, visual acuity is 20/70. (From Shingleton BJ, Hersh PH, Kenyon KR (eds): Eye Trauma. St. Louis, Mosby-Year Book, 1991, color plate 16–2.)

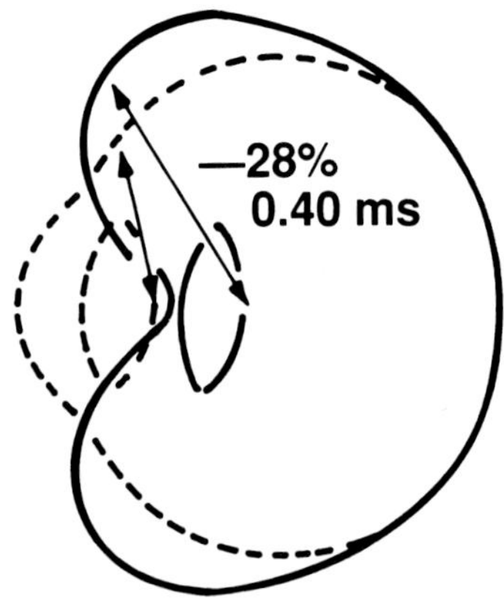

FIGURE 11–30 **Mechanism of blunt injury.** Shape of the globe at maximum deformation (0.40 msec after impact), heavy line; of eye at rest, dashed line. Distance between vitreous base and posterior pole of lens is increased by 28%. (From Schepens CL: Pathogenesis of traumatic rhegmatogenous retinal detachment. *In* Schepens CL: Retinal Detachment and Allied Diseases. Philadelphia, WB Saunders, 1983.)

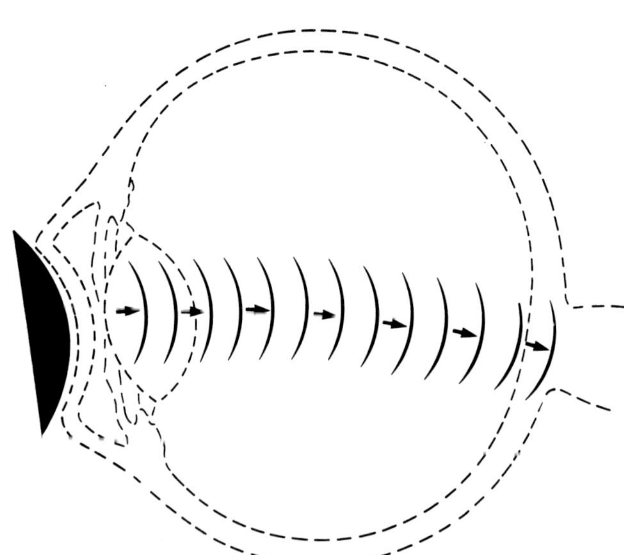

FIGURE 11–31 **Mechanism of blunt injury.** Transmission of force from an anterior blunt injury to the posterior segment. (Modified from Benson WE: The effects of blunt trauma on the posterior segment of the eye. Trans Pa Acad Ophthalmol Otolaryngol 37:26, 1984.)

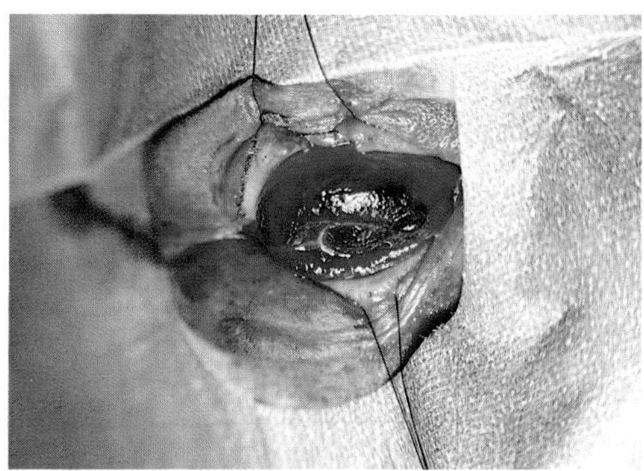

FIGURE 11–32 **Scleral rupture.** Ruptured globe after blunt trauma.

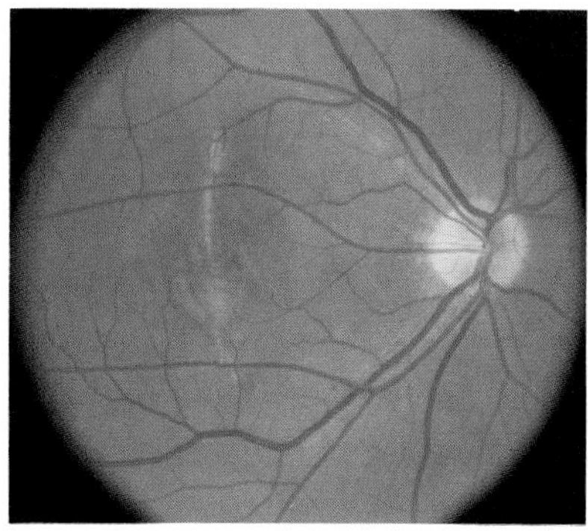

FIGURE 11–35 **Choroidal rupture.** Choroidal rupture 2 years after initial trauma.

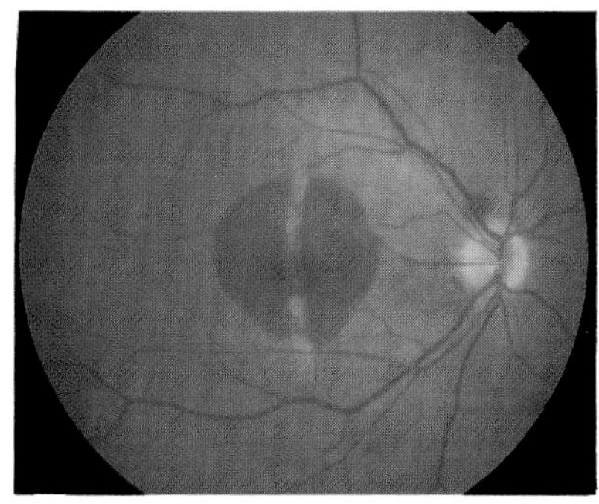

FIGURE 11–33 **Choroidal rupture.** Acute subfoveal choroidal rupture with subretinal hemorrhage.

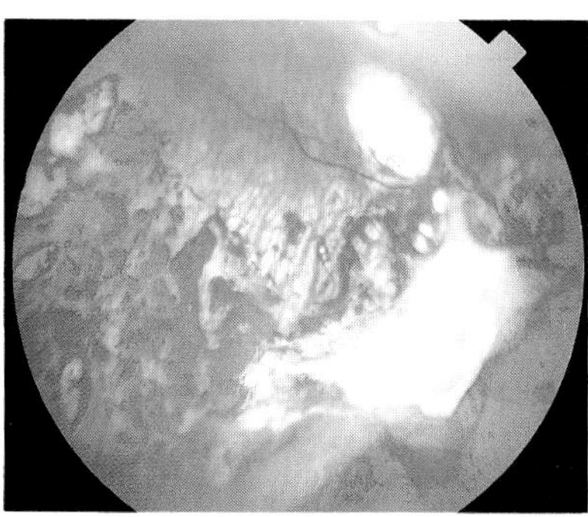

FIGURE 11–36 **Choroidal rupture.** Retinitis sclopetaria with late atrophy of choroid and retina and fibrous intraocular proliferation.

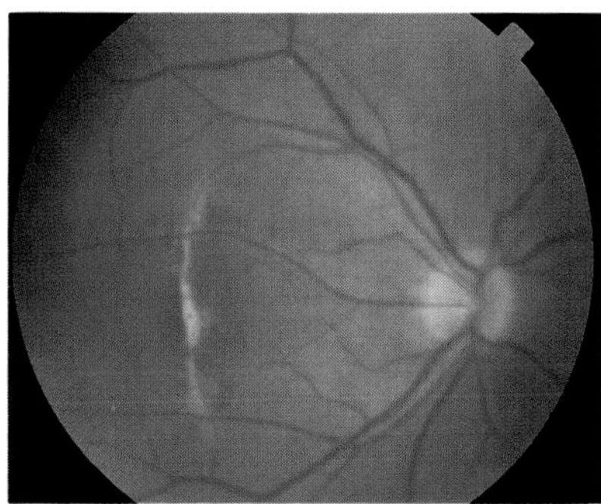

FIGURE 11–34 **Choroidal rupture.** Choroidal rupture 1 month after hemorrhage clears.

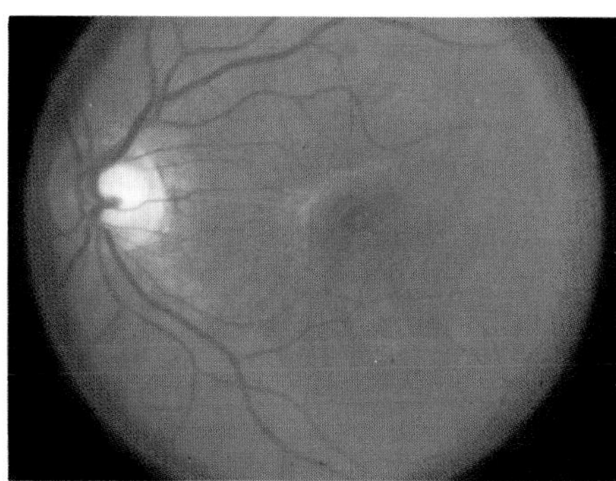

FIGURE 11–37 **Traumatic retinal breaks.** Macular hole and macular fibrosis after blunt ocular trauma.

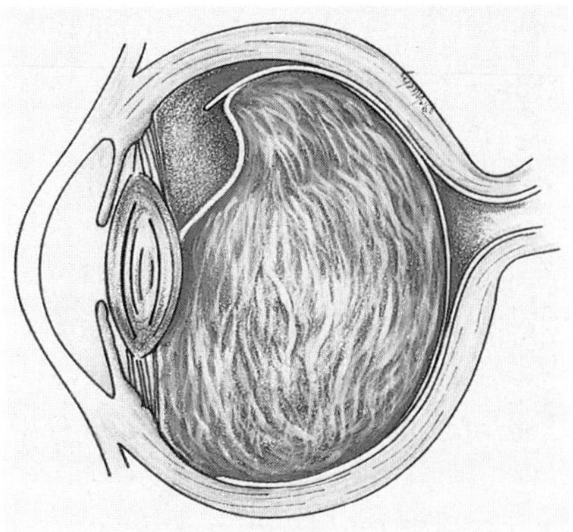

FIGURE 11–38 **Retinal dialysis.** Traumatic retinal dialysis with vitreous base disinserted and lying loosely in the vitreous cavity. Note the vitreous attachment to the posterior dialysis flap.

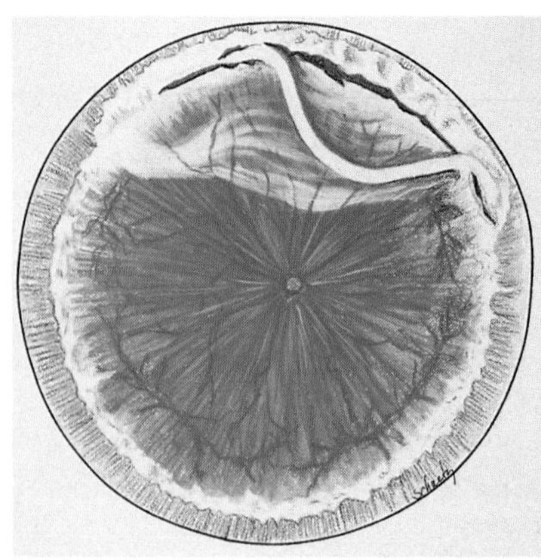

FIGURE 11–41 **Retinal dialysis.** Fundoscopic appearance of retinal dialysis with vitreous base disinserted and loosely hanging in vitreous cavity. (Modified from Weidenthal DJ, Schepens CL: Peripheral fundus changes associated with ocular contusion. Am J Ophthalmol 62:465, 1966. Copyright by The Ophthalmic Publishing Company.)

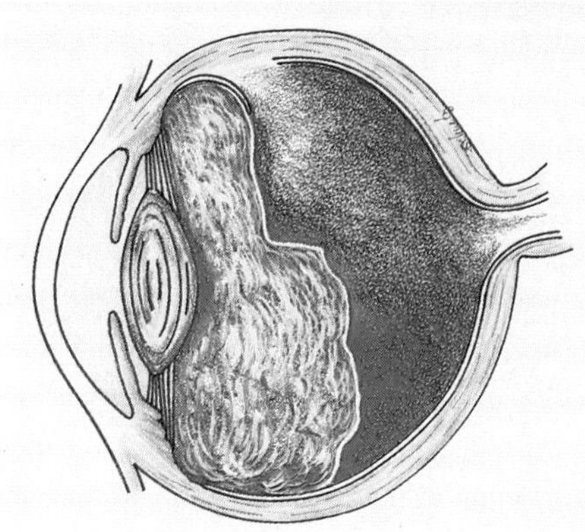

FIGURE 11–39 **Retinal dialysis.** Traumatic retinal tear with the vitreous attached to anterior flap and disinserted posteriorly.

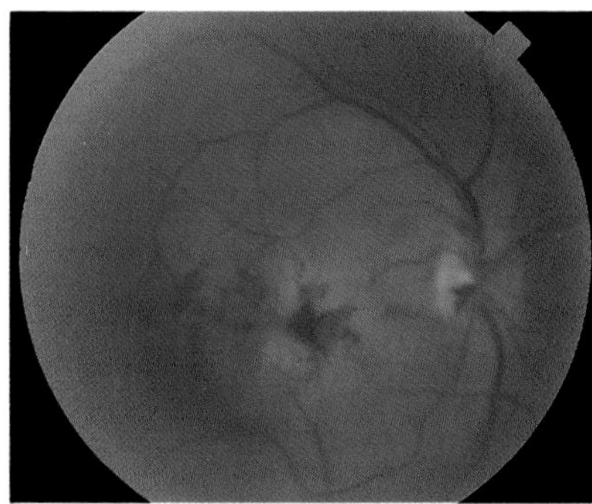

FIGURE 11–42 **Commotio retinae.** Acute commotio retinae with intraretinal hemorrhage.

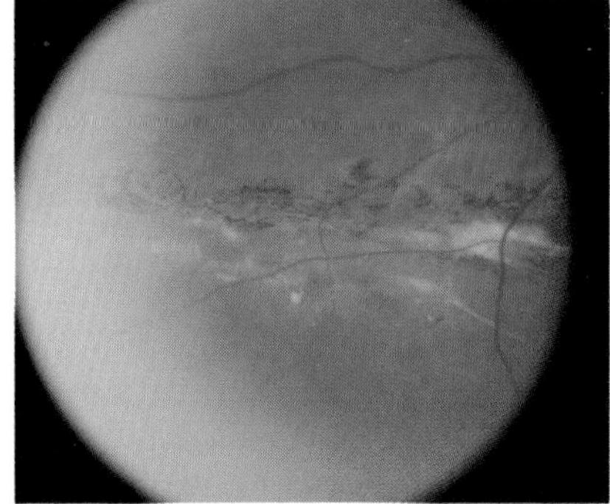

FIGURE 11–40 **Retinal dialysis.** Chronic retinal detachment secondary to retinal dialysis with a demarcation line.

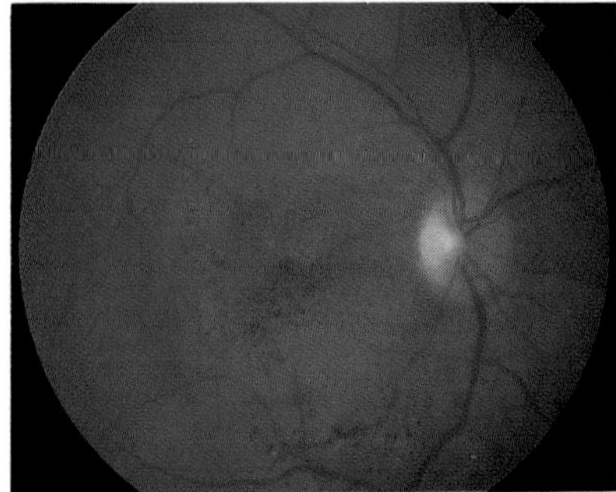

FIGURE 11–43 **Commotio retinae.** Extensive retinal pigment epithelial disorganization after resolution of acute commotio retinae.

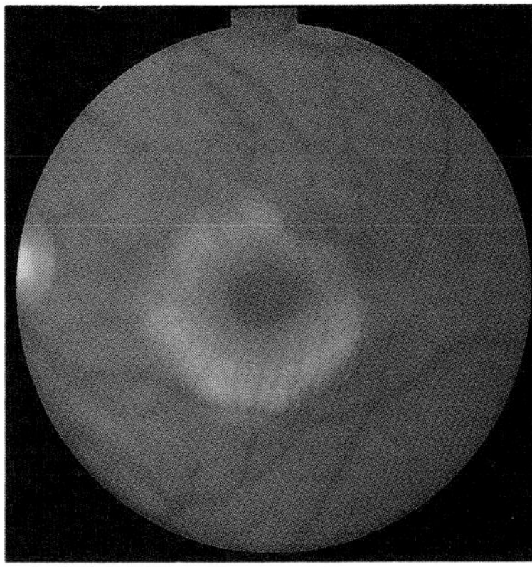

FIGURE 11–44 **Commotio retinae.** Commotio retinae with primarily retinal pigment epithelial opacification.

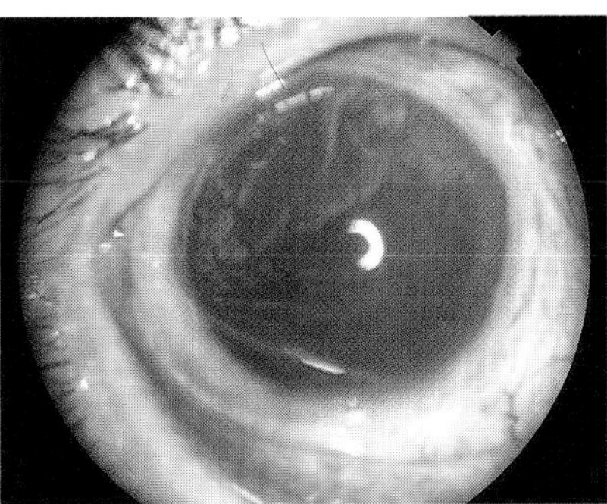

FIGURE 11–47 **Penetrating trauma.** Perforating trauma in the posterior segment. Recurrent retinal detachment after traumatic scleral rupture with evulsion of the lens and iris.

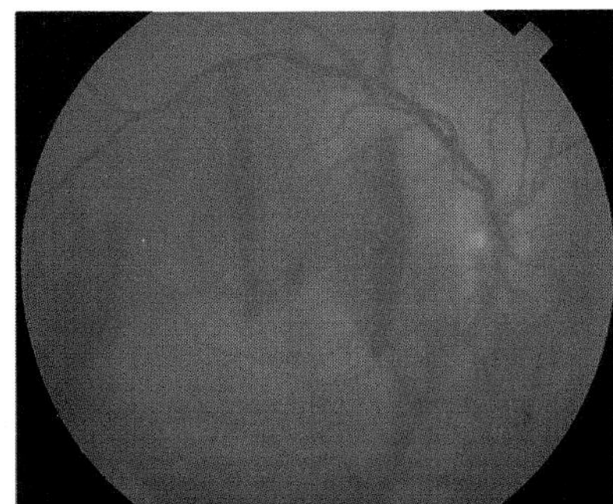

FIGURE 11–45 **Vitreous changes in blunt trauma.** Traumatic vitreous hemorrhage.

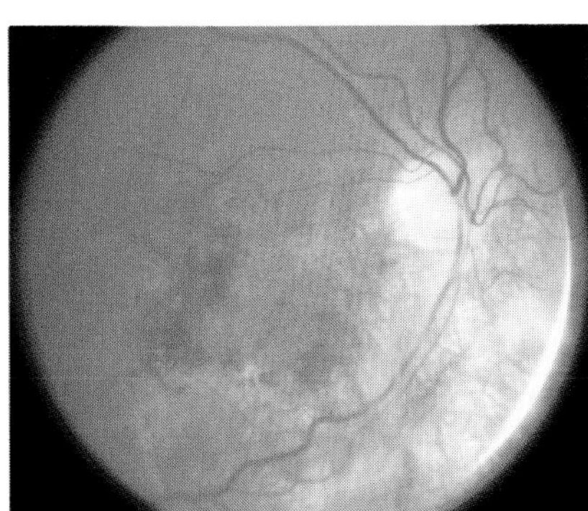

FIGURE 11–46 **Optic nerve injury.** Extensive retinal pigment epithelial disruption, choroidal atrophy, and optic atrophy after blunt ocular trauma with war games projectile.

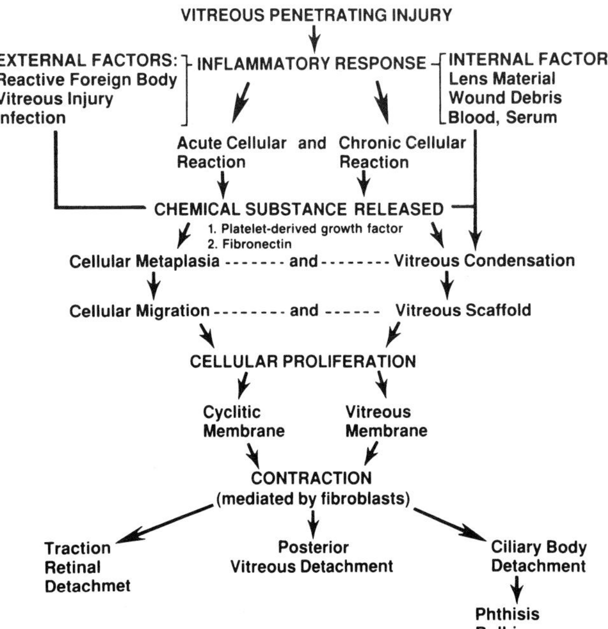

FIGURE 11–48 **Penetrating trauma.** Sequelae of vitreous penetrating injury. (Modified from Tolentio FI: The vitreous in ocular trauma. Bull Soc Belg Ophthalmol 223:179, 1987.)

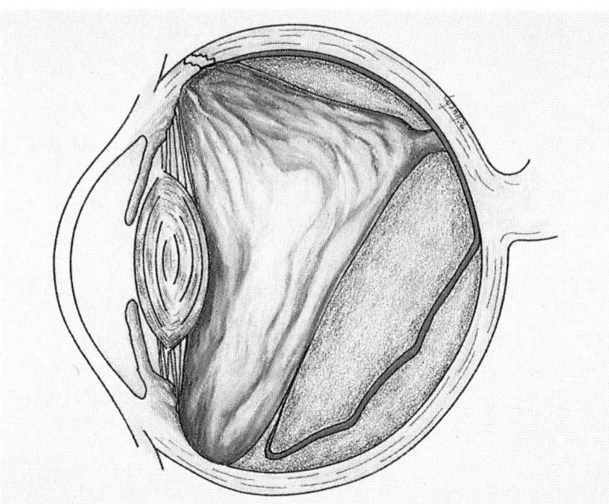

FIGURE 11–49 **Sequelae of penetrating injury.** Intraocular proliferation and retinal detachment after perforating injury involving posterior segment. (Modified from Conway BP, Michels RG: Vitrectomy techniques in the management of selected penetrating ocular injuries. Ophthalmology 85:560, 1978.)

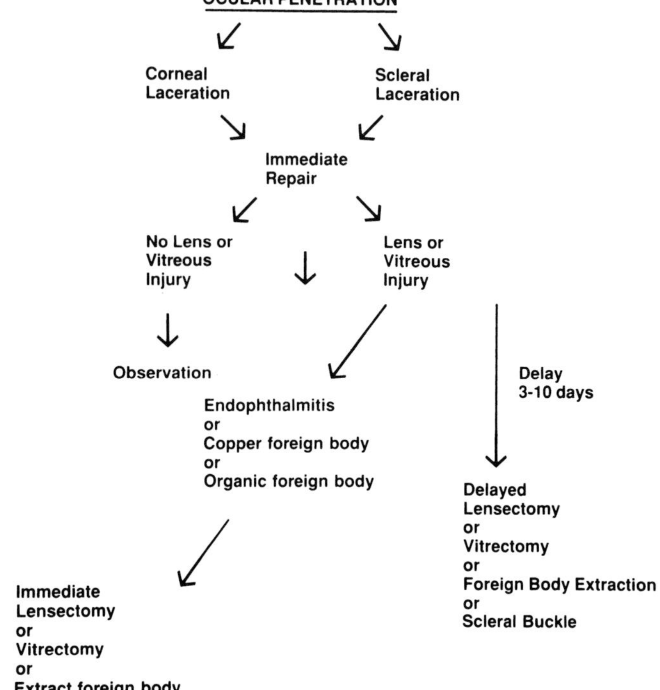

FIGURE 11–50 **Repair of perforating trauma.** Algorithm depicting planning of repair of ocular penetrating injury.

Early (0-72 hours)	Late (3-14 days)	Delayed >3 weeks
Endophthalmitis	Retinal Detachment	Pupillary membrane
Toxic Intraocular foreign body	Lens - Vitreous Injury	Dislocated lens
Retinal detachment	Severe Vitreous Hemorrhage	Ghost Cell glaucoma
	Double perforating injury	Retinal detachment with PVR
	Intraocular foreign body	Macular pucker
		Vitreous Opacity

FIGURE 11–51 **Repair of perforating trauma.** Indications for early, late, and delayed vitrectomy after ocular trauma.

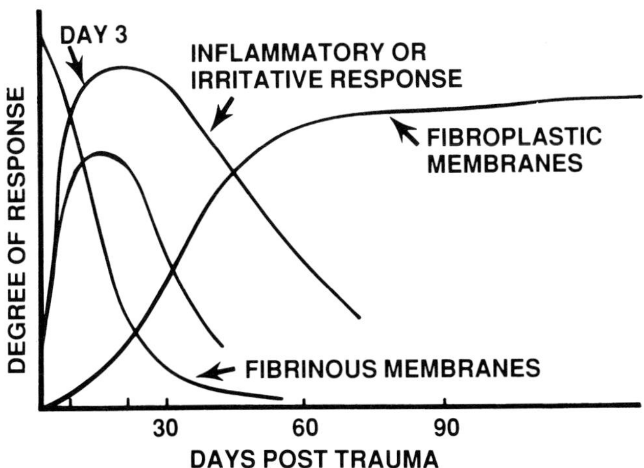

FIGURE 11–52 **Repair of perforating trauma.** Relative timing of intraocular fibrinous, inflammatory, and fibroplastic responses after ocular trauma. (Modified from Coleman DJ: The role of vitrectomy in traumatic vitreopathy. Trans Am Acad Ophthalmol Otolaryngol 108:48, 1990.)

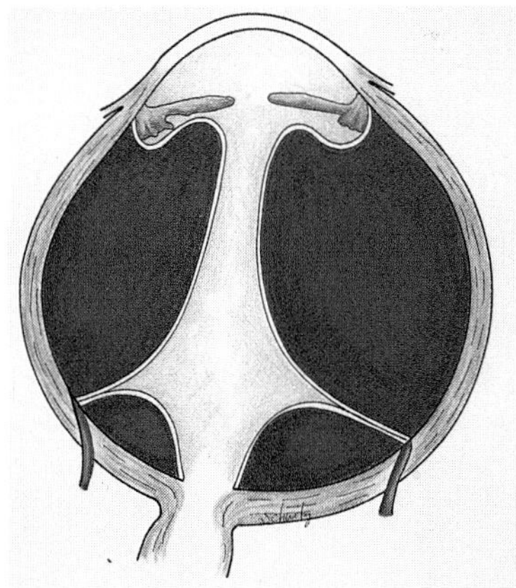

FIGURE 11–53 **Secondary repair of scleral perforation.** Traumatic hemorrhage into suprachoroidal space. Note tethering of choroid at vortex veins.

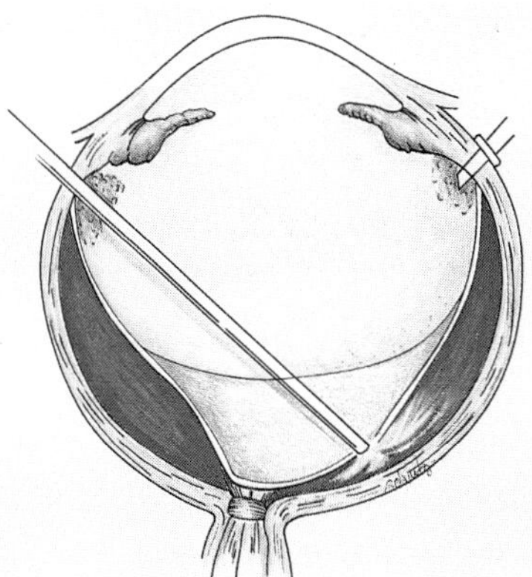

FIGURE 11–54 **Secondary repair of scleral perforation.** Final air-fluid exchange and endodrainage through retinal break after vitrectomy and lensectomy for penetrating ocular trauma. (Modified from Conway BP, Michels RG: Vitrectomy techniques in the management of selected penetrating ocular injuries. Ophthalmology 85:560, 1978.)

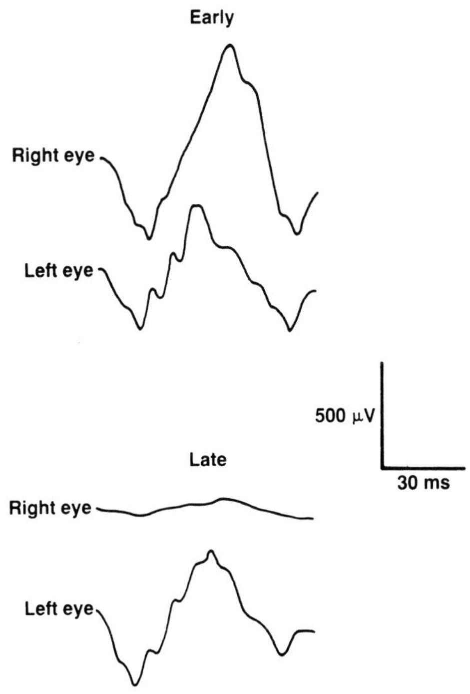

FIGURE 11–55 **Intraocular foreign body.** Electroretinographic changes secondary to iron toxicity (ms, milliseconds). (Modified from Good P, Gross K: Electrophysiology and metallosis: Support for an oxidative (free radical) mechanism in the human eye. Ophthalmologica 196:204, 1988.)

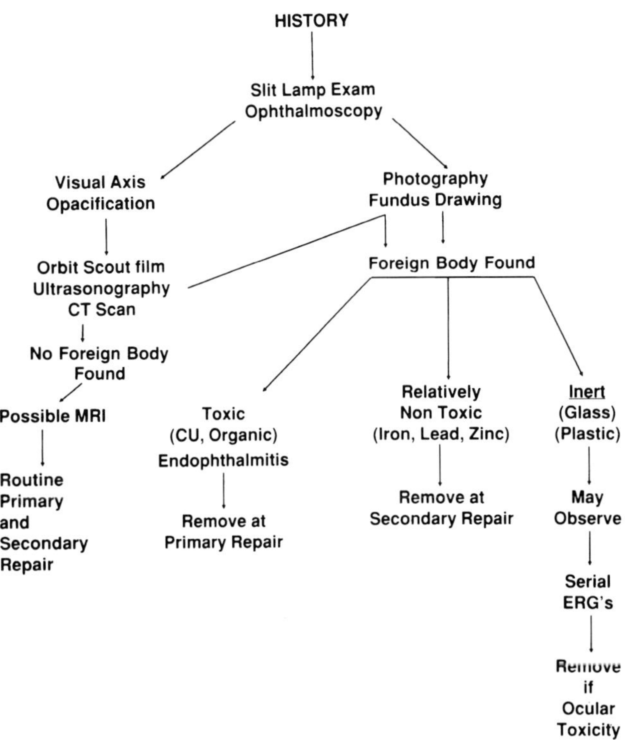

FIGURE 11–56 **Intraocular foreign body.** Algorithm of management of intraocular foreign body.

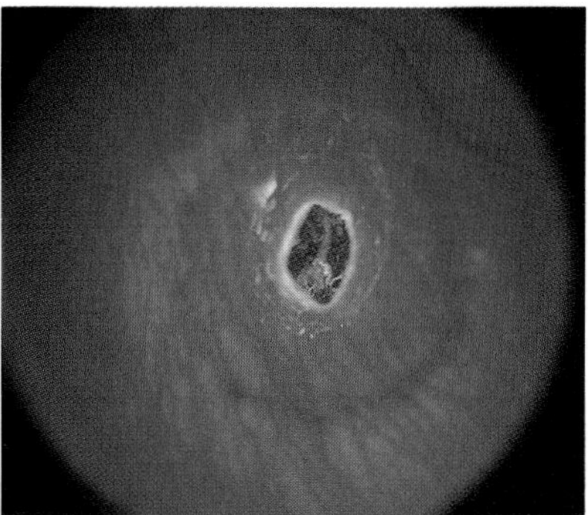

FIGURE 11–57 **Intraocular foreign body.** Intraocular foreign body imbedded in the retina.

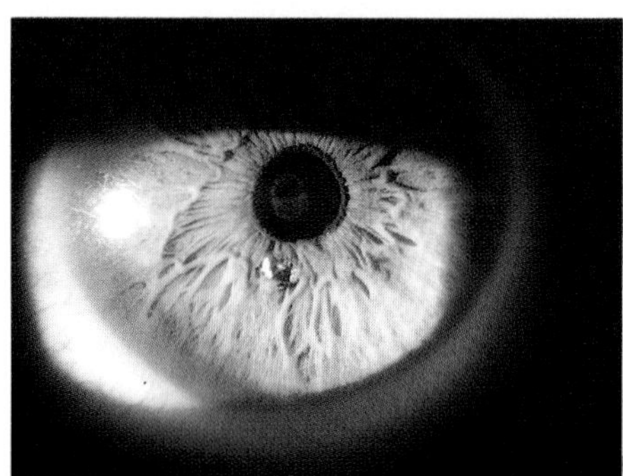

FIGURE 11–58 **Intraocular foreign body.** Metallic intraocular foreign body on the iris.

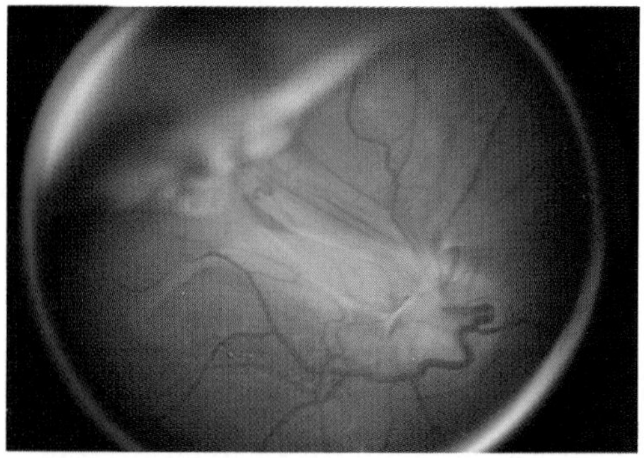

FIGURE 11–59 **Extraction of intraocular foreign body.** Chronic traction retinal detachment and macular fibrosis after removal of an intraocular foreign body.

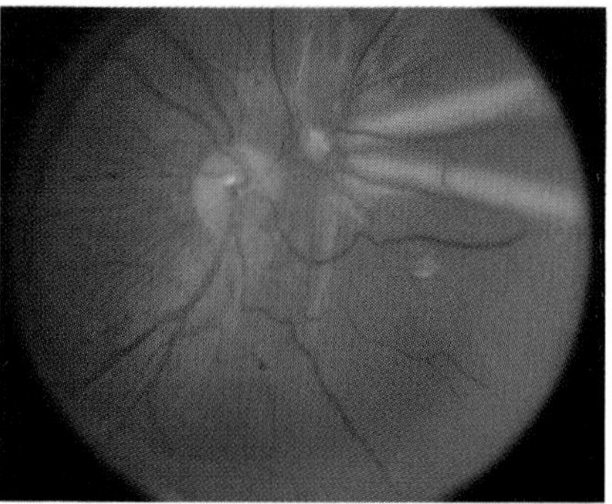

FIGURE 11–60 **Extraction of intraocular foreign body.** Star fold and retinal detachment 1 year after removal of neglected intraocular foreign body.

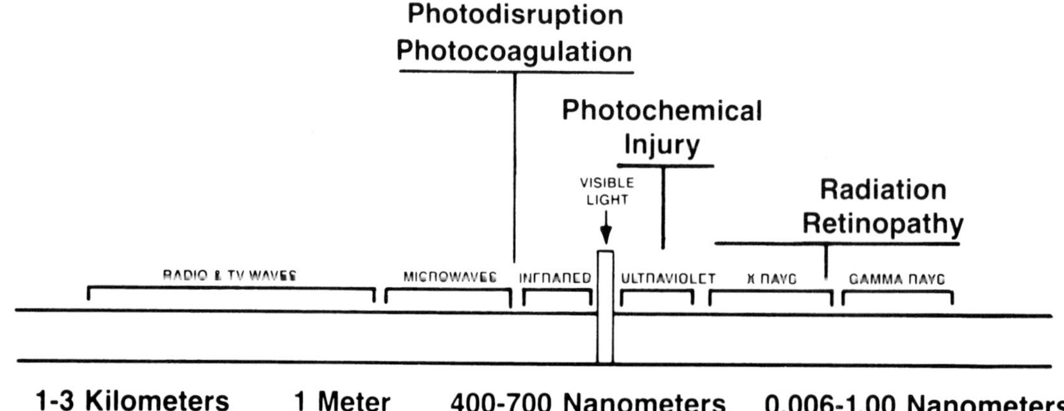

FIGURE 11–61 **Manifestations of electromagnetic trauma on the posterior segment.** Electromagnetic spectrum and its relationship to posterior segment injury.

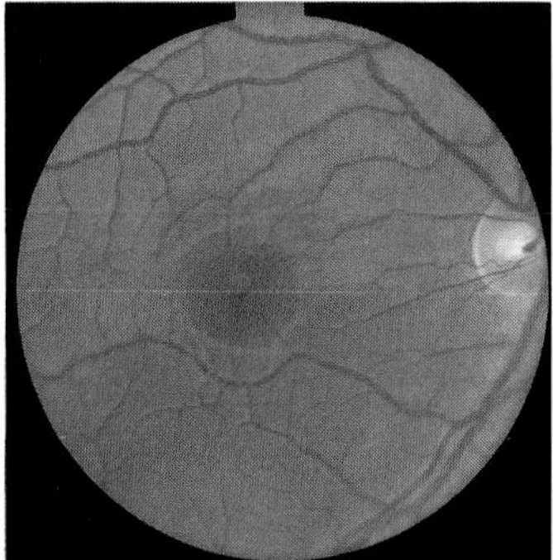

FIGURE 11-62 Solar retinopathy.

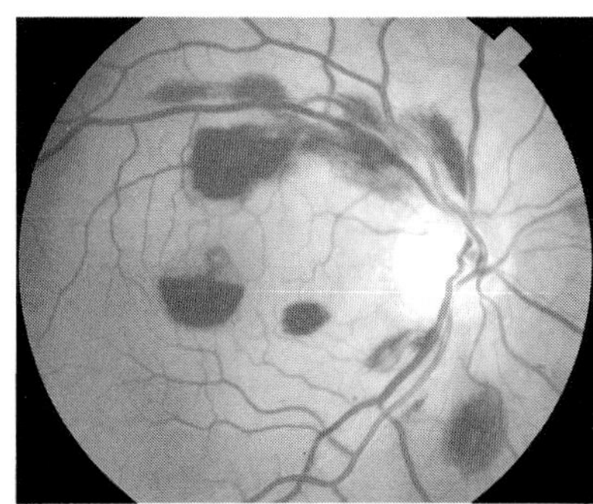

FIGURE 11-64 **Manifestations in the posterior segment of remote trauma.** Valsalva retinopathy.

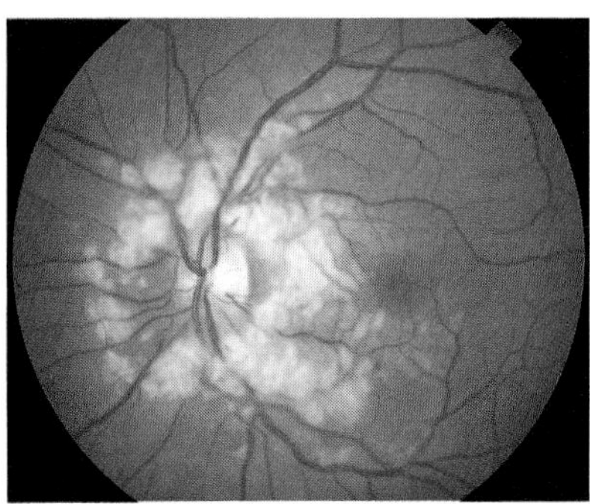

FIGURE 11-63 **Manifestations in the posterior segment of remote trauma.** Purtscher's retinopathy after a motor vehicle accident.

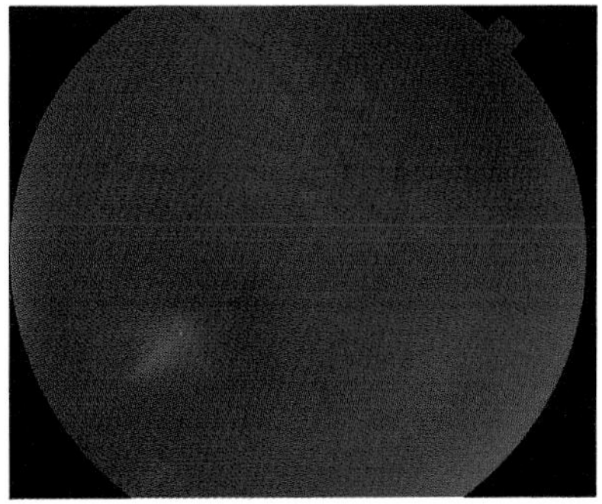

FIGURE 11-65 **Child abuse.** Intraretinal hemorrhages secondary to shaken baby syndrome.

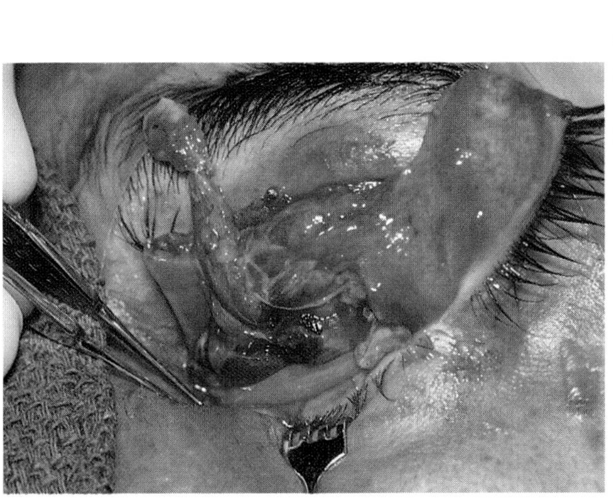

A

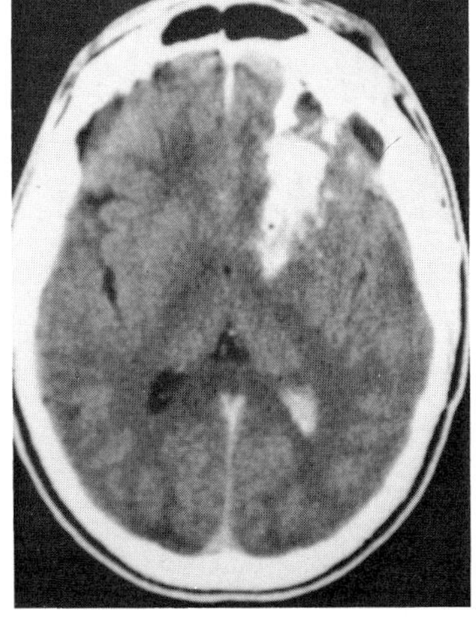

B

FIGURE 11-66 **Imaging.** This patient sustained a penetrating gear shift injury to the left orbit. *A,* The clinical photograph demonstrates an obviously significant injury to the upper eyelid and globe. *B,* The CT scan, however, reveals the deep penetration into the frontal lobe. This finding highlights the need for a thorough local and systemic evaluation in all patients with apparently "isolated" orbital trauma.

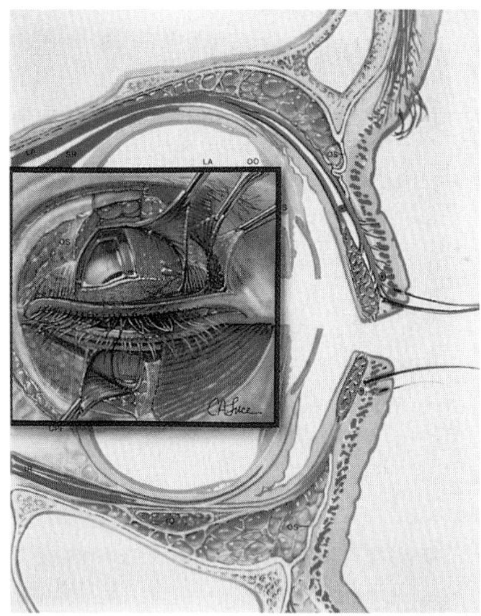

FIGURE 11–67 **Periocular lacerations.** This diagram relates the orbital surface anatomy to the potentially traumatized structures located subcutaneously and within the anterior orbit.

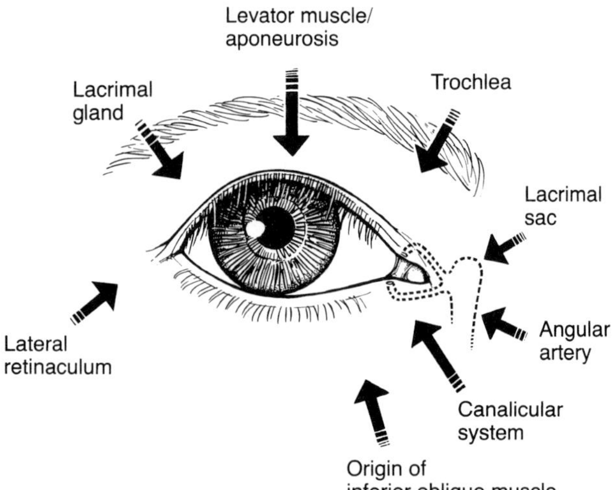

FIGURE 11–68 **Periocular lacerations.** An anatomic cross-sectional view of the orbit demonstrates the thinness of the eyelids and the relatively superficial location of the underlying orbital septum and levator aponeurosis. (From Zide BM, Jelks GW: Surgical Anatomy of the Orbit. New York, Raven Press, 1985.)

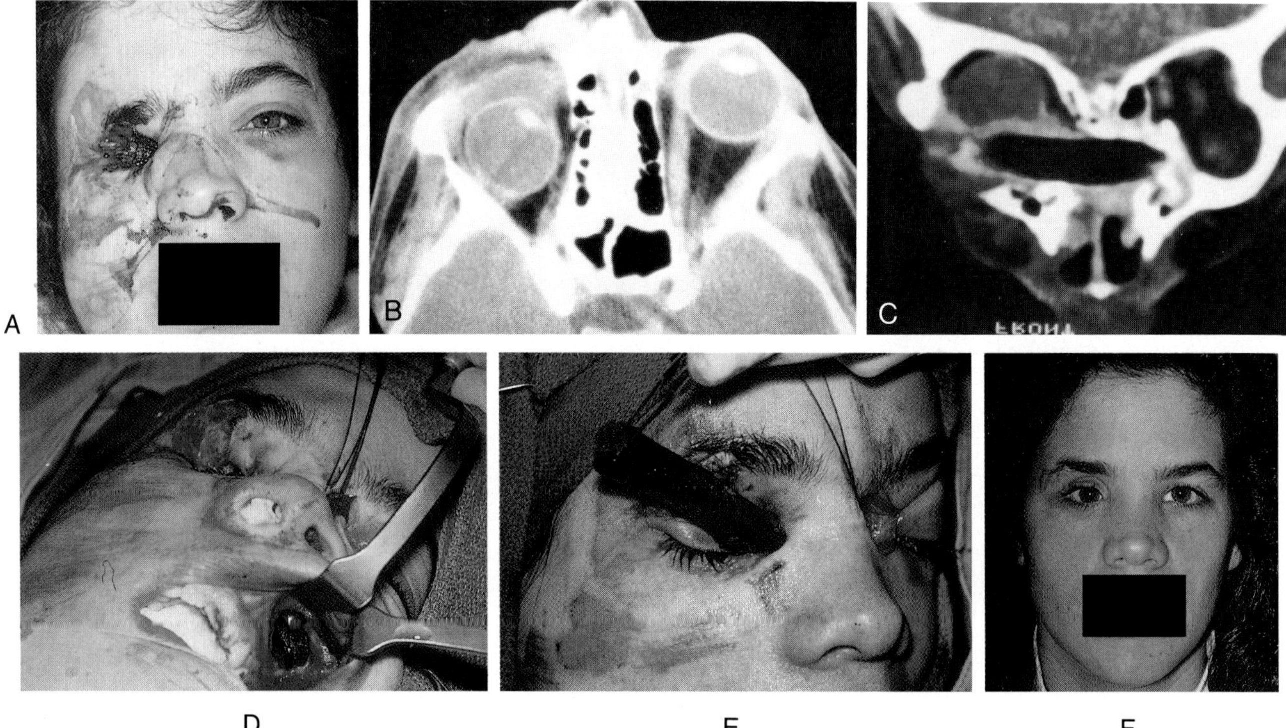

FIGURE 11–69 **Foreign body.** *A,* This patient struck her head against a tree stump while sledding, sustaining a deeply penetrating wooden branch foreign body injury. On initial examination, the right globe could not be visualized. *B,* An axial CT scan demonstrates that the globe appeared intact, yet retrodisplaced within the orbit. *C,* A coronal CT scan is essential to localize accurately the position of the foreign body. The direct coronal CT image reveals that the path of the stick passed extracranially just beneath the cribriform plate, through the superior nasal cavity, disrupting a portion of the anteromedial left orbital floor and entering the left maxillary antrum. *D,* Before removal, the branch was maximally exposed along its tract of penetration through a left transoral gingival sulcus and left external ethmoidectomy approach. *E,* The 7.5-cm branch was then removed under direct visualization and maximal control. *F,* Ten months following the repair, the patient's vision was 20/20, and her appearance was remarkably improved. Yet, there was significant posttraumatic telecanthus and enophthalmos, which required secondary surgical repair. This highlights the need for close follow-up of patients postoperatively to detect, monitor, and manage anticipated secondary problems.

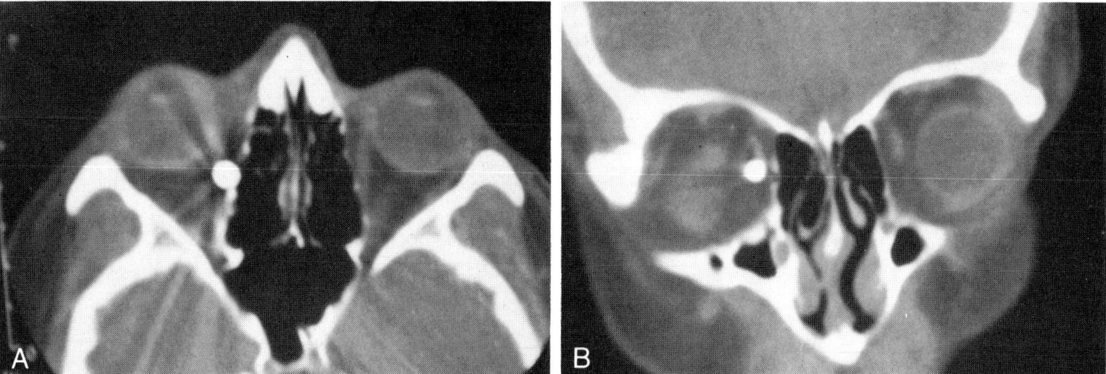

FIGURE 11–70 **Foreign body.** This deep orbital foreign body (BB shot), well localized by both axial *(A)* and coronal *(B)* CT scans, was causing no functional deficit and was not easily accessible surgically. Therefore, the patient was managed conservatively, without surgical intervention.

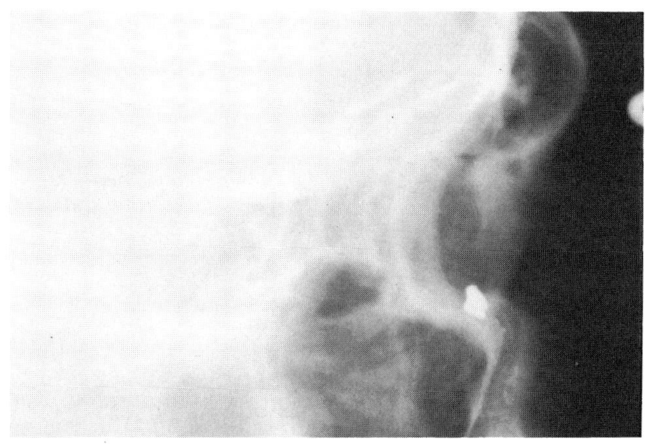

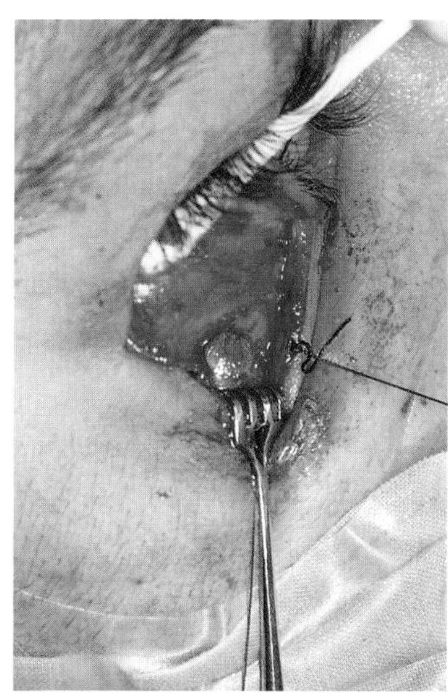

FIGURE 11–71 **Foreign body.** This symptomatic pellet foreign body was easily palpable and located just posterior to the infraorbital rim. The pellet was uneventfully exposed and removed through a right subciliary approach.

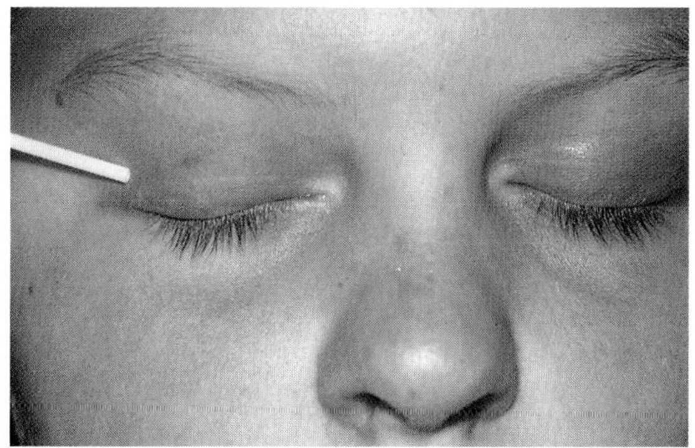

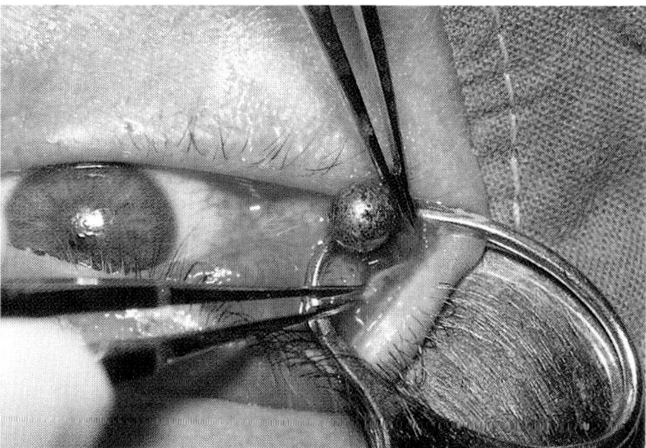

FIGURE 11–72 **Foreign body.** *A,* A BB shot injury to the upper eyelid resulted in a retained foreign body in the anterior orbit. The BB was palpable at the site indicated, and its position was confirmed radiologically. *B,* At surgery, the BB was "captured" with a chalazion clamp and excised transconjunctivally.

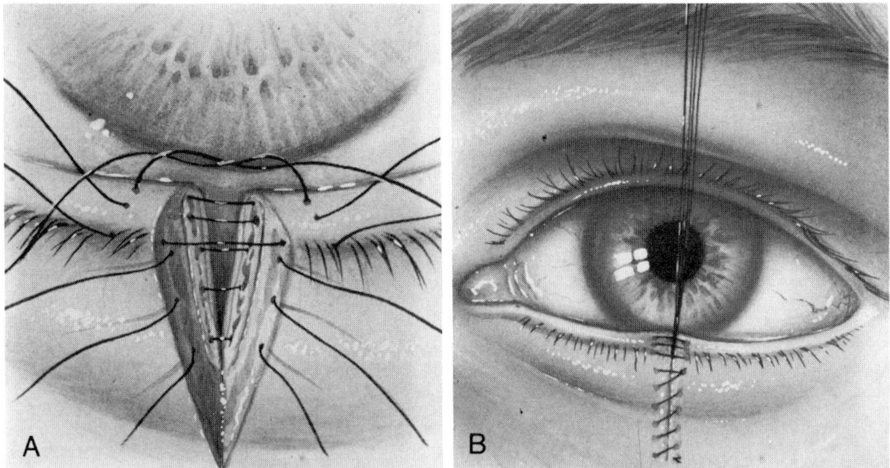

FIGURE 11–73 **Marginal full-thickness laceration repair.** *A,* Schematic view of a full-thickness eyelid laceration repair. Buried sutures within the tarsus reduce the tension across the wound. The eyelid marginal anatomy is approximated accurately using the local anatomic landmarks of meibomian glands, gray line, and lash line. *B,* The eyelid marginal sutures are incorporated within the skin sutures to minimize the risk of suture contact with the globe.

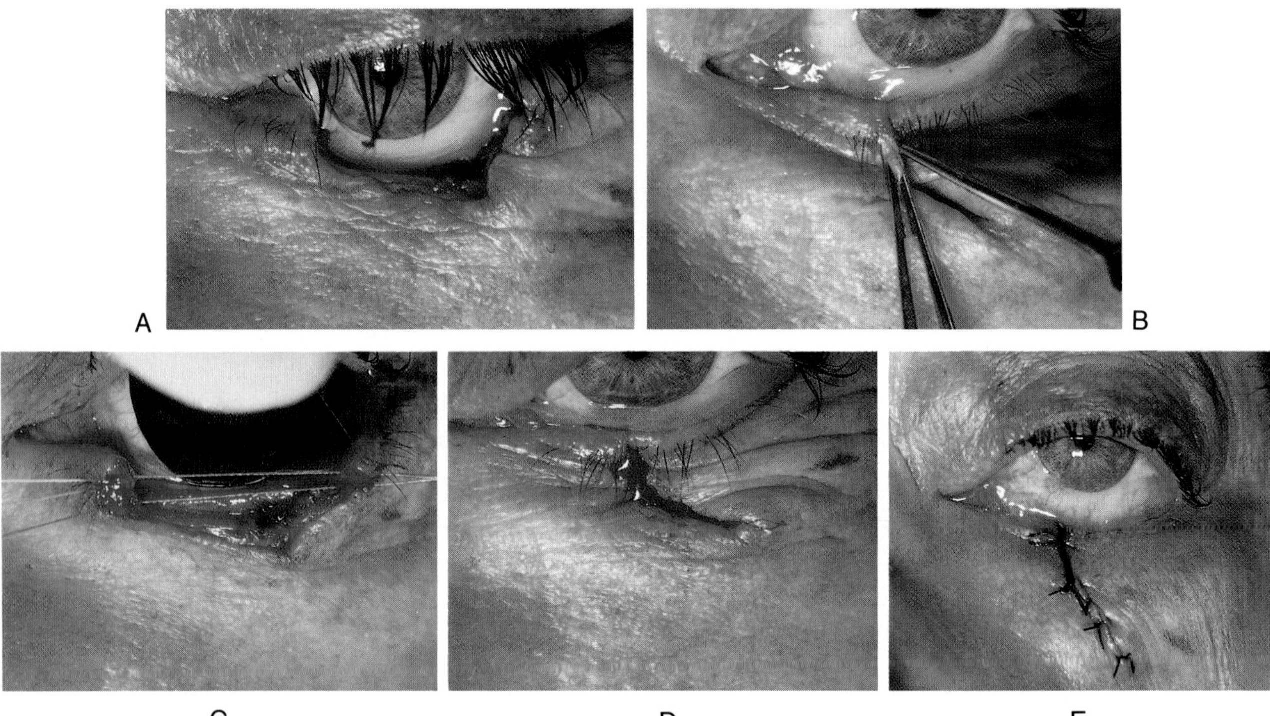

FIGURE 11–74 **Marginal full-thickness laceration repair.** *A,* Clinical photograph of a full-thickness repair. This defect resulted from an excision of an eyelid tumor. *B,* Although the wound appears to gape widely, manipulation with forceps demonstrates that it could be closed without excessive tension. *C,* Vicryl sutures through the inferior tarsus are initially placed to reduce the tension of the wound. *D,* Following tying of the tarsal sutures, the lid margin is well approximated and repaired with minimal tension. *E,* Final repair with silk marginal sutures incorporated into the lower eyelid skin sutures.

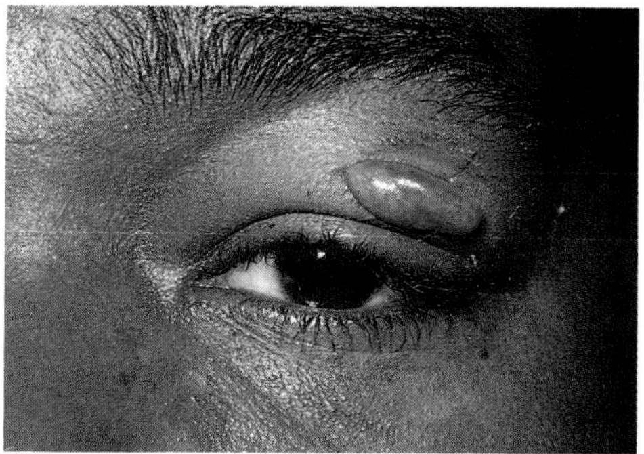

FIGURE 11–75 **Levator laceration repair.** Orbital fat was noted to be prolapsing from this upper eyelid stab wound. The presence of the fat implies perforation of the orbital septum and raises the suspicion of an underlying levator injury.

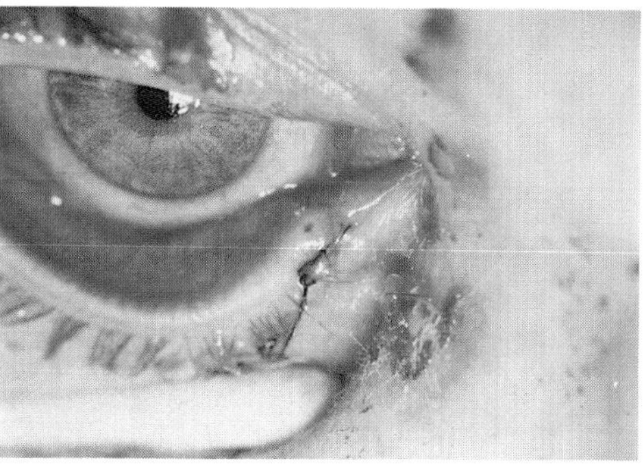

FIGURE 11–76 **Canalicular repair.** A full-thickness eyelid marginal laceration medial to the punctum is a pathognomonic location for a canalicular laceration, yet it was missed by the surgeon who performed the primary repair.

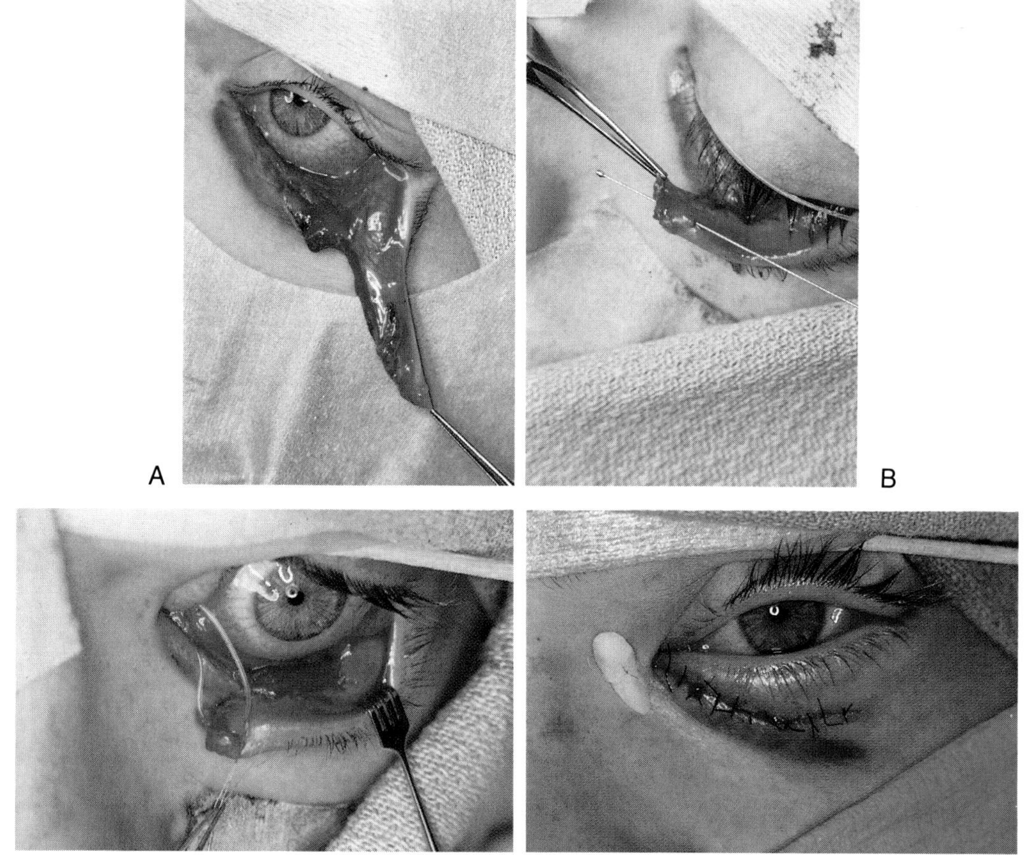

FIGURE 11–77 **Canalicular repair.** Clinical photographs of a canalicular repair. *A,* The medial portion of the eyelid, involving the canaliculus, was avulsed following a blunt shearing injury. *B,* A Crawford-type tube is passed through the lateral portion of the canaliculus, then the medial cut end of the canaliculus, and into the nasolacrimal duct. *C,* The appearance of the eyelid following the polymeric silicone tube cannulation of the entire nasolacrimal drainage system, before repair of the lacerations. *D,* Immediate postoperative appearance of the repair with a bolstered medial canthus suture in place.

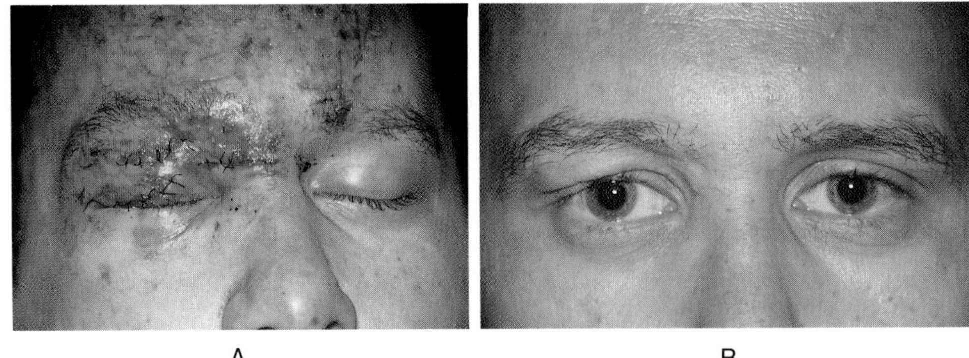

FIGURE 11–78 **Superficial avulsions.** *A,* This diffuse superficial avulsion injury sustained in a motor vehicle accident was allowed to granulate after the wounds were aggressively irrigated and debrided of superficial glass foreign bodies. Small focal lacerations were sutured. *B,* At 6 months, the wounds appeared to have healed well with minimal scarring.

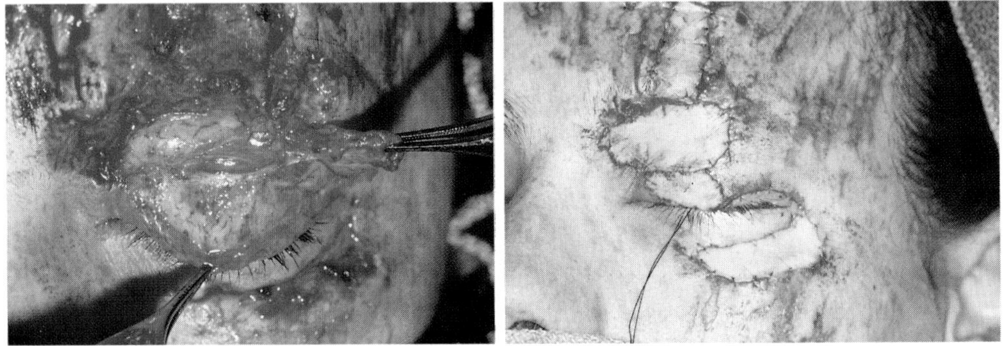

FIGURE 11–79 **Deep tissue loss.** *A,* Deeper avulsion injuries and associated tissue loss, with exposed orbital fat or septum, often require full-thickness skin grafts to accomplish the repair. *B,* The immediate postoperative appearance with full-thickness skin grafts in place.

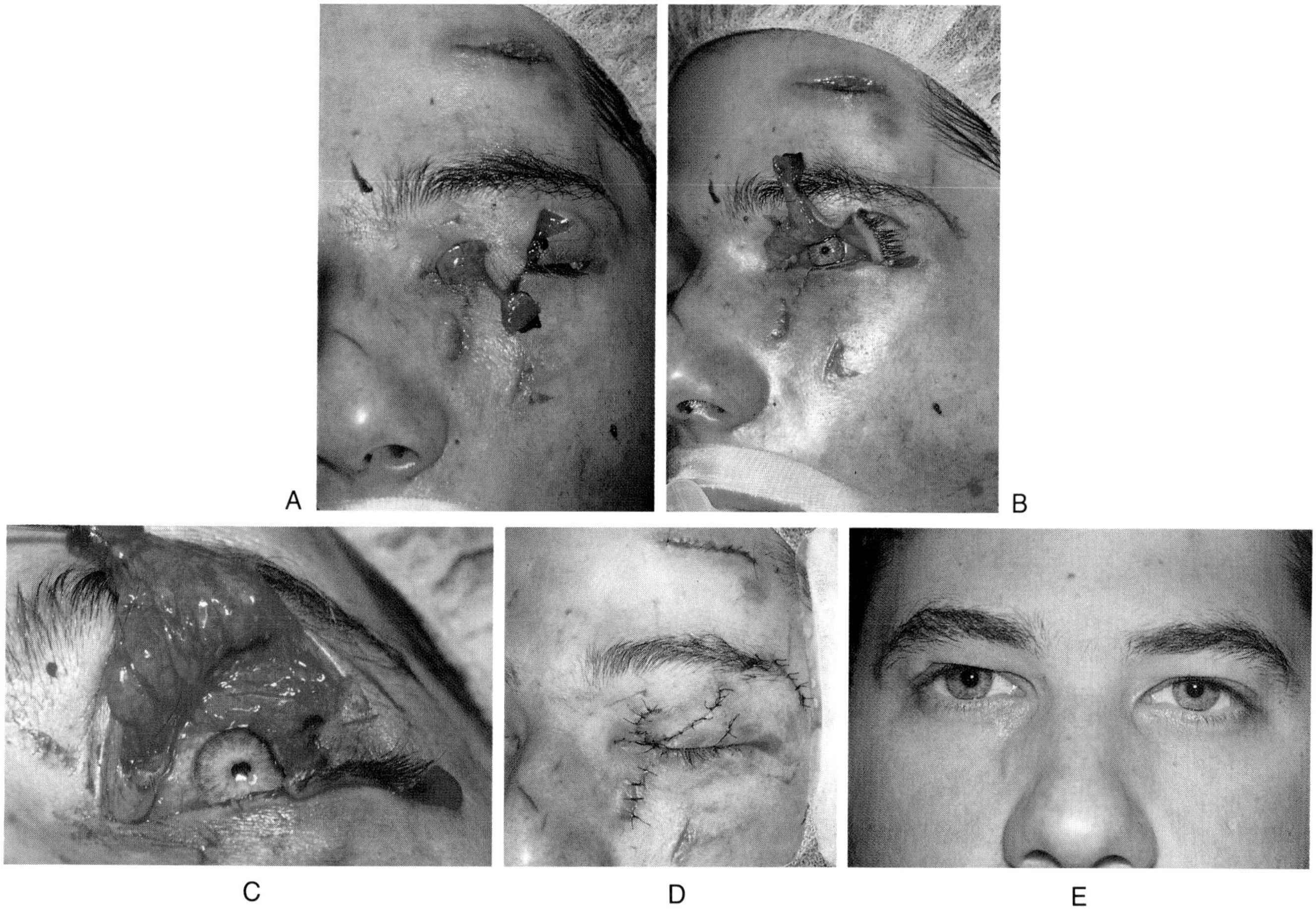

FIGURE 11–80 **Deep tissue loss.** *A* and *B,* This patient was struck with a glass object that shattered on his face, resulting in complex eyelid and facial lacerations. The initial appearance of the wounds suggested the possibility of significant tissue loss. *C,* The exposed orbital fat in the upper eyelid was representative of the deeper orbital injury involving the levator aponeurosis. *D,* Systematic repair of the wounds to the tarsus, levator aponeurosis, eyelid margin, and eyelids and brow resulted in intraoperative restoration of the severely disorganized anatomy. *E,* The 7-months' postoperative appearance demonstrates the excellent functional and cosmetic result.

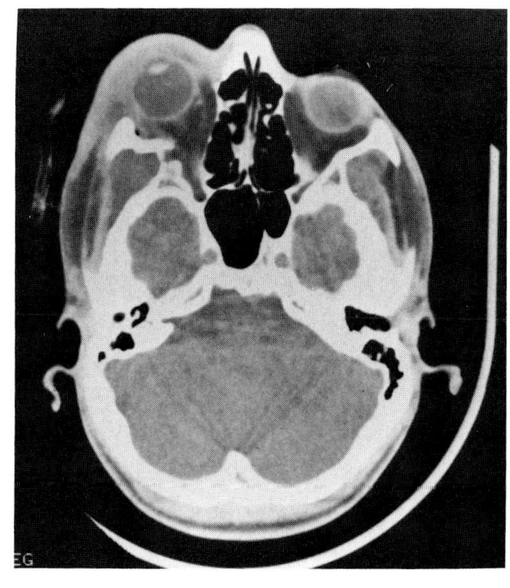

FIGURE 11–81 **CT imaging.** Axial CT scan showing bilateral LeFort III fractures. Soft tissue windows show impingement of lateral orbital wall on lateral rectus muscle.

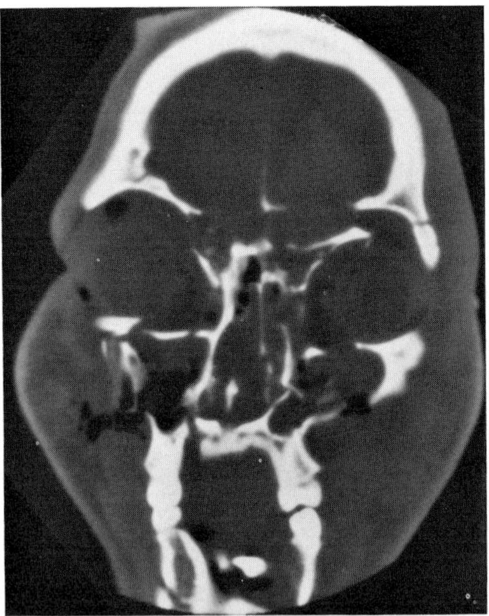

FIGURE 11–82 **CT imaging.** Coronal CT scan shows panfacial fracture including bilateral four-wall orbital injuries.

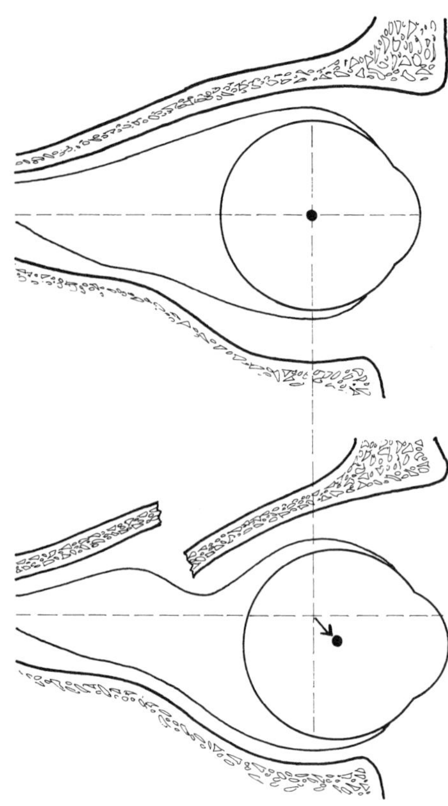

FIGURE 11–84 **Signs and symptoms of supraorbital frontal fractures.** Mechanism of proptosis and downward globe displacement with certain supraorbital fractures.

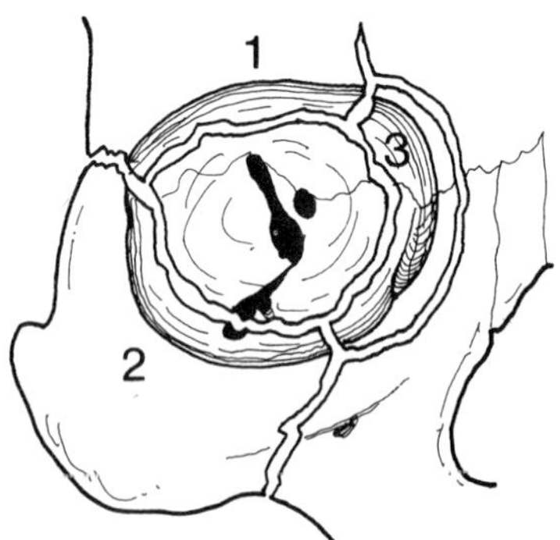

FIGURE 11–83 **Zones of the orbit.** The orbit can be conceptually divided into thirds based on patterns of fracture. These consist of supraorbital *(1)*, zygomatic *(2)*, and nasoethmoid (medial wall) *(3)* segments. The internal orbit is a fourth zone.

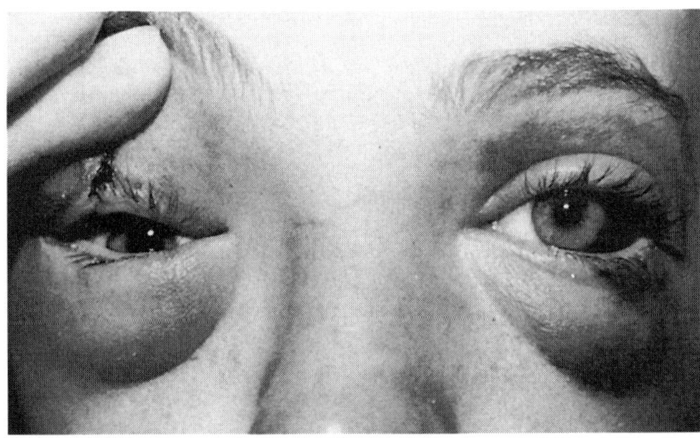

FIGURE 11–85 **Superior orbital fissure syndrome.** Patient with superior orbital fissure syndrome.

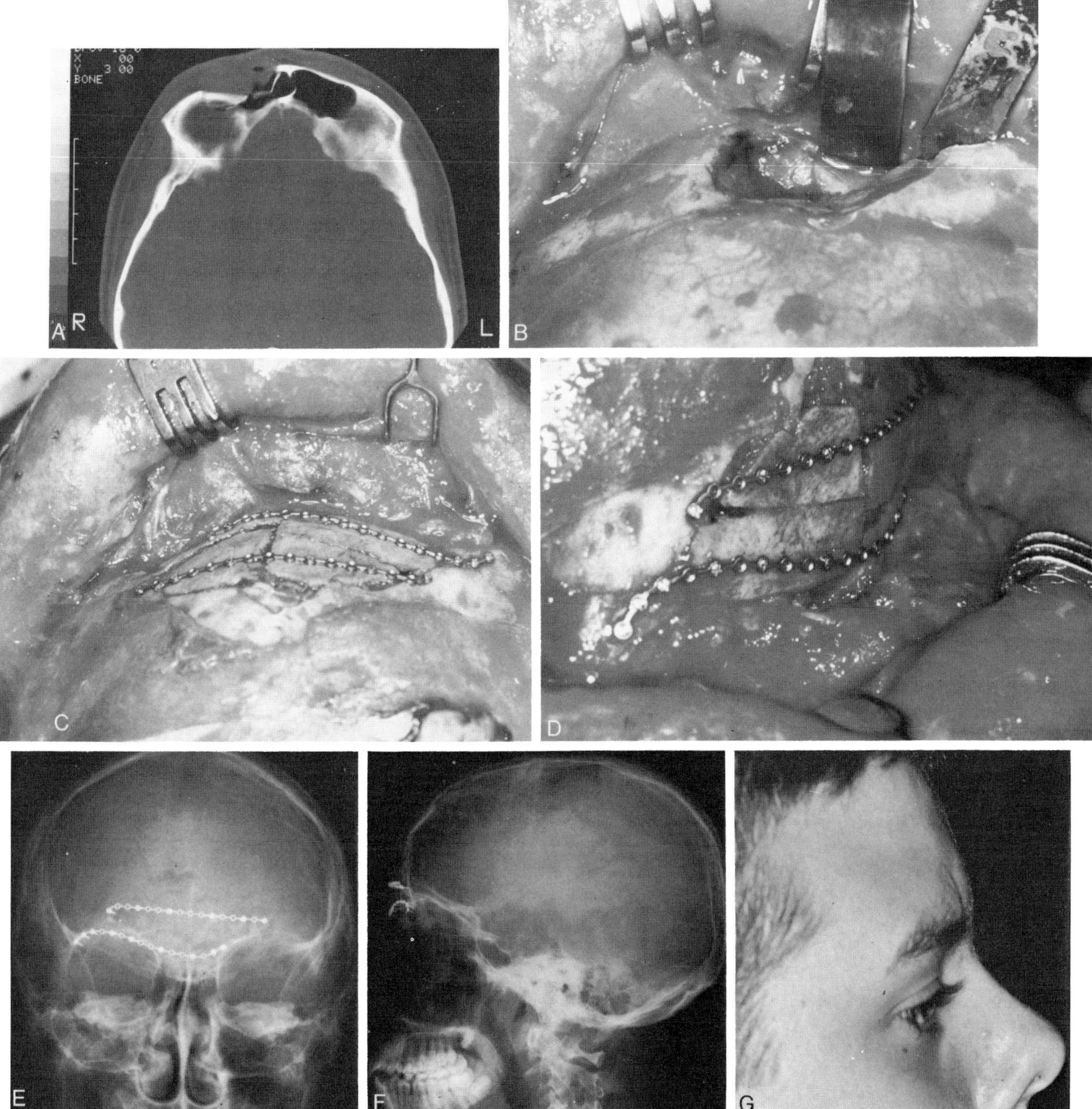

FIGURE 11–86 **Management of frontal fracture.** *A,* Axial CT scan shows fracture involvement of anterior wall of frontal sinus, supraorbital rim, and orbital roof. *B,* Intraoperative view through coronal exposure shows depressed comminuted fracture. *C,* Postreduction view from above. Supraorbital rim was aligned and fixated with microplates. Frontal sinus mucosa was exenterated and frontal sinus obliterated. Anterior wall of left sinus was removed for exposure and then replaced. Comminuted bone of right anterior wall of frontal sinus was replaced with cranial bone harvested from parietal area. *D,* Lateral view of reconstructed supraorbital rim. *E,* Postoperative plain film, anteroposterior view. *F,* Postoperative plain film, lateral view. Shows restoration and maintenance of supraorbital and frontal projection obtained with plate and screw fixation. *G,* Postoperative lateral view. Only contour deformity results from indented posttraumatic scar.

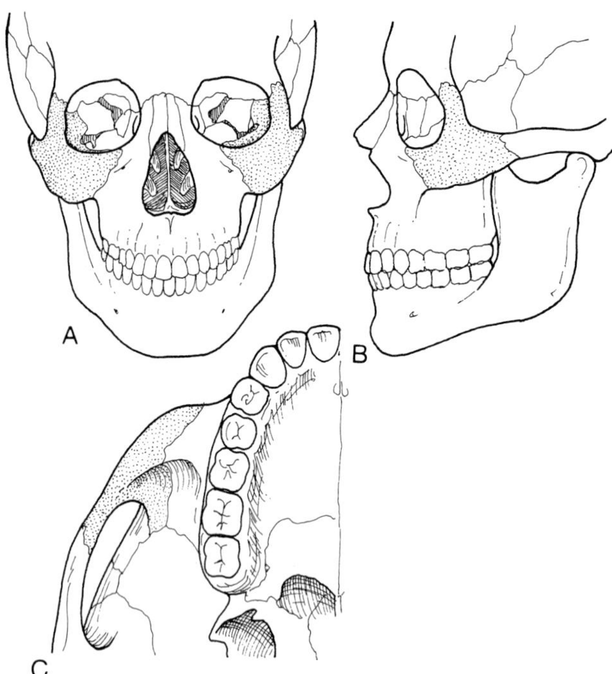

FIGURE 11–87 **Zygoma.** The zygoma composes the majority of the lateral and lower portions of the orbit. It has five major articulations. Superiorly with the frontal bone at the zygomaticofrontal articulation and with the greater wing of the sphenoid, it articulates with the maxilla at the infraorbital rim and the lateral buttresses. Articulation with the zygomatic process of the temporal bone is the point at which it forms the arch. *A,* Frontal view. *B,* Lateral view. *C,* Inferior view.

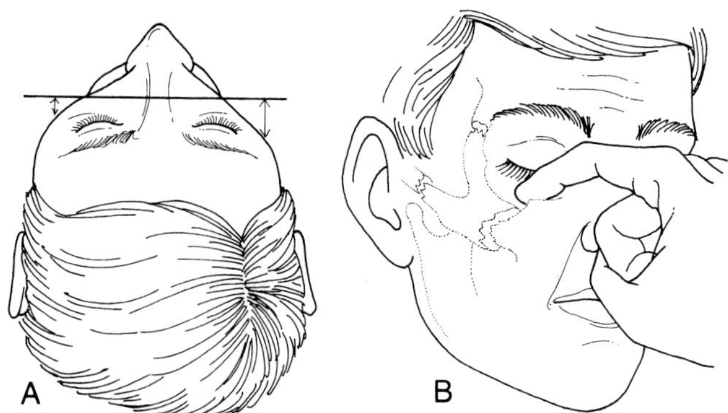

FIGURE 11–88 **Examination of zygomatic fracture.** *A,* Loss of malar prominence is best appreciated by looking down from above. *B,* Palpation of step deformity at zygomaticomaxillary suture of infraorbital rim.

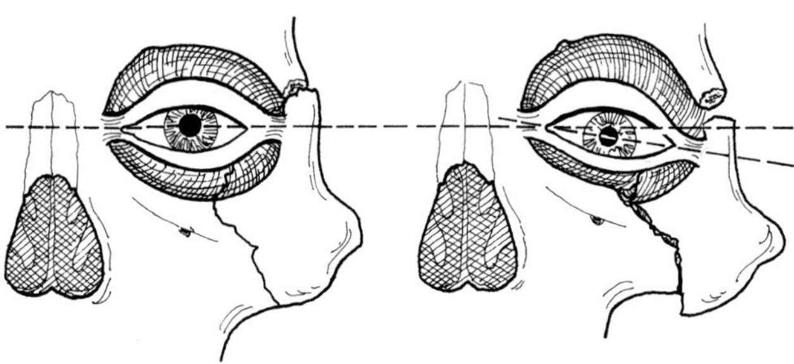

FIGURE 11–89 **Diagnosis of zygomatic fractures.** Downwardly displaced zygoma results in lateral canthal dystopia because lateral canthus is attached to Whitnall's tubercule in lateral orbital wall. *A,* Normal position. *B,* Interior canthal displacement with inferiorly based zygomatic body.

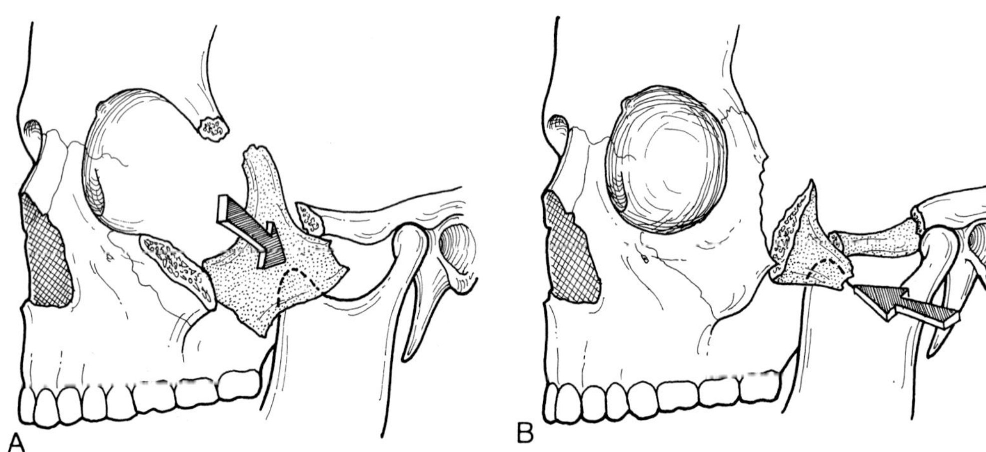

FIGURE 11–90 **Diagnosis of zygomatic fracture.** Impaction of zygoma or zygomatic arch may result in trismus by impinging on coronoid process of mandible. *A,* Impacted zygomatic body fracture. *B,* Impacted zygomatic arch fracture.

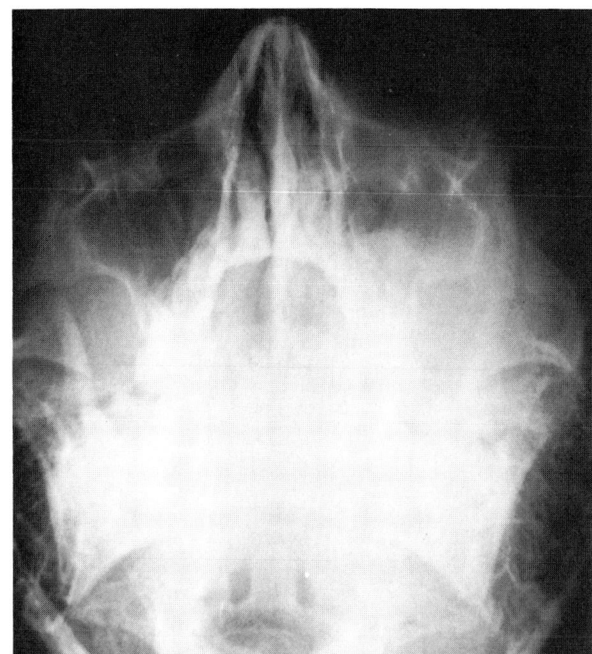

FIGURE 11–91 **Fracture of the zygoma.** Plain x-ray (Waters') film of patient with fracture of the zygoma.

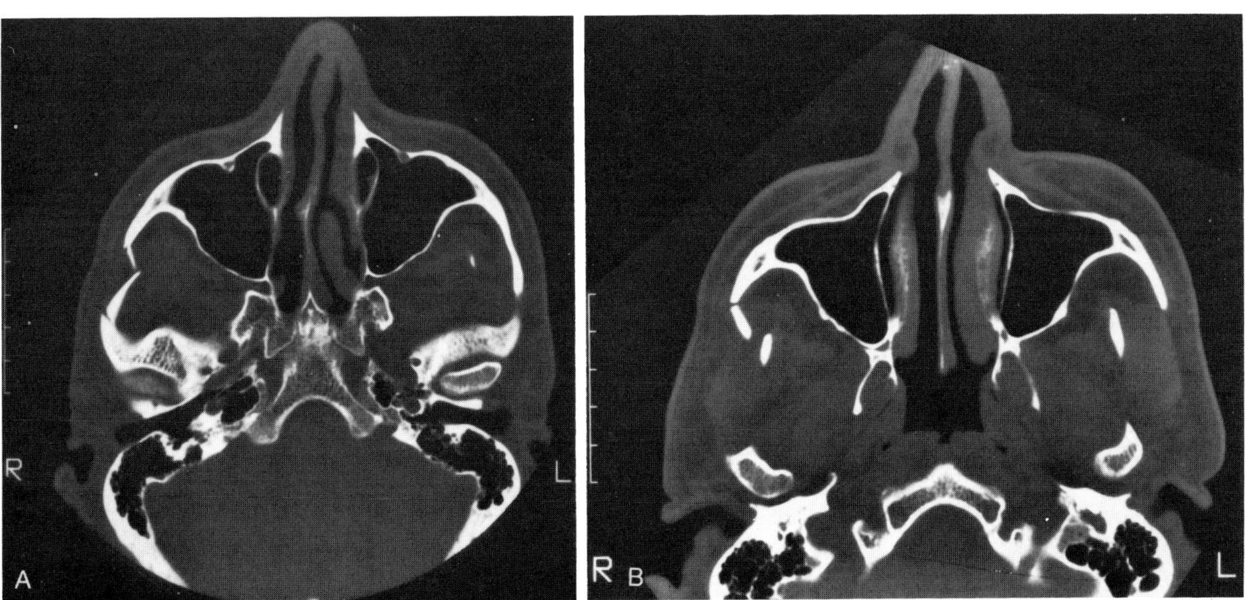

FIGURE 11–92 **Comminuted fractures.** *A,* Axial CT scan shows isolated arch fracture. *B,* On lower cut, note proximity of fracture segments to coronoid process of mandible with potential for trismus.

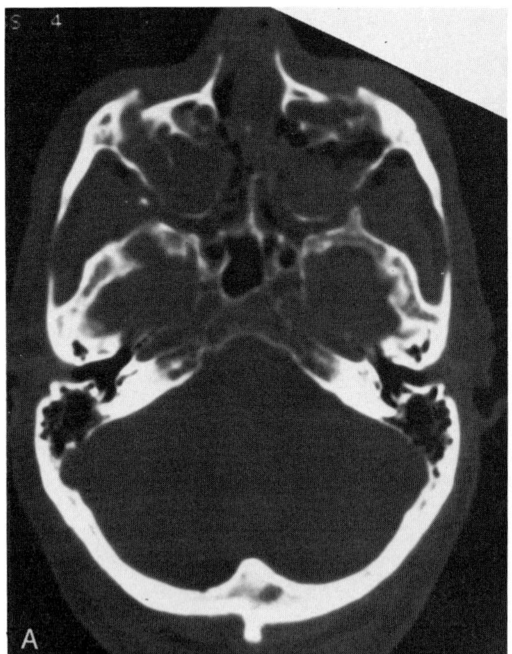

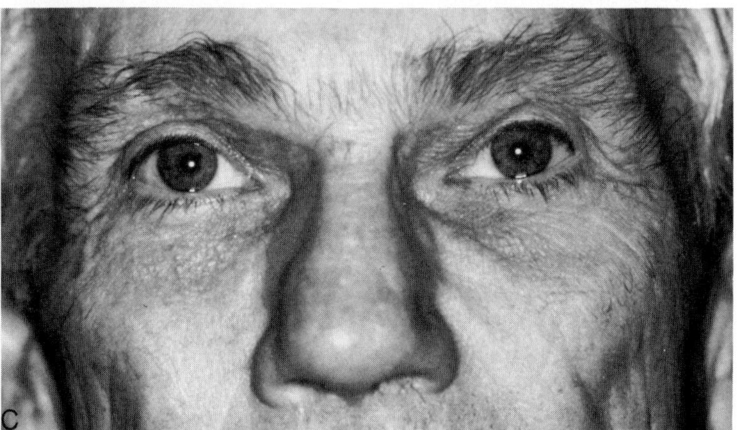

FIGURE 11–93 **Nasoethmoid fractures.** Patient with nasoethmoidal orbital fracture and frontal sinus fracture. *A,* Preoperative axial CT scan shows fractures of the medial orbital rims. *B,* All fixation of orbital rims was done using microplates and screws. "Loose" canthal bearing segment was fixated with transnasal canthopexy. Medial orbital rim position was further stabilized with mini reduction plates brought across the bridge of the nose. Nasomaxillary buttresses were not stabilized from below. Cranial bone graft was used to augment the nasal dorsum. *C,* Postoperative appearance at 6 months.

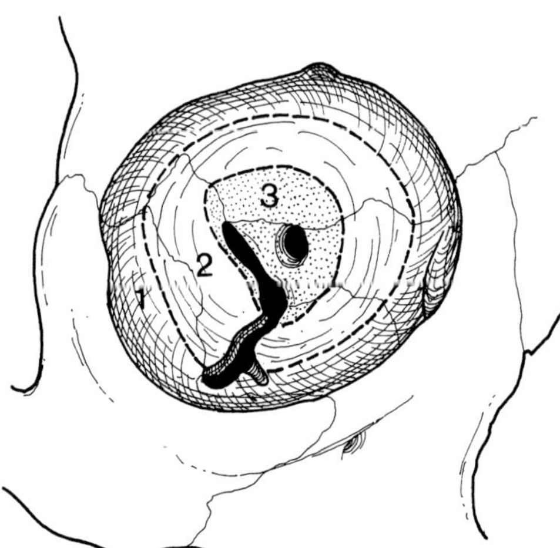

FIGURE 11–94 **Anatomy of the internal orbit.** Internal orbit divided into concentric thirds *(1, 2, 3)* based on bone thickness.

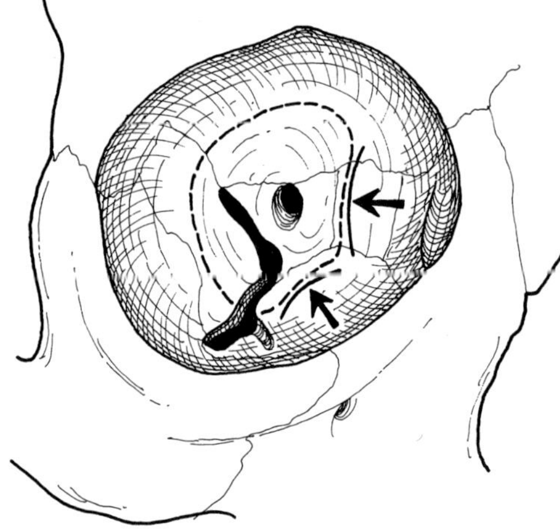

FIGURE 11–95 **Anatomy of the internal orbit.** Orbital wall cross section showing convex shape of medial floor and medial wall and middle third of orbit. *Arrows* point to areas of convexity.

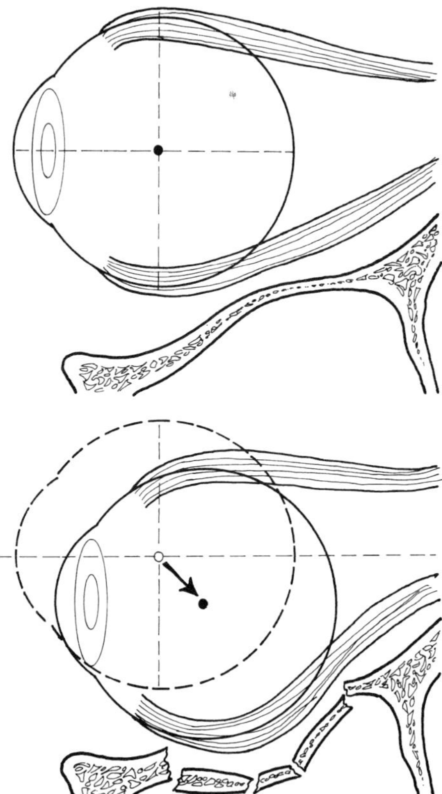

FIGURE 11-96 **Sagittal section of orbit.** Loss of convexity of floor increases orbital volume and tends toward enophthalmos.

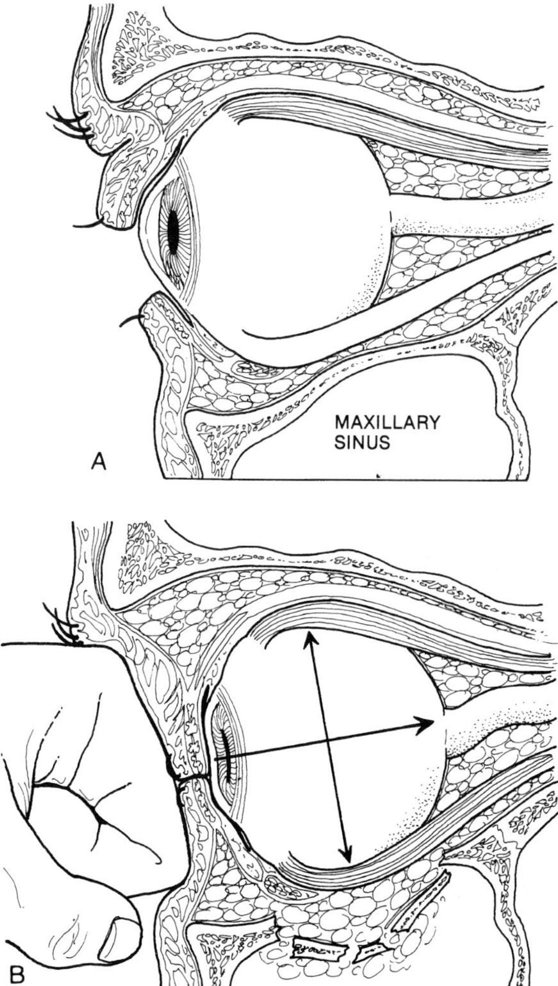

FIGURE 11-97 **Blowout fractures.** Diagrammatic representation of hydraulic theory of blowout fracture. Increase in intraorbital pressures results in fracture of weakest portion of orbital floor. *A,* Sagittal view of intact orbit. *B,* Sagittal view showing hydraulic force *(arrows)* through globe fracturing floor.

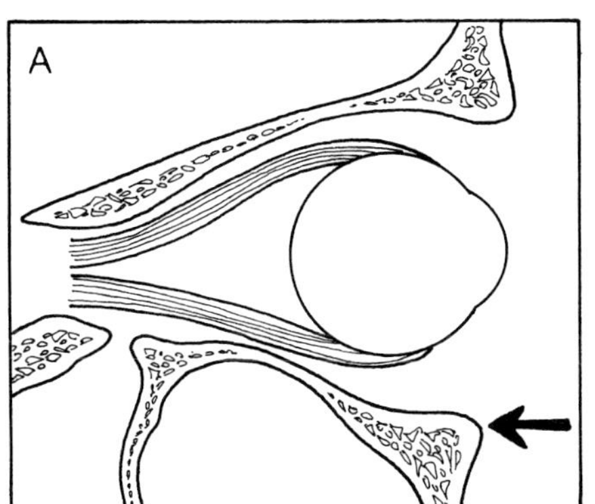

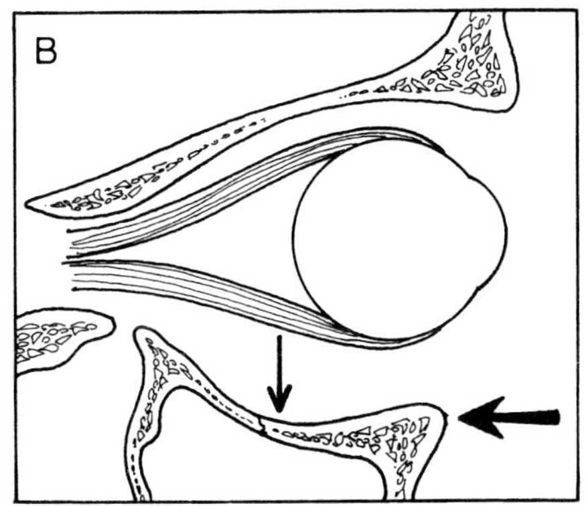

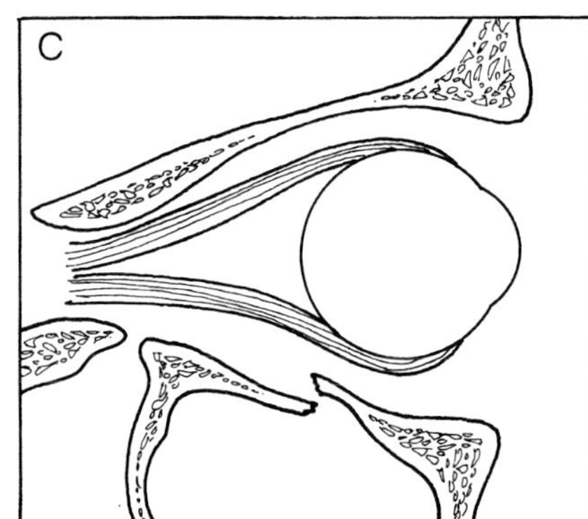

FIGURE 11-98 **Blowout fractures.** Diagrammatic representation of transmission theory as proposed by Fujino. Force to orbital rim, which is deformed but not fractured, is transmitted to weaker orbital floor, which is disrupted. *A, Arrow* shows impact at infraorbital rim. *B, Small arrow* shows deformation that results in fracture of orbital floor. *C,* Resulting displacement of orbital floor.

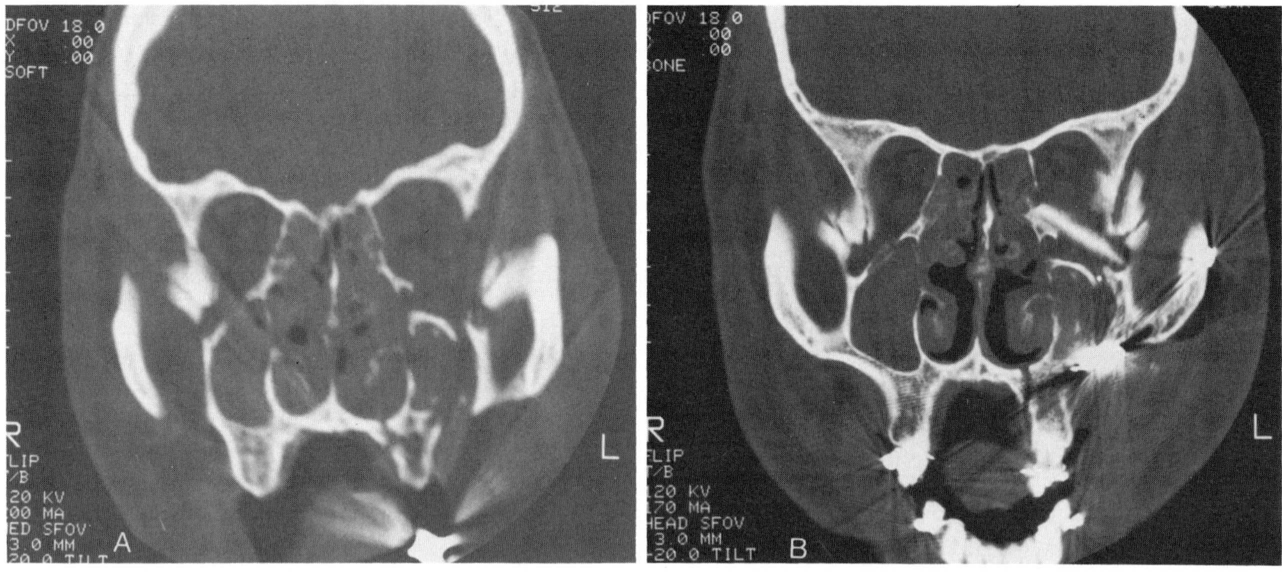

FIGURE 11–99 **Reconstruction.** LeFort II and III fracture patterns with marked disruption of left orbit and less involvement of right side. Left orbit was reconstructed with cranial bone grafts after reduction and fixation of orbital rims and maxillary buttresses. *A,* Preoperative CT scan. *B,* Postoperative CT scan shows placement of grafts to mimic anatomy of less involved right side.

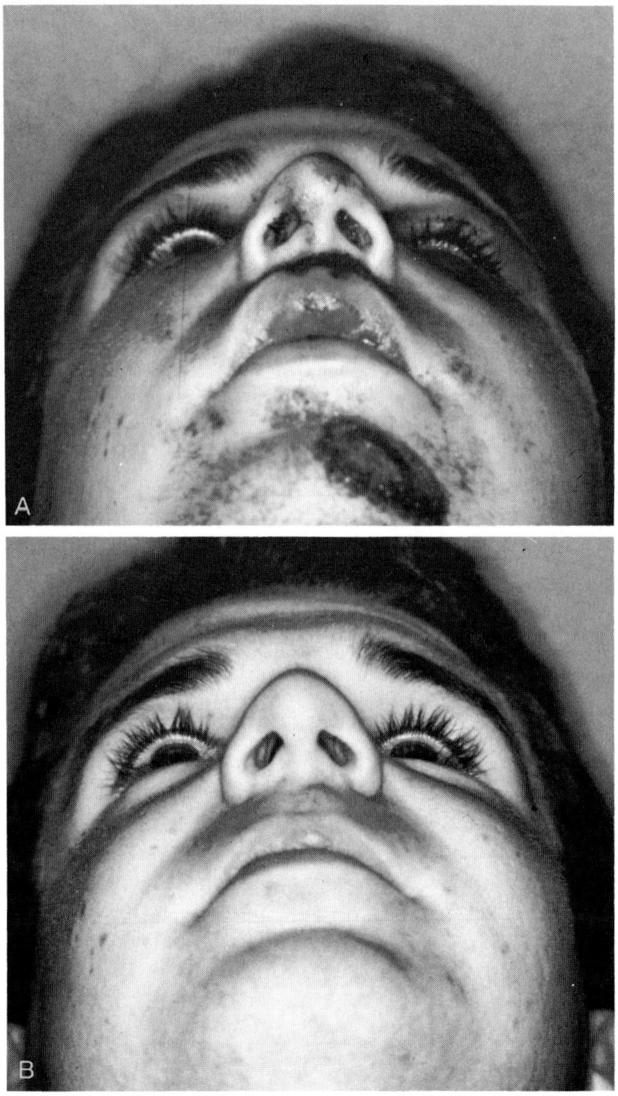

FIGURE 11–100 **Reconstruction.** Fracture with acute enophthalmos resulting from zygoma, heminasoethmoidorbital, and disruption of medial orbital floor. Vitallium mesh was used together with bone grafts to reconstruct the internal orbit. *A,* Preoperative worm's eye view. *B,* Postoperative worm's eye view. *C,* Lateral plain film showing method of fixation.

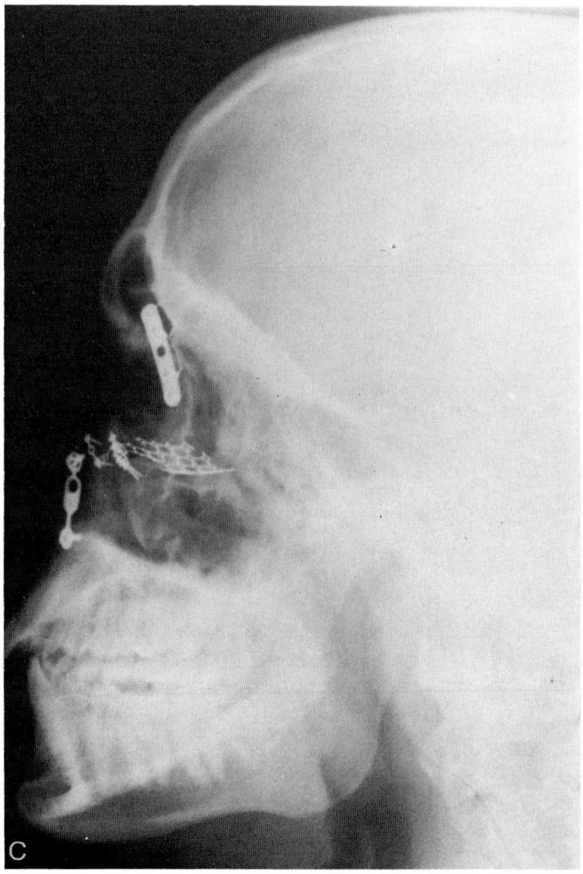

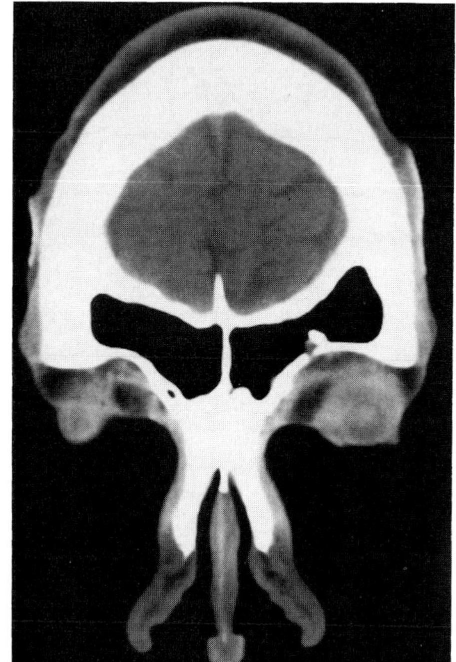

FIGURE 11-101 **Injury to orbital structures.** A 36-year-old man was struck in the left eye from below with a metal bar and was treated for minor conjunctival injury. The patient had a persistent left frontal headache. Coronal CT scan demonstrates orbital roof fracture. Views posterior to the fracture showed frontal sinus opacification. His symptoms resolved following systemic antibiotic therapy.

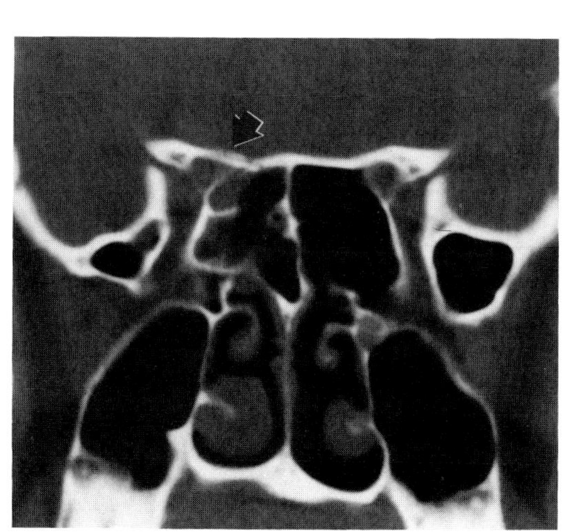

FIGURE 11-102 **Optic nerve trauma.** Coronal CT scan demonstrating a fracture in the roof of the ethmoid sinus involving the optic canal.

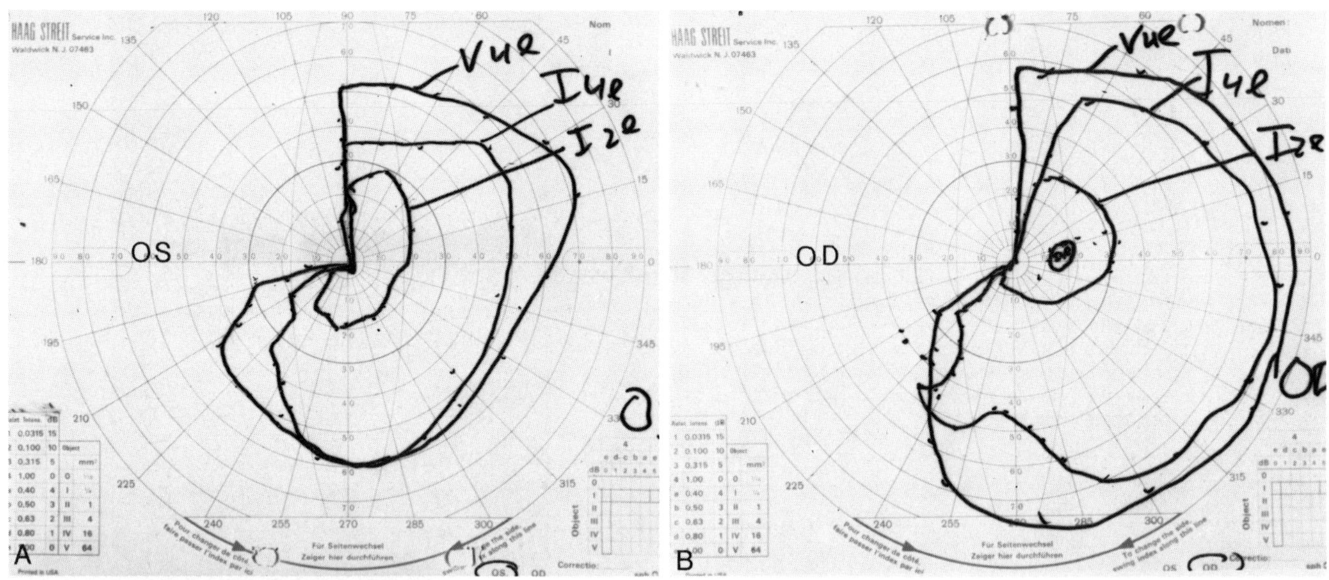

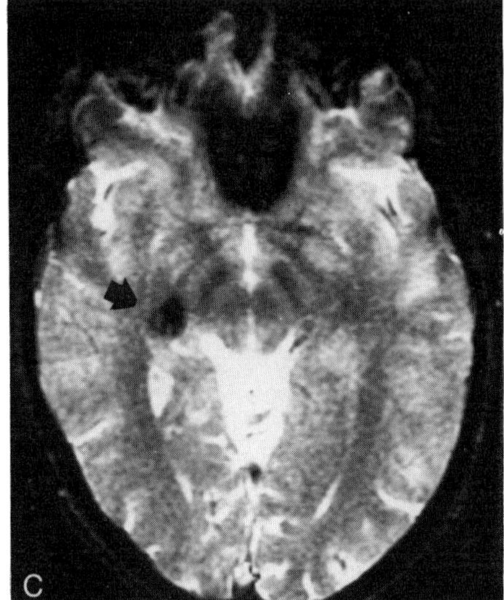

FIGURE 11–103 **Retrichiasmal lesions.** A 29-year-old woman walked into a thin wire antenna protruding from a sailboat mast and experienced acute pain in the right eye (O.D.) and a headache. The physical examination was normal except for a small superonasal conjunctival wound and a visual field defect. *A* and *B,* Visual fields, showing an incomplete left homonymous hemianopic defect. *C,* Magnetic resonance imaging scan demonstrating a lesion in the region of the right lateral geniculate body.

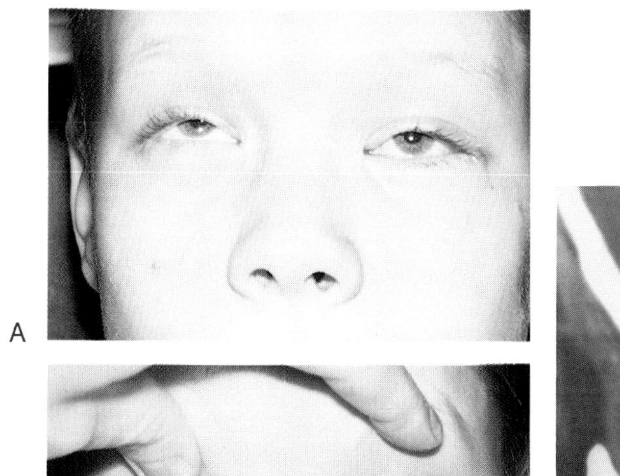
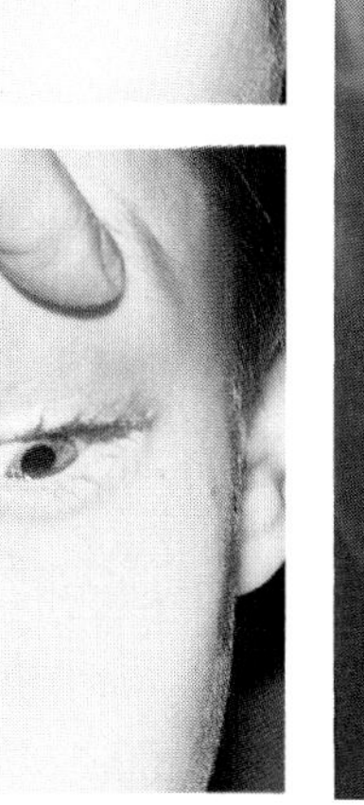
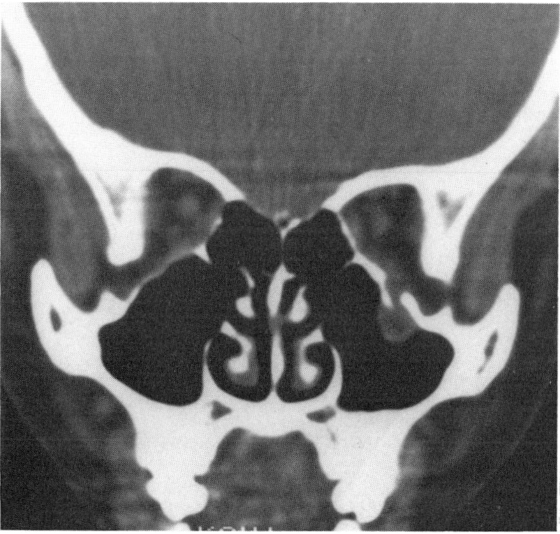

A B C

FIGURE 11-104 **Ocular motor dysfunction.** An 11-year-old boy was struck by a knee in the left eye (O.S.) while wrestling. Limited elevation *(A)* and depression *(B)* in the O.S.; forced ductions positive. *C,* CT scan of the orbit, demonstrating blowout fracture of the floor with soft tissue and inferior rectus entrapment.

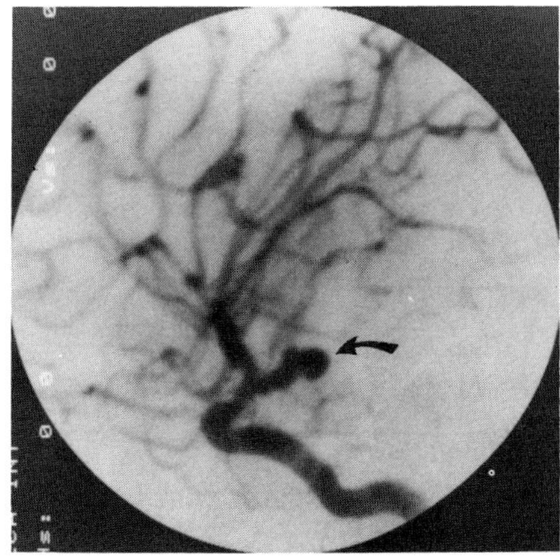

FIGURE 11-105 **Ocular motor dysfunction.** A 38-year-old woman was struck by a fist in the left eye (O.S.), suffering periorbital contusion, lid edema with complete ptosis, and brow laceration without loss of consciousness. When sutures were removed 1 week later, she complained of inability to open the O.S. and worsening headache. Examination showed complete left oculomotor nerve palsy. Contrast-enhanced CT scan was normal. Cerebral angiography revealed posterior communicating arterial aneurysm *(arrow).*

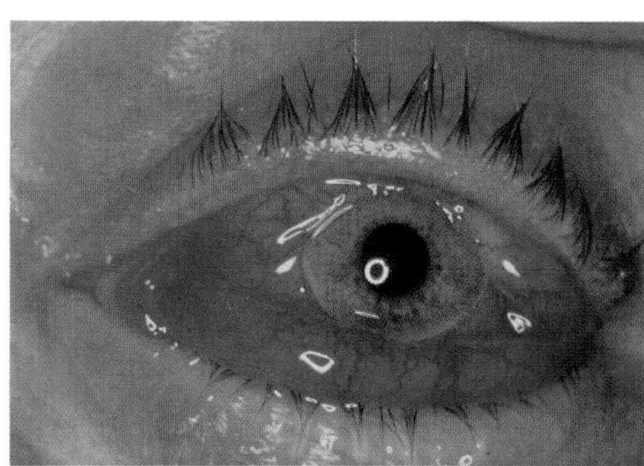

FIGURE 11-106 **Multiple cranial neuropathy.** Carotid–cavernous sinus fistula with marked conjunctival chemosis and "arterialization" of conjunctival vessels in a characteristic corkscrew pattern.

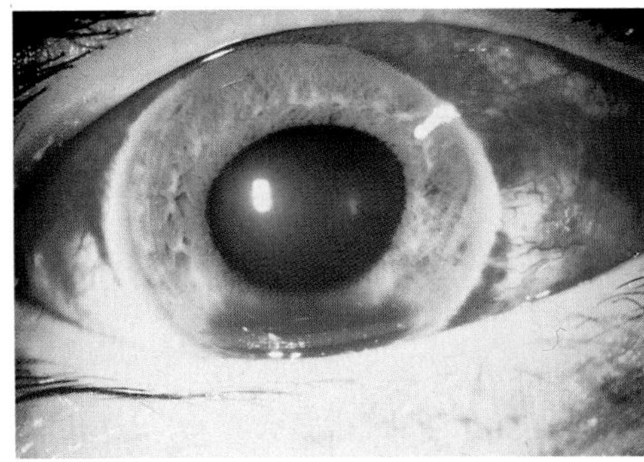

FIGURE 11–107 **Pupillary dysfunction in trauma.** Traumatic mydriasis following blunt trauma to the globe. A small hyphema is also present.

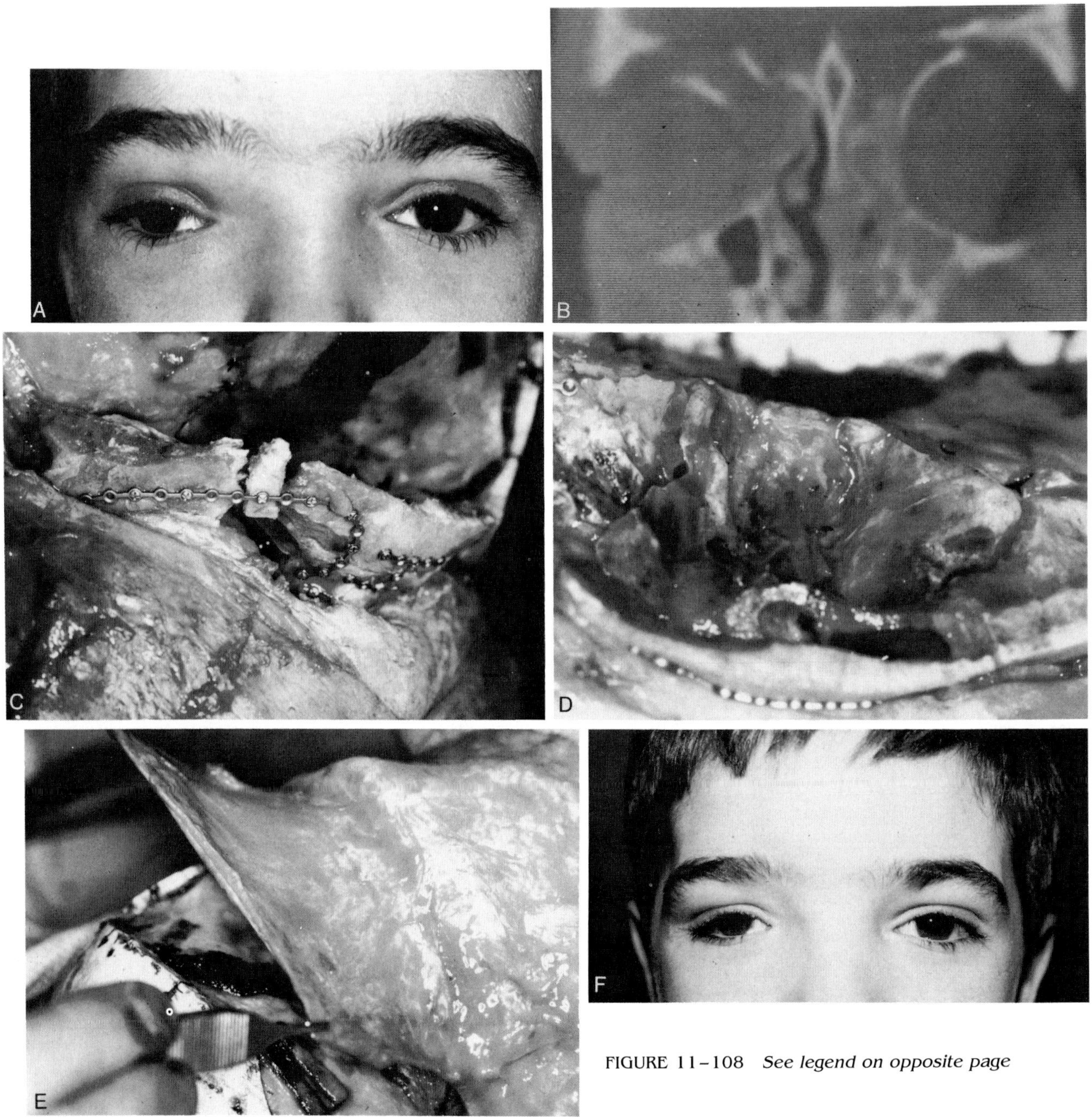

FIGURE 11–108 *See legend on opposite page*

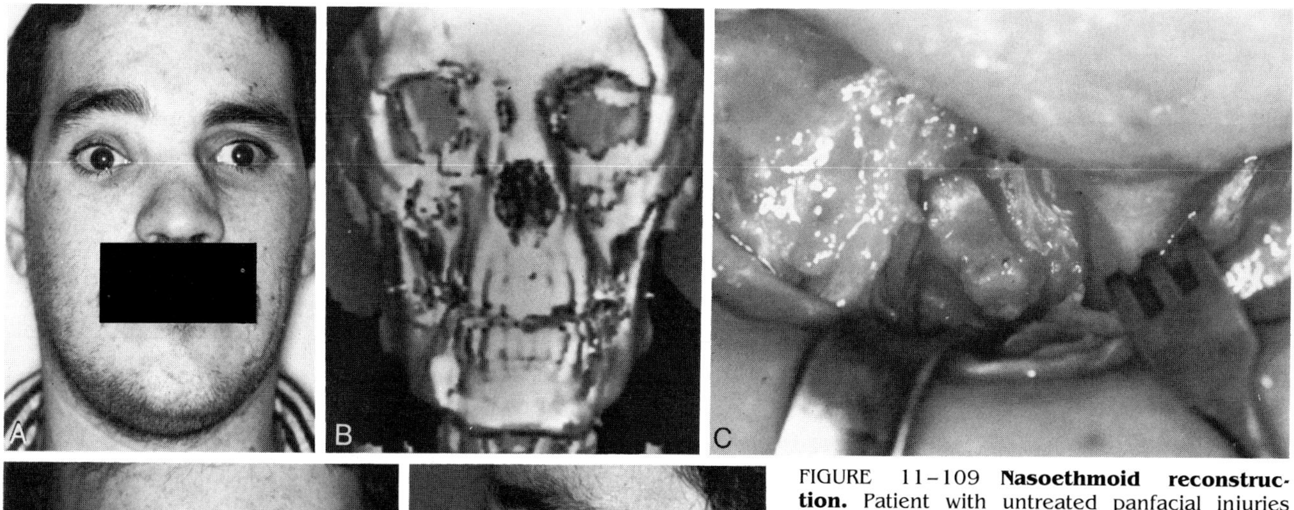

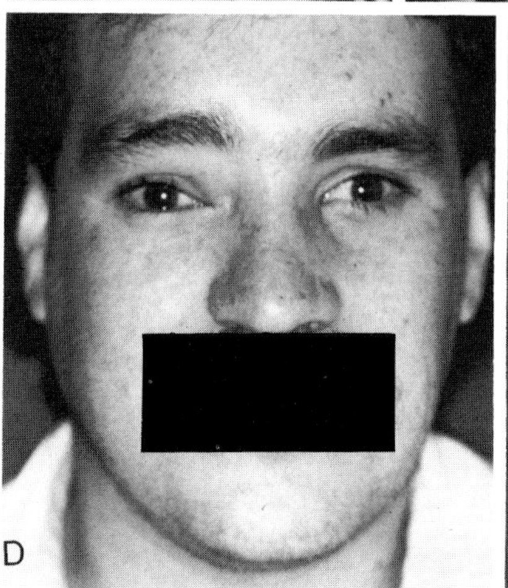

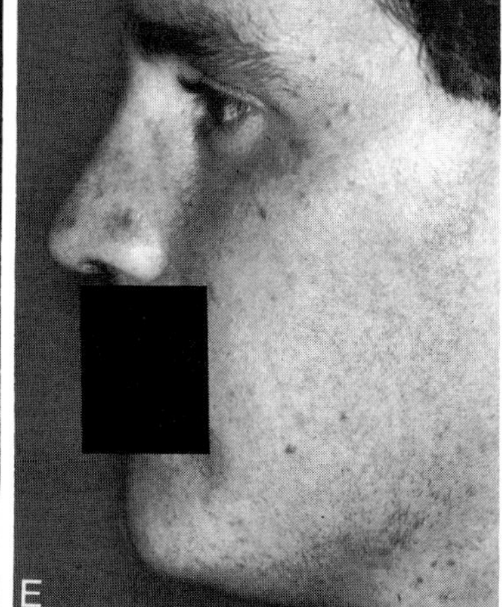

FIGURE 11–109 **Nasoethmoid reconstruction.** Patient with untreated panfacial injuries including four-wall orbital injury. Neurosurgical injury had left him in prolonged coma. *A,* Preoperative appearance. *B,* Preoperative three-dimensional CT scan demonstrates well-marked outward splaying of right medial orbital wall responsible for most obvious portion of orbital deformity. *C,* Intraoperative view shows marked lateral displacement of medial orbital wall, which was segmentally osteotomized and repositioned. Supraorbital osteotomy was not performed after neurosurgical consultation. The medial supraorbital rim was subsequently contoured. A cranial bone graft fixated with a lag screw was used to restore dorsal nasal contour. A transzygomatic deformity was not addressed. A submucosal resection was subsequently performed. Strabismus requires future surgery. *D,* Frontal view 2 years after surgery. *E,* Lateral view 2 years after surgery.

◀ FIGURE 11–108 **Supraorbital reconstruction.** An 8-year-old boy with untreated bilateral frontal and nasoethmoidal injury complicated by recurrent meningitis. Only the right side was addressed. (Surgery performed with neurosurgeon Brooke Swearingen, M.D.). *A,* Preoperative appearance. Note lateral and inferior displacement of right globe. *B,* Coronal CT scan shows marked displacement of medial wall and supraorbital area. *C,* Intraoperative view of right reconstructed supraorbital rim. Rim was osteotomized, repositioned, and fixated with microplates and screws. Note gaps between osteotomized segments. Medial orbital rim was also repositioned. A transnasal canthopexy was also performed. *D,* View from above the cranial base exposed by the neurosurgeon to identify all areas of communication and to allow adequate dural repair. Reconstructed supraorbital rim at bottom of photograph. *E,* Galeal frontalis flap elevated. This flap was used to line the cranial base and isolate the cranial cavity from the nasal cavity. *F,* Postoperative appearance at 1 year.

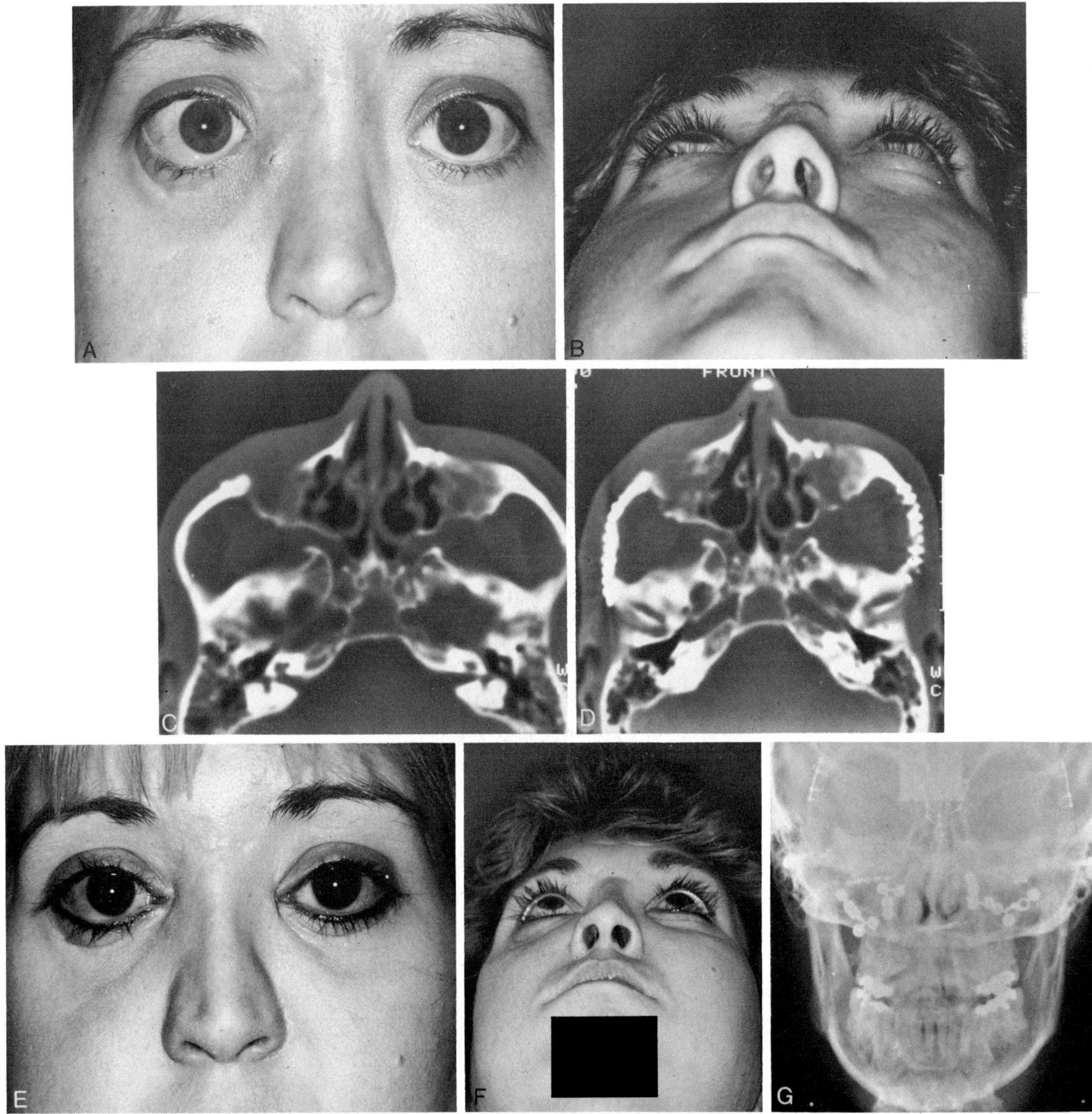

FIGURE 11-110 **Nasoethmoid reconstruction.** Patient who underwent limited treatment of a LeFort III fracture and a central midfacial fracture. *A,* Preoperative appearance. *B,* Preoperative worm's eye view. Note loss of anterior posterior projection and increased facial width as well as telecanthus and relative proptosis. *C,* Preoperative axial CT scan shows bowed zygomatic arch and impacted midface. The orbital deformities were treated with a subcranial LeFort III, LeFort I, and central midfacial osteotomies; bilateral transnasal canthopexy; bilateral lateral canthopexy; and cantilevered cranial bone graft for the nose. *D,* Postoperative axial CT scan. *E,* Appearance 1 year postoperatively. *F,* Postoperative worm's eye view. *G,* Postoperative plain film shows miniplate fixation at LeFort I level and microplate fixation of orbital segments.

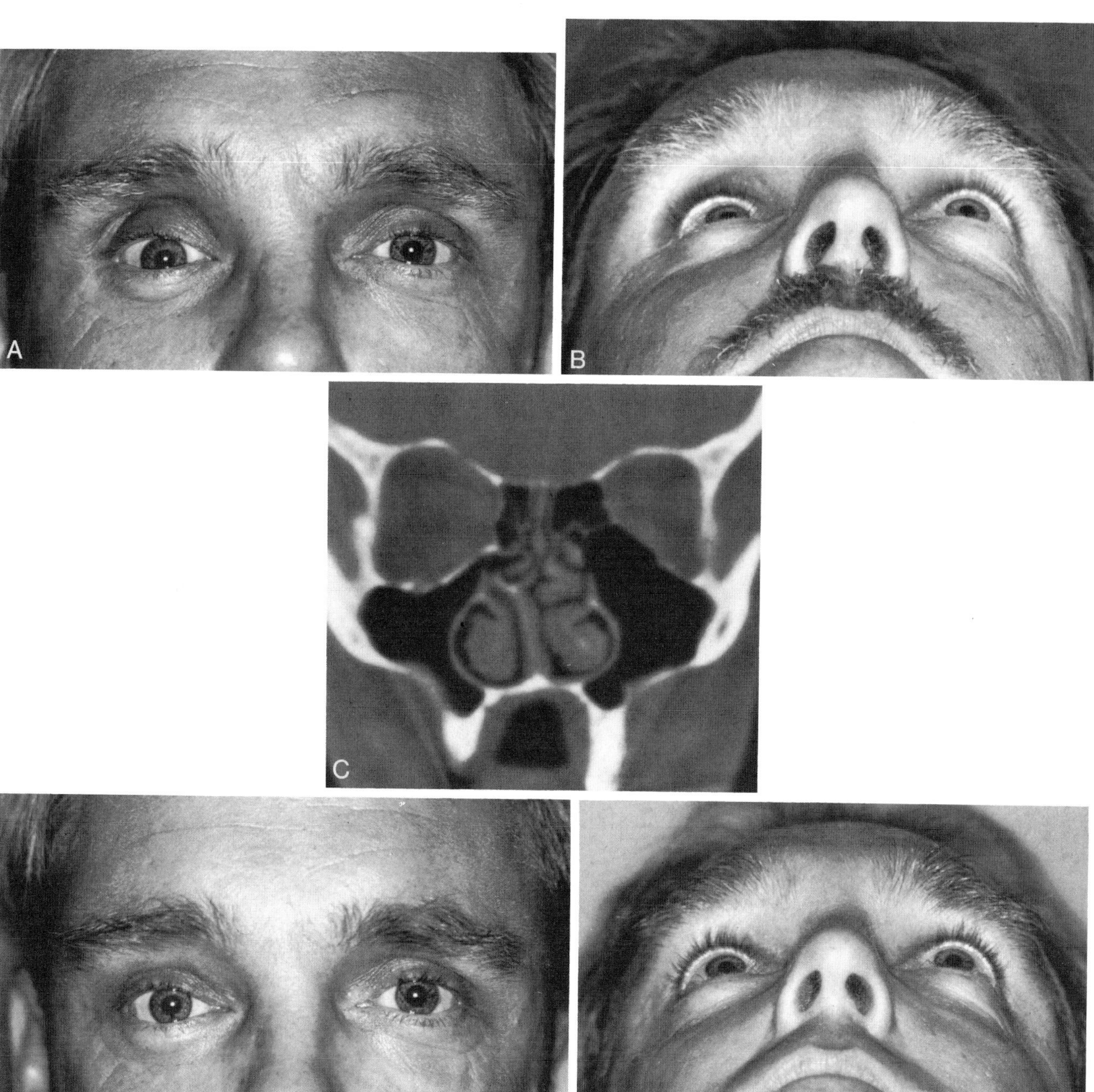

FIGURE 11-111 **Internal orbital reconstruction.** Patient with significant posttraumatic enophthalmos and minimal zygomatic contour deformity. Reconstruction was performed through transconjunctival incision. A rim osteotomy was used to gain access to the deep internal orbit. Vitallium mesh was used to support polyethylene (Medpor) implants and the orbital contents. *A,* Preoperative anteroposterior view. *B,* Preoperative worm's eye view. *C,* Preoperative coronal CT scan shows marked expansion of orbital floor and medial orbital wall. *D,* Postoperative anteroposterior view. *E,* Postoperative worm's eye view at 1 year.

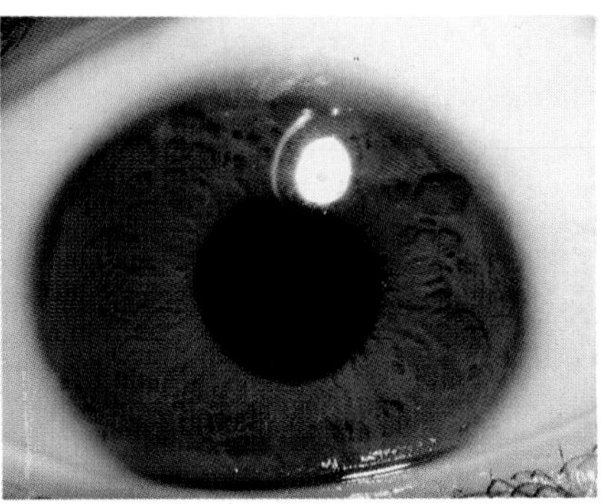

FIGURE 11–112 **Prenatal and birth trauma.** A vertical rupture in Descemet's membrane and corneal edema following forceps delivery.

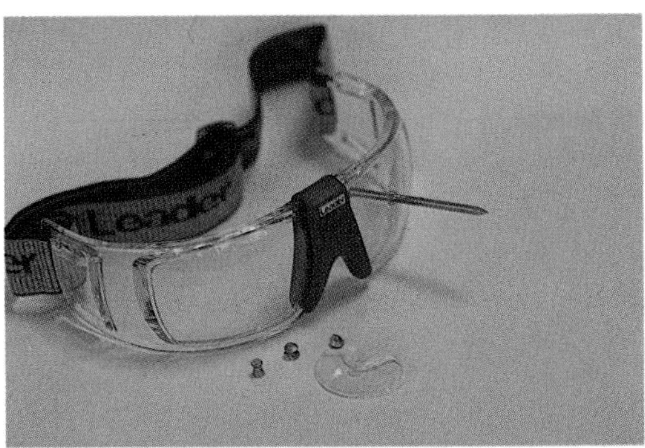

FIGURE 11–115 **Eye protectors.** The resistance of a polycarbonate racquetsport eye protector to having a nail driven through the lens. The pellets were driven at a similar protector at various speeds, and the protector did not shatter until the pellet flattened, as is seen in the third pellet from the left. *Note:* The pellet did not penetrate the protector and actually broke a piece out of it.

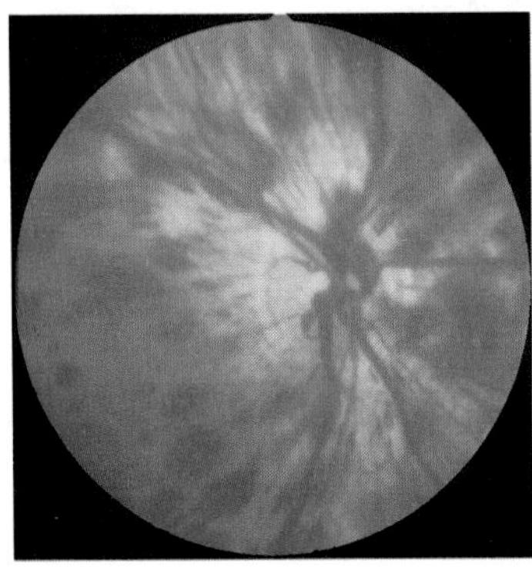

FIGURE 11–113 **Child abuse.** Extensive retinal hemorrhages in a shaken infant.

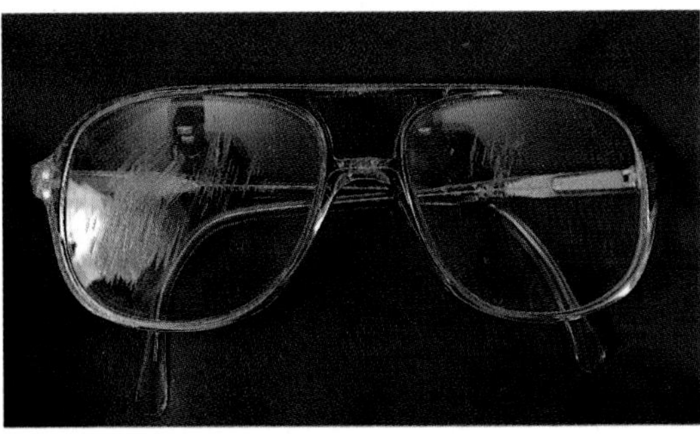

FIGURE 11–116 **Eye protectors.** A child fell from a bicycle and scratched the polycarbonate lens in his street-wear glasses. The lenses did not shatter, possibly saving him from further injury.

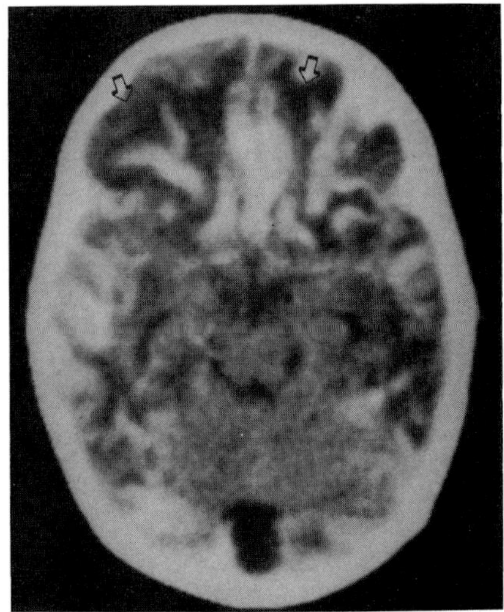

FIGURE 11–114 **Child abuse.** Prominent subdural effusions *(arrows)* are seen in this CT scan obtained during the tenth day of hospitalization of a shaken infant. The CT scan obtained on the day of admission failed to demonstrate these subdural hemorrhages.

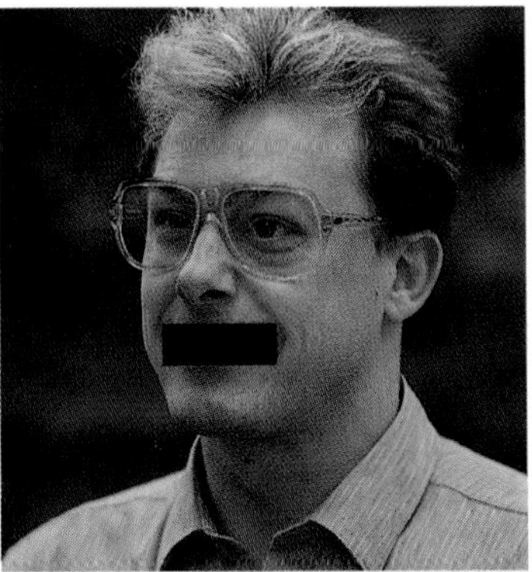

FIGURE 11–117 **Eye protectors.** A racquetsport eye protector into which a prescription polycarbonate lens can be inserted.

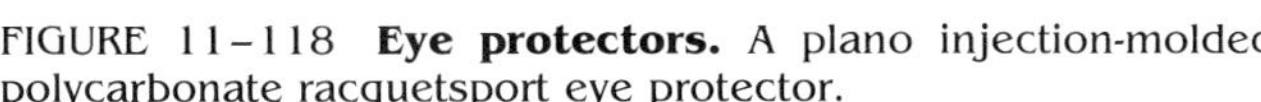

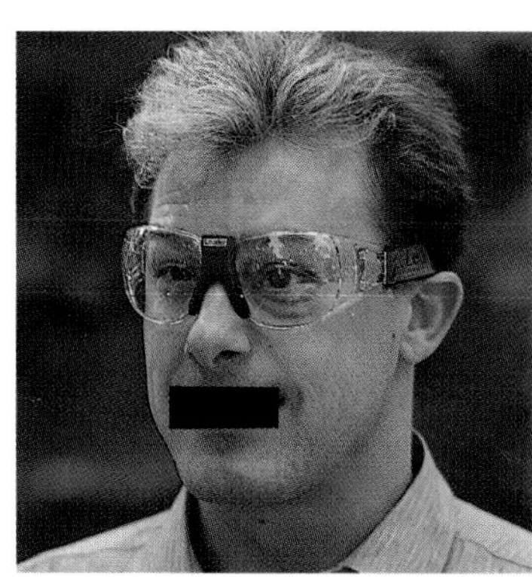

FIGURE 11–118 **Eye protectors.** A plano injection-molded polycarbonate racquetsport eye protector.

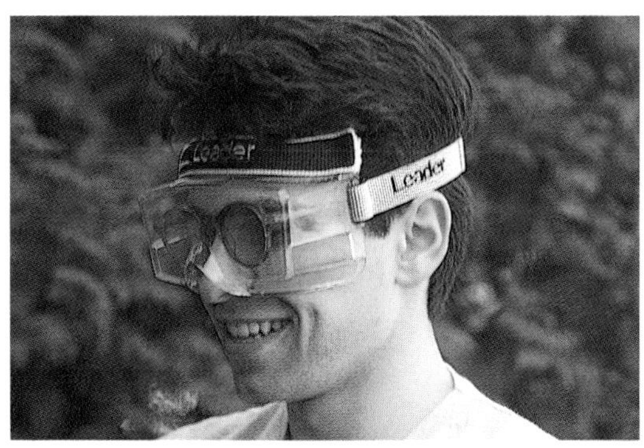

FIGURE 11–119 **Eye protectors.** An eye protector that can be worn over street-wear spectacles.

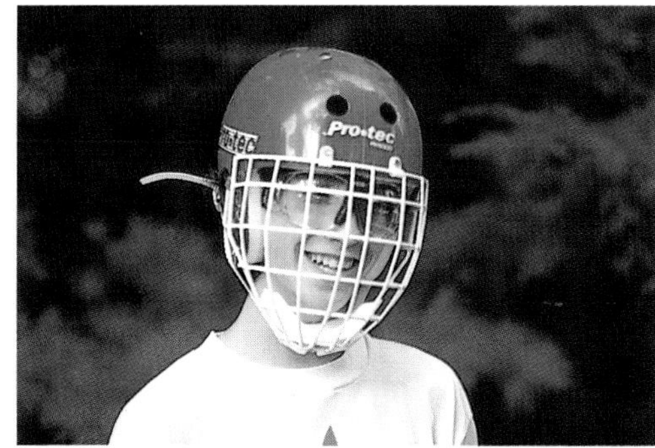

FIGURE 11–120 **Eye protectors.** A hockey face protector.

Index

A

B

C

D

E

F

I

J

K

N

O

W

X

Z